Evidence classification schemes

Evidence classification scheme for a therapeutic intervention

---

Class I An adequately powered prospective, randomized, controlled clinical trial with masked outcome assessment in a representative population or an adequately powered systematic review of prospective randomized controlled clinical trials with masked outcome assessment in representative populations. The following are required:

(a) randomization concealment;
(b) primary outcome(s) is/are clearly defined;
(c) exclusion/inclusion criteria are clearly defined;
(d) adequate accounting for dropouts and crossovers with numbers sufficiently low to have minimal potential for bias; and
(e) relevant baseline characteristics are presented and substantially equivalent among treatment groups or there is appropriate statistical adjustment for differences.

Class II Prospective matched-group cohort study in a representative population with masked outcome assessment that meets a–e above *or* a randomized, controlled trial in a representative population that lacks one criteria a–e.

Class III All other controlled trials (including well-defined natural history controls or patients serving as own controls) in a representative population, where outcome assessment is independent of patient treatment.

Class IV Evidence from uncontrolled studies, case series, case reports, or expert opinion.

Rating of recommendations
Level A (established as effective, ineffective, or harmful) requires at least one convincing class I study or at least two consistent, convincing class II studies.

Level B (probably effective, ineffective, or harmful) requires at least one convincing class II study or overwhelming class III evidence.

Level C (possibly effective, ineffective, or harmful) rating requires at least two convincing class III studies.

Evidence classification scheme for a diagnostic measure

Class I A prospective study in a broad spectrum of persons with the suspected condition, using a 'gold standard' for case definition, where the test is applied in a blinded evaluation, and enabling the assessment of appropriate tests of diagnostic accuracy.

Class II A prospective study of a narrow spectrum of persons with the suspected condition, or a well-designed retrospective study of a broad spectrum of persons with an established condition (by 'gold standard') compared to a broad spectrum of controls, where test is applied in a blinded evaluation, and enabling the assessment of appropriate tests of diagnostic accuracy.

Class III Evidence provided by a retrospective study where either persons with the established condition or controls are of a narrow spectrum, and where test is applied in a blinded evaluation.

Class IV Any design where test is not applied in blinded evaluation or evidence provided by expert opinion alone or in descriptive case series (without controls).

Rating of recommendations
Level A (established as useful/predictive or not useful/predictive) requires at least one convincing class I study or at least two consistent, convincing class II studies.

Level B (established as probably useful/predictive or not useful/predictive) requires at least one convincing class II study or overwhelming class III evidence.

Level C (established as possibly useful/predictive or not useful/predictive) requires at least two convincing class III studies.

FIRST EDITION

European Handbook of Neurological Management

Richard Hughes
Professor of Neurology
Department of Clinical Neuroscience
King's College London
London, UK

Michael Brainin
Professor of Clinical Neurology
Donauklinikum Gugging and Donau-Universität
Krems, Austria

Nils Erik Gilhus
Professor of Neurology
University of Bergen and
Haukeland University Hospital
Bergen, Norway

Blackwell
Publishing

© 2006 Blackwell Publishing Ltd

Blackwell Publishing, Inc., 350 Main Street, Malden, Massachusetts 02148-5020, USA
Blackwell Publishing Ltd, 9600 Garsington Road, Oxford OX4 2DQ, UK
Blackwell Publishing Asia Pty Ltd, 550 Swanston Street, Carlton, Victoria 3053, Australia

The right of the Author to be identified as the Author of this Work has been asserted in accordance with the Copyright, Designs and Patents Act 1988.

First published 2006

2 2007

Library of Congress Cataloging-in-Publication Data

European handbook of neurological management/[edited by] Richard Hughes, Michael Brainin, Nils Erik Gilhus. – 1st ed.
    p. ; cm.
    Includes bibliographical references and index.
    ISBN 978-1-4051-3050-9 (alk. paper)

    1. Nervous system–Diseases–Treatment–Europe–Handbooks, manuals, etc.
I. Hughes, R. A. C. (Richard Anthony Cranmer) II. Brainin, M. (Michael)
III. Gilhus, Nils Erik.
    [DNLM: 1. Nervous System Diseases–Practice Guideline. WL 140 E885 2006]
RC346.E97 2006
616.8–dc22

                                                                2006001142

    ISBN 978-1-4051-3050-9

A catalogue record for this title is available from the British Library

Set in 9/12pt Stone Serif by Newgen Imaging Systems (P) Ltd., Chennai, India
Printed and bound in Singapore by COS Printers Pte Ltd

Commissioning Editor: Stuart Taylor
Development Editor: Rob Blundell
Production Controller: Kate Charman

For further information on Blackwell Publishing, visit our website:
www.blackwellpublishing.com

The publisher's policy is to use permanent paper from mills that operate a sustainable forestry policy, and which has been manufactured from pulp processed using acid-free and elementary chlorine-free practices. Furthermore, the publisher ensures that the text paper and cover board used have met acceptable environmental accreditation standards.

Contents

Section 1: Introductory Chapters

1   Introduction: background to the book   1
     R. Hughes, M. Brainin, N.E. Gilhus

2   Foreword   3
     Christopher Gardner-Thorpe

3   Guidance for development, refereeing and dissemination of guidelines   7
     M. Brainin, M. Barnes, J.-C. Baron, N.E. Gilhus, R. Hughes, K. Selmaj, G. Waldemar

Section 2: Investigation

4   Routine cerebrospinal fluid (CSF) analysis   14
     F. Deisenhammer, A. Bartos, R. Egg, N.E. Gilhus, G. Giovannoni, S. Rauer, F. Sellebjerg

5   Use of imaging in acute stroke   28
     J.C. Masdeu, P. Irimia, S. Asenbaum, J. Bogousslavsky, M. Brainin, H. Chabriat, K. Herholz,
     H.S. Markus, E. Martínez-Vila, K. Niederkorn, P.D. Schellinger, R.J. Seitz

6   Use of imaging in multiple sclerosis   45
     M. Filippi, M.A. Rocca, D.L. Arnold, R. Bakshi, F. Barkhof, N. De Stefano, F. Fazekas,
     E. Frohman, J.S. Wolinsky

7   Neurophysiological tests and neuroimaging procedures in non-acute headache   63
     G. Sandrini, L. Friberg, W. Jänig, R. Jensen, D. Russell, M. Sanchez del Rìo, T. Sand, J. Schoenen,
     M. van Buchem, J.G. van Dijk

8   Use of anti-interferon beta antibody measurements in multiple sclerosis   72
     P. Soelberg Sørensen, F. Deisenhammer, P. Duda, R. Hohlfeld, K.-M. Myhr, J. Palace, C. Polman,
     C. Pozzilli, C. Ross

9   Use of anti-nerve antibodies   87
     H.J. Willison, N.E. Gilhus, F. Graus, B.C. Jacobs, R. Liblau, C. Vedeler, A. Vincent

10   Use of skin biopsy in the diagnosis of peripheral neuropathy   94
     G. Lauria, D.R. Cornblath, O. Johansson, J.C. McArthur, S.I. Mellgren, M. Nolano,
     N. Rosenberg, C. Sommer

11   Assessment of neuropathic pain   109
     G. Cruccu, P. Anand, N. Attal, L. Garcia-Larrea, M. Haanpää, E. Jørum, J. Serra, T.S. Jensen

Section 3: Major Neurological Diseases

12 Acute stroke   123
    W. Hacke, M. Kaste, J. Bogousslavsky, M. Brainin, A. Chamorro, K. Lees, D. Leys, H. Kwiecinski,
    D. Toni, T. Olsen, P. Langhorne, H. Diener, M. Hennerici, J. Ferro, J. Sivenius, N. Wahlgren, P. Bath

13 Migraine   159
    S. Evers, J. Áfra, A. Frese, P.J. Goadsby, M. Linde, A. May, P.S. Sándor

14 Cluster headache   177
    S. Evers, J. Áfra, A. Frese, P.J. Goadsby, M. Linde, A. May, P.S. Sándor

15 Dystonia   191
    A. Albanese, M.P. Barnes, K.P. Bhatia, E. Fernandez-Alvarez, G. Filippini, T. Gasser, J.K. Krauss,
    A. Newton, I. Rektor, M. Savoiardo, J. Valls-Solè

16 Mild traumatic brain injury   207
    P.E. Vos, Yuri Alekseenko, L. Battistin, G. Birbamer, F. Gerstenbrand, A. Potapov, T. Prevec,
    Ch.A. Stepan, P. Traubner, A. Twijnstra, L. Vecsei, K. von Wild

17 Early (uncomplicated) Parkinson's disease   224
    M. Horstink, E. Tolosa, U. Bonuccelli, G. Deuschl, A. Friedman, P. Kanovsky, J.P. Larsen, A. Lees,
    W. Oertel, W. Poewe, O. Rascol, C. Sampaio

18 Late (complicated) Parkinson's disease   245
    M. Horstink, E. Tolosa, U. Bonuccelli, G. Deuschl, A. Friedman, P. Kanovsky, J.P. Larsen, A. Lees,
    W. Oertel, W. Poewe, O. Rascol, C. Sampaio

19 Alzheimer's disease and other disorders associated with dementia   266
    G. Waldemar, B. Dubois, M. Emre, J. Georges, I.G. McKeith, M. Rossor, P. Scheltens, P. Tariska,
    B. Winblad

Section 4: Neuromuscular Diseases

20 Amyotrophic lateral sclerosis   299
    P.M. Andersen, G.D. Borasio, R. Dengler, O. Hardiman, K. Kollewe, P.N. Leigh, P.-F. Pradat,
    V. Silani, B. Tomik

21 Post-polio syndrome   322
    E. Farbu, N.E. Gilhus, M.P. Barnes, K. Borg, M. de Visser, A. Driessen, R. Howard, F. Nollet,
    J. Opara, E. Stalberg

22 Autoimmune neuromuscular conduction disorders   332
    G.O. Skeie, S. Apostolski, A. Evoli, N.E. Gilhus, I.K. Hart, L. Harms, D. Hilton-Jones, A. Melms,
    J. Verschuuren, H.W. Horge

23 Chronic inflammatory demyelinating polyradiculoneuropathy   344
    R.A.C Hughes, P. Bouche, D.R. Cornblath, E. Evers, R.D.M. Hadden, A. Hahn, I. Illa, C.L. Koski,
    J.M. Léger, E. Nobile-Orazio, J. Pollard, C. Sommer, P. Van den Bergh, P.A. van Doorn,
    I.N. van Schaik

24 Multifocal motor neuropathy   354
    I.N. van Schaik, P. Bouche, I. Illa, J.M. Léger, P. Van den Bergh, D.R. Cornblath, E. Evers,
    R.D.M. Hadden, R.A.C. Hughes, C.L. Koski, E. Nobile-Orazio, J. Pollard, C. Sommer,
    P.A. van Doorn

25   Paraproteinaemic demyelinating neuropathy   362
     R.D.M. Hadden, E. Nobile-Orazio, C. Sommer, A. Hahn, I. Illa, E. Morra, J. Pollard, R. Hughes,
     P. Bouche, D. Cornblath, E. Evers, C.L. Koski, J.M. Léger, P. Van den Bergh, P. van Doorn,
     I.N. van Schaik

26   Limb girdle muscular dystrophies   376
     F. Norwood, M. de Visser, B. Eymard, H. Lochmüller, K. Bushby

Section 5: Infections

27   Neurological complications of HIV infection   386
     P. Portegies, L. Solod, P. Cinque, A. Chaudhuri, J. Begovac, I. Everall, T. Weber, M. Bojar,
     P. Martinez-Martin, P.G.E. Kennedy

28   Encephalitis   396
     I. Steiner, H. Budka, A. Chaudhuri, M. Koskiniemi, K. Sainio, O. Salonen, P.G.E. Kennedy

Section 6: Neurological Problems

29   Treatment of neuropathic pain   412
     N. Attal, G. Cruccu, M. Haanpää, P. Hansson, T.S. Jensen, T. Nurmikko, C. Sampaio, S. Sindrup,
     P. Wiffen

30   Acute relapses of multiple sclerosis   433
     F. Sellebjerg, D. Barnes, G. Filippini, R. Midgard, X. Montalban, P. Rieckmann, K. Selmaj,
     L.H. Visser, P. Soelberg Sørensen

31   Status epilepticus   443
     H. Meierkord, P. Boon, B. Engelsen, K. Göcke, S. Shorvon, P. Tinuper, M. Holtkamp

32   Alcohol-related seizures   451
     G. Bråthen, E. Ben-Menachem, E. Brodtkorb, R. Galvin, J.C. Garcia-Monco, P. Halasz,
     M. Hillbom, M.A. Leone, A.B. Young

33   Brain metastases   461
     R. Soffietti, P. Cornu, J.Y. Delattre, R. Grant, F. Graus, W. Grisold, J. Heimans, J. Hildebrand,
     P. Hoskin, M. Kalljo, P. Krauseneck, C. Marosi, T. Siegal, C. Vecht

34   Paraneoplastic syndromes   472
     C.A. Vedeler, J.C. Antoine, B. Giometto, F. Graus, W. Grisold, I.K. Hart, J. Honnorat,
     P.A.E. Sillevis Smitt, J.J.G.M. Verschuuren, R Voltz

35   Nystagmus and oscillopsia   484
     A. Straube, R.J. Leigh, A. Bronstein, W. Heide, P. Riordan-Eva, C.C. Tijssen, I. Dehaene,
     D. Straumann

36   Orthostatic hypotension   493
     H. Lahrmann, P. Cortelli, M. Hilz, C.J. Mathias, W. Struhal, M. Tassinari

37   Cerebral venous and sinus thrombosis   501
     K. Einhäupl, M.-G. Bousser, S.F.T.M. de Bruijn, J.M. Ferro, I. Martinelli, F. Masuhr, J. Stam

38   Cerebral vasculitis   510
     N.J. Scolding, H. Wilson, R. Hohlfeld, C. Polman, I. Leite, N.E. Gilhus

39   Neurological problems in liver transplantation   516
     M. Guarino, J. Benito-Leon, J. Decruyenaere, E. Schmutzhard, K. Weissenborn,
     A. Stracciari

40 Fatty acid mitochondrial disorders   526
    C. Angelini, A. Federico, H. Reichmann, A. Lombes, P. Chinnery, D. Turnbull

Section 7: Sleep Disorders
41 Narcolepsy   534
    M. Billiard, C. Bassetti, Y. Dauvilliers, L. Dolenc-Grošelj, G.J. Lammers, G. Mayer, T. Pollmächer,
    P. Reading, K. Sonka

42 Sleep disorders in neurologic disease   552
    P. Jennum, J. Santamaria, C. Bassetti, P. Clarenbach, B. Högl, I. Arnulf, R. Poirrier, K. Sonka,
    E. Svanborg, L.D.-Grosels, D. Kaynack, M. Kruger, A. Papavasiliou, P. Reading, Z. Zahariev

43 Restless legs syndrome and periodic limb movement disorder   569
    L. Vignatelli, M. Billiard, P. Clarenbach, D. Garcia-Borreguero, D. Kaynak, V. Liesiene,
    C. Trenkwalder, P. Montagna

Section 8: Rehabilitation
44 Cognitive rehabilitation   592
    S.F. Cappa, T. Benke, S. Clarke, B. Rossi, B. Stemmer, C.M. van Heugten

Index   613

Colour plates appear after p. 120

CHAPTER 1

Introduction: background to the book

R. Hughes,[a] M. Brainin,[b] N.E. Gilhus[c]

The word Handbook means variously a manual of mediaeval ecclesiastical offices and ritual, a bookmaker's betting book or a book containing concise information on a particular subject. We hope that the European Handbook of Neurological Management is more than any of these. It is a unique endeavour to bring together peer-reviewed guidelines for the treatment and management of neurological diseases, based where possible on evidence and where not by the consensus of a range of experts drawn from different European countries. We do not think that this has been attempted before. There have been times during the past two years when we have understood why not, and also why our politicians have such difficulty in reaching consensus in the European Parliament.

Less than ten years have gone by since the first EFNS task force on the preparation of neurological management guidelines prepared guidance for the preparation of such guidelines. This was revised in 2004 and the revised version is presented in Chapter 3 of this Handbook. The word guidance is appropriate, because it has been reassuringly difficult to persuade colleagues in the different neurological subspecialties to follow guidance bureaucratically. Serious departures from the guidance have been explained in individual chapters when necessary. Often, of course, the evidence on which to base recommendations has been inadequate and task forces have necessarily had to make up their minds on the basis of limited evidence. In such cases, they have offered opinions about best practice as 'Good Practice Points'. The Handbook therefore goes beyond the evidence-based guidelines preferred by some authorities and extends to offering advice in evidence-free areas. The least common denominator is that each chapter is based on the consensus of neurologists from several different European centres. The international European nature of the consensus offers some protection against inappropriate bias. It also means that a broader set of experiences has been taken into account, including national guideline documents from several countries. The multinational European authorship has made it even clearer how important aspects of common neurological practice are not evidence-based, or even not in accordance with best available evidence. The broad geographical authorship will hopefully facilitate the implementation of the recommendations in all European countries, as well as outside Europe.

Where possible, task forces have linked up with other European organisations to produce a guideline which therefore has the imprimatur not only

[a]Department of Clinical Neuroscience, King's College London School of Medicine, United Kingdom; [b]Department of Neurology, Donauklinikum Gugging and Donau-Universität, Krems, Austria; [c]Department of Neurology, University of Bergen and Haukeland University Hospital, Bergen, Norway.

of the European Federation of Neurological Societies but also of another European or international organisation. For instance, the chapter on Acute Stroke is the official policy of the European Stroke Initiative. Chapters on Parkinson's Disease and Dystonia have been produced as collaborative efforts with The Movement Disorder Society – European Section. The chapter on Amyotrophic Lateral Sclerosis was produced in concert with the European Amyotrophic Lateral Sclerosis Consortium. The chapters on Chronic Inflammatory Demyelinating Polyradiculoneuropathy, Multifocal Motor Neuropathy and Paraproteinaemic Demyelinating Neuropathy were produced as collaborative efforts with the International Peripheral Nerve Society, to which North American and Australian co-authors willingly co-opted.

The coverage of the book has necessarily been opportunistic, being based on areas of particular interest and enthusiasm to European authors. The titles fall naturally into sections. The investigation section includes chapters on cerebrospinal fluid analysis, imaging, diagnostic antibodies and skin biopsy. The section on major neurological diseases includes stroke, migraine, Parkinson's disease, dystonia, mild traumatic brain injury and Alzheimer's disease. The section on neuromuscular diseases covers motor neuron disease, inflammatory neuropathy and limb girdle muscular dystrophy and myasthenia, leaving diabetic and other neuropathies and myopathies for the future. The section on infections covers HIV infection and encephalitis, but not meningitis. Specific neurological problems include the treatment of neuropathic pain, acute relapses of multiple sclerosis and status epilepticus, to name but a few. There are three guidelines on sleep disorders. The Handbook concludes appropriately with a section on cognitive rehabilitation.

Inevitably there are numerous possibilities for future volumes. We have made a start, but this is really only the end of the beginning.

This Handbook illustrates how more and better research is necessary in clinical neurology. Well-controlled studies with sufficient quality, size and follow-up time are needed for many drug and non-drug treatments and procedures. Such studies are usually multicentre, and often need to be multinational. The EFNS provides a wonderful platform for multinational collaboration. We hope that the guidelines in this Handbook will stimulate more high-quality European studies to fill the gaps in knowledge that have been identified. The Handbook is an expression of the willingness and ability of the EFNS to play an important role in initiating and supporting multinational European projects.

Guidelines are just that. They are not regulations. They are for the guidance of wise men and the obedience of no-one. They have to be interpreted in the light of local facilities and the needs of the individual patients. They are not intended to have legal and binding implications in individual cases. They are offered as a service to the European and even the wider international community and as an aid on which local guidelines may be formulated and decisions about treatment made.

Acknowledgement

Construction of this Handbook has been an enormous task which many have shared. We thank in particular the Guideline authors who have given their time and expertise without financial reward, Lisa Müller, Executive Director of the EFNS, Mary Mathias at King's College London School of Medicine and Rob Blundell at our publishers, Blackwell's.

CHAPTER 2

Foreword

Christopher Gardner-Thorpe[a]

This handbook of the European Federation of Neurological Societies (EFNS) provides a compendium of those areas where in particular the EFNS is promoting good practice and good fellowship among neurologists throughout Europe. To be forward looking, it is often necessary to look carefully at the past. This is important to help avoid exploring once again the ground over which earlier workers have trod to avoid misrouting, blind alleys and the mistakes that inevitably are committed from time to time by all human beings.

This then forms the study of the history of our subject – neurology. The study of the past is important for at least three reasons – to educate and plan for the future, as an academic discipline and because it is fun.

The EFNS has many Panels. The Panel on the History of Neurology in one sense provides an umbrella for the work of the rest of the other Panels. It seeks representation from each and every country in Europe. At each EFNS meeting the Panel runs a series of lectures, often based primarily upon the history of neuroscience in the country in which the meeting is held. A distinguished speaker delivers the annual Clifford Rose Lecture and a neurohistory tour provides a view of the development of the subject based on sites of particular importance and interest in that area.

This handbook presents guidelines for the management of important disorders of the nervous system. By looking to the investigations and treatments used in former years, often it is possible to understand better, and to devise new strategies for, the management of conditions with which neurologists deal.

The Scientific Committee of the EFNS provides a broad overview of the functions of the organization. But when did neuroscience really begin? Who were the instigators of the various ideas that guide us in our everyday neurological activities? A review of the work of those who went before us might help answer these questions.

A major change in the emphasis of the management of chronic disease states is demonstrated by the greater emphasis now placed upon reduction in disability in contrast to a former approach in which the cure of disease and the prolongation of life were paramount – matters that remain of the greatest importance but which may need to be secondary to disability management.

Stroke is of worldwide importance as a major cause of disability and death. Galen of Pergamon (c130–201) described some of the vasculature of the brain and the great vein that bears his name is witness to this fact. Venous occlusion is widely recognized now, largely due to the ready availability of magnetic resonance (MR) imaging that has also led to a better understanding of the

[a]Chairperson, EFNS Panel on the History of Neurology, Exeter, UK, cgardnerthorpe@doctors.org.uk

so-called benign intracranial hypertension, benign in so few ways for the sufferer. However, it is to Thomas Willis (1621–1675) that the proper recognition of the arterial supply is due, illustrated for Willis so delicately by that great British architect, Christopher Wren (1632–1723). The study of the anatomy of the brain has contributed to the understanding of the pathophysiology of stroke in its acute form and in later management, once again, rehabilitation becomes important. More recently, the association of migraine with cerebral infarction has shown the relationship between an apparently benign yet common cause of headache and the more devastating effects of cerebral arterial occlusion. Do the theories that migraine is of electrical origin or due to a channelopathy help us to understand this? The study of inflammatory processes underlying occlusion has led to the beginnings of an understanding of cerebral vasculitis, lupus and other immune pathology, seemingly separate from temporal or giant cell arteritis.

After Willis, Charles Bell (1774–1842), whose name is associated with the commonest form of lower motor neurone facial palsy, drew and annotated tinted images to teach the anatomy of the nervous system and to illustrate surgical procedures for the treatment of those injured in the Iberian Peninsular War of 1807–1814 and at the Battle of Waterloo in 1815. Like his older brother John Bell (1763–1820), also an experienced surgeon in Edinburgh, Charles augmented his knowledge and understanding of anatomy and physiology. They were both superb teachers to whom, in our differing times and with different tools, we aspire in introducing our successors to important concepts in medicine and surgery. Charles Bell's oil paintings and watercolours are still fresh and captivating, as are so many paintings of medical subjects made available to us all now with Alan Emery's annotations in the *Journal of the Royal College of Physicians* and elsewhere.

If these subjects seem tame, then there is the exciting work on movement disorders that has progressed by leaps and bounds. The treatment of that disorder was described in 1817 by James Parkinson (1755–1824) in his famous *An Essay on the Shaking Palsy*. The enormity of his work was not

recognized by that eponymous writer – or perhaps it would, for he was a polymath with interests in the church, politics, chemistry, geology and many areas of medicine. He witnessed rabies, tetanus and lightning strike, and in the dingy courtyards of London he saw social conditions that spelt disease. That Parisian master, perhaps the first true neurologist, Jean-Martin Charcot (1825–1893) who was born the year after Parkinson died, gave the latter's name to paralysis agitans, now known as Parkinson Disease (not Parkinson's Disease, for we try to forgo the possessive 's' which seems to suggest the describer was also a sufferer of the disease). Charcot taught to distinguish between multiple sclerosis and motor neurone disease, and much else besides. A long time was to pass before disease-modifying therapy became available for the former and some less horrifying differential diagnoses for the latter, including the post-polio syndrome, and the curious multifocal motor neuropathy with conduction block that may respond to the use of intravenous infusions of gamma globulin. These expensive treatments are important for those who suffer. Sadly, not all conditions are amenable to modification but we must be confident they will be so in due course: George Sumner Huntington (1851–1916) and George-Edmond-Albert-Brutus Gilles de la Tourette (1857–1904) would have been pleased if that happens.

Neurosurgery has something to offer those with movement disorders, as indeed it has an increasing place in the management of epilepsy and other conditions. Functional techniques introduce a new approach to disability management and have become possible through innovative technology, good engineering and miniaturization. The coiling of intracranial aneurysms is a good example of this. Exploration of the sites that may help alleviate the effects of movement disorders has led to increased understanding of the hard wiring of the brain and the gradual acceptance that what is hard wired can actually change its function. We tend to think of the brain as working in the ways that we can invent to use our own technology; because a computer has different memory systems, we might say so must the brain; because binary code is a way in which at present we can develop technology easily, so the brain must work by switching.

The lessons of history tell us that we shall almost certainly abandon these theories as newer, better ones come along. Those who judge us in the future will ask how we could possibly believe what we do now. After all, we do that in respect of our predecessors and then realize how naïve we are. Our techniques have descended the neuraxis and functional surgery is proving helpful in the management of spinal cord and peripheral nerve disorders too.

Just as Robert Koch (1843–1910) introduced us to ideas of infection and his successors found means of eradicating smallpox, so shall those who proclaim that AIDS and Creutzfeld–Jakob disease will never be treated find in due course, let us hope, that eradication has been possible – only to be replaced by other initially inexplicable problems, resulting from the natural selection process in which the infecting agents indulge. And so to genetics and the work of Gregor Johann Mendel (1822–1884) and others who were the right persons in the right place at the appropriate time. Mendel's arithmetical bent combined with his painstaking work led to the theory that has stood the test of time, albeit better understood in molecular biological terms in the twentieth century. Not so fast though, for modifier genes have entered the arena and then new theory fuses with the old as the dialectic allows thesis, antithesis and the synthesis of new ideas. To this we may attribute our better understanding of muscle disease, studied at first by gross microscopic technique and then by ultrastructural means: stains, chemistry, metabolic approaches and mitochondrial studies.

Why are different muscle groups affected in different varieties of muscular dystrophy? Perhaps it is better that we reframe the question and ask why our classification of the disorders was based upon observation of which muscles are involved. The answer is that it was the best approach available before newer molecular and genetic techniques became available. We create the classification and then ask why the disorders are grouped in a certain way. We only name certain structures as muscles because of the similarities between them – microscopic, chemical and so on; but the closer we look, the more differences we see. Why should a structure that flexes one joint always

develop anatomically in that way? If it does so, it has differences from other structures that move other parts; and if there are differences then there may well be different disease states that disrupt function. Perhaps it is our classification that is not sufficiently comprehensive. What is disease anyway? Is it just that which is socially unacceptable to the majority?

Much of the new neuroscience studies itself on the basis of cognitive phenomena. Can a brain ever understand itself fully? Is it a contradiction in terms to believe it can ever do so? Those who classify by lumping conditions together will speak of dementia whereas those who split will speak of the disorders described by Alois Alzheimer (1864–1915) and Arnold Pick (1851–1924), and by Hans-Gerhardt Creutzfeldt (1885–1964) and Alfons Maria Jakob (1884–1931). Some will classify anatomically, as in the fronto-temporal dementias, and others by functional magnetic resonance or by neurochemistry. Cognitive rehabilitation and neurosexology are covered in the collection of papers in this volume. Cognition requires sensory input from visual, cochlear and labyrinthine sources, increasingly areas of interest to clinicians who study the nervous system, structures that are extensions of the brain some might say. That enigmatic condition of benign positional vertigo is now attributed to otolith dislocation, such an obvious and straightforward explanation that has led to treatment. Why did you not think of it, or I? Which other conditions are due to some apparently simple process? Some of the lesions of another curious condition, multiple sclerosis, may well represent not a destructive process but rather the important areas of repair where axonal degeneration may be overcome by judicious nurturing of the extent of the inflammatory process that surrounds them. Should we measure success by the extent to which we can suppress MR lesions or, by doing just that, are we worsening the outcome? We do not know but perhaps our successors will; and they might criticize us initially and then realize that the lessons of history apply to each and every generation.

It is in the arena of imaging, however, that such striking advances have been made. Logic led to the development of tomography in the imaging of tuberculous lesions of the lungs, contrast studies in the exploration of body cavities including the spaces in and around the brain and spinal cord, and the development of computing led to the computerized tomographic (CT) scanner. In a sense, the foundations of MR were laid by the computer analysis of X-ray images but MR went several stages further for it uses different physics techniques. Clinicians have learned that for much (but not for all) of the time they may not get the diagnosis right; in embarrassing fashion, a clinical diagnosis may be shattered by the judicious use of MR. What will be the next major advance in technique? If we knew that then we should all be using it and wondering what would be the next advance, and the next, and so on. Older isotope imaging techniques have led to positron emission tomography (PET) scanning which may well be used in routine practice in the very near future; and what is used frequently often becomes cheaper.

Developments in basic chemistry have led to new physical chemical techniques to identify immunological disorders and, hence, understanding of various autoimmune processes has paralleled the introduction of techniques to measure antibodies. Vasculitis, chronic inflammatory demyelinating neuropathy (CIDP) and disorders of the neuromuscular junction all come under this category. The treatments for such conditions come and go – yesterday it was steroids, steroid-sparing drugs and plasmapheresis, whereas today we use gamma globulin and tomorrow perhaps stem cell therapy and somatic cell nucleus transfer. Many of these procedures require critical care skills. The intensive care units of the latter part of the twentieth century have paved the way for ever more sophisticated care and for more adventurous neurosurgical techniques. Anaesthetic techniques have enabled artificial sleep and relaxation in order that the structure we believe mediates sleep can rest while surgeons explore it. Sleep studies are a fairly new approach to the disabling disorders that upset our patients, the restless legs and restless minds that can beset us all.

We must not sleep in the study of our subject of neurology. The vigilance we need, the executive drive and the relentless search to advance studies of the nervous system in form and function, must be fostered. This volume provides a basis for this and in many important subjects it goes further; it provides pointers to further study, something that can unite those working in Europe, one to another, and all of us to the wider world in the hope that neuroscience can point to a peaceful and rewarding way ahead.

CHAPTER 3

Guidance for development, refereeing and dissemination of guidelines

M. Brainin,[a] M. Barnes,[b] J.-C. Baron,[c]
N.E. Gilhus,[d] R. Hughes,[e] K. Selmaj,[f]
G. Waldemar[g]

Introduction

Since the publication of the first EFNS task force reports in 1997, a total of 20 evidence-based guidelines for the treatment and management of neurological diseases have been published by the EFNS (www.efns.org/guidelines). In 2001, recommendations for the preparation of neurological guidelines were issued by the EFNS Scientific Committee (Eur J Neurol 2001; 8: 549–550). These have now been updated and revised. More unified criteria for standards of reporting have been set up which include classes of scientific evidence and predefined levels of recommendation. These criteria as well as others listed below should be used for all working groups that aim at recommending treatment, diagnostic procedures or other interventions within the framework of the EFNS.

Neurological treatment guidelines/management recommendations on a European scale by EFNS

Neurological diseases and disability are a primary concern worldwide. A global survey revealed that of the leading ten disabling diseases, eight were caused by diseases of the brain (Üstün *et al.*, 1999). In Europe, brain diseases cause a loss of 23% of the years of healthy life and 50% of years lived with disability. Thus 35% of the total burden of disability-adjusted life years is caused by brain diseases alone (Olesen and Leonardi, 2003). In Europe, both mortality and morbidity due to neurological causes are increasing and the health expenditure for this burden is also growing rapidly. In reality, part of the cost is due to treatments that have become established without scientific evidence. Although the situation varies from country to country, this is the case not only for many treatments for common diseases such as stroke, migraine and other headaches, Parkinsonism and epilepsy, but also for other conditions including many areas of neurological prevention and neurorehabilitation.

[a]Department of Neurology, Donauklinikum and Donau-Universität, Maria Gugging, Austria; [b]Hunters Moor Regional Neurorehabilitation Centre, Newcastle upon Tyne, UK; [c]Department of Neurology, Addenbrooke's Hospital, Cambridge, UK; [d]Department of Neurology, University of Bergen, Norway; [e]Department of Clinical Neurosciences, King's College London, UK; [f]Department of Neurology, Medical University of Lodz, Poland; [g]Rigshospitalet, Copenhagen University Hospital, Denmark.

European Journal of Neurology 2001, 8:549–550

The European Federation of Neurological Societies (EFNS) has recognized the demands for the development of European standards for the management and treatment of neurological diseases and has – since 1997 – published some 20 such guidelines. They have been distributed widely on the web and as printed material. Several of them have been translated into other European languages for use of national neurological societies. The task force applications and practice recommendations published within the framework of the EFNS (http://www.efns.org) have increased and have therefore undergone critical review. To meet the needs of future task forces preparing guidelines, instructions more specific than the previous guidance (Hughes *et al.*, 2001) seemed necessary and this paper responds to that need.

Aim of guidelines

The aim of an EFNS neurological management guideline is to provide evidence-based guidance for clinical neurologists, other health care professionals and health care providers about important aspects of the management of neurological diseases. It provides the view of an expert task force appointed by the Scientific Committee of the EFNS. It represents a peer-reviewed statement of the minimum number of desirable standards for the guidance of practice based on the best available evidence. It is not intended to have legally binding implications in individual cases.

Scientific basis of guidelines

The increasing burden of neurological diseases and disability can only be met by implementing measures of prevention and treatment that are scientifically proven and based upon evidence-based criteria. Sets of treatment recommendations and management guidelines have been prepared by the EFNS as well as by the American Academy of Neurology (AAN), Quality Standards Subcommittee (1999). The critical standards used

in both organizations aim to:

1. Evaluate the scientific evidence according to pre-specified levels of certainty.
2. Grade the recommendations according to the strength of available scientific evidence.

This Subcommittee of the EFNS recommends the use of such classes of evidence and grades of recommendations as those developed by the AAN that were applied for a therapeutic measure (Hirtz *et al.*, 2003) and a diagnostic measure (Shevell *et al.*, 2003) within the AAN practice guidelines groups. The definitions and requirements for the classes of evidence and levels of recommendations from the AAN were adapted and modified slightly and are listed in Tables 3.1 and 3.2.

Some of the issues under discussion include the question of classifying secondary endpoints from large, randomized, controlled trials as either first or second class evidence. The Subcommittee members agree that these secondary endpoints should generally not have the same scientific weight as the primary ones. This becomes relevant when the primary and secondary endpoints are both positive (or negative), implying that they both bear statistically significant results in favour of (or contrary to) the intervention under investigation. To name but one example: many intervention trials with cardiovascular endpoints (e.g. myocardial infarction) also have a secondary neurological endpoint (e.g. stroke). Assuming that both are positive, this does not imply that the treatment is effective for both cardiac and cerebral endpoints with equal scientific certainty, because the inclusion parameters, endpoint definitions and the diagnostic work-up regularly differ in precision and in absolute numbers of cases for both endpoints and usually heavily favour the primary one. These issues have not been handled uniformly in the past and therefore the need for these new, extended guidelines.

One other issue to be discussed within the framework of each task force when evaluating scientific evidence refers to important clinical areas for which no high class evidence is available or likely to become available in the near future. In such cases that should be marked as exceptional it may be possible to recommend best practice

Table 3.1 Evidence classification scheme for a therapeutic intervention

Class I An adequately powered prospective, randomized, controlled clinical trial with masked outcome assessment in a representative population or an adequately powered systematic review of prospective randomized controlled clinical trials with masked outcome assessment in representative populations. The following are required:

(a) randomization concealment;
(b) primary outcome(s) is/are clearly defined;
(c) exclusion/inclusion criteria are clearly defined;
(d) adequate accounting for dropouts and crossovers with numbers sufficiently low to have minimal potential for bias; and
(e) relevant baseline characteristics are presented and substantially equivalent among treatment groups or there is appropriate statistical adjustment for differences.

Class II Prospective matched-group cohort study in a representative population with masked outcome assessment that meets a–e above *or* a randomized, controlled trial in a representative population that lacks one criteria a–e.

Class III All other controlled trials (including well-defined natural history controls or patients serving as own controls) in a representative population, where outcome assessment is independent of patient treatment.

Class IV Evidence from uncontrolled studies, case series, case reports, or expert opinion.

Rating of recommendations

Level A (established as effective, ineffective, or harmful) requires at least one convincing class I study or at least two consistent, convincing class II studies.

Level B (probably effective, ineffective, or harmful) requires at least one convincing class II study or overwhelming class III evidence.

Level C (possibly effective, ineffective, or harmful) rating requires at least two convincing class III studies.

Table 3.2 Evidence classification scheme for a diagnostic measure

Class I A prospective study in a broad spectrum of persons with the suspected condition, using a 'gold standard' for case definition, where the test is applied in a blinded evaluation, and enabling the assessment of appropriate tests of diagnostic accuracy.

Class II A prospective study of a narrow spectrum of persons with the suspected condition, or a well-designed retrospective study of a broad spectrum of persons with an established condition (by 'gold standard') compared to a broad spectrum of controls, where test is applied in a blinded evaluation, and enabling the assessment of appropriate tests of diagnostic accuracy.

Class III Evidence provided by a retrospective study where either persons with the established condition or controls are of a narrow spectrum, and where test is applied in a blinded evaluation.

Class IV Any design where test is not applied in blinded evaluation or evidence provided by expert opinion alone or in descriptive case series (without controls).

Rating of recommendations

Level A (established as useful/predictive or not useful/predictive) requires at least one convincing class I study or at least two consistent, convincing class II studies.

Level B (established as probably useful/predictive or not useful/predictive) requires at least one convincing class II study or overwhelming class III evidence.

Level C (established as possibly useful/predictive or not useful/predictive) requires at least two convincing class III studies.

based on the experience of the guideline development group. An example of such an important area is the problem of recommendations for driving after a stroke where it is not easily conceivable to gather a large body of randomized evidence. Such 'Good Practice Points' have been used by the Scottish Intercollegiate Guidelines Network (SIGN) and make the recommendations more useful for health workers (SIGN, 2002). But such 'Good Practice Points' should not imply that they are based on more than class IV evidence that indicates large clinical uncertainty. This is not to indicate that a randomized trial to test the intervention can be avoided by assigning such points to a specific recommendation.

Critical review of guidelines

Current methods of developing guidelines have progressed from the informal consensus (TOBSAT = the old boys sat at a table; see Grilli *et al.*, 2000) to formal consensus methods, which use a systematic approach to assess the experts' opinion and reach an agreement on recommendation. The evidence-based consensus links its work directly to scientific evidence (Shaneyfelt *et al.*, 1999). According to the AAN, the strength of the guideline development process is that it 'aims at the evidence-based category, with little use for expert opinion' to reduce the likelihood of severe bias when relying on informal consensus alone (Franklin and Zahn, 2002). Consequently, guideline development has also been subjected to systematic evaluation. Following a systematic search, practice guidelines published in peer-reviewed medical literature between 1985 and 1997 were assessed with a 25-item measurement instrument that included the use of levels of evidence. From the 279 guidelines investigated, the mean overall adherence to such levels of evidence was 43% but improved significantly between 1985 and 1997 (36.9% versus 50.4%; $P < 0.001$) (Shaneyfelt *et al.*, 1999). Grilli *et al.* (2000) found similar discrepancies when investigating 431 guidelines between 1988 and 1998. The authors suggest the development of common standards of reporting, similar to the CONSORT statement for reporting the results of clinical trials

(Moher *et al.*, 2001). A more recent review of guidelines for stroke prevention has shown that there are significant differences in information about panel selection, funding source and consensus methods. Thus, it concludes that current stroke prevention guidelines do not provide adequate information to permit assessment of their quality (Hart and Bailey, 2002).

Guideline recommendations should also include the description of the methods used for synthesizing individual judgements. The development of the consensus reached is important but minority statements should also be included when necessary (Black *et al.*, 1999). All critical reviews are recommended to make use of a systematic and formal procedure of establishing guidelines. One recent and major effort was published by a Conference on Guideline Standardization (COGS) that produced a checklist to be used prospectively by developers to enable standardized recommendations (Shiffman *et al.*, 2003). This was achieved by means of a reiterative method (mostly several rounds of balloting by panel experts who gave differing weights to different pieces of scientific evidence). This method has reproducible results and is less likely to be biased by individual opinion. It involves stricter definitions for collecting and synthesizing evidence about potential harms, benefits and patients' preferences, and more effective considerations for implementation. Unfortunately, this COGS method is very laborious. The EFNS guidance proposed here captures the most important elements of the COGS proposals.

In addition to management guidelines, appropriate methods are needed to develop expert consensus on the process of care. Examples include the timely referral for diagnostic procedures (e.g. nerve conduction velocity testing in carpal tunnel syndrome?) and measures to improve patient satisfaction (Franklin and Zahn, 2002). Such process-related guidelines must take patient preferences into account and are no less important than treatment guidelines. Finally, there is evidence that adherence to guidelines improves patient outcome. This has been shown, for example, for post-acute rehabilitation following stroke indicating that such guidelines can also be used as quality of care indicators (Duncan *et al.*, 2002).

As a result of these quality issues, the goals and the process of the task force work are described in more detail below. These will be reviewed every 4 years and updated if necessary by the Subcommittee.

Collection of scientific data

1 The Cochrane Library should be consulted by every person or group planning to develop a guideline. There is little randomized evidence for many therapeutic options, and non-randomized studies also have to be considered. Authors of treatment guidelines should liaise with the coordinating editors of the appropriate Cochrane review group and review the list of registered titles of the Cochrane systematic reviews that have not yet been converted into protocols (www.cochrane.no/titles). The EFNS and the AAN have agreed to share their list of practice parameters or management guidelines under preparation.

2 Collection of data from original scientific papers in referee-based scientific journals is the cornerstone for evaluation of scientific evidence. Such papers can be identified from several bibliographic databases. It is important to use specific and sensitive keywords as well as combinations of keywords. A single keyword is rarely sufficient. Both older and new scientific papers should be included. It is imperative that the data are collected from the primary paper itself, and not from secondary literature. The full paper should always be read and not the abstract alone. Data can be included from papers that have been accepted but not yet published, but not usually before acceptance. In accordance with the Cochrane Library, unpublished data from randomized trials can be used provided they are of high quality. Such exceptions should be explained in the synthesizing evidence section of the report.

3 Collection of papers containing any previous meta-analyses of the same or similar topics should always be undertaken. Such papers are always helpful, but they usually do not give the full and final conclusion for a task force.

4 Collection of review/overview papers is done from the same bibliographic databases. Such reviews are usually well known by the experts in the field, and may be included in the work of the task force. The conclusions of such papers should never be used without independently evaluating the scientific evidence of the papers from the original data.

5 Scientific data from papers published in refereed journals not included in the main databases may be included. As such papers are more difficult to identify, it is not a prerequisite for a task force to collect them.

6 Scientific data from non-refereed journals, books or other publications should usually not influence recommendations and conclusions. They are therefore not important to collect.

7 Previous guideline documents and recommendations should be sought from MEDLINE, EMBASE and other sources including national and international neurology organizations, patient organizations, and national or supranational health-related bodies. Although task force conclusions should rely on quality-assured scientific data alone, it is appropriate to discuss previous guidelines and recommendations (which may be registered by the International Network of Agencies for Health Technology Assessment, www.inahta.org).

The process of proposing, planning and writing a guideline

1 Neurological Management Guidelines will be produced by Task Forces appointed by the Scientific Committee.

2 Proposals for Task Forces concerning neurological management should be submitted to the Scientific Committee. The proposal should include the title, objectives, membership, conflict of interests, short (100–300 words) explanation of why the guideline is needed, already existing guidelines on the same or related topic, search strategy, method for reaching consensus, and time frame for accomplishment. Task Forces will usually be appointed following a proposal from the chairperson of a Scientific Panel to the Scientific Committee.

3 The Task Force will consist of a chairperson and at least six but not usually more than 12 members. No more than two members should usually come from any one country. Conflicts of interest must be declared by members at the time of the formation of the Task Force. The chairperson should be free from conflicts of interest. If feasible, the group should include a patient advocate (normally an officer from a European patient organization if the Task Force deals with a clinically relevant topic) and other relevant specialists (such as a statistician) and health professionals. If Task Forces have a budget, they must nominate a secretary and treasurer and submit an annual account to the Management Committee.

4 The Task Force will review the available evidence and include within its report the search strategy employed. Where appropriate, the evidence concerning health care interventions must be based on a thorough systematic literature search and review. The report should include a structured summary that contains the main conclusions. Irreconcilable differences between group members should be referred to the Scientific Committee through its chairman.

5 Existing guidelines prepared by other organizations (including European neurology subspecialty societies, European national neurological societies, non-European neurological societies, and other organizations) will be sought and where appropriate adopted in part or whole with appropriate acknowledgement and respect for copyright rules.

6 The format of the guidelines will use the style of the *European Journal of Neurology* and follow a template with these sections:

  (1) Title. This should read: EFNS Guideline on Report of an EFNS Task Force on (title of Task Force, if different from the topic of the guideline);
  (2) Structured abstract;
  (3) Membership of task force;
  (4) Objectives;
  (5) Background;
  (6) Search strategy;
  (7) Method for reaching consensus;
  (8) Results;
  (9) Recommendations;
  (10) Statement of the likely time when the guidelines will need to be updated;
  (11) Conflicts of interest;
  (12) References.

7 The length of the guideline report should not be more than eight printed pages including references (4000 words). Supplementary material may be published on the EFNS website. The authors will be the EFNS Task Force on *management/diagnosis/other of condition*. The authors will be listed as Members of the Task Force with the chairman first and the other authors in alphabetical order.

8 The task force should submit the completed guideline for approval to the chairperson of the Scientific Committee.

9 The Scientific Committee will have the proposed management guideline reviewed by its members, the president of the EFNS and the chairpersons of any Scientist Panel that might be affected by the guidelines but which is not involved in the preparation of them. Additional external peer reviewing may be sought especially in areas where few neurological experts are available. Within 8 weeks of submission, the chairperson of the Scientific Committee will advise the chairperson of the Task Force whether the guidelines have been accepted or not as the official guidelines of the EFNS. If revision is needed, the Task Force will prepare a revised version and submit this to the review process again, highlighting the revisions and documenting the responses to each of the referees' comments.

10 Following approval, the management guidelines will be submitted by the chairperson of the Task Force to the editor/s of the *European Journal of Neurology* with a view to publication. The editor will have the power to accept or reject the guidelines for publication and may make minor editorial changes.

11 The validity of the published guidelines will be reviewed by the chairpersons of the Task Force and the relevant Scientist Panel at least every 2 years.

12 Guidelines will be published on the EFNS web and in the *European Journal of Neurology*.
13 National societies will be encouraged to translate guidelines for dissemination in their own countries.

References

American Academy of Neurology, Quality Standards Subcommittee (1999). *Process for Developing Practice Parameters*. Saint Paul, MN: American Academy of Neurology.

Black N, Murphy M, Lauping D *et al*. (1999). Consensus developing methods: a review of best practices creating clinical guidelines. *J Health Serv Res Policy* **4:**236–238.

Cochrane Collaboration. http://www.cochrane.org .

Duncan PW, Horner RD, Reker DM *et al*. (2002). Adherence to postacute rehabilitation guidelines is associated with functional recovery in stroke. *Stroke* **33:**167–178.

Franklin GM, Zahn CA (2002). AAN clinical practice guidelines. *Neurology* **59:**975–976.

Grilli R, Magrini N, Penna A, Mura G, Liberati A (2000). Practice guidelines developed by specialty societies: the need for a critical appraisal. *The Lancet* **355:**103–106.

Hart RG, Bailey RD (2002). An assessment of guidelines for prevention of ischemic stroke. *Neurology* **59:**977–982.

Hirtz D, Berg A, Bettis D *et al*. (2003) Practice parameter: treatment of the child with a first unprovoked seizure. Report of the Quality Standards Subcommittee of the American Academy of Neurology and the Practice Committee of the Child Neurology Society. *Neurology* **60:**166–175.

Hughes RAC, Barnes MP, Baron J-C, Brainin M (2001). Guidance for the preparation of neurological management guidelines by EFNS scientific task forces. *Eur J Neurol* **8:**549–550.

Moher D, Schulz KF, Altman DG, for the CONSORT Group (2001). The CONSORT statement: revised recommendations for improving the quality of reports of parallel-group randomised trials. *The Lancet* **357:** 1191–1194.

Olesen J, Leonardi M (2003). The burden of brain diseases in Europe. *Eur J Neurol* **10:**471.

Scottish Intercollegiate Guidelines Network (SIGN) (2002). Management of patients with stroke. A national clinical guideline. http://www.sign.ac.uk.

Shaneyfelt TM, Mayo-Smith MF, Rothwange J (1999). Are guidelines following guidelines? The methodological quality of clinical practice guidelines in the peer-reviewed medical literature. *JAMA* **281:** 1900–1905.

Shevell M, Ashwal S, Donley D *et al*. (2003). Practice parameter: evaluation of the child with global developmental delay. Report of the Quality Standards Subcommittee of the American Academy of Neurology and The Practice Committee of the Child Neurology Society. *Neurology* **60:**367–380.

Shiffman RN, Shekelle P, Overhage M, Slutsky J, Grimshaw J, Deshpande AM (2003). Standardized reporting of clinical practice guidelines: a proposal from the Conference on Guideline Standardization. *Ann Intern Med* **139:**493–498.

Üstün TB, Rehm J, Chatterji S *et al*. (1999). Multiple-informant ranking of the disabling effects of different health conditions in 14 countries. *The Lancet* **354:**111–115.

CHAPTER 4

Routine cerebrospinal fluid (CSF) analysis

F. Deisenhammer,[a] A. Bartos,[b] R. Egg,[a]
N. E. Gilhus,[c] G. Giovannoni,[d] S. Rauer,[e]
F. Sellebjerg[f]

Background A great variety of neurological diseases require investigation of the cerebrospinal fluid (CSF) to prove the diagnosis or to rule out relevant differential diagnoses.

Objectives To evaluate the theoretical background and provide guidelines for clinical use in routine CSF analysis including total protein, albumin, immunoglobulins, glucose, lactate, cell count, cytological staining, and investigation of infectious CSF.

Methods Systematic Medline search for the above mentioned variables. Review of appropriate publications by one or more of the task force members. Grading of evidence and recommendations was based on consensus by all task force members.

CSF should be analysed immediately after collection. If storage is needed 12 ml of CSF should be partitioned into three to four sterile tubes.

Albumin CSF/serum ratio (Q_{alb}) should be preferred to total protein measurement and normal upper limits should be related to patients' age. Elevated Q_{alb} is a non-specific finding but occurs mainly in bacterial, cryptococcal, and tuberculous meningitis, leptomeningeal metastases as well as acute and chronic demyelinating polyneuropathies.

Pathological decrease of the CSF/serum glucose ratio or an increase in lactate concentration indicates bacterial or fungal meningitis or leptomeningeal metastases.

Intrathecal immunoglobulin G synthesis is best demonstrated by isoelectric focusing followed by specific staining.

Cellular morphology (cytological staining) should be evaluated whenever pleocytosis is found or leptomeningeal metastases or pathological bleeding is suspected. Computed tomography-negative intrathecal bleeding should be investigated by bilirubin detection.

Introduction

The cerebrospinal fluid (CSF) is a dynamic, metabolically active substance that has many

---

[a]Department of Neurology, Innsbruck Medical University, Austria; [b]Department of Neurology, Charles University, Prague, Czech Republic; [c]Department of Clinical Medicine, University of Bergen, Bergen, Norway, and Department of Neurology, Haukeland University Hospital, Bergen, Norway; [d]Department of

Neuroinflammation, Institute of Neurology, University College London, Queen Square, London, UK; [e]Department of Neurology and Clinical Neurophysiology, Albert-Ludwigs University, Freiburg, Germany; [f]Department of Neurology, Copenhagen University Hospital, Denmark.

Table 4.1 Typical constellation of CSF parameters in some neurological diseases.

	Total protein (g/l)	Glucose ratio	Lactate (mmol/l)	Cell count (per 3.2 μl)	Typical cytology
Normal values[a]	<0.45	>0.4–0.5	<1.0–2.9	<15	MNC
Disease					
Acute bacterial meningitis	↑	↓	↑	>1000	PNC
Viral neuro-infections (meningo/encephalitis)	=/↑	=/↓	=	10–1000	PNC/MNC
Autoimmune polyneuropathy	↑	=	=	=	
Infectious polyneuropathy	↑	=	=	↑	MNC
Subarachnoidal haemorrhage	↑	=	=	↑	erythrocytes, macrophages, siderophages MNC
Multiple sclerosis	=	=	=	=/↑	MNC
Leptomeningeal metastases	↑	=/↓	NA	=/↑	malignant cells, mononuclears

CSF, cerebrospinal fluid; MNC, mononuclear cells; PNC, polymorphonuclear cells. ↑/↓, increased/decreased; =, within normal limits; NA, evidence not available. [a]Normal values are given for lumbar CSF in adults.

important functions. It is invaluable as a diagnostic aid in the evaluation of inflammatory conditions, infectious or non-infectious, involving the brain, spinal cord, and meninges as well as in CT-negative subarachnoidal haemorrhage and in leptomeningeal metastases. CSF is obtained with relative ease by lumbar puncture (LP). Alterations in CSF constituents may be similar in different pathologic processes and cause difficulties in interpretation. Combining a set of CSF variables referred to as routine parameters (i.e. determination of protein, albumin, immunoglobulin, glucose, lactate, and cellular changes, as well as specific antigen and antibody testing for infectious agents) will increase the diagnostic sensitivity and specificity.

The aim of this guideline paper was to produce recommendations on how to use this set of CSF parameters in different clinical settings and to show how different constellations of these variables correlate with diseases of the nervous system (table 4.1) (Brainin *et al.*, 2004).

Search strategy

A Medline search using the search terms cerebrospinal fluid (CSF), immunoglobulin G (IgG) immunoglobulin M (IgM), immunoglobulin A (IgA), and albumin was conducted. Also, the key words 'cerebrospinal fluid' or 'CSF' were cross-referenced with 'glucose', 'lactate', 'cytology', 'cell* in title' excluding 'child*'. Furthermore, a search for 'cerebrospinal fluid' and 'immunoglobulin' and 'diagnosis' and 'electrophoresis' or 'isoelectric focusing' was performed limited to the time between 1 January 1980 and 1 January 2005, and returned only items with abstracts, and English language (274 references). A search for 'cerebrospinal fluid' AND 'infectious' limited for time (1 January 1980 until now) returned 560 abstracts. Abstracts that primarily did not deal with diagnostic issues and infectious CSF (e.g. non-infectious inflammatory diseases, vaccination, general CSF parameters, pathophysiology, cytokines and therapy) were excluded resulting in 60 abstracts.

Searching the items 'cerebrospinal fluid' AND 'serology' limited for time (1 January 1980 until now) and excluding abstracts not directly related to the topic returned 35 abstracts and a search for 'cerebrospinal fluid' AND 'bacterial culture' limited for time (1 Jan 1980 until now) resulted in 28 abstracts.

The abstracts were selected by the author who was in charge of the respective topic.

In addition, text books and articles identified in reference lists of individual papers were selected if considered appropriate.

There are no guidelines for CSF analysis published by the American Academy of Neurology (AAN). Individual task force members prepared draft statements for various parts of the manuscript. Evidence was classified as Class I–IV and recommendations as Level A–C according to the scheme agreed for EFNS guidelines (Brainin et al., 2004). When only Class IV evidence was available but consensus could be reached, the Task Force has offered advice as Good Practice Points (Brainin et al., 2004). The statements were revised and adapted into a single document that was then revised until consensus was reached.

Quantitative analysis of total protein and albumin

The blood–CSF barrier is a physical barrier, consisting of different anatomical structures, for the diffusion and filtration of macromolecules from blood to CSF. The integrity of these barriers and CSF bulk flow determine the protein content of the CSF (Thompson, 1988; Reiber, 1994). In newborns, CSF protein concentrations are high, but decrease gradually during the first year of life, and are maintained at low levels in childhood. In adults, CSF protein concentrations increase with age (Eeg-Olofson et al., 1981; Statz and Felgenhauer, 1983) (Class I). The CSF to serum albumin concentration quotient (Q_{alb}) can also be used to evaluate blood–CSF barrier integrity (Andersson et al., 1994). The Q_{alb} is not influenced by intrathecal protein synthesis, is corrected for the plasma concentration of albumin, and is an integral part of intrathecal immunoglobulin synthesis

formulae. The Q_{alb} is a method-independent measure, allowing the use of the same reference values in different laboratories (Blennow et al., 1993; Reiber, 1995). However, there are no conclusive data on how the Q_{alb} performs compared to total protein as a measure of blood–CSF barrier function in large cohorts of unselected patients.

There is a concentration gradient for total protein and the Q_{alb} along the neuraxis with the lowest concentrations in the ventricular fluid and the highest concentrations in the lumbar sac (Thompson, 1988; Fishman, 1992). A significant decrease of the Q_{alb} was observed from the first 0–4 ml of CSF to the last 21–24 ml of CSF obtained by LP (Blennow et al., 1993) (Class I). The Q_{alb} is also influenced by body weight, sex, degenerative lower back disease, hypothyroidism, alcohol consumption (Class II) and smoking (Class III) (Kornhuber et al., 1987; Skouen et al., 1994; Nyström et al., 1997; Seyfert et al., 2002). Posture and physical activity may influence the CSF protein concentration, resulting in higher CSF protein concentrations in inactive, bed-ridden patients (Seyfert et al., 2002) (Class III). Elevated CSF protein concentrations can be found in the majority of patients with bacterial (0.4–4.4 g/l), cryptococcal (0.3–3.1 g/l), tuberculous (0.2–1.5 g/l) meningitis and neuroborreliosis (Stockstill and Kauffman, 1983; Sabeta, 1985; Kaiser, 1998; Negrini et al., 2000) (Class II). A concentration of >1.5 g/l is specific (99%), but insensitive (55%) for bacterial meningitis as compared to a variety of other inflammatory diseases (Lindquist et al., 1988) (Class I).

In viral neuroinfections CSF protein concentrations are raised to a lesser degree (usually <0.95 g/l) (Negrini et al., 2000) (Class II). The concentration in herpes simplex virus encephalitis is normal in half of the patients during the first week of illness (Koskiniemi et al., 1984) (Class IV).

Non-infectious causes for an increased CSF protein and sometimes with an increased cell count include subarachnoidal haemorrhage, central nervous system (CNS) vasculitis, and CNS neoplasm (Jerrard et al., 2001) (Class IV). Elevated total protein concentration with normal CSF cell count (albuminocytologic dissociation) is a hallmark in acute and chronic inflammatory demyelinating polyneuropathies but protein levels may be normal during the first week (Segurado *et al.*, 1986; Senevirante, 2000) (Class IV). Total CSF protein is elevated in 80% of patients with leptomeningeal metastases to a median concentration of 1 g/l with a wide range (Twijnstra *et al.*, 1989) (Class III).

In conclusion, there is Class I evidence that increased Q_{alb} and total CSF protein concentrations are mainly supportive of bacterial, cryptococcal, and tuberculous meningitis as well as leptomingeal metastases. As Q_{alb} or protein is usually not the only CSF investigation the combination with other CSF variables will increase the diagnostic specificity, like albuminocytologic dissociation in Gullain–Barré syndrome.

Quantitative intrathecal immunoglobulin synthesis

Intrathecal Ig synthesis is found in various, mainly inflammatory CNS diseases (table 4.2). There is a close correlation between the Q_{alb} and the CSF-serum IgG concentration quotient (Q_{IgG}) which led to the development of the IgG index (Q_{IgG} /Q_{alb}) (Delpech and Lichtblau, 1972; Ganrot and Laurell, 1974; Link and Tibbling, 1977). Reiber's hyperbolic formula and Öhman's extended immunoglobulin indices are based on the demonstration of non-linear relationships between the Q_{alb} and CSF-serum concentration quotients for IgG, IgA and IgM (Öhman *et al.*, 1989 and 1993; Reiber, 1994).

Table 4.2 Percentage of patients in different categories of disease with elevated IgA-index, IgG-index, IgM-index, or non-linear intrathecal synthesis formula values (data from Schipper *et al.*, 1988; McLean *et al.* 1990; Öhman *et al.*, 1992; Sellebjerg *et al.*, 1996; Korenke *et al.*, 1997). Unexpected increases are more common with the IgA index, IgG index and IgM index than with corresponding non-linear formulae.

	IgG (%)	IgA (%)	IgM (%)
No inflammatory and no CNS disease	<5	<5	<5
Non-inflammatory CNS disease (including degenerative and vascular diseases)	<25[a]	<5	<5
Infections of the nervous system	25–50	25	25
Bacterial infections	25–50	25–50	<25
Viral infections	25–50	<25	<25
Lyme neuroborreliosis	25–50	<25	75
Multiple sclerosis	70–80	<25	<25
Clinically isolated syndromes	40–60	<10	<25
Inflammatory neuropathies	25–50[a]	25–50[a]	25–50[a]
Neoplastic disorders (in general)	<25[a]	ND	ND
Paraneoplastic syndromes	<25	ND	ND
Meningeal carcinomatosis	25–50	ND	ND
Other neuroinflammatory diseases	25–50[b]	ND[c]	ND

CNS, central nervous system; ND, not determined in larger studies using non-linear immunoglobulin formulae. [a]Usually not associated with oligoclonal bands (artefact in presence of barrier impairment); [b]rare in biopsy-proven neurosarcoidosis; [c]prominent IgA synthesis in adrenoleukodystrophy.

For the detection of intrathecal IgG synthesis, the detection of IgG oligoclonal bands is superior to the IgG index and the non-linear formulae both in terms of diagnostic sensitivity and specificity. However, the detection of IgG oligoclonal bands is technically more demanding than the quantitative measures, and it has been suggested that in the setting of suspected multiple sclerosis (MS), oligoclonal bands analysis may be omitted in patients with an IgG-index value above 1.1, as almost 100% of such patients turn out to have intrathecally synthesized IgG oligoclonal bands (F. Deisenhammer, unpublished data).

In studies comparing CSF findings in patients with MS and other neurological diseases, non-linear formulae were superior (Öhman *et al.*, 1992; Sellebjerg *et al.*, 1996). Intrathecal IgA, IgG and IgM synthesis formulae may be helpful in discriminating between different infectious diseases of the nervous system (Felgenhauer, 1982; Felgenhauer and Schädlich, 1987) (Class III). However, one study suggested that increased values of the Reiber formula do not always reflect intrathecal IgM synthesis as increased values were observed in several patients with non-inflammatory diseases without IgM oligoclonal bands in CSF (Sharief *et al.*, 1990) (Class II). In conclusion, there is no evidence to support the routine use of quantitative assessment of intrathecal immunoglobulin synthesis in the diagnosis of neurological diseases, but in the setting of suspected MS the IgG index may be used as a screening procedure to determine intrathecal IgG synthesis.

Qualitative (oligoclonal) intrathecal IgG synthesis

The detection of intrathecal oligoclonal IgG in the CSF is useful diagnostically, particularly as it is one of the laboratory criteria supporting the clinical diagnosis of MS (McDonald *et al.*, 2001). In addition, it can be used to assist in the diagnosis of other putative autoimmune disorders of the CNS, such as paraneoplastic disorders and CNS infections (Rauer and Kaiser, 2000; Stich *et al.*, 2003; Storstein *et al.*, 2004).

Using electrophoresis techniques it is possible to classify the humoral responses according to the number of antibody clones produced (i.e. monoclonal, oligoclonal and polyclonal responses; figure 4.1). Earlier methods have now been superseded by the development of the more

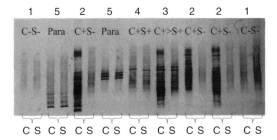

Figure 4.1. IEF immunoblots of the five consensus patterns of various CSF and serum isoelectric focusing patterns for local/systemic synthesis. The pattern number is given above the paired samples.

Type 1 (C-S-): No bands in CSF and serum. Normal.

Type 2 (C+S-): Oligoclonal IgG is present in the CSF with no apparent corresponding abnormality in serum, indicating local intrathecal synthesis of IgG. Typical example: MS.

Type 3 (C+>S+): There are IgG bands in both the CSF and serum, with additional bands present in the CSF. The oligoclonal bands that are common to both CSF and serum imply a systemic inflammatory response, whereas the bands that are restricted to the CNS suggest that there is an additional CNS-only response. Typical examples: MS, systemic lupus erythematodes (SLE), sarcoid etc.

Type 4 (C+S+): There are oligoclonal bands present in the CSF, which are identical to those in serum. This is not indicative of local synthesis, but rather, the pattern is consistent with passive transfer of oligoclonal IgG from a systemic inflammatory response. Typical examples: Guillain–Barre syndrome, acute disseminated encephalomyelitis (ADEM) and systemic infections.

Type 5 (Para): There is a monoclonal IgG pattern in both CSF and serum, the source of which lies outside the CNS. Typical examples: Myeloma, monoclonal gammopathy of undetermined significance (MGUS).

sensitive technique of isoelectric focusing (IEF) and immunofixation (Andersson *et al.*, 1994).

Isoelectric focusing uses a pH gradient to separate IgG populations on the basis of charge, which are then transferred onto a nitro-cellulose or other membrane before immunostaining using an anti-human immunoglobulin (Keir *et al.*, 1990). Some laboratories continue to use silver staining to detect oligoclonal bands (OCBs) with good results (Blennow and Fredman, 1995).

As CSF is an ultrafiltrate of plasma, it contains immunoglobulins that are passively transferred from the plasma, as well as immunoglobulins synthesized locally. Any systemic pattern of immunoglobulin production seen in plasma or serum will therefore be mirrored in the CSF. It is imperative that any CSF analysis for oligoclonal bands is accompanied by a paired blood analysis.

An oligoclonal intrathecal IgG antibody response is not specific. Table 4.3 provides a list with the proportion of cases with oligoclonal bands (for a more detailed list please see McLean *et al.* (1990)). Local synthesis of oligoclonal bands is therefore not diagnostic and has to be interpreted in the clinical context. A recently published recommendation regarding detection of oligoclonal bands concluded as follows (Freedman *et al.*, 2005):

> The single most informative analysis is a qualitative assessment of CSF for IgG, best performed using IEF together with some form of immunodetection (blotting or fixation). This qualitative analysis should be performed using unconcentrated CSF and must be compared directly with serum run simultaneously in the same assay in an adjacent track. Optimal runs utilize similar amounts of IgG from paired serum and CSF. Recognised positive and negative controls should be run with each set of samples.

In putative non-infectious inflammatory disorders of the CNS there is Class I evidence to support the use of CSF IEF for both predictive and diagnostic testing in the diagnosis of MS. In other non-infectious inflammatory disorders of the CNS Class II and III evidence exists to support the use of CSF IEF to supplement other diagnostic tests (table 4.3).

CSF glucose concentration, CSF/serum glucose ratio and lactate

As glucose is actively transported across the blood–brain barrier the CSF glucose levels are directly proportional to the plasma levels and therefore simultaneous measurement in CSF and blood is required. Normal CSF glucose concentration is 50–60% of serum values (Jerrard *et al.*, 2001) (Class IV). A CSF/serum glucose ratio less than 0.4–0.5 is considered to be pathological (Feigin *et al.*, 1992) (Class IV). CSF glucose takes several hours to equilibrate with plasma glucose; therefore, in unusual circumstances levels of CSF glucose can actually be higher than plasma levels for several hours. During CSF storage glucose is degraded. Therefore, glucose determination must be performed immediately after CSF collection.

A high CSF glucose concentration has no specific diagnostic importance and is related to an elevated blood glucose concentration, for example, in diabetics.

The behaviour of the CSF/serum glucose ratio in different neurological diseases is shown in table 4.1.

The relevance of CSF lactate is similar to that of CSF/serum glucose ratio. CSF lactate is independent of blood concentration (Watson and Scott, 1995) (Class IV). The normal value is considered to be <2.8–3.5 mmol/l (Jordan, 1983) (Class II). Except for mitochondrial disease CSF lactate correlates inversely with CSF/serum glucose ratio. An increased level can be detected earlier than the reduced glucose concentration.

Decreased CSF/serum glucose ratio or increased CSF lactate indicate bacterial and fungal infections or leptomeningeal metastases.

Cytological examination

Cytological evaluation should be performed within 2 h after puncture, preferably within 30 min because of a lysis of both red blood cells and white blood cells (Steele *et al.*, 1986) (Class IV).

Cerebrospinal fluid leukocytes are usually counted in a Fuchs-Rosenthal chamber (volume 3.2 μl) and therefore, counts are reported as '/3'

Table 4.3 Inflammatory diseases of the CNS associated with CSF oligoclonal IgG bands (McLean *et al.*, 1990).

Disorder	Incidence of oligoclonal bands (%)	Evidence
Multiple sclerosis	95	Class I[a]
Auto-immune		
Neuro-SLE	50	Class III
Neuro-Behcet's	20	Class II
Neuro-sarcoid	40	Class III
Harada's meningitis-uveitis	60	Class III
Infectious		
Acute viral encephalitis (<7 days)	<5	Class II
Acute bacterial meningitis (<7 days)	< 5	Class II
Subacute sclerosing panencephalitis (SSPE)	100	Class I
Progressive rubella panencephalitis	100	Class I
Neurosyphilis	95	Class I
Neuro-AIDS	80	Class II
Neuro-borrelliosis	80	Class I
Tumour	<5	Class III
Hereditary		
Ataxia-telangiectasia	60	Class III
Adrenoleukodystrophy (encephalitic)	100	Class II

CNS, central nervous system; CSF, cerebrospinal fluid; IgG, immunoglobulin G; SLE, systemic lupus erythematodes. [a]This is based on studies using the Poser diagnostic criteria (Poser *et al.*, 1983) that were validated against the original Schumacher criteria (Schumacher *et al.*, 1965). None of these criteria have been validated using population-based studies. Therefore, it could be argued that the diagnostic 'gold standard' is a flawed standard.

cells to correct for a standard volume of 1 μl. A cytocentrifuge (cytospin), the Sayk sedimentation chamber, or membrane filtration can be used to obtain a sufficient number of cells for cytology (Lamers and Wevers, 1995). For cellular differentiation May–Gruenwald–Giemsa staining is widely used but specific methods may be performed, especially for the detection of malignant cells (Roma *et al.*, 2002; Adam *et al.*, 2001) (Class II).

Lymphocytes and monocytes at the resting phase and occasionally ependymal cells are found in normal CSF.

An increased number of neutrophilic granulocytes can be found in bacterial and acute viral CNS infections (Spanos *et al.*, 1989; Adam, 2001)

(Class II). In the postacute phase a mononuclear transformation occurs.

Upon activation lymphocytes can enlarge or become plasma cells indicating an unspecific inflammatory reaction (Adam, 2001; Zeman *et al.*, 2001) (Class IV). Resting monocytes enlarge and display vacuoles when activated. Macrophages are the most activated monocytes. These cell forms can occur in a great variety of diseases.

Erythrophages occur 12–18 h after haemorrhage. Siderophages containing haemosiderin are seen as early as 1–2 days after haemorrhage and may persist for weeks. Macrophages containing haematoidin (crystallized bilirubin) degraded from haemoglobin may appear about 2 weeks after bleeding and are a sign of a previous subarachnoid

Table 4.4 List of infectious agents responsible for the vast majority of infectious CNS diseases.

Pathogen	Symptoms, Comments	Recommended diagnostic method*
Bacteria		
Should be considered in first line		
Neisseria meningitides		Microscopy, culture
Streptococcus pneumoniae		Microscopy, culture
Haemophilus influenzae	Rare due to vaccination	Microscopy, culture
Staphylococcus aureus	Neurosurgical intervention, trauma	Microscopy, culture
Escherichia coli	Newborns	Microscopy, culture
Borrelia burgdorferi sensu lato		Serology
Treponema pallidum	Syphilis in the past	Serology
Mycobacterium tuberculosis		PCR[a], culture, positive tuberculin test
Should be considered especially in immunosuppressed patients		
Actinobacter species		Culture
Bacteroides fragilis		Culture
JC-virus	Progressive multifocal leukoencephalopathy	PCR
Listeria monocytogenes		Microscopy, culture
Nocardia asteroides		Microscopy (modified Ziehl-Neelsen stain and culture from brain biopsy)
Pasteurella multocida		Culture
Streptococcus mitis		Culture
Should be considered in special situations		
Brucella spp.	Ingestion of raw milk (products) from cows, sheep or goats	Culture
Campylobacter fetus		Microscopy, culture
Coxiella burnetti (Q-fever)	Contact with infected parturient animals (sheep, goat, cattle) or inhalation of dust contaminated by the excrements of infected animals or ticks	Serology
Leptospira interrogans	Exposure to contaminated water or rodent urine	Culture, serology
Mycoplasma pneumoniae	Children and young adults	Serology
Rickettsia	Tick exposure, exanthema	Serology
coagulase-negative staphylococci	Patients with ventricular shunts or drainages	Culture
group B streptococci	(preterm) newborns	Microscopy, culture
Tropheryma whipplei (M. Whipple)	Patients with gastrointestinal symptoms (malabsorption)	PCR
Viruses		
Should be considered in first line		
Herpes simplex virus (HSV) type 1 and 2		PCR, serology
Varicella–Zoster virus (VZV)		PCR, serology
Enteroviruses (Echovirus, Coxsackievirus A, B)		PCR, serology
Human immunodeficiency virus (HIV) type 1 and 2		PCR, serology

Continued

Table 4.4 Continued.

Pathogen	Symptoms, Comments	Recommended diagnostic method*
Epstein–Barr virus (EBV)	Lymphadenitis, splenomegaly	PCR
Cytomegalovirus (CMV)	Very rare in immunocompetent patients	PCR
Should be considered in special situations		
Adenovirus	Children and young adults	PCR, culture, antigen detection
Human T-cell leukaemia virus type I (HTLV-I)	Spastic paraparesis	Serology
Influenza - and		Serology
Parainfluenza virus		
Lymphocytic chorio-meningitis (LCM)		Serology
Mumps virus		Serology
Poliovirus	Flaccid paresis	PCR
Rabies virus	Contact with rabies-infected animals	PCR from CSF, root of hair, cornea
Rotavirus	Diarrhoea, febrile convulsions in children	Antigen detection in stool specimens
Rubella virus		Serology
Sandfly Fever	Endemic region: Italy	Serology
Fungi		
Aspergillus fumigatus		Antigen detection in CSF, where required culture from brain biopsy
Cryptococcus neoformans		Antigen detection in CSF, india ink stain, less sensitive than antigen detection, culture
Parasites		
Toxoplasma gondii		CSF: PCR, serology; brain biopsy: PCR
Strongyloides stercoralis		Pathogen detection in stool

The following pathogens should be considered in acute myelitis [Recommendation Level B]: HSV type 1 and 2 (PCR), VZV (PCR), Enteroviruses (PCR), *Borrelia burgdorferi sensu latu* (serology, AI), HIV (serology), tick-borne encephalitis virus (only in endemic areas) (serology, AI). [a]Nested PCR technique has been shown to be substantially more sensitive and specific than conventional single step PCR techniques (Takahashi *et al.*, 2005).

bleeding (Adam, 2001) (Class IV). However, spectrophotometry of CSF involving bilirubin quantitation has been recommended as the method of choice to prove CT-negative subarachnoid bleeding up to 2 weeks after onset (UK National External Quality Assessment Scheme for Immunochemistry Working Group, 2003).

Lipophages indicate CNS tissue destruction. The presence of macrophages without detectable intracellular material is a non-specific finding,

occurring in disc herniation, malignant meningeal infiltration, spinal tumours, head trauma, stroke, MS, vasculitis, infections and subarachnoid haemorrhage (Adam, 2001) (Class IV).

Eosinophils are normally not present in CSF. The presence of 10 or more eosinophils/μl in CSF or eosinophilia of at least 10% of the total CSF leukocyte count is associated with a limited number of diseases, including parasitic infections, and coccidioiodomycosis. It can occur in malignancies and react to medication and ventriculoperitoneal shunts (Lo Re, 2003). Malignant CSF cells indicate leptomeningeal metastases. False positive results often occur when inflammatory cells are mistaken for tumour cells or due to contamination with peripheral blood (Twijnstra *et al.*, 1987). False negative detection of malignant cells on cytologic examination of CSF is common. Factors increasing the detection rate of malignant cells include a volume of at least 10.5 ml and repeating this procedure once if the cytology is negative. The detection rate of 50–70% after the first investigation can be increased to 85–92% after a second puncture (Glantz *et al.*, 1998) (Class III). Further LPs will only slightly increase the diagnostic sensitivity (Wasserstrom *et al.*, 1982; Kaplan *et al.*, 1990) (Class III).

In conclusion, cell count is generally useful because most of the indications for CSF analysis include diseases that are associated with elevated numbers of various cells. Cytological staining can be helpful in distinguishing CNS diseases when the cell count is increased.

Investigation of infectious CSF

There are many small to medium-sized studies investigating the diagnostic sensitivity and specificity of tests for various infectious agents but no controlled study evaluating a work-up of infectious CSF in general. Therefore, there are no valid data on the indication, sensitivity and specificity of microbiological procedures in general (i.e. how to proceed with CSF in obvious CNS infections). Existing proposals for the general work-up of infectious CSF are based on clinical practice and theoretically plausible procedures (Schlossberg, 1990; Kniehl *et al.*, 2001; Kaiser, 2002).

There are a great number of methods for antigen or specific antibody detection and their use depend mainly on the type of antigen (table 4.4).

In neuroinfections specific antigen or antibody detection should be performed depending on the clinical presentation and the results of basic CSF analysis. The formula for the estimation of the relative intrathecal synthesis of specific antibodies in the CSF (Antibody Index [AI]) is as

follows:

Estimation of intrathecal synthesis of specific antibodies in the CSF (Antibody Index [AI])

$$\text{Antibody ratio} = \frac{\text{Antibody} - \text{concentration}_{\text{CSF}}}{\text{Antibody} - \text{concentration}_{\text{serum}}}$$

$$\text{IgG ratio} = \frac{\text{IgG} - \text{concentration}_{\text{CSF}}}{\text{IgG} - \text{concentration}_{\text{serum}}}$$

$$\text{AI} = \text{Antibody ratio}/\text{IgG ratio}(\text{positive} > 1,5)$$

Cerebrospinal fluid polymerase chain reaction can be performed rapidly and inexpensively and has become an integral component of diagnostic medical practice. A patient with a positive PCR result is 88 times more likely to have a definite diagnosis of viral infection of the CNS as compared to a patient with a negative PCR result. A negative PCR result can be used with moderate confidence to rule out a diagnosis of viral infection of the CNS (the probability of a definite viral CNS infection was 0.1 in case of a negative PCR result compared to a positive PCR result) (Jeffery *et al.*, 1997). It should be considered that false negative results are most likely if the CSF sample is taken within the first 3 days after the illness or 10 days and more after the onset of the disease (Davies *et al.*, 2005; Kennedy, 2005).

In general, PCR is indicated in the following situations:

when microscopy, culture or serology is insensitive or inappropriate;
when culture does not yield a result despite clinical suspicion of infectious meningitis/meningoencephalitis; and
in immunodeficient patients.

RECOMMENDATIONS

CSF should be analysed immediately (i.e. <1 h) after collection. If storage is required for later investigation this can be done at 4–8°C (short term) or at −20°C (long term). Only

continued

protein components and RNA (after appropriate preparation) can be analysed from stored CSF (Good Practice Point).

The Level B recommendation regarding CSF partitioning and storage states that 12 ml of CSF should be partitioned into three to four sterile tubes. It is important that the CSF is not allowed to sediment before partitioning. Store 3–4 ml at 4°C for general investigations, cultivation and microscopic investigation of bacteria and fungi, antibody testing, polymerase chain reaction (PCR), and antigen detection. Larger volumes (10–15 ml) are necessary for certain pathogens like *Mycobacterium tuberculosis*, fungi or parasites.

Normal CSF protein concentration should be related to the patient's age (higher in the neonate period and after age of 60 years) and the site of LP (Level B). Exact upper normal limits of protein concentration differ according to the technique and the examining laboratory.

The Q_{alb} should be preferred to total protein concentrations, partly because reference levels are more clearly defined and partly because it is not confounded by changes in other CSF proteins (Level B).

The glucose concentration in CSF should be related to the blood concentration. Therefore CSF glucose/serum ratio is preferable. Pathological changes in this ratio or in lactate concentration are supportive for bacterial or fungal meningitis or leptomeningeal metastases (Level B).

Intrathecal IgG synthesis can be measured by various quantitative methods, but at least for the diagnosis of MS the detection of oligoclonal bands by appropriate methods is superior to any existing formula (Level A). Patients with other diseases associated with intrathecal inflammation, for example, patients with CNS infections, may also have intrathecal IgA and IgM synthesis as assessed by non-linear formulae (Reiber hyperbolic formulae or extended indices), which should be preferred to the linear IgA and IgM indices (Level B).

Cellular morphology (cytological staining) should be evaluated whenever pleocytosis is found or leptomeningeal metastases or pathological

bleeding is suspected (Level B). If cytology is inconclusive in case of query CSF bleeding measurement of bilirubin is recommended up to 2 weeks after the clinical event.

For standard microbiological examination sedimentation at $3000 \times g$ for 10 min is recommended (Level B). Microscopy should be performed using Gram or methylene blue, Auramin O or Ziehl-Nielsen (*M. tuberculosis*), or Indian ink stain (*Cryptococcus*). Depending on the clinical presentation incubation with bacterial and fungal culture media can be useful. Anaerobic culture media are recommended only if there is suspicion of brain abscess. A viral culture is generally not recommended. A list of infectious agents and their association with different diseases as well as the recommended method of detection is provided in table 4.4. The results of bacterial antigen detection have to be interpreted with respect to the microscopical CSF investigation and culture results. It is not routinely recommended in cases of negative microscopy. A diagnosis of bacterial nervous system infection based on antigen detection alone is not recommended (risk of contamination).

Conflicts of interest

The authors have reported no conflicts of interest.

Acknowledgment

We are grateful to Professor Christian Bogdan (Director of the Department for Microbiology and Hygiene, Albert Ludwigs-Universität Freiburg, Germany) and to Professor Rüdiger Dörries (Head of the Department of Virology, Institute of Medical Microbiology und Hygiene Ruprecht-Karls-Universität Heidelberg, Germany) for critical review of the microbiological part of the manuscript (infectious CSF).

References

Adam P, Taborsky L, Sobek O *et al.* (2001). Cerebrospinal fluid. *Adv. Clin. Chem.* **36**:1–62.

Andersson M, Alvarez-Cermeño J, Bernadi G *et al.* (1994). Cerebrospinal fluid in the diagnosis of multiple sclerosis: a consensus report. *J Neurol Neurosurg Psychiatry* **57:**897–902.

Blennow K, Fredman P, Wallin A, Gottfries C-G, Långström G, Svennerholm L (1993). Protein analyses in cerebrospinal fluid. I. Influence of concentration gradients for proteins on cerebrospinal fluid/serum albumin ratio. *Eur Neurol* **33:**126–128.

Blennow K, Fredman P (1995). Detection of cerebrospinal fluid leakage by isoelectric focusing on polyacrylamide gels with silver staining using the PhastSystem. *Acta Neurochir* **136:**135–139.

Brainin M, Barnes M, Baron JC, Gilhus NE, Hughes R, Selmaj K, Waldemar G (2004). Guidance for the preparation of neurological management guidelines by EFNS scientific task forces–revised recommendations 2004. *Eur J Neurol* **11:**577–581.

Davies NW, Brown LJ, Gonde J, Irish D, Robinson RO, Swan AV, Banatvala J, Howard RS, Sharief MK, Muir P (2005). Factors influencing PCR detection of viruses in cerebrospinal fluid of patients with suspected CNS infections. *J Neurol Neurosurg Psychiatry* **76:**82–87.

Delpech B, Lichtblau E (1972). Étude quantitative des immunoglobulines G et de l'albumine du liquide cephalo rachidien. *Clin Chim Acta* **37:**15–23.

Donald PR, Malan C, van der Walt A (1983). Simultaneous determination of cerebrospinal fluid glucose and blood glucose concentrations in the diagnosis of bacterial meningitis. *J Pediatr* **103:**413–415.

Eeg-Olofson O, Link H, Wigertz A (1981). Concentrations of CSF proteins as a measure of blood brain barrier function and synthesis of IgG within the CNS in 'normal' subjects from the age of 6 months to 30 years. *Acta Paediatr Scand* **70:**167–170.

Feigin RD, McCracken GH Jr, Klein JO (1992). Diagnosis and management of meningitis. *Pediatr Infect Dis J* **11:**785–814.

Felgenhauer K (1982). Differentiation of the humoral immune response in inflammatory diseases of the central nervous system. *J Neurol* **228:**223–237.

Felgenhauer K, Schädlich H-J (1987). The compartmental IgM and IgA response within the central nervous system. *J Neurol Sci* **77:**125–135.

Freedman MS, Thompson EJ, Deisenhammer F *et al.* (2005) Recommended standard of cerebrospinal fluid analysis in the diagnosis of multiple sclerosis. *Arch Neurol* **62:**865–870.

Fishman RA (1992). *Cerebrospinal Fluid in Diseases of the Nervous System.* Philadelphia, PA: W.B. Saunders, 1992.

Ganrot K, Laurell C-B (1974). Measurement of IgG and albumin content of cerebrospinal fluid, and its interpretation. *Clin Chem* **20:**571–573.

Genton B, Berger JP (1990). Cerebrospinal fluid lactate in 78 cases of adult meningitis. *Intensive Care Med* **16:**196–200.

Glantz MJ, Cole BF, Glantz LK, Cobb J, Mills P, Lekos A, Walters BC, Recht LD (1998). Cerebrospinal fluid cytology in patients with cancer: minimizing false-negative results. *Cancer* **82:**733–739.

Jeffery KJ, Read SJ, Peto TE, Mayon-White RT, Bangham CR (1997). Diagnosis of viral infections of the central nervous system: clinical interpretation of PCR results. *Lancet* **349:**313–317.

Jerrard DA, Hanna JR, Schindelheim GL (2001). Cerebrospinal fluid. *J Emerg Med* **21:**171–178.

Jordan GW, Statland B, Halsted C (1983). CSF lactate in diseases of the CNS. *Arch Intern Med* **143:**85–87.

Kaiser R (1998). Neuroborreliosis. *J Neurol* **245:**247–255.

Kaiser R (2002). Entzündliche und infektiöse Erkrankungen. In: Hufschmidt A, Lücking CH, eds. *Neurologie Compact, Leitlinie für Klinik und Praxis.* Georg Thieme Verlag, Stuttgart.

Kaplan JG, DeSouza TG, Farkash A, Shafran B, Pack D, Rehman F, Fuks J, Portenoy R (1990). Leptomeningeal metastases: comparison of clinical features and laboratory data of solid tumors, lymphomas and leukemias. *J Neurooncol* **9:**225–229.

Keir G, Luxton RW, Thompson EJ (1990). Isoelectric focusing of cerebrospinal fluid immunoglobulin G: an annotated update. *Ann Clin Biochem* **27:**436–443.

Kennedy PG (2005). Viral encephalitis. *J Neurol* **252:**268–272.

Kniehl ER, Dörries HK, Geiss B, Matz D, Neumann-Häfelin HW, Pfister H, Prange D, Schlüter B, Spellerberg FB, Specker (2001). *MiQ 17: Qualitätsstandards in der mikrobiologisch-infektiologischen Diagnostik.* Mauch H, Lütticken R eds. München, Jena: Urban & Fischer, 2001.

Korenke GC, Reiber H, Hunneman DH, Hanefeld F (1997). Intrathecal IgA synthesis in X-linked cerebral adrenoleukocystrophy. *J Child Neurol* **12:**314–320.

Kornhuber J, Kaiserauer, CH, Kornhuber AW, Kornhuber ME (1987). Alcohol consumption and blood-cerebrospinal fluid barrier dysfunction in man. *Neurosci Lett* **79:**218–222.

Koskiniemi M, Vaheri A, Taskinen E (1984). Cerebrospinal fluid alterations in herpes simplex virus encephalitis. *Rev Infect Dis* **6:**608–618.

Lamers KJB, Wevers RA (1995). Cerebrospinal fluid diagnostics: biochemical and clinical aspects. *Klin Biochem Metab* **3**:63–75.

Lindquist L, Linne T, Hansson LO, Kalin M, Axelsson G (1988). Value of cerebrospinal fluid analysis in the differential diagnosis of meningitis: a study in 710 patients with suspected central nervous system infection. *Eur J Clin Microbiol Infect Dis* **7**:374–380.

Link H, Tibbling G (1977). Principles of albumin and IgG analyses in neurological disorders. III. Evaluation of IgG synthesis within the central nervous system in multiple sclerosis. *Scand J Clin Lab Invest* **37**:397–401.

Lo Re V 3rd, Gluckman SJ (2003). Eosinophilic meningitis. *Am J Med* **114**:217–223.

McDonald WI, Compston A, Edan G et al. (2001). Recommended diagnostic criteria for multiple sclerosis: guidelines from the international panel on the diagnosis of multiple sclerosis. *Ann Neurol* **50**:121–127.

McLean BN, Luxton RW, Thompson EJ (1990). A study of immunoglobulin G in the cerebrospinal fluid of 1007 patients with suspected neurological disease using isoelectric focusing and the Log IgG-Index. A comparison and diagnostic applications. *Brain* **113**:1269–1289.

Negrini B, Kelleher KJ, Wald ER (2000). Cerebrospinal fluid findings in aseptic versus bacterial meningitis. *Pediatrics* **105**:316–319.

Nyström E, Hamberger A, Lindstedt G, Lundquist C, Wikkelsö (1997). Cerebrospinal fluid proteins in subclinical and overt hypothyroidism. *Acta Neurol Scand* **95**:311–314.

Öhman S, Forsberg P, Nelson N, Vrethem M (1989). An improved formula for the judgement of intrathecally produced IgG in the presence of blood brain barrier damage. *Clin Chim Acta* **181**:265–272.

Öhman S, Ernerudh J, Forsberg P, Henriksson A, von Schenck H, Vrethem M (1992). Comparison of seven formulae and isoelectrofocusing for determination of intrathecally produced IgG in neurological diseases. *Ann Clin Biochem* **29**:405–410.

Öhman S, Ernerudh J, Forsberg P, von Schenck H, Vrethem M (1993). Improved formulae for the judgement of intrathecally produced IgA and IgM in the presence of blood CSF barrier damage. *Ann Clin Biochem* **30**:454–462.

Poser CM, Paty W, Scheinberg LC et al. (1983). New diagnostic criteria for multiple sclerosis: guidelines for research protocols. *Ann Neurol* **13**:227–231.

Rauer S, Kaiser R (2000). Demonstration of anti-HuD specific oligoclonal bands in the cerebrospinal fluid from patients with paraneoplastic neurological syndromes. Qualitative evidence of anti-HuD specific IgG-synthesis in the central nervous system. *J Neuroimmunol* **111**:241–244.

Reiber H (1994). Flow rate of cerebrospinal fluid (CSF) – a concept common to normal blood-CSF barrier function and to dysfunction in neurological diseases. *J Neurol Sci* **122**:189–203.

Reiber H (1995). External quality assessment in clinical neurochemistry: survey of analysis for cerebrospinal fluid (CSF) proteins based on CSF/serum quotients. *Clin Chem* **41**:256–263.

Reiber H, Thompson EJ, Grimsley G et al. (2003). Quality Assurance for Cerebrospinal Fluid Protein Analysis: International Consensus by an Internet-Based Group Discussion. *Clin Chem Lab Med* **41**:331–337. Available at: www.teamspace.net/CSF.

Roma AA, Garcia A, Avagnina A, Rescia C, Elsner B (2002). Lymphoid and myeloid neoplasms involving cerebrospinal fluid: comparison of morphologic examination and immunophenotyping by flow cytometry. *Diagn Cytopathol* **27**:271–275.

Sabetta JR, Andriole VT (1985). Cryptococcal infection of the central nervous system. *Med Clin North Am* **69**:333–344.

Schipper HI, Bardosi A, Jacobi C, Felgenhauer K (1988). Meningeal carcinomatosis: origin of local IgG production in the CSF. *Neurology* **38**:413–416.

Schlossberg D (1990). *Infections of the Nervous System.* Springer-Verlag, Berlin.

Schumacher FA, Beebe GW, Kibler RF et al. (1965). Problems of experimental trials of therapy in multiple sclerosis. *Ann NY Acad Sci* **122**:552–568.

Segurado OG, Kruger H, Mertens HG (1986). Clinical significance of serum and CSF findings in the Guillain-Barre syndrome and related disorders. *J Neurol* **233**:202–208.

Sellebjerg F, Christiansen M, Rasmussen LS, Jaliachvili I, Nielsen PM, Frederiksen JL (1996). The cerebrospinal fluid in multiple sclerosis. Quantitative assessment of intrathecal immunoglobulin synthesis by empirical formulae. *Eur J Neurol* **3**:548–559.

Seneviratne U (2000). Guillain-Barre syndrome. *Postgrad Med J* **76**:774–782.

Seyfert S, Kunzmann V, Schwertfeger N, Koch HC, Faulstich A (2002). Determinants of lumbar CSF protein concentration. *J Neurol* **249**:1021–1026.

Sharief MK, Keir G, Thompson EJ (1990). Intrathecal synthesis of IgM in neurological diseases: a comparison between detection of oligoclonal bands and quantitative estimation. *J Neurol Sci* **96**:131–143.

Skouen JS, Larsen JL, Vollset SE (1994). Cerebrospinal fluid protein concentrations related to clinical findings in patients with sciatica caused by disk herniation. *J Spinal Disord* **7:**12–18.

Spanos A, Harrell FE Jr, Durack DT (1989). Differential diagnosis of acute meningitis. An analysis of the predictive value of initial observations. *JAMA* **262:** 2700–2707.

Statz A, Felgenhauer K (1983). Development of the blood-CSF barrier. *Develop Med Child Neurol* **25:**152–161.

Steele RW, Marmer DJ, O'Brien MD, Tyson ST, Steele CR (1986). Leukocyte survival in cerebrospinal fluid. *J Clin Microbiol* **23:**965–966.

Stich O, Graus F, Rasiah C, Rauer S (2003). Qualitative evidence of anti-Yo-specific intrathecal antibody synthesis in patients with paraneoplastic cerebellar degeneration. *J Neuroimmunol* **141:**165–169.

Stockstill MT, Kauffman CA (1983). Comparison of cryptococcal and tuberculous meningitis. *Arch Neurol* **40:**81–85.

Storstein A, Monstad SE, Honnorat J, Vedeler CA (2004). Paraneoplastic antibodies detected by isoelectric focusing of cerebrospinal fluid and serum. *J Neuroimmunol* **155:**150–154.

Takahashi T, Nakayama T, Tamura M, Ogawa K, Tsuda H, Morita A, Hara M, Togo M, Shiota H, Suzuki Y, Minami M, Ishikawa H, Miki K, Shikata E, Takahashi S, Kuragano T, Matsumoto K, Sawada S, Mizutani T (2005). Nested polymerase chain reaction for assessing the clinical course of tuberculous meningitis. *Neurology* **64:**1789–1793.

Thompson EJ (1988). *The CSF Proteins: A Biochemical Approach*. Amsterdam, Netherlands: Elsevier.

Twijnstra A, Ongerboer de Visser BW, van Zanten AP (1987). Diagnosis of leptomeningeal metastasis. *Clin Neurol Neurosurg* **89:**79–85.

Twijnstra A, Ongerboer de Visser BW, van Zanten AP, Hart AA, Nooyen WJ (1989). Serial lumbar and ventricular cerebrospinal fluid biochemical marker measurements in patients with leptomeningeal metastases from solid and hematological tumors. *J Neurooncol* **7:**57–63.

UK National External Quality Assessment Scheme for Immunochemistry Working Group. (2003) National guidelines for analysis of cerebrospinal fluid for bilirubin in suspected subarachnoid haemorrhage. *Ann Clin Biochem* **40:**481–488.

van Oostenbrugge RJ, Twijnstra A (1999). Presenting features and value of diagnostic procedures in leptomeningeal metastases. *Neurology* **53:**382–385.

Wasserstrom WR, Glass JP, Posner JB (1982). Diagnosis and treatment of leptomeningeal metastases from solid tumors: experience with 90 patients. *Cancer* **49:**759–772.

Watson MA, Scott MG (1995). Clinical utility of biochemical analysis of cerebrospinal fluid. *Clin Chem* **41:**343–360.

Zeman D, Adam P, Kalistova H, Sobek O, Andel J, Andel M (2001). Cerebrospinal fluid cytologic findings in multiple sclerosis. A comparison between patient subgroups. *Acta Cytol* **45:**51–59.

CHAPTER 5

Use of imaging in acute stroke

J.C. Masdeu,[a] P. Irimia,[a] S. Asenbaum,[b]
J. Bogousslavsky,[c] M. Brainin,[d] H. Chabriat,[e]
K. Herholz,[f] H.S. Markus,[g] E. Martínez-Vila,[a]
K. Niederkorn,[h] P.D. Schellinger,[i] R.J. Seitz,[j]

Abstract

Objective To develop and publish an EFNS Guideline on the use of neuroimaging for the management of acute stroke.

Background Neuroimaging techniques are necessary for the evaluation of stroke, one of the leading causes of death and neurological impairment in developed countries. The multiplicity of techniques available has increased the complexity of decision making for physicians.

Methods We performed a comprehensive review of the literature in English for the period 1959 to 2005 and critically assessed the relevant publications. The members of the Panel reviewed and corrected an initial draft, until a consensus was reached on recommendations stratified according to the EFNS criteria.

Results and recommendations Non-contrast CT scan is the established imaging procedure for the initial evaluation of stroke patients. However, magnetic resonance imaging (MRI) has a higher sensitivity than computerised tomography (CT) for the demonstration of infarcted or ischemic areas and depicts well acute and chronic intracerebral haemorrhage. Perfusion and diffusion MRI together with MR angiography are very helpful for the acute evaluation of patients with ischemic stroke. MRI and MRA are the recommended techniques for the screening of cerebral aneurysms and for the diagnosis of cerebral venous thrombosis and arterial dissection. For the non-invasive study of extracranial vessels, MR angiography is less portable and more expensive than ultrasonography but it has higher sensitivity and specificity for carotid stenosis. Transcranial Doppler (TCD) is very useful for monitoring arterial reperfusion after thrombolysis, for the diagnosis of intracranial stenosis

[a]Department of Neurology and Neurosurgery, University of Navarra, Spain; [b]Department of Neurology, Medical University of Vienna, Vienna, Austria; [c]Department of Neurology, Centre Hospitalier Universitaire Vaudois, Lausanne, Switzerland; [d]Department of Neurology, Donauklinikum and Donau-Universität, Maria Gugging, Austria; [e]Department of Neurology, Lariboisiere Hospital, University of Paris, Paris, France; [f]Wolfson Molecular Imaging Centre, University of Manchester, Manchester, United Kingdom; [g]Department of Neurology and Clinical Neuroscience, St George's Hospital Medical School, London, United Kingdom; [h]Department of Neurology, Karl Franzens University, Graz, Austria; [i]Department of Neurology, University Clinic at Heidelberg, Germany; [j]Department of Neurology, University Hospital Düsseldorf, Düsseldorf, Germany.

and of right-to-left shunts, and for monitoring vasospasm after subarachnoid haemorrhage. Currently, SPECT and PET have a more limited role in the evaluation of the acute stroke patient.

Objectives

The objective of the Task Force is to develop and publish an EFNS Guideline on the use of neuroimaging for the management of acute stroke. The Guideline is based on published scientific evidence as well as the consensus of experts. The resulting report is intended to provide updated and evidence-based recommendations regarding the use of diagnostic neuroimaging techniques, including cerebrovascular ultrasonography, in patients with stroke and thus guide neurologists, other health care professionals and health care providers in clinical decision making and in the elaboration of clinical protocols. It is not intended to have legally binding implications in individual situations.

This guideline evaluates neuroimaging in acute stroke. Neuroimaging is also very important in the management of cerebrovascular disease in a more elective setting, for instance for the performance of angioplasty or the placement of an arterial stent. These procedures will be covered in future guidelines.

Background

Stroke is the second cause of death and one of the major determining factors of hospital admission and permanent disability (World Health Organization. The World Health Report 1999. Geneva, Switzerland: WHO 1999). In the developed countries, the proportion of the population over the age of 65 years is growing and this trend is likely to increase stroke incidence in the next decades. Major advances in the understanding of the mechanisms of stroke and its management have been made thanks to the substantial progress in neuroimaging techniques. However, the multiplicity of neuroimaging techniques available for the evaluation of stroke patients has increased

the complexity of decision making for physicians. Neurologists, who have been educated to manage acute stroke patients, should be trained in the use of neuroimaging, which allows for the development of a pathophysiologically oriented treatment.

Successful care of acute stroke patients requires a rapid and accurate diagnosis because the time window for treatment is narrow. In the case of intravenous thrombolysis for ischemic stroke, the treatment is safer and more effective the earlier it is given (Hacke *et al.*, 2004). Current recommendations call for a 3-h time limit for intravenous thrombolysis (Tissue plasminogen activator for acute ischemic stroke. The National Institute of Neurological Disorders and Stroke rt-PA Stroke Study Group, 1995) that can be extended to 6 h for intra-arterial thrombolysis (Furlan *et al.*, 1999). Thus, the neuroimaging protocol designed to determine the cause of stroke should delay treatment as little as possible. Neuroimaging can not only separate ischemic from haemorrhagic stroke, but also provide information about the presence of ischemic but still viable and thus salvageable tissue (penumbra tissue) and vessel occlusion in the hyperacute phase of ischemic stroke. Therefore, neuroimaging is critical for an improved selection of patients who could be treated with thrombolysis up to the 3-h limit and beyond (Schellinger *et al.*, 2003). Thus, neuroimaging criteria have been used for patient selection and outcome in the *Desmoteplase in Acute Stroke* (DIAS) trial, using thrombolysis between 3 and 9 h after stroke onset (Hacke *et al.*, 2005). Determining stroke type using neuroimaging goes well beyond separating ischemic from haemorrhagic stroke. For instance, the depiction of multiple cortical infarcts may lead to a fuller work-up for cardiogenic emboli (Shinokawa *et al.*, 2000). The characteristic semilunar high-intensity signal in the vessel wall on MRI alerts to the presence of arterial dissection as the cause of stroke (Lanczik *et al.*, 2005).

Search strategy

The Cochrane Library was consulted and no studies were found regarding the use of neuroimaging techniques in stroke. A comprehensive literature review using the MEDLINE database was conducted by searching for the period 1959 to 2005. Relevant literature in English including existing guidelines, meta-analyses, systematic reviews, randomised controlled trials, and observational studies have been critically assessed. Selected articles have been rated based on the quality of study design, and clinical practice recommendations have been developed and stratified to reflect the quality and the content of the evidence according to EFNS criteria (Brainin *et al.*, 2004) (see table 3.2).

Method for reaching consensus

The author panel critically assessed the topic through analysis of the medical literature. A proposed guideline with specific recommendations was drafted for circulation to all panel members. Each panelist studied and commented in writing on each successive guideline draft, revised to progressively accommodate the panel consensus. After the approval of the panelists, a final version was submitted to the chairperson of the Scientific Committee.

Results

Imaging of the brain

The primary objectives of brain imaging in acute stroke are to exclude a non-vascular lesion as the cause of the symptoms and to determine whether the stroke is caused by an ischemic infarction or a haemorrhage. It is not possible to exclude stroke mimics, such as a neoplasm, and distinguish between ischemic and haemorrhagic stroke based exclusively on the history and physical examination (Britton *et al.*, 1984). Determining the nature of the lesion by brain imaging is necessary before starting any treatment, particularly thrombolysis and antithrombotic drugs (Class I, Level A).

Computed tomography

Conventional CT of the head is the examination most frequently used for the emergent evaluation of patients with acute stroke because of its wide availability and usefulness (Class II, Level B). It has

been utilized as a screening tool in most of the major therapeutic trials conducted to date (Hacke *et al.*, 2004). It is useful to distinguish between ischemic stroke and intracerebral or subarachnoid haemorrhage, and can also rule out other conditions that could mimic stroke such as brain tumours. Signs of early ischemia may be identified as early as 2 h from stroke onset, although they may appear much later (von Kummer *et al.*, 1996). Early infarct signs include the hyperdense middle cerebral artery (MCA) sign (Gacs *et al.*, 1983; Bastianello *et al.*, 1991) (indicative of a thrombus or embolus in the M1 segment of the vessel), the MCA dot sign (Barber *et al.*, 2001; Leary *et al.*, 2003) (indicating thrombosis of M2 or M3 MCA branches), the loss of the gray-white differentiation in the cortical ribbon (Truwit *et al.*, 1990) or the lentiform nucleus (Tomura *et al.*, 1988), and sulcal effacement (Moulin *et al.*, 1996). The presence of some of these signs has been associated with poor outcome (Moulin *et al.*, 1996). In the European Cooperative Acute Stroke Study (ECASS I) trial those patients with signs of early infarction involving more than one third of the territory of the middle cerebral artery had an increased risk of haemorrhagic transformation following treatment with thrombolysis (Hacke *et al.*, 1995). A secondary analysis of other thrombolytic trials with a 6-h time window (ECASS II and MAST-E) demonstrated that the presence of early CT changes was a risk factor for intracerebral haemorrhage (Jaillard *et al.*, 1999; Larrue *et al.*, 2001) and similar results have been observed in larger series of patients (Tanne, *et al.* 2002). However, in the National Institute of Neurological Disorders and Stroke (NINDS) trial and the Australian Streptokinase Trial (ASK) there was no relation between intracranial haemorrhage and early CT changes (Patel *et al.*, 2001; Gilligan *et al.*, 2002), and it has been argued that the poorer outcome in patients with CT changes may have more to do with delayed treatment than with the changes themselves, with additional damage of the potentially salvageable tissue in the larger, CT visible infarcts (Grotta, 2003). As ischemic changes are difficult to detect for clinicians without adequate training in reading CT (von Kummer *et al.*, 1996; von Kummer, 1998), scoring systems have been developed to quantify early CT changes, like the Alberta Stroke Programme Early CT Score (ASPECTS). More extensive early changes using ASPECTS correlate with high rates of intracranial haemorrhage and poor outcome at long term, and therefore might improve identification of ischemic stroke patients who particularly benefit from thrombolysis and those at risk of symptomatic haemorrhage (Barber *et al.*, 2000; Hill *et al.*, 2003). However, given the conflicting evidence, the presence of hipodensity on early CT, even affecting more than one third of the MCA territory, cannot be construed to be an absolute contraindication to the use of thrombolytic therapy in the first 3 h after stroke (Class IV, Level GPP).

Conventional CT contrast enhancement is not indicated for the acute diagnosis of stroke, but may be helpful to show the infarcted area in the subacute stage (2–3 weeks after stroke onset) when there may be obscuration of the infarction by the 'fogging effect' (Wing *et al.*, 1976; Becker *et al.*, 1979) (Class IV, Level C).

CT identifies the vast majority of *intracerebral haemorrhages* in the acute phase of stroke as a hyperdense area, except petechial haemorrhages and bleedings in patients with very low haemoglobin levels (New and Aronow, 1976), because the high density of blood on CT is a function of the haemoglobin concentration. CT demonstrates the size and topography of the haemorrhage and gives information about the presence of mass effect, hydrocephalus, and intraventricular extension of the bleeding. In addition, it may identify (although not as well as MRI) possible structural abnormalities (aneurysms, arteriovenous malformations or tumours) that caused the haemorrhage. The characteristic hyperdensity of intracerebral haemorrhage on CT disappears with time, becoming hypodense after approximately 8–10 days (Dennis *et al.*, 1987; Wardlaw *et al.*, 2004). For this reason CT is not a useful technique to distinguish between old haemorrhage and infarction.

Subarachnoid haemorrhage (SAH) can be detected in 98–100% of patients with newer CT helical units in the first 12 h from the onset of symptoms (van der Rinkel *et al.*, 1995; Sidman *et al.*, 1996) and in 93% of patients studied within the first 24 h (Sames *et al.*, 1996; Morgenstern *et al.*, 1998). CT is the imaging procedure of choice to diagnose SAH (Class I, Level A). Some experts recommend performing the study with thin cuts (3 mm in thickness) through the base of the brain, because small collections of blood may be missed with thicker cuts (Edlow and Caplan, 2000) (Class IV, Level GPP). CT cannot identify subarachnoid haemorrhage in patients with low haemoglobin levels, because blood may appear isodense, and in those scanned after 3 weeks of the bleeding when blood has usually been metabolized (van Gijn and van Dongen, 1982).

Cerebral venous thrombosis (CVT) is an uncommon cause of stroke (Bogousslavsky and Pierre, 1992; Arboix *et al.*, 2001). CT can show direct signs of venous thrombosis and other indirect nonspecific signs, but in about one third of cases CT is normal (Bousser *et al.*, 1985; Renowden, 2004). Direct signs on unenhanced CT are the cord sign, corresponding to thrombosed cortical veins, and the dense triangle sign, corresponding to a thrombus in the superior sagital sinus, and, on enhanced CT of the sagital sinus, the delta sign (Virapongse *et al.*, 1987). Indirect signs such as local hypodensities due to oedema or infarction, hyperdensities secondary to haemorrhagic infarction, or brain swelling and small ventricles suggest the diagnosis of CVT. CT venography has emerged as a good procedure to detect CVT (Casey *et al.*, 1996).

Perfusion-CT techniques, such as slow-infusion/whole-brain perfusion-CT and dynamic perfusion-CT, may help distinguish between reversible and irreversible areas of ischemia. Slow-infusion perfusion-CT is useful to evaluate the perfusion of the entire brain, but only provides qualitative information related to cerebral blood volume and therefore cannot be used to differentiate reversible from irreversible ischemia (Hunter *et al.*, 1998; Lev *et al.*, 2001). Dynamic perfusion-CT (PCT) involves dynamic acquisition of sequential CT slices during the intravenous administration of iodinated contrast media (Wintermark *et al.*, 2002; 2005). PCT allows the estimation of cerebral blood flow (CBF), cerebral blood volume (CBV), and mean transit time (MTT) in a limited volume of brain tissue, currently 20- to 48-mm in thickness, but faster CT equipment is now becoming available to permit the study of larger regions of the brain. Areas with prolonged MTT are haemodynamically compromised. In these areas, the regions with increased CBV resulting from vasodilatation and collateral recruitment are considered to have preserved autoregulation and to represent 'tissue at risk', whereas regions with decreased CBV correspond to the infarct core (Wintermark *et al.*, 2002; Schramm *et al.*, 2004). PCT overestimates brain haemodynamic values in pixels including large vessels (Kudo *et al.*, 2003). PCT can be performed and analysed in less than 15 min (Schramm *et al.*, 2004). However, there are no studies to date demonstrating that perfusion CT is useful for the selection of candidates to thrombolysis. Pregnancy, diabetes, renal failure, and allergy to contrast material are relative contraindications to perform a perfusion brain CT. Perfusion CT is particularly helpful for the study of stroke patients for whom MRI is contraindicated, such as those with pacemakers (Class IV, Level GPP).

Magnetic resonance imaging
MRI has a higher sensitivity than conventional CT and results in lower interrater variability in the diagnosis of ischemic stroke within the first hours of stroke onset (Bryan *et al.*, 1991; Shuaib *et al.*, 1992; Culebras *et al.*, 1997; Masaryk *et al.*, 2000; Fiebach *et al.*, 2002; Hacke *et al.*, 2003) (Class I, Level A). MRI is particularly useful to show lesions in the brain stem or cerebellum, identify lacunar infarcts, and document vessel occlusion and brain oedema (Bryan *et al.*, 1991; Culebras *et al.*, 1997). In addition, new MRI techniques can provide information about tissue viability. Diffusion-weighted (DWI) and perfusion-weighted (PWI) MRI studies may inform about the presence of reversibly and irreversibly damaged ischemic tissues in the hyperacute phase of stroke (Sorensen *et al.*, 1996; Warach *et al.*, 1996; Barber *et al.*, 1998; Beaulieu *et al.*, 1999; Schlaug *et al.*, 1999; Rohl *et al.*, 2001). DWI may demonstrate deeply ischemic or infarcted brain tissue within minutes of onset of symptoms (Warach *et al.*, 1992). PWI requires the intravenous administration of gadolinium and provides information about brain tissue perfusion at a given time. The

most widely used indicator of brain perfusion is the time-to-peak, being the time until the intravenous gadolinium bolus reaches brain tissue. This model-independent measure allows an estimation of the severity of ischemia in comparison to the non-affected hemisphere in an objective manner (Wittsack *et al.*, 2002). The absolute volume difference or ratio of the PWI area and the DWI area (diffusion–perfusion mismatch) is a useful method to estimate the presence of ischemic penumbra tissue (Latchaw *et al.*, 2003; Davis and Donnan, 2004). Not only the volume of abnormal perfusion but also its degree predicts the extent of ischemic brain damage (Seitz *et al.*, 2005). PWI/DWI-mismatch has been evaluated in several studies as a selection tool for thrombolytic therapy beyond 3 h (Rother *et al.*, 2002) and in a recent phase II trial it was used as a selection tool and surrogate parameter for thrombolysis within 3–9 h (Hacke *et al.*, 2005). However, the extent of DWI/PWI mismatch has not predicted outcome after thrombolysis in an open label study (Rother *et al.*, 2002).

MRI can help identify occluded intracranial arteries by the loss of the normal intravascular flow voids (Bryan *et al.*, 1991). Some sequences, such as T2*-weighted MRI or fluid attenuated inversion recovery (FLAIR) (hyperintense artery sign), may demonstrate acute MCA thromboembolism with a higher sensitivity than CT, but the type of arterial change on MRI does not predict recanalisation, clinical outcome or intracerebral haemorrhage (ICH) after intravenous thrombolysis (Flacke *et al.*, 2000; Schellinger *et al.* 2005).

Intracranial haemorrhage with acute stroke is easily detectable on MRI using T2*-weighted images (Linfante *et al.*, 1999; Schellinger *et al.*, 1999; Fiebach *et al.*, 2004). MRI can identify intraparenchymal haemorrhage within the first 6 h after symptom onset as accurately as CT (Fiebach *et al.*, 2004; Kidwell *et al.*, 2004). Susceptibility-weighted T2*-sequences (gradient echo) can also detect clinically silent parenchymal microbleeds, not visible on CT, which may leave enough local haemosiderin to remain detectable for months or years after the bleeding. Although microbleeds are associated with a history of ICH and prospectively have been shown to pose a 3% risk of

ICH (Tsushima *et al.*, 2003), the risk of bleeding after thrombolysis in patients with microbleeds has not been established. While some retrospective studies reported an increased risk of symptomatic haemorrhage after thrombolysis (Kidwell *et al.*, 2002; Nighoghossian *et al.*, 2002), a more recent publication from one of the same groups failed to document it (Derex *et al.*, 2004). MRI is also useful to date the haemorrhagic event accurately and to detect lesions (as tumours, vascular malformations or aneurysms) that may underlie the ICH (Dul and Drayer, 1994). To detect these lesions, repeated studies may be needed after some of the swelling and vasospasm have subsided.

Subarachnoid haemorrhage can be detected using T2* (Fiebach *et al.*, 2004) and FLAIR (Noguchi *et al.*, 1995, 1997). MR sequences, but at present CT remains the imaging method of choice for this diagnosis (Class I, Level A).

Arterial dissection is a leading cause of stroke in young persons (Bogousslavsky and Pierre, 1992). MRI is the initial procedure of choice (Culebras *et al.*, 1997; Kasner *et al.*, 1997; Oelerich *et al.*, 1999), replacing conventional angiography as the gold standard (Class II, Level B), because MRI can show the mural haematoma of the dissected vessel on the axial images (Kirsch *et al.*, 1998) (high signal in the wall). Visualisation of these changes in the vertebral artery is more difficult than for the larger carotid artery, making diagnosis of vertebral dissection less reliable. The study can be completed with MR angiography to visualise occlusion of the artery, pseudoaneurysms or a long stenotic segment with tapered ends (Levy *et al.*, 1994; Bousson *et al.*, 1999). Other techniques, including ultrasonography (de Bray *et al.*, 1994; Bartels and Flugel, 1996) or CT angiography (Levy *et al.*, 1994; Bousson *et al.*, 1999), may be useful for the non-invasive diagnosis of arterial dissection.

Cerebral venous thrombosis (CVT). MR combined with MR angiography is the method of choice for the diagnosis and follow-up of CVT (Mattle *et al.*, 1991; Ameri and Bousser, 1992; Renowden, 2004). MR is more sensitive than CT to show parechymal abnormalities and the presence of thrombosed veins.

In summary, MRI is very helpful in the clinical setting for the management of acute stroke and to guide decisions regarding thrombolysis (Schellinger *et al.*, 2003) (Class I, Level A). It is particularly helpful for the study of stroke patients for whom perfusion CT may be dangerous, such as those with renal failure or diabetes. However, MRI in the acute phase of stroke is not widely available in European hospitals (Thomassen *et al.*, 2003). Other limitations and contraindications for the use of MRI are: claustrophobia, agitation, morbid obesity, the presence of intracranial ferromagnetic elements, an aneurysm recently clipped or coiled, otic or cochlear implants, some old prosthetic heart valves, pacemakers, and some, not all, neurostimulators.

SPECT and PET

Single photon emission computed tomography (SPECT) and positron emission tomography (PET) are functional neuroimaging techniques based on the principles of tracer technology using radio-labeled substances as systemically administered tracers. In the setting of stroke SPECT has been used for the evaluation of cerebral perfusion. Earlier perfusion SPECT studies failed to show any advantage of SPECT over the structured clinical evaluation (NIH, Canadian, Scandinavian stroke scales) in the prediction of the evolution of acute stroke (Bowler *et al.*, 1996). However, using ECD SPECT in the first 6 h after stroke, Barthel and co-workers were able to determine which patients would develop massive MCA-territory necrosis, with hemispheric herniation (Barthel *et al.*, 2001). These patients have a high risk of haemorrhage following thrombolysis and could potentially be helped by early decompressive hemicraniectomy (Berrouschot *et al.*, 1998). Complete MCA infarctions were predicted with significantly higher accuracy with early SPECT compared with early CT and clinical parameters. The predictive value increased when the findings on CT, clinical examination and SPECT were considered (Barthel *et al.*, 2001). Other studies have found SPECT to add predictive value to the clinical score on admission (Alexandrov *et al.*, 1997; Hirano *et al.*, 2001; Mahagne *et al.*, 2004). Those studies suggest that a patient with a normal SPECT study performed within 3 h of stroke onset, will most likely recover spontaneously and therefore may not benefit from thrombolysis. A patient with a dense deficit in the entire MCA distribution has a high risk of haemorrhage with thrombolysis, and, depending on age and other factors, should be considered for decompressive hemicraniectomy. The patients most likely to benefit from thrombolysis are the ones with less massive lesions (Alexandrov *et al.*, 1997; Barthel *et al.*, 2001). Thus, SPECT is helpful in the evaluation of acute stroke (Class III, Level C). Unfortunately, the need to perform either CT or MRI in acute stroke renders the performance of SPECT difficult within the time frame allotted for the evaluation of these patients. SPECT is also helpful in the evaluation of cerebral perfusion in non-acute cerebrovascular disease, for instance in the days after a subarachnoid haemorrhage (Sviri *et al.*, 2004) (Class III, Level C).

PET allows to measure a large variety of physiological variables including the cerebral blood flow, the cerebral blood volume, the cerebral glucose metabolism as well as neurotransmitters and neuroreceptors, such as benzodiazepine receptors with flumazenil, an accurate marker of neuronal loss (Heiss *et al.*, 2004). As PET has been considered the gold standard for these kinds of measurements in humans, it is also extremely well suited to help identify the degree of ischemic damage in the brain. However, it does not allow for the reliable identification of lesions in the vessels or non-vascular lesions giving rise to the stroke syndrome. This, coupled with the cost and current lack of availability of this technique, renders it less useful than MRI and CT for most practising neurologists.

Imaging of the extracranial vessels
Imaging of the extracranial and intracranial vessels will help identify the underlying mechanism of the stroke (atherothrombotic, embolic, dissection or other). Non-invasive imaging methods are increasingly accepted as replacements for digital substraction angiography (DSA) in carotid stenosis evaluation prior to endarterectomy, to avoid the risks of DSA (Hankey *et al.*, 1990) (Class IV, GPP). Ultrasonography (US), comprising Doppler sonography and colour-coded duplex sonography, is probably the most common non-invasive imaging examination performed to aid in the diagnosis

of carotid disease. The peak systolic velocity and the presence of plaque on grey-scale and/or colour Doppler/Duplex US images are the main parameters that should be used when diagnosing and grading ICA stenosis (Grant *et al.*, 2003). The examination may be limited by the presence of extensive plaque calcifications, vessel tortuosity and in patients with tandem lesions. In addition, Doppler US is both technician- and equipment-dependent and all sonographers should be able to demonstrate that they have validated their testing procedures.

MR angiography (MRA) using time of flight angiography (TOF) and contrast enhanced MRA (CEMRA) are powerful means to assess vascular pathology. Either technique provides specific information: while TOF visualizes changes of flow in the arteries or veins depending on imaging parameters, CEMRA visualizes the vascular lumen. MRA and US have yielded comparable findings. Two meta-analysis (Blakeley *et al.*, 1995; Kallmes *et al.*, 1996) and several reviews (Westwood *et al.*, 2002; Nederkoorn *et al.*, 2003) have compared the diagnostic value of Doppler US, MR angiography (MRA), and conventional digital subtraction angiography (DSA) for the diagnosis of carotid artery stenosis. The meta-analysis published by Blakeley *et al.* (1995) concluded that Doppler US and MRA had similar diagnostic performance in predicting carotid artery occlusion and >70% stenosis. In the systematic review performed by Nederkoorn PJ, *et al.* (Nederkoorn *et al.*, 2003) for the diagnosis of 70–99% stenosis, MRA had a pooled sensitivity of 95% and a pooled specificity of 90%, and US 86% and 87% respectively. For recognizing occlusion, MRA had a sensitivity of 98% and a specificity of 100%, and DUS had a sensitivity of 96% and a specificity of 100%. Thus, contrast-enhanced MRA is slightly more precise than US and appears to achieve a higher sensitivity for the detection of stenosis, and to allow improved differentiation of tight stenosis from occlusion. However, the difference is minimal and other factors such as availability and quality of US performance may render one procedure more useful than the other (Class II, Level B).

CT angiography, a contrast-dependent technique, has been compared with DSA for the detection and quantification of carotid stenosis and occlusions (Schwartz *et al.*, 1992; Cumming and Morrow, 1994; Leclerc *et al.*, 1995; Cinat *et al.*, 1998; Sameshima *et al.*, 1999; Koelemay *et al.*, 2004). A recent systematic review concludes that this technique has demonstrated a good sensitivity and specificity for occlusion (97%), but the pooled sensitivity and specificity for detection of a 70–99% stenosis by CTA were 85% and 93% respectively (Koelemay *et al.*, 2004) (Class II, Level B).

DSA is the reference method to determine the degree of carotid stenosis because endarterectomy trials for symptomatic (NASCET Collaborators 1991; Barnett *et al.*, 1998; Randomised trial of endarterectomy for recently symptomatic carotid stenosis: final results of the MRC European Carotid Surgery Trial (ECST) 1998) and asymptomatic (Executive Committee for the Asymptomatic Carotid Atherosclerosis Study 1995) patients were performed using this method. However, angiography carries the risk of stroke and death (Hankey *et al.*, 1990; Willinsky *et al.*, 2003) and many centres are not using DSA prior to carotid endarterectomy (Dawson *et al.*, 1997; Grant *et al.*, 2003), particularly when non-invasive methods are concordant (Class IV, GPP). When non-invasive methods are inconclusive or there is a discrepancy between them, DSA is necessary.

Imaging of the intracranial vessels

Transcranial Doppler (TCD) is a non-invasive ultrasonographic procedure that measures local blood flow velocity and direction in the proximal portions of large intracranial arteries (Babikian *et al.*, 2000; Sloan *et al.*, 2004). It is useful for screening for intracranial stenosis (Rorick *et al.*, 1994; Demchuk *et al.*, 2000) and occlusion (Zanette *et al.*, 1989) in patients with cerebrovascular disease (Class II, Level B). In children with sickle cell disease, detection of asymptomatic intracerebral stenoses using TCD allows selection of a group at high risk of future stroke, who benefit from exchange transfusion (Adams *et al.*, 1998) (Class I, Level A). It is also useful for the detection and monitoring of intracranial artery vasospasm after subarachnoid haemorrhage, particularly in the middle cerebral artery (Lysakowski *et al.*, 2001) (Class I, Level A). TCD can be used to monitor

recanalisation during thrombolysis in acute MCA occlusions (Burgin *et al.*, 2000) (Class II, Level B). There is increasing interest in its therapeutic use. In vitro studies demonstrate it has an additive effect on clot lysis when used with rtPA, and clinical studies have suggested that continuous TCD monitoring in patients with acute middle cerebral artery occlusion treated with intravenous thrombolysis may improve both early recanalisation and clinical outcome (Eggers *et al.*, 2003; Alexandrov *et al.*, 2004). TCD allows for the documentation of a right-to-left shunt in patients with ischemic stroke (Class II, Level A). TCD discloses a shower of air bubbles in the MCA after the intravenous injection of saline mixed with air bubbles (Job *et al.*, 1994; Klotzsch *et al.*, 1994; Serena *et al.*, 1998).

Even in asymptomatic patients, TCD is the only imaging technique that allows detection of circulating emboli (Class II, Level A). These appear as short duration high intensity signals, because they reflect and backscatter more ultrasound than the surrounding red blood cells. Studies have shown that asymptomatic embolisation is common in acute stroke, particularly in patients with carotid artery disease (Siebler *et al.*, 1993; Markus *et al.*, 1995). In this group the presence of embolic signals has been shown to predict the combined stroke and TIA risk (Siebler *et al.*, 1995; Valton *et al.*, 1997; Molloy and Markus, 1999; Censori *et al.*, 2000; Goertler *et al.*, 2002) and more recently the risk of stroke alone (Markus and MacKinnon, 2005) (Class II, Level A). Embolic signals have also been used as surrogate markers to evaluate antiplatelet agents in both single centre studies (Kaposzta *et al.*, 2002) and recently in the multicentre international CARESS trial (Markus *et al.*, 2005). Embolic signal monitoring is used to monitor for embolisation following carotid endarterectomy; the presence of frequent embolic signals in this setting predicts early post-operative stroke (Levi *et al.*, 1997) and can be reduced by more aggressive antiplatelet treatment, including dextran (Levi *et al.*, 2001) and clopidogrel (Payne *et al.*, 2004). TCD can also be used to determine cerebrovascular reserve by determining the extent to which MCA flow velocity can increase in response to the vasodilator carbon dioxide or acetazolamide. Reserve is reduced in a proportion of patients with carotid occlusion and tight stenosis, and impaired reserve predicts recurrent TIA and stroke risk particularly in the group with carotid occlusion (Silvestrini *et al.*, 2000; Markus and Cullinane, 2001) (Class III, Level B).

TCD examination cannot be performed in about 10–15% of patients, particularly older women, because they lack a transtemporal window due to the thickness of the skull (Jarquin-Valdivia *et al.*, 2004). The use of intravenous echo contrast agents may improve detection of flow velocities in patients with limited transtemporal window (Hansberg *et al.*, 2002). TCD velocities may be altered in patients with cardiac pump failure (low velocities) or anaemia (increased velocities).

MR angiography can identify intracranial steno-occlusive lesions mainly in the proximal segments. Compared with DSA, the diagnostic accuracy of MR angiography for the identification of the proximal intracranial arterial stenosis has a high sensitivity and specificity (superior to 80%) (Korogi *et al.*, 1997; Hirai *et al.*, 2002; Alvarez-Linera *et al.*, 2003) (Class II, Level B). CT angiography is another useful technique but with less sensitivity and specificity than MRI, because it does not allow for assessment of stenosis in the cavernous portion of the internal carotid artery or in arteries with circumferential wall calcification (Skutta *et al.*, 1999; Hirai *et al.*, 2002).

MR and CT angiography can be used to show large aneurysms (Class II, Level B), but these techniques fail to identify aneurysm of less than 5 mm in diameter, those located in the intracranial carotid artery, and cannot clearly establish the critical relationship of the neck of the aneurysm(s) with arterial branches (Chung *et al.*, 1999; White *et al.*, 2001; Villablanca *et al.*, 2002). DSA is needed to demonstrate small aneurysms and before surgery or endovascular treatment (Class I, Level A). MR and CT angiography have been used for screening of individuals with a history of intracranial aneurysm or SAH in first degree relatives (Masaryk *et al.*, 2000) (The Magnetic Resonance Angiography in Relatives of Patients with Subarachnoid Hemorrhage Study Group, 1999). Despite relatively limited sensitivity, CT angiography is indicated for suspected or confirmed aneurysms that demand further verification of their presence, geometry, or relationship to parent artery branches and osseous anatomic landmarks. Low-volume high-density contrast media have substantially increased the ability of CT angiography to depict small aneurysms, small branches and collateral vessels (Schuknecht, 2004).

RECOMMENDATIONS

Imaging of the brain Non-contrast computed tomography (CT) scan is the established imaging procedure for the initial evaluation of patients with stroke to document or exclude intracerebral haemorrhage (ICH) and subarachnoid haemorrhage (SAH) (Class II, Level C). However, CT use has been consecrated more by availability than by randomized studies comparing its effectiveness with magnetic resonance imaging (MRI). Either CT or MRI should be used for the definition of stroke type and treatment of stroke (Class I, Level A).

Given the controversial nature of data on early CT infarct signs involving more than one third of the territory of the middle cerebral artery as predictors of the outcome of IV rtPA treatment, the presence of such signs cannot be construed as an absolute contraindication to thrombolysis in the first 3 h after stroke (Class IV, Level GPP).

Perfusion CT is helpful when MRI is not available and for the study of stroke patients for whom MRI is contraindicated (Class IV, Level GPP).

MRI has a higher sensitivity than conventional CT for the documentation of infarction within the first hours of stroke onset, lesions in the posterior fossa, identification of small lesions, and documentation of vessel occlusion and brain oedema (Class I, Level A).

In conjunction with MRI and MR angiography, perfusion and diffusion MR are very helpful for the acute evaluation of patients with ischemic stroke (Class I, Level A).

Perfusion and diffusion MR are helpful to select patients for intravenous thrombolysis beyond 3 h (Class III, Level C).

MRI with MR angiography is the method recommended for the diagnosis and follow-up of arterial dissection (Class II, Level B).

Single photon emission computed tomography (SPECT) is helpful to predict the malignant course of brain swelling with large hemispheric infarctions (Class III, Level C). SPECT is also helpful in the evaluation of cerebral perfusion in non-acute cerebrovascular disease, for instance in the days after a subarachnoid haemorrhage (Class III, Level C).

Detection of haemorrhagic stroke In stroke, MRI can detect acute and chronic intracerebral haemorrhage (Class I, Level A).

Although the detection of subarachnoid haemorrhage is possible with MRI, currently CT scan is the diagnostic procedure of choice (Class I, Level A).

Imaging of extracranial vessels Ultrasonography (US) is the non-invasive *screening* technique indicated for the study of vessels involved in causing symptoms of carotid stenosis (Class IV, GPP).

MR angiography has slightly higher sensitivity and specificity than US to determine carotid stenosis and occlusion, but other factors, such as availability, may render one procedure more useful than the other (Class II, Level B).

CT angiography (CTA) has a sensitivity and specificity similar to MR for carotid occlusion and similar to US for the detection of severe stenosis (Class II, Level B).

Digital substraction angiography (DSA) is generally recommended for grading carotid stenosis prior to endarterectomy (Class I, Level A), but when there is concordance of non-invasive methods cerebral arteriography may not be necessary (Class IV, Level GPP).

Imaging of intracranial vessels Transcranial Doppler (TCD) is very useful for assessing stroke risk of children aged 2–16 years with sickle cell disease (Class I, Level A), detection and monitoring of vasospasm after subarachnoid haemorrhage (Class I, Level A), diagnosis of intracranial steno-occlusive disease (Class II, Level B), diagnosis of right-to-left shunts (Class II, Level A), and for monitoring arterial reperfusion after thrombolysis of acute middle cerebral artery (MCA) occlusions (Class II, Level B).

TCD can detect cerebral emboli and impaired cerebral haemodynamics. The presence of embolic signals with carotid stenosis predicts early recurrent stroke risk (Class II, Level A). The detection of impaired cerebral haemodynamics in carotid occlusion may identify a group at high risk of recurrent stroke (Class III, Level B).

MRA and CT angiography are very useful for the diagnosis of intracranial stenosis and cerebral aneurysms larger than 5 mm (Class II, Level B). MRA is the recommended technique for screening of cerebral aneurysms in individuals with a history of aneurysms or SAH in a first degree relative (Class II, Level B).

DSA is the recommended technique for the diagnosis of cerebral aneurysm as the cause of SAH (Class I, Level A).

MRI with MR angiography is the method recommended for the diagnosis and follow-up of cerebral venous thrombosis (Class II, Level B).

Conflicts of interest

None of the authors has a conflict of interest with regard to the contents of this manuscript.

References

Adams RJ, McKie VC, Hsu L, Files B, Vichinsky E, Pegelow C *et al.* (1998). Prevention of a first stroke by transfusions in children with sickle cell anemia and abnormal results on transcranial Doppler ultrasonography. *N Engl J Med* **339**:5–11.

Alexandrov AV, Masdeu JC, Devous M, Sr., Black SE, Grotta JC (1997). Brain single-photon emission CT with HMPAO and safety of thrombolytic therapy in acute ischemic stroke. Proceedings of the meeting of the SPECT Safe Thrombolysis Study Collaborators and the members of the Brain Imaging Council of the Society of Nuclear Medicine. *Stroke* **28**:1830–1834.

Alexandrov AV, Molina CA, Grotta JC, Garami Z, Ford SR, Alvarez-Sabin J *et al.* (2004). Ultrasound-enhanced systemic thrombolysis for acute ischemic stroke. *N Engl J Med* **351**:2170–2178.

Alvarez-Linera J, Benito-Leon J, Escribano J, Campollo J, Gesto R (2003). Prospective evaluation of carotid artery stenosis: elliptic centric contrast-enhanced MR angiography and spiral CT angiography compared with digital subtraction angiography. *AJNR Am J Neuroradiol* **24**:1012–1019.

Ameri A, Bousser MG (1992). Cerebral venous thrombosis. *Neurol Clin* 10:87–111.

Arboix A, Bechich S, Oliveres M, Garcia-Eroles L, Massons J, Targa C (2001). Ischemic stroke of unusual cause: clinical features, etiology and outcome. *Eur J Neurol* **8**:133–139.

Babikian VL, Feldmann E, Wechsler LR, Newell DW, Gomez CR, Bogdahn U *et al.* (2000). Transcranial Doppler ultrasonography: year 2000 update. *J Neuroimaging* **10**:101–115.

Barber PA, Darby DG, Desmond PM, Yang Q, Gerraty RP, Jolley D *et al.* (1998). Prediction of stroke outcome with echoplanar perfusion- and diffusion-weighted MRI. *Neurology* **51**:418–426.

Barber PA, Demchuk AM, Zhang J, Buchan AM (2000). Validity and reliability of a quantitative computed tomography score in predicting outcome of hyperacute stroke before thrombolytic therapy. ASPECTS Study Group. Alberta Stroke Programme Early CT Score. *Lancet* **355**:1670–1674.

Barber PA, Demchuk AM, Hudon ME, Pexman JH, Hill MD, Buchan AM (2001). Hyperdense sylvian fissure MCA 'dot' sign: a CT marker of acute ischemia. *Stroke* **32**:84–88.

Barnett HJ, Taylor DW, Eliasziw M, Fox AJ, Ferguson GG, Haynes RB *et al.* (1998). Benefit of carotid endarterectomy in patients with symptomatic moderate or severe stenosis. North American Symptomatic Carotid Endarterectomy Trial Collaborators. *N Engl J Med* **339**:1415–1425.

Bartels E, Flugel KA (1996). Evaluation of extracranial vertebral artery dissection with duplex color-flow imaging. *Stroke* **27**:290–295.

Barthel H, Hesse S, Dannenberg C, Rossler A, Schneider D, Knapp WH *et al.* (2001). Prospective value of perfusion and x-ray attenuation imaging with single-photon emission and transmission computed tomography in acute cerebral ischemia. *Stroke* **32**:1588–1597.

Bastianello S, Pierallini A, Colonnese C, Brughitta G, Angeloni U, Antonelli M *et al.* (1991). Hyperdense middle cerebral artery CT sign. Comparison with angiography in the acute phase of ischemic supratentorial infarction. *Neuroradiology* **33**:207–211.

Beaulieu C, de Crespigny A, Tong DC, Moseley ME, Albers GW, Marks MP (1999). Longitudinal magnetic resonance imaging study of perfusion and diffusion in stroke: evolution of lesion volume and correlation with clinical outcome. *Ann Neurol* **46**:568–578.

Becker H, Desch H, Hacker H, Pencz A (1979). CT fogging effect with ischemic cerebral infarcts. *Neuroradiology* **18**:185–192.

Berrouschot J, Barthel H, von Kummer R, Knapp WH, Hesse S, Schneider D (1998). 99m technetium-ethyl-cysteinate-dimer single-photon emission CT can predict fatal ischemic brain edema. *Stroke* **29**:2556–2562.

Blakeley DD, Oddone EZ, Hasselblad V, Simel DL, Matchar DB (1995). Noninvasive carotid artery testing. A meta-analytic review. *Ann Intern Med* **122**:360–367.

Bogousslavsky J, Pierre P (1992). Ischemic stroke in patients under age 45. *Neurol Clin* **10**:113–124.

Bousser MG, Chiras J, Bories J, Castaigne P (1985). Cerebral venous thrombosis–a review of 38 cases. *Stroke* **16**:199–213.

Bousson V, Levy C, Brunereau L, Djouhri H, Tubiana JM (1999). Dissections of the internal carotid artery: three-dimensional time-of-flight MR angiography and MR imaging features. *AJR Am J Roentgenol* **173**:139–143.

Bowler JV, Wade JP, Jones BE, Nijran K, Steiner TJ (1996). Single-photon emission computed tomography using hexamethylpropyleneamine oxime in the prognosis of acute cerebral infarction. *Stroke* **27**:82–86.

Brainin M, Barnes M, Baron JC, Gilhus NE, Hughes R, Selmaj K *et al.* (2004).Guidance for the preparation of neurological management guidelines by EFNS scientific task forces–revised recommendations 2004. *Eur J Neurol* **11**:577–581.

Britton M, Hindmarsh T, Murray V, Tyden SA (1984). Diagnostic errors discovered by CT in patients with suspected stroke. *Neurology* **34**:1504–1507.

Bryan RN, Levy LM, Whitlow WD, Killian JM, Preziosi TJ, Rosario JA (1991). Diagnosis of acute cerebral infarction: comparison of CT and MR imaging. *AJNR Am J Neuroradiol* **12**:611–620.

Burgin WS, Malkoff M, Felberg RA, Demchuk AM, Christou I, Grotta JC *et al.* (2000). Transcranial doppler ultrasound criteria for recanalization after thrombolysis for middle cerebral artery stroke. *Stroke* **31**:1128–1132.

Casey SO, Alberico RA, Patel M, Jimenez JM, Ozsvath RR, Maguire WM *et al.* (1996). Cerebral CT venography. *Radiology* **198**:163–170.

Censori B, Partziguian T, Casto L, Camerlingo M, Mamoli A (2000). Doppler microembolic signals predict ischemic recurrences in symptomatic carotid stenosis. *Acta Neurol Scand* **101**:327–331.

Chung TS, Joo JY, Lee SK, Chien D, Laub G (1999). Evaluation of cerebral aneurysms with high-resolution MR angiography using a section-interpolation technique: correlation with digital subtraction angiography. *AJNR Am J Neuroradiol* **20**:229–235.

Cinat M, Lane CT, Pham H, Lee A, Wilson SE, Gordon I (1998). Helical CT angiography in the preoperative evaluation of carotid artery stenosis. *J Vasc Surg* **28**:290–300.

Culebras A, Kase CS, Masdeu JC, Fox AJ, Bryan RN, Grossman CB *et al.* (1997). Practice guidelines for the use of imaging in transient ischemic attacks and acute stroke. A report of the Stroke Council, American Heart Association. *Stroke* **28:**1480–1497.

Cumming MJ, Morrow IM (1994). Carotid artery stenosis: a prospective comparison of CT angiography and conventional angiography. *AJR Am J Roentgenol* **163:**517–523.

Davis SM, Donnan GA (2004). Advances in penumbra imaging with MR. *Cerebrovasc Dis* **17(Suppl 3):**23–27.

Dawson DL, Roseberry CA, Fujitani RM (1997). Preoperative testing before carotid endarterectomy: a survey of vascular surgeons' attitudes. *Ann Vasc Surg* **11:**264–272.

de Bray JM, Lhoste P, Dubas F, Emile J, Saumet JL (1994). Ultrasonic features of extracranial carotid dissections: 47 cases studied by angiography. *J Ultrasound Med* **13:**659–664.

Demchuk AM, Christou I, Wein TH, Felberg RA, Malkoff M, Grotta JC et al. (2000). Accuracy and criteria for localizing arterial occlusion with transcranial Doppler. *J Neuroimaging* **10:**1–12.

Dennis MS, Bamford JM, Molyneux AJ, Warlow CP (1987). Rapid resolution of signs of primary intracerebral haemorrhage in computed tomograms of the brain. *Br Med J (Clin Res Ed)* **295:**379–381.

Derex L, Nighoghossian N, Hermier M, Adeleine P, Philippeau F, Honnorat J et al. (2004). Thrombolysis for ischemic stroke in patients with old microbleeds on pretreatment MRI. *Cerebrovasc Dis* **17:**238–241.

Dul K, Drayer BP (1994). CT and MRI imaging of intracerebral hemorrhage. In Kase CS, Caplan LR, editors. *Intracerebral Hemorrhage*. Boston, Massachusetts, Butterworth-Heinemann. pp. 73–93.

ECST Collaborators (1998). Randomised trial of endarterectomy for recently symptomatic carotid stenosis: final results of the MRC European Carotid Surgery Trial (ECST). *Lancet* **351:**1379–1387.

Edlow JA, Caplan LR (2000). Avoiding pitfalls in the diagnosis of subarachnoid hemorrhage. *N Engl J Med* **342:**29–36.

Eggers J, Koch B, Meyer K, Konig I, Seidel G (2003). Effect of ultrasound on thrombolysis of middle cerebral artery occlusion. *Ann Neurol* **53:**797–800.

Executive Committee (1995). Endarterectomy for asymptomatic carotid artery stenosis. *JAMA* **273:**1421–1428.

Fiebach JB, Schellinger PD, Jansen O, Meyer M, Wilde P, Bender J et al. (2002). CT and diffusion-weighted MR imaging in randomized order: diffusion-weighted imaging results in higher accuracy and lower interrater variability in the diagnosis of hyperacute ischemic stroke. *Stroke* **33:**2206–2210.

Fiebach JB, Schellinger PD, Geletneky K, Wilde P, Meyer M, Hacke W et al. (2004). MRI in acute subarachnoid haemorrhage; findings with a standardised stroke protocol. *Neuroradiology* **46:**44–48.

Fiebach JB, Schellinger PD, Gass A, Kucinski T, Siebler M, Villringer A et al. (2004). Stroke magnetic resonance imaging is accurate in hyperacute intracerebral hemorrhage: a multicenter study on the validity of stroke imaging. *Stroke* **35:**502–506.

Flacke S, Urbach H, Keller E, Traber F, Hartmann A, Textor J et al. (2000). Middle cerebral artery (MCA) susceptibility sign at susceptibility-based perfusion MR imaging: clinical importance and comparison with hyperdense MCA sign at CT. *Radiology* **215:**476–482.

Furlan A, Higashida R, Wechsler L, Gent M, Rowley H, Kase C et al. (1999). Intra-arterial prourokinase for acute ischemic stroke. The PROACT II study: a randomized controlled trial. Prolyse in Acute Cerebral Thromboembolism. *JAMA* **282:**2003–2011.

Gacs G, Fox AJ, Barnett HJ, Vinuela F (1983). CT visualization of intracranial arterial thromboembolism. *Stroke* **14:**756–762.

Gilligan AK, Markus R, Read S, Srikanth V, Hirano T, Fitt G et al. (2002). Baseline blood pressure but not early computed tomography changes predicts major hemorrhage after streptokinase in acute ischemic stroke. *Stroke* **33:**2236–2242.

Goertler M, Blaser T, Krueger S, Hofmann K, Baeumer M, Wallesch CW (2002). Cessation of embolic signals after antithrombotic prevention is related to reduced risk of recurrent arterioembolic transient ischaemic attack and stroke. *J Neurol Neurosurg Psychiatry* **72:**338–342.

Grant EG, Benson CB, Moneta GL, Alexandrov AV, Baker JD, Bluth EI et al. (2003). Carotid artery stenosis: gray-scale and Doppler US diagnosis–Society of Radiologists in Ultrasound Consensus Conference. *Radiology* **229:**340–346.

Grotta J (2003). NIHSS/EIC mismatch explains the >1/3 MCA conundrum. *Stroke* **34:**e148–e149.

Hacke W, Kaste M, Fieschi C, Toni D, Lesaffre E, von Kummer R et al. (1995). Intravenous thrombolysis with recombinant tissue plasminogen activator for acute hemispheric stroke. The European Cooperative Acute Stroke Study (ECASS). *JAMA* **274:**1017–1025.

Hacke W, Kaste M, Bogousslavsky J, Brainin M, Chamorro A, Lees K et al. (2003). European Stroke Initiative Recommendations for Stroke Management-update 2003. *Cerebrovasc Dis* **16:**311–337.

Hacke W, Donnan G, Fieschi C, Kaste M, von Kummer R, Broderick JP et al. (2004). Association of outcome with early stroke treatment: pooled analysis of ATLANTIS, ECASS, and NINDS rt-PA stroke trials. *Lancet* **363:**768–774.

Hacke W, Albers G, Al Rawi Y, Bogousslavsky J, Davalos A, Eliasziw M *et al.* (2005). The Desmoteplase in Acute Ischemic Stroke Trial (DIAS): a phase II MRI-based 9-hour window acute stroke thrombolysis trial with intravenous desmoteplase. *Stroke* **36:**66–73.

Hankey GJ, Warlow CP, Sellar RJ (1990). Cerebral angiographic risk in mild cerebrovascular disease. *Stroke* **21:**209–222.

Hansberg T, Wong KS, Droste DW, Ringelstein EB, Kay R (2002). Effects of the ultrasound contrast-enhancing agent Levovist on the detection of intracranial arteries and stenoses in chinese by transcranial Doppler ultrasound. *Cerebrovasc Dis* **14:**105–108.

Heiss WD, Sobesky J, Smekal V, Kracht LW, Lehnhardt FG, Thiel A *et al.* (2004). Probability of Cortical Infarction Predicted by Flumazenil Binding and Diffusion-Weighted Imaging Signal Intensity. A Comparative Positron Emission Tomography/Magnetic Resonance Imaging Study in Early Ischemic Stroke. *Stroke* **35:**1892–1898.

Hill MD, Rowley HA, Adler F, Eliasziw M, Furlan A, Higashida RT *et al.* (2003). Selection of acute ischemic stroke patients for intra-arterial thrombolysis with pro-urokinase by using ASPECTS. *Stroke* **34:**1925–1931.

Hirai T, Korogi Y, Ono K, Nagano M, Maruoka K, Uemura S *et al.* (2002). Prospective evaluation of suspected stenoocclusive disease of the intracranial artery: combined MR angiography and CT angiography compared with digital subtraction angiography. *AJNR Am J Neuroradiol* **23:**93–101.

Hirano T, Read SJ, Abbott DF, Baird AE, Yasaka M, Infeld B *et al.* (2001). Prediction of the Final Infarct Volume within 6 h of Stroke Using Single Photon Emission Computed Tomography with Technetium-99m Hexamethylpropylene Amine Oxime. *Cerebrovasc Dis* **11:**119–127.

Hunter GJ, Hamberg LM, Ponzo JA, Huang-Hellinger FR, Morris PP, Rabinov J *et al.* (1998). Assessment of cerebral perfusion and arterial anatomy in hyperacute stroke with three-dimensional functional CT: early clinical results. *AJNR Am J Neuroradiol* **19:**29–37.

Jaillard A, Cornu C, Durieux A, Moulin T, Boutitie F, Lees KR *et al.* (1999). Hemorrhagic transformation in acute ischemic stroke. The MAST-E study. MAST-E Group. *Stroke* **30:**1326–1332.

Jarquin-Valdivia AA, McCartney J, Palestrant D, Johnston SC, Gress D (2004). The thickness of the temporal squama and its implication for transcranial sonography. *J Neuroimaging* **14:**139–142.

Job FP, Ringelstein EB, Grafen Y, Flachskampf FA, Doherty C, Stockmanns A *et al.* (1994). Comparison of transcranial contrast Doppler sonography and transesophageal contrast echocardiography for the detection of patent foramen ovale in young stroke patients. *Am J Cardiol* **74:**381–384.

Kallmes DF, Omary RA, Dix JE, Evans AJ, Hillman BJ (1996). Specificity of MR angiography as a confirmatory test of carotid artery stenosis. *AJNR Am J Neuroradiol* **17:**1501–1506.

Kaposzta Z, Martin JF, Markus HS (2002). Switching off embolization from symptomatic carotid plaque using S-nitrosoglutathione. *Circulation* **105:**1480–1484.

Kasner SE, Hankins LL, Bratina P, Morgenstern LB (1997). Magnetic resonance angiography demonstrates vascular healing of carotid and vertebral artery dissections. *Stroke* **28:**1993–1997.

Kidwell CS, Saver JL, Villablanca JP, Duckwiler G, Fredieu A, Gough K *et al.* (2002). Magnetic resonance imaging detection of microbleeds before thrombolysis: an emerging application. *Stroke* **33:**95–98.

Kidwell CS, Chalela JA, Saver JL, Starkman S, Hill MD, Demchuk AM *et al.* (2004). Comparison of MRI and CT for detection of acute intracerebral hemorrhage. *JAMA* **292:**1823–1830.

Kirsch E, Kaim A, Engelter S, Lyrer P, Stock KW, Bongartz G *et al.* (1998). MR angiography in internal carotid artery dissection: improvement of diagnosis by selective demonstration of the intramural haematoma. *Neuroradiology* **40:**704–709.

Klotzsch C, Janssen G, Berlit P (1994). Transesophageal echocardiography and contrast-TCD in the detection of a patent foramen ovale: experiences with 111 patients. *Neurology* **44:**1603–1606.

Koelemay MJ, Nederkoorn PJ, Reitsma JB, Majoie CB (2004). Systematic review of computed tomographic angiography for assessment of carotid artery disease. *Stroke* **35:**2306–2312.

Korogi Y, Takahashi M, Nakagawa T, Mabuchi N, Watabe T, Shiokawa Y *et al.* (1997). Intracranial vascular stenosis and occlusion: MR angiographic findings. *AJNR Am J Neuroradiol* **18:**135–143.

Kudo K, Terae S, Katoh C, Oka M, Shiga T, Tamaki N *et al.* (2003). Quantitative cerebral blood flow measurement with dynamic perfusion CT using the vascular-pixel elimination method: comparison with H2(15)O positron emission tomography. *AJNR Am J Neuroradiol* **24:**419–426.

Lanczik O, Szabo K, Hennerici M, Gass A (2005). Multiparametric MRI and ultrasound findings in patients with internal carotid artery dissection. *Neurology* **65:**469–471.

Larrue V, von Kummer RR, Muller A, Bluhmki E (2001). Risk factors for severe hemorrhagic transformation in ischemic stroke patients treated with recombinant tissue plasminogen activator: a secondary analysis of the European-Australasian Acute Stroke Study (ECASS II). *Stroke* **32:**438–441.

Latchaw RE, Yonas H, Hunter GJ, Yuh WT, Ueda T, Sorensen AG *et al.* (2003). Guidelines and recommendations for perfusion imaging in cerebral ischemia: A scientific statement for healthcare professionals by the writing group on perfusion imaging, from the Council on Cardiovascular Radiology of the American Heart Association. *Stroke* **34:**1084–1104.

Leary MC, Kidwell CS, Villablanca JP, Starkman S, Jahan R, Duckwiler GR *et al.* (2003). Validation of computed tomographic middle cerebral artery "dot"sign: an angiographic correlation study. *Stroke* **34:**2636–2640.

Leclerc X, Godefroy O, Pruvo JP, Leys D (1995). Computed tomographic angiography for the evaluation of carotid artery stenosis. *Stroke* **26:**1577–1581.

Lev MH, Segal AZ, Farkas J, Hossain ST, Putman C, Hunter GJ *et al.* (2001). Utility of perfusion-weighted CT imaging in acute middle cerebral artery stroke treated with intra-arterial thrombolysis: prediction of final infarct volume and clinical outcome. *Stroke* **32:**2021–2028.

Levi CR, O'Malley HM, Fell G, Roberts AK, Hoare MC, Royle JP *et al.* (1997). Transcranial Doppler detected cerebral microembolism following carotid endarterectomy. High microembolic signal loads predict postoperative cerebral ischaemia. *Brain* **120(Pt 4):**621–629.

Levi CR, Stork JL, Chambers BR, Abbott AL, Cameron HM, Peeters A *et al.* (2001). Dextran reduces embolic signals after carotid endarterectomy. *Ann Neurol* **50:**544–547.

Levy C, Laissy JP, Raveau V, Amarenco P, Servois V, Bousser MG *et al.* (1994). Carotid and vertebral artery dissections: three-dimensional time-of-flight MR angiography and MR imaging versus conventional angiography. *Radiology* **190:**97–103.

Linfante I, Llinas RH, Caplan LR, Warach S (1999). MRI features of intracerebral hemorrhage within 2 hours from symptom onset. *Stroke* **30:**2263–2267.

Lysakowski C, Walder B, Costanza MC, Tramer MR (2001). Transcranial Doppler versus angiography in patients with vasospasm due to a ruptured cerebral aneurysm: A systematic review. *Stroke* **32:**2292–2298.

Mahagne MH, David O, Darcourt J, Migneco O, Dunac A, Chatel M *et al.* (2004). Voxel-based mapping of cortical ischemic damage using Tc 99m L,L-ethyl cysteinate dimer SPECT in acute stroke. *J Neuroimaging* **14:**23–32.

Markus HS, Thomson ND, Brown MM (1995). Asymptomatic cerebral embolic signals in symptomatic and asymptomatic carotid artery disease. *Brain* **118(Pt 4):**1005–1011.

Markus H, Cullinane M (2001). Severely impaired cerebrovascular reactivity predicts stroke and TIA risk in patients with carotid artery stenosis and occlusion. *Brain* **124:**457–467.

Markus HS, MacKinnon A (2005). Asymptomatic embolization detected by Doppler ultrasound predicts stroke risk in symptomatic carotid artery stenosis. *Stroke* **36:**971–975.

Markus HS, Droste DW, Kaps M, Larrue V, Lees KR, Siebler M *et al.* (2005). Dual antiplatelet therapy with clopidogrel and aspirin in symptomatic carotid stenosis evaluated using doppler embolic signal detection: the Clopidogrel and Aspirin for Reduction of Emboli in Symptomatic Carotid Stenosis (CARESS) trial. *Circulation* **111:**2233–2240.

Masaryk T, Drayer BP, Anderson RE, Braffman B, Davis PC, Deck MD *et al.* (2000). Cerebrovascular disease. American College of Radiology. ACR Appropriateness Criteria. *Radiology* **215(Suppl):**415–435.

Mattle HP, Wentz KU, Edelman RR, Wallner B, Finn JP, Barnes P *et al.* (1991). Cerebral venography with MR. *Radiology* **178:**453–458.

Molloy J, Markus HS (1999). Asymptomatic embolization predicts stroke and TIA risk in patients with carotid artery stenosis. *Stroke* **30:**1440–1443.

Morgenstern LB, Luna-Gonzales H, Huber JC, Jr., Wong SS, Uthman MO, Gurian JH *et al.* (1998). Worst headache and subarachnoid hemorrhage: prospective, modern computed tomography and spinal fluid analysis. *Ann Emerg Med* **32:**297–304.

Moulin T, Cattin F, Crepin-Leblond T, Tatu L, Chavot D, Piotin M *et al.* (1996). Early CT signs in acute middle cerebral artery infarction: predictive value for subsequent infarct locations and outcome. *Neurology* **47:**366–375.

NASCET Collaborators (1991). Beneficial effect of carotid endarterectomy in symptomatic patients with high-grade carotid stenosis. *N Engl J Med* **325:**445–453.

Nederkoorn PJ, van der GY, Hunink MG (2003). Duplex ultrasound and magnetic resonance angiography compared with digital subtraction angiography in carotid artery stenosis: a systematic review. *Stroke* **34:**1324–1332.

New PF, Aronow S (1976). Attenuation measurements of whole blood and blood fractions in computed tomography. *Radiology* **121:**635–640.

NINDS rt-PA Stroke Study Group (1995). Tissue plasminogen activator for acute ischemic stroke. *N Engl J Med* **333:**1581–1587.

Nighoghossian N, Hermier M, Adeleine P, Blanc-Lasserre K, Derex L, Honnorat J *et al.* (2002). Old microbleeds are a potential risk factor for cerebral bleeding after ischemic stroke: a gradient-echo T2*-weighted brain MRI study. *Stroke* **33:**735–742.

Noguchi K, Ogawa T, Inugami A, Toyoshima H, Sugawara S, Hatazawa J et al. (1995). Acute subarachnoid hemorrhage: MR imaging with fluid-attenuated inversion recovery pulse sequences. *Radiology* **196:**773–777.

Noguchi K, Ogawa T, Seto H, Inugami A, Hadeishi H, Fujita H et al. (1997). Subacute and chronic subarachnoid hemorrhage: diagnosis with fluid-attenuated inversion-recovery MR imaging. *Radiology* **203:**257–262.

Oelerich M, Stogbauer F, Kurlemann G, Schul C, Schuierer G (1999). Craniocervical artery dissection: MR imaging and MR angiographic findings. *Eur Radiol* **9:**1385–1391.

Patel SC, Levine SR, Tilley BC, Grotta JC, Lu M, Frankel M et al. (2001). Lack of clinical significance of early ischemic changes on computed tomography in acute stroke. *JAMA* **286:**2830–2838.

Payne DA, Jones CI, Hayes PD, Thompson MM, London NJ, Bell PR et al. (2004). Beneficial effects of clopidogrel combined with aspirin in reducing cerebral emboli in patients undergoing carotid endarterectomy. *Circulation* **109:**1476–1481.

Renowden S (2004). Cerebral venous sinus thrombosis. *Eur Radiol* **14:**215–226.

Rohl L, Ostergaard L, Simonsen CZ, Vestergaard-Poulsen P, Andersen G, Sakoh M et al. (2001). Viability thresholds of ischemic penumbra of hyperacute stroke defined by perfusion-weighted MRI and apparent diffusion coefficient. *Stroke* **32:**1140–1146.

Rorick MB, Nichols FT, Adams RJ (1994). Transcranial Doppler correlation with angiography in detection of intracranial stenosis. *Stroke* **25:**1931–1934.

Rother J, Schellinger PD, Gass A, Siebler M, Villringer A, Fiebach JB et al. (2002). Effect of intravenous thrombolysis on MRI parameters and functional outcome in acute stroke <6 hours. *Stroke* **33:**2438–2445.

Sames TA, Storrow AB, Finkelstein JA, Magoon MR (1996). Sensitivity of new-generation computed tomography in subarachnoid hemorrhage. *Acad Emerg Med* **3:**16–20.

Sameshima T, Futami S, Morita Y, Yokogami K, Miyahara S, Sameshima Y et al. (1999). Clinical usefulness of and problems with three-dimensional CT angiography for the evaluation of arteriosclerotic stenosis of the carotid artery: comparison with conventional angiography, MRA, and ultrasound sonography. *Surg Neurol* **51:**301–308.

Schellinger PD, Jansen O, Fiebach JB, Hacke W, Sartor K (1999). A standardized MRI stroke protocol: comparison with CT in hyperacute intracerebral hemorrhage. *Stroke* **30:**765–768.

Schellinger PD, Fiebach JB, Hacke W (2003). Imaging-based decision making in thrombolytic therapy for ischemic stroke: present status. *Stroke* **34:**575–583.

Schellinger PD, Chalela JA, Kang DW, Latour LL, Warach S (2005). Diagnostic and prognostic value of early MR imaging vessel signs in hyperacute stroke patients imaged <3 hours and treated with recombinant tissue plasminogen activator. *AJNR Am J Neuroradiol* **26:**618–624.

Schlaug G, Benfield A, Baird AE, Siewert B, Lovblad KO, Parker RA et al. (1999). The ischemic penumbra: operationally defined by diffusion and perfusion MRI. *Neurology* **53:**1528–1537.

Schramm P, Schellinger PD, Klotz E, Kallenberg K, Fiebach JB, Kulkens S et al. (2004). Comparison of perfusion computed tomography and computed tomography angiography source images with perfusion-weighted imaging and diffusion-weighted imaging in patients with acute stroke of less than 6 hours' duration. *Stroke* **35:**1652–1658.

Schuknecht B (2004). Latest techniques in head and neck CT angiography. *Neuroradiology* **46(Suppl 2):**s208–s213.

Schwartz RB, Jones KM, Chernoff DM, Mukherji SK, Khorasani R, Tice HM et al. (1992). Common carotid artery bifurcation: evaluation with spiral CT. Work in progress. *Radiology* **185:**513–519.

Seitz RJ, Meisel S, Weller P, Junghans U, Wittsack HJ, Siebler M (2005). Initial ischemic event: Perfusion-weighted MR imaging and apparent diffusion coefficient for stroke evolution. *Radiology* **237:**1020–1028.

Serena J, Segura T, Perez-Ayuso MJ, Bassaganyas J, Molins A, Davalos A (1998). The need to quantify right-to-left shunt in acute ischemic stroke: a case-control study. *Stroke* **29:**1322–1328.

Shinokawa N, Hirai T, Takashima S, Kameyama T, Obata Y, Nakagawa K et al. (2000). Relation of transesophageal echocardiographic findings to subtypes of cerebral infarction in patients with atrial fibrillation. *Clin Cardiol* **23:**517–522.

Shuaib A, Lee D, Pelz D, Fox A, Hachinski VC (1992). The impact of magnetic resonance imaging on the management of acute ischemic stroke. *Neurology* **42:**816–818.

Sidman R, Connolly E, Lemke T (1996). Subarachnoid hemorrhage diagnosis: lumbar puncture is still needed when the computed tomography scan is normal. *Acad Emerg Med* **3:**827–831.

Siebler M, Sitzer M, Rose G, Bendfeldt D, Steinmetz H (1993). Silent cerebral embolism caused by neurologically symptomatic high-grade carotid stenosis. Event rates before and after carotid endarterectomy. *Brain* **116(Pt 5):**1005–1015.

Siebler M, Nachtmann A, Sitzer M, Rose G, Kleinschmidt A, Rademacher J et al. (1995). Cerebral microembolism and the risk of ischemia in asymptomatic high-grade internal carotid artery stenosis. *Stroke* **26:**2184–2186.

Silvestrini M, Vernieri F, Pasqualetti P, Matteis M, Passarelli F, Troisi E et al. (2000). Impaired cerebral vasoreactivity and risk of stroke in patients with asymptomatic carotid artery stenosis. *JAMA* **283:** 2122–2127.

Skutta B, Furst G, Eilers J, Ferbert A, Kuhn FP (1999). Intracranial stenoocclusive disease: double-detector helical CT angiography versus digital subtraction angiography. *AJNR Am J Neuroradiol* **20:**791–799.

Sloan MA, Alexandrov AV, Tegeler CH, Spencer MP, Caplan LR, Feldmann E et al. (2004). Assessment: transcranial Doppler ultrasonography: report of the Therapeutics and Technology Assessment Subcommittee of the American Academy of Neurology. *Neurology* **62:**1468–1481.

Sorensen AG, Buonanno FS, Gonzalez RG, Schwamm LH, Lev MH, Huang-Hellinger FR et al. (1996). Hyperacute stroke: evaluation with combined multisection diffusion-weighted and hemodynamically weighted echo-planar MR imaging. *Radiology* **199:**391–401.

Sviri GE, Lewis DH, Correa R, Britz GW, Douville CM, Newell DW (2004). Basilar artery vasospasm and delayed posterior circulation ischemia after aneurysmal subarachnoid hemorrhage. *Stroke* **35:**1867–1872.

Tanne D, Kasner SE, Demchuk AM, Koren-Morag N, Hanson S, Grond M et al. (2002). Markers of increased risk of intracerebral hemorrhage after intravenous recombinant tissue plasminogen activator therapy for acute ischemic stroke in clinical practice: the Multicenter rt-PA Stroke Survey. *Circulation* **105:**1679–1685.

The Magnetic Resonance Angiography in Relatives of Patients with Subarachnoid Hemorrhage Study Group (1999). Risks and benefits of screening for intracranial aneurysms in first-degree relatives of patients with sporadic subarachnoid hemorrhage. *N Engl J Med* **341:**1344–1350.

Thomassen L, Brainin M, Demarin V, Grond M, Toni D, Venables GS (2003). Acute stroke treatment in Europe: a questionnaire-based survey on behalf of the EFNS Task Force on acute neurological stroke care. *Eur J Neurol* **10:**199–204.

Tomura N, Uemura K, Inugami A, Fujita H, Higano S, Shishido F (1988). Early CT finding in cerebral infarction: obscuration of the lentiform nucleus. *Radiology* **168:**463–467.

Truwit CL, Barkovich AJ, Gean-Marton A, Hibri N, Norman D (1990). Loss of the insular ribbon: another early CT sign of acute middle cerebral artery infarction. *Radiology* **176:**801–806.

Tsushima Y, Aoki J, Endo K (2003). Brain microhemorrhages detected on T2*-weighted gradient-echo MR images. *AJNR Am J Neuroradiol* **24:**88–96.

Valton L, Larrue V, Pavy LT, Geraud G (1997). Cerebral microembolism in patients with stroke or transient ischaemic attack as a risk factor for early recurrence. *J Neurol Neurosurg Psychiatry* **63:**784–787.

van der Wee N, Rinkel GJ, Hasan D, van Gijn J (1999). Detection of subarachnoid haemorrhage on early CT: is lumbar puncture still needed after a negative scan? *J Neurol Neurosurg Psychiatry* **58:**357–359.

van Gijn J, van Dongen KJ (1982). The time course of aneurysmal haemorrhage on computed tomograms. *Neuroradiology* **23:**153–156.

Villablanca JP, Jahan R, Hooshi P, Lim S, Duckwiler G, Patel A et al. (2002). Detection and characterization of very small cerebral aneurysms by using 2D and 3D helical CT angiography. *AJNR Am J Neuroradiol* **23:**1187–1198.

Virapongse C, Cazenave C, Quisling R, Sarwar M, Hunter S (1987). The empty delta sign: frequency and significance in 76 cases of dural sinus thrombosis. *Radiology* **162:**779–785.

von Kummer R, Holle R, Gizyska U, Hofmann E, Jansen O, Petersen D et al. (1996a). Interobserver agreement in assessing early CT signs of middle cerebral artery infarction. *AJNR Am J Neuroradiol* **17:** 1743–1748.

von Kummer R, Nolte PN, Schnittger H, Thron A, Ringelstein EB (1996b). Detectability of cerebral hemisphere ischaemic infarcts by CT within 6 h of stroke. *Neuroradiology* **38:**31–33.

von Kummer R (1998). Effect of training in reading CT scans on patient selection for ECASS II. *Neurology* **51:**S50–S52.

Warach S, Chien D, Li W, Ronthal M, Edelman RR (1992). Fast magnetic resonance diffusion-weighted imaging of acute human stroke. *Neurology* **42:**1717–1723.

Warach S, Dashe JF, Edelman RR (1996a). Clinical outcome in ischemic stroke predicted by early diffusion-weighted and perfusion magnetic resonance imaging: a preliminary analysis. *J Cereb Blood Flow Metab* **16:**53–59.

Warach S, Mosley M, Sorensen AG, Koroshetz W (1996b). Time course of diffusion imaging abnormalities in human stroke. *Stroke* **27:**1254–1256.

Wardlaw JM, Keir SL, Seymour J, Lewis S, Sandercock PA, Dennis MS et al. (2004). What is the best imaging strategy for acute stroke? *Health Technol Assess* **8**:iii, ix–iii, 180.

Westwood ME, Kelly S, Berry E, Bamford JM, Gough MJ, Airey CM *et al.* (2002). Use of magnetic resonance angiography to select candidates with recently symptomatic carotid stenosis for surgery: systematic review. *BMJ* **324**:198.

White PM, Teasdale EM, Wardlaw JM, Easton V (2001). Intracranial aneurysms: CT angiography and MR angiography for detection prospective blinded comparison in a large patient cohort. *Radiology* **219**: 739–749.

Willinsky RA, Taylor SM, TerBrugge K, Farb RI, Tomlinson G, Montanera W (2003). Neurologic complications of cerebral angiography: prospective analysis of 2,899 procedures and review of the literature. *Radiology* **227**:522–528.

Wing SD, Norman D, Pollock JA, Newton TH (1976). Contrast enhancement of cerebral infarcts in computed tomography. *Radiology* **121**:89–92.

Wintermark M, Reichhart M, Cuisenaire O, Maeder P, Thiran JP, Schnyder P *et al.* (2002a). Comparison of admission perfusion computed tomography and qualitative diffusion- and perfusion-weighted magnetic resonance imaging in acute stroke patients. *Stroke* **33**:2025–2031.

Wintermark M, Reichhart M, Thiran JP, Maeder P, Chalaron M, Schnyder P *et al.* (2002b). Prognostic accuracy of cerebral blood flow measurement by perfusion computed tomography, at the time of emergency room admission, in acute stroke patients. *Ann Neurol* **51**:417–432.

Wintermark M, Sesay M, Barbier E, Borbely K, Dillon WP, Eastwood JD *et al.* (2005). Comparative overview of brain perfusion imaging techniques. *Stroke* **36**: 2032–2033.

Wittsack HJ, Ritzl A, Fink GR, Wenserski F, Siebler M, Seitz RJ *et al.* (2002). MR imaging in acute stroke: diffusion-weighted and perfusion imaging parameters for predicting infarct size. *Radiology* **222**:397–403.

World Health Organization. The World Health Report 1999 (1999). Geneva, Switzerland: WHO.

Zanette EM, Fieschi C, Bozzao L, Roberti C, Toni D, Argentino C *et al.* (1989). Comparison of cerebral angiography and transcranial Doppler sonography in acute stroke. *Stroke* **20**:899–903.

CHAPTER 6

Use of imaging in multiple sclerosis

M. Filippi,[a] M.A. Rocca,[a] D.L. Arnold,[b] R. Bakshi,[c]
F. Barkhof,[d] N. De Stefano,[e] F. Fazekas,[f]
E. Frohman,[g] J.S. Wolinsky[h]

Background Magnetic resonance (MR)-based techniques are widely used for the assessment of patients with suspected and definite multiple sclerosis (MS). However, despite the publication of several position papers, which attempted to define the utility of MR techniques in the management of MS, their application in everyday clinical practice is still suboptimal. This is probably related not only to the fact that the majority of published guidelines focused on the optimization of MR technology in clinical trials, but also to the continuing development of modern, quantitative MR-based techniques that have not as yet entered the clinical arena.

Aims The present report summarizes the conclusions of the 'EFNS Expert Panel of Neuroimaging of MS' on the application of conventional and non-conventional MR techniques to the clinical management of patients with MS. These guidelines are intended to assist in the use of conventional MRI for the diagnosis and longitudinal monitoring of patients with MS. In addition, they should provide a foundation for the development of more widespread but rational clinical applications of non-conventional MR-based techniques in studies of MS patients.

Introduction

Conventional magnetic resonance imaging (cMRI) has proven to be sensitive for detecting multiple sclerosis (MS) lesions and their changes over time (Filippi *et al.*, 2003a; Bakshi *et al.*, 2004). This exquisite sensitivity has made cMRI the most important paraclinical tool in diagnosing MS and establishing a prognosis at the clinical onset of the disease. These are the main reasons why cMRI findings have a major role in the recently developed International Panel (IP) diagnostic criteria for MS (McDonald *et al.*, 2001). Many research groups have subsequently taken steps to validate and refine these recommendations (Barkhof *et al.*, 2003; Dalton 2003a; Frohman *et al.*, 2003;

[a]Neuroimaging Research Unit, Department of Neurology, Scientific Institute and University Ospedale San Raffaele, Milan, Italy; [b]McConnell Brain Imaging Centre, Montreal Neurological Institute, Montreal, Canada; [c]Center for Neurological Imaging, Partners MS Center, Departments of Neurology and Radiology, Brigham and Women's Hospital, Harvard Medical School, Boston, MA, USA; [d]Image Analysis Centre, VU medical Centre, Amsterdam, The Netherlands; [e]Institute of Neurological Sciences, University of Siena, Siena, Italy; [f]Department of Neurology, Karl Frenzens University, Graz, Austria; [g]University of Texas Southwestern Medical Center at Dallas, Dallas, USA; [h]Department of Neurology, University of Texas Health Science Center, Houston, USA.

European Journal of Neurology 2006, 13:313–325

Tintore *et al.*, 2003; Polman *et al.*, 2005). However, for clinicians, it still remains unclear how and when cMRI should be used, not only at the onset of the disease, but also during the subsequent disease phases. In addition, despite the sensitivity of cMRI for detecting MS lesions, the correlation between cMRI metrics (i.e. hyperintense lesions on T2- and post-contrast T1-weighted images, hypointense lesions on T1-weighted images and atrophy measurements) and clinical findings of MS is still limited (Filippi *et al.*, 2003a). Among the likely reasons for this clinical/MRI discrepancy, a major one is the low pathological specificity of the abnormalities seen on cMRI scans and the inability of cMRI metrics to detect and quantify the extent of damage in normal-appearing brain tissues (Rovaris and Filippi, 1999; Filippi *et al.*, 2003a). These inherent limitations of cMRI have prompted the development and application of modern quantitative MR techniques (MR spectroscopy [^{1}H-MRS], magnetization transfer [MT] MRI, diffusion weighted [DW] MRI and functional MRI [fMRI]) to the study of MS. Although these techniques have provided important insight into the pathobiology of MS, their practical value in the assessment of MS patients in clinical practice has yet to be realized.

Aim of the European Federation of Neurological Science (EFNS) Task Force

The aim of the 'EFNS Expert Panel of Neuroimaging of MS' is to define guidelines for the application of conventional and non-conventional MR techniques for the diagnosis and monitoring of patients with MS in clinical practice. In addition, they should clarify the current status and clinical role of non-conventional MR techniques.

Search strategy: data for this review were identified by searches of Medline and references from relevant articles from 1965 to 2005. The search terms 'Multiple Sclerosis', 'Magnetic Resonance Imaging', 'Diagnosis', 'Prognosis', 'Atrophy', 'Magnetization Transfer MRI', 'Diffusion Weighted MRI', 'Diffusion Tensor MRI', 'Proton Magnetic Resonance Spectroscopy', 'Disability' and 'Treatment'

were used. Only papers published in English were reviewed.

MRI assessment of patients at presentation with clinically isolated syndromes suggestive of MS

In about 85% of patients with MS, the clinical onset of the disease is a clinically isolated syndrome (CIS) involving the optic nerve, brainstem or spinal cord (Noseworthy *et al.*, 2000). Approximately 50–80% of these patients already have lesions on cMRI, consistent with prior disease activity (Filippi *et al.*, 1994; Barkhof *et al.*, 1997a; O'Riordan *et al.*, 1998; Brex *et al.*, 2002). As recent randomized controlled trials (Jacobs *et al.*, 2000; Comi *et al.*, 2001; Achiron *et al.*, 2004) have shown a treatment effect in patients with a CIS and MRI abnormalities suggestive of MS, it has become critical to expedite the identification of those patients at high risk to a multiphasic inflammatory demyelinating disorder consistent with MS. Equally compelling has been the desire to characterize those factors that have the ability to prospectively predict which patients will be at highest risk for precocious and substantial disability accrual.

Conventional MRI

All of the diagnostic criteria proposed for MS (Schumacher *et al.*, 1965; Poser *et al.*, 1983; McDonald *et al.*, 2001) require the demonstration of disease dissemination in space and time. The central principle advanced in each of these diagnostic schemes involves the confirmation of two or more clinical attacks, separated in time, which involve at least two distinct areas of the central nervous system (CNS). Another key requirement in each of the diagnostic criteria is the exclusion of alternative diagnostic considerations that can mimic MS by appropriate tests. The Poser criteria, published in 1983, were the first set of criteria that integrated findings from paraclinical and laboratory tests (including cerebro-spinal fluid [CSF] analysis, evoked potentials [EP] and MRI) to demonstrate spatial dissemination of the disease and to increase diagnostic confidence.

A critical feature in the diagnostic evaluation of patients suspected of having MS is the characterization of lesions profiles that are suggestive of the disease. Brain MS lesions are frequently located in the periventricular regions, the corpus callosum and infratentorial areas (with the pons and cerebellum more frequently affected than the medulla and midbrain), and are characterized by oval or elliptical shapes (Ormerod et al., 1987). In addition, consensus has been reached on criteria useful to identify T2-hyperintense (Filippi et al., 1998a) and T1-enhancing lesions (Barkhof et al., 1997b). As MS frequently affects the spinal cord, some characteristics of MS cord lesions have also been identified. Cord MS lesions are more frequently observed within the cervical than in the thoracic regions, are usually peripheral, limited to two vertebral segments in length or less, occupy less than half the cross-sectional area of the cord, and are not seen as T1-hypointensities (Gass et al., 1998). Acute plaques typically produce swelling of the cord and enhancement after gadolinium (Gd) administration (Tartaglino et al., 1995; Rocca et al., 1999).

The optic nerve is also frequently involved in the course of MS. When an optic neuritis (ON) is suspected to be the onset manifestation of MS, the principal role of MRI is to assess the brain for asymptomatic lesions (Optic Neuritis Study Group, 1997; 2003; Brex et al., 2002; Hickman et al., 2002), whereas optic nerve MRI can be useful in ruling out alternative diagnosis. The sensitivity of MRI for detecting optic nerve lesions in patients with ON is high: a seminal study using a short-tau inversion recovery (STIR) sequence showed lesions in 84% of symptomatic nerves and 20% of asymptomatic nerves (Miller et al., 1988a). The use of fat-saturated fast spin echo (Gass et al., 1996) and selective partial inversion recovery pre pulse (SPIR)-FLAIR (Jackson et al., 1998) sequences has led to increases in sensitivity for detecting lesions in patients with an ON. In MS patients, increased T2 signal can be seen for a long time after an episode of ON, despite improvements in vision and visual EP, and even in the absence of acute attacks of ON (Davies et al., 1998). T1-hypointense lesions are not seen in the optic nerve (Gass et al., 1998), whereas Gd enhancement is a consistent feature of acute ON (Kupersmith et al., 2002; Hickman et al., 2004).

In the past two decades, a number of MRI criteria have been proposed (Fazekas et al., 1988; Paty et al., 1988; Barkhof et al., 1997a) to increase the confidence in rendering a diagnosis of MS:

- Criteria of Paty et al. (1988): presence of at least four T2-hyperintense lesions, or three T2 lesions, of which one is periventricular. These criteria are characterized by high sensitivity but relatively low specificity (Lee et al., 1991) (class I evidence).
- Criteria of Fazekas et al. (1988): presence of at least three T2-hyperintense lesions with two of the following characteristics: an infratentorial lesion, a periventricular lesion and a lesion larger than 6 mm. These criteria showed both high sensitivity and high specificity when evaluated retrospectively in definite MS (Offenbacher et al., 1993), but have limited predictive value when applied prospectively in patients with CIS (Tas et al., 1995) (class II evidence).
- Criteria of Barkhof et al. (1997a): presence of at least three of the four following features: presence of at least one Gd enhancing lesion, at least one juxtacortical lesion, at least one infratentorial lesion and three or more periventricular lesions (class I evidence). In 2000, Tintorè et al. slightly modified these criteria by allowing for nine T2 lesions to be an alternative for the presence of an enhancing lesion and reported a high specificity of these criteria to predict conversion from CIS to clinically definite (CD) MS (class I evidence).

In the most recent diagnostic criteria (McDonald et al., 2001) proposed by an IP of MS specialists, demonstration of dissemination in space was based on the modified Barkhof-Tintoré criteria. For the first time, these criteria underpinned the role of spinal cord lesions in demonstrating disease dissemination in space. When these more stringent imaging criteria are not fulfilled, the IP criteria allow the presence of at least two T2 lesions when oligoclonal bands are detected in the CSF. However, Tintoré et al. (2003) recently showed that this alternative criterion may result in a decreased diagnostic accuracy as they reported in CIS patients followed for 3 years a specificity of only 63% for the development of CDMS (class III evidence). In the IP criteria (McDonald *et al.*, 2001), temporal dissemination can be demonstrated either by the presence of at least one enhancing lesion on an MRI scan performed 3 months or more after the onset of the clinical event or by the presence of one new T2 or enhancing lesion on an MRI scan performed 6 months or more after the onset of the clinical event (only if there is a previous scan at least 3 months after the event in case of a T2 lesion).

The major advantage of the IP criteria (McDonald *et al.*, 2001) is that they facilitate the early diagnosis of MS in patients with a clinically isolated attack before a second clinical relapse has occurred. In a 3-year follow-up study of CIS patients, Dalton *et al.* (2002a) showed a sensitivity, specificity and accuracy of 83% of the IP criteria to predict conversion to CDMS (class III evidence). These results were confirmed by Tintoré *et al.* (2003), who reported a sensitivity of 74%, specificity of 86% and accuracy of 80% (class III evidence). In the placebo arm of a trial of patients at the earliest clinical stage of MS, the IP criteria for dissemination in space were similarly effective in predicting subsequent evolution to CDMS (Barkhof *et al.*, 2003) (class II evidence). However, it is worth noting that the MRI spatial dissemination criteria are less specific in predicting conversion to CDMS when applied to patients presenting with a CIS of the brain stem (Sastre-Garriga *et al.*, 2004) (class II evidence). The presence of asymptomatic cord lesions was helpful in demonstrating spatial dissemination in recently diagnosed MS patients (Bot *et al.*, 2002) (class IV evidence), but the substitution of a brain lesion with a cord lesion did not impact significantly on the subsequent diagnosis in patients presenting with ON (Dalton *et al.*, 2003b) (class III evidence). When a new T2-lesion was allowed as evidence for dissemination in time, one study showed that 82% of CIS patients who fulfilled the IP MRI criteria for MS after 3 months had developed CDMS within 3 years (Dalton *et al.*, 2003a) (class III evidence), and another found that 80% of those CIS who fulfilled the same criteria after 1 year developed CDMS within 3 years (Tintore *et al.*, 2003) (class III evidence).

Several authors have investigated the prognostic role of MR-derived metrics in patients presenting with CIS. The MRI findings that showed the strongest predictive value for the subsequent development of definite MS on short- to medium-term follow up were the number and extent of T2-visible brain lesions at disease onset (Filippi *et al.*, 1994; O'Riordan *et al.*, 1998; Brex *et al.*, 2002; Minneboo *et al.*, 2004) (class II evidence), the presence of infratentorial lesions (Minneboo *et al.*, 2004) (class III evidence) and the presence of Gd-enhancing lesions (Barkhof *et al.*, 1997a, class I evidence; Jacobs *et al.*, 2000, class IV evidence).

During the last decades, several quantitative MR techniques have been developed for the assessment of brain damage in patients with MS. Even if the application of these techniques in everyday clinical practice is, at the moment, still premature, as these techniques often require dedicated personnel and specific softwares for the analysis, it is likely that with their progressive availability their use in clinical practice will increase.

The progressive development of brain and spinal cord atrophy is a well-known radiographic feature of MS (Miller *et al.*, 2002, Lin *et al.*, 2004). Objective quantification of CNS atrophy has been recognized as a potentially useful marker of the destructive and irreversible components of MS-related tissue damage. Recent MRI studies have confirmed that irreversible tissue loss/damage occurs early in the course of the disease and it is likely that the extent of such irreversible tissue damage conveys important prognostic information. Three studies (Dalton *et al.*, 2002b, 2004a; Filippi *et al.*, 2004a) showed the development of regional or global brain atrophy over a period up to 3 years in CIS patients who evolved to MS. In one of these studies (Dalton *et al.*, 2004a), progressive gray matter atrophy in the brain was also observed. A recent study has shown that in CIS patients a low dose of interferon (IFN) beta-1a given subcutaneously once a week reduces the rate of brain atrophy by about 30% over 2 years (Filippi *et al.*, 2004a). On the contrary, compared to normal controls, cord area was found to be only slightly reduced in patients presenting with CIS and an abnormal MRI scan, and cord area remained stable over 1 year after disease onset (Brex *et al.*, 2001a).

Non-conventional MRI

(1) MT-MRI. Reduced MT ratio (MTR) values have been detected in the normal-appearing brain tissue (NABT) from patients at presentation with CIS (Iannucci *et al.*, 2000; Traboulsee *et al.*, 2002). The extent of these abnormalities appears to be an independent predictor of subsequent disease evolution (Iannucci *et al.*, 2000). However, these observations were not confirmed by later studies (Kaiser *et al.*, 2000; Brex *et al.*, 2001b). No abnormalities have been detected in the cervical cord of CIS patients using this technique (Rovaris *et al.*, 2004).

(2) DT MRI. DT MRI has disclosed subtle abnormalities in the normal-appearing white matter (NAWM) of patients at presentation with CIS (Gallo *et al.*, 2005). However, these abnormalities were not found to be predictive of temporal lesion dissemination in time (as defined by McDonald criteria) at 3 and 12 months (Gallo *et al.*, 2005).

(3) ^{1}H-MRS. Metabolic abnormalities, consisting in a reduction of the concentration of N-acetylasparate (NAA) of the whole brain (Filippi *et al.*, 2003b) and in an increase of myo-inositol (mI) and creatine (Cr) in NAWM (Fernando *et al.*, 2004) have been shown in patients at the earliest clinical stage of MS. These findings suggest that widespread axonal pathology, glial injury and an increase in cell turnover or metabolism are rather early phenomenon in the course of the disease. (4) Functional MRI. Using fMRI, an abnormal pattern of movement-associated cortical activation has also been described in CIS patients within 3 months of disease onset (Rocca *et al.* 2003; Filippi *et al.* 2004b). In a 1-year follow-up study of CIS patients (Rocca *et al.*, 2005), those who developed CDMS had a different motor fMRI response at first presentation when compared with those who did not, suggesting that, in CIS patients, the extent of early cortical reorganization following tissue injury might be a factor associated to a different disease evolution.

RECOMMENDATIONS

In patients at presentation with CIS suggestive of MS (i.e. neurological findings typically seen in

the setting of MS) (Frohman *et al.*, 2003), after appropriate exclusion of alternative diagnostic considerations that can mimic MS, the following recommendations should be considered:

(1) cMRI of the brain (dual-echo, pre- and post-contrast T1-weighted scans) should be obtained as soon as possible in all patients presenting with an isolated demyelinating syndrome involving the CNS, not only to collect additional evidence for lesion dissemination in space, but also to exclude other possible neurological conditions. As suggested by recent guidelines from the American Academy of Neurology (Frohman *et al.*, 2003), the finding in these patients of three or more T2-hyperintense lesions with the imaging characteristics underlined by the IP guidelines (McDonald *et al.*, 2001) (Type A) and the presence of two or more Gd-enhancing lesions at baseline are sensitive predictors of the subsequent development of CDMS within the next 7–10 years (Type B).

(2) The presence of three or more white matter lesions on brain T2-weighted MRI in patients suspected of having MS is not diagnostic, especially when their location and appearance is non-characteristic for demyelination. In this context, the IP criteria (McDonald *et al.*, 2001) should be applied. Incidental white matter lesions are not an infrequent observation even in the young normal population. Note that with ageing (at least >50 years) incidental white matter lesions may also show progression (Schmidt *et al.*, 2003; Longstreth *et al.*, 2005) (Good Practice Point).

(3) In the case of steroids treatment, which is known to dramatically suppress Gd enhancement, one of the possible markers of inflammation, cMRI should be performed before treatment or, at least, 1 month after treatment termination (Good Practice Point).

(4) cMRI of the spinal cord is useful in those circumstances when brain MRI is normal or equivocal, and in patients with non-specific brain

continued

T2-abnormalities (especially when older than 50 years), because, contrary to what happens for the brain, cord lesions rarely develop with ageing *per se* (Kidd *et al.*, 1993). In patients presenting with a spinal cord syndrome, spinal cord MRI is highly recommended to rule out other conditions that may mimic MS, such as compressive lesions (Good Practice Point).

(5) In patients with acute ON, MRI of the optic nerve can be useful in ruling out alternative diagnosis. In this case, STIR sequences should be used (Good Practice Point).

(6) Follow-up MRIs are required to demonstrate disease dissemination in time. In this perspective, the appearance of Gd-enhancing lesions 3 months after the clinical episode (and after a baseline MRI assessment) or new T2 or Gd-enhancing lesions 6 months after the clinical episode (and after a baseline MRI assessment) is highly predictive of the subsequent development of definite MS in the near term (Frohman *et al.*, 2003) (Type A). Follow-up scans need to be performed with the same machinery and scanning parameters and identical slice positions are required for exact comparison.

(7) Repeat scanning beyond the two initial studies need to be considered by individual neurologists considering the clinical circumstances that are appropriate for each patient [is not routinely recommended as the disease becomes more likely to manifest clinically in the longer term (Dalton *et al.*, 2002a; Miller *et al.*, 2004)] (Good Practice Point).

(8) Even though non-conventional MRI techniques may provide essential and critical information about patients with CIS and their application for monitoring treatment might provide a more accurate assessment of efficacy on inflammation, axonal protection and demyelination/remyelination, their use in clinical practice is, currently, not recommended. All these techniques are yet to be adequately compared to cMRI for sensitivity and specificity in detecting tissue damage in MS and for predicting the development of MS and disability.

At present, these quantitative techniques show differences at a group level, but do not allow inferences at an individual level.

(9) In patients with insidious neurological progression suggestive of MS, according to published criteria (Thompson *et al.*, 2000), an abnormal CSF finding with evidence of inflammation and immune abnormality is another important finding to corroborate the diagnostic suspicion.

MRI in patients with established MS

In patients with relapsing-remitting (RR) and secondary progressive (SP) MS, disease activity is detected five to ten times more frequently on cMRI scans than with clinical assessment of relapses (McDonald *et al.*; 1994). This coupled with the fact that cMRI provides objective and sensitive measures of disease activity, led to the use of cMRI as an established tool for assessing the natural history of MS progression and for monitoring response to treatment. In a clinical trial context, cMRI is used as a primary outcome measure in phase II studies, where serial scans (usually monthly) are acquired to detect disease activity (new or enlarged T2-lesion counts, total enhancing and new enhancing lesion counts and enhancing lesion volume) (Barkhof *et al.*, 1997c). In phase III trials, given the uncertainty of cMRI in predicting clinical benefit, surrogate imaging methods are used as secondary outcome measures to detect disease progression, usually on yearly scans, specifically in terms of increase in total T2-hyperintense lesion load (Filippi *et al.*; 1998b).

Conventional MRI

The cMRI sequences typically used for studying MS patients are dual-echo and post-contrast T1-weighted scans. Lesion burden on T2 MRI increases by 5–10% per year (IFNB Multiple Sclerosis Study Group, 1995). Several cross-sectional studies evaluated differences in T2-lesion load among different MS phenotypes. T2-lesion load is higher in SPMS in comparison to benign (Thompson *et al.*, 1990; Filippi *et al.*, 1995a), RRMS and primary progressive (PP) MS (Thompson *et al.*, 1990). However, the magnitude of the correlation between T2-lesion measures and disability within various disease phenotypes in cross-sectional studies has been rather disappointing (Filippi *et al.*, 1995b; Gasperini *et al.*, 1996; Miller *et al.*, 1998; Kappos *et al.*, 1999). This poor relationship is likely related to the many limitations of the clinical scales used to measure impairment and disability in MS and to the inability of cMRI to character-ize and quantify the extent and severity of MS pathology beyond T2-visible lesions (Filippi and Grossman; 2002). Furthermore, a plateauing rela-tionship between dual-echo lesion load and dis-ability has recently been demonstrated indicating that for EDSS higher than 4.5, metrics different from T2-lesion loads should be taken into account (Li *et al.*, 2003). Serial MRI studies have shown that enhancement occurs in almost all new lesions in patients with RRMS or SPMS (Miller *et al.*, 1988b; Tortorella *et al.*, 1999) and can be some-times detected even before the onset of clinical symptoms (Kermode *et al.*, 1990). The burden of MRI activity can be stratified on the basis of clinical phenotype, being higher in RRMS (Thomp-son *et al.*, 1992) and SPMS (Thompson *et al.*, 1991) in comparison with PPMS (Thompson *et al.*, 1991) and benign MS (Thompson *et al.*, 1992). It is conspicuous that severely disabled SPMS patients exhibit a substantially lower incidence of enhancing lesions when compared to those with mildly disabled RRMS (Filippi *et al.*, 1997a). Several studies have investigated the prognostic role of enhancing MRI on corresponding clini-cal parameters. The number of enhancing lesions increases shortly before and during clinical relapses and predicts subsequent MRI activity (Koudriavt-seva *et al.*, 1997; Molyneux *et al.*, 1998; Simon, 1999; Zivadinov and Zorzon, 2002). A moder-ate correlation has been demonstrated between the degree of clinical disability and the mean frequency of enhancing lesions in patients with RRMS (Stone *et al.*, 1995) and SPMS (Losseff *et al.*, 1996a).

A rigorous and valid strategy for the MR-based longitudinal monitoring of MS (either natural or modified by treatment) must involve the use of standardized imaging protocols (including consis-tency in slice thickness and imaging planes, field strength and patient repositioning). Several guide-lines have emphasized the importance of accurate patient positioning inside the magnet to define landmarks for achieving effective coregistration on serial scans. Such procedures facilitate the accu-rate interpretation of follow-up studies. Several reviews provide detailed analysis of the advantages and disadvantages of the application of different pulse sequences for characterizing the disease bur-den in MS (Filippi *et al.*, 1998b; Miller *et al.*, 1998). In addition, considering the importance of active lesion detection for assessing disease activity, several strategies have been suggested to increase enhancing lesion detection, including increased post-injection delay, increased Gd dose, and the application of MT saturation pulses to reduce back-ground signal and increase lesion identification (Rovaris and Filippi, 1999; Filippi and Rocca, 2003). However, despite the increased sensitiv-ity of these strategies, the application of higher doses of Gd and MT pulsing in the routine assess-ment of MS patients is still not advisable due to an unfavourable cost–benefit ratio. However, there is general agreement that an interval of 5–7 min between the injection of contrast material and the acquisition of post-contrast sequences should be maintained routinely to optimize the sensitivity and create standardization within and between centres (Fazekas *et al.*, 1999).

Over the past decade, a large number of paral-lel group, placebo-controlled and baseline-versus-treatment trials have clearly shown the ability of several immunomodulating and immunosup-pressive treatments to reduce both MRI-measured inflammation and the consequent increase of accu-mulated lesion burden in patients with CIS (Comi *et al.*, 2001a; Achiron *et al.* 2004; Jacobs *et al.* 2004) (class I evidence), RRMS (Simon *et al.*, 1998; Sorensen *et al.*, 1998; Comi *et al.*, 2001b; Miller *et al.*, 2003; Metz *et al.*, 2004; Rizvi and Agius, 2004; Rose *et al.*, 2004; Vollmer *et al.*, 2004) (class I evidence) and SPMS (Miller *et al.*, 1999; Paolillo *et al.*, 1999; Rice *et al.*, 2000) (class I evidence). Recently, the long-term effects of some of these treatments on MRI-accumulated disease burden have also been documented (The North American Study Group on IFNβ-1b in SPMS, 2004; Li and Abdalla, 2004; Coles *et al.*, 2004) (class I evidence). Two different studies, conducted on patients treated with IFN-β1a, have recently explored whether MRI disease activity measured with Gd or new T2 lesions at the beginning of the treatment identifies better subsequent IFN-beta therapeutic response than clinical activity (Giugni *et al.*, 2003; Rudick, *et al.*, 2004, class I evidence). Even if these data suggest that MRI classification may facilitate rational therapeutic decisions, they need to be replicated before being applied in clinical practice. Persistently hypointense lesions on enhanced T1-weighted images (known as 'black holes') correspond to areas where chronic severe tissue disruption has occurred. At present, there is a general tendency to consider the assessment of the extent of chronic black holes as a surrogate marker to monitor MS evolution. T1-hypointense lesion load is higher (Lycklama à Nijeholt *et al.*, 1998; Stevenson *et al.*, 1999; van Walderveen *et al.*, 1999, 2001) and increases more rapidly over time in SPMS and PPMS than in RRMS (Paolillo *et al.*, 1999; van Walderveen *et al.*, 1999). Cross-sectional (Truyen *et al.*, 1996; Lycklama à Nijeholt *et al.*, 1998; Iannucci *et al.*, 1999; van Walderveen *et al.*, 1995, 1999) and longitudinal studies (Losseff *et al.*, 1996b; Paolillo *et al.*, 1999) have shown that T1-hypointense lesion load correlates better with clinical disability than T2-lesion load, particularly in SPMS patients.

A few trials have investigated the effect of treatment in preventing the accumulation of T1 black holes (Simon *et al.*, 2000; Barkhof *et al.*, 2001; Filippi *et al.*, 2000a; Patti *et al.*, 2004) in RRMS and SPMS and have consistently shown that the effect, if any, of all the tested treatments in reducing the rate of accumulation of black holes was moderate at best. Several studies have also evaluated the effects of available treatments (Brex *et al.*, 2001c; Filippi *et al.*, 2001; Dalton *et al.*, 2004b) on the probability of newly formed MS lesions to evolve into chronically T1-hypointense lesions. Although this approach is highly time consuming, it is promising for assessing in a relatively short time the ability of a given treatment to favourably alter the mechanisms leading to irreversible tissue loss.

Measurement of brain and cord atrophy has also been applied to assess the extent of tissue loss in MS (Miller *et al.*, 2002). In MS patients with different disease phenotypes, on average, brain volume decreases by about 1% yearly (Miller *et al.*, 2002), despite evidence of highly variable disease activity. Although it appears to be more pathologically specific than T2-lesion load, brain atrophy is at best only moderately correlated with disability in RRMS and SPMS (Miller *et al.*, 2002; Benedict *et al.*, 2004; Zivadinov *et al.*, 2004). The strength of the correlation increases when neuropsychological impairment is considered (Benedict *et al.*, 2004) and with a longitudinal study design (Hohol *et al.*, 1997; Fisher *et al.*, 2002). Also, in patients with MS, particularly in those with the progressive phenotypes of the disease, changes at a given time point and over time of cord cross-sectional area correlate better with clinical disability than changes in cord T2-visible lesions (Losseff *et al.*, 1996b; Filippi *et al.*, 1997b).

Alternately, good correlations have recently been found between regional brain atrophy and disability in MS patients. Cross-sectional studies (Chard *et al.*, 2002; De Stefano *et al.*, 2003) demonstrated grey matter atrophy in early RRMS. In addition, brain atrophy appears to evolve by involving different structures in different phases of the disease, with ventricular enlargement predominant in RRMS, and cortical atrophy more important in the progressive forms of the disease (Pagani *et al.*, 2005). Furthermore, regional brain atrophy shows a better correlation with cognitive impairment than global atrophy or T1 and T2-lesion assessments (Bermel *et al.*, 2002; Benedict *et al.*, 2005).

As shown for T1-hypointense lesions, the effect of treatment in preventing the development of brain atrophy in patients with RRMS and SPMS was at best moderate and not seen at all in some studies (Paolillo *et al.*, 1999; Rudick *et al.*, 1999; Simon 1999; Filippi *et al.*, 2000b; Molyneux *et al.*, 2000; Rovaris *et al.*, 2001; Coles *et al.*, 2004; Smith 2004; Sormani *et al.*, 2004). To refine the reproducibility of brain atrophy measurements, several recommendations have been provided (Miller *et al.*, 2002; Pelletier *et al.*, 2004; Sormani *et al.*, 2004), including: (1) the acquisition of 3D T1-weighted sequences; (2) the use of automated segmentation algorithms for images segmentation; (3) the development of a quality assurance programme to confirm the stability of the measurement system over time.

Non-conventional MRI

MT-MRI, DT-MRI and ^{1}H-MRS provide quantitative and continuous measures that can assess global (whole brain), as well as specific CNS structures, including the optic nerve and spinal cord, and various compartments (i.e. macroscopic lesions, NABT, NAWM and grey matter) (Filippi and Grossman, 2002; Filippi *et al.*, 2003a). Using these techniques, microscopic abnormalities beyond the resolution of cMRI have been detected in patients with different disease phenotypes and have been shown to correlate better with the degree of disability and cognitive impairment than cMRI measures (Filippi and Grossman, 2002; Filippi *et al.*, 2003a). Longitudinal studies have shown significant worsening of non-conventional MRI metrics over time in MS patients. These techniques provide useful prognostic information for the medium-term clinical disease evolution (Rovaris *et al.*, 2003).

Several recent MS clinical trials have incorporated MT-MRI to assess the impact of treatment on demyelination and axonal loss. MT-MRI has been used in phase II and phase III trials for RRMS (injectable and oral IFNβ-1a, IFNβ-1b, oral GA) (Richert *et al.*, 1998; 2001; Kita *et al.*, 2000) and SPMS (IFNβ-1b and immunoglobulins) (Inglese *et al.*, 2003; Filippi *et al.*, 2004c). The studies on RRMS patients were conducted at single centres with a small number of patients, and, as a consequence, they were not confronted with problems of standardization of MT acquisition and post-processing. In contrast, those conducted on SPMS patients included larger samples of patients, recruited from several centres. The results of these multicentre trials have shown a lack of effect of IFNβ-1b (Inglese *et al.*, 2003) and intravenous immunoglobulins (Filippi *et al.*, 2004c) on MT-MRI-derived quantities of the whole brain tissue and NAWM from SPMS patients.

An international consensus conference of the White Matter Study Group of the International Society for MR in Medicine has provided several guidelines for using MT-MRI for monitoring treatment in MS (Horsfield *et al.*, 2003). Among the suggestions provided in these guidelines, it is recommended the use of scanners with field strength of 1.5 T, gradient-echo sequences and the standardization of magnetization saturation among centres. Corrections for scanner properties like variations in the B_1 field may also serve to reduce the variability of MT measurements between sites (Ropele *et al.*, 2005). Quality assurance procedures and centralized analysis of the data represent additional important requirements.

^{1}H-MRS studies are relatively technically challenging and time-consuming and require calibration among centres, post-processing, and information from cMRI, as well as knowledgeable and experienced personnel. As a consequence, high-quality ^{1}H-MRS technology and operators are still confined to relatively few centres. Sampling and reposition errors and scanner drift are also likely to occur in serial studies. This inevitably reduces the reproducibility of ^{1}H-MRS measures. The use of whole brain NAA measurements overcomes these limitations, at the price of losing information on specific brain regions or tract systems (Gonen *et al.*, 2000). Preliminary studies have been conducted to evaluate the effect of disease-modifying treatments on ^{1}H-MRS-derived parameters (Sarchielli *et al.*, 1998; Narayanan *et al.*, 2001; Schubert *et al.*, 2002; Parry *et al.*, 2003; Khan *et al.*, 2003). Recently, Narayana *et al.* (2004) demonstrated the feasibility of applying ^{1}H-MRS in multicentre clinical trials of MS, by showing the between-centres stability of NAA/Cr ratios.

RECOMMENDATIONS

In patients with established MS, the following recommendations should be considered:

(1) cMRI scans (dual-echo and post-contrast T1-weighted images) should be obtained using standardized protocols and accurate procedures for patients' repositioning to facilitate

continued

the interpretation of follow-up studies. Post-contrast T1-weighted scans should be acquired after an interval of 5–7 min from the injection of contrast material (Fazekas *et al.*, 1999). Considering the weak correlation with clinical finding and the low predictive value of cMRI metrics for the subsequent worsening of clinical disability, the use of surveillance MRI for the purpose of making treatment decisions can not be generally recommended (Fazekas *et al.*, 1999). Serial MRI scans should be considered when diagnostic issues arise.

(2) Repetition of MRI of the spinal cord is advisable only if suspicion arises concerning the evolution of an alternate process (e.g. mechanical compression) or atypical symptoms develop.

(3) Although preliminary work based on clinical trial data has suggested that the presence (Giugni *et al.*, 2003) and amount (Rudick *et al.*, 2004) of MRI-detected disease activity may identify IFN β response status in terms of relapse rate (Giugni *et al.*, 2003) and accumulated disability (Rudick *et al.*, 2004) in MS patients at a group level, there are no validated methods for monitoring disease-modifying therapy in individual patients.

(4) Metrics derived from cMRI are not enough to provide a complete picture of the MS pathological process. Although cMRI has undoubtedly improved our ability to assess the efficacy of experimental MS therapies and, at least partially, our understanding of MS evolution, it provides only limited information on MS pathology in terms of accuracy and specificity and it has limited correlations with clinical metrics. This implies that the ability of a given treatment to modify metrics derived from cMRI does not mean that the treatment will necessarily be able to prevent the progressive accumulation of clinical disability, especially at an individual patient level.

(5) Measurements of T1-hypointense lesions loads and brain and cord atrophy in clinical practice continue to be considered at a preliminary stage of development, as they need to be standardized in terms of acquisition and post-processing. Conversely, these metrics should be included as an end-point in disease-modifying agents trials (Miller *et al.*, 2002), to further elucidate the mechanisms responsible for disability.

(6) The application of non-conventional MRI techniques in monitoring patients with established MS in clinical practice is, at the moment, not advisable. All these techniques still need to be evaluated for sensitivity and specificity in detecting tissue damage in MS and its changes over time.

(7) MT-MRI should be incorporated into new clinical trials to gain additional insights into disease pathophysiology and into the value of this technique in the assessment of MS. The performance and contribution of DT-MRI and ^{1}H-MRS in multi-centre trials still have to be evaluated.

Conflict of interest

These guidelines are provided as an educational service of the EFNS task force. It is based on current scientific and clinical information.

Acknowledgements

The authors declare that they have no conflict of interest in regard to this manuscript. We are grateful to Prof. D. H. Miller (Institute of Neurology, London, UK) for his helpful and thoughtful comments to the manuscript.

References

Achiron A, Kishner I, Sarova-Pinhas I, Raz H, Faibel M, Stern Y, Lavie M, Gurevich M, Dolev M, Magalashvili D, Barak Y (2004). Intravenous immunoglobulin treatment following the first demyelinating event suggestive of multiple sclerosis: a randomized, double-blind, placebo-controlled trial. *Arch Neurol* **61**:1515–1520.

Bakshi R, Hutton GJ, Miller JR, Radue EW (2004). The use of magnetic resonance imaging in the diagnosis and long-term management of multiple sclerosis. *Neurology* **63**:S3–S11.

Barkhof F, Filippi M, Miller DH, Scheltens P, Campi'A, Polman CH, Comi G, Ader HJ, Losseff N, Valk J (1997a). Comparison of MRI criteria at first presentation to predict conversion to clinically definite multiple sclerosis. *Brain* **120**:2059–2069.

Barkhof F, Filippi M, van Waesberghe JH, Molyneux P, Rovaris M, Lycklama à Nijeholt GJ, Tubridy N, Miller DH, Yousry TA, Radü EW, Ader HJ (1997b). Improving interobserver variation in reporting gadolinium-enhanced MRI lesions in multiple sclerosis. *Neurology* **49:**1682–1688.

Barkhof F, Filippi M, Miller DH, Tofts P, Kappos L, Thompson AJ (1997c). Strategies for optimizing MRI techniques aimed at monitoring disease activity in multiple sclerosis treatment trials. *J Neurol* **244:**76–84.

Barkhof F, van Waesberghe JH, Filippi M, Yousry T, Miller DH, Hahn D, Thompson AJ, Kappos L, Brex P, Pozzilli C, Polman CH; European Study Group on Interferon beta-1b in Secondary Progressive Multiple Sclerosis (2001). T1 hypointense lesions in secondary progressive multiple sclerosis: effect of interferon beta-1b treatment. *Brain* **124:** 1396–1402.

Barkhof F, Rocca M, Francis G, Van Waesberghe JH, Uitdehaag BM, Hommes OR, Hartung HP, Durelli L, Edan G, Fernandez O, Seeldrayers P, Sorensen P, Margrie S, Rovaris M, Comi G, Filippi M; Early Treatment of Multiple Sclerosis Study Group (2003). Validation of diagnostic magnetic resonance imaging criteria for multiple sclerosis and response to interferon beta1a. *Ann Neurol* **53:**718–724.

Benedict RH, Carone DA, Bakshi R (2004). Correlating brain atrophy with cognitive dysfunction, mood disturbances, and personality disorder in multiple sclerosis. *J Neuroimaging* **14:**36S–45S.

Benedict RHB, Zivadinov R, Carone DA, Weinstock-Guttman B, Gaines J, Maggiore C, Sharma J, Antonietta Tomassi M, Bakshi R (2005). Regional lobar atrophy predicts memory impairment in multiple sclerosis. *AJNR Am J Neuroradiol;* **26:**1824–1831.

Bermel R, Bakshi R, Tjoa C, Puli S, Jacobs L (2002). Bicaudate ratio as an MRI marker of brain atrophy in multiple sclerosis. *Arch Neurol* **59:**275–280.

Bot JC, Barkhof F, Lycklama a Nijeholt G, van Schaardenburg D, Voskuyl AE, Ader HJ, Pijnenburg JA, Polman CH, Uitdehaag BM, Vermeulen EG, Castelijns JA (2002). Differentiation of multiple sclerosis from other inflammatory disorders and cerebrovascular disease: value of spinal MR imaging. *Radiology* **223:**46–56.

Brex PA, Leary SM, O'Riordan JI, Miszkiel KA, Plant GT, Thompson AJ, Miller DH (2001a). Measurement of spinal cord area in clinically isolated syndromes suggestive of multiple sclerosis. *J Neurol Neurosurg Psychiatry* **70:**544–547.

Brex PA, Leary SM, Plant GT, Thompson AJ, Miller DH (2001b). Magnetization transfer imaging in patients with clinically isolated syndromes suggestive of multiple sclerosis. *AJNR Am J Neuroradiol* **22:**947–951.

Brex PA, Molyneux PD, Smiddy P, Barkhof F, Filippi M, Yousry TA, Hahn D, Rolland Y, Salonen O, Pozzilli C,

Polman CH, Thompson AJ, Kappos L, Miller DH; European Study Group on Interferon beta-1b in Secondary Progressive MS (2001c). The effect of IFNβ-1b on the evolution of enhancing lesions in secondary progressive MS. *Neurology* **57:**2185–2190.

Brex PA, Ciccarelli O, O'Riordan JI, Sailer M, Thompson AJ, Miller DH (2002). A longitudinal study of abnormalities on MRI and disability from multiple sclerosis. *N Engl J Med* **346:**158–164.

Chard DT, Griffin CM, Parker GJ, Kapoor R, Thompson AJ, Miller DH (2002). Brain atrophy in clinically early relapsing-remitting multiple sclerosis. *Brain* **125:**327–337.

Coles A, Deans J, Compston A (2004). Campath-1H treatment of multiple sclerosis: lessons from the bedside for the bench. *Clin Neurol Neurosurg* **106:**270–274.

Comi G, Filippi M, Barkhof F, Durelli L, Edan G, Fernandez O, Hartung H, Seeldrayers P, Sorensen PS, Rovaris M, Martinelli V, Hommes OR; Early Treatment of Multiple Sclerosis Study Group (2001a). Effect of early interferon treatment on conversion to definite multiple sclerosis. *Lancet* **357:**1576–1582.

Comi G, Filippi M, Wolinsky JS (2001b). European/Canadian multicenter, double-blind, randomized, placebo-controlled study of the effects of glatiramer acetate on magnetic resonance imaging–measured disease activity and burden in patients with relapsing multiple sclerosis. European/Canadian Glatiramer Acetate Study Group. *Ann Neurol* **49:**290–297.

Dalton CM, Brex PA, Miszkiel KA, Hickman SJ, MacManus DG, Plant GT, Thompson AJ, Miller DH (2002a). Application of the new McDonald criteria to patients with clinically isolated syndromes suggestive of multiple sclerosis. *Ann Neurol* **52:**47–53.

Dalton CM, Brex PA, Jenkins R, Fox NC, Miszkiel KA, Crum WR, O'Riordan JI, Plant GT, Thompson AJ, Miller DH (2002b). Progressive ventricular enlargement in patients with clinically isolated syndromes is associated with the early development of multiple sclerosis. *J Neurol Neurosurg Psychiatry* **73:**141–147.

Dalton CM, Brex PA, Miszkiel KA, Fernando K, MacManus DG, Plant GT, Thompson AJ, Miller DH (2003a). New T2 lesions enable an earlier diagnosis of multiple sclerosis in clinically isolated syndromes. *Ann Neurol* **53:**673–676.

Dalton CM, Brex PA, Miszkiel KA, Fernando K, MacManus DG, Plant GT, Thompson AJ, Miller DH (2003b). Spinal cord MRI in clinically isolated optic neuritis. *J Neurol Neurosurg Psychiatry* **74:**1386–1389.

Dalton CM, Chard DT, Davies GR, Miszkiel KA, Altmann DR, Fernando K, Plant GT, Thompson AJ, Miller DH (2004a). Early development of multiple sclerosis is associated with progressive grey matter atrophy in patients presenting with clinically isolated syndromes. *Brain* **127**:1101–1107.

Dalton CM, Miszkiel KA, Barker GJ, MacManus DG, Pepple TI, Panzara M, Yang M, Hulme A, O'Connor P, Miller DH (2004b). Effect of natalizumab on conversion of gadolinium enhancing lesions to T1 hypointense lesions in relapsing multiple sclerosis. *J Neurol* **251:** 407–413.

Davies MB, Williams R, Haq N, Pelosi L, Hawkins CP (1998). MRI of optic nerve and postchiasmal visual pathways and visual evoked potentials in secondary progressive multiple sclerosis. *Neuroradiology* **40:** 765–770.

De Stefano N, Matthews PM, Filippi M, Agosta A, De Luca M, Bartolozzi ML, Guidi L, Ghezzi A, Montanari E, Cifelli A, Federico A, Smith SM (2003). Evidence of early cortical atrophy in MS: relevance of white matter changes and disability. *Neurology* **60**:1157–1162.

Fazekas F, Offenbacher H, Fuchs S, Schmidt R, Niederkorn K, Horner S, Lechner H (1988). Criteria for an increased specificity of MRI interpretation in elderly subjects with suspected multiple sclerosis. *Neurology* **38:** 1822–1825.

Fazekas F, Barkhof F, Filippi M, Grossman RI, Li DK, McDonald WI, McFarland HF, Paty DW, Simon JH, Wolinsky JS, Miller DH (1999). The contribution of magnetic resonance imaging to the diagnosis of multiple sclerosis. *Neurology* **53**:448–456.

Fernando KT, McLean MA, Chard DT, MacManus DG, Dalton CM, Miszkiel KA, Gordon RM, Plant GT, Thompson AJ, Miller DH (2004). Elevated white matter myo-inositol in clinically isolated syndromes suggestive of multiple sclerosis. *Brain* **127**:1361–1369.

Filippi M, Grossman RI (2002). MI techniques to monitor MS evolution. The present and the future. *Neurology* **58**:1147–1153.

Filippi M, Rocca MA (2003). MRI aspects of the "inflammatory phase" of multiple sclerosis. *Neurol Sci* **24**: S275–278.

Filippi M, Horsfield MA, Morrissey SP, MacManus DG, Rudge P, McDonald WI, Miller DH (1994). Quantitative brain MRI lesion load predicts the course of clinically isolated syndromes suggestive of multiple sclerosis. *Neurology* **44**:635–641.

Filippi M, Campi A, Mammi S, Martinelli V, Locatelli T, Scotti G, Amadio S, Canal N, Comi G (1995a). Brain magnetic resonance imaging and multimodal evoked potentials in benign and secondary progressive multiple sclerosis. *J Neurol Neurosurg Psychiatry* **58**:31–37.

Filippi M, Paty DW, Kappos L, Barkhof F, Compston DA, Thompson AJ, Zhao GJ, Wiles CM, McDonald WI, Miller DH (1995b). Correlations between changes in disability and T2-weighted brain MRI activity in multiple sclerosis. *Neurology* **45**:255–260.

Filippi M, Rossi P, Colombo B, Pereira C, Comi G (1997a). Serial contrast-enhanced MR in patients with multiple sclerosis and varying levels of disability. *AJNR Am J Neuroradiol* **18**:1549–1556.

Filippi M, Colombo B, Rovaris M, Pereira C, Martinelli V, Comi G (1997b). A longitudinal magnetic resonance imaging study of the cervical cord in multiple sclerosis. *J Neuroimaging* **7**:78–80.

Filippi M, Gawne-Cain ML, Gasperini C, van Waesberghe JH, Grimaud J, Barkhof F, Sormani MP, Miller DH (1998a). Effect of training and different measurement strategies on the reproducibility of brain MRI lesion load measurements in multiple sclerosis. *Neurology* **50**:238–244.

Filippi M, Horsfield MA, Ader HJ, Barkhof F, Bruzzi P, Evans A, Frank JA, Grossman RI, McFarland HF, Molyneux P, Paty DW, Simon J, Tofts PS, Wolinsky JS, Miller DH (1998b). Guidelines for using quantitative measures of brain magnetic resonance imaging abnormalities in monitoring the treatment of multiple sclerosis. *Ann Neurol* **43**:499–506.

Filippi M, Rovaris M, Rice GPA, Sormani MP, Iannucci G, Giacomotti L, Comi G (2000a). The effect of Cladribine on T1 'black hole' changes in progressive MS. *J Neurol Sci* **176**:42–44.

Filippi M, Rovaris M, Iannucci G, Mennea S, Sormani MP, Comi G (2000b). Whole brain volume changes in patients with progressive MS treated with cladribine. *Neurology* **55**:1714–1718.

Filippi M, Rovaris M, Rocca MA, Sormani MP, Wolinsky JS, Comi G; European/Canadian Glatiramer Acetate Study Group (2001). Glatiramer acetate reduces the proportion of new MS lesions evolving into "black holes". *Neurology* **57**:731–733.

Filippi M, Rocca MA, Comi G (2003a). The use of quantitative magnetic-resonance-based techniques to monitor the evolution of multiple sclerosis. *Lancet Neurol* **2**:337–346.

Filippi M, Bozzali M, Rovaris M, Gonen O, Kesavadas C, Ghezzi A, Martinelli V, Grossman RI, Scotti G, Comi G, Falini A (2003b). Evidence for widespread axonal damage at the earliest clinical stage of multiple sclerosis. *Brain* **126**:433–437.

Filippi M, Rovaris M, Inglese M, Barkhof F, De Stefano N, Smith S, Comi G (2004a). Interferon beta-Ia for brain tissue loss in patients at presentation with syndromes suggestive of multiple sclerosis: a randomised, double-blind, placebo-controlled trial. *Lancet* **364:**1489–1496.

Filippi M, Rocca MA, Mezzapesa DM, Ghezzi A, Falini A, Martinelli V, Scotti G, Comi G (2004b). Simple and complex movement-associated functional MRI changes in patients at presentation with clinically isolated syndromes suggestive of MS. *Hum Brain Map* **21:**106–115.

Filippi M, Rocca MA, Pagani E, Iannucci G, Sormani MP, Fazekas F, Ropele S, Hommes OR, Comi G (2004c). European study on intravenous immunoglobulin in multiple sclerosis: results of magnetization transfer magnetic resonance imaging analysis. *Arch Neurol* **61:**1409–1412.

Fisher E, Rudick RA, Simon JH, Cutter G, Baier M, Lee JC, Miller D, Weinstock-Guttman B, Mass MK, Dougherty DS, Simonian NA (2002). Eight-year follow-up study of brain atrophy in patients with MS. *Neurology* **59:**1412–1420.

Frohman EM, Goodin DS, Calabresi PA, Corboy JR, Coyle PK, Filippi M, Frank JA, Galetta SL, Grossman RI, Hawker K, Kachuck NJ, Levin MC, Phillips JT, Racke MK, Rivera VM, Stuart WH; Therapeutics and Technology Assessment Subcommittee of the American Academy of Neurology (2003). The utility of MRI in suspected MS: report of the Therapeutics and Technology Assessment Subcommittee of the American Academy of Neurology. *Neurology* **61:**602–611.

Gallo A, Rovaris M, Riva R, Ghezzi A, Benedetti B, Martinelli V, Falini A, Comi G, Filippi M (2005). Diffusion tensor MRI detects normal-appearing white matter damage unrelated to short-term disease activity in patients at the earlier clinical stage of multiple sclerosis. *Arch Neurol* **62:**803–808.

Gasperini C, Horsfield MA, Thorpe JW, Kidd D, Barker GJ, Tofts PS, MacManus DG, Thompson AJ, Miller DH, McDonald WI (1996). Macroscopic and microscopic assessment of disease burden by MRI in multiple sclerosis: relationship to clinical parameters. *J Magn Reson Imaging* **6:**580–584.

Gass A, Moseley IF, Barker GJ, Jones S, MacManus D, McDonald WI, Miller DH (1996). Lesion discrimination in optic neuritis using high-resolution fat- suppressed fast spin-echo MRI. *Neuroradiology* **38:**317–321.

Gass A, Filippi M, Rodegher ME, Schwartz A, Comi G, Hennerici MG (1998). Characteristics of chronic MS lesions in the cerebrum, brainstem, spinal cord, and optic nerve on T1-weighted MRI. *Neurology* **50:**548–550.

Giugni E, Paolillo A, Tomassini V, Mainero C, Gasperini C, Russo PL, Bagnato F, Bastianello S, Pozzilli C (2003). An active scan at 12th month of therapy is associated with a worse response to IFN beta over the subsequent five years of treatment in RRMS. *Neurology* **60:**A251–A252.

Gonen O, Catalaa I, Babb JS, Ge Y, Mannon LJ, Kolson DL, Grossman RI (2000). Total brain N-acetylaspartate: a new measure of disease load in MS. *Neurology* **54:**15–19.

Hickman SJ, Dalton CM, Miller DH, Plant GT (2002). Management of acute optic neuritis. *Lancet* **360:**1953–1962.

Hickman SJ, Toosy AT, Jones SJ, Altmann DR, Miszkiel KA, MacManus DG, Barker GJ, Plant GT, Thompson AJ, Miller DH (2004). Serial magnetization transfer imaging in acute optic neuritis. *Brain* **127:**692–700.

Hohol MJ, Guttmann CR, Orav J, Mackin GA, Kikinis R, Khoury SJ, Jolesz FA, Weiner HL (1997). Serial neuropsychological assessment and magnetic resonance imaging analysis in multiple sclerosis. *Arch Neurol* **54:**1018–1025.

Horsfield MA, Barker GJ, Barkhof F, Miller DH, Thompson AJ, Filippi M (2003). Guidelines for using quantitative magnetization transfer magnetic resonance imaging for monitoring treatment of multiple sclerosis. *J Magn Reson Imaging* **17:**389–3897.

Iannucci G, Minicucci L, Rodegher M, Sormani MP, Comi G, Filippi M (1999). Correlations between clinical and MRI involvement in multiple sclerosis: assessment using T1, T2 and MT histograms. *J Neurol* **171:**121–129.

Iannucci G, Tortorella C, Rovaris M, Sormani MP, Comi G, Filippi M (2000). Prognostic value of MR and magnetization transfer imaging findings in patients with clinically isolated syndromes suggestive of multiple sclerosis at presentation. *AJNR Am J Neuroradiol* **21:**1034–1038.

IFNB Multiple Sclerosis Study Group and the University of British Columbia MS/MRI Analysis Group (1995). Interferon beta 1b in the treatment of multiple sclerosis: final outcome of the randomized controlled trial. *Neurology* **45:**1277–1285.

Inglese M, van Waesberghe JH, Rovaris M, Beckmann K, Barkhof F, Hahn D, Kappos L, Miller DH, Polman C, Pozzilli C, Thompson AJ, Yousry TA, Wagner K, Comi G, Filippi M (2003). The effect of interferon beta-1b on quantities derived from MT MRI in secondary progressive MS. *Neurology* **60:**853–860.

Jackson A, Sheppard S, Laitt RD, Kassner A, Moriarty D (1998). Optic neuritis: MR imaging with combined fat- and water-suppression techniques. *Radiology* **206:**57–63.

Jacobs L, Beck R, Simon J, Kinkel RP, Brownscheidle CM, Murray TJ, Simonian NA, Slasor PJ, Sandrock AW (2000). Intramuscular interferon beta-1a therapy initiated during the first demyelinating event in multiple sclerosis. *N Engl J Med* **343:**898–904.

Kaiser JS, Grossman RI, Polansky M, Udupa JK, Miki Y, Galetta SL (2000). Magnetization transfer histogram analysis of monosymptomatic episodes of neurologic dysfunction: preliminary findings. *Am J Neuroradiol* **21**:1043–1047.

Kappos L, Moeri D, Radue EW, Schoetzau A, Barkhof F, Miller DH, Guttmann CRG, Hohol MJ, McFarland HF, Gasperini C, Filippi M for the Gadolinium MRI Meta-analysis Group (1999). Predictive value of gadolinium-enhanced MRI for relapse rate and changes in disability/impairment in multiple sclerosis: a metaanalysis. *Lancet* **353**:964–969.

Kermode AG, Thompson AJ, Tofts P, MacManus DG, Kendall BE, Kingsley DP, Moseley IF, Rudge P, McDonald WI (1990). Breakdown of the blood brain barrier precedes symptoms and other MRI signs of new lesion in multiple sclerosis: pathogenetic and clinical implication. *Brain* **113**:1477–1489.

Kidd D, Thorpe JW, Thompson AJ, Kendall BE, Moseley IF, MacManus DG, McDonald WI, Miller DH (1993). Spinal cord MRI using multi-array coils and fast spin echo. II. Findings in multiple sclerosis. *Neurology* **43**:2632–2637.

Kita M, Goodkin DE, Bacchetti P, Waubant E, Nelson SJ, Majumdar S (2000). Magnetization transfer ratio in new MS lesions before and during therapy with IFNß-1a. *Neurology* **54**:1741–1745.

Khan O, Shen Y, Ching W, Caon C, Sonenvirth E, Latif Z, Hu J, Sehgal V (2003). Combining immunomodulation and neuroprotection: cerebral axonal recovery in relapsing-remitting multiple sclerosis patients treated with glatiramer acetate. *Mult Scler* **9(Suppl 1)**:S63.

Koudriavtseva T, Thompson AJ, Fiorelli M, Gasperini C, Bastianello S, Bozzao A, Paolillo A, Pisani A, Galgani S, Pozzilli C (1997). Gadolinium enhanced MRI disease activity in relapsing-remitting multiple sclerosis. *J Neurol Neurosurg Psychiatry* **62**:285–287.

Kupersmith MJ, Alban T, Zeiffer B, Lefton D (2002). Contrast-enhanced MRI in acute optic neuritis: relationship to visual performance. *Brain* **125**:812–822.

Lee KH, Hashimoto SA, Hooge JP, Kastrukoff LF, Oger JJ, Li DK, Paty DW (1991). Magnetic resonance imaging of the head in the diagnosis of multiple scelrosis: a prospective 2-year follow-up with comparison of clinical evaluation, evoked potentials, oligoclonal banding and CT. *Neurology* **41**:657–660.

Li D, Abdalla JA (2004). Long-term observational follow-up of the PRISMS cohort: analyses of MRI BOD shows benefit of high dose, high frequency IFN beta-1° (Rebif). *Neurology* **62**:A153–A154.

Li DKB, Filippi M, Petkau J, Held U, Daumer M (2003). T2 lesion burden on MRI plateaus as MS disability accumulates. *Mult Scler* **9**:S58.

Lin X, Tench CR, Evangelou N, Jaspan T, Constantinescu CS (2004). Measurement of spinal cord atrophy in multiple sclerosis. *J Neuroimaging* **14**:20S–26S.

Longstreth WT, Arnold AM, Beauchamp NJ Jr, Manolio TA, Lefkowitz D, Jungreis C, Hirsch CH, O'Leary DH, Furberg CD (2005). Incidence, manifestations, and predictors of worsening white matter on serial cranial magnetic resonance imaging in the elderly: the Cardiovascular Health Study. *Stroke* **36**:56–61.

Losseff N, Kingsley D, McDonald WI, Miller DH, Thompson AJ (1996a). Clinical and magnetic resonance imaging predictors in primary and secondary progressive MS. *Mult Scler* **1**:218–222.

Losseff NA, Wang L, Lai HM, Yoo DS, Gawne-Cain ML, McDonald WI, Miller DH, Thompson AJ (1996b). Progressive cerebral atrophy in multiple sclerosis: a serial MRI study. *Brain* **119**:2009–2019.

Lycklama à Nijeholt GJ, van Walderveen MAA, van Waesberghe JH, Polman C, Scheltens P, Rosier PF, Jongen PJ, Barkhof F (1998). Brain and spinal cord abnormalities in multiple sclerosis. Correlation between MRI parameters, clinical subtypes and symptoms. *Brain* **121**:687–697.

McDonald WI, Miller DH, Thompson AJ (1994). Are magnetic resonance findings predictive of clinical outcome in therapeutic trials in multiple sclerosis? The dilemma of interferon-beta. *Ann Neurol* **36**:14–18.

McDonald WI, Compston A, Edan G, Goodkin D, Hartung HP, Lublin FD, McFarland HF, Paty DW, Polman CH, Reingold SC, Sandberg-Wollheim M, Sibley W, Thompson A, van den Noort S, Weinshenker BY, Wolinsky JS (2001). Recommended diagnostic criteria for multiple sclerosis: guidelines from the International Panel on the diagnosis of multiple sclerosis. *Ann Neurol* **50**:121–127.

Metz LM, Zhang Y, Yeung M, Patry DG, Bell RB, Stoian CA, Yong VW, Patten SB, Duquette P, Antel JP, Mitchell JR (2004). Minocycline reduces gadolinium-enhancing magnetic resonance imaging lesions in multiple sclerosis. *Ann Neurol* **55**:756.

Miller DH, Newton MR, van der Poel JC, du Boulay EP, Halliday AM, Kendall BE, Johnson G, MacManus DG, Moseley IF, McDonald WI (1988a). Magnetic resonance imaging of the optic nerve in optic neuritis. *Neurology* **38**:175–179.

Miller DH, Rudge P, Johnson J, Kendall BE, MacManus DG, Moseley IF, Barnes D, McDonald WI

(1988b). Serial gadolinium-enhanced magnetic resonance imaging in multiple sclerosis. *Brain* **111:**927–939.

Miller DH, Grossman RI, Reingold SC, McFarland HF (1998). The role of magnetic resonance techniques in understanding and managing multiple sclerosis. *Brain* **121:**3–24.

Miller DH, Molyneux PD, Barker GJ, MacManus DG, Moseley IF, Wagner K (1999). Effect of interferon-beta1b on magnetic resonance imaging outcomes in secondary progressive multiple sclerosis: results of a European multicenter, randomized, double-blind, placebo-controlled trial. European Study Group on Interferon-beta1b in secondary progressive multiple sclerosis. *Ann Neurol* **46:**850–859.

Miller DH, Barkhof F, Frank JA, Parker GJM, Thompson AJ (2002). Measurement of atrophy in multiple sclerosis: pathological basis, methodological aspects and clinical relevance. *Brain* **125:**1676–1695.

Miller DH, Khan OA, Sheremata WA, Blumhardt LD, Rice GP, Libonati MA, Willmer-Hulme AJ, Dalton CM, Miszkiel KA, O'Connor PW; International Natalizumab Multiple Sclerosis Trial Group (2003). A controlled trial of natalizumab for relapsing multiple sclerosis. *N Engl J Med* **348:**15–23.

Miller DH, Filippi M, Fazekas F, Frederiksen JL, Matthews PM, Montalban X, Polman CH (2004). Role of magnetic resonance imaging within diagnostic criteria for multiple sclerosis. *Ann Neurol* **56:**273–278.

Minneboo A, Barkhof F, Polman CH, Uitdehaag BM, Knol DL, Castelijns JA (2004). Infratentorial lesions predict long term disability in patients with initial findings suggestive of multiple sclerosis. *Arch Neurol* **61:**217–221.

Molyneux PD, Filippi M, Barkhof F, Gasperini C, Yousry TA, Truyen L, Lai HM, Rocca MA, Moseley IF, Miller DH (1998). Correlations between monthly enhanced MRI lesion rate and changes in T2 lesion volume in multiple sclerosis. *Ann Neurol* **43:**332–339.

Molyneux PD, Kappos L, Polman C, Pozzilli C, Barkhof F, Filippi M, Yousry T, Hahn D, Wagner K, Ghazi M, Beckmann K, Dahlke F, Losseff N, Barker GJ, Thompson AJ, Miller DH (2000). The effect of interferon beta-1b treatment on MRI measures of cerebral atrophy in secondary progressive multiple sclerosis. *Brain* **123:**2256–2263.

Narayana PA, Wolinsky JS, Rao SB, He R, Mehta M; PROMiSe Trial MRSI Group (2004). Multicentre proton magnetic resonance spectroscopy imaging of primary progressive multiple sclerosis. *Mult Scler* **10:**S73–S78.

Narayanan S, De Stefano N, Francis GS, Arnaoutelis R, Caramanos Z, Collins DL, Pelletier D, Arnason BGW, Antel JP, Arnold DL (2001). Axonal metabolic recovery in multiple sclerosis patients treated with interferon beta-1b. *J Neurol* **248:**979–986.

Noseworthy JH, Lucchinetti C, Rodriguez M, Weinshenker BG (2000). Multiple sclerosis. *N Engl J Med* **343:**938–952.

Offenbacher H, Fazekas F, Schmidt R, Freidl W, Flooh E, Payer F, Lechner H (1993). Assessment of MRI criteria for a diagnosis of MS. *Neurology* **43:**905–909.

Optic Neuritis Study Group (1997). The 5-year risk of MS after optic neuritis. Experience of the optic neuritis treatment trial. *Neurology* **49:**1404–1413.

Optic Neuritis Study Group (2003). High- and low-risk profiles for the development of multiple sclerosis within 10 years after optic neuritis. Experience of the Optic Neuritis Treatment Trial. *Arch Ophthalmol* **121:**944–949.

O'Riordan JI, Thompson AJ, Kingsley DP, MacManus DG, Kendall BE, Rudge P, McDonald WI, Miller DH (1998). The prognostic value of brain MRI in clinically isolated syndromes of the CNS. A 10-year follow-up. *Brain* **121:**495–503.

Ormerod IE, Miller DH, McDonald WI, du Boulay EP, Rudge P, Kendall BE, Moseley IF, Johnson G, Tofts PS, Halliday AM (1987). The role of NMR imaging in the assessment of multiple sclerosis and isolated neurological lesions. A quantitative study. *Brain* **110:**1579–1616.

Pagani E, Rocca MA, Gallo A, Rovaris M, Martinelli V, Comi G, Filippi M (2005). Regional brain atrophy evolves differently in patients with multiple sclerosis according to clinical phenotype. *AJNR Am J Neuroradiol* **26:**341–346.

Paolillo A, Coles AJ, Molyneux PD, Gawne-Cain M, MacManus D, Barker GJ, Compston DA, Miller DH (1999). Quantitative MRI in patients with secondary progressive MS treated with monoclonal antibody Campath 1H. *Neurology* **53:**751–757.

Parry A, Corkill R, Blamire AM, Palace J, Narayanan S, Arnold D, Styles P, Matthews PM (2003). Beta-interferon treatment does not always slow the progression of axonal injury in multiple sclerosis. *J Neurol* **250:**171–178.

Patti F, Amato MP, Filippi M, Gallo P, Trojano M, Comi G (2004). A double blind, placebo-controlled, phase II, add-on study of cyclophosphamide (CTX) for 24 months in patients affected by multiple sclerosis on a background therapy with interferon-beta study denomination: CYCLIN. *J Neurol Sci* **223:**69–71.

Paty DW, Oger JJ, Kastrukoff LF, Hashimoto SA, Hooge JP, Eisen AA, Eisen KA, Purves SJ, Low MD, Brandejs V, *et al*. (1988). MRI in the diagnosis of MS: a prospective study with comparison of clinical evaluation, evoked

potentials, oligoclonal banding, and CT. *Neurology*
38:180–185.

Pelletier D, Garrison K, Henry R (2004). Measurement of
whole-brain atrophy in multiple sclerosis. *J Neuroimaging* **14:**11S–19S.

Polman CH, Wolinsky JS, Reingold SC (2005). Multiple
sclerosis diagnostic criteria three years later. *Mult Scler*
11:5–12.

Poser CM, Paty DW, Scheinberg L, McDonald WI,
Davis FA, Ebers GC, Johnson KP, Sibley WA,
Silberberg DH, Tourtellotte WW (1983). New diagnostic criteria for multiple sclerosis: guidelines for research
protocols. *Ann Neurol* **13:**227–231.

Rice GPA, Filippi M, Comi G (2000). Cladribine and
progressive MS. Clinical and MRI outcomes of a multicenter controlled trial. *Neurology* **54:**1145–1155.

Richert ND, Ostuni JL, Bash CN, Duyn JH, McFarland HF,
Frank JA (1998). Serial whole-brain magnetization
transfer imaging in patients with relapsing-remitting
multiple sclerosis at baseline and during treatment
with interferon beta-1b. *AJNR Am J Neuroradiol*
19:1705–1713.

Richert ND, Ostuni JL, Bash CN, Leist TP, McFarland HF,
Frank JA (2001). Interferon beta-1b and intravenous
methylprednisolone promote lesion recovery in multiple sclerosis. *Mult Scler* **7:**49–58.

Rizvi SA, Agius MA (2004). Current approved options
for treating patients with multiple sclerosis. *Neurology*
63:S8–S14.

Rocca MA, Mastronardo G, Horsfield MA, Pereira C,
Iannucci G, Colombo B, Moiola L, Comi G, Filippi M
(1999). Comparison of three MR sequences for the
detection of cervical cord lesions in patients with multiple sclerosis. *AJNR Am J Neuroradiol* **20:**1710–1716.

Rocca MA, Mezzapesa DM, Falini A, Ghezzi A,
Martinelli V, Scotti G, Comi G, Filippi M (2003).
Evidence for axonal pathology and adaptive cortical reorganization in patients at presentation with
clinically isolated syndromes suggestive of multiple
sclerosis. *NeuroImage* **18:**847–855.

Rocca MA, Mezzapesa DM, Ghezzi A, Falini A,
Martinelli V, Scotti G, Comi G, Filippi M (2005).
A widespread pattern of cortical activations in patients
at presentation with CIS is associated with evolution
to definite MS. *AJNR Am J Neuroradiol* in press.

Ropele S, Filippi M, Valsasina P, Korteweg T, Barkhof F,
Tofts PS, Samson R, Miller DH, Fazekas F (2005). Assessment and correction of B1-induced errors in magnetization transfer ratio measurements. *Magn Reson Med*
53:134–140.

Rose JW, Watt HE, White AT, Carlson NG
(2004). Treatment of multiple sclerosis with an
anti-interleukin-2 receptor monoclonal antibody. *Ann
Neurol* **56:**864–867.

Rovaris M, Filippi M (1999). Magnetic resonance techniques to monitor disease evolution and treatment
trial outcomes in multiple sclerosis. *Curr Opin Neurol*
12:337–344.

Rovaris M, Comi G, Rocca MA, Wolinsky JS, Filippi M
and the European/Canadian Glatiramer Acetate Study
Group (2001). Short-term brain volume change in
relapsing-remitting multiple sclerosis: effect of glatiramer acetate and implications. *Brain* **124:**1803–1812.

Rovaris M, Agosta F, Sormani MP, Inglese M, Martinelli V,
Comi G, Filippi M (2003). Conventional and magnetization transfer MRI predictors of clinical multiple
sclerosis evolution: a medium-term follow-up study.
Brain **126:**2323–2332.

Rovaris M, Gallo A, Riva R, Ghezzi A, Bozzali M,
Benedetti B, Martinelli V, Falini A, Comi G, Filippi M
(2004). An MT MRI study of the cervical cord in clinically isolated syndromes suggestive of MS. *Neurology*
63:584–585.

Rudick RA, Fisher E, Lee JC, Simon J, Jacobs L (1999).
Use of the brain parenchymal fraction to measure
whole brain atrophy in relapsing-remitting MS. Multiple Sclerosis Collaborative Research Group. *Neurology*
53:1698–1704.

Rudick RA, Lee JC, Simon J, Ransohoff RM, Fisher E
(2004). Defining interferon beta response status in
multiple sclerosis patients. *Ann Neurol* **56:**548–555.

Sarchielli P, Presciutti O, Tarducci R, Gobbi G, Alberti A,
Pelliccioli GP, Orlacchio A, Gallai V (1998). 1H-MRS in
patients with multiple sclerosis undergoing treatment
with interferon beta-1a: results of a preliminary study.
J Neurol Neurosurg Psychiatry **64:**204–212.

Sastre-Garriga J, Tintore M, Rovira A, Nos C, Rio J,
Thompson AJ, Montalban X (2004). Specificity of
Barkhof criteria in predicting conversion to multiple
sclerosis when applied to clinically isolated brainstem
syndromes. *Arch Neurol* **61:**222–224 pp. 7–15.

Schmidt R, Enzinger C, Ropele S, Schmidt H, Fazekas F;
Austrian Stroke Prevention Study (2003). Progression
of cerebral white matter lesions: 6-year results of
the Austrian Stroke Prevention Study. *Lancet* **361:**
2046–2048.

Schubert F, Seifert F, Elster C, Link A, Walzel M, Mientus S,
Haas J, Rinneberg H (2002). Serial 1H-MRS in relapsing-remitting multiple sclerosis: effects of interferon-beta therapy on absolute metabolite concentrations.
MAGMA **14:**213–222.

Schumacher FA, Beeve GW, Kibler RF (1965). Problems of
experimental trails of therapy in multiple sclerosis. *Ann
NY Acad Sci* **122:**552–568.

Simon JH (1999). From enhancing lesions to brain atrophy in MS. *J Neuroimmunol* **98:**7–15l.

Simon JH, Jacobs LD, Campion M, Wende K, Simonian N, Cookfair DL, Rudick RA, Herndon RM, Richert JR, Salazar AM, Alam JJ, Fischer JS, Goodkin DE, Granger CV, Lajaunie M, Martens-Davidson AL, Meyer M, Sheeder J, Choi K, Scherzinger AL, Bartoszak DM, Bourdette DN, Braiman J, Brownscheidle CM, Whitham RH (1998). Magnetic resonance studies of intramuscular interferon beta-1a for relapsing multiple sclerosis. The Multiple Sclerosis Collaborative Research Group. *Ann Neurol* **43:**79–87.

Simon JH, Lull J, Jacobs LD, Rudick RA, Cookfair DL, Herndon RM, Richert JR, Salazar AM, Sheeder J, Miller D, McCabe K, Serra A, Campion MK, Fischer JS, Goodkin DE, Simonian N, Lajaunie M, Wende K, Martens-Davidson A, Kinkel RP, Munschauer FE 3rd (2000). A longitudinal study of T1 hypointense lesions in relapsing MS: MSCRG trial of interferon beta-1a. *Neurology* **55:**185–192.

Smith D (2004). Preliminary analysis of a trial of pulse cyclophosphamide in OFN-beta-resistant active MS. *J Neurol Sci* **223:**73–79.

Sorensen PS, Wanscher B, Jensen CV, Schreiber K, Blinkenberg M, Ravnborg M, Kirsmeier H, Larsen VA, Lee ML (1998). Intravenous immunoglobulin G reduces MRI activity in relapsing multiple sclerosis. *Neurology* **50:**1273–1281.

Sormani MP, Rovaris M, Valsasina P, Wolinsky JS, Comi G, Filippi M (2004). Measurement error of two different techniques for brain atrophy assessment in multiple sclerosis. *Neurology* **62:**1432–1434.

Stevenson VL, Miller DH, Rovaris M, Barkhof F, Brochet B, Dousset V, Dousset V, Filippi M, Montalban X, Polman CH, Rovira A, de Sa J, Thompson AJ (1999). Primary and transitional progressive MS, a clinical and MRI cross-sectional study. *Neurology* **52:**839–845.

Stone LA, Smith E, Albert PS, Bash CN, Maloni H, Frank JA, McFarland HF (1995). Blood-brain barrier disruption on contrast enhanced MRI in patients with mild relapsing-remitting multiple sclerosis: relationship to course, gender and age. *Neurology* **45:**1122–1126.

Tartaglino LM, Friedman DP, Flanders AE, Lublin FD, Knobler RL, Liem M (1995). Multiple sclerosis in the spinal cord: MR appearance and correlation with clinical parameters. *Radiology* **195:**725–732.

Tas MW, Barkhof F, van Walderveen MA, Polman CH, Hommes OR, Valk J (1995). The effect of gadolinium on the sensitivity and specificity of MR in the initial diagnosis of multiple sclerosis. *Am J Neuroradiol* **2:**259–264.

The North American Study Group on Interferon beta-1b in Secondary Progressive MS (2004). Interferon beta-1b in secondary progressive MS: Results from a 3-year controlled study. *Neurology* **63:**1788–1795.

Tintoré M, Rovira A, Martinez MJ, Rio J, Diaz-Villoslada P, Brieva L, Borras C, Grive E, Capellades J, Montalban X (2000). Isolated demyelinating syndromes: comparison of different MRI criteria to predict conversion to clinically definite multiple sclerosis. *Am J Neruoradiol* **21:**702–706.

Tintoré M, Rovira A, Rio J, Nos C, Grive E, Sastre-Garriga J, Pericot I, Sanchez E, Comabella M, Montalban X (2003). New diagnostic criteria for multiple sclerosis: application in first demyelinating episode. *Neurology* **60:**27–30.

Thompson AJ, Kermode AG, MacManus DG, Kendall BE, Kingsley DP, Moseley IF, McDonald WI (1990). Patterns of disease activity in multiple sclerosis: clinical and magnetic resonance imaging study. *BMJ* **300:**631–634.

Thompson AJ, Kermode AG, Wicks D, MacManus DG, Kendall BE, Kingsley DP, McDonald WI (1991). Major differences in the dynamics of primary and secondary progressive multiple sclerosis. *Ann Neurol* **29:**53–62.

Thompson AJ, Miller DH, Youl BD, MacManus D, Moore S, Kingsley D, Kendall B, Feinstein A, McDonald WI (1992). Serial gadolinium-enhanced MRI in relapsing/remitting multiple sclerosis of varying disease duration. *Neurology* **42:**60–63.

Thompson AJ, Montalban X, Barkhof F, Brochet B, Filippi M, Miller DH, Polman CH, Stevenson VL, McDonald WI (2000). Diagnostic criteria for primary progressive multiple sclerosis: a position paper. *Ann Neurol* **47:**831–835.

Tortorella C, Rocca MA, Codella C, Gasperini C, Capra R, Bastianello S, Filippi M (1999). Disease activity in multiple sclerosis studied with weekly triple dose magnetic resonance imaging. *J Neurol* **246:**689–692.

Traboulsee A, Dehmeshki J, Brex PA, Dalton CM, Chard D, Barker GJ, Plant GT, Miller DH (2002). Normal-appearing brain tissue MTR histograms in clinically isolated syndromes suggestive of MS. *Neurology* **59:**126–128.

Truyen L, van Waesberghe JHTM, van Walderveen MAA, van Oosten BW, Polman CH, Hommes OR, Ader HJ, Barkhof F (1996). Accumulation of hypointense lesions (black holes) on T1 spin-echo MRI correlates with disease progression in multiple sclerosis. *Neurology* **47:**1469–1476.

Vollmer T, Key L, Durkalski V, Tyor W, Corboy J, Markovic-Plese S, Preiningerova J, Rizzo M, Singh I (2004). Oral simvastatin treatment in relapsing-remitting multiple sclerosis. *Lancet* **363:**1607–1608.

van Walderveen MAA, Barkhof F, Hommes OR, Polman CH, Tobi H, Frequin ST, Valk J (1995). Correlating MRI and clinical activity in multiple sclerosis: relevance of hypointense lesions on short TR/short TE (T1-weighted) spin-echo images. *Neurology* **45:**1684–1690.

van Walderveen MA, Truyen L, van Osten BW, Castelijns JA, Lycklama a Nijeholt GJ, van Waesberghe JH, Polman C, Barkhof F (1999). Development of hypointense lesion on T1-weighted spin echo magnetic resonance images in multiple sclerosis: relation to inflammatory activity. *Arch Neurol* **56:**345–351.

van Walderveen MAA, Lycklama à Nijeholt GJ, Adèr HJ, Jongen PJ, Polman CH, Castelijns JA, Barkhof F (2001). Hypointense lesions on T1 weighted SE MRI: relation to clinical characteristic in subgroups of multiple sclerosis patients. *Arch Neurol* **58:** 76–81.

Zivadinov R, Bakshi R (2004). Central nervous system atrophy and clinical status in multiple sclerosis. *J Neuroimaging* **14:**27S–35S.

Zivadinov R, Zorzon M (2002). Is gadolinium enhancement predictive of the development of brain atrophy in multiple sclerosis? A review of literature. *J Neuroimaging* **12:**302–309.

CHAPTER 7

Neurophysiological tests and neuroimaging procedures in non-acute headache

G. Sandrini,[a] L. Friberg,[b] W. Jänig,[c] R. Jensen,[d]
D. Russell,[e] M. Sanchez del Rìo,[f] T. Sand,[g]
J. Schoenen,[h] M. van Buchem,[i] J.G. van Dijk[j]

Abstract

Background The use of instrumental examinations in headache patients varies widely.

Methods To evaluate their usefulness, the most common instrumental procedures were evaluated, on the basis of evidence from the literature, by an EFNS Task Force (TF) on neurophysiological tests and imaging procedures in non-acute headache patients.

1 Interictal electroencephalography (EEG) is not routinely indicated in the diagnostic evaluation of headache patients. Interictal EEG is, however, indicated if the clinical history suggests a possible diagnosis of epilepsy (differential diagnosis). Ictal EEG could be useful in certain patients suffering from hemiplegic and basilar migraine.

2 Recording of *evoked potentials* is not recommended for the diagnosis of headache disorders.

3 There is no evidence to justify the recommendation of autonomic tests for the routine clinical examination of headache patients.

4 *Manual palpation* of pericranial muscles, with standardized palpation pressure, can be recommended for subdividing patient groups but not for diagnosis. Pressure algometry and electromyography (EMG) cannot be recommended as clinical diagnostic tests.

5 In adult and paediatric patients with migraine, with no recent change in attack pattern, no history of seizures, and no other focal neurological signs or symptoms, the routine use of *neuroimaging* is not warranted. In patients with atypical headache patterns, a history of seizures and focal neurological signs or symptoms, magnetic resonance imaging (MRI) may be indicated.

6 If attacks can be fully accounted for by the standard headache classification [International Headache Society (IHS)], a positron emission tomography (PET) or single-photon emission

[a]University Centre for Adaptive Disorders and Headache, IRCCS C. Mondino Foundation, Pavia, Italy; [b]Department of Clinical Physiology and Nuclear Medicine, Bispebjerg Hospital, Copenhagen, Denmark; [c]Physiologisches Institut, Christian-Albrechts-Universität, Kiel, Germany; [d]Department of Neurology, Glostrup Hospital, University of Copenhagen, Glostrup, Denmark; [e]Department of Neurology, Rikshospitalet, Oslo, Norway; [f]Department of Neurology, Hospital Ruber Internacional, Madrid, Spain; [g]Department of Neurology, Norwegian University of Science and Technology, Trondheim, Norway; [h]University Department of Neurology, CHR Citadelle, Liege, Belgium; [i]Department of Radiology, Leiden University Medical Centre, Leiden, The Netherlands; and [j]Department of Neurology and Clinical Neurophysiology, Leiden University Medical Centre, Leiden, The Netherlands.

computerized tomography (SPECT) and scan will generally be of no further diagnostic value.

7 Nuclear medicine examinations of the cerebral circulation and metabolism can be carried out in subgroups of headache patients for diagnosis and evaluation of complications, when patients experience unusually severe attacks, or when the quality or severity of attacks has changed.

8 *Transcranial Doppler* examination is not helpful in headache diagnosis.

Although many of the examinations described are of little or no value in the clinical setting, most of the tools have a vast potential for further exploring the pathophysiology of headaches and the effects of pharmacological treatment.

Introduction

The most important tools in the diagnosis and treatment of headache disorders are, without doubt, careful clinical neurological examinations and the compilation of detailed reports on the patient's history and symptoms. By applying the diagnostic criteria of the International Headache Society (IHS Classification, 1988), there can be a probable diagnosis that allows adequate treatment. However, in many cases, particularly when the headache presents as atypical with changing clinical features or as a symptom of another primary illness, neurologists find it necessary to supplement the clinical work up of the patient with para-clinical tests. The differential diagnosis of acute headache (e.g. primary thunderclap headache) versus symptomatic headache presents several difficulties and neuroimaging investigations are mandatory. This report is a critical review of the literature on the application of neurophysiological tests and imaging procedures in non-acute headache patients. In addition to evaluating the clinical usefulness of these tests and procedures in the diagnostic setting, we have also attempted to outline the guidelines for their use, as attempted by various authors (Silberstein, 2000; Lewis *et al.*, 2002). Of all the available techniques, neuroimaging, particularly magnetic resonance imaging (MRI), is the most suitable and cost-effective para-clinical testing method used in

headache patients, with the highest rate of diagnosis. Finally, we consider the potential use of these methods in headache research. An extensive review of the main references in the literature, together with an update on the most important contributions made by neurophysiological studies to our understanding of the pathogenesis of primary headache, is being published elsewhere (Friberg *et al.*, 2003).

Aims and methods

The intention in compiling the information in this document was to develop guidelines to help physicians make appropriate choices regarding the use of instrumental tests in non-acute headache patients. Reviews of published clinical evidence (from 1988 to 2002) were evaluated. Key literature references pre-dating the IHS Classification (1988) were particularly carefully examined as these studies applied different diagnostic criteria for headache.

The guidelines were prepared according to the EFNS criteria (Hughes *et al.*, 2001; Brainin *et al.*, 2004) and the level of evidence and grade of recommendation were expressed in accordance with this reference. These guidelines were originally published in the *European Journal of Neurology* 2004; 11: 577–581.

Main findings for the different techniques

Electroencephalography

The usefulness of electroencephalography (EEG) in the diagnosis of headache is debated. Although early EEG studies of migraine emphasized the frequent abnormal recordings, contemporary reviewers have criticized most of them for various methodological omissions and flaws (Sand, 1991). The American Academy of Neurology concludes, 'EEG is not useful in the routine evaluation of patients with headache (guideline)', admitting, however, that EEG may be used in headache patients with associated symptoms suggesting a seizure disorder (Rosenberg *et al.*, 1995).

EEG is the best laboratory technique to support the clinical diagnosis of epilepsy, showing good sensitivity (80–90% in serial recordings) and specificity (false positive rates in 0.2–3.5% of healthy subjects) (Walczak and Jayakar, 1998). It also plays an important role in the evaluation of other focal and diffuse central nervous system (CNS) disorders.

Quantitative frequency analysis of EEG (QEEG), with or without topographic mapping, is a more objective method than conventional EEG interpretation, although there are a number of possible methodological pitfalls that should be avoided. The use of QEEG is generally recommended only in conjunction with visual EEG interpretation performed by a skilled observer (Nuwer, 1997).

Evoked potentials

Evoked potentials (EPs) are cortical EEG potentials temporally linked to a specific sensory input. Although all sensory stimuli contribute to the overall EEG activity, EPs cannot be identified in the normal EEG because they are not separable from ongoing EEG activity. However, when clear temporal definition of the stimulus is possible (i.e. in the case of a sudden onset), short stretches of post-stimulus EEG can be averaged. Any activity that is not time-locked to the stimulus disappears from the average, while the EEG response to the stimulus remains. In this way, the cortical response to very specific stimuli can be investigated in spatial and temporal detail. In migraine, much attention has been paid to visual stimuli, which is not surprising given the presence of visual auras and photophobia in this disorder. EPs have made it possible to document cortical excitability, as well as habituation and gating phenomena in migraine (Ambrosini *et al.*, 2003).

Reflex responses

Several electrophysiological techniques have been used to explore polysynaptic reflexes in headache patients. The blink reflex (BR) and corneal reflex (CR) are reflected in the bilateral closure of the eyelids in response to a stimulus, usually, in laboratory settings, that is an electrical stimulation of the supraorbital nerve. The BR consists of three components: an ipsilateral early component (R1), a bilateral late component (R2) and a bilateral ultralate component (R3). The precise nature of R1 and R2

is still debated, while R3 is considered to be a nociceptive component. The CR is composed of two late bilateral symmetrical components, probably equivalent to the R2 component.

Several BR and CR abnormalities have been described in primary headaches, but data documenting the specificity and sensitivity of these tests (Sandrini *et al.*, 1991, 2002, 2003; Proietti Cecchini *et al.*, 2003) are scarce. The exteroceptive suppression (ES) of masticatory muscle activity is a trigemino–trigeminal reflex consisting of biphasic (ES1 and ES2) inhibition of voluntary contraction (of variable duration) that occurs bilaterally in response to various exteroceptive stimuli. The inhibitory effect is mediated by interneurones located in the propriobulbar and pontine reticular formation, close to the trigeminal motor nucleus on each side. The literature contains conflicting data on ES abnormalities in tension-type headaches (Schoenen and Bendtsen, 2000).

Nociceptive flexion reflexes (NFRs), evoked at the biceps femoral muscle by electrical stimulation of the sural nerve, are thought to constitute a useful tool for exploring the pain control system in human beings, but only a few NFR studies have been conducted in headache patients (Sandrini *et al.*, 1993).

Autonomic tests

The autonomic nervous system (ANS) consists of three parts: the sympathetic, parasympathetic and enteric nervous systems. Each of these is divided into subsystems according to the effector organs innervated by the terminal neurones. 'Sympathetic' and 'parasympathetic' neurones are actually defined on the basis of anatomical rather than functional criteria; thus, afferent neurones innervating visceral organs are not denoted as sympathetic or parasympathetic, but visceral (Jänig and McLachlan, 1999; Jänig, 2003a). When considering the role of the ANS in the different types of headache, there are three different questions that should be borne in mind (Jänig, 2003b):

1 Is the ANS involved in the generation and maintenance of pain? Hypotheses regarding the mechanisms of possible sympathetic nervous system involvement in the generation and maintenance of pain have been formulated and tested

in animal and human experimental models (Jänig, 1999; Jänig and Baron, 2001, 2002).

2 Are functional autonomic abnormalities associated with different types of headache, the consequence of and therefore secondary to headache? This question addresses the observation that all pain is accompanied by autonomic reactions that are based on central reflex pathways in the neuraxis, and on the central integration of nociceptive with autonomic systems. In normal biological conditions, these autonomic reactions are primarily protective for the organism, but this may not necessarily continue to be the case in pathobiological conditions.

3 Are headache and functional autonomic abnormalities parallel events and therefore the consequence of possible central abnormalities? If they are, it could be useful to investigate these autonomic abnormalities in an attempt to elucidate the central pathophysiological changes that may underlie both headache and autonomic disturbances.

The diagnosis and management of autonomic disorders are highly dependent on the testing procedures used (Mathias and Bannister, 1999). Neurophysiological techniques have revealed several autonomic disturbances in primary headache, in cluster headache in particular (Saunte *et al.*, 1983; Salvesen *et al.*, 1988), but the clinical relevance of these findings remains to be verified (Schoenen and Thomsen, 2000).

Pericranial muscle tenderness evaluation

The tension-type headache (TTH) was divided into two subgroups in the IHS classification, to study the pathophysiological relevance of pericranial muscles in this disorder. This subdivision was necessitated by the clinical observation that many TTH patients have increased tension, tenderness and stiffness in their neck and shoulder muscles, and that some, a smaller group and much more difficult to treat, lack muscle tenderness. The IHS classification did not lay down specific diagnostic methods and, at the time, no scientific basis for this subdivision had been established. Although several studies have been carried out since then (Schoenen

et al., 1991; Jensen *et al.*, 1993, 1994; Jensen and Rasmussen, 1996), it is still not clear whether different pathophysiological mechanisms subtend the headache in these two subgroups. The recording of tenderness has been a widely debated subject as it has been difficult to compare the results of different observers. A fairly recent methodological study showed manual palpation to be an easy and reliable method of studying myofascial pain sensitivity in a clinical setting, provided the intensity of the applied pressure is controlled (Bendtsen *et al.*, 1995).

Pressure pain threshold (PPT) recording is also recommended in the IHS Classification (1988), although the methodology to be used and the locations to be examined are not specified. Pressure algometry, not requiring specific skills and having no particular technical requirements, is easy and safe for clinical use. The PPT, as a quantitative measure of pain, can be recorded either from a localized tender spot, or from a fixed spot in all subjects, regardless of findings on palpation. Previous studies have demonstrated that the latter method gives highly reliable and reproducible results within the same subject, but considerably varying results between subjects (Jensen *et al.*, 1993).

Neuroimaging

Radiological examinations are often sought in patients with headache. Most headache sufferers seeking medical attention fear they may have a serious illness and often request a radiological investigation. As radiological examinations are not particularly invasive or uncomfortable, and as they detect any intracranial diseases present, the threshold for requesting them is low. However, when deciding whether or not to use radiological techniques, one should consider the likelihood of the detection of underlying diseases in headache patients (Mitchell *et al.*, 1993). In the medical literature, studies that use radiological techniques in populations of headache patients can be divided into three categories. First, studies investigating the aetiology and pathophysiological mechanisms of headache; second, studies focusing on the pathological sequelae of headache; and third, studies on the role of radiological techniques in the work up of headache patients. As the aim of this

paper was to provide guidelines on the usefulness of radiological techniques in the evaluation
of headache patients with normal neurological
examinations, we reviewed a subset of the third
category.

The current literature has been reviewed with
a view to establishing guidelines for the future
use of radiological methods in headache patients
(Frishberg, 1994), and the methods were found
to present certain limitations. Although there is a
need for further systematic studies on this topic,
some conclusions can, nevertheless, be drawn
(Frishberg, 1994).

There is no role for conventional roentgen techniques (skull films) in the work up of headache
patients, as the conditions underlying headache in
these subjects are generally located inside the skull
and therefore not detectable using these methods. Digital subtraction angiography (DSA) is an
invasive procedure associated with a significant
morbidity and mortality rate. DSA still seems
to be superior to other radiological techniques
in detecting intracranial arterio-venous malformations (AVMs) and fistulas. However, it is relatively
rare for any of these conditions to underlie the
headache, and, furthermore, some lesions of this
kind are also visible using non-invasive techniques
[computerized tomography (CT) and MRI]. Therefore, it is not appropriate to use DSA in the screening of headache patients for intracranial disease.

Both CT and MRI can be performed with and
without the application of intravenous contrast
agents. MRI is more sensitive to the presence of
intracranial disease than CT, and the sensitivity of
both techniques is increased when they are used in
conjunction with intravenous contrast agents.

Detection of the presence of a recent intracranial
haemorrhage is straightforward on CT. However,
it has been demonstrated that MRI is at least as
sensitive as CT in detecting bleeding in the subarachnoid space, if adequate sequences such as
fluid attended inversion recovery (FLAIR) are used
(Noguchi et al., 1997). Recently, functional MRI
(fMRI) of the brain also allowed very interesting
studies of brain time perfusion, water molecular
diffusion and cerebral cortical activation. However, these techniques and applications are still
in a state of evolution. The extent to which they

can be applied in the examination of headache is
not yet clear, although they may prove to be helpful in differentiating between ischaemic insult and
prolonged migraine aura in select patients during
migraine attacks (Ay et al., 1999).

SPECT and PET

Single-photon emission computerized tomography (SPECT) and positron emission tomography
(PET) are nuclear medicine imaging methods (De
Deyn et al., 1997), both of which require the
administration of radioactive tracers to the patient.
SPECT involves the sampling of emitted radiation,
by means of a gamma camera with the camera
heads or their collimators moving around the subject's head during data acquisition. Because SPECT
cameras are versatile, less expensive and less costly
to run than PET cameras, SPECT brain scans are
carried out at most large hospitals.

The most commonly performed type of brain
SPECT reveals regional cerebral blood flow (rCBF)
changes. Following inhalation or i.v. injection of
Xe^{133}, it is possible to quantify the rCBF, although
at the expense of spatial resolution (Croft, 1990).
Tc^{99m}-labelled rCBF tracers are the ones most
frequently used because Tc^{99m} is readily available in all nuclear medical departments. SPECT
rCBF investigations can provide information about
acute changes in regional perfusion that often arise
in relation to the neurological symptoms associated with the aura phase of migraine (Friberg,
1999; Friberg et al., 2003). SPECT combined
with transcranial Doppler (TCD) can, further,
provide information about changes in diameter
of the larger intracranial arteries (Friberg et al.,
1991).

Positron emission tomography is a cumbersome and more expensive technique than SPECT.
With the exception of F^{18}-labelled tracers ($t_{1/2} =$
110 min), most isotopes for PET decay very quickly.
Therefore PET requires an in-house cyclotron and
online radiochemistry production unit (Saha et al.,
1992). The positron emitting isotopes, such as C^{11},
O^{15} and F^{18}, are naturally incorporated into bio-
logically active molecules. This has facilitated the
synthesis of a large number of radioactive labelled
tracers for PET, for example, receptor-specific

ligands and metabolism markers. However, only a fraction of these are used in clinical scans. As a result of the high cost of establishing and running a PET unit, the availability of PET scans is limited. Most countries in Europe have only a few PET centres, located in university hospitals.

Transcranial Doppler

The Doppler principle is utilized in medicine in the following way: an ultrasound signal is transmitted into the body and the changes in sound frequency that occur when it is reflected or scattered from the moving blood cells are observed. The accuracy of TCD velocity recordings is influenced by the angle of insonation, which, in turn, is determined by the technique adopted and the local vessel anatomy. Assuming the angle of insonation is constant, velocity (V) is dependent on volume flow (F) through the vessel and on the vessel cross-sectional area (A), according to the formula $F = V \times A$. It will, therefore, be influenced by factors that cause changes in CBF, vessel diameter, or both. Simultaneous TCD and rCBF measurements may contribute to determining vascular changes in headache patients, as each cerebral vessel supplies a defined volume of cerebral tissue (Dahl *et al.*, 1990). TCD is mainly used to evaluate vascular reactivity in migraine (Friberg *et al.*, 2003).

RECOMMENDATIONS

Electroencephalogram
Routine EEG with standard visual interpretation
Interictal EEG is not routinely indicated in the diagnostic evaluation of headache patients.

Interictal EEG is only indicated if the clinical history suggests a possible diagnosis of epilepsy, for example, in the case of: (i) unusually brief headache episodes; (ii) unusual aura symptoms (e.g. gastric/olfactory sensations, circular visual symptoms); (iii) headache associated with unusually brief auras or aura-like phenomena; (iv) headache associated with severe neurological deficits; and (v) other risk factors for epilepsy. Ictal EEG is indicated during episodes suggesting

complicated aura and during auras associated with decreased consciousness or confusion.

Quantitative EEG methods (frequency analysis with or without topographic mapping). Current QEEG methods are not routinely indicated in the diagnostic evaluation of headache patients.

Quantitative frequency analysis of EEG must always be recorded with raw EEG data and interpreted by a skilled physician to avoid misinterpretation of technical artefacts, normal state fluctuations and various physiological rhythms.

Analysis of photic driving

Photic driving may be increased in migraine and tension-type headache patient groups as compared with headache-free subjects. The specificity of the method is not yet sufficiently documented.

RECOMMENDATIONS

There is not enough evidence to suggest that the photic driving methods that are currently in use can reliably discriminate either between migraine and non-migraine primary headache patients or between primary headache patients and headache-free subjects (Class II, Level B).

Evoked potentials

The literature data, often conflicting, failed to demonstrate the usefulness of EPs as a diagnostic tool in migraine. Findings should therefore be replicated before visually evoked potentials (VEPs) can be recommended in the diagnosis of migraine (not enough data are available for other types of headache). In conclusion, we do not recommend the use of EPs in the diagnosis of headache disorders.

This is a class II level of evidence, but the literature contains contrasting data and the clinical significance of abnormalities is poorly understood. The grade of recommendation is B.

Reflex responses

Most of the neurophysiological investigation techniques have only limited usefulness in the diagnosis of headache. Further research in large populations is needed to establish which electro-physiological markers could be relevant in clinical practice.

This is a class IV level of evidence for nociceptive flexion reflex (not blinded studies), and class III for corneal reflex and blink reflex. The grade of recommendation is C for corneal and blink reflex. As for exteroceptive suppression of masticatory muscle activity, only few blinded studies (class III) fail to confirm previous investigations. The grade of recommendation is C.

Autonomic tests

Studies of autonomic functions in migraine and cluster headache were mostly focused on autonomic systems innervating specific target organs which, anatomically and functionally, are not necessarily related to the supposed autonomic origin of the pain. Autonomic parameters are confounded by effector organ response characteristics.

RECOMMENDATIONS

Therefore, there is no clear evidence justifying the recommendation of autonomic tests for the routine clinical examination of headache patients (Class IV, Level C).

Clinical tests, PPTs and EMG (with special reference to TTH)

Tenderness recorded by manual palpation is the most specific and sensitive test in patients with TTH, and can therefore be recommended as a routine clinical test in contrast to EMG and PPTs. However, this manual palpation is non-specific and cannot be used to discriminate between different coexisting primary or secondary headaches.

This is a class III level of evidence and the grade of recommendation is C (few blinded studies mainly concerning methodology in healthy volunteers).

Neuroimaging

When neuroimaging is warranted, the most sensitive method should be used, and we recommend MRI and not CT in these cases.

The grade of recommendation is C, as most studies are non-analytical and although there exist a few randomized clinical trials, some of them are not directly relevant to these recommendations (class IV).

RECOMMENDATIONS

1 In adult and paediatric patients with migraine, with no recent change in pattern, no history of seizures, and no other focal neurological signs or symptoms, the routine use of neuroimaging is not warranted.
2 In patients with atypical headache patterns, a history of seizures, or neurological signs or symptoms, or symptomatic illness such as tumours, acquired immunodeficiency syndrome (AIDS) and neurofibromatosis, MRI may be indicated (to be carefully evaluated in each case).

SPECT and PET

If attacks can be fully accounted for by the standard headache classification (IHS), a PET or SPECT scan will generally be of no further diagnostic value.

Nuclear medicine examinations of cerebral circulation and metabolism can be carried out in subgroups of headache patients for diagnosis and evaluation of complications. rCBF can be of particular value in patients in whom the standard classification (IHS) cannot be fully applied, when patients experience unusually severe attacks, or the quality or severity of attacks has changed. rCBF recordings should then be carried out both during an attack (if possible several repeated scans) and interictally (at a time interval of >5 days after an attack). Quantifiable rCBF measurements are preferable to distribution images.

This is a class IV level of evidence, that is, most studies are case reports or case series. There is insufficient evidence to make specific recommendations.

Transcranial Doppler

Transcranial Doppler examination is not helpful in headache diagnosis. It is, however, a non-invasive examination with an excellent temporal resolution that is useful for studying the vascular aspects of the headache pathophysiology and the vascular effects of anti-headache medication. The information obtained using this method is easier to interpret if side-to-side comparisons are made or if it is combined with rCBF measurements.

This is a class IV level of evidence.

Acknowledgements

We wish to thank Dr Alberto Proietti Cecchini, and secretaries Heidi Ulm and Cristina Rivieccio for their valuable help in preparing this paper, and Ms Catherine Wrenn for the linguistic revision of the manuscript. We are also grateful for the comments and suggestions given by Prof. Jes Olesen and Prof. Peer Tfelt-Hansen. We thank Pfizer, Inc. and GlaxoSmithKline, Inc. for their financial support of the work of this Task Force.

This is a Continuing Medical Education paper and can be found with corresponding questions on the Internet at: http://www.blackwellpublishing.com/products/journals/ene/mcqs. Certificates for correctly answering the questions will be issued by the EFNS.

This work was partially supported by a grant from the Eurohead project (LSHM-CT-2004-504837).

References

Ambrosini A, Maertens de Noordhout A, Sandor P, Schoenen J (2003). Electrophysiological studies in migraine: a comprehensive review of their interest and limitations. *Cephalalgia* **23(Suppl 1):**13–31.

Ay H, Buonanno FS, Rordorf G *et al.* (1999). Normal diffusion-weighted MRI during stroke-like deficits. *Neurology* **52:**1784–1792.

Bendtsen L, Jensen R, Jensen NK, Olesen J (1995). Pressure-controlled palpation: a new technique which increases the reliability of manual palpation. *Cephalalgia* **15:**205–210.

Brainin M, Barnes M, Baron J-C *et al.* (2004). Guidance for the preparation of neurological management guidelines by EFNS scientific task forces. *Eur J Neurol* **1:**577–581.

Croft BY (1990). Instrumentation and computers for brain single photon emission computed tomography. *J Nucl Med* **20:**281–289.

Dahl A, Russell D, Nyberg-Hansen R, Rootwelt K (1990). Cluster headache: transcranial Doppler ultrasound and rCBF studies. *Cephalalgia* **10:**87–94.

De Deyn PP, Nagels G, Pickut BA *et al.* (1997). SPECT in neurology and psychiatry. In: De Deyn PP, Dierckx RA, Alavi A, Pickut BA, eds. *SPECT in Headache with Special Reference to Migraine*, vol. 54, 1st edn. John Libbey & Co. Ltd, London, pp. 455–466.

Friberg L (1999). Migraine pathophysiology and its relation to cerebral hemodynamic changes. In: Edvinsson L, ed. *Migraine and Headache Pathophysiology*. Martin Dunitz Ltd, London, pp. 133–140.

Friberg L, Olesen J, Iversen HK, Sperling B (1991). Migraine pain associated with middle cerebral artery dilatation: reversal by sumatripan. *Lancet* **338:**13–17.

Friberg L, Sandrini G, Jänig W *et al.* (2003). Instrumental investigations in primary headache. An updated review and new perspectives. *Funct Neurol* **8:**27–44.

Frishberg BM (1994). The utility of neuroimaging in the evaluation of headache in patients with normal neurological examinations. *Neurology* **44:**1191–1197.

Hughes RAC, Barnes MP, Baron JC, Brainin M (2001). Guidance for the preparation of neurological management guidelines by EFNS scientific task forces. *Eur J Neurol* **8:**549–550.

Headache Classification Subcommittee of the International Headache Society (2004). The International Classification of Headache Disorders, 2nd Edition. *Cephalalgia*. **24(Suppl 1)**.

Jänig W (1999). Pain and the sympathetic nervous system: pathophysiological mechanisms. In: Bannister R, Mathias CJ, eds. *Autonomic Failure*, 4th edn. Oxford University Press, Oxford, pp. 99–108.

Jänig W (2003a). The autonomic nervous system and its co-ordination by the brain. In: Davidson RJ, Scherer KR, Goldsmith HH, eds. *Handbook of Affective Sciences. Part II Autonomic Psychophysiology*. Oxford University Press, New York, pp. 135–186.

Jänig W (2003b). Relationship between pain and autonomic phenomena in headache and other pain syndromes. *Cephalalgia* **23(Suppl 1):**43–48.

Jänig W, Baron R (2001). The role of the sympathetic nervous system in neuropathic pain: clinical observations and animal models. In: Hansson PT, Fields HL, Hill RG, Marchettini P, eds. *"Neuropathic Pain: Pathophysiology and Treatment"*. *Progress in Pain Research and Management*, Vol. 21. IASP Press, Seattle, WA, pp. 125–149.

Jänig W, Baron R (2002). Complex regional pain syndrome is a disease of the central nervous system. *Clin Auton Res* **12:**150–164.

Jänig W, McLachlan EM (1999). Neurobiology of the autonomic nervous system. In: Bannister R, Mathias CJ, eds.

Autonomic Failure, 4th edn. Oxford University Press, Oxford, pp. 315.

Jensen R, Rasmussen BK (1996). Muscular disorders in tension-type headache. *Cephalalgia* **16:**97–103.

Jensen R, Rasmussen BK, Pedersen B, Olesen J (1993). Muscle tenderness and pressure pain thresholds in headache. A population study. *Pain* **52:**193–199.

Jensen R, Fuglsang-Frederiksen A, Olesen J (1994). Quantitative surface EMG of pericranial muscles in headache. A population study. *Electroencephalogr Clin Neurophysiol* **93:**335–344.

Lewis DW, Ashwal S, Dahl G *et al.* (2002). Practice parameter. Evaluation of children and adolescents with recurrent headaches: report of the Quality Standards Subcommittee of the American Academy of Neurology and the Practice Committee of the Child Neurology Society. *Neurology* **59:**490–498.

Mathias CJ, Bannister R (1999). Investigation of autonomic disorders. In: Bannister R, Mathias CJ, eds. *Autonomic Failure*, 4th edn. Oxford University Press, Oxford.

Mitchell CS, Osborn RE, Grosskreutz SR (1993). Computed tomography in the headache patient: is routine evaluation really necessary? *Headache* **33:**82–86.

Noguchi K, Ogawa T, Seto H *et al.* (1997). Subacute and chronic subarachnoid hemorrhage: diagnosis with fluid-attenuated inversion-recovery MR imaging. *Radiology* **203:**257–262.

Nuwer M (1997). Assessment of digital EEG, quantitative EEG and EEG brain mapping. Report of the American Academy of Neurology and the American Clinical Neurophysiology Society. *Neurology* **49:**277–292.

Proietti Cecchini A, Sandrini G, Fokin IV, Moglia A, Nappi G. (2003). Trigemino-facial reflexes in primary headaches. *Cephalalgia* **23(Suppl 1):**33–42.

Rosenberg J, Alter M, Byrne TD *et al.* (1995). Practice parameter: the electroencephalogram in the evaluation of headache. Report of the Quality Standards Subcommittee of the American Academy of Neurology. *Neurology* **45:**1411–1413.

Saha GB, MacIntyre WJ, Go RT (1992). Cyclotrons and positron emission tomography radiopharmaceuticals for clinical imaging. *Semin Nucl Med* **22:**150–161.

Salvesen R, Sand T, Sjaastad O (1988). Cluster headache: combined assessment with pupillometry and evaporimetry. *Cephalalgia* **8:**211–218.

Sand T (1991). EEG in migraine: a review of the literature. *Funct Neurol* **6:**722.

Sandrini G, Alfonsi E, Ruiz L *et al.* (1991). Impairment of corneal pain perception in cluster headache. *Pain* **3:**299–304.

Sandrini G, Arrigo A, Bono G, Nappi G (1993). The nociceptive flexion reflex as a tool for exploring pain control systems in headache and other pain syndromes. *Cephalalgia* **13:**21–27.

Sandrini G, Proietti Cecchini A, Milanov I, Tassorelli C, Buzzi MG, Nappi G (2002). Electrophysiological evidence for trigeminal neuron sensitization in patients with migraine. *Neurosci Lett* **317:**135–138.

Sandrini G, Friberg L, Schoenen J, Nappi G (2003). Exploring pathophysiology of headache. *Cephalalgia* **23(Suppl 1):**152.

Saunte C, Russell D, Sjaastad O (1983). Cluster headache: on the mechanisms behind attack-related sweating. *Cephalalgia* **3:**175–185.

Schoenen J, Bendtsen L (2000). Neurophysiology of tension-type headache. In: Olesen J, Tfelt-Hansen P, Welch KMA, eds. *The Headaches*, 2nd edn. Lippincott Williams & Wilkins, Philadelphia, PA.

Schoenen J, Thomsen LL (2000). Neurophysiology and autonomic dysfunction in migraine. In: Olesen J, Tfelt-Hansen P, Welch KMA, eds. *The Headaches*, 2nd edn. Lippincott Williams & Wilkins, Philadelphia, PA.

Schoenen J, Gerard P, de Pasqua V, Sianard-Gainko J (1991). Multiple clinical and paraclinical analyses of chronic tension-type headache associated or unassociated with disorder of pericranial muscles. *Cephalalgia* **11:**135–139.

Silberstein SD (2000). Practice parameter: evidence-based guidelines for migraine headache (an evidence-based review): report of the Quality Standards Subcommittee of the American Academy of Neurology. [Erratum appears in *Neurology* 2000 Jan 9;**56(1):**142]. *Neurology* **55:**754–762.

Walczak T, Jayakar P (1998). Interictal EEG in epilepsy. In: Engel J, Pedley T, eds. *A Comprehensive Textbook*. Lippincott Raven, Philadelphia, New York, pp. 831–848.

CHAPTER 8

Use of anti-interferon beta antibody measurements in multiple sclerosis

P. Soelberg Sørensen,[a] F. Deisenhammer,[b]
P. Duda,[c] R. Hohlfeld,[d] K.-M. Myhr,[e] J. Palace,[f]
C. Polman,[g] C. Pozzilli,[h] C. Ross[i]

Abstract

Background Therapy-induced binding and neutralizing of antibodies is a major problem in IFNβ treatment of multiple sclerosis.

Objectives To provide guidelines outlining the methods and clinical use of the measurements of binding and neutralizing antibodies.

Methods Systematic search of the Medline database for available publications on binding and neutralizing antibodies. Review of appropriate publications by one or more of the task force members. Grading of evidence and recommendations was based on consensus by all task force members.

Measurements of binding antibodies (BABs) can be reliably used for interferon (IFN)β antibody screening before performing a neutralizing antibody (NAB) assay (Recommendation Level A).

Measurement of NABs should be performed in specialized laboratories with a validated cytopathic effect (CPE) assay or Myxovirus resistance protein A (MxA) production assay using serial dilution of the test sera. The NAB titre should be calculated using the Kawade formula (Recommendation Level A). Tests for the presence of NABs should be carried out during the first 24 months of therapy (Recommendation Level A). In patients who remain NAB negative during this period measurements of NABs can be discontinued (Recommendation Level B). In patients with NABs, measurements should be repeated, and therapy with IFNβ should be discontinued in patients with high titres of NABs sustained at repeated measurements with 3–6 months intervals (Recommendation Level A).

Background and objectives

Interferon (IFN)β is a first line therapy for relapsing–remitting multiple sclerosis (MS). In recent years, several publications have concordantly reported that binding antibodies (BABs) and neutralizing antibodies (NABs) occur during

[a]Copenhagen Danish Multiple Sclerosis Research Center, Neuroscience Centre, Copenhagen University Hospital, Rigshospitalet, Copenhagen, Denmark; [b]Department of Neurology, University of Innsbruck, Innsbruck, Austria; [c]Outpatient Clinic Neurology-Neurosurgery, University Hospitals, Basel, Switzerland; [d]Institute for Clinical Neuroimmunology, University of Munich, Klinikum Grosshadern, Munich, Germany; [e]Department of Neurology, Haukeland University Hospital, Bergen, Norway; [f]Multiple Sclerosis Group, Radcliffe Infirmary, Oxford, UK; [g]Department of Neurology, VU University Medical Center, Amsterdam, The Netherlands; [h]Department of Neurological Sciences, II Faculty of Medicine, University "La Sapienza", Rome, Italy; [i]Institute for Inflammation Research, Copenhagen University Hospital, Rigshospitalet, Copenhagen, Denmark.

European Journal of Neurology 2005, 12:817–827

treatment with recombinant IFNβ products. The frequencies and titres of anti-IFNβ antibodies vary considerably depending on the IFNβ preparation, the frequency and route of administration, and the type of assay being used. There is no generally accepted standardized assay for measuring BABs and NABs. Clinical studies in patients with MS have demonstrated that when NABs to IFNβ develop, the therapeutic benefits of IFNβ are reduced or abolished.

The objectives of our task force were to: (i) evaluate differences in immunogenicity of IFNβ products, (ii) evaluate the reliability and give recommendations on BABs and NABs assays, (iii) evaluate the impact of NABs on clinical efficacy and give recommendation on the clinical use of measurement of IFNβ antibodies and (iv) review the evidence on prevention of NAB development and the management of patients with NABs.

Search strategy and consensus

The task force systematically searched the Medline database for available information published in English up to September 2004. Key words included: interferon beta, multiple sclerosis, immunogenicity, antibodies, binding antibody assays, NAB assays. Articles related to this topic from the authors' personal literature databases were also included. For each specific issue at least one member of the task force assessed all published papers and omitted those that did not fulfil given criteria, and read and rated the remaining articles according to the guidance for preparation of neurological management guidelines by EFNS Scientific task forces-revised recommendations 2004 (Brainin et al., 2004). Each paragraph of the guidelines was drafted by one member of the task force and circulated to the other members. After appropriate revision the guidelines were finalized and consensus was reached among all task force members at a meeting.

Immunogenicity

It is entirely predictable that patients treated with long-term recombinant IFNβ produce antibodies against the product. This observation follows in the wake of other biological products troubled by the production of antibodies including IFN-α, erythropoietin, factor VIII and human insulin. Understandably, the closer a product is to the species' natural antigen the less likely it is to provoke antibodies.

Immunogenicity of IFNβ products

The three commercially available IFNβ products vary substantially in their immunogenicity. The first licensed product, FNβ-1b, is produced from *Escherichia. coli* and it differs from the natural human product by methionin-1 deletion, cystein-17 to serine mutation, and lack of glycosylation. There is about a tenfold increase in the weight of protein present in a single IFNβ-1b dose compared to the IFNβ-1a versions to reach a suitable specific activity level. This is likely to lead to increased aggregation (Runkel et al., 1998) which may enhance its antigenicity. IFNβ-1a in contrast is identical in primary and secondary structure to the native form and is produced in mammalian cells - a system associated with less host cell contaminants. The proportion of patients reported to have neutralizing antibodies range from 2% to greater than 40% and Table 8.1 summarizes the data from the initial pivotal relapsing–remitting and secondary progressive placebo controlled trials. The immunogenicity of Avonex after the initial studies was profoundly reduced for reasons that either are not clear or confidential, but it is possible that the tendency for aggregation was reduced.

Dynamics of NABs

The majority of patients destined to become NAB-positive do so within 6–18 months of treatment. Patients on IFNβ-1b tend to become positive earlier than those on IFNβ-1a. However the percentage becoming positive on IFNβ-1a (Rebif) has been reported to catch up in frequency (Ross et al., 2000; Dubois et al., 2003). It is likely that tolerance may occur over the long-term during continued IFNβ therapy (Rice et al., 1999; Sorensen et al., 2005). For NAB-positive patients, the probability of reverting to NAB-negative status was significantly higher in patients treated with IFNβ-1b than in

Table 8.1 Frequency of NAB-positive patients in initial pivotal placebo controlled trials.

Study	IFNβ product and dosage
IFNB MS Study Group (RRMS), 1993	IFNβ-1b (Betaferon) 250 μg/2. day
European IFNB MS Study Group (SPMS), 1998	IFNβ-1b (Betaferon) 250 μg/2. day
Jacobs et al., 1996	IFNβ-1a (Avonex) 30 μg weekly
PRISMS, 1998	IFNβ-1a (Rebif) 22 μg 3 × weekly
PRISMS, 1998	IFNβ-1a (Rebif) 44 μg 3 × weekly
SPECTRIMS, 2001	IFNβ-1a (Rebif) 22 μg 3 × weekly
SPECTRIMS, 2001	IFNβ-1a (Rebif) 44 μg 3 × weekly
Clanet et al. 2002	IFN-beta 1a (Avonex) 60 μg weekly
The North American Study Group on Interferon beta-1b in Secondary Progressive MS, 2004	IFN-beta 1b 160 μg /m^2 /2. day IFN-beta 1b 250 μg /2. day

patients treated with IFNβ-1a (Rebif) when followed over 36–48 months (Gneiss et al., 2004; Sorensen et al., 2005). Thus it seems that tolerance is an earlier feature with the IFNβ-1b formulation than with the IFNβ-1a formulation. Antibody titre appears to be predictive, with lower NAB titres more likely to revert to a NAB-negative state (Rice et al., 1999; Gneiss et al., 2004).

Influence of dosage and route of administration

It is difficult to separate the relative influence of the (i) dosage frequency, (ii) total weekly dosage and (iii) method of administration from the present available evidence.

Intramuscular administration (im) of IFNβ-1b once weekly at 250 μg delayed the appearance and reduced the levels of BABs detected by ELISA when compared to the standard regime (Perini et al., 2001). However, NABs were present in 41% of patients treated with repeated im IFNβ-1b and 38% of those treated by the subcutaneous route (The IFNB Multiple Sclerosis Study Group, 1993; The IFNB Multiple Sclerosis Study Group and The University of British Columbia MS/MRI Analysis Group, 1996). IFNβ-1a (Rebif) 22 μg administered subcutaneously (sc) once weekly was significantly less immunogenic than three times weekly (Ross et al., 2000). However, IFNβ-1a (Rebif) 22 μg im once or twice weekly was not obviously different to conventional treatment (Perini et al., 2001; Bertolotto A et al., 2002). No effect on antibody

frequency was seen with two different doses of IFNβ-1b (1.6 and 8 MIU). An increase in NAB frequency was seen with an increased dose of Avonex (Clanet et al., 2002). However, the higher dose of IFNβ-1a (Rebif 44 μg) was associated with a lower proportion of patients developing NABs than on the lower dose (22 μg) in the pivotal relapsing–remitting and secondary progressive studies (see Table 8.1). The presence of a drug in the serum tested could reduce the sensitivity of the assay leading to an apparent but false reduction in antibody positive rates (von Wussow et al., 1989; Ross et al., 2000). Oddly, this Rebif dose effect was not noted in those two-year placebo patients who were subsequently randomized to either IFNβ-1a (Rebif) 22 or 44 μg, nor in the EVIDENCE study where IFNβ-1a (Rebif) 44 μg three times weekly was associated with a high rate of NAB-positive patients (>20%) (Panitch et al., 2002). Thus doubt exists as to whether Rebif 44 μg really does stimulate less antibody production than 22 μg three times weekly.

Evidence regarding immmunogenicity

Overall, the immunogenicity of the recombinant IFNβ appears to be most influenced by the formulation itself although increasing the frequency of injections also appears to be important. The influence of the intramuscular versus the subcutaneous route appears minimal. The effect of different doses is less clear. There is general agreement that the IFNβ-1a (Avonex) is the least immunogenic. There is class I evidence that the majority of patients with two consecutive NAB-positive tests remain NAB-positive for more than 2 years, although a substantial number of patients, who become NAB-positive, may revert to NAB-negative status during continuous IFNβ 1b therapy.

Measurements of binding and neutralizing antibodies

Binding antibodies
A Pub-Med search using 'binding antibodies assay interferon beta' found that 21 of the 55 articles were relevant for detection of BABs with IFNβ treatment.

Although BABs against IFNβ are induced in a majority of such treated patients, only a subset develop NABs causing loss of bioactivity. As the method of NAB detection is cumbersome many laboratories use a simpler binding assay for screening purposes and only BAB-positive samples are further analysed by the NAB assay. The different assays can be divided into three basic methods: ELISA, Western Blotting (WB), and radio-immunoprecipitation (RIPA) or affinity chromatography (ACA) assays (Table 8.2).

ELISA methods
The ELISA methods most commonly used are direct binding (i.e. direct coating of test wells with IFNβ) assays or capture (i.e. coating of test wells with a capture anti-IFNβ antibody) assays. ELISA titres generally correlated only weakly with NAB titres, but BAB-negative samples measured by ELISA reliably predict NAB-negativity. Only one study compared different BAB assays and demonstrated that cELISA is superior to dELISA with respect to specificity for NABs and the correlation between the BAB and NAB titre.

Western blot
This method gave similar results to the ELISA and had a low false negative rate when screening for NAB positivity. BAB titres cannot be calculated using WB.

Affinity chromatography and radio-immunoprecipitation assay
The advantage of affinity chromatography assay (ACA) and radio-immunoprecipitation assay (RIPA) is that the antigen is in solution and, therefore, no epitopes are obscured by binding to a solid phase. Radioactive isotopes usage limits the use of these assays. Affinity chromatography was very sensitive with up to 97% of treated patients being BAB positive depending on the IFNβ preparation and time on treatment. In the RIPA no NAB-positive sample was negative and there was a moderate correlation with the NAB titre. RIPA state correlated better with MRI lesion burden change than NAB titres (Table 8.2).

Conclusion and recommendations
There are no existing recommendations on BAB assays. There is class 1 evidence that IFNβ BAB assays have a very high sensitivity and specificity, and can be reliably used for IFNβ antibody screening before performing a NAB assay (Recommendation Level A). Different BAB assays should be evaluated and compared using a large number of serum samples to identify the method with the best sensitivity and specificity for NAB detection (Recommendation Level B).

Neutralizing antibodies
PubMed was searched using the terms 'neutralizing antibodies interferon beta assay'. Thirty-four of 54 articles covered methods of NAB detection and were included. About 50% of patients who develop BABs also develop NABs. There is no standardized assay for NAB detection and, although the principle of NAB measurement is more or less unique, the materials used vary immensely between different laboratories.

Test systems
Almost all reported NAB assays used cultured cell lines responsive to IFNβ. Test samples are incubated with IFNβ prior to addition of the cells. If the test samples contain NABs, receptor activation is blocked and antiviral proteins will not be induced.

Table 8.2 Methods used for BAB detection: the ELISA method, the Western Blot (WB) method and the radio-immunoprecipitation (RIPA) or affinity chromatography (ACA) assays.

Method	Type* and concentration of IFN	Validation/cut-off	Reference
dELISA	IFNβ-1a or 1b/0.2 μg	Mean + 3x SD of normal	(Perini et al., 2004)
ELISA	IFNβ-1b/concentration not given	NAB (MxA induction)	(Kremenchutzky, 2003)
dELISA, cELISA	IFNβ-1a and 1b/1.5 μg/ml	NAB assay	(Pachner et al., 2004)
dELISA	IFNβ-1a/1b/human IFNβ	Mean + 3x SD of normal	(Bellomi et al., 2003)
dELISA	IFNβ-1b/1000 IU per ml	NAB assay	(Mayr et al., 2003)
dELISA	IFNβ/1 μg/ml	2x background of uncoated wells	(Slavikova et al., 2003)
dELISA	IFNβ-1a/1 μg/ml IFNβ/1.2 μg/ml	Mean + 3 $\times$ SD of baseline sera	(Monzani et al., 2002)
dELISA	IFNβ-1a/1 μg/ml	3x OD of background	(Vallittu et al., 2002)
dELISA	IFNβ-1a and 1b/1 μg/ml	Arbitrary (OD > 0.5)	(Fernandez et al., 2001)
Affinity chromatography	Radio-labelled IFNβ-1a/3000 cpm	Mean + 3x SD of controls	(Ross et al., 2000)
cELISA	IFNβ-1a and 1b/10^4 U/ml	Standard curve†	(Kivisakk et al., 2000)
dELISA	IFNβ-1a and 1b/1–312ng per well	Mean + 2x SD of controls	(Antonelli et al., 1999)
WB, dELISA	IFNβ-1b/5000IU/well (ELISA) IFNβ-1b/2.5 μg per gel	NAB assay/detection limit of WB	(Deisenhammer et al., 1999)
dELISA	IFNβ-1b/2 μg/ml	Control placebo samples/ 39 binding units	(Pungor et al., 1998)
dELISA	IFNβ-1a and 1b/1000 IU per ml	Mean of control + 2x SD	(Khan and Dhib-Jalbut1998)
dELISA	IFNβ-1b/1 μg/ml	Mean of control + 3x SD	(Ferrarini et al., 1998)
RIPA	Radio-labelled IFNβ-1a and 1b/10 μg	NAB assay/mean of control + 3x SD	(Lawrence et al., 2003) (Lampasona et al., 2003)

dELISA: direct enzyme-linked immunosorbent assay; cELISA: capture ELISA; WB: western blot; RIPA: Radio-immunoprecipitation assay. *This column refers to the antigen used in the assay. IFNβ-1a is a recombinant human glycosilated IFNβ preparation whereas IFNβ-1b is not glycosilated. †For the standard curve an internal positive control was used which in turn was compared to a WHO reference antibody (G038-501-572).

In most cases, one of two different methods are used: either to measure the antiviral effect of IFNβ by challenging the cells with viruses, that is, the CPE, or to measure IFNβ induced gene products, namely the MxA protein (a specific marker of class 1 IFNs), that is, the MxA induction assay. The assays vary with respect to several variables including the cell line, the virus, the IFNβ preparations and dosage, the incubation times, and the methods of MxA detection (Table 8.3).

A few alternative methods have been reported. Measurement of IFNβ bioactivity showed that NAB-positive patients had significantly lower levels of in vivo IFNβ inducible genes at the mRNA and protein level. Although the different markers were not compared to each other directly, MxA

mRNA appears to be the most sensitive and specific marker of NABs. Low MxA levels indicated the presence of NABs.

Validation

The MxA induction assay is one of the most thoroughly validated NAB assays and has been used by several authors. It was validated using a CPE assay as gold-standard and two different IFNβ preparations for cell stimulation were compared. Most laboratories use internal standards for quality controls. One of these standards is the reference IFNβ antibody (NIH code GO38-501 572) which has a defined neutralizing titre of 1:1700 against ten Laboratory Units (LU) of human IFNβ. In CPE

Table 8.3 Overview of assays for NAB detection showing cell lines, viruses, IFNβ preparations and doses, incubation times, and methods of MxA detection.

Type of assay (read-out)	Cells/Virus	IFNβ type/ concentration	Titer calculation/Cut-off for NAB positivity	Validation/QC	Reference
MxA protein	Human whole blood	Betaferon/1000IU/ml	MxA increase < 22.5ng/ml	NAB assay (Pungor et al., 1998) Standard curve with rMxA	(Kob et al., 2003)
MxA RNA	Human PBMC	Avonex, Betaferon, Rebif, therapeutic dose	MxA RNA < 132fg/ pgGAPDH	CPE assay (Bertolotto 2000)	(Bertolotto et al., 2003)
MxA protein (Meditest)	Human lung carcinoma cells (A549)	Betaferon 10 IU	>20 neutralizing units	CPE assay (Pungor et al., 1998)	(Polman et al., 2003a)
CPE	A549/EMCV	rIFNβ1a and 1b/10 LU	Kawade titer > 80	Internal positive and negative controls	(Monzani et al., 2002)
CPE/MxA protein by FACS	WISH/VSV PBMC	IFNβ-1a/10 experimental units	Titer > 20 for bioassay MxA protein < 2 × mean of baseline	Not stated	(Vallittu et al., 2002)
CPE	A549/EMCV	IFN type?/ 3,10,100 LU	% reduction of IFN activity		(Ross et al, 2000)
CPE	A549/EMCV	Avonex, Betaferon, Rebif/10 IU/ml	Kawade titer > 20	Internal positive and negative controls	(Bertolotto et al., 2000)
CPE	A549/EMCV	IFNβ-1a	Kawade/50% CPE		(Zang et al., 2000)
CPE	WISH/VSV	IFNβ-1b/100 IU/ml	Kawade titer > 20	Reference ab G038-501-572	(Kivisakk et al., 2000)
CPE	Sindbis virus	IFNβ-1a and 1b/ 20 U/ml	Kawade/10LU	Not stated	(Antonelli et al., 1999)
CPE	FL-cells/Sindbis virus	IFNβ?/10 U/ml	6 × serum dilution of EC50	Not stated	(Kageshita et al., 1999)
MxA protein	A549	IFNβ-1b (Betaser) 10 LU	Kawade > 20	CPE assay using EMCV	(Pungor et al., 1998)
CPE	Human fibroblasts/VSV	IFNβ1-a and 1-b/ 100U/ml	50% of CPE	Not stated	(Khan and Dhib-Jalbut, 1998)
CPE	A549/EMCV	IFNβ-1a/10 IU	Kawade, different cut-off values compared to neopterin as bioactivity marker	Internal positive and negative controls	(Rudick et al., 1998)
CPE	WISH/VSV	IFNβ-1a /10 EU/ml	Kawade/ titer > 4	Controlled for cell survival	(Abdul-Ahad et al., 1997)

Table 8.3 Contd.

Type of assay (read-out)	Cells/Virus	IFNβ type/ concentration	Titer calculation/Cut-off for NAB positivity	Validation/QC	Reference
CPE	FS-4 fibroblasts/ EMCV	Fiblaferon (natural IFNβ) and IFNβ-1a	NU as difference between original and remaining IFNβ activity	Not stated	(Fierlbeck *et al.*, 1994)
Cell proliferation	Melanoma cells		Relative reduction of proliferation		
Cell proliferation	Daudi cells	IFNβ 10IU	50% inhibition of proliferation	CPE	(Prummer *et al.*, 1996)
CPE	FS-4 fibroblasts/ EMCV	Fiblaferon (natural IFNβ)/100 U/ml	Neutralizing unit = one unit of neutralized IFNβ	Not stated	(Dummer *et al.*, 1991)
CPE	A549/EMCV	Betaser	Kawade		(Redlich and Grossberg 1989)
CPE	Human fibroblasts	Betaser	Serum dilution that reduces activity of 3 to 1 LU/ml/Once > 100 NU/ml or 3 consecutive times > 20 NU	Reference antibody no G023-902-527	

CPE: cytopathic effect; FACS: fluorescence activated cell sorter; LU: laboratory unit; NU: neutralizing unit; PBMC: peripheral blood mononuclear cells; EMCV: encephalomyocarditis virus; VSV: vesicular stomatitis virus.

assays cell viability and viral CPE controls are widely used.

Existing recommendations

The WHO expert committee on biological standardization published informal recommendations on measurement of antibodies to interferon in the technical report series No. 725 in 1985. The reference assay in this international study group used A549 cells and the encephalomyocarditis (EMC) virus but recommended development of simpler assays. For NAB assays the expert committee recommended that the following details should be reported: (1) final concentration of interferon and serum in the reaction mixture; (2) final volume in the reaction mixture; (3) the lowest final dilution of serum tested. For the calculation of the neutralizing titre the Kawade method was recommended. This method calculates the serum dilution that reduces the IFN potency from 10 LU/ml to 1 LU/ml (Grossberg *et al.*, 2001a).

Conclusion and recommendations

Measurements of binding and neutralizing antibodies against IFNβ should be performed in specialized laboratories (Recommendation Level A). Measurement of NABs with a validated CPE assay is still the gold standard. It is recommended that A549 cells are used with a fixed amount of IFNβ (the preparation used by the patient) for stimulation and serial dilution of the test sera. The stimulated cells can either be challenged with EMC viruses or MxA production determined. Standard curves should be obtained using increasing amounts of IFNβ until saturation is reached. The NAB titre should be calculated using the Kawade formula (Recommendation Level A).

Titres above 20–60 (depending on the IFNβ preparation used in the assay) are associated with a loss of IFNβ bioactivity (class I evidence). As the EMEA currently validates a NAB assay based upon the MxA production of A549 cells (MxA induction assay), it is recommended to use the EMEA protocol. (This recommendation is only based on class IV evidence, but consensus was reached to offer this advice as good practice). Validation of

simpler NAB assay methods is strongly recommended such as the vivo biological response to IFNβ administration (Recommendation Level A).

Clinical use of measurements of antibodies against IFNβ

PubMed was searched for 'IFNβ antibodies and multiple sclerosis'. Of the 236 articles searched 103 were original articles or review articles on antibodies against IFNβ or controlled clinical trials of IFNβ in which measurements of antibodies were performed. For assessment of the impact of NABs we selected controlled randomized trials of IFNβ in MS with blindly analysed NABs and controlled non-randomized studies with blind evaluation of NABs of at least 3 years' duration (Table 8.4). NABs usually appear as low affinity antibodies in small concentrations and later as higher affinity antibodies in larger concentrations. Therefore, whereas the effect on antibodies on the biologic response to IFNβ may be apparent after 9–12 months, the clinical consequences of neutralizing antibodies are usually not seen until 12–18 moths after start of IFNβ therapy. Hence, only trials of sufficient duration ($\geq$3 years) and blind evaluation of NAB status were graded as class I evidence for effects of NABs. Trials of less sufficient duration (2–3 years) and blind evaluation of NAB status were graded as class II evidence, and trials of inappropriate duration (<2 years) and/or no blind evaluation of NAB status were classified as class III evidence regarding clinical effects of NABs.

It has been common to classify patients as NAB-positive after two consecutive serum samples containing NABs in a titre of 20 or more ('once positive, always positive'). (The IFNB Multiple Sclerosis Study Group, 1993; The IFNB Multiple Sclerosis Study Group and The University of British Columbia MS/MRI Analysis Group, 1996). The use of this approach will invariably result in an underestimation of the clinical consequences of NABs in studies of 2 years or shorter. Therefore, methods that account for switches between NAB-positive and NAB-negative periods ('interval positive') theoretically provide a more accurate assessment of the clinical impact of NABs on relapse rate and MRI activity (Sorensen *et al.*, 2003).

Table 8.4 Effect of NABs to IFNβ on clinical and MRI outcomes in MS therapeutic trials†.

Study	IFNβ product	No. of patients	Duration	Relapse rate‡	MRI Activity‡	Disease progression‡	MRI Severity‡	Class (primary end-point)	Class (NAB evaluation)§
IFNB MS Study Group, 1996	Betaferon		3 years	+(*)	+(ns)	+(ns)	+(ns)	I	I
Rudick et al., 1998	Avonex		2 years	−(ns)	+(ns)	+(ns)	ND	I	II
PRISMS-4, 2001	Rebif		4 years	+(**)	+(***)	−(ns)	ND	I	I
SPECTRIMS 2001	Rebif		3 years	+(ns)	ND	ND	ND	I	I
Durelli et al., 2002	Betaferon/Avonex		2 years	+(ns)	ND	ND	ND	III	II
Panitch et al., 2002	Rebif/Avonex		48 weeks	+(ns)	+(***)	ND	ND	I	III
Polman et al., 2003a	Betaferon		3 years	+(**)	ND	+(ns)	+(**)	−	−
Sorensen et al., 2003	Betaferon/ Avonex/Rebif		5 years	+(**)	ND	+(ns)	+(ns)	III	−

†See text for selection of trials and for definition of the different clinical and MRI outcomes.

‡+ =outcome worse in the NAB-positive group than in the NAB-negative group.

− = outcome better in the NAB-positive group than in the NAB-negative group.

ND = not done

Statistical significance is given in parentheses (ns = not significant; * = $p < 0.05$;

** = $p < 0.01$; *** = $p < 0.001$)

§ I = trials of sufficient duration (>3 years) and blind evaluation of NAB status

II = trials of less sufficient duration (2–3 years) and blind evaluation of NAB status

III = trials of inappropriate duration (<2 years) and/or no blind evaluation of NAB status.

Effect of NABs on relapses

In the pivotal phase III trial of IFNβ-1b NAB-positive patients had significantly higher annual relapse rates during years 2 and 3 (1.08) than NAB-negative patients (0.56) ($p < 0.01$) and equivalent to patients given placebo (1.06). (The IFNB Multiple Sclerosis Study Group, 1993). In the pivotal phase III IFNβ-1a (Rebif) trial no significant difference in relapse rate was seen over the study duration of 2 years between NAB-positive and NAB-negative patients (PRISMS Study Group, 1998). But in the 2-year extension phase, NABs caused a clear reduction in efficacy on relapses (PRISMS Study Group, 2001).

There was no correlation observed between NAB status and relapse rate in patients treated for 2 years in the pivotal phase III trial of IFNβ-1a (Avonex) (Rudick *et al.*, 1998).

In the secondary progressive Betaferon study (Polman *et al.*, 2003a) the 'once positive, always positive' method showed that NAB-positive patients had a 45% increase in relapse rates ($p = 0.009$) when they switched to being NAB-positive compared to their prior NAB-negative state. However, relapse rates in NAB-positive patients showed only a trend ($p = 0.07$) to increase when the 'all switches considered' method was applied. Higher titres seemed to reduce the treatment effect more. In the secondary progressive IFNβ-1a (Rebif) study the relapse effect was reduced in NAB-positive patients (44 μg) such that the difference between NAB-positive and placebo patients was no longer statistically significant (SPECTRIMS Study Group, 2001). The INCOMIN-study (an open randomized study comparing IFNβ-1b (Betaferon) with IFNβ-1a (Avonex) reported that the frequency of NABs in patients with relapses was a little higher than in patients without relapses (Durelli *et al.*, 2002). The EVIDENCE study (open randomized comparison of IFNβ-1a (Rebif) with IFNβ-1a (Avonex)) continued only for 48 weeks making this study inadequate for assessing the clinical impact of NABs (Panitch *et al.*, 2002).

In a Danish nationwide prospective study, NABs were measured blinded for up to 60 months in 541 randomly selected patients (Sorensen *et al.*, 2003). The presence of NABs had a significant effect on relapse rates. In NAB-positive periods the annual relapse rate increased more than 50% compared with NAB-negative periods. Comparing NAB-positive to NAB-negative patients the median time to first relapse was significantly reduced by 244 days ($p = 0.009$), and the proportion of relapse free patients was significantly lower ($p = 0.0064$).

Effect on MRI outcomes

The pivotal study of IFNβ-1b (Betaferon) showed significantly more enlarging lesions in NAB-positive patients compared with NAB-negative patients during years 2 ($p = 0.03$) and 3 ($p = 0.01$) (The IFNB Multiple Sclerosis Study Group, 1993; The IFNB Multiple Sclerosis Study Group and The University of British Columbia MS/MRI Analysis Group, 1996). In the PRISMS study there was a trend over the first two years towards more MRI activity in NAB-positive patients (PRISMS Study Group, 1998). Over 4 years (PRISMS Study Group, 2001), NAB-positive patients compared to NAB-negative patients had a nearly fivefold increase in the median number of T2 active lesions ($p < 0.001$), and a 17.6% increase compared to an 8.5% decrease in MRI burden of disease ($p < 0.001$). In the pivotal study of IFNβ-1a (Avonex) a trend was seen towards more gadolinium-enhanced lesions in NAB-positive patients ($p = 0.062$) (Rudick *et al.*, 1998). Secondary progressive patients on IFNβ-1b (Betaferon) showed a higher percentage increase from baseline in T2 lesion volume in NAB-positive patients compared with NAB-negative patients ($p = 0.004$) (Polman *et al.*, 2003a). Despite the short duration of the EVIDENCE study it was apparent that NAB-positive patients had more T2 active lesions than NAB-negative patients ($p = 0.0004$) (Panitch *et al.*, 2002).

Effect of NABs on disease progression

None of the randomized studies were powered to detect a NAB effect on disease progression. In the pivotal IFNβ-1b study (Betaferon), however, a strong trend was seen towards an effect of NABs on the mean change in EDSS from baseline in the third year ($p = 0.083$) (The IFNB Multiple Sclerosis Study Group, 1993; The IFNB Multiple Sclerosis Study Group and The University of

British Columbia MS/MRI Analysis Group, 1996). NAB positive patients on high dose Rebif showed a near significant ($p = 0.051$) increase in the mean number of EDSS progressions compared with NAB negative patients in the 4-year PRISMS trial (Rice GPA, personal communication, poster presentation ECTRIMS 2000). The Danish study also showed a strong trend towards a higher mean EDSS in NAB-positive patients compared to NAB-negative patients at month 42 and 48, and towards shorter time to disease progression in NAB-positive patients ($p = 0.10$) (Sorensen *et al.*, 2003). Neither the SPECTRIMS study (IFNβ-1a (Rebif) (Li *et al.*, 2001), nor the study of IFNβ-1b (Betaferon) in secondary progressive patients found a significant difference between NAB-positive and NAB-negative patients (Polman *et al.*, 2003b).

Safety issues

The presence of NABs has not been reported to be associated with adverse events or toxicity.

Conclusions and Recommendations regarding the clinical use of NAB measurements

It is recommended that patients treated with IFNβ are tested for the presence of NABs during the first 24 months of therapy (Recommendation Level A). Measurement of NABs can be discontinued in those patients remaining NAB-negative during this period but should be resumed if disease activity increases (Recommendation Level B). There is class I evidence that the presence of NABs significantly hampers the effect of IFNβ on the relapse rate and on both active lesions and burden of disease seen on MRI. In patients with NABs, NAB measurements should be repeated at intervals of 3–6 months and therapeutic options should be re-evaluated (Recommendation Level A). Therapy with IFNβ should be discontinued in patients with high titres of NABs (e.g. titres >100 in patients using IFNβ-1b) and sustained at repeated measurements with 3–6 months intervals (Recommendation Level A).

Prevention and treatment of NABs

Steroids

Short pulses of steroids have been demonstrated to be safe, well tolerated and clinically effective for patients with MS. A clinical trial randomly assigned 161 patients to receive IFNβ-1b, either alone or in combination with 1 g of methylprednisolone (MP) administered monthly intravenously (iv) (Pozzilli *et al.*, 2002). Using an MxA assay it was found that there was a significant reduction in NAB development in patients treated with MP, when defined as titres $\geq 1 : 20$ on one occasion but not when defined as twice consecutively positive. There was no difference in the frequency of patients that developed NABs at high titres ($>1 : 100$). The development of NAB-positivity was significantly delayed in the MP group (Kaplan Meyer analysis, log-Rank test; $p < 0.05$ by month 6 of therapy). These results suggest that the chronic administration of steroids prevents or delays the formation of NABs, but does not reduce the titre in NAB-positive patients.

Other immunosuppressive agents

A number of clinical trials have been performed with either RR-MS or SP-MS patients to evaluate the use of IFNβ in association with an immunosuppressive agent (Patti *et al.*, 2001; Calabresi *et al.*, 2002; Fernandez *et al.*, 2002). However, the NAB data originating from these small studies are inconsistent and do not allow any definitive conclusion as to whether additional immunosuppression reduces NAB formation.

Switching IFNβ preparations or increasing the dose of IFNβ

One of the possible strategies to overcome the formation of NABs in MS could be the switching from one preparation of IFNβ to another, but unfortunately many studies have showed that NABs are cross-reactive between IFNβ-1a and IFNβ-1b (Khan and Dhib-Jalbut, 1998; Bertolotto *et al.*, 2000; Kivisakk *et al.*, 2000). Thus, switching to an alternative IFNβ preparation is not of clinical benefit for a NAB-positive MS patient.

It is well known that the amount of antigen to which an individual is exposed influences the magnitude of the immune response and that very large doses or repeated administrations of small amounts of antigen are often inhibitory in the production of antibodies (Dresser and Mitchison,

1968). However, at present, there is no evidence that increasing the dosage of IFNβ is of benefit to NAB-positive patients.

Other strategies

Plasmapheresis and immunoglobulins (IgG) might be considered as possible procedures to diminish NAB generation. At present, the effects of the IgG on blocking antibody production are widely accepted in patients with autoimmune diseases. However, IgG and plasmapheresis do not affect memory plasma cells (Rudick and Goodkin, 1999). Therefore, the concomitant administration of IgG or plasmapheresis may be useful in eliminating circulating NABs, but it would not be expected to impede the production of NABs once it has been triggered.

Conclusions and future considerations on prevention of NABs formation

Limited evidence is available on managements that reduce NAB formation to IFNβ in MS. One gram iv MP administration every month has been revealed to be safe and able to minimize the formation of NABs over time (Recommendation Level C). However, no effect has been observed in reducing the amplitude of NABs titres once NABs have been formed. Further studies are warranted to strengthen these results and to expand our knowledge in such an intriguing matter.

Principal recommendations regarding measurements of antibodies against IFNβ and the clinical use of NAB measurements

- BAB assays can be reliably used for IFNβ antibody screening before performing a NAB assay (Recommendation Level A).
- Measurements of binding and neutralizing antibodies against IFNβ should be performed in specialized laboratories (Recommendation Level A).
- Measurement of NABs should be performed with a validated CPE assay or an MxA production assay using serial dilution of the test sera. The NAB titre should be calculated using the Kawade formula (Recommendation Level A).

- Tests for the presence of NABs should be performed during the first 24 months of therapy (Recommendation Level A).
- Measurements of NABs can be discontinued in those patients remaining NAB-negative during this period but should be resumed if disease activity increases (Recommendation Level B).
- In patient with NABs, measurements should be repeated after 3–6 months (Recommendation Level A).
- Therapy with IFNβ should be discontinued in patients with high titres of NABs and sustained at repeated measurements with 3-6 months intervals (Recommendation Level A).

Conflicts of Interest

P.S. Sorensen has received honoraria for lecturing and advisory councils, travel expenses for attending meetings, and financial support for his department from Biogen Idec, Schering, Serono, TEVA, Sanofi-Aventis, Baxter, and Bayer. F. Deisenhammer has received personal compensation and research support from Biogen Idec, Schering, Serono, Aventis, and Medacorp. P. Duda has nothing to declare. R. Hohlfeld has received grant support and consutancy fees from Serono, Biogen Idec, Schering, and TEVA. K.-M. Myhr has received personal compensation from Schering, Biogen Idec, Serono, and Aventis. J. Palace has received honoraria for lecturing and advisory councils, travel expenses for attending meetings, and financial support for her department from Biogen Idec, Schering, Serono, and TEVA. C. Polman has received honoraria for consutancy, and for delivering lectures at scientific meetings from Biogen Idec, Schering, and Serono. C. Pozzilli has nothing to declare. C. Ross has nothing to declare.

References

Abdul-Ahad AK, Galazka AR, Revel M, Biffoni M, Borden EC (1997). Incidence of antibodies to interferon-beta in patients treated with recombinant human interferon-beta 1a from mammalian cells. *Cytokines Cell Mol Ther* **3**:27–32.

Antonelli G, Simeoni E, Bagnato F *et al.* (1999). Further study on the specificity and incidence of neutralizing antibodies to interferon (IFN) in relapsing remitting multiple sclerosis patients treated with IFN beta-1a or IFN beta-1b. *J Neurol Sci* **168:**131–136.

Bellomi F, Scagnolari C, Tomassini V *et al.* (2003). Fate of neutralizing and binding antibodies to IFN beta in MS patients treated with IFN beta for 6 years. *J Neurol Sci* **215:**3–8.

Bertolotto A, Malucchi S, Milano E, Castello A, Capobianco M, Mutani R (2000). Interferon beta neutralizing antibodies in multiple sclerosis: neutralizing activity and cross-reactivity with three different preparations. *Immunopharmacology* **48:**95–100.

Bertolotto A, Malucchi S, Sala A, *et al.* (2002). Differential effects of three interferon betas on neutralising antibodies in patients with multiple sclerosis: a follow up study in an independent laboratory. *J Neurol Neurosurg Psychiatry* **73:**148–153.

Bertolotto A, Gilli F, Sala A *et al.* (2003). Persistent neutralizing antibodies abolish the interferon beta bioavailability in MS patients. *Neurology* **60:**634–639.

Brainin M, Barnes M, Baron JC *et al.* (2004). Guidance for the preparation of neurological management guidelines by EFNS scientific task forces–revised recommendations 2004. *Eur J Neurol* **11:**577–581.

Calabresi PA, Wilterdink JL, Rogg JM, Mills P, Webb A, Whartenby KA (2002). An open-label trial of combination therapy with interferon beta-1a and oral methotrexate in MS. *Neurology* **58:**314–317.

Clanet M, Radue EW, Kappos L *et al.* (2002). A randomized, double-blind, dose-comparison study of weekly interferon beta-1a in relapsing MS. *Neurology* **59:**1507–1517.

Deisenhammer F, Reindl M, Harvey J, Gasse T, Dilitz E, Berger T (1999). Bioavailability of interferon beta 1b in MS patients with and without neutralizing antibodies. *Neurology* **52:**1239–1243.

Dresser DW, Mitchison NA (1968). The mechanism of immunological paralysis. *Adv Immunol* **8:** 129–181.

Dubois BD, Keenan E, Porter BE *et al.* (2003). Interferon beta in multiple sclerosis: experience in a British specialist multiple sclerosis centre. *J Neurol Neurosurg Psychiatry* **74:**946–949.

Dummer R, Muller W, Nestle F *et al.* (1991). Formation of neutralizing antibodies against natural interferon-beta, but not against recombinant interferon-gamma during adjuvant therapy for high-risk malignant melanoma patients. *Cancer* **67:**2300–2304.

Durelli L, Verdun E, Barbero P *et al.* (2002). Every-other-day interferon beta-1b versus once-weekly interferon beta-1a for multiple sclerosis: results of a 2-year prospective randomised multicentre study (INCOMIN). *Lancet* **359:**1453–1460.

European Study Group on interferon beta-1b in secondary progressive MS (1998). Placebo-controlled multicentre randomised trial of interferon beta-1b in treatment of secondary progressive multiple sclerosis. *Lancet* **352:**1491–1497.

Fernandez O, Mayorga C, Luque G *et al.* (2001). Study of binding and neutralising antibodies to interferon-beta in two groups of relapsing-remitting multiple sclerosis patients. *J Neurol* **248:**383–388.

Fernandez O, Guerrero M, Mayorga C *et al.* (2002). Combination therapy with interferon beta-1b and azathioprine in secondary progressive multiple sclerosis. A two-year pilot study. *J Neurol* **249:**1058–1062.

Ferrarini AM, Sivieri S, Buttarello M, Facchinetti A, Perini P, Gallo P (1998). Time-course analysis of CD25 and HLA-DR expression on lymphocytes in interferon-beta 1b-treated multiple sclerosis patients. *Mult Scler* **4:**174–177.

Fierlbeck G, Schreiner T, Schaber B, Walser A, Rassner G (1994). Neutralizing interferon beta antibodies in melanoma patients treated with recombinant and natural interferon beta. *Cancer Immunol Immunother* **39:**263–268.

Gneiss C, Reindl M, Lutterotti A *et al.* (2004). Interferon-beta: the neutralizing antibody (NAb) titre predicts reversion to NAb negativity. *Mult Scler* **10:** 507–510.

Grossberg SE, Kawade Y, Kohase M, Klein JP (2001a). The neutralization of interferons by antibody. II. Neutralizing antibody unitage and its relationship to bioassay sensitivity: the tenfold reduction unit. *J Interferon Cytokine Res* **21:**743–755.

Grossberg SE, Kawade Y, Kohase M, Yokoyama H, Finter N (2001b). The neutralization of interferons by antibody. I. Quantitative and theoretical analyses of the neutralization reaction in different bioassay systems. *J Interferon Cytokine Res* **21:**729–742.

Jacobs LD, Cookfair DL, Rudick RA *et al.* (1996). Intramuscular interferon beta-1a for disease progression in relapsing multiple sclerosis. The Multiple Sclerosis Collaborative Research Group (MSCRG). Ann Neurol **39:**285–294.

Kageshita T, Yamamoto A, Yamazaki N, Ishihara K, Ono T (1999). Low frequency of neutralizing antibodies against natural interferon-beta during adjuvant therapy for Japanese patients with melanoma. *J Dermatol Sci* **19:**208–212.

Khan OA, Dhib-Jalbut SS (1998). Neutralizing antibodies to interferon beta-1a and interferon beta-1b in MS patients are cross-reactive. *Neurology* **51:**1698–1702.

Kivisakk P, Alm GV, Fredrikson S, Link H (2000). Neutralizing and binding anti-interferon-beta (IFN-beta) antibodies. A comparison between IFN-beta-1a and IFN-beta-1b treatment in multiple sclerosis. *Eur J Neurol* **7:**27–34.

Kob M, Harvey J, Schautzer F *et al.* (2003). A novel and rapid assay for the detection of neutralizing antibodies against interferon-beta. *Mult Scler* **9:**32–35.

Kremenchutzky M (2003). Long-term evolution of anti-INFbeta antibodies in IFNbeta-treated MS patients: the London, Canada, MS Clinic experience. *Neurology* **61:**S29–S30.

Larocca AP, Leung SC, Marcus SG, Colby CB, Borden EC (1989). Evaluation of neutralizing antibodies in patients treated with recombinant interferon-beta ser. *J Interferon Res* **9(Suppl 1):**S51–S60.

Lampasona V, Rio J, Franciotta D, Furlan R, Avolio C, Fazio R, Lavolpe V, Vincent A, Comi G, Trojano M, Montalban X, Martino G (2003). Serial immunoprecipitation assays for interferon–(IFN)-beta antibodies in multiple sclerosis patients. *Eur Cytokine Netw* **14:**154–157.

Lawrence N, Oger J, Aziz T, Palace J, Vincent A (2003). A sensitive radioimmunoprecipitation assay for assessing the clinical relevance of antibodies to IFN beta. *J Neurol Neurosurg Psychiatry* **74:**1236–1239.

Li DK, Zhao GJ, Paty DW (2001). Randomized controlled trial of interferon-beta-1a in secondary progressive MS: MRI results. *Neurology* **56:**1505–1513.

Mayr M, Berek K, Deisenhammer F (2003). Evolution of interferon-beta binding antibodies in MS patients may predict development of neutralizing antibodies. *Eur J Neurol* **10:**462–464.

Monzani F, Meucci G, Caraccio N *et al.* (2002). Discordant effect of IFN-beta1a therapy on anti-IFN antibodies and thyroid disease development in patients with multiple sclerosis. *J Interferon Cytokine Res* **22:**773–781.

Pachner AR, Narayan K, Price N, Hurd M, Dail D (2004). MxA Gene Expression Analysis as an Interferon-beta Bioactivity Measurement in Patients with Multiple Sclerosis and the Identification of Antibody-Mediated Decreased Bioactivity. *Mol Diag* **7:**17–25.

Panitch H, Goodin DS, Francis G *et al.* (2002). Randomized, comparative study of interferon beta-1a treatment regimens in MS: The EVIDENCE Trial. *Neurology* **59:**1496–1506.

Patti F, Cataldi ML, Nicoletti F *et al.* (2001). Combination of cyclophosphamide and interferon-beta halts progression in patients with rapidly transitional multiple sclerosis. *J Neurol Neurosurg Psychiatry* **71:**404–407.

Perini P, Facchinetti A, Bulian P *et al.* (2001). Interferon-beta (INF-beta) antibodies in interferon-beta1a- and interferon-beta1b-treated multiple sclerosis patients. Prevalence, kinetics, cross-reactivity, and factors enhancing interferon-beta immunogenicity in vivo. *Eur Cytokine Netw* **12:**56–61.

Perini P, Calabrese M, Biasi G, Gallo P (2004). The clinical impact of interferon beta antibodies in relapsing-remitting MS. *J Neurol* **251:**305–309.

Polman C, Kappos L, White R *et al.* (2003a). Neutralizing antibodies during treatment of secondary progressive MS with interferon beta-1b. *Neurology* **60:**37–43.

Polman CH, Kappos L, Petkau J, Thompson A (2003b). Neutralising antibodies to interferon beta during the treatment of multiple sclerosis. *J Neurol Neurosurg Psychiatry* **74:**1162–1163.

Pozzilli C, Antonini G, Bagnato F *et al.* (2002). Monthly corticosteroids decrease neutralizing antibodies to IFN-beta1b: a randomized trial in multiple sclerosis. *J Neurol* **249:**50–56.

PRISMS (Prevention of Relapses and Disability by Interferon beta-1a Subcutaneously in Multiple Sclerosis) Study Group (1998). Randomised double-blind placebo-controlled study of interferon beta-1a in relapsing/remitting multiple sclerosis. *Lancet* **352:**1498–1504.

PRISMS Study Group (2001). PRISMS-4: Long-term efficacy of interferon-beta-1a in relapsing MS. *Neurology* **56:**1628–1636.

Prummer O, Bunjes D, Wiesneth M *et al.* (1996). Antibodies to interferon-alpha: a novel type of autoantibody occurring after allogeneic bone marrow transplantation. *Bone Marrow Transplant* **17:**617–623.

Pungor E, Files JG, Gabe JD*et al.* (1998). A novel bioassay for the determination of neutralizing antibodies to IFN-ß1b. *J Interferon Cytokine Res* **18:**1025–1030.

Redlich PN, Grossberg SE (1989). Analysis of antigenic domains on natural and recombinant human IFN-ß by the inhibition of biologic activities with monoclonal antibodies. *J Immunol* **143:**1887–1893.

Rice GP, Paszner B, Oger J, Lesaux J, Paty D, Ebers G (1999). The evolution of neutralizing antibodies in multiple sclerosis patients treated with interferon beta-1b. *Neurology* **52:**1277–1279.

Ross C, Clemmesen KM, Svenson M *et al.* (2000). Immunogenicity of interferon-beta in multiple sclerosis patients: influence of preparation, dosage, dose frequency, and route of administration. Danish Multiple Sclerosis Study Group. *Ann Neurol* **48:**706–712.

Rudick RA, Goodkin DE (1999). *Multiple Sclerosis Therapeutics*. Martin Dunitz, London, pp. 309–333.

Rudick RA, Simonian NA, Alam JA *et al.* (1998). Incidence and significance of neutralizing antibodies to interferon beta-1a in multiple sclerosis. Multiple Sclerosis Collaborative Research Group (MSCRG). *Neurology* **50:**1266–1272.

Runkel L, Meier W, Pepinsky RB *et al.* (1998). Structural and functional differences between glycosylated and non-glycosylated forms of human interferon-beta (IFN-beta). *Pharm Res* **15**:641–649.

Secondary Progressive Efficacy Clinical Trial of Recombinant Interferon-beta-1a in MS (SPECTRIMS) Study Group (2001). Randomized controlled trial of interferon- beta-1a in secondary progressive MS: Clinical results. *Neurology* **56**:1496–1504.

Slavikova M, Schmeisser H, Kontsekova E, Mateicka F, Borecky L, Kontsek P (2003). Incidence of autoantibodies against type I and type II interferons in a cohort of systemic lupus erythematosus patients in Slovakia. *J Interferon Cytokine Res* **23**:143–147.

Sorensen PS, Ross C, Clemmesen KM *et al.* (2003). Clinical importance of neutralising antibodies against interferon beta in patients with relapsing-remitting multiple sclerosis. *Lancet* **362**:1184–1191.

Sorensen PS, Koch-Henriksen N, Ross C, Clemmesen KM, Bendtzen K (2005). Appearance and disappearance of neutralizing antibodies during interferon-beta therapy. *Neurology* **65**:33–99.

The IFNB Multiple Sclerosis Study Group (1993). Interferon beta-1b is effective in relapsing-remitting multiple sclerosis. I. Clinical results of a multicenter, randomized, double-blind, placebo-controlled trial. *Neurology* **43**:655–661.

The IFNB Multiple Sclerosis Study Group and The University of British Columbia MS/MRI Analysis Group (1996). Neutralizing antibodies during treatment of multiple sclerosis with interferon beta-1b: experience during the first three years. *Neurology* **47**:889–894.

The North American Study Group on interferon beta-1b in Secondary Progressive MS (2004). Interferon beta-1b in secondary progressive MS: Results from a 3-year controlled study. *Neurology* **63**:1788–1795.

Vallittu AM, Halminen M, Peltoniemi J *et al.* (2002). Neutralizing antibodies reduce MxA protein induction in interferon- beta-1a-treated MS patients. *Neurology* **58**:1786–1790.

von Wussow P, Jakschies D, Freund M, Deicher H (1989). Humoral response to recombinant interferon-alpha 2b in patients receiving recombinant interferon-alpha 2b therapy. *J Interferon Res* **9(Suppl 1):**S25–S31.

Zang YC, Yang D, Hong J, Tejada-Simon MV, Rivera VM, Zhang JZ (2000). Immunoregulation and blocking antibodies induced by interferon beta treatment in MS. *Neurology* **55**:397–404.

CHAPTER 9

Use of anti-nerve antibodies

H.J. Willison,[a] N.E. Gilhus,[b] F. Graus,[c]
B.C. Jacobs,[d] R. Liblau,[e] C. Vedeler,[b] A. Vincent[f]

Abstract

Background Autoantibodies to a wide variety of neural components are frequently sought in the sera of patients with neurological diseases suspected to have an antibody-associated autoimmune basis. This is especially so for peripheral nerve and neuromuscular disorders, although recently there has been considerable growth in the application of anti-nerve antibody tests to central nervous system (CNS) disorders. Variations in assay methodology and availability are likely to exist throughout European diagnostic immunology centres, and inter-laboratory discrepancies in performance for some assays have been reported.

Objectives To investigate the availability of quality assurance schemes in monitoring assay performance that is currently largely unknown.

Methods In 1999, the European Federation of Neurological Societies (EFNS) commissioned a task force to conduct a questionnaire-based survey of assay availability, methodology and quality control issues amongst a sample of European centres. All 18 national representatives of the Neuroimmunology Panel within the EFNS were invited to estimate the service provision within their country, to which 12 panel members responded.

Results From these responses, it emerged that many different assays using a broad array of immunological detection techniques were being performed throughout European centres, involving over 20 separate antigens. With the exception of the estimation of anti-acetylcholine receptor (anti-AChR) antibodies for the diagnosis of myasthenia gravis, in 2000, there were no systematic quality assurance schemes available, this being conducted on an ad hoc basis, or not at all.

As quality is a central component of assay sensitivity and specificity, the task force concluded that there was an urgent need to introduce pan-European quality assurance schemes, based on provision of positive and negative test sera from a central source, in which all neuroimmunology laboratories should participate. Progress in this area since 2000 is reported. In addition, a summary table of tests with established methodology that

[a]University Department of Neurology, Institute of Neurological Sciences, Southern General Hospital, Glasgow, UK; [b]Department of Neurology, Haukeland University Hospital and University of Bergen, Bergen, Norway; [c]Service of Neurology, Hospital Clinic de Barcelona, Barcelona, Spain; [d]Erasmus Medical Center, Rotterdam, The Netherlands; [e]Hopital de la Salpetriere, Paris, France; [f]Department of Clinical Neurology, Institute of Molecular Medicine, John Radcliffe Hospital, Oxford, UK.

are widely regarded as clinically useful is appended to the report.

Objective

To evaluate service provision and quality assurance schemes for clinically useful autoantibody tests in neurology.

Background

Over the last 20 years there has been a steady increase in the use of anti-nerve antibody assays to aid diagnosis or research into neurological diseases thought to have an antibody-associated or antibody-mediated autoimmune basis (Quarles et al., 1990; Pestronk, 1998; Vincent et al., 1998, 1999; Giometto et al., 1999; Vincent, 1999; Willison and Yuki, 2002; Lang and Vincent, 2003; Honnorat and Cartalat-Carel, 2004). The range of antigens tested and their associated diseases includes nerve and neuromuscular junction disorders and paraneoplastic disorders affecting the central nervous system, as listed and referenced in Table 9.1. With respect to the use of the anti-AChR antibody assay to aid in the diagnosis in myasthenia gravis, the radioimmunoassay in standard use has been thoroughly validated for many years (Vincent and Newsom-Davis, 1985). Both non-commercial and commercial quality assurance schemes for laboratories to participate in are available. However, the procedures in place for quality assurance in the identification of antibodies that mark paraneoplastic syndromes and for anti-ganglioside antibodies are less well developed. Efforts have been made to produce standard protocols, exchange samples and run workshops in both these latter areas, as manifested by the Immune Neuropathy Cause and Treatment (INCAT) group (Willison et al., 1999) and the Paraneoplastic Neurological Syndrome Euronetwork (Coordinator B Giometti). Such studies have principally involved researchers and laboratories with a specialized interest in these fields rather than clinical laboratories performing routine screening.

The anti-neuronal antibodies associated with paraneoplastic syndromes, antiHu anti-Yo and anti-Ri (ANNA-1, PCA-1, ANNA-2 respectively), were initially demonstrated by immunohistochemistry of brain sections and more recently by blotting of recombinant proteins, as listed in Table 9.1. The clinical utility of these investigations is considerable, and the importance of accurate identification paramount to clinical decision-making. In addition, this spectrum of autoantibodies is the subject of important research developments. This has recently been discussed in a detailed workshop report (Graus et al., 2004).

The determination of anti-ganglioside and glycolipid antibodies has increasingly entered clinical practice over recent years (Willison and Yuki, 2002). Anti-glycolipid antibodies are associated with acute and chronic peripheral neuropathies and may be useful in the diagnosis of clinical subtypes of neuropathy. They are extensively measured by enzyme-linked immunosorbent assay, dot blot, and thin layer chromatography overlay (Zielasek et al., 1994; Willison et al., 1999; Alaedini et al., 2002).

Both anti-neuronal and anti-glycolipid antibody assays are being conducted in laboratories throughout Europe. Until recently, this has been without any externally or independently monitored quality assurance, although such a scheme is now available through Instand eV. (http://www.instand-ev.de/). To investigate the scale of this issue and to identify the perceived needs of neuroimmunology laboratories in assay availability and quality, we conducted a questionnaire-based survey of European neuroimmunology centres and here report and discuss the findings.

Methods

Under the auspices of the EFNS Scientific Panel on Neuroimmunology, an anti-nerve antibody Task Force was established to conduct the review. Eighteen national representatives were invited to participate in a questionnaire-based survey. The questionnaire requested information on (i) the availability of tests both within the individual's institution and nationally, (ii) an approximation of the number of tests conducted annually, (iii) the

Table 9.1 Range of antigens tested and their associated diseases.

Antibody specificity	Associated neurological disorders	Detection method	References
Anti-Hu (ANNA-1)	Subacute sensory neuronopathy, limbic encephalitis, brain stem encephalitis, paraneoplastic encephalomyelitis, chronic pseudo-obstruction	IMH/IMF, confirmed by WB on recombinant protein or neuronal extracts	(Dalmau et al., 1992; Lucchinetti et al., 1998)
Anti-Yo (PCA-1)	Paraneoplastic cerebellar degeneration	IMH/IMF, confirmed by WB as above	(Furneaux et al., 1990; Peterson et al., 1992)
Anti-Ri (ANNA-2)	Myoclonus/opsoclonus	IMH/IMF, confirmed by WB as above	(Luque et al., 1991)
Anti-Tr	Paraneoplastic cerebellar degeneration	IMH/IMF (requires fixed tissue),	(Graus et al., 1997)
Anti-amphiphysin	Stiff person syndrome, encephalomyelitis, subacute sensory neuronopathy	IMH/IMF (requires fixed tissue), confirmed by WB as above	(Folli et al., 1993; Saiz et al., 1997)
Anti-CV2/CRMP5	Cerebellar degeneration, encephalomyelitis, limbic encephalitis	IMH/IMF (requires fixed tissue), confirmed by WB as above	(Honnorat et al., 1996)
Anti-VGKC	Acquired neuromyotonia Limbic encephalitis (usually not paraneoplastic)	RIA	(Hart et al., 1997)
Anti-VGCC	Lambert-Eaton myasthenic syndrome, paraneoplastic cerebellar degeneration	RIA	(Motomura et al., 1995; Mason et al., 1997)
Anti-(TA) Ma2	Limbic encephalitis	IMH/IMF, confirmed by WB as above	(Voltz et al., 1999; Dalmau et al., 2004)
Anti-AChR, MuSK	Myasthenia gravis	RIA	(Vincent and Newsom-Davis 1985; Hoch et al., 2001)
Anti-GM1, GD1b (IgM) Anti-GM1 (IgG/IgM) Anti-GM2 (IgM)	Multifocal motor neuropathy, Motor forms of Guillain Barre syndrome Chronic motor neuropathy	ELISA, TLC	(Yuki et al., 1990; Pestronk 1998; O'Hanlon et al., 2000)
Anti-GD1a (IgG)	Acute motor axonal neuropathy	ELISA, TLC	(Ho et al., 1999)
Anti-GD1b and other disialylated gangliosides (IgM)	Paraproteinaemic neuropathies CANOMAD	ELISA, TLC	(Willison et al., 2001; Serrano-Munuera et al., 2002)
Anti-MAG/SGPG (IgM)	IgM paraproteinaemic neuropathy	WB of CNS myelin, ELISA	(Weiss et al., 1999)
Anti-GAD	Stiff person syndrome/cerebellar ataxia	IMH/IMF (requires fixed tissue), confirmed by WB, RIA	(Solimena et al., 1990; Saiz et al., 1997)

IMH/IMF: immunohistochemistry/immunofluorescence; WB: western blot; requires fixed tissue: requires paraformaldehyde fixed tissue; RIA: radioimmunoassay; TLC: thin layer chromatography overlay; ELISA: enzyme-linked immunosorbent assay; MAG: myelin associated glycoprotein; SGPG: sulphated glucuronyl paragloboside; CANOMAD: chronic ataxic neuropathy, ophthalmoplegia, M protein, cold agglutinins, anti-disialosyl antibodies; VGCC: voltage-gated calcium channels; VGKC: voltage-gated potassium channel; Ach-R: acetyl-choline receptor; MuSK: muscle specific kinase; GAD: glutamic acid decarboxylase.

methodology used, (iv) the availability of quality assurance schemes, (v) the availability of positive and negative control sera, and (vi) the interest in setting up and participating in a pan-European quality assurance scheme. Communication in the task force group was mainly through e-mail and consensus was obtained through e-mail revisions and modifications of the manuscript.

Results

The questionnaire was distributed to 18 national members of the EFNS Scientific Panel on Neuroimmunology, of which 12 responded. The range of assays being conducted is summarized in Table 9.1, as are the associated neurological disorders and key references. Antibody assays for anti-AChR antibodies are widely available, being conducted in at least one centre in most of the countries that responded (10 of 12). Quality assurance schemes were used either nationally or internationally and the exclusive method used was the standard radioimmunoassay, using iodinated bungarotoxin bound to acetylcholine receptors extracted either from muscle or from muscle-like cell lines. Commercial kits are available for AChR and MuSK antibodies from RSR Ltd, Cardiff, UK.

Antibodies to glutamic acid decarboxylase (GAD), found in autoimmune stiff person syndrome (Saiz et al., 1997), were conducted in 5 of 12 neuroimmunology laboratories in responding countries and estimated using a variety of methods including immunohistology, ELISA, radioimmunoassay and Western blot. At present it is difficult to compare values between different laboratories despite the use of International Units in some cases. Because these assays are designed principally for use in investigation of diabetes, and because titres are much higher in stiff person syndrome and some cases of cerebellar ataxia than in diabetes, it will be important to ensure that laboratories performing this test for neurological disorders use techniques designed to measure high titres.

Antibody assays to voltage gated calcium channels (VGCC) and potassium channels (VGKC) were rarely conducted, being available in three and one surveyed centres, respectively. A commercial kit for the VGCC test is now available (RSR Ltd, Cardiff, UK) and results from different laboratories should be comparable.

Antibody assays for Hu (ANNA-1) and Yo (APCA-1) were widely available and frequently conducted in many centres in most countries (9 of 12), using a combination of immunohistochemistry and western blot analysis. Anti-Ri (ANNA-2), -Tr and -amphiphysin antibodies were sought less frequently. The less frequent paraneoplastic antibodies, anti-Ma, anti-Ta and anti-CV2/CRMP5, can also be detected by immunohistochemistry, but in many cases fixed rather than fresh frozen tissue is required, and not all laboratories do this routinely. There is a need to distribute positive sera to help in the recognition of these antibodies. It is likely that there will be increasing use of comprehensive commercial immunoblots such as that marketed by Ravo-Diagnostika (Freiburg, Germany) that detects six different paraneoplastic antibodies.

Anti-myelin-associated glycoprotein (MAG) antibodies were determined in laboratories in at least one centre in 7 of 12 countries, using a commercial kit that has good standardization (Buhlmann Laboratories, Basel, Switzerland), or using western blot of myelin. Measurement of anti-ganglioside antibodies was also widely available in many centres and included a wide range of gangliosides and glycolipids (e.g. GM1, GM2, GA1, GD1a, GD1b, GQ1b and sulphatides), but the details of the ELISAs used differ considerably between laboratories (Zielasek et al., 1994; Willison et al., 1999; Alaedini et al., 2002; Kaida et al., 2004; Hirakawa et al., 2005).

In response to questions on quality assurance, most of the centres reported that they conducted in-house quality assurance, although information on their precise nature was not sought. However, the only assay in which national or international quality assurance was extensively followed was the anti-AChR antibody assay. With respect to quality assurance schemes for other antigens, all laboratories indicated that they would join a quality assurance scheme for at least some, if not all, the investigations they were conducting.

Discussion and Good Practice Points

It is evident from this survey that a wide variety of antibody assays used in the diagnosis of neuroimmunological diseases are being conducted in many centres throughout Europe. This survey was restricted to major antigens and their respective antibodies, but did not consider the very wide array of emerging tests that have yet to be fully validated for clinical utility. This represents a healthy perception of the value of such investigations amongst clinical neurologists, but also highlights the need for a high degree of inter-laboratory uniformity and standards of practice.

A number of co-operative inter-laboratory studies have previously been conducted through distribution of coded positive and negative samples to participating laboratories. These have demonstrated marked variations in the ability to detect accurately positive or negative samples for both anti-ganglioside antibodies and antibodies marking paraneoplastic syndromes, particularly for borderline samples. This particular issue was not addressed in this survey. However, information was sought on methodology and in this context it is evident that methodologies being used vary quite widely amongst different laboratories.

The most striking finding of this survey was the lack of organized quality assurance schemes for the great majority of these autoantibodies, the exception being for anti-AChR antibodies, and more recently some anti-neuronal and anti-glycolipid antibodies. The survey indicated a very strong demand for such quality assurance schemes to be instituted. The mechanism by which such schemes should be organized is a matter for debate. Our Good Practice Points are thus summarized as follows:

GOOD PRACTICE POINTS

1. The determination of anti-neuronal antibodies should be conducted using protocols agreed during the course of multi-centre comparative studies, such as the INCAT study for anti-glycolipid antibodies.

2. Laboratories conducting immunoassays for anti-AChR antibodies should join existing quality assurance schemes.

3. Where no official scheme is available (i.e. for the majority of assays covered in this survey) laboratories should develop arrangements for exchanging coded positive and negative samples at least biannually, to ensure sensitivity and specificity are being maintained.

4. A quality assurance scheme for the most commonly measured anti-glycolipid antibodies (GM1 and GQ1b) and paraneoplastic antibodies (Hu and Yo) should be established as a matter of priority (this has now been done).

5. The EFNS should consider how open access quality control schemes in Europe are best established, both for laboratory and other measures, and should actively promote such schemes.

Conflict of interest

Angela Vincent and Clinical Neurology, Oxford, receive royalties from the sale of AChR, VGCC and MuSK antibody kits, and VGCC, MuSK and VGKC antibody tests by Athena Diagnostics. No other conflict of interest was reported.

References

Alaedini A, Briani C, Wirguin I, Siciliano G, D'Avino C, Latov N (2002). Detection of anti-ganglioside antibodies in Guillain–Barre syndrome and its variants by the agglutination assay. *J Neurol Sci* **196(1–2):**41–44.

Chiba A, Kusunoki S, Shimizu T, Kanazawa I (1992). Serum IgG antibody to ganglioside GQ1b is a possible marker of Miller Fisher syndrome. *Ann Neurol* **31(6):**677–679.

Dalmau J, Graus F, Rosenblum MK, Posner JB (1992). Anti-Hu–associated paraneoplastic encephalomyelitis/sensory neuronopathy. A clinical study of 71 patients. *Medicine (Baltimore)* **71(2):**59–72.

Dalmau J, Graus F, Villarejo A, Posner JB, Blumenthal D, Thiessen B, Saiz A, Meneses P, Rosenfeld MR (2004). Clinical analysis of anti-Ma2-associated encephalitis. *Brain* **127(Pt 8):**1831–1844.

Folli F, Solimena M, Cofiell R, Austoni M, Tallini G, Fassetta G, Bates D, Cartlidge N, Bottazzo GF, Piccolo G (1993). Autoantibodies to a 128-kd synaptic protein in three women with the stiff-man syndrome and breast cancer. *N Engl J Med* **328(8):**546–551.

Furneaux HM, Rosenblum MK, Dalmau J, Wong E, Woodruff P, Graus F, Posner JB (1990). Selective expression of Purkinje-cell antigens in tumor tissue from patients with paraneoplastic cerebellar degeneration. *N Engl J Med* **322(26):**1844–1851.

Giometto B, Taraloto B, Graus F (1999). Autoimmunity in paraneoplastic neurological syndromes. *Brain Pathol* **9(2):**261–273.

Graus F, Dalmau J, Valldeoriola F, Ferrer I, Rene R, Marin C, Vecht CJ, Arbizu T, Targa C, Moll JW (1997). Immunological characterization of a neuronal antibody (anti-Tr) associated with paraneoplastic cerebellar degeneration and Hodgkin's disease. *J Neuroimmunol* **74(1–2):**55–61.

Graus F, Delattre JY, Antoine JC, Dalmau J, Giometto B, Grisold W, Honnorat J, Smitt PS, Vedeler C, Verschuuren JJ, Vincent A, Voltz R (2004). Recommended diagnostic criteria for paraneoplastic neurological syndromes. *J Neurol Neurosurg Psychiatry* **75(8):**1135–1140.

Hart IK, Waters C, Vincent A, Newland C, Beeson D, Pongs O, Morris C, Newsom-Davis J (1997). Autoantibodies detected to expressed K+ channels are implicated in neuromyotonia. *Ann Neurol* **41(2):**238–246.

Hirakawa M, Morita D, Tsuji S, Kusunoki S (2005). Effects of phospholipids on antiganglioside antibody reactivity in GBS. *J Neuroimmunol* **159(1–2):**129–132.

Ho TW, Willison HJ, Nachamkin I, Li CY, Veitch J, Ung H, Wang GR, Liu RC, Cornblath DR, Asbury AK, Griffin JW, McKhann GM (1999). Anti-GD1a antibody is associated with axonal but not demyelinating forms of Guillain–Barre syndrome. *Ann Neurol* **45(2):**168–173.

Hoch W, McConville J, Helms S, Newsom-Davis J, Melms A, Vincent A (2001). Auto-antibodies to the receptor tyrosine kinase MuSK in patients with myasthenia gravis without acetylcholine receptor antibodies. *Nat Med* **7(3):**365–368.

Honnorat J, Antoine JC, Derrington E, Aguera M, Belin MF (1996). Antibodies to a subpopulation of glial cells and a 66 kDa developmental protein in patients with paraneoplastic neurological syndromes. *J Neurol Neurosurg Psychiatry* **61(3):**270–278.

Honnorat J, Cartalat-Carel S (2004). Advances in paraneoplastic neurological syndromes. *Curr Opin Oncol* **16(6):**614–620.

Kaida K, Morita D, Kanzaki M, Kamakura K, Motoyoshi K, Hirakawa M, Kusunoki S (2004). Ganglioside complexes as new target antigens in Guillain–Barre syndrome. *Ann Neurol* **56(4):**567–571.

Lang B, Vincent A (2003). Autoantibodies to ion channels at the neuromuscular junction. *Autoimmun Rev* **2(2):**94–100.

Lucchinetti CF, Kimmel DW, Lennon VA (1998). Paraneoplastic and oncologic profiles of patients seropositive for type 1 antineuronal nuclear autoantibodies. *Neurology* **50(3):**652–657.

Luque FA, Furneaux HM, Ferziger R, Rosenblum MK, Wray SH, Schold SC, Jr., Glantz MJ, Jaeckle KA, Biran H, Lesser M (1991). Anti-Ri: an antibody associated with paraneoplastic opsoclonus and breast cancer. *Ann Neurol* **29(3):**241–251.

Mason WP, Graus F, Lang B, Honnorat J, Delattre JY, Valldeoriola F, Antoine JC, Rosenblum MK, Rosenfeld MR, Newsom-Davis J, Posner JB, Dalmau J (1997). Small-cell lung cancer, paraneoplastic cerebellar degeneration and the Lambert–Eaton myasthenic syndrome. *Brain* **120(Pt 8):**1279–1300.

Motomura M, Johnston I, Lang B, Vincent A, Newsom-Davis J (1995). An improved diagnostic assay for Lambert–Eaton myasthenic syndrome. *J Neurol Neurosurg Psychiatry* **58(1):**85–87.

O'Hanlon GM, Veitch J, Gallardo E, Illa I, Chancellor AM, Willison HJ (2000). Peripheral neuropathy associated with anti-GM2 ganglioside antibodies: clinical and immunopathological studies. *Autoimmunity* **32(2):**133–144.

Pestronk A (1998). Multifocal motor neuropathy: diagnosis and treatment. *Neurology* **516(Suppl 5):**S22–S24.

Peterson K, Rosenblum MK, Kotanides H, Posner JB (1992). Paraneoplastic cerebellar degeneration. I. A clinical analysis of 55 anti-Yo antibody-positive patients. *Neurology* **42(10):**1931–1937.

Quarles RH, Ilyas AA, Willison HJ (1990). Antibodies to gangliosides and myelin proteins in Guillain–Barre syndrome. *Ann Neurol* **27(Suppl):**S48–S52.

Saiz A, Arpa J, Sagasta A, Casamitjana R, Zarranz JJ, Tolosa E, Graus F (1997). Autoantibodies to glutamic acid decarboxylase in three patients with cerebellar ataxia, late-onset insulin-dependent diabetes mellitus, and polyendocrine autoimmunity. *Neurology* **49(4):**1026–1030.

Serrano-Munuera C, Rojas-Garcia R, Gallardo E, De Luna N, Buenaventura I, Ferrero M, Garcia T, Garcia-Merino JA, Gonzalez-Rodriguez C, Guerriero A, Marco M, Marquez C, Grau JM, Graus F, Illa I (2002). Antidisialosyl antibodies in chronic idiopathic ataxic neuropathy. *J Neurol* **249(11):**1525–1528.

Solimena M, Folli F, Aparisi R, Pozza G, De Camilli P (1990). Autoantibodies to GABA-ergic neurons and pancreatic beta cells in stiff-man syndrome. *N Engl J Med* **322(22):**1555–1560.

Vincent A (1999). Antibodies to ion channels in paraneoplastic disorders. *Brain Pathol* **9(2):**285–291.

Vincent A, Newsom-Davis J (1985). Acetylcholine receptor antibody as a diagnostic test for myasthenia gravis: results in 153 validated cases and 2967 diagnostic assays. *J Neurol Neurosurg Psychiatry* **48(12):**1246–1252.

Voltz R, Gultekin SH, Rosenfeld MR, Gerstner E, Eichen J, Posner JB, Dalmau J (1999). A serologic marker of paraneoplastic limbic and brain-stem encephalitis in patients with testicular cancer. *N Engl J Med* **340(23):**1788–1795.

Weiss MD, Dalakas MC, Lauter CJ, Willison HJ, Quarles RH (1999). Variability in the binding of anti-MAG and anti-SGPG antibodies to target antigens in demyelinating neuropathy and IgM paraproteinemia. *J Neuroimmunol* **95(1–2):**174–184.

Willison HJ, O'Leary CP, Veitch J, Blumhardt LD, Busby M, Donaghy M, Fuhr P, Ford H, Hahn A, Renaud S, Katifi HA, Ponsford S, Reuber M, Steck A, Sutton I, Schady W, Thomas PK, Thompson AJ, Vallat JM, Winer J (2001). The clinical and laboratory features of chronic sensory ataxic neuropathy with anti-disialosyl IgM antibodies. *Brain* **124(Pt 10):** 1968–1977.

Willison HJ, Veitch J, Swan AV, Baumann N, Comi G, Gregson NA, Illa I, Zielasek J, Hughes RA (1999). Inter-laboratory validation of an ELISA for the determination of serum anti-ganglioside antibodies. *Eur J Neurol* **6(1):**71–77.

Willison HJ, Yuki N (2002). Peripheral neuropathies and anti-glycolipid antibodies. *Brain* **125(Pt 12):** 2591–2625.

Yuki N, Yoshino H, Sato S, Miyatake T (1990). Acute axonal polyneuropathy associated with anti-GM1 antibodies following Campylobacter enteritis. *Neurology* **40(12):**1900–1902.

Zielasek J, Ritter G, Magi S, Hartung HP, Toyka KV (1994). A comparative trial of anti-glycoconjugate antibody assays: IgM antibodies to GM1. *J Neurol* **241(8):**475–480.

CHAPTER 10

Use of skin biopsy in the diagnosis of peripheral neuropathy

G. Lauria,[a] D.R. Cornblath,[b] O. Johansson,[c]
J.C. McArthur,[b] S.I. Mellgren,[d] M. Nolano,[e]
N. Rosenberg,[f] C. Sommer[g]

Abstract

Background Skin biopsy has become a widely used tool to investigate small calibre sensory nerves including somatic unmyelinated intraepidermal nerve fibres (IENF), dermal myelinated nerve fibres, and autonomic nerve fibres in peripheral neuropathies and other conditions. Different techniques for tissue processing and nerve fibre evaluation have been used. In March 2004, a Task Force was set up under the auspices of the European Federation of Neurological Societies (EFNS) with the aim of developing guidelines on the use of skin biopsy in the diagnosis of peripheral neuropathies.

Methods We searched the Medline database from 1989, the year of the first publication describing the innervation of human skin using immunostaining with anti-protein-gene-product 9.5 (PGP 9.5) antibodies to 31 March 2005. All pertinent papers were rated according to the EFNS guidance. The final version of the guidelines was elaborated after consensus among members of the Task Force was reached.

Results and Conclusions For diagnostic purposes in peripheral neuropathies, we recommend performing a 3-mm punch skin biopsy at the distal leg and quantifying the linear density of IENF in at least three 50-μm thick sections *per* biopsy, fixed in 2% PLP or Zamboni's solution, by bright-field immunohistochemistry or immunofluorescence with anti-PGP 9.5 antibodies (Recommendation Level A). Quantification of IENF density closely correlated with warm and heat-pain threshold, and appeared more sensitive than sensory nerve conduction study and sural nerve biopsy in diagnosing small-fibre sensory neuropathy. Diagnostic efficiency and predictive values of this technique were very high (Recommendation Level A). Confocal microscopy may be particularly useful to investigate myelinated nerve fibres, dermal receptors, and dermal annexes innervation. In the future, the diagnostic yield of dermal myelinated nerve fibre quantification and of sweat

[a]Immunology and Muscular Pathology Unit, Department of Clinical Neurosciences, National Neurological Institute "Carlo Besta", Milan, Italy; [b]Department of Neurology, The Johns Hopkins University School of Medicine, Baltimore, MD, USA; [c]Experimental Dermatology Unit, Department of Neuroscience, Karolinska Institute, Stockholm, Sweden; [d]Department of Neurology, University of Tromsø, Norway; [e]Department of Neurology, Salvatore Maugeri Foundation, IRCCS, Center of Telese Terme, Italy; [f]Department of Neurology, Academic Medical Center (AMC), University of Amsterdam, The Netherlands; [g]Department of Neurology, University of Würzburg, Germany.

European Journal of Neurology 2005, 12:747–758

gland innervation should be addressed. Longitu-dinal studies of IENF density and regeneration rate are warranted to correlate neuropathologi-cal changes to progression of neuropathy and to assess the potential usefulness of skin biopsy as an outcome measure in peripheral neuropathy trials (Recommendation Level B). In conclusion, punch skin biopsy is a safe and reliable tech-nique (Recommendation Level A). Training in an established cutaneous nerve laboratory is recom-mended before using skin biopsy as a diagnostic tool in peripheral neuropathies. Quality control at all levels is mandatory.

Objectives

In the last decade skin biopsy has gained widespread use as a method to investigate small-diameter nerve fibres in human epidermis and dermis. In particular, this technique may be used to evaluate either qualitatively or quantitatively somatic unmyelinated intraepidermal nerve fibres (IENF). Skin biopsy can be used to evaluate abnor-malities in cutaneous innervation for diagnosis of neuropathy including those with the so-called 'pure' small fibre sensory neuropathy (SFSN), at dif-ferent stages of neuropathy, and in different types of peripheral neuropathies, including autonomic and demyelinating neuropathies.

A growing number of laboratories in Europe and the United States have been using skin biopsy in the diagnostic evaluation of patients with periph-eral neuropathy. However, different techniques for tissue processing and nerve fibre evaluation have developed.

The objectives of our Task Force were: (i) to eval-uate the techniques for performing skin biopsy and the choice of biopsy location; (ii) to eval-uate the methods for tissue processing and for quantification of IENF; (iii) to assess the diag-nostic performance of skin biopsy in periph-eral neuropathies; (iv) to compare skin biopsy with clinical, neurophysiological, psychophysical, autonomic, and sural nerve biopsy examination; (v) to recommend EU standards; and (vi) to pro-pose, if needed, new studies to address unresolved issues.

Search strategy

The Task Force systematically searched the Medline database from 1989, the year when the first papers reporting immunostaining of human skin with anti-protein-gene-product 9.5 (PGP 9.5) antibod-ies were published (Dalsgaard et al., 1989; Wang et al., 1990), to 31 March 2005. For each specific issue, we stored all the articles sorted by the Med-line search, omitted those that were not pertinent, and read and rated the remaining articles according to EFNS guidelines (Brainin et al., 2004). In some cases, the investigators were asked for original data and methodological details.

Method for reaching consensus

Data extraction was carried out and compared among each member of the Task Force. Discrep-ancies in each topic were discussed and settled during a consensus meeting held in Milan on 8 January 2005. The revised and final version of the guidelines is presented here.

Results

Methods to perform skin biopsy and choice of biopsy location

Skin biopsy was most commonly performed using a 3-mm disposable circular punch under sterile technique, after topical anaesthesia with lido-caine. No suture was required, and no side effects were reported. Healing was reported to occur within 7–10 days. Epidermis and superficial der-mis, including sweat glands, were taken. This technique was first developed at the Karolinska Institute (Wang et al., 1990), and later standard-ized at the University of Minnesota (Kennedy and Wendelschafer-Crabb, 1993) and at the Johns Hopkins University (McCarthy et al., 1995).

A less invasive sampling method is removal of the epidermis alone by applying a suction capsule to the skin. With this method, there is no bleed-ing, and local anaesthesia is not needed. How-ever, the method does not provide information on dermal and sweat gland nerve fibres. More-over, thus far it has not been systematically used to investigate patients with peripheral neuropathy.

This technique was developed at the University of Minnesota (Kennedy *et al.*, 1999).

In most studies on peripheral neuropathies, skin biopsies were obtained from the distal part of the leg (10 cm above the external malleolus), in some from the calf, and in many of them also from the upper lateral aspect of the thigh (20 cm below the anterior iliac spine). These locations were chosen to detect the length-dependent loss of cutaneous nerve fibres, which is typical of axonal polyneuropathy.

RECOMMENDATIONS

We emphasize that a 3-mm punch skin biopsy is a minimally invasive technique. It requires training and is safe as long as sterile procedures and haemostasis are correctly performed. For diagnostic purposes in peripheral neuropathies, we recommend performance of a 3-mm punch skin biopsy. In polyneuropathies, we recommend skin biopsy at the distal leg for quantification of epidermal innervation density. An additional biopsy from the proximal thigh may provide information about a length-dependent process (Level A).

Methods to process tissue and to quantify IENF

In neurology, punch skin biopsy was primarily developed to evaluate both qualitatively and quantitatively IENF immunostained by the cytoplasmatic neuronal marker PGP 9.5, an ubiquitin carboxyl-terminal hydrolase. Antibodies against specific cytoskeletal (i.e. tubules and microtubules) (Lauria *et al.*, 2004) and axonal membrane (i.e. $G_{\alpha 0}$) epitopes (Polydefkis *et al.*, 2004) label the same number of PGP 9.5-positive IENF, suggesting that targeted markers could be used to investigate sensory endings in peripheral neuropathies.

After the biopsy, the specimen is immediately fixed in cold fixative for up to 24 h at 4°C, then kept in a cryoprotective solution for one night, and serially cut with a freezing microtome or a cryostat. Each biopsy yields about 55 vertical 50-μm sections. However, the first and the last few

sections should not be used for cutaneous nerve examination because of possible artefacts.

In most studies, either 2% paraformaldehyde-lysine-periodate (2% PLP) or Zamboni's (2% paraformaldehyde, picric acid) fixative were used. In earlier studies (McCarthy *et al.*, 1996; McArthur *et al.*, 1998) tissue was fixed in formalin, which produced a more fragmented appearance of nerve fibres compared with PLP, without affecting the innervation density (Herrmann *et al.*, 1999; Lauria *et al.*, 1999). No study systematically compared IENF evaluations in peripheral neuropathies using the different fixatives, though Ljungberg and Johansson (1993) studied the influence of the immunohistochemical method, including the choice of fixative, on the procedure for visualizing neuronal markers in human skin.

Two immunostaining methods have been used: bright-field immunohistochemistry (Wang *et al.*, 1990; Hilliges *et al.*, 1995; McCarthy *et al.*, 1995; Holland *et al.*, 1997, 1998; McArthur *et al.*, 1998, 2000; Karanth *et al.*, 1989; Lauria *et al.*, 1998, 1999, 2001, 2003; Johansson *et al.*, 1999; Hilliges and Johansson 1999; Scott *et al.*, 1999; Herrmann *et al.*, 1999, 2004a, b; Polydefkis *et al.*, 2000, 2002, 2004; Hirai *et al.*, 2000; Chien *et al.*, 2001; Pan *et al.*, 2001, 2003; Smith *et al.*, 2001; Omdal *et al.*, 2002; Rajan *et al.*, 2003; Nodera *et al.*, 2003; Chiang *et al.*, 2002, 2003; Sumner *et al.*, 2003; Singer *et al.*, 2004; Shun *et al.*, 2004; Gøransson *et al.*, 2004; Li *et al.*, 2005; Koskinen *et al.*, 2005) and indirect immunofluorescence with or without confocal microscopy (Kennedy *et al.*, 1996, 1999; Kawakami *et al.*, 2001; Reilly *et al.*, 1997; Facer *et al.*, 1998; Periquet *et al.*, 1999; Novak *et al.*, 2001; Nolano *et al.*, 2001, 2003; Sommer *et al.*, 2002; Hoitsma *et al.*, 2002; Besné *et al.*, 2002; Perretti *et al.*, 2003; Pittenger *et al.*, 2004; Moura *et al.*, 2004; Hilz *et al.*, 2004).

In most studies using bright-field immunohistochemistry, at least three sections of 50-μm thickness from each biopsy were examined (figure 10.1). In confocal microscope studies, usually sections of 80–100 μm thickness were immunostained. Confocal microscopy allows analysing double, triple, and even quadruple stained sections, for example, with antibodies against PGP 9.5 and collagen IV to visualize axons and basement membrane to

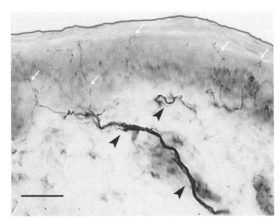

Figure 10.1. Quantification of IENF density using bright-field immunohistochemistry with anti-protein-gene-product 9.5 antibodies.
Arrows indicate IENF and arrowheads indicate dermal nerve bundles. The red line marks the length of the section. Linear IENF density (IENF/mm) is obtained dividing the number of IENF by the length of the section. Bar = 30 μm. See also Plate 10.1, pp. 120–121.

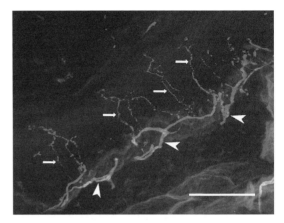

Figure 10.2. Projection of a stack of 16 optical sections of 2-μm thickness obtained by confocal microscopy from a triple-stained skin section.
Nerve fibres are stained in green (protein-gene-product 9.5), basement membrane and the blood vessels are stained in red (collagen IV), and endothelium and epidermis are stained in blue (ULEX-Europaeus agglutinin I). Arrows indicate IENF and arrowheads indicate dermal nerve bundles. The quantification is performed in 3D on the stack of optical sections using Neurolucida software. Bar = 50 μm. See also Plate 10.2, pp. 120–121.

trace IENF from the site where they penetrate the basement membrane to their endings (figure 10.2). Quantification of IENF density was performed on images based on the stack of consecutive 2-μm optical sections (usually 16 sections) for a standard linear length of epidermis (usually 1–3 mm). IENF may be evaluated either qualitatively or quantitatively.

For quantitative analysis, IENF are counted either under the light microscope at high magnification, that is, 40×, or using software for image analysis. In both methods, single IENF crossing the dermal–epidermal junction are counted, whereas secondary branching is excluded from quantification. No study provided information on the rules for counting IENF fragments. The length of the section is measured with computerized software (i.e., freely available at http://rsb.info.nih.gov/nih-image/index.html) and the linear epidermal innervation density is therefore calculated. IENF density is reported as IENF *per* millimetre (IENF/mm). A comprehensive review on methods and rules for IENF counting is available (Kennedy *et al.*, 2005) (figure 10.3).

Significant correlation with a stereologic technique (Stocks *et al.*, 1996) supported the reliability

of linear IENF density quantification under light microscopy (McArthur *et al.*, 1998). No systematic study comparing light and confocal microscope method was carried out. However, a recent meta-analysis (N. Rosenberg, 2005, personal communication) emphasized that sensitivity and specificity of IENF quantification in patients with SFSN were not influenced by different microscopy techniques and suggested that, for diagnostic purposes, confocal microscopy that is more complicated, expensive, and time-consuming is not required.

An alternative estimation method based on simple 'counting and calculating', without the aid of an image analysis system, has been used under light microscopy (Chien *et al.*, 2001; Pan *et al.*, 2001; Herrmann *et al.*, 2004b). This is based on the hypothesis that the epidermal length of specifically defined sections (i.e. the 19th, 25th, 31st) is close to the maximum diameter of the skin punch, namely 3 mm. The 'ocular IENF density' in the section is therefore calculated dividing the number of IENF by 3 mm. This method significantly correlated with conventional quantification

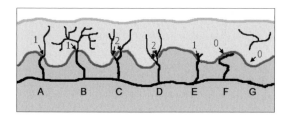

Figure 10.3. Intraepidermal nerve fiber counting rules
Diagram of skin innervation:
Nerves–black; Basement membrane–darkgray;
Dermis–medium gray; Epidermis–light gray

A. Count nerve as it crosses the basement membrane of the epidermis.
B. Nerves that branch after crossing the basement membrane are counted as a single unit.
C. Nerves that split below the basement membrane are counted as two units.
D. Nerves that appear to branch within the basement membrane are counted as two units.
E. Nerve fragments that do cross the basement membrane are counted.
F. Nerve fibers that approach the basement membrane but do not cross it are not counted.
G. Nerves fragments in epidermis that do not cross the basement membrane in the section are not counted.

From: Kennedy WR, Wendelschafer-Crabb G, Polydefkis M, McArthur J (2005). Pathology and quantitation of cutaneous nerves. In: Dyck PJ, Thomas PK. eds., Peripheral Neuropathy 4th edition Philadelphia: Saunders, 869–896.

of epidermal innervation density obtained by measuring the length of the section (Chien *et al.*, 2001).

One study (Hilliges and Johansson, 1999) compared three methods to quantify IENF density per projected area (IENF/mm^2) in 14-μm thick sections in 45 biopsies from healthy subjects: (1) the unbiased nerve fibre profile and nerve fibre fragment estimation methods, (2) the traditional method of counting whole nerve fibres, and (3) the nerve fibre estimation method. Comparative analysis showed a good correlation ($R > 0.96$) between the three numerical methods. It was emphasized that section thickness and nerve fibre shape could affect the count, and therefore always need to be separately analysed and corrected for in a pilot run before commencing any larger comparative study. This study is one of the very few examples where

an unbiased, correct, and efficient counting rule on vertical sections by design-based stereology and with a fixed reference space was utilized within this specific area of interest. Hilliges and Johansson (1999) concluded that reporting nerve fibre profiles counted per projected surface area is very useful for comparing results from different laboratories regardless of section thickness, shape or form.

Recently, Koskinen and co-workers (2005) compared the epidermal innervation density at the distal leg estimated per epidermal length with that calculated per epidermal area using a volume-corrected mitotic index that might correct the variations caused by optic factors, such as different high power microscopic fields between microscopes. The two methods showed a significant correlation coefficient.

The 'skin blister' method has also been used to quantify the innervation of the epidermis (Kennedy *et al.*, 1999). Blisters are obtained by applying to skin surface a suction capsule with single or multiple 2 or 3 mm holes depending upon the number and size of samples desired. A negative pressure induces the epidermis to separate at the dermal–pidermal junction without damaging the basement membrane and the underlying capillary loops. After removing the capsule, the blister roof is excised, fixed, and immunostained. Epidermal nerve fibre density is calculated in sampling areas (IENF/mm^2) using a grid to reduce the chance of double counting IENF. Counting includes secondary branching of fibres. This technique allows quantifying IENF in an area several times larger (up to 7 mm^2) than the surface of a single 3 mm section and offers a horizontal perspective that makes immediately apparent an uneven distribution of nerve fibres. The 'skin blister' method has been used in a limited number of patients and controls.

RECOMMENDATIONS

For diagnostic purposes in peripheral neuropathies, we recommend bright-field immunohistochemistry or immunofluorescence with anti-PGP 9.5 antibodies in 2% PLP or Zamboni's fixed sections of 50-μm thickness. For methodological issues on bright-field immunohistochemistry we refer to McCarthy *et al.*, (1995), on immunofluorescence to Wang *et al.*, (1990), and on confocal microscopy to Kennedy and Weldelschafer-Crabb (1993). IENF should be counted at high magnification (i.e. 40×) in at least three sections per biopsy. We emphasize that only single IENF crossing the dermal–epidermal junction should be counted, excluding secondary branching from quantification. The length of the section should be measured to calculate the exact linear epidermal innervation density (IENF/mm) (Level A).

Further studies are warranted to establish the reliability of the 'ocular' method (Level B) and the 'blister technique' (Level C) for quantification of IENF density in peripheral neuropathies.

Diagnostic performances of skin biopsy

Different normative range and cut-off values of IENF density in neuropathy patients have been reported using either bright-field immunohistochemistry or confocal microscope technique (Kennedy *et al.*, 2005). No systematic study comparing the two methods has been carried out. Therefore, data are presented separately. Skin biopsy was also used to investigate dermal myelinated nerve fibres in healthy subjects, and subjects with immune-mediated neuropathy (Lombardi *et al.*, 2005) and inherited neuropathies (Li *et al.*, 2005).

Bright-field immunohistochemistry

Normative data

Three large studies estimated the density of IENF in 98 (McArthur *et al.*, 1998), 106 (Gøransson *et al.*, 2004), and 55 (Pan *et al.*, 2001) healthy subjects ranging from 13 to 92 years. The density ranged from 13.8 ± 6.7/mm (mean ± standard deviation [SD]; lower 5th percentile 3.8) (McArthur *et al.*, 1998) to 12.4 ± 4.6/mm (mean ± SD) (Gøransson *et al.*, 2004) and 12.9 ± 5.3/mm (mean ± SD) (Pan *et al.*, 2001). Increasing age and male gender was independently associated with decreasing IENF density at the distal leg on multivariate analysis (Gøransson *et al.*, 2004). Similarly, Hsieh

and colleagues (Pan *et al.*, 2001; Chien *et al.*, 2001; Shun *et al.*, 2004) reported different normative values between subjects aged <60 years (11.1 ± 3.7/mm [mean± SD]; lower 5th percentile 5.8/mm) and >60 years (7.6 ± 3.0/mm [mean ± SD]; lower 5th percentile 2.5/mm). Conversely, McArthur and colleagues (1998) found no sex or age effect (except for higher values in the youngest subjects aged 10–19 years).

Mean IENF density at the proximal thigh, estimated in one of these normative studies (McArthur *et al.*, 1998), was 21.1 ± 10.4/mm (mean ± SD; lower 5th percentile 5.2/mm). This value did not differ from that found in smaller series (Holland *et al.*, 1997; Lauria *et al.*, 1999, 2003; Scott *et al.*, 1999; Smith *et al.*, 2001), which confirmed the presence of a decreasing gradient of epidermal innervation in the lower limb, with a density approximately 60% higher at the proximal thigh than at the distal leg. All these studies used the same method to estimate the linear epidermal innervation density, namely count of single IENF and measurement of exact section length. Overall, inter- and intraobserver agreement was generally high and supported the reliability of the method, as recently confirmed by an inter-laboratory study (Smith *et al.*, 2005).

Diagnostic yield

Two studies (McArthur *et al.*, 1998; Chien *et al.*, 2001) were specifically designed to assess the diagnostic performances of skin biopsy in peripheral neuropathies of different aetiology. Moreover, several smaller studies including 537 patients (McCarthy *et al.*, 1995; Holland *et al.*, 1997; Herrmann *et al.*, 1999, 2004a,b; Scott *et al.*,1999; Lauria *et al.*, 1999, 2001, 2003; Smith *et al.*, 2001; Chiang *et al.*, 2002; Omdal *et al.*, 2002; Polydefkis *et al.*, 2002; Pan *et al.*, 2003; Sumner *et al.*, 2003; Shun *et al.*, 2004) investigated the density of IENF in patients with peripheral neuropathies using the same technique. Most of them described a length-dependent loss of IENF with significantly lower density at the distal leg, reflecting the dying-back process typical of axonal neuropathies. A non-length pattern of skin denervation was found in sensory ganglionopathies (Lauria *et al.*, 2001).

McArthur and colleagues (1998) compared 98 healthy subjects (age 13–82 years) and 20 patients with neuropathy (diagnosis was based on a composite measure using the Total Neuropathy Score [Cornblath *et al.*, 1999]), whereas Chien and colleagues (2001) investigated 55 healthy subjects (age 25–73 years) and 35 patients with SFSN (diagnosis was based on clinical grounds and elevated sensory thresholds to warm and cold stimuli). Density of IENF below the lower 5th percentile was considered abnormal. Specificity (percentage of true negative) did not differ between the two studies (97 and 95%, respectively), whereas sensitivity (percentage of true positive) was higher in Chien *et al.* (80%) than in McArthur *et al.* (45%) study. The lower sensitivity in McArthur *et al.* (1998) might be due to the non-homogeneous group of patients in the study. The high specificity suggests that quantification of IENF density is a good tool to verify the presence of a neuropathy. This may apply to pure SFSN, in which clinical and electrophysiological examinations can be normal. Conversely, normal IENF density does not rule out the presence of sensory neuropathy.

A recent meta-analysis (N. Rosenberg, 2005, personal communication) focused on patients with possible SFSN and normal electrophysiological examination, including 161 patients from 9 studies (two of them based on confocal microscope technique). Using the cut-off values of the different studies, the sensitivity of IENF density assessment for the diagnosis of SFSN ranged from 69 to 82% with a specificity of 97%.

Koskinen and co-workers (2005) reported a diagnostic efficiency of 93% for idiopathic or secondary (diabetic,cytotoxic or amyloid)SFN (sensitivity of both methods was 90%, specificity 95%, positive predictive value 95% and negative predictive value 91%).

Immunofluorescence technique

Normative data

No study was specifically designed to assess the normative range of epidermal innervation density by indirect immunofluorescence with or without confocal microscopy. Overall, values were higher than those found using light microscopy technique. Normal values have been reviewed by Kennedy and colleagues in the new Dyck and Thomas textbook on peripheral neuropathies (Kennedy *et al.*, 2005).

Density of IENF at the distal leg, quantified in 81 healthy subjects included in five studies (Kennedy *et al.*, 1996; Periquet *et al.*, 1999; Nolano *et al.*, 2001; Hoitsma *et al.*, 2002; Pittenger *et al.*, 2004), ranged between 17.4 ± 7.4/mm and 33.0 ± 7.9/mm (mean $\pm$ SD) in subjects with age 20–59 years (lower 5th percentile 20.0) and was 20.1 ± 5.0/mm (mean $\pm$ SD) in subjects over 60 years (lower 5th percentile 11.8). The thickness of the skin sections analysed in these studies varied from 32 to 60 μm. With confocal microscopy, the most important variable that may account for the different results in IENF density is the number of optical sections used to create the image on which quantification is performed. Analysis of sixteen 2-μm optical sections taken by confocal microscopy from fresh fixed 60-μm frozen sections corresponded to the analysis of 50-μm sections after correction for shrinkage and compression.

One study (Nolano *et al.*, 2003) estimated the density of 11.3 ± 2.9 IENF/mm (mean $\pm$ SD) in the glabrous skin of fingertip in 14 healthy subjects (age 22–53). The authors also estimated a density of 59.0 ± 29.3 (mean $\pm$ SD) myelinated endings *per* square millimeter, with a mean diameter of 3.3 ± 0.5 (SD) μm and an internodal length of 79.1 ± 13.8 (SD) μm. The mean density of Meissner corpuscles in the fingertip of digit III was 33.02 ± 13.2 (SD) *per* square millimeter. No age effect was found, but a higher number of neural structures was observed in females related to a smaller fingertip surface, suggesting that spatial distribution of nerve endings might depend also on body growth.

Diagnostic yield

Data on IENF density in neuropathies come from a more limited number of studies, including 198 patients from five studies (Kennedy *et al.*, 1996; Periquet *et al.*, 1999; Novak *et al.*, 2001; Hoitsma *et al.*, 2002; Pittenger *et al.*, 2004). In all studies, IENF density was significantly lower in neuropathy patients than in controls. In 89 patients with SFSN and no electrophysiological abnormalities reported in two studies from the same laboratory (Periquet *et al.,* 1999; Novak *et al.,* 2001), density ranged between 9.2±6.2 and 14.9 ± 11.0 (mean ± SD). Median density was 5.4/mm in 7 patients with sarcoidosis-associated SFSN and no electrophysiological abnormalities (Hoitsma *et al.,* 2002). In 48 diabetic and non-diabetic neuropathy patients, IENF density was 17.5±3.3 (Pittenger *et al.,* 2004). IENF density was not altered in patients with diabetes of <5 years duration (37.4 ± 7.1/mm; mean ± SD), whereas it was significantly decreased in patients with >5 years duration (7.8 ± 7.1/mm; mean ± SD). These data are in contrast with previous studies showing reduced IENF density in patients with neuropathy and impaired glucose tolerance (Smith *et al.,* 2001; Sumner *et al.,* 2003).

Overall, cut-off values and mean densities quantified using confocal microscopy were higher than in light microscope studies. Nevertheless, sensitivity and specificity of skin biopsy in the diagnosis of SFSN, separately examined in the meta-analysis by Rosenberg and colleagues (2005, personal communication), were not influenced by different microscope techniques.

The median density of dermal nerve fibres in healthy subjects quantified by stereological methods at hand, upper arm, shoulder, back and thigh was 23.7/mm, with no significant differences between sites (Liang *et al.,* 1996). Dermal nerve fibres were never quantified in patients with peripheral neuropathy.

Morphological changes reflecting axonal derangement were reported in several case series. One study (Lombardi *et al.,* 2005) examined 14 patients with neuropathy associated with anti-myelin-associated glycoprotein (MAG) antibodies. All patients showed specific IgM deposits on dermal myelinated fibres, with a higher prevalence at the distal site of the extremities. Conversely, no patient with chronic inflammatory demyelinating polyradiculoneuropathy (CIDP) or IgM paraproteinemic neuropathy had deposits of IgM. These results suggest that skin biopsies can be a potential tool for investigating immune-mediated demyelinating neuropathies.

Recently, ultrastructure and myelin gene protein expression of dermal nerve fibres from finger and forearm of healthy subjects and patients with Charcot Marie Tooth disease (CMT) and hereditary neuropathy with liability to pressure palsies (HNPP) were investigated. This study demonstrated that dermal myelinated nerves not only show abnormalities previously detected in sural nerve biopsies, but also detect abnormal features not previously reported. Results suggest that biopsy of glabrous skin may be a potential tool to investigate the morphological markers of disease progression and the genotype–phenotype correlations in patients with demyelinating or dysmyelinating neuropathies (Li *et al.,* 2005).

RECOMMENDATIONS

Diagnostic efficiency and predictive values of skin biopsy with linear quantification of IENF in the diagnosis of peripheral neuropathy were very high (Level A). Immunohistochemical technique does not seem to influence the ability of skin biopsy to demonstrate SFSN. For diagnostic purposes or as outcome measure in clinical trials we recommend rigorous quantitative assessment with appropriate quality controls (Level B). Cut-off values for epidermal densities in studies based on immunofluorescence microscopy appeared to be higher than in bright-field microscopy studies. Thus far, only the bright-field microscope method was used to establish normative reference range and diagnostic performances. For quantitative purposes in evaluating peripheral neuropathies, we recommend determination of IENF density using either immunohistochemistry with bright-field microscopy or immunofluorescence (Level A). Appropriate normative data from healthy subjects matched for age, gender, ethnicity, and anatomical site should be used. Quality control should include all the steps of the procedure, in particular the aspect of intra- and inter-observer ratings.

Studies comparing the diagnostic yield of bright-field microscopy and immunofluorescence with

continued

and without confocal microscopy in homogeneous groups of neuropathy patients are warranted. We emphasize that confocal microscope technique may be useful to investigate cutaneous nerve fibres in demyelinating neuropathies. Furthermore, the diagnostic yield of dermal nerve fibre quantification needs to be addressed. Confocal microscope technique applied to glabrous skin allows investigation of dermal receptors and their myelinated endings and might provide morphological information that potentially enlarges the usefulness of skin biopsy in sensory neuropathies.

Assessment of morphological changes

Besides estimation of epidermal innervation density, several papers included morphological changes of both IENF (i.e. axonal swellings and branching) and dermal nerve bundles (i.e. weaker and fragmented immunoreactivity to PGP 9.5) among pathologic features in patients with peripheral neuropathy. Recently, two studies including 72 patients (Lauria *et al.*, 2003; Herrmann *et al.*, 2004b) investigated the diagnostic yield of IENF swellings in sensory neuropathies. Swellings were defined as enlargements either above 1.5 μm or twice the diameter of the parent IENF. Both studies found a significantly higher prevalence of swellings at the distal leg in neuropathies, including patients with normal IENF density and persisting painful symptoms in the feet, than in controls. Increased swellings at the distal leg correlated with impaired heat-pain threshold, development of symptomatic neuropathy, and progression of neuropathy.

Increased branching of IENF was also considered as a common feature in peripheral neuropathies (Kennedy *et al.*, 1996; Scott *et al.*, 1999; Herrmann *et al.*, 1999; Smith *et al.*, 2001). One study reported a significantly higher branching ratio (number of branch points/density) and normal density of IENF at the proximal thigh in patients with sensory neuropathy (Lauria *et al.*, 1999). Increased branching complexity in unaffected sites suggested that predegenerative changes might precede the loss of fibres. These data need to be confirmed by further studies.

Morphological abnormalities of dermal nerve bundles, such as fragmented immunoreactivity to PGP 9.5, were described in most patients with peripheral neuropathy. Nevertheless, no study designed to quantify the changes of either unmyelinated or small-myelinated nerve fibres was performed.

RECOMMENDATIONS

Quantification of IENF swellings at the lower limb could have a predictive value to the progression of neuropathy, especially if large (Level B). Further studies are warranted to establish whether increased IENF swellings could support the diagnosis of sensory neuropathy and whether this morphological change occurs earlier than decreased IENF density. Further studies are also needed to verify whether increased branching is an early diagnostic finding in peripheral neuropathy.

Quantification of sweat gland innervation

Several studies (Karanth *et al.*, 1989; McCarthy *et al.*, 1995; Kennedy *et al.*, 1996; Facer *et al.*, 1998; Nolano *et al.*, 2000, 2001; Perretti *et al.*, 2003; Pan *et al.*, 2003) described reduced innervation of sweat glands in patients with peripheral neuropathies using both PGP 9.5 and neuropeptide (substance P, calcitonin gene-related peptide, vasointestinal peptide) immunostaining. Two studies (Hirai *et al.*, 2000; Sommer *et al.*, 2002) quantified the density of sweat gland nerve fibres using different methods. Hirai and colleagues found decreased nerve fibre length around sweat glands in 32 patients with diabetic neuropathy. Sommer and colleagues reported significant correlation between anhidrosis and reduced sweat gland innervation *per* area in four patients with Ross syndrome.

Hilz and colleagues (2004) used a semi-quantitative approach based on a 5-degree rating scale (0 = normal, 1 = reduction <50% of normal density [mild], 2 = reduction >50% of normal density [moderate], 3 = sparse innervation, 4 = no nerve fibres) to classify sweat gland innervation in 10 patients with familial dysautonomia. One study

(Facer *et al.*, 1998) focused on leprosy neuropathy and found a correlation between reduced nicotine-induced axon-reflex sweating and decreased innervation of sweat glands. One study (Pan *et al.*, 2003) examined cutaneous innervation in Guillain-Barré syndrome (GBS). Though about 60% of patients had clinical manifestations of autonomic dysfunction, no correlation between sweat gland innervation and RR interval variability or sympathetic skin response was observed.

RECOMMENDATIONS

Data on sweat gland innervation density in healthy subjects and in patients with peripheral neuropathy as well as data on correlation between sweat gland nerve fibre density and autonomic assessment are limited (class III evidence). Although part of the neuropathologic examination of skin biopsy, assessment of sweat gland innervation still lacks extensive validation.

Correlation between IENF density and clinical, neurophysiological, psycho-physical, autonomic, and sural nerve biopsy examinations
Correlation with clinical measures of neuropathy

Only a few studies correlated epidermal innervation density to validated clinical scales. Decrease in IENF density correlated with progression of neuropathy and duration of diabetes (Holland *et al.*, 1997; Lauria *et al.*, 2003; Shun *et al.*, 2004). In HIV-associated sensory neuropathy, IENF density inversely correlated with severity of neuropathic pain measured by patient and physician evaluation score, but not by the Gracely Pain Scale (Polydefkis *et al.*, 2002). Another study (Herrmann *et al.*, 2004b) showed that assessment of IENF density could not differentiate between patients with symptomatic or asymptomatic HIV neuropathy. However, IENF densities at the distal leg showed a non-significant trend toward an inverse correlation with overall pain intensity among patients with symptomatic neuropathy.

In patients with diabetic neuropathy, a negative correlation between IENF density and duration of diabetes, neurological impairment score, and the results of sensory evaluation was reported (Shun *et al.*, 2004; Pittenger *et al.*, 2004). However, no correlation between IENF density and the presence of neuropathic pain was found (Pittenger *et al.*, 2004).

In patients with GBS, reduced IENF values were significantly associated with higher disability grade, need of ventilatory support, and dysautonomia (Pan *et al.*, 2003).

Correlation with sensory nerve conduction studies

Concordance between sural sensory nerve action potential (SNAP) amplitude and IENF density was investigated in several studies with different results. This is likely in keeping with the different types of neuropathy examined (i.e. large fibre vs. small fibre). Overall, concordance between sural SNAP amplitude and IENF density was found in patients with clinical impairment of large nerve fibres, whereas skin biopsy appeared more sensitive than nerve conduction study (NCS) in diagnosing SFSN (Holland *et al.*, 1997; Periquet *et al.*, 1999; Herrmann *et al.*, 1999; Smith *et al.*, 2001; Lauria *et al.*, 2003; Shun *et al.*, 2004). One study (Herrmann *et al.*, 2004a) described a linear correlation between medial plantar SNAP amplitude and IENF density in patients with normal sural NC values. Another study (Hirai *et al.*, 2000) reported significant correlation between sural nerve conduction velocity and length of dermal nerve fibres in patients with diabetic neuropathy.

Correlation with non-conventional neurophysiological examinations

No study was specifically designed to correlate skin innervation with non-conventional methods for assessing small fibre nerve conduction, such as laser-evoked potentials, microneurography, and nociceptive reflex recording. Available data rely on single case studies. In a patient with congenital insensitivity to pain, microneurography revealed absent sensory and skin sympathetic C fibre activity that correlated with loss of IENF and sweat gland nerves (Nolano *et al.*, 2000). In two patients with generalized anhidrosis, microneurography and skin biopsy allowed differentiation between specific postganglionic autonomic nerve fibre impairment and eccrine gland dysfunction (Donadio *et al.*, 2005). In two patients with Ross syndrome, abnormal laser-evoked potentials correlated with decreased IENF density and increased thermal thresholds (Perretti *et al.*, 2003).

Correlation with quantitative sensory testing and autonomic nervous system testing

Psychophysical assessment of thermal, heat-pain, and vibratory thresholds provides information on Aδ, C and Aβ fibres, respectively. IENF density inversely correlated more closely with warm and heat-pain threshold (Pan *et al.*, 2001, 2003; Chiang *et al.*, 2002; Pittenger *et al.*, 2004; Shun *et al.*, 2004) than with cooling threshold (Holland *et al.*, 1997; Periquet *et al.*, 1999; Novak *et al.*, 2001). The size of the QST probe is likely to affect the analysis (Khalili *et al.*, 2001). Correlation with impaired vibratory threshold is more likely when patients have clinical and electrophysiological evidence of large fibre neuropathy (Lauria *et al.*, 2003).

Significant correlation was found between decrease in IENF density and abnormal autonomic function assessed by quantitative sudomotor axonal reflex test (QSART) in patients with painful neuropathy (Novak *et al.*, 2001). However, no correlation with other measures of autonomic dysfunction, such as RR interval variability and sympathetic skin response, was found in GBS patients.

Correlation with sural nerve biopsy

One study (Herrmann *et al.*, 1999) compared IENF density at the distal leg and sural nerve morphometry in 26 patients with peripheral neuropathy. IENF density correlated with total myelinated, small myelinated, and large myelinated fibres, whereas there was a trend toward correlation with unmyelinated fibres. IENF and sural nerve small myelinated fibre density were concordant in 73% of patients. Decreased IENF density was the only indicator of SFSN in 23% patients. Similar findings were reported in smaller case series (Holland *et al.*, 1998; Scott *et al.*, 1999).

RECOMMENDATIONS

Correlation between IENF density and the severity of neuropathic pain needs extensive validation. Decrease in IENF density might represent a further index to predict poorer outcome in patients with GBS.

Quantification of IENF density can assess better than sural NCS and sural nerve biopsy the diagnosis of SFSN (Level A). Concordance between IENF quantification and medial plantar SNAP amplitude in patients with normal sural NCS suggests that distal sensory nerve recording might be more sensitive than sural NCS in diagnosis of sensory neuropathy.

Inverse correlation between IENF density and warm threshold assessed by QST in patients with SFSN demonstrates that both methods can reliably assess the impairment of unmyelinated nerve fibres in peripheral neuropathies (Level A). Correlation with heat-pain and cooling thresholds as well as measures of autonomic dysfunction needs more extensive validation (Level C).

Studies on skin reinnervation

Two distinct patterns of skin reinnervation have been described. After transecting the subepidermal plexus ('incision' or intracutaneous axotomy model), Wallerian degeneration is followed by fast collateral sprouting from the epidermal axons outside the incision line, leading to complete reinnervation of the epidermis by 30–75 days. Conversely, removal of the incised cylinder of skin ('excision' model) leaves a denervated area in which Schwann cells are absent and causes a slower reinnervation rate, which is not achieved after 23 months (Rajan *et al.*, 2003). These findings suggest that skin biopsy might be used to study the effect of growth factors on small fibre reinnervation in peripheral neuropathies.

Previous studies showed that cutaneous nerve fibres could spontaneously regenerate after nerve injury (Lauria *et al.*, 1998; Nodera *et al.*, 2003) or following chemical denervation with topical capsaicin. Parallel to the disappearance of IENF and dermal nerves, capsaicin induced loss of heat-pain and pinprick sensation that recovered after skin reinnervation (Simone *et al.*, 1998; Nolano *et al.*, 1999).

A recent study (Polydefkis *et al.*, 2004) investigated the regeneration rate of IENF after capsaicin treatment in 31 healthy and 20 diabetic subjects. The authors found that IENF regeneration rate was lower in diabetic patients irrespective of the presence or absence of neuropathy, suggesting that diabetes per se causes a functional impairment of peripheral axonal regrowth. The relationship of this finding to the eventual development of peripheral neuropathy is uncertain.

RECOMMENDATIONS

Skin biopsy with quantification of IENF density can be used to assess the regeneration rate of sensory axons in peripheral neuropathies and could represent a potential outcome measure in clinical trials (Level B).

EU standards

Skin biopsy is a reliable technique to assess loss and regeneration of sensory nerve fibres in peripheral neuropathies. For diagnostic purposes, we endorse a 3-mm punch skin biopsy at the distal leg, and quantification of linear epidermal innervation density in at least three 50-μm thick sections per biopsy, fixed in 2% PLP or Zamboni's solution, by immunohistochemistry using anti-PGP 9.5 antibodies and bright-field microscopy or immunofluorescence with or without confocal microscopy.

We strongly recommend training in an established cutaneous nerve laboratory before performing and processing skin biopsies in the diagnosis of peripheral neuropathies. Appropriate normative data from healthy subjects matched for age, gender, ethnicity, and anatomical site should be always used. Quality control should include all the steps of the procedure, in particular the aspect of intra- and inter-observer ratings for qualitative assessments and for quantitative analysis of epidermal densities.

Proposal for new studies

Collaborative studies should be designed to compare the diagnostic predictive values of IENF quantification by light and confocal microscopy technique in homogeneous groups of patients with peripheral neuropathy of different pathogenesis (i.e. axonal vs. demyelinating). Standardization of methods for quantification of dermal and sweat gland nerve fibres with both the techniques should be addressed.

Correlation studies of IENF density to clinical measures, QST, nerve conductions, and non-conventional neurophysiological tests should be designed to assess the relative diagnostic values to the progression of neuropathy.

Longitudinal studies of IENF density and regeneration rate should be performed both in healthy subjects and in patients with early neuropathy to confirm the potential usefulness of skin biopsy as an outcome measure in peripheral neuropathy trials.

Conflicts of interest

No member of the Task Force has any conflict of interest in this report.

References

Besne I, Descombes C, Breton L (2002). Effect of age and anatomical site on density of sensory innervation in human epidermis. *Arch Dermatol* **138**:1445–1450.

Brainin M, Barnes M, Baron JC, Gilhus NE, Hughes R, Selmaj K, Waldemar G (2004). Guideline Standards Subcommittee of the EFNS Scientific Committee. Guidance for the preparation of neurological management guidelines by EFNS scientific task forces-revised recommendations 2004. *Eur J Neurol* **11**:577–581.

Cornblath DR, Chaudhry V, Carter K, Lee D, Seysedadr M, Miernicki M, Joh T (1999). Total neuropathy score. Validation and reliability study. *Neurology.* **53**:1660–1664.

Chiang MC, Lin YH, Pan CL, Tseng TJ, Lin WM, Hsieh ST (2002). Cutaneous innervation in chronic inflammatory demyelinating polyneuropathy. *Neurology* **59**:1094–1098.

Chien HF, Tseng TJ, Lin WM, Yang CC, Chang YC, Chen RC, Hsieh ST (2001). Quantitative pathology of cutaneous nerve terminal degeneration in the human skin. *Acta Neuropathol* **102**:455–461.

Dalsgaard CJ, Rydh M, Haegerstrand A (1989). Cutaneous innervation in man visualized with protein gene product 9.5 (PGP 9.5) antibodies. *Histochemistry* **92:**385–390.

Donadio V, Montagna P, Nolano M, Cortelli P, Misciali C, Pierangeli G, Provitera V, Casano A, Baruzzi A, Liguori R (2005). Generalised anhidrosis: different lesion sites demonstrated by microneurography and skin biopsy. *J Neurol Neurosurg Psychiatry,***76:**588–591.

Facer P, Mathur R, Pandya SS, Ladiwala U, Singhal BS, Anand P (1998). Correlation of quantitative tests of nerve and target organ dysfunction with skin immuno-histology in leprosy. *Brain* **121:**2239–2247.

Gøransson LG, Mellgren SI, Lindal S, Omdal R (2004). The effect of age and gender on epidermal nerve fiber density. *Neurology* **62:**774–777.

Herrmann DN, Griffin JW, Hauer P, Cornblath DR, McArthur JC (1999). Epidermal nerve fibre density and sural nerve morphometry in peripheral neuropathies. *Neurology* **53:**1634–1640.

Herrmann DN, Ferguson ML, Pannoni V, Barbano RL, Stanton M, Logigian EL (2004a). Plantar nerve AP and skin biopsy in sensory neuropathies with normal routine conduction studies. *Neurology* **63:**879–885.

Herrmann DN, Griffin JW, Hauer P, Cornblath DR, McArthur JC (1999). Epidermal nerve fiber density and sural nerve morphometry in peripheral neuropathies. *Neurology* **53:**1634–1640.

Herrmann DN, McDermott MP, Henderson D, Chen L, Akowuah K, Schifitto G, and The North East Aids Dementia (Nead) Consortium (2004b) Epidermal nerve fiber density, axonal swellings and QST as predictors of HIV distal sensory neuropathy. *Muscle Nerve* **29:**420–427.

Hilliges M, Wang L, Johansson O (1995). Ultrastructural evidence for nerve fibers within all vital layers of the human epidermis. *J Invest Dermatol* **104:**134–137.

Hilliges M, Johansson O (1999). Comparative analysis of numerical estimation methods of epithelial nerve fibers using tissue sections. *J Peripher Nerv Syst* **4:** 53–57.

Hilz MJ, Axelrod FB, Bickel A, Stemper B, Brys M, Wendelschafer-Crabb G, Kennedy WR (2004). Assessing function and pathology in familial dysautonomia: assessment of temperature perception, sweating and cutaneous innervation. *Brain* **127:**2090–2098.

Hirai A, Yasuda H, Yoko M, Maeda T, Kikkawa R (2000). Evaluation of diabetic neuropathy through the quanti-tation of cutaneous nerves. *J Neurol Sci* **172:**55–62.

Hoitsma E, Marziniak M, Faber CG, Reulen JP, Sommer C, De Baets M, Drent M (2002). Small fibre neuropathy in sarcoidosis. Lancet **359:**2085–2086.

Holland NR, Stocks A, Hauer P, Cornblath DR, Griffin JW, McArthur JC (1997). Intraepidermal nerve fibre density

in patients with painful sensory neuropathy. *Neurology* **48:**708–711.

Holland NR, Crawford TO, Hauer P, Cornblath DR, Griffin JW, McArthur JC (1998). Small-fibre sensory neuropathies: clinical and neuropathology of idio-pathic cases. *Ann Neurol* **44:** 47–59.

Karanth SS, Springall DR, Lucas S, Levy D, Ashby P, Levene MM, Polak JM (1989). Changes in nerves and neuropeptides in skin from 100 leprosy patients inves-tigated by immunocytochemistry. *J Pathol* **157:**15–26.

Kawakami T, Ishihara M, Mihara M (2001). Distribu-tion density of intraepidermal nerve fibers in normal human skin. *J Dermatol* **28:**63–70.

Kennedy WR, Wendelschafer-Crabb G (1993) The inner-vation of human epidermis. *J Neurol Sci* **115:**184–190.

Kennedy WR, Wendelschafer-Crabb G (1996) Utility of skin biopsy in diabetic neuropathy. In: Goldblatt D, Younger D, eds., *Seminars in Neurology; Diabetic neuropa-thy*. New York: G. Thieme, **16:**163–171.

Kennedy WR, Wendelschafer-Crabb G, Johnson T (1996). Quantitation of epidermal nerves in diabetic neuropa-thy. *Neurology* **47:**1042–1048.

Kennedy WR, Nolano M, Wendelschafer-Crabb G, Johnson TL, Tamura E (1999) A skin blister method to study epidermal nerves in peripheral nerve disease. *Muscle Nerve* **22:**360–371.

Kennedy WR, Wendelschafer-Crabb G, Polydefkis M, McArthur J (2005). Pathology and quantitation of cuta-neous nerves. In: Dyck PJ, Thomas PK. eds., *Periph-eral Neuropathy*, 4th edition Philadelphia: Saunders, pp. 869–896.

Khalili N, Wendelschafer-Crabb G, Kennedy WR, Simone DA (2001) Influence of thermode size for detecting heat pain dysfunction in a capsaicin model of epidermal nerve fiber loss. Pain **91:**241–250.

Koskinen M, Hietaharju A, Kyläniemi M, Peltola J, Rantala I, Udd B, Haapasalo H (2005). A quantitative method for the assessment of intraepidermal nerve fibers in small-fiber neuropathy. *J Neurol* **252:**789–794.

Johansson O, Wang L, Hilliges M, Liang Y (1999). Intraepidermal nerves in human skin: PGP 9.5 immunohistochemistry with special reference to the nerve density in skin from different body regions. *J Peripher Nerv Syst* **4:**43–52.

Lauria G, McArthur JC, Hauer PE, Griffin JW, Cornblath DR (1998). Neuropathologic alterations in diabetic truncal neuropathy: evaluation by skin biopsy. *J Neurol Neurosurg Psychiatry* **65:**762–766.

Lauria G, Holland N, Hauer PE, Cornblath DR, Griffin JW, McArthur JC (1999). Epidermal innervation: changes with aging, topographic location, and in sensory neu-ropathy. *J Neurol Sci* **164:**172–178.

Lauria G, Sghirlanzoni A, Lombardi R, Pareyson D (2001). Epidermal innervation in sensory ganglionopathies – Clinical and neurophysiological correlations. *Muscle Nerve* 24:1034–1039.

Lauria G, Morbin M, Lombardi R, Borgna M, Mazzoleni G, Sghirlanzoni A, Pareyson D (2003). Axonal swellings predict the degeneration of epidermal nerve fibers in painful neuropathies. *Neurology* 61:631–636.

Lauria G, Borgna M, Morbin M, Lombardi R, Mazzoleni G, Sghirlanzoni A, Pareyson D (2004). Tubule and neurofilament immunoreactivity in human hairy skin: markers for intraepidermal nerve fibers. *Muscle Nerve* 30:310–316.

Li J, Bai Y, Ghandour K, Qin P, Grandis M, Trostinskaia A, Ianakova E, Wu X, Schenone A, Vallat JM, Kupsky WJ, Hatfield J, Shy ME (2005). Skin biopsies in myelin-related neuropathies: bringing molecular pathology to the bedside. *Brain*, 128:1168–1177.

Liang Y, Heilborn JD, Marcusson JA, Johansson O (1996). Increased NGFr immunoreactive dermal nerve fibers in prurigo nodularis. *Eur J Dermatol* 6:563–567.

Lombardi R, Erne B, Lauria G, Pareyson D, Borgna M, Morbin M, Arnold A, Czaplinski A, Fuhr P, Schaeren-Wiemers N, Steck AJ (2005). Anti-MAG neuropathy patients show specific IgM deposits in cutaneous nerve fibers. *Ann Neurol*, 57:180–187.

Ljungberg A, Johansson O (1993). Methodological aspects on immunohistochemistry in
dermatology with special reference to neuronal markers. *Histochem J* 25:735–745.

McArthur JC, Stocks EA, Hauer P, Cornblath DR, Griffin JW (1998). Epidermal nerve fiber density: normative reference range and diagnostic efficiency. *Arch Neurol* 55:1513–1520.

McArthur JC, Yiannoutsos C, Simpson DM, Adornato BT, Singer EJ, Hollander H, Marra C, Rubin M, Cohen BA, Tucker T, Navia BA, Schifitto G, Katzenstein D, Rask C, Zaborski L, Smith ME, Shriver S, Millar L, Clifford DB, Karalnik IJ (2000). A phase II trial of nerve growth factor for sensory neuropathy associated with HIV infection. AIDS Clinical Trials Group Team. *Neurology* 54:1080–1088.

McCarthy BG, Hsieh ST, Stocks A, Hauer P, Macko C, Cornblath DR, Griffin JW, McArthur JC (1995). Cutaneous innervation in sensory neuropathies: evaluation by skin biopsy. *Neurology* 45:1848–1855.

Moura L, Oliveira ASB, Zanoteli E, Cardoso R, Schmidt B, Gabbai AA (2004) Padronização normal das fibras nervosas intraepidérmicas em 30 voluntários saudáveis com PGP 9,5. *Arq Neuropsiquiatr* 62:271–275.

Nodera H, Barbano RL, Henderson D, Herrmann DN (2003). Epidermal reinnervation concomitant with symptomatic improvement in a sensory neuropathy. *Muscle Nerve* 27:507–509.

Nolano M, Crisci C, Santoro L, Barbieri F, Casale R, Kennedy WR, Wendelschafer-Crabb G, Provitera V, Di Lorenzo N, Caruso G (2000). Absent innervation of skin and sweat glands in congenital insensitivity to pain with anhidrosis. *Clin Neurophysiol* 111:1596–1601.

Nolano M, Provitera V, Crisci C, Saltalamacchia AM, Wendelschafer-Crabb G, Kennedy WR, Filla A, Santoro L, Caruso G (2001). Small fibers involvement in Friedreich's ataxia. *Ann Neurol* 50:17–25.

Nolano M, Provitera V, Crisci C, Stancanelli A, Wendelschafcr-Crabb G, Kennedy WR, Santoro L (2003). Quantification of myelinated endings and mechanoreceptors in human digital skin. *Ann Neurol* 54:197–205.

Nolano M, Simone DA, Wendelschafer-Crabb G, Johnson TL, Hazen E, Kennedy WR (1999). Topical capsaicin in humans: parallel loss of epidermal nerve fibers and pain sensation. *Pain* 81:135–145.

Novak V, Freimer ML, Kissel JT, Sahenk Z, Periquet IM, Nash SM, Collins MP, Mendell JR (2001). Autonomic impairment in painful neuropathy. *Neurology* 56:861–868.

Omdal R, Mellgren SI, Gøransson L, Skjesol A, Lindal S, Koldingsnes W, Husby G (2002). Small nerve fiber involvement in SLE: a controlled study. *Arthritis Rheumatol* 46:1228–1232.

Pan CL, Lin YH, Lin WM, Tai TY, Hsieh ST (2001). Degeneration of nociceptive nerve terminals in human peripheral neuropathy. *Neuroreport* 12:787–792.

Pan CL, Tseng TJ, Lin YH, Chiang MC, Lin WM, Hsieh ST (2003). Cutaneous innervation in Guillain-Barré syndrome: pathology and clinical correlations. *Brain* 126:386–397.

Periquet IM, Novak V, Collins MP, Nagaraja HN, Erdem S, Nash SM, Freimer ML, Sahenk Z, Kissel JT, Mendell JR (1999). Painful sensory neuropathy. Prospective evaluation using skin biopsy. *Neurology* 53:1641–1647.

Perretti A, Nolano M, De Joanna G, Tugnoli V, Iannetti G, Provitera V, Cruccu G, Santoro L (2003). Is Ross syndrome a dysautonomic disorder only? An electrophysiologic and histologic study *Clinical Neurophysiology* 114:7–16.

Pittenger GL, Ray M, Burcus NI, Mcnulty P, Basta B, Vinik AI (2004). Intraepidermal nerve fibers are indicators of small-fiber neuropathy in both diabetic and nondiabetic patients *Diabetes Care* 27:1974–1979.

Polydefkis M, Allen RD, Hauer P, Earley CJ, Griffin JW, Mc Arthar JC (2000). Sub clinical sensory neuropathy in late-onset restless legs syndrome. *Neurology* **55:**1115–1121.

Polydefkis M, Yiannoutsos CT, Cohen BA, Hollander H, Schifitto G, Clifford DB, Simpson DM, Katzenstein D, Shriver S, Hauer P, Brown A, Haidich AB, Moo L, McArthur JC (2002). Reduced intraepidermal nerve fibre density in HIV-associated sensory neuropathy. *Neurology* **58:**115–119.

Polydefkis M, Hauer P, Sheth S, Sirdofsky M, Griffin JW, McArthur JC (2004). The time course of epidermal nerve fibre regeneration: studies in normal controls and in people with diabetes, with and without neuropathy. *Brain* **127:**1606–1615.

Rajan B, Polydefkis M, Hauer P, Griffin JW, McArthur JC (2003). Epidermal reinnervation after intracutaneous axotomy in man. *J Comp Neurol* **457:**24–36.

Reilly DM, Ferdinando D, Johnston C, Shaw C, Buchanan KD, Green MR (1997). The epidermal nerve fibre network: characterization of nerve fibres in human skin by confocal microscopy and assessment of racial variations. *Br J Dermatol* **137:**163–170.

Scott LJ, Griffin JW, Luciano C, Barton NW, Banerjee T, Crawford T, McArthur JC, Tournay A, Schiffmann R (1999). Quantitative analysis of epidermal innervation in Fabry disease. *Neurology* **52:**1249–1254.

Shun CT, Chang YC, Wu HP, Hsieh SC, Lin WM, Lin YH, Tai TY, Hsieh ST (2004). Skin denervation in type 2 diabetes: correlations with diabetic duration and functional impairments. *Brain* **127:**1593–1605.

Simone DA, Nolano M, Johnson T, Wendelschafer-Crabb G, Kennedy WR (1998). Intradermal injection of capsaicin in human produces degeneration and subsequent reinnervation of epidermal nerve fibres: correlation with sensory function. *J Neurosci* **18:**8947–8959.

Singer W, Spies JM, McArthur J, Low J, Griffin JW, Nickander KK, Gordon V, Low PA (2004). Prospective evaluation of somatic and autonomic small fibers in selected autonomic neuropathies. *Neurology* **62:**612–618.

Smith AG, Howard JR, Kroll R, Ramachandran P, Hauer P, Singleton JR, McArthur J (2005). The reliability of skin biopsy with measurement of intraepidermal nerve fiber density. *J Neurol Sci* **228:**65–69.

Smith GA, Ramachandran P, Tripp S, Singleton RJ (2001). Epidermal nerve innervation in impaired glucose tolerance and diabetes-associated neuropathy. *Neurology* **57:**1701–1704.

Sommer C, Lindenlaub T, Zillikens D, Toyka KV (2002). Selective loss of cholinergic sudomotor fibers causes anhidrosis in Ross syndrome. *Ann Neurol* **52:**247–250.

Stocks EA, McArthur JC, Griffin JW, Mouton PR (1996). An unbiased method for estimation of total epidermal nerve fibre length. *J Neurocytology* **25:**637–644.

Sumner CJ, Sheth S, Griffin JW, Cornblath DR, Polydefkis M (2003). The spectrum of neuropathy in diabetes and impaired glucose tolerance. *Neurology* **60:**108–111.

Wang L, Hilliges M, Jernberg T, Wieberg-Edstrom D, Johansson O (1990). Protein gene product 9.5-immunoreactive nerve fibers and cells in human skin. *Cell Tissue Res* **261:**25–33.

CHAPTER 11

Assessment of neuropathic pain

G. Cruccu,[a,b] P. Anand,[c] N. Attal,[d]
L. Garcia-Larrea,[a,e] M. Haanpää,[a,f] E. Jørum,[a,g]
J. Serra,[a,h] T.S. Jensen[a,i]

Abstract

Background Although there are very many published and ongoing controlled trials about the efficacy of drugs for relieving neuropathic pain, there is uncertainty about the definition and classification of neuropathic pain, the necessary diagnostic procedures and the outcome measures. Existing recommendations or guidelines only deal with a few specific aspects or diseases.

Aim To produce neurological guidelines on the methods of assessing neuropathic pain and response to treatment.

Methods We systematically searched the Medline database from 1986 to 2004 and studied existing, authoritative recommendations, looking for evidence-based studies.

Results Common notions about most of the issues were not supported by evidence-based studies. We were able to produce the following grade B recommendations: although quantitative sensory testing (QST) is not conclusive to demonstrate neuropathic pain, it is helpful to quantify the effects of treatments on allodynia and hyperalgesia; laser-evoked potentials are the most reliable laboratory diagnostic tool; punch skin biopsy should be preferred to nerve biopsy; SF-36 and Nottingham Health Profile are the suggested quality-of-life scales.

Conclusions The whole field of neuropathic pain needs a reappraisal, to begin with its own definition and classification and end with new studies on dedicated laboratory measures.

Background and objectives

Neuropathic pain is a major disability in common neurological diseases, such as neuropathy, myelopathy, multiple sclerosis, or stroke. Pain is a complex sensation, strongly modulated by

[a]EFNS Panel on Neuropathic Pain; [b]Department of Neurological Sciences, La Sapienza University, Rome, Italy; [c]Peripheral Neuropathy Unit, Imperial College London, Hammersmith Hospital, UK; [d]INSERM E-332, Centre d'Evaluation et de Traitement de la Douleur, Hôpital Ambroise Paré and Université Versailles Saint-Quentin, Versailles, France; [e]INSERM and Laboratoire de neurophysiologie humaine du CERMEP, Lyon, France; [f]Pain Clinic, Department of Anaesthesiology and Department of Neurosurgery, Helsinki University Hospital, Helsinki, Finland; [g]Department of Neurology, The National Hospital, Oslo, Norway; [h]Neuropathic Pain Unit, Hospital General de Catalunya, Barcelona, Spain; [i]Department of Neurology and Danish Pain Research Center, Aarhus University Hospital, Aarhus, Denmark.

cognitive influences, and understanding nociceptive function and dysfunction is a hard task for all pain specialists. Neuropathic pain is a neurological disorder with a high prevalence, thus it is essential that neurologists get involved in its diagnosis and management. Because of lack of neurological guidelines for the assessment of neuropathic pain and its treatment, the objectives of our Task Force were: (i) to re-examine the definitions of neuropathic pain proposed by the International Association for the Study of Pain (IASP), (ii) to evaluate the sensitivity of the various methods of assessing neuropathic pains (e.g. pain quality and intensity scales, quantitative sensory testing, nociceptive reflexes, pain-related evoked potentials, functional neuroimaging), (iii) to evaluate the reliability of the above methods in assessing standard treatments and (iv) to propose, if necessary, new experiments that may help to clarify unsolved issues. Search and analysis were concluded in 2004 (Cruccu *et al.* 2004).

Search strategy

The Task Force systematically searched the Medline database from 1986 (i.e. the year when IASP published the first 'Classification of chronic pain'), though for some issues the search went back to the 1960s and also used major textbooks and existing guidelines on some partial issues (American Diabetes Association and American Academy of Neurology 1988; Peripheral Neuropathy Association 1993; Merskey and Bogduk 1994; Deuschl and Eisen 1999; Rolke *et al.*, 2003). For each specific issue, we stored all the articles sorted by the Medline search, omitted those that were not pertinent, and read and rated the remaining articles according to the guidance for European Federation of Neurological Societies (EFNS) guidelines (Brainin *et al.*, 2004).

Definitions

Neuropathic (= neurogenic) pain is defined by IASP as pain caused by a lesion or dysfunction of the nervous system (Merskey and Bogduk, 1994). The IASP definition does not mention which kind of lesions. It is generally understood, however, that

the lesion must involve the somatosensory pathways with damage to small fibres in peripheral nerves or to the spino-thalamo-cortical system in the central nervous system (CNS). Previous classifications of neuropathic pain have been based on underlying disease (e.g. diabetic neuropathy, multiple sclerosis, etc.) or site of lesion (e.g. peripheral nerve, spinal cord, etc.). Traditionally, neurologists have considered neuropathic pains to be present only when there are *definite* signs of a nervous lesion. The issue about definition became even more demanding following the suggestion of a mechanism-based classification (Woolf and Max, 2001). Some characteristics of neuropathic pain such as sensitized nociceptors, allodynia, abnormal temporal summation, or extraterritorial spread of pain, are also shared by less clear chronic pain conditions (Hansson *et al.*, 2001; Jensen *et al.*, 2001). The inclusion of the word 'dysfunction' in the definition of neuropathic pain implies that other conditions such as complex regional pain syndromes or even musculoskeletal disorders associated with signs of hypersensitivity may be considered neuropathic pains. Although the *narrow* definition (referring to lesion) is easier to understand and complies with the current disease-based treatment indications, the *broad* definition (referring to dysfunction) may be rewarding for some reasons. By focusing on the mechanism, it makes clear that hyperexcitability and plasticity of the nervous system are key phenomena in chronic pain, and that treatment efficacy depends more on the underlying mechanism than aetiology (Sindrup and Jensen, 1999).

Comment

Testing the validity of a *narrow* vs. a *broad* definition of neuropathic pain should be a major goal for future studies. In the meanwhile, however, we suggest the *narrow* definition and classification is retained, because of risk of overestimating neuropathic pain and because it is easy to understand. Indeed a subcommittee on definition and classification of neuropathic pain of the IASP taxonomy committee is now proposing a *narrow* definition and a grading of neuropathic pain patients where the level 'definite' requires objective demonstration of disease or injury of the somatosensory system (Rasmussen *et al.*, 2004).

Clinical examination and psychophysiological measures

Bedside examination

The examination of a pain patient aims at clarifying underlying disease and understanding whether the pain is nociceptive, neuropathic, psychogenic, or a combination of such. In case of neuropathic pain, abnormal sensory findings should be neuroanatomically logical, compatible with a definite lesion site.

Location, quality and intensity of pain should be assessed. A clear understanding of the possible types of negative (e.g. sensory loss) and positive (e.g. paresthesia) symptoms and signs is necessary. Neuropathic pain can be spontaneous (*stimulus-independent* or *spontaneous pain*) or elicited by a stimulus (*stimulus-dependent* or *stimulus-evoked pain*). Spontaneous pain is often described as a constant burning sensation, but may also include intermittent shooting, lancinating sensations, electric shock-like pain and *dysesthesias* (i.e. abnormal, unpleasant sensations). *Paresthesias* are abnormal, though not unpleasant, sensations. Stimulus-evoked pains are elicited by mechanical, thermal, or chemical stimuli. *Hyperalgesia* is an increased pain response to a stimulus that normally provokes pain, whereas *allodynia* is a pain sensation induced by a stimulus that normally does not provoke pain, and thus implies a change in the quality of a sensation. Mechanical allodynia, which is most easily tested, is further classified as dynamic (brush-evoked) or static (pressure-evoked).

Neurological examination in suspected neuropathic pain should include quantification and mapping of motor, sensory and autonomic phenomena to identify all signs of neurological dysfunction. It is advisable to end a neurological examination with the sensory assessment. It is helpful to maintain a detailed record, preferably a diagram, of any sensory disorder to allow immediate comparison on re-testing. Although difficult for the non-specialist and time-consuming for everybody, tattooing the sensory abnormality on the patient's skin (and possibly obtaining photographical records) provides valuable information. With experience, the territory of each sensory deficit or pain can be mapped separately to reflect different areas of impairment. Tactile sense is best assessed by a piece of cotton wool, pinprick sense by a wooden cocktail-stick, thermal sense by warm and cold objects (e.g. metal thermorollers), and vibration sense by a 128-Hz tuning fork (Table 11.1). The intensity, quality and spatial-temporal aspects of the evoked sensations should be noted, as there may be aberrations in all of them (Hansson, 1994). Standardized terms must be used in patient documents, as many cultural and medical traditions differ in the meaning of similar words (Merskey and Bogduk, 1994).

RECOMMENDATIONS

Although there are no validated studies on bedside examination, good clinical practice teaches that in pain patients a thorough neurological examination is invaluable – the sensory testing being the most important part of it – and is preliminary to any quantitative assessment.

Quantitative sensory testing

Quantitative sensory testing (QST) may be defined as the analysis of perception in response to external stimuli of controlled intensity (figure 11.1). Detection and pain thresholds are determined by applying stimuli to the skin in an ascending and descending order of magnitude. Mechanical sensitivity for tactile stimuli is measured using von Frey hairs or Semmes-Weinstein monofilaments (Waylett-Rendall, 1988), pin-prick sensation with weighted needles (Chan *et al.*, 1992), and vibration sensitivity with an electronic vibrameter (Goldberg and Lindblom, 1979). Thermal perception and thermal pain are measured using a probe that operates on the Peltier principle (Fruhstorfer *et al.*, 1976, Claus *et al.*, 1990, Yarnitsky *et al.*, 1995).

QST has been used for the early diagnosis and follow up of small-fibre neuropathies that cannot be assessed by standard nerve conduction studies (see below) and its usefulness is now agreed

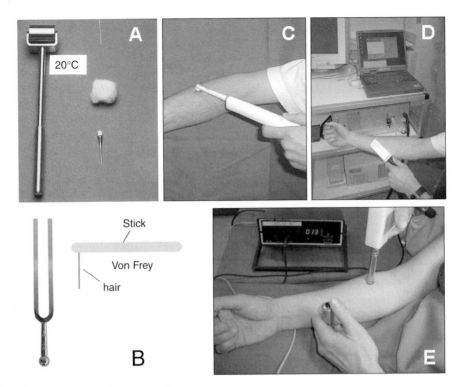

Figure 11.1. Psychophysiological assessment.
From the classical tools of bedside examination (A), through the von Frey hairs (B), to the devices of quantitative sensory testing, such as electrical brush (C), thermotest (D), and pressure algometer (E).(Courtesy by TS Jensen)

Table 11.1 Summary of choice methods of assessing nerve function per sensation.

Fibres	Sensation	Testing Clinical	[1]QST	Laboratory
Aβ	Touch	Piece of cotton wool	von Frey filaments	Nerve conduction
	Vibration	Tuning fork (128 Hz)	[2]Vibrameter	studies, [3]SEPs
Aδ	Pinprick, sharp pain	Wooden cocktail stick	Weighted needles	Nociceptive reflexes, [4]LEPs
	Cold	Thermorollers	[5]Thermotest	–
C	Warmth	Thermorollers	[5]Thermotest	[4]LEPs
	Burning	–	[5]Thermotest	

[1]Quantitative Sensory Testing; [2]or other device providing graded vibratory stimuli; [3]Somatosensory-evoked potentials; [4]Laser-evoked potentials; [5]or other device providing graded thermal stimuli.

in the early diagnosis of diabetic neuropathies (Consensus Statement 1988, 1993). QST is also particularly appropriate to quantify mechanical and thermal allodynia and hyperalgesia, which may help characterize painful neuropathic syndromes and clarify some of their pathophysiological mechanisms.

This method, however, has never been used to make a differential diagnosis between neuropathic and non-neuropathic pains. Indeed QST changes are also found in non-neuropathic pain states, such as rheumatoid arthritis and inflammatory arthromyalgias (Leffler *et al.*, 2000, 2002, class 2).

QST has been used in many trials to assess the absence of deleterious effects of treatments on sensory perception and less commonly to measure the treatment efficacy on evoked pains. Whereas most studies failed to detect treatment effects on *pain thresholds* in response to mechanical or thermal stimuli, treatments did significantly modulate *brush-induced allodynia* (intensity or area), *hyperalgesia* and other less common components of neuropathic pain (*temporal summation, aftersensation, radiating pain*) (class 2: Leung *et al.*, 2001; Marchettini *et al.*, 1992; Watson *et al.*, 1992; Baranowski *et al.*, 1999; Eide *et al.*, 1994, 1995; Belfrage *et al.*, 1995; Felsby *et al.*, 1996; Rowbotham *et al.*, 1995, 1996; Pud *et al.*, 1998; Sindrup *et al.*, 1999; Attal *et al.*, 2000, 2002; Wallace *et al.*, 2000, 2002; Sjölund *et al.*, 2001; Vestegaard *et al.*, 2001).

Differential effects of treatments on allodynia/hyperalgesia in comparison to spontaneous pain and modality-specific effects have been reported (class 2: Eide *et al.*, 1994, 1995; Belfrage *et al.*, 1995; Attal *et al.*, 2000, 2002; Wallace *et al.*, 2000, 2002; Leung *et al.*, 2001; Sjölund *et al.*, 2001; Vestegaard *et al.*, 2001).

As QST abnormalities are also found in non-neuropathic pains, they cannot be taken as a conclusive demonstration of neuropathic pain (Recommendation Level B); furthermore QST depends on expensive equipment, it is time-consuming and thus difficult to use in clinical practice. In contrast, QST is helpful to quantify the effects of treatments on allodynia and hyperalgesia and can reveal a differential efficacy of treatments on different pain components (Recommendation Level B). To evaluate mechanical allodynia/hyperalgesia, we recommend the use of simple tools such as a brush and at least one high-threshold von Frey filament. The evaluation of pain in response to thermal stimuli is best performed using the thermotest, but we do not recommend the systematic measure of thermal stimuli except for pathophysiological research or treatment trials. A simple and sensitive tool to quantify pain induced by thermal stimuli in clinical practice should be developed.

Pain quality and intensity scales

To assess ongoing pain, but also paroxysmal and evoked pains, the pain intensity can be measured by visual analog (VAS), numerical rating (NRS), or verbal rating (VRS) scales. VAS is one of the oldest, easiest and best-validated measures to assess pain (Huskisson, 1974). Among the numerical scales the 11-point Likert scale (0 = no pain, 10 = worst possible pain) has been most widely used in recent neuropathic pain studies. In verbal rating the patients choose one of the given verbal descriptors of the intensity of pain they feel. VRS can be used for both intensity and unpleasantness. A combination of verbal and numeral rating is the Gracely Pain Scale with 13 words describing pain intensity and the numbers from 0 to 20 (Gracely *et al.*, 1978).

The McGill Pain Questionnaire (MPQ; Melzack, 1975), and its shorter version (SF-MPQ; Melzack, 1987) are the most frequently used self-rating instruments for pain measurement and also often used in treatment trials. Both MPQ and SF-MPQ provide data on the various sensory and affective dimensions of pain, but they are not specifically designed to assess neuropathic pain and their translations in languages other than English need further validations.

Of the scales designed for neuropathic pain assessment, the Symptom Score Scale (Kvinesdal *et al.*, 1984) has only been used in diabetic neuropathy and the Neuropathic Pain Scale (Galer and Jensen, 1997) does not include important items such as paroxysmal pain and numbness and its validation was mainly based on analysis of the discriminant validity and predictive values of its descriptors. Both the Leeds assessment of neuropathic symptoms and signs (LANSS scale) and Neuropathic Pain Questionnaire (NPQ) were developed to differentiate neuropathic from nociceptive pain patients, rather than as tools for quantitative assessment (Bennett, 2001; Krause and Backonja, 2003); these scales have only been preliminary and currently are not widely used. The Neuropathic Pain Symptom Inventory (NPSI) (Bouhassira *et al.*, 2004) has been designed to evaluate specifically the different symptoms of neuropathic pain and allows the user to discriminate and quantify five distinct dimensions of neuropathic pains (burning pain, deep pressure pain, paroxysmal pain, paresthesia/dysesthesia and evoked pains). It has been properly validated and is currently used in large multicentric trials.

RECOMMENDATIONS

It is recommended to rate the intensity and the unpleasantness of pain separately (Smith *et al.*, 1998). The intensity of the different pain components that the patient may report (spontaneous ongoing pain, spontaneous paroxysmal pain, dysesthesiae, paresthesiae) or the evoked pains (allodynia and hyperalgesia), as well as pain worsening with movement, should be rated separately, but using the same scale, as is the case in the NPSI. If different pain components involve different territories, these can be documented on a template body map. The simplest scales are probably the best. Whereas VRS is found to be easier by many patients, VAS is more apt to treatment trials because it permits parametric statistics. The Likert 0–10 NRS is a good compromise (Level C).

Methods specifically designed to assess treatment efficacy

Although changes in the pain level can be and are often measured with the questionnaires or scales described above, some methods have been specifically conceived for assessing treatment efficacy, for example, VAS for pain relief or the six-item Pain Relief Scale (Devers and Galer, 2000). As the interventions may improve the patient's well-being also in other respects, or may have adverse effects, the validated measure, Global Impression of Change (GIC), is recommended. It consists of seven verbal descriptors from 'very much improved' to 'very much worse', either reported by the patient (PGIC) or evaluated by the physician (CGIC). The proportion of responders, need of rescue medication, or patient's preference of treatment have also been used in pharmacological studies and these have shown their ability to reveal treatment effects in neuropathic pain.

'Number Needed to Treat' (NNT) (McQuay and Moore, 1998) has been used both in meta-analyses and single studies (Sindrup *et al.*, 1999, 2003) to express how many patients should be treated to have at least 50% pain relief in one patient. A 50% pain relief has been the 'gold standard' criterion used in meta-analyses to calculate the NNT. With data from 2700 patients participating in a Phase-III study, Farrar *et al.* (2001) compared the 11-point Likert NRS and PGIC. They found that a 50% pain reduction in the NRS corresponded to 'very much improved' in the PGIC, whereas even a 30% reduction in the NRS was clinically important.

RECOMMENDATIONS

All the psychometric instruments assessing treatment in neuropathic pain have been shown to be sensitive in several class 2 randomized controlled trials (RCTs). We recommend the use of unidimensional pain scales, particularly the NRS and pain relief scales and the evaluation of specific pain symptoms (such as burning pain, pain paroxysms, or allodynia) as this may reveal preferential effects of treatments (Level B). We do not favour the systematic use of non-specific multidimensional scales (e.g. MPQ). Although interesting, the multidimensional scales specific for neuropathic pain still lack extensive validation as tools for treatment assessment (Level C).

Other outcome measures

Pain reduction is most commonly used as the primary end point in the intervention studies. It is recommended to use assessment of sleep, mood, functional capacity and quality-of-life (QoL) as secondary endpoints. Sleep can be assessed with VAS, 11-point Likert scale for sleep interference or verbal rating (good, fair or poor). Some scales for QoL, for example, Nottingham Health Profile (NHP), also assess sleep. The Beck Depression Scale (BDI; Beck *et al.*, 1961) or the Zung Self-Rating Depression Scale (ZDS; Zung 1965) is used to evaluate depression. For evaluation of anxiety, the Hospital

Anxiety and Depression Scale (HADS; Zigmond and Snaith, 1983) or the State, Trait and Anxiety (STAIT; Spielberg, 1975) and the Pain Anxiety Symptom Scale (PASS; McCracken *et al.*, 1992) are available. The QoL scales NHP and SF-36 Health Survey (SF-36) evaluate also mood.

Neuropathic patients' functional capacity (physical, cognitive, emotional and social) can be impaired by the underlying neurological disease, sensory disturbances and treatment. The Sickness Impact Profile (SIP), a generic measure of functional status (Follick *et al.*, 1985) has been used for neuropathic pain patients.

Improvement of QoL has been regarded as the final aim of pain treatment. QoL is measured either by the 0-10 scale or by specific scales such as SF-36 (Ware *et al.*, 1992), NHP (Hunt *et al.*, 1980) or QoL Index (Ferrans, 1990). In a comparison study in neuropathic pain patients, SF-36 showed a higher internal consistency reliability than NHP (class 2: Meyer-Rosberg *et al.*, 2001a,b).

RECOMMENDATIONS

In clinical studies, QoL should be assessed with a validated and comprehensive scale such as SF-36 or NHP (Level B). Mood, sleep, anxiety and depression, if not included in the chosen QoL measure, should be assessed separately.

Laboratory tests

As pain is a complex experience, strongly influenced by cultural, social and emotional factors, it would be of paramount importance to rely on techniques that provide its laboratory measure.

Standard electrodiagnostic studies

Large-size, non-nociceptive afferents have a lower electrical threshold than small-size, nociceptive afferents. Unless special techniques are adopted (experimental blocks) or special organs are stimulated (cornea, tooth pulp, glans), electrical stimuli unavoidably also excite large, non-nociceptive afferents. The large-afferent input inhibits the nociceptive input at central synapses and hinders the nociceptive signals (IFCN Recommendations for the Practice of Clinical Neurophysiology).

RECOMMENDATIONS

Standard neurophysiological responses to electrical stimuli, such as *nerve conduction studies* and *somatosensory evoked potentials*, are useful to demonstrate, locate and quantify damage along the peripheral or central sensory pathways. But they do not assess the function of nociceptive pathways (Level B).

Microneurography

Microneurography is a minimally invasive technique that allows single-fibre recordings from nerve fibres in awake subjects (Torebjork *et al.*, 1993). Microneurography provides useful information on the physiology of nociceptors and their behaviour in various experimental pain models and has proven useful, by correlating abnormal discharges to perception, in understanding the pathophysiology of positive sensory symptoms in neuropathic pain patients (Torebjork *et al.*, 1993; Campero *et al.*, 1996, 1998). Microneurography, however, is time-consuming and difficult, requiring both an expert investigator and a collaborative patient; hence it is unsuitable for the clinical setting.

Nociceptive reflexes

The RIII flexion reflex in the biceps femoris (RIII) and the corneal reflex are purely nociceptive reflexes, in that they are exclusively mediated by nociceptive afferents and are suppressed by the antinociceptive systems and analgesic drugs (Willer *et al.*, 1984, 1989; Willer 1985; Cruccu *et al.*, 1991; Sandrini *et al.*, 2000). Although the cutaneous silent period in the hand muscles (CSP) is probably a nociceptive reflex, a few studies contradict this notion and one study showed that CSP is insensitive to opiates (Serrao *et al.*, 2001; Inghilleri *et al.*, 2002). Even though the main electrically elicited trigeminal reflexes (blink reflex and exteroceptive suppression) have been often used in pain studies, their nature is strongly controversial: evidence has been provided that large-myelinated, non-nociceptive fibres predominantly contribute to these reflexes, and that these reflexes are suppressed more by benzodiazepines than opiates (Cruccu *et al.*, 1990, 1991, class 2).

As diagnostic tools, the use of the nociceptive RIII flexion reflex, corneal reflex and CSP in neuropathic pain is extremely rare (Boureau *et al.*, 1991, class 2). The trigeminal blink reflex and exteroceptive suppression have been consistently found to be normal in essential trigeminal neuralgia and abnormal in trigeminal pains secondary to neuropathy, cerebello-pontine angle tumours and multiple sclerosis (IFCN Recommendations for the practice of Clinical Neurophysiology, class 2).

Although the RIII reflex has been used to assess the efficacy of opiates, NSAIDs, hypnosis and neurostimulation procedures (class 2: Willer *et al.*, 1985, 1989; Garcia-Larrea *et al.*, 1989, 1999; Boureau *et al.*, 1991; Sandrini *et al.*, 2000, 2002), there is little experience in neuropathic pain patients.

RECOMMENDATIONS

The electrically elicited trigeminal reflexes (blink reflex and masseter inhibitory reflex) are diagnostically useful to differentiate essential trigeminal neuralgia from symptomatic trigeminal pains (Level B). The other nociceptive reflexes have little diagnostic value. The nociceptive reflex that is most used and appears to be most reliable in assessing treatment efficacy is the RIII flexion reflex (Level B).

Laser-evoked potentials

For many years a number of techniques have been tried for the selective activation of pain afferents (figure 11.2). The best method now appears to be provided by radiant-heat pulse stimuli delivered by laser stimulators, which selectively excite the free nerve endings (A-delta and C) in the superficial skin layers (Bromm and Treede, 1984; Treede *et al.*, 1995). That laser-evoked potentials (LEPs) are nociceptive responses is now widely agreed by over 200 studies. *Late* LEPs reflect activity of the A-delta

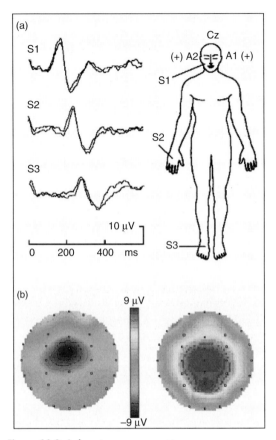

Figure 11.2. Laboratory assessment.
Laser-evoked potentials (LEPs) can be easily elicited from all body dermatomes and recorded from scalp electrodes. This figure, showing LEPs after face, hand, and foot stimulations and their brain maps, is modified from a normative study in 100 subjects (modified from Truini *et al.*, 2005). See also Plate 11.1, pp. 120–121.

and *ultralate* LEPs of the unmyelinated nociceptive pathway (Bromm and Treede, 1984, 1987, 1991; Bragard *et al.*, 1996; Magerl *et al.*, 1999).

Late LEPs have proved reliable in assessing damage to the peripheral and central nociceptive system in peripheral neuropathies, idiopathic and symptomatic trigeminal neuralgia, syringomyelia, multiple sclerosis, Wallenberg syndrome and brain infarction (class 2: Kakigi *et al.*, 1991,1992; Agostino *et al.*, 2000; Cruccu *et al.*, 2001, 2003; Garcia-Larrea *et al.*, 2002; Truini *et al.*, 2003). In peripheral and central neuropathic pains, LEPs are more sensitive than any other neurophysiological test and the finding of a LEP suppression helps to diagnose neuropathic pain (class 2: Kakigi *et al.*, 1992; Casey *et al.*, 1996; Agostino *et al.*, 2000; Garcia-Larrea *et al.*, 2002; Truini *et al.* 2003). In fibromyalgia and myofascial syndromes, chronic fatigue syndrome, chronic inflammatory pains and psychogenic pain, LEPs have been found facilitated (mostly increased amplitude) (Lorenz *et al.*, 1997; Granot *et al.*, 2001; Wendler *et al.*, 2001). Late LEPs are suppressed by aspirin, morphine and carbamazepine (Lorenz *et al.*, 1997; Cruccu *et al.*, 2001).

Ultralate LEPs related to C-fibre activation are technically more difficult. Only a few studies have been carried out in patients (Bromm and Treede 1991; Lankers *et al.*, 1991; Granot *et al.*, 2001; Cruccu *et al.*, 2003).

RECOMMENDATIONS

Laser-evoked potentials are the easiest and most reliable neurophysiological method of assessing the function of nociceptive pathways; in clinical practice their main limit is that they are currently available in too few centres. *Late* LEPs (which assess A-delta pathways) are diagnostically useful in peripheral and central neuropathic pains (Level B). The experience as a tool for assessing treatments is so far insufficient. More studies on *ultralate* LEPs in patients with neuropathic pain are encouraged.

Functional Neuroimaging (PET, fMRI)

Positron emission tomography (PET) and functional magnetic resonance imaging (fMRI) measure with different methods cerebral blood flow (rCBF) or metabolic changes that reflect local synaptic activity in defined brain regions. 'Activation' studies investigate changes specifically associated to a given task or a particular stimulus by comparing statistically 'activated' and 'control' conditions.

In *experimental pain*, fMRI and PET studies have disclosed a network of brain regions that are activated by noxious stimuli. These regions constantly include the secondary somatosensory cortex (SII), the insular cortex, the anterior cingulate cortex (ACC) and with slightly less consistency the contralateral thalamus and primary somatosensory cortex (SI) (Peyron *et al.*, 2000). Activation of the lateral thalamus, SI, SII and insula are thought to be related to the sensory-discriminative aspects of pain processing, while ACC, and also the posterior parietal and prefrontal cortices, appear to participate in the affective and attentional concomitants of pain sensation, as well as in response selection.

In patients with *chronic spontaneous neuropathic pain*, there is converging evidence from several independent groups (but for a total of 41 patients only) that unilateral pain is associated with decreased resting rCBF in contralateral thalamus, and that such rCBF decrease can be reverted by analgesic procedures (Iadarola *et al.*, 1995; Hsieh *et al.*, 1995; Garcia-Larrea *et al.*, 1999). This suggests that thalamic hypoperfusion contralateral to pain might be used in the future as a marker of neuropathic pain, and that restoration of thalamic blood flow could be used to monitor treatment. Although analgesic procedures including opiates and neurostimulation have induced rCBF increase in ACC, the number of patients tested is still too small to decide whether this can be a marker of efficacy. In patients with *provoked neuropathic pain*, allodynia and hyperalgesia have been associated with amplification of the thalamic, insular, SI and SII responses, but not ACC (Iadarola *et al.*, 1997; Peyron *et al.*, 2000; Baron *et al.*, 1999). Again the number of patients examined is still too small (Peyron *et al.*, 2000). We encourage imaging studies in patients with allodynia.

The combination of administration of drugs with fMRI to elucidate pharmacological effects on brain function (*pharmacological functional magnetic resonance imaging*, phMRI) has been recently proposed. The assessment of the effect of analgesic drugs on pain-related brain activity would provide a better understanding of pain and analgesia and hence the development of novel therapeutic strategies. Data in patients, however, are still lacking.

Comment

There is converging evidence that chronic spontaneous neuropathic pain is associated with decreased activity in contralateral thalamus, whereas provoked neuropathic pain is associated with increased activity in the thalamic, insular and somatosensory regions. In view of the potential relevance of these data, we encourage functional neuroimaging studies in patients with neuropathic pain.

Biopsy

Painful neuropathies are characterized by preferential involvement of unmyelinated and thinly myelinated nerve fibres.

Nerve biopsy may not be useful in the early detection or monitoring the progression of small fibre neuropathy as small fibres are difficult to quantify, and require the use of an electron microscope (Llewelyn *et al.*, 1991). There is growing evidence that simple unmyelinated-fibre counts in nerve biopsies fail to reflect the degree of unmyelinated-fibre degeneration (class 2: Hermann *et al.*, 1999; Periquet *et al.*, 1999).The procedure itself may cause considerable discomfort and may occasionally be associated with complications like pain, infection and permanent sensory loss. However, nerve biopsy is indicated if diagnostic considerations include amyloidosis or vasculitis.

Punch skin biopsy was suggested as an alternative approach to the assessment of small fibre involvement allowing the quantification of C fibres and Aδ nerve fibres through the measure of the density of intra-epidermal nerve fibres (IENF). The loss of IENF was demonstrated in a variety of neuropathies including small fibre sensory neuropathies (class 2: McCarthy *et al.*, 1995; Holland *et al.*, 1997, 1998). Skin biopsy has recently been proved able to investigate mechanoreceptors and their myelinated afferents (Nolano *et al.*, 2003). Punch skin biopsy is easy to perform, is minimally invasive and most suitable for follow-up. However, it is currently available in only a few research centres.

RECOMMENDATIONS

Often the cause for an underlying neuropathy may not be found despite extensive investigations, and careful evaluation is needed before such cases are considered as idiopathic or 'psychogenic'. Punch skin biopsy, which can detect changes when sural nerve biopsy is still normal, is emerging as a minimally invasive tool for detecting small fibre involvement; in pain patients it should be preferred to nerve biopsy (Level B).

Conflicts of Interest

We do not have any conflict of interest.

References

Agostino R, Cruccu G, Romaniello A, Innocenti P, Inghilleri M, Manfredi M (2000). Dysfunction of small myelinated afferents in diabetic polyneuropathy, as assessed by laser evoked potentials. *Clin Neurophysiol* **111**:270–276.

American Diabetes Association and American Academy of Neurology (1988) Consensus Statement. Report and recommendations of the San Antonio Conference on diabetic neuropathy. *Diabetes* **37**:1000–1004.

Attal N, Gaude V, Dupuy M (2000). Intravenous lidocaine in central pain. A double-blind placebo-controlled psycho-physical study. *Neurology* **544**:564–574.

Attal N, Guirimand F, Brasseur L, Gaude V, Chauvin M, Bouhassira D (2002). Effects of IV morphine in central pain: A randomized placebo-controlled study. *Neurology* **58**:554–563.

Baranowski AP, De Courcey J, Bonello E (1999). A trial of intravenous lidocaine on the pain and allodynia of postherpetic neuralgia. *J Pain Symptom Manage* **17**:429–434.

Baron R, Baron Y, Disbrow E *et al.* (1999). Brain processing of capsaicin-induced secondary hyperalgesia: a functional MRI study. *Neurology* **53**:548–57.

Beck A, Ward C, Mendelson M, Mock J, Erbaugh J (1961). An inventory to measure depression. *Arch Gen Psychiatry* **4**:561–567.

Belfrage M, Sollevi A, Segerdahl M, Sjolund KF, Hansson P (1995). Systemic adenosine infusion alleviates spontaneous and stimulus evoked pain in patients with peripheral neuropathic pain. *Anesth Analg* **81**:713–717.

Bennett M (2001). The LANSS Pain Scale: the Leeds assessment of neuropathic symptoms and signs. *Pain* **92**:147–57.

Bouhassira D, Attal N, Fermanian J, *et al.* (2004) Development and validation of the Neuropathic Pain Symptom Inventory. *Pain* **108**:248–257.

Boureau F, Luu M, Doubrere JF (1991). Study of experimental pain measures and nociceptive reflex in chronic pain patients and normal subjects. *Pain* **44:** 131–138.

Bragard D, Chen AC, Plaghki L (1996). Direct isolation of ultra-late (C-fibre) evoked brain potentials by CO_2 laser stimulation of tiny cutaneous surface areas in man. *Neurosci Lett* **209:**81–84.

Brainin M, Barnes M, Baron JC, Gilhus NE, Hughes R, Selmaj K, Waldemar G (2004). Guideline Standards Subcommittee of the EFNS Scientific Committee. Guidance for the preparation of neurological management guidelines by EFNS scientific task forces–revised recommendations 2004. *Eur J Neurol* **11:**577–581.

Bromm B, Treede RD (1984). Nerve fibre discharges, cerebral potentials and sensations induced by CO_2 laser stimulation. *Hum Neurobiol* **3:**33–40.

Bromm B, Treede RD (1987). Human cerebral potentials evoked by CO_2 laser stimuli causing pain. *Exp Brain Res* **67:**153–162.

Bromm B, Treede RD (1991). Laser-evoked cerebral potentials in the assessment of cutaneous pain sensitivity in normal subjects and patients. *Rev Neurol (Paris)* **147:**625–643.

Campero M, Serra J, Ochoa JL (1996). C-polymodal nociceptors activated by noxious low temperature in human skin. *J Physiol* **497:**565–572.

Campero M, Serra J, Marchettini P, Ochoa JL (1998). Ectopic impulse generation and autoexcitation in single myelinated afferent fibers in patients with peripheral neuropathy and positive sensory symptoms. *Muscle Nerve* **21:**1661–1667.

Casey KL, Beydoun A, Boivie J, Sjolund B, Holmgren H, Leijon G, Morrow TJ, Rosen I (1996). Laser-evoked cerebral potentials and sensory function in patients with central pain. *Pain* **64:**485–491.

Chan AW, McFarlane IA, Bowsher D, Campbell JA (1992). Weighted needle pinprick sensory thresholds: a simple test of sensory function in diabetic peripheral neuropathy. *J Neurol Neurosurg Psychiatry* **55:** 56–59.

Claus D, Hiltz MJ, Neundorfer B (1990). Thermal discrimination thresholds: a comparison of different methods. *Acta Neurol Scand* **76:**288–96

Cruccu G, Leandri M, Feliciani M, Manfredi M (1990). Idiopathic and symptomatic trigeminal pain. *J Neurol Neurosurg Psychiatry* **53:**1034–1042.

Cruccu G, Ferracuti S, Leardi MG, Fabbri A, Manfredi M (1991). Nociceptive quality of the orbicularis oculi reflexes as evaluated by distinct opiate- and benzodiazepine-induced changes in man. *Brain Res* **556:**209–217.

Cruccu G, Leandri M, Iannetti GD, Mascia A, Romaniello A, Truini A, Galeotti F, Manfredi M (2001). Small-fiber dysfunction in trigeminal neuralgia: carbamazepine effect on laser-evoked potentials. *Neurology* **56:**1722–1726.

Cruccu G, Pennisi E, Truini A, *et al.* (2003) Unmyelinated trigeminal pathways as assessed by laser stimuli in humans. *Brain* **126:**2246–2256.

Cruccu G, Anand P, Attal N, Garcia-Larrea L, Haanpaa M, Jorum E, Serra J, Jensen TS (2004) EFNS guidelines on neuropathic pain assessment. *Eur J Neurol* **11:**153–162.

Deuschl G, Eisen A (1999) Recommendations for the Practice of Clinical Neurophysiology. IFCN Guidelines. *Electroencephalogr Clin Neurophysiol* suppl. 52.

Devers A, Galer BS (2000). Topical lidocaine patch relieves a variety of neuropathic pain conditions: an open-label study. *Clin J Pain* **16:**205–208.

Eide PK, Jorum E, Stubhaub A, Bremmes J, Breivik H (1994). Relief of post-herpetic neuralgia with the N-methyl-D-aspartic acid receptor antagonist ketamine: a double-blind, cross-over comparison with morphine and placebo. *Pain* **58:**347–354.

Eide PK, Stubhaug A, Stenehjem AE (1995). Central dysesthesia pain after traumatic spinal cord injury is dependent on N-methyl-D-aspartate receptor activation. *Neurosurgery* **37:**1080–1087.

Farrar JT, Young JP Jr, LaMoreaux L, Werth JL, Poole MR (2001). Clinical importance of change in chronic pain intensity measured on an 11-point numerical pain rating scale. *Pain* **94:**149–158.

Felsby S, Nielsen J, Arendt Nielsen L, Jensen TS (1996). NMDA receptor blockade in chronic neuropathic pain: a comparison of ketamine and magnesium chloride. *Pain* **64:**283–291.

Ferrans C (1990). Development of a quality of life index for patients with cancer. *Oncol Nurs Forum* **17** (suppl 3)**:**15–19.

Follick MJ, Smith TW, Ahern DK (1985). The sickness impact profile: a global measure of disability in chronic low back pain. *Pain* **21:**67–76.

Fruhstorfer H, Lindblom U, Schmidt WG (1976). Method for quantitative estimation of thermal threshold in patients. *J Neurol Neurosurg Psychiatry* **39:**1071–1075.

Galer BS, Jensen MP (1997). Development and preliminary validation of a pain measure specific to neuropathic pain: The Neuropathic Pain Scale. *Neurology* **48:**332–338.

Garcia-Larrea L, Sindou M, Mauguiere F (1989). Nociceptive flexion reflexes during analgesic neurostimulation in man. *Pain* **39:**145–156.

Garcia-Larrea L, Peyron R, Mertens P, Gregoire MC, Lavenne F, Le Bars D, Convers P, Mauguiere F, Sindou M, Laurent B (1999). Electrical stimulation of motor cortex for pain control: a combined PET-scan and electrophysiological study. *Pain* **83:**259–273.

Garcia-Larrea L, Convers P, Magnin M, Andre-Obadia N, Peyron R, Laurent B, Mauguiere F (2002). Laser-evoked potential abnormalities in central pain patients: the influence of spontaneous and provoked pain. *Brain* **125:**2766–2781.

Goldberg JM, Lindblom U (1979). Standardised method of determining vibratory perception thresholds for diagnosis and screening in neurological investigation. *J Neurol Neurosurg Psychiatry* **42:**793–803.

Gracely RH, McGrath F, Dubner R (1978). Ratio scales of sensory and affective verbal pain descriptors. *Pain* **5:**5–18.

Granot M, Buskila D, Granovsky Y, Sprecher E, Neumann L, Yarnitsky D (2001). Simultaneous recording of late and ultra-late pain evoked potentials in fibromyalgia. *Clin Neurophysiol.* **112:**1881–1887.

Hansson P (1994). Possibilities and potential pitfalls of combined bedside and quantitative somatosensory analysis in pain patients. In: Boivie J, Hansson P, Lindblom U, eds., *Progress in Pain Research and Management, Vol 3, Touch, Temperature and Pain in Health and Disease,* Seattle: IASP Press. pp. 113–132.

Hansson PT, Fields HL, Hill RG, Marchettini P (2001). *Progress in Pain Research and Management, Vol. 21, Neuropathic Pain: Pathophysiology and Treatment.* Seattle: IASP Press.

Hermann DN, Griffin JW, Hauer BS, Cornblath DR, McArthur JC (1999). Epidermal nerve fibre density and sural nerve morphometry in peripheral neuropathies. *Neurology* **53:**1634–1640.

Holland NR, Stocks A, Hauer P, Cornblath DR, Griffin JW, McArthur JC (1997). Intraepidermal nerve fiber density in patients with painful sensory neuropathy. *Neurology* **48:**708–711.

Holland NR, Crawford TO, Hauer P, Cornblath DR, Griffin JW, McArthur JC (1998). Small fiber sensory neuropathies: clinical course and neuropathology of idiopathic cases. *Ann Neurol* **44:**47–59.

Hsieh JC, Belfrage M, Stone-Elander S, Hansson P, Ingvar M (1995). Central representation of chronic ongoing neuropathic pain studied by positron emission tomography. *Pain* **63:**225–236.

Hunt SM, McKenna SP, McEwen J, Backett EM, Williams J, Papp E (1980). A quantitative approach to perceived health status: a validation study. *J Epidemiol Comm Health* **34:**281–286.

Huskisson EC (1974). Measurement of pain. *Lancet* **2:**1127–1131.

Iadarola MJ, Max MB, Berman KF, Byas-Smith MG, Coghill RC, Gracely RH, Bennett GJ (1995). Unilateral decrease in thalamic activity observed with positron emission tomography in patients with chronic neuropathic pain. *Pain* **63:**55–64.

Inghilleri M, Conte A, Frasca V, et al. (2002). Is the cutaneous silent period an opiate-sensitive reflex? *Muscle Nerve* **25:**695–9.

Jensen TS, Gottrup H, Bach FW, Sindrup SH (2001). The clinical picture of neuropathic pain. *Eur J Pharmacol* **429:**1–11.

Krause SJ, Backonja MM (2003). Development of a neuropathic pain questionnaire. *Clin J Pain* **19:**306–314.

Kakigi R, Shibasaki H, Kuroda Y, Neshige R, Endo C, Tabuchi K, Kishikawa T (1991). Pain-related somatosensory evoked potentials in syringomyelia. *Brain* **114:**1871–1889.

Kakigi R, Shibasaki H, Ikeda T, Neshige R, Endo C, Kuroda Y (1992). Pain-related somatosensory evoked potentials following CO2 laser stimulation in peripheral neuropathies. *Acta Neurol Scand.* **85:**347–352.

Kvinesdal B, Molin J, Froland A, Gram LF (1984). Imipramine treatment of painful diabetic neuropathy. *JAMA* **251:**1727–1730.

Lankers J, Frieling A, Kunze K, Bromm B (1991). Ultralate cerebral potentials in a patient with hereditary motor and sensory neuropathy type I indicate preserved C-fibre function. *J Neurol Neurosurg Psychiatry* **54:**650–652.

Leffler AS, Kosek E, Hansson P (2000). The influence of pain intensity on somatosensory perception in patients suffering from subacute/chronic lateral epicondylalgia. *Eur J Pain* **4:**57–71.

Leffler AS, Kosek E, Lerndal T, Nordmark B, Hansson P (2002). Somatosensory perception and function of diffuse noxious inhibitory controls (DNIC) in patients suffering from rheumatoid arthritis. *Eur J Pain* **6:**161–176.

Leung A, Wallace MS, Ridgeway B, Yaksh T (2001). Concentration-effect relationship of intravenous alfentanil and ketamine on peripheral neurosensory thresholds, allodynia and hyperalgesia of neuropathic pain. *Pain* **91:**177–187.

Llewelyn JG, Gilbey SG, Thomas PK, King RHM, Muddle JR, Watkins PJ (1991). Sural nerve morphometry in diabetic autonomic and painful sensory neuropathy: a clinicopathological study. *Brain* **114:**867–892.

Lorenz J, Beck H, Bromm B (1997). Cognitive performance, mood and experimental pain before and during morphine-induced analgesia in patients with chronic non-malignant pain. *Pain* **73:**369–375.

Magerl W, Ali Z, Ellrich J, Meyer RA, Treede RD (1999). C- and A delta-fiber components of heat-evoked

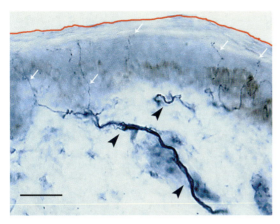

Plate 10.1. Quantification of IENF density using bright-field immunohistochemistry with anti-protein-gene-product 9.5 antibodies.
Arrows indicate IENF and arrowheads indicate dermal nerve bundles. The red line marks the length of the section. Linear IENF density (IENF/mm) is obtained dividing the number of IENF by the length of the section. Bar = 30 μm.

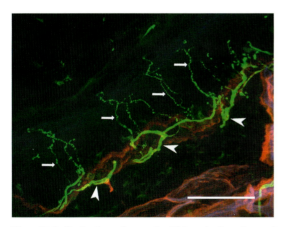

Plate 10.2. Projection of a stack of 16 optical sections of 2-μm thickness obtained by confocal microscopy from a triple-stained skin section.
Nerve fibres are stained in green (protein-gene-product 9.5), basement membrane and the blood vessels are stained in red (collagen IV), and endothelium and epidermis are stained in blue (ULEX-Europaeus agglutinin I). Arrows indicate IENF and arrowheads indicate dermal nerve bundles. The quantification is performed in 3D on the stack of optical sections using Neurolucida software. Bar = 50 μm.

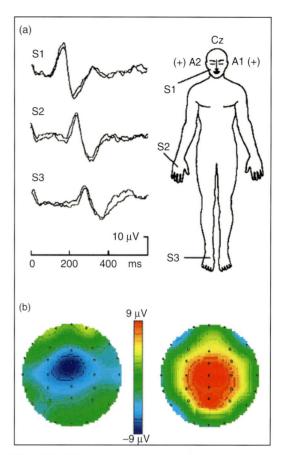

Plate 11.1. Laboratory assessment.
Laser-evoked potentials (LEPs) can be easily elicited from all body dermatomes and recorded from scalp electrodes. This figure, showing LEPs after face, hand, and foot stimulations and their brain maps, is modified from a normative study in 100 subjects. (modified from Truini et al., 2005)

cerebral potentials in healthy human subjects. *Pain* **82:**127–137.

Marchettini P, Lacerenza M, Marangoni C, Pellegata G, Sotgiu ML, Smirne S (1992). Lidocaine test in neuralgia. *Pain* **48:**377–382.

Max MB, Kishore-Kumar R, Schafer SC, Meister B (1991). Efficacy of desipramine in painful diabetic neuropathy: a placebo-controlled trial. *Pain* **45:**3–9.

McCarthy BG, Hsieh ST, Stocks A, Hauer P, Macko C, Cornblath DR, Griffin JW, McArthur JC (1995). Cutaneous innervation in sensory neuropathies: Evaluation by skin biopsy. *Neurology* **45:**1848–1855.

McCracken LM, Zayfert C, Gross T (1992). The Pain Anxiety Symptoms Scale: development and validation of a scale to measure fear of pain. *Pain* **50:**67–73.

McQuay H, Moore A (1998). *An Evidence-based Resource for Pain Relief.* Oxford: Oxford University Press.

Melzack R (1975). The McGill Pain Questionnaire: major properties and scoring methods. *Pain* **1:**275–299.

Melzack R (1987). The short-form McGill Pain Questionnaire. *Pain* **30:**191–197.

Merskey H, Bogduk N (1994). *Task Force on Taxonomy of the International Association for the Study of Pain: Classification of Chronic Pain. Description of Pain Syndromes and Definitions of Pain Terms.* Seattle: IASP Press.

Meyer-Rosberg K, Kvarnström A, Kinnman E, Gordh T, Nordfors L, Kristofferson A (2001a). Peripheral neuropathic pain - multidimensional burden for patients. *Eur J Pain* **5:**379–389.

Meyer-Rosberg K, Bruckhardt CS, Huizar K, Kvarnström A, Nordfors L, Kristofferson A (2001b). A comparison of the SF-36 and Nottingham Health Profile in patients with chronic neuropathic pain. *Eur J Pain* **5:**391–403.

Nolano M, Provitera V, Crisci C, Stancanelli A, Wendelschafer-Crabb G, Kennedy WR, Santoro L (2003). Quantification of myelinated endings and mechanoreceptors in human digital skin. *Ann Neurol* **54:**197–205.

Peripheral Neuropathy Association (1993) Quantitative sensory testing: a consensus report from the peripheral neuropathy association. *Neurology* **43:**1050–1052.

Periquet MI, Novak V, Collins MP, Nagaraja HN, Erdem S, Nash SM, Freimer ML, Sahenk Z, Kissel JT, Mendell JR (1999). Painful sensory neuropathy- prospective evaluation using skin biopsy. *Neurology* **53:**1641–1647.

Peyron R, Laurent B, Garcia-Larrea L (2000). Functional imaging of brain responses to pain. A review and meta-analysis. *Neurophysiol Clin* **30:**263–288.

Pud D, Eisenberg E, Spitzer A, Adler R, Fried G, Yarnitsky D (1998). The NMDA receptor antagonist amantadine reduces surgical neuropathic pain in cancer patients: a double-blind randomized, placebo controlled trial. *Pain* **75:**349–354.

Rasmussen PV, Sindrup SH, Jensen TS, Bach FW (2004) Symptoms and signs in patients with suspected neuropathic pain. *Pain* **110:**461–469.

Rolke R, Andrews K, Magerl W, Treede R-D (2003) *German Research Network on Neuropathic Pain. Quantitative Sensory Testing. A Standardised Battery of Sensory Testing.* Institute of Physiology and Pathophysiology, University of Mainz, Germany.

Rowbotham MC, Davies PS, Fields HL (1995). Topical lidocaine gel relieves postherpetic neuralgia. *Ann Neurol* **37:**246–253.

Rowbotham MC, Davies PS, Verkempinck C, Galer BS (1996). Lidocaine patch: double-blind controlled study of a new treatment method for postherpetic neuralgia. *Pain* **65:**38–44.

Sandrini G, Milanov I, Malaguti S, Nigrelli MP, Moglia A, Nappi G (2000). Effects of hypnosis on diffuse noxious inhibitory controls. *Physiol Behav* **69:**295–300.

Sandrini G, Tassorelli C, Cecchini AP, Alfonsi E, Nappi G (2002). Effects of nimesulide on nitric oxide-induced hyperalgesia in humans – neurophysiological study. *Eur J Pharmacol* **450:**259–262.

Serrao M, Parisi L, Pierelli F, Rossi P (2001). Cutaneous afferents mediating the cutaneous silent period in the upper limbs: evidence for a role of low-threshold sensory fibres. *Clin Neurophysiol* **112:**2007–2014.

Sindrup SH, Jensen TS (1999) Effects of pharmacological treatment of neuropathic pain: an update and effect related to mechanism of drug action. *Pain* **83:**389–400.

Sindrup SH, Andersen G, Madsen C, Smith T, Brosen K, Jensen TJ (1999). Tramadol relieves pain and allodynia in polyneuropathy : a randomised double blind controlled trial. *Pain* **83:**85–90.

Sindrup SH, Bach FW, Madsen C, Gram LF, Jensen TS (2003). Venlafaxine versus imipramine in painful polyneuropathy: A randomized, controlled trial. *Neurology* **60:**1284–1289.

Sjolund KF, Belfrage M, Karlsten R, Segerdahl M, Arner S, Gordh T, Solevi A (2001). Systemic adenosine infusion reduces the area of tactile allodynia in neuropathic pain following peripheral nerve injury: a multi-centre, placebo-controlled study. *Eur J Pain* **5:**199–207.

Smith WB, Gracely RH, Safer MA (1998). The meaning of pain: cancer patient's rating and recall of pain intensity and affect. *Pain* **78:**123–129.

Spielberg CD (1975). The measurement of state and trait anxiety; conceptual and methodological issues. In: Levi L, ed. *Emotions: Their Parameters and Measurement.* New York: Raven Press, pp. 713–725.

Torebjork E (1993). Human microneurography and intra-neural microstimulation in the study of neuropathic pain. *Muscle Nerve* **16**:1063–1065.

Treede R-D, Meyer RA, Raja SN, Campbell JN (1995). Evidence for two different heat transduction mechanisms in nociceptive primary afferents innervating monkey skin. *J Physiol* **483**:747–758.

Truini A, Haanpaa M, Zucchi R, Galeotti F, Iannetti GD, Romaniello A, Cruccu G (2003). Laser-evoked potentials in post-herpetic neuralgia. *Clin Neurophysiol* 114:702–709.

Truini A, Galeotti F, Romaniello A, *et al.* (2005) Laser evoked potentials: normative values. *Clin Neurophysiol* 116:821–826.

Vestergaard K, Andersen G, Gottrup H, Kristensen BT, Jensen TS (2001). Lamotrigine for central post-stroke pain: a randomized controlled trial. *Neurology* **56**:184–190.

Wallace MS, Magnuson S, Ridgeway B (2000). Efficacy of oral mexiletine for neuropathic pain with allodynia: a double blind placebo controlled cross over study. *Reg Anesthesia and Pain Med* **25**:459–467.

Wallace MS, Rowbotham MC, Katz NP, Dworkin RH, Dotson RM, Galer BS, Rauck RL, Backonja MM, Quessy SN, Meisner PD (2002). A randomized, double-blind, placebo-controlled trial of a glycine antagonist in neuropathic pain. *Neurology* **59**:1694–1700.

Ware JE Jr, Sherbourne CD (1992). The MOS 36-item Short-Form Health Survey. *Med Care* 30:473–483.

Watson CPN, Chipman M, Reed K, Evans RJ, Birkett N (1992). Amitriptyline versus maprotiline in postherpetic neuralgia: a randomised, double blind, cross over study. *Pain* **48**:29–36.

Waylett-Rendall J (1988). Sensibility evaluation and rehabilitation. *Orthop Clin North Am* **19**:43–56.

Wendler J, Hummel T, Reissinger M, Manger B, Pauli E, Kalden JR, Kobal G (2001). Patients with rheumatoid arthritis adapt differently to repetitive painful stimuli compared to healthy controls. *J Clin Neurosci* **8**:272–277.

Willer JC (1985). Studies on pain. Effects of morphine on a spinal nociceptive flexion reflex and related pain sensation in man. *Brain Res* **331**:105–114.

Willer JC, Roby A, Le Bars D (1984). Psychophysical and electrophysiological approaches to the pain-relieving effects of heterotopic nociceptive stimuli. *Brain* **107**:1095–1112.

Willer JC, De Broucker T, Bussel B, Roby-Brami A, Harrewyn JM (1989). Central analgesic effect of ketoprofen in humans: electrophysiological evidence for a supraspinal mechanism in a double-blind and cross-over study. *Pain* **38**:1–7.

Woolf CJ, Max M (2001). Mechanism based pain diagnosis. *Anesthesiology* **95**:241–249.

Yarnitsky D, Sprecher E, Zaslansky R, Hemli JA (1995). Heat pain thresholds: normative data and repeatability. *Pain* **60**:329–332.

Zigmond AS, Snaith RP (1983). The hospital anxiety and depression scale. *Acta Psychiatr Scand* **67**:361–370.

Zung WWK (1965). A self-rating depression scale. *Arch Gen Psychiatry* **12**:63–70.

CHAPTER 12

Acute stroke*

W. Hacke,[a,c] M. Kaste,[a,d] J. Bogousslavsky,[a,e]
M. Brainin,[a,f] A. Chamorro,[a,g] K. Lees,[a,h]
D. Leys,[a,i] H. Kwiecinski,[a,j] D. Toni,[a,k] T. Olsen,[b,l]
P. Langhorne,[b,m] H. Diener,[b,n] M. Hennerici,[b,o]
J. Ferro,[b,p] J. Sivenius,[b,q] N. Wahlgren,[b,r] P. Bath,[b,s]

Abstract

The guideline 'Recommendations for Stroke Management' was originally published in 2003 in *Cerebrovascular Diseases* (Hack *et al.*, 2003). Although already widely distributed, this guideline is included in this handbook because it has remained the most important one in its field. It covers all important areas of stroke management including acute therapy, prevention and rehabilitation. It represents a collaborative effort of a writing group of the European Stroke Initiative that was endorsed by the three European Societies, which are represented in the EUSI: the European Stroke Council (ESC), the European Neurological Society (ENS) and the European Federation of Neurological Societies (EFNS). In the meantime, this guideline has been translated into numerous languages including Spanish, Russian and Chinese. Updates and

slide kits are available on the internet. An extended version was also published in 2003 (Hack *et al.*, 2003). A study comparing these guidelines with North American ones has in the meantime been published (Klijn and Hankey, 2004). The ratings for recommendations follow an evidence classification scheme that complies with an earlier version of the EFNS guidance for guideline document (Hughes *et al.*, 2001), but do not consider the more comprehensive ratings of the later classification (Brainin *et al.*, 2004) used for the other guidelines in this book.

Introduction

The European Stroke Initiative Recommendations for Stroke Management were first published in the Journal *Cerebrovascualr Diseases* in 2000. The first publication was well received and was followed by a lengthier supplement. After 3 years, the European Stroke Initiative (EUSI) Executive Committee felt that there were enough new data to justify a complete revision of the recommendations. The EUSI Executive Committee also decided that the consensus for the recommendations should

*The authors have prepared this guideline on behalf of the European Stroke Council (ESC), The European Neurological Society (ENS) and the European Federation of Neurological Societies (EFNS).

[a]European Stroke Initiative Executive Committee; [b]EUSI Writing Committee; [c]University of Heidelberg, Germany; [d]Helsinki, Finland; [e]Lausanne, Switzerland; [f]Department of Neurology, Donauklinikum and Donau-Universität, Austria; [g]Barcelona, Spain; [h]Glasgow, UK; [i]Lille, France; [j]Warsaw, Poland; [k]Rome, Italy; [l]Copenhagen, Denmark; [m]Glasgow, UK; [n]Essen, Germany; [o]Mannheim, Germany; [p]Lisbon, Portugal; [q]Kuopiu, Finland; [r]Stockholm, Sweden; [s]Nottingham, UK.

Table 12.1 Definitions of levels of evidence for these recommendations (EUSI 2000; modified after Adams *et al.*, 1994).

Level I: highest level of evidence
Source
 primary endpoint from randomised, double-blinded study with adequate sample size
 properly performed meta-analysis of qualitatively outstanding randomised trials

Level II: intermediate level of evidence
Source
 randomised, non-blinded studies
 small, randomised trials
 pre-defined secondary end-points of large, randomised trials

Level III: lower level of evidence
Source
 prospective case series with concurrent or historical control
 post-hoc analyses of randomised trials

Level IV: undetermined level of evidence
Source
 small case series without control, case reports
 general agreement despite of lack of evidence from controlled trials

---

have a broader base and therefore invited several European stroke neurologists from different countries to join the writing group. The members of both, Writing Group and Executive Committee, met for 3 days in December 2002 in Heidelberg and prepared the new recommendations. The recommendations from the EUSI published in 2000 (European Stroke Initiative, 2000) have now been completely revised and updated. In accordance with the European Neurological Society (ENS), the European Federation of Neurological Society (EFNS) and the European Stroke Council (ESC), which also represents the European Stroke Conference, provide an overview of established or widely used therapeutic strategies as well as an evaluation of evolving, but not yet proven, strategies. These are discussed in detail as well as classified according to their scientific levels of evidence. On the basis of such evidence, specific recommendations are made. Experts' opinions on several issues on stroke prevention and treatment can be assessed at the EUSI website free of charge at www.eusi-stroke.com. These lectures represent an extension of many issues discussed in these recommendations but have not passed the consensus process

of the EUSI documents and therefore only reflect the opinion of the lecturing experts.

The levels of evidence in this article are defined by the same criteria as in the previous recommendations. They correspond to those published by the EFNS (Hughes *et al.*, 2001) and are listed in table 12.1.

Organisation of stroke care: education, referral, stroke units and rehabilitation

Acute stroke is one of the leading factors of morbidity and mortality worldwide. After cardiovascular disease, stroke ranks as either the second or third most common cause of death in industrialised countries. In Europe, the crude death rate ranges from 63.5/100,000 (males, Switzerland 1992) to 273.4/100,000 (females, Russia 1991). Such large differences in mortality between the east and the west in Europe have been noted (Stegmayr *et al.*, 2000) and attributed to differences in risk factor expression with higher levels of hypertension and other risks in eastern countries as compared to the west, thus resulting in more severe strokes in Eastern Europe (Ryglewicz *et al.*, 2000; Brainin *et al.*, 2000). Also, within Western Europe notable regional variations have been found (Wolfe *et al.*, 2000). Stroke as the most important cause of morbidity and long-term disability in Europe imposes an enormous economic burden. The average cost from first stroke to death has been calculated for several European countries (Kaste *et al.*, 1998) and has, for example, in Sweden been shown to approximate 79,000 Ł (Asplund *et al.*, 1993).

Over the past decades, acute stroke has increasingly been recognised as a medical emergency. Acute, post-acute, and rehabilitation care of stroke patients in specialised wards as well as revascularising therapies have been proven to be effective in acute ischaemic stroke. The establishment of a network consisting of acute stroke units, seamless continuation to post-acute care and rehabilitation, as well as further care in the community has become standard treatment in many European countries. Systems of care have emerged that include nationwide concepts of stroke care units that focus on acute care such as in Austria or Germany (Weimar *et al.*, 2002; Brainin and Steiner, 2003), and systems of stroke units that focus on comprehensive care including rehabilitation as in the United Kingdom or Scandinavia (Jorgensen *et al.*, 1995; Kalra, 1995; Indredavik, 1997).

Several publications of European guidelines and consensus papers have been published over the past years: these include reports from the Pan European Consensus Meeting on Stroke Management (Aboderin *et al.*, 1996), the European Ad Hoc Consensus Group (The European Ad Hoc Consensus Group, 1996, 1997), the Task Force on Acute Neurological Stroke Care of the European Federation of Neurological Societies (Brainin *et al.*, 1997, 2000; Thomassen *et al.*, in press), and the European Stroke Initiative (2000). Among North American guidelines and treatment recommendations issued by the American Academy of Neurology are those for acute treatment (Adams *et al.*, 1994, 2003), carotid surgery (Biller *et al.*, 1998), management of transient ischaemic attacks (TIAs) (Feinberg *et al.*, 1994; Albers *et al.*, 1999) and primary prevention of stroke (Goldstein *et al.*, 2001). Earlier recommendations have been issued

by the WHO (WHO Task Force on Stroke and other Cerebrovascular Disorders, 1989).

Education

Many patients and relatives do not recognise the symptoms of stroke and do not realise that seeking treatment is urgent. Reasons for this shortcoming include a poor awareness of stroke by the victim or family, reluctance to seek immediate medical help, incorrect diagnosis by the paramedical service and perceiving stroke not as an emergency by medical personnel and the family physician (Evenson *et al.*, 2000; Becker *et al.*, 2001; Yoon and Byles, 2002;). These facts emphasise the need for continuous education. The aims of public education initiatives are to enable and encourage the general population to recognise immediately the symptoms of stroke, to realise that urgent medical attention is needed, and to use the emergency transportation services and go immediately to an adequately equipped hospital. Primary contact with general practitioners may cause delays and prevent early start of adequate therapy (Evenson *et al.*, 2000). Educational efforts should be directed at patients at risk for stroke, their families, caregivers or co-workers and to large employers (Wein *et al.*, 2000). Teaching the public about symptoms and signs of stroke is one of the highest priorities of public medical education.

Inaccurate initial diagnosis by professional groups represents a major problem. Ambulance dispatchers may have false positive assessment rate of up to 50%, and even in trained paramedics, this rate is about 25% (Kothari *et al.*, 1997). However, this result can be improved by adequate training (Kothari *et al.*, 1997).

Physicians also need to be trained in the recognition of symptoms and signs of acute stroke and the necessity of immediate transportation to an adequately equipped unit. The medical personnel should be trained in recognising the acute presentations of ischaemic stroke and should be able to cope with the early complications after stroke. Training should include the ability to conduct a medical examination that focuses on the level of consciousness, presence of focal weakness, presence of seizure activity and recognition of aphasia and other major cognitive disturbances. The concept of 'Time is Brain' should be understood by all involved in the 'Stroke Chain of Survival'. No time should be wasted when the patient has arrived at the hospital and written standards for in-hospital delays should be available in hospitals receiving patients with acute stroke. Although such measures have not been shown to be effective by themselves (Kwan and Sandercock, 2003) they can be considered effective in preventing in-hospital delays. One example is that set by the National Institute of Neurological Disorders and Stroke in 1997.

Referral

Stroke is a medical and occasionally also a surgical emergency. Successful care of the acute stroke victim begins with the recognition both by the public and the health professional that stroke is an emergency, like acute myocardial infarction and trauma. The majority of stroke patients do not receive adequate therapy because they do not reach the hospital soon enough (Barber et al., 2001). Successful care of the acute stroke victim as an emergency depends on a 4-step chain:

1 Rapid recognition of and reaction to stroke warning signs
2 Immediate use of emergency medical system (EMS) services
3 Priority transport with notification of the receiving hospital
4 Rapid and accurate diagnosis and treatment at the hospital.

Failure to recognise stroke symptoms and consulting a primary physician delay the interval between stroke onset and arrival at the hospital (Ferro et al., 1994; Derex et al., 2002; Harraf et al., 2002).

Once stroke symptoms are suspected, patients or their proxies should call the emergency medical system. Ambulance transportation decreases the delay onset of stroke hospital arrival (Level III). Helicopter transport is playing an increasing role in transfer of patients with stroke between hospitals and should be activated earlier (Thomas et al., 2002). The EMS system should have an electronic validated algorithm of questions to diagnose stroke during the phone interview with the patient/proxy (Porteus et al., 1999; Camerlingo et al., 2001). Patients with onset of stroke symptoms within

less than 3 h should be given priority in evaluation/transportation by EMS. The EMS ambulance dispatchers should be able to recognise stroke symptoms and signs (Kothari et al., 1997) and identify and provide appropriate help for patients who need emergent care because of impaired consciousness, seizures, vomiting, haemodynamic instability or other early complication or co-morbidity of stroke.

If a general practitioner or other doctor receives a call or consults a patient with suspected stroke, he/she should recommend/arrange emergent transportation, preferably through the EMS system, to the nearest emergency room of a hospital providing organized acute stroke care or stroke unit if available. The EMS ambulance dispatchers should inform the stroke unit personnel that they are going to refer a stroke patient and describe the clinical status. The initial evaluation of stroke patients can be made by emergency room doctors. In fact, emergency room doctors can correctly make the diagnosis of stroke in about 90% of cases (Ferro et al., 1998).

Patients with subarachnoid haemorrhage should be referred urgently to a hospital where neurosurgical treatment, neuroradiological interventions and intensive care are available (Level I).

RECOMMENDATIONS

1 Stroke patients should be treated in stroke units (Level I).* Therefore, suspected stroke victims should be transported without delay to the nearest medical centre with an available stroke unit, or to a hospital providing organised acute stroke care if a stroke unit is not available.
2 Once stroke symptoms are suspected, patients or their proxies should call the EMS or a similar emergency medical system (Level III)
3 Patients with subarachnoid haemorrhage should be referred urgently to a centre with facilities for neurosurgical treatment, neuroradiological interventions and neurointensive care (Level I).

*The recommendations in this chapter follow Table 12.1 and not Level A–C, Good Practice Point system used in the rest of the book.

Stroke units

Stroke care should take place in a stroke unit. A meta-analysis by the Stroke Unit Trialist's collaboration (Stroke Unit Trialists' Collaboration, 2002) showed a 18% relative reduction in mortality, a reduction in death or dependence and a reduction in death or need of institutional care when treated in a stroke unit in comparison to a general medical ward (Level I). The absolute changes indicated a 3% reduction in all cause mortality (numbers needed to treat [NNT] 33), a 3% reduction in the need for nursing home care, and a 6% increase in the number of independent survivors (NNT 16). All types of patients with stroke benefit from treatment and rehabilitation in stroke units: males and females, young and elderly stroke patients and patients with mild, moderate and severe strokes.

A stroke unit consists of a hospital unit or part of a hospital unit that exclusively or nearly exclusively takes care of stroke patients. A survey across Europe showed that various forms of stroke unit care exist (Brainin *et al.*, 2000). Most of such stroke units provide a co-ordinated multidisciplinary approach to treatment and care. The core disciplines of such a multidisciplinary team are: medical treatment, nursing, physiotherapy, occupational therapy, speech and language therapy and social work. The multidisciplinary team should have a specialist interest in stroke management and work in a coordinated way (through regular meetings to plan patient care). Programmes of regular staff education and training should be in place.

The typical components of care in the stroke unit trials (Langhorne *et al.*, 2002) were as follows:

1 Assessment–medical assessment and diagnosis including computerised tomography (CT) scanning, early assessment of nursing and therapy needs.
2 Early management policies - early mobilisation, prevention of complications, treatment of hypoxia, hyperglycaemia, pyrexia and dehydration.
3 Ongoing rehabilitation policies (coordinated multidisciplinary team care, early assessments of needs after discharge).

Stroke units fall into several categories:

1 The acute stroke unit admitting patients acutely and continuing treatment for several days but usually for less than 1 week.
2 The comprehensive stroke unit admitting patients acutely and continuing treatment and rehabilitation for several weeks if necessary.
3 The rehabilitation stroke unit admitting patients after a delay of 1 or 2 weeks and continuing treatment and rehabilitation for several weeks or months if necessary.
4 A mobile stroke team is a mobile team offering stroke care and treatment to stroke patients at a variety of wards. Such teams are usually established in hospitals where stroke units are not available.

Of these only the comprehensive stroke unit and the rehabilitation stroke unit have proven to be effective in terms of reduced mortality and handicap (Stroke Unit Trialists' Collaboration, 2002).

The size of a stroke unit should be adequate to provide specialist multidisciplinary stroke care for the whole duration of hospital admission. In practice, this is often achieved with a single comprehensive unit (in smaller hospitals) or a combination of acute unit and rehabilitation units (in larger hospitals). Further evidence is needed to recommend the type and size of the most effective stroke units in more detail (table 12.2).

RECOMMENDATIONS

1 Stroke patients should be treated in stroke units (Level I).
2 Stroke units should provide coordinated multidisciplinary care provided by medical, nursing and therapy staff who specialise in stroke care (Level I).

Emergency management

The time window for treatment of patients with acute stroke is narrow. Acute emergency management of stroke therefore requires parallel processes at different levels of patient management. For example, acute assessment of neurological and

Table 12.2 Requirements.

Minimum requirements for centres managing acute stroke patients

1   Availability of 24 h CT scanning
2   Established stroke treatment guidelines and operational procedures
3   Close cooperation of neurologists, internists and rehabilitation experts
4   Specially trained nursing personnel
5   Early multidisciplinary rehabilitatio including speech therapy, occupational therapy and physical therapy
6   Established network of rehabilitation facilities to provide a continuous process of care
7   Neurosonological investigations within 24 h (extracranial vessels, colour-coded duplex sonography)
8   ECG, Echocardiography
9   Laboratory examinations (including coagulation parameters)
10 Monitoring of blood pressure, ECG, oxygen saturation, blood glucose, body temperature

Additional facilities recommended

1   MRI/MRA
2   Diffusion and perfusion MR
3   CT angiography
4   Echocardiography (transoesophageal)
5   Cerebral angiography
6   Transcranial Doppler sonography
7   Specialised neuroradiological, neurosurgical and vascular surgical consultation

---

vital functions parallels treatment of acutely life-threatening conditions. The selection of special treatment strategies may already be ongoing before the final decision on the subtype of acute stroke has been made. Time is the most important factor, especially the minutes and first hours after stroke onset.

The acute stroke patient, even the one with milder symptoms, must be recognised as an urgently ill medical patient (Brott and Reed, 1989; Adams *et al.*, 1994; Brott *et al.*, 1994). The patient has to be transported to an emergency unit, and the examining physician must assess the stroke patient with the priority due to a life-threatening and disabling illness. Only a minority of the stroke patients present with an immediate life-threatening condition, but many have severe abnormalities in basic physiological functions. Symptoms and signs that may predict later complications such as space-occupying infarction or bleeding, recurrent stroke, and medical conditions

such as hypertensive crisis, co-existing myocardial infarction, aspiration pneumonia and renal failure must be recognised early. Also, early assessment of stroke subtypes based on the physical and neurological evaluation as well as on skilled interpretation of the results of CT- and MRI-scanning is essential for the prediction of a high risk of early recurrence.

The initial examination includes observation of breathing and pulmonary function, concomitant heart disease, assessment of blood pressure and heart rate, and determination of arterial oxygen saturation using infrared pulse-oximetry if available. Simultaneously, blood samples for clinical chemistry, coagulation and haematology studies are drawn, and a venous line is inserted. Standard electrolyte solutions are given until clinical chemistry results are available. After the emergency assessment, which in part will be done by emergency nurses or other emergency room (ER) personnel, the neurologist should perform

Table 12.3 Emergent diagnostic tests in acute stroke.

1	CT
2	ECG and chest X-ray
3	Clinical chemistry
	Complete blood count and platelet count, prothrombin time, INR, PTT
	Serum electrolytes
	Blood glucose
	CRP, sedimentation rate
	Arterial blood gas analysis, if hypoxia is suspected
	Hepatic and renal chemical analyses
4	Pulse oxymetry
5	Lumbar puncture (only if CT is negative and subarachnoidal haemorrhage is clinically suspected)
6	Duplex and transcranial ultrasound
7	EEG*
8	MRI* and MRA*/CTA*
9	Diffusion MR* and perfusion MR*
10	Echocardiography (transthoracic and transoesophageal)*

*In selected cases.

a targeted neurological examination. The examination is supplemented, if possible, by a careful medical history focussing on risk factors for arterisclerosis and cardiac disease. Especially in young patients, a history of drug abuse, oral contraceptive use, infection, trauma or migraine may give important clues (table 12.3).

Diagnostic imaging

Cranial CT is widely available and it not only reliably distinguishes between haemorrhage and ischaemic stroke or subarachnoid haemorrhage but can also rule out many other brain diseases. Signs of early ischaemia can sometimes be detected as early as 2 h after stroke onset, but this may be difficult even for the trained examiner, in particular in very early studies. Early infarct signs include sulcus effacement, swelling of the basal ganglia and the hyper-intense middle cerebral artery sign. Early signs of extensive infarction with intracranial midline shifts indicate a very serious event and a high risk, both for secondary haemorrhage and large malignant oedema formation and may justify repeated imaging after a short interval. Parenchymal haemorrhage can be identified

almost immediately either in deep structures in patients with hypertension or in atypical areas in patients without hypertension or under adequate treatment, usually due to cerebral amyloid angiopathy. Infratentorial haemorrhage or cerebellar infarcts can be identified similar to supratentorial lesions, but smaller haemorrhages/ischaemic infarcts, in particular in the brain stem, may easily be missed. In addition, CT may detect subarachnoid blood in the majority of cases with subarachnoid haemorrhage. Sometimes haemorrhages may even be interpreted as primary, but indeed are secondary to ischaemic events. Involvement of clearly defined vascular territories are indicative of such conditions, which are easier to identify in MRI studies. Brain haemorrhages tend to grow in the first 6–12 h after stroke in about 40–50% of all patients even without clinical deterioration, which makes a second early CT study necessary. CT angiography (CTA) is a reliable tool to obtain information on extra- and intracranial arterial patency, and its use in clinical practice often adds value to the diagnostic work-up (Schellinger *et al.*, 2003).

Magnetic resonance imaging (MRI) is more sensitive and is increasingly used in referral hospitals with stroke unit expertise as a standard procedure. Recent objections because of a suspected lower sensitivity to identify brain haemorrhages have been overcome by modern MRI techniques such as T2*–weighted imaging, which indeed are even more sensitive than CT scanning for the display of intracerebral haemorrhage. Diffusion-weighted MR is very sensitive for early detection of the damaged brain tissue and combined with perfusion-weighted MR may help in identifying patients who benefit from early thrombolysis. In fact, current concepts suggest that patients with a significant perfusion–diffusion mismatch may benefit from restoration of the ischaemic penumbra surrounding an already necrotic core of infarction, whereas those with overlapping areas of diffusion and perfusion deficits have a less favourable benefit risk ratio. These MR techniques are not yet available on a large scale but do seem promising tools for future routine applications. MR angiography can be used to identify occlusions of major intracranial arteries but should carefully be interpreted if studies from extracranial cerebral arteries are missing. In this case, ultrasound can be useful to identify severe haemodynamical relevant carotid obstructions, which are likely to produce significant perfusion deficits in small embolic or lacunar strokes and may thus mimic falsely a remarkable perfusion–diffusion mismatch. MR angiography also has a role in evaluating the venous system and aneurysms down to a 3-mm diameter.

Ultrasound studies are routinely performed in stroke centres. The major goal is to identify large obstructive lesions in the extracranial as well as in the intracranial basal arteries. In addition, transcranial Doppler may be useful to monitor spontaneous or drug-induced thrombolysis in the majority of patients. In about one quarter of the patients it is not possible or is very difficult to get adequate signals through the temporal bone window without application of contrast agents. The detection of rare causes of ischaemic stroke, such as dissections, intimal hyperplasia and other less frequent aetiologies is facilitated by the systematic use of ultrasound studies. Transoesophageal and transthoracic echocardiography is frequently indicated in suspected cardio-embolic stroke but usually is not performed on an emergency basis.

It seems useful to have these studies available within the first 24 h after onset of stroke to choose the best available secondary prevention, in particular in the presence of cardiac sources of embolism. They can also sometimes be identified by means of middle cerebral artery (MCA) monitoring if high intensity transient signals are observed.

RECOMMENDATIONS

1 A head CT is the most important diagnostic tool in patients with suspected stroke to differentiate between ischaemia and haemorrhage.
2 Vascular imaging (ultrasound, CTA and magnetic resonance angiography (MRA)) in the acute condition gives additional information about the vessel patency in the brain and neck vessels and should supplement all imaging procedures already in the acute phase.
3 MRI/MRA can replace CT if performed appropriately and in particular T2*–weighted imaging is necessary to identify even small haemorrhages.
4 Diffusion and perfusion MR may be of additional help for assessing the risk/benefit ratio for early revascularization therapy.

Quality management and control of process quality

It is mandatory to establish a documentation system for all strokes in a way that allows evaluation of the major characteristics of the patients treated in stroke units. Items chosen must also allow case-mix analyses across units, regions, or even countries. These should include major predictors of outcome such as age, National Institute of Health (NIH) scale values at onset, and diabetes. Several systems of documentations have been developed and recommended for use. It is important to help young colleagues understand that such documentation has to be performed concurrently by either the treating physicians or the stroke nurses themselves and should not be left to additional staff that otherwise do not participate in the work of the stroke unit. It is essential to have follow-up data at least 3 months following the stroke onset to enable benchmarking. These data should at least include

Table 12.4 Recommendations for the quality control of time frames for treatment of acute stroke.

Time frame prolonged	Recommendation
Time from stroke onset to calling emergency service	Increase public information and support stroke awareness campaigns
Time from stroke onset to hospital door	Training of paramedics necessary
Time from hospital door to CT	Screening and revision of intrahospital organization

mortality and Rankin scale. In addition, process quality should also be monitored and evaluated on a regular basis. Some recommendations are listed in table 12.4.

Rehabilitation

Forty percent of stroke patients need active rehabilitation services. Rehabilitation of a stroke victim is started as soon as the patient is clinically stable. The intensity of the actual rehabilitation programme depends on the status of the patient and the degree of the disability. In patients incapable of active training, passive methods may be used to prevent contractions and joint pain and to prevent distress for the patient when active movement is possible. Passive rehabilitation measures also minimise the risk of bedsores and pneumonia. All joints on the paralysed side are moved through the full range of motion several times a day (3–4 times at least). Cooperative patients are encouraged to take an active part in the rehabilitation programme. Prolonged immobilisation and hemiplegia carry the risk of deep venous thrombosis and pulmonary embolism.

Treatment in dedicated stroke rehabilitation wards is based on multidisciplinary team-work consisting of a physician, physiotherapist, speech therapist, occupational therapist, neuropsychologist, social worker and nurse (Stroke Unit Trialists' Collaboration, 2002). In such a unit there is a motivating and encouraging attitude that maintains the patient's desire to improve. Important is a milieu of an 'enriched environment', where patients feel comfortable, and which supports patient's efforts and encourages the patient to practise even beyond working hours (Johansson, 2000). Elderly stroke patients may equally benefit from the well-organised management of stroke (Kaste et al., 1995; Jørgensen et al., 2000).

As soon as the patient is stable, the patient should be carefully assessed for the degree of disability. The extent and distribution of motor weakness and the accompanying sensory and proprioceptive deficits should be noted in detail. The assessment should include evaluation of intellectual impairment especially specific cognitive deficits such as aphasia, apraxia, agnosia, disorders of memory and attention, and the broad range of emotional distress and motivational disturbances. When the patient is transferred to a rehabilitation hospital it is of the utmost importance that all members of the stroke team transfer documentation of the patient's progress to the stroke team of the rehabilitation hospital (Kaste et al., 1995). After institutional rehabilitation the rehabilitation programme can be taken over by an outpatient rehabilitation clinic. This ensures the smooth transfer of the patient to the next rehabilitation step back to normal. The length of the rehabilitation period in the acute stage depends upon the severity of the stroke, and locally available stroke rehabilitation services. Under usual circumstances, rehabilitation following the acute phase of ischaemic stroke should not last longer than 6–12 weeks and rarely more than 24 weeks.

There are recent reports of rehabilitation methods that are based on developing muscle strength and increasing the width of movements with plentiful repetition and enhanced resistance training of the affected limb. These methods are called 'forced use'. Novel restorative programmes that focus on the functional improvement of the upper extremity (Taub et al., 1993; Miltner et al., 1999) or on the recovery of gait (Hesse et al., 2001; Werner et al., 2002) have provided promising tools for the treatment of stroke patients with residual disability.

The fastest recovery of neurological deficit occurs during the first 3 months after the onset of symptoms. Active rehabilitation, however, should be administered as long as objective improvement in the neurological function is observed.

In addition to national organisations involved in providing information to stroke survivors, the role of locally based self-help groups is important in supporting stroke patients and their caregivers. Well-integrated social and medical care with case management programmes may be one way to reduce admission to institutions and prevent functional decline in the elderly (Bernabei *et al.*, 1998). Supporting the patient in his/her social environment is important. Keeping up social contacts is perhaps something that offers the best opportunity to influence the patient's quality of life. Every chronic stroke patient with a marked disability should have regular contact with a family physician, who can encourage the patient, notice possible impairment of clinical state, and take care of secondary prevention.

With focused rehabilitation programmes stroke patients can become ambulatory and largely independent. Of major importance is that the majority of survivors are able to live at home and do not require nursing-home care. That such results can be achieved with systematic stroke management and not by chance is verified by identical results from University Hospitals of Umeå, Sweden (Strand *et al.*,1985), Copenhagen, Denmark, Kuopio, Finland (Sivenius *et al.*, 1985) and Trondheim, Norway (Indredavik *et al.*, 1991).

RECOMMENDATIONS

1 Every patient should have access to evaluation for rehabilitation.
2 In patients with a clear indication for rehabilitation, treatment should be initiated early after stroke (Level I). Disabled patients should have access to structured care including institutional care.
3 Rehabilitation should be provided by a multidisciplinary team in a stroke unit (Level I).
4 The intensity and duration of rehabilitation should be optimal for each patient; new methods of rehabilitation should be used (e.g. repetitive training and forced use), ideally supplementary to established methods (Level II).
5 Patients with chronic symptomatic stroke should be supported in their social environment. This includes access to a family physician, evaluation of outpatient rehabilitation services, secondary prevention and support in psychosocial functioning (Level II).

Prevention

Primary prevention

Primary prevention aims to reduce the risk of stroke in asymptomatic people. Recommendations concerning patients with TIAs are considered here as secondary prevention. Relative risk reduction (RRR), absolute risk reduction (ARR) and numbers needed to treat (NNT) to avoid one major vascular event per year, are provided for each therapy in tables 12.5, 12.6 and 12.7.

Arterial hypertension (high blood pressure)

Elevated blood pressure is strongly and directly related to vascular and overall mortality without any evidence of a threshold (Prospective Studies Collaboration, 2002). Lowering high blood pressure substantially reduces this risk, depending on the magnitude by which blood pressure is lowered (Neal *et al.*, 2000; Staessen *et al.*, 2001). Most studies comparing different drugs have not suggested that any class is superior (Neal *et al.*, 2000; Staessen *et al.*, 2001), except Losartan (50–100 mg) v.s. Atenolol (Dahlof *et al.*, 2002) and Chlorthalidone v.s. Amlodipine and Lisinopril (ALLHAT investigators, 2002).

Diabetes mellitus (DM)

As there are other good reasons to treat diabetes appropriately, it seems prudent to do so in those at risk for stroke. Blood pressure should be lowered more aggressively in diabetics to achieve levels below 135/80 mmHg (Turner *et al.*, 1999).

The American Diabetes Association recommends using aspirin in primary prevention for anyone with diabetes older than 30 years with no known

Table 12.5 Relative risk reduction (RRR), Absolute risk reduction (ARR) and numbers needed to treat (NNT) to avoid one stroke per year in patients who undergo surgery for internal carotid artery stenosis. Modified from (Hankey and Warlow 1999).

Disease(%)	RRR(%)	ARR/year(%)	NNT to avoid 1 stroke/year
Asymptomatic (60–99)	53	1.2	85
Symptomatic (70–99)	65	3.8	27
Symptomatic (50–69)	29	1.3	75
Symptomatic (<50)	No benefit	No benefit	No benefit

Table 12.6 Relative risk reduction (RRR), Absolute risk reduction (ARR) and numbers needed to treat (NNT) to avoid 1 major vascular event per year in patients with antithrombotic therapy. Modified from (Hankey and Warlow 1999).

Disease	Treatment	RRR (%)	ARR/ year (%)	NNT to avoid 1 major vascular event/year
Non-cardioembolic ischaemic stroke or TIA	ASA/placebo	13	1.0	100
	ASA + DYP/ aspirin	15	0.9	111
	ASA+DYP/ placebo	19	1.2	53
	Clopidogrel/ ASA	13	0.6	166
Atrial fibrillation (primary prevention)	Warfarin/ placebo	62	2.7	37
	ASA/placebo	22	1.5	67
Atrial fibrillation (secondary prevention)	Warfarin/ placebo	67	8	13
	ASA/placebo	21%	2.5%	40

Table 12.7 Relative risk reduction (RRR), Absolute risk reduction (ARR) and numbers needed to treat (NNT) to avoid 1 major vascular event per year in patients with risk factors modification. Modified from (Hankey and Warlow 1999).

Clinical condition	Treatment	RRR (%)	ARR (%)	NNT to avoid 1 stroke/year
General population with increased blood pressure	Antihypertensive	42	0.2	94
Post stroke/TIA with increased blood pressure	Antihypertensive	31	2.2	45
Post stroke/TIA with normal blood pressure	Antihypertensive	28	4	42
Post stroke/TIA	Statins	24		59
	Smoking cessation	33	1.7	43
			2.3	

contra-indications (American Diabetes Association, 2000).

Hyperlipidaemia

Three primary or combined primary/secondary prevention trials were unable to show a significant reduction in stroke rate under Pravastatin (WOSCOP study group, 1998; ALLHAT investigators, 2002; Shepherd *et al.*, 2002), despite a tendency (minus 11%) in men (WOSCOP study group, 1998). In the larger Heart Protection Study (2002), the reduction in the event rate under simvastatin was significant even in those with LDL cholesterol below 3.0 mmol/L (116 mg/dL), or total cholesterol below 5.0 mmol/L (193 mg/dL). The annual excess of myopathies was of 1 per 10,000 patients treated (Heart Protection Study, 2002).

Cigarette smoking

Cohort studies have shown cigarette smoking to be an independent risk factor for ischaemic stroke in men (Abbott *et al.*, 1986) and women (Colditz *et al.*, 1988). A meta-analysis of 22 studies indicates that smoking doubles the risk of ischaemic stroke (Shinto *et al.*, 1989). Subjects who stop smoking reduce this risk by 50% (Colditz *et al.*, 1988).

Alcohol consumption

Heavy alcohol drinking (more than 60 g/d) increases the risk of stroke, while light or moderate alcohol consumption may be protective against all strokes including ischaemic strokes (Reynolds *et al.*, 2003). Consumption of up to 12 g of alcohol per day was associated with a reduced relative risk (RR) of all strokes (RR: 0.83), and of ischaemic stroke (RR: 0.80) [13]. Moderate consumption (12 to 24 g. per day) was associated with a reduced risk of ischaemic stroke (RR: 0.72) (Reynolds *et al.*, 2003).

Life-style modification

In men, vigorous exercise was associated with a decreased risk of stroke (Lee *et al.*, 1999). The data suggested that this association was mediated through beneficial effects on body weight, blood pressure, serum cholesterol, and glucose tolerance, and that, apart from these effects, physical activity had no influence on stroke incidence. Substantial

evidence supports the use of diets high in non-hydrogenated unsaturated fats, whole grains, fruits and vegetables, and fish once a month, and adequate omega-3-fatty acids, to reduce the risk of ischaemic heart disease, and probably stroke (Hu *et al.*, 2002; He *et al.*, 2002).

Postmenopausal oestrogen-replacement therapy

Stroke rates rise rapidly in women once they become menopausal. However, in an analysis based on a 16-year follow-up of 59,337 postmenopausal women participating in a Nurses' Health Study, there was only a weak association between stroke and oestrogen replacement (Grodstein *et al.*, 2001). According to the HERS II trial, hormone replacement in healthy women is associated with an increased risk of ischaemic stroke (Grady *et al.*, 2002).

RECOMMENDATIONS

1 Blood pressure measurement is an essential component of regular health care visits. Blood pressure should be lowered to normal levels (<140/ < 90 mm Hg, or <135/80 mm Hg in diabetics) by means of life-style modification. Most hypertensive patients will also need pharmacological treatment to achieve normal blood pressure (Level I).

2 Although strict control of glucose levels in DM has not been proven to be associated with a decreased risk of stroke, it should be encouraged because of benefits in terms of other diabetic complications (Level III).

3 Cholesterol lowering therapy (Simvastatin) is recommended for high-risk patients (Level I).

4 Cigarette smoking should be discouraged (Level II).

5 Heavy use of alcohol should be discouraged, light or moderate alcohol consumption may be protective against stroke (Level I).

6 Regular physical activity is recommended (Level II).

7 A low salt, low saturated fat, high fruit and vegetable diet rich in fibre is recommended (Level II).

8 Subjects with an elevated body mass index should take a weight reducing diet (Level II).
9 Hormone replacement therapy (oestrogen / progesterol) should not be used for primary prevention of stroke (Level I).

Antithrombotic therapy

A meta-analysis (Hart *et al.*, 2000) of the five trials (Peto *et al.*, 1988; Physicians Health research group, 1989; EDTRS investigators, 1992; Hanson *et al.*, 1998; Mead, 1998) comparing aspirin with no aspirin in 52,251 subjects after a mean follow-up of 4.6 years, found no effect on stroke rate. A further trial found that aspirin (100 mg per day) was associated with a non-significant reduction in stroke of 33% (de Gaetano, 2001). No data are available on the use of other antiplatelet agents in primary prevention. There is no proof that aspirin is beneficial in patients with asymptomatic internal artery stenosis, but these patients being at increased risk for MI, there is a consensus to use aspirin.

Warfarin reduces the rate of ischaemic stroke by 70% in patients with atrial fibrillation (AF), with an optimal International Normalised Ratio (INR) level between 2.0 and 3.0 (EAFT group, 1995). In this group, aspirin (300 mg per day) reduces stroke by 21% and is significantly less efficacious than warfarin (Hart *et al.*, 1998). As the annual rate of stroke among people with AF is very wide, risk stratification should be used to determine whether patients should be given oral anticoagulation, aspirin or nothing (Fuster *et al.*, 2001). Oral anticoagulation has a higher chance to be effective in patients with AF who have one or more risk factors, such as a previous ischaemic stroke, or TIA or a previous systemic embolism, age over 75 years, high blood pressure, or poor left ventricular function (Fuster *et al.*, 2001). In patients over 75 years, warfarin used with high INR values (range 3.0–4.5) increases the risk of haemorrhage (The Stroke Prevention in Reversible Ischaemia Trial Study Group, 1997).

Patients with AF who have prosthetic heart valves should receive long-term anticoagulation with a target INR based on the prosthesis type, but not less than INR 2 to 3 (Fuster *et al.*, 2001).

RECOMMENDATIONS

1 Although aspirin does not reduce the risk of stroke in healthy subjects, it does reduce the risk of MI and can be recommended in subjects with one or more vascular risk factors (Level I).
2 Clopidogrel, ticlopidine, trifusal and dipyridamole have not been studied in asymptomatic subjects and therefore cannot be recommended for primary stroke prevention (Level IV).
3 Asymptomatic patients with a greater than 50% ICA stenosis should receive aspirin in order to reduce the risk of MI (Level IV).
4 Long-term oral anticoagulation therapy (target INR 2.5; range 2.0–3.0) should be considered for all AF patients at high risk of embolism: age >75 years, or age >60 years plus risk factors such as high BP, left ventricular dysfunction, DM (Level I).
5 Long-term aspirin (325 mg per day) or warfarin is recommended for patients with non-valvular AF at moderate risk for embolism: age 60–75 years without additional risk factors (Level I).
6 Warfarin is recommended for AF patients aged 60–75 with diabetes or coronary heart disease (Level I).
7 Although not yet established by randomised studies, in patients over 75 years, warfarin may be used with a lower INR (target INR of 2.0; range 1.6–2.5) to decrease the risk of haemorrhage (Level III).
8 Patients with AF unable to receive oral anticoagulants should be offered aspirin (Level I).
9 Long-term aspirin (325 mg per day) or no therapy are recommended for patients with nonvalvular AF at low risk for embolism: age <60 years without additional risk factors (Level I).
10 Patients with AF who have prosthetic heart valves should receive long-term anticoagulation with a target INR based on the prosthesis type, but not less than INR 2 to 3 (Level II).

Carotid surgery and endovascular treatment for asymptomatic carotid stenosis

The Asymptomatic Carotid Athero-sclerosis Study (ACAS), reported that patients with an asymptomatic carotid stenosis greater than 60% had a 5-year RR reduction of 53% of ipsilateral stroke if carotid surgery was performed (ACAS Executive Committee, 1995). However, the absolute risk reduction was small (5.9% in 5 years), as was the rate of ipsilateral stroke in the medically treated group (11.0% in 5 years, or 2.3% annually). Moreover, these results were achieved with a perioperative rate of complications (stroke or death) of only 2.3%. A meta-analysis of five trials of carotid surgery for asymptomatic carotid stenosis concluded that, although surgery reduces the incidence of ipsilateral stroke, the absolute benefit of carotid surgery is small, as the rate of stroke in medically treated patients is low (Benavente *et al.* 1998). Medical management alone is the best alternative for many asymptomatic subjects.

Specific issues

1 Patients with an occlusion of the ICA contralateral to the operated carotid artery do not benefit from endarterectomy (Baker *et al.*, 2000; Straus *et al.*, 2002).
2 The ipsilateral stroke risk increases with the degree of the stenosis (ECST group, 1995; Inzitari *et al.*, 2000).
3 A subgroup analysis of ACAS indicates that women have significantly lower benefit from surgery than men.
4 There are no prospective trials investigating the benefit of antiplatelet drugs in patients with asymptomatic carotid stenosis (Chambers *et al.*, 2002).

Carotid artery angioplasty and stenting for asymptomatic stenosis

There are no data from randomised trials about the benefit and risk of carotid angioplasty compared to endarterectomy in asymptomatic patients (Roubin *et al.*, 2001).

RECOMMENDATIONS

1 Carotid surgery may be indicated for some asymptomatic patients with a 60–99% stenosis

of the ICA. The carotid endarterectomy (CEA)-related risk for stroke or death must be less than 3%, and patients with a life expectancy of at least 5 years (or under the age of 80) may benefit from surgery (Level II).
2 Carotid angioplasty, with or without stenting, is not routinely recommended for patients with asymptomatic carotid stenosis. It may be considered in the context of randomised clinical trials.

Secondary prevention

Antiplatelet therapy

A meta-analysis of 287 trials (Antiplatelet Trialists Collaboration, 2002), showed a 25% relative reduction of serious vascular events (non-fatal myocardial infarction, non-fatal stroke, or vascular death) under antiplatelet therapy in patients with previous ischaemic stroke or TIA: when 1000 patients are treated for 2 years, 36 events are prevented among those with previous stroke or TIA, and this benefit substantially outweighs the absolute risks of major extra-cranial bleeding (Antiplatelet Trialists Cooperation, 2002). Another meta-analysis has attributed a more modest 13% RRR under antiplatelet therapy (Algra *et al.*, 2000)

Aspirin: studies directly comparing the effects of different doses of aspirin failed to show differences in stroke recurrences (Dutch TIA group, 1991; Farrell *et al.*, 1991). The risk benefit ratio of adding another antithrombotic drug to aspirin has not been fully studied.

Clopidogrel is slightly more effective than aspirin in preventing vascular events (CAPRIE Steering Committee, 1996). It is the agent of choice in patients with contraindications, or adverse effects, to aspirin, and may be more effective in higher risk patients (i.e. with a previous stroke, peripheral artery disease, symptomatic coronary disease and diabetes) and after coronary surgery (Bhatt *et al.*, 2000).

Dipyridamole plus aspirin: the ESPS II study (Diener *et al.*, 1996), a randomised, double blind, placebo-controlled trial showed that the combination of aspirin (50 mg) plus dipyridamole (400 mg) doubles the effect of aspirin alone, and of dipyridamole alone: the RRR versus placebo were 37%, 18% and 16% respectively.

Specific issues
1 The incidence of major bleeding complications is independent of the dose of aspirin.
2 The incidence of gastro-intestinal disturbances with aspirin is dose-dependent. Lower doses are safer.
3 The treatment of patients who have a recurrent vascular event on antithrombotic therapy remains unsettled. Such patients should be re-evaluated for pathophysiology and risk factors. Patients without cardiac sources of embolism who suffered a recurrent event while under aspirin do not benefit from warfarin.

RECOMMENDATIONS

1 Appropriate antiplatelet therapy should be given to prevent stroke recurrence and further vascular events (Level I). There are three treatment options that may all be considered as first choice depending on patient characteristics.
2 Aspirin 50–325 mg should be given to reduce stroke recurrence (Level I).
3 Where available, the combination of aspirin (50 mg) and long release dipyridamole (200 mg twice daily) can be given as first choice to reduce the risk of stoke recurrence (Level I).
4 Clopidogrel is slightly more effective than aspirin in the prevention of further vascular events (Level I). It may also be prescribed as first choice or when aspirin and dipyridamole are not tolerated (Level IV), and in high risk patients (Level III).
5 Patients with TIA or ischaemic stroke and unstable angina or non Q wave myocardial infarction should be treated with a combination of clopidogrel 75 mg and aspirin 75 mg (Level III).
6 Patients starting treatment with thienopyridine derivatives should receive clopidogrel instead of ticlopidine because it has fewer side-effects (Level III).
7 In patients who cannot be treated by aspirin or thienopyridine derivatives, long release dipyridamole alone (200 mg twice daily) may be used as an alternative (Level II).

Anticoagulation

Oral anticoagulation (INR 2.0–3.0) reduces the risk of recurrent stroke in patients with non-valvular AF and recent ischaemic stroke (EAF study group, 1995; Fuster *et al.*, 2001).

Although evidence from randomised trials is lacking, long-term anticoagulation is routinely used for patients with mechanical prosthetic valves, with a target INR between 3.0 and 4.0 (Cannegieter, 1995). There is no argument supporting oral anticoagulation in non-cardiac ischaemic strokes (Mohr *et al.*, 2001), and an excessive mortality and major bleeding in excessively anticoagulated patients (target INR 3.0–4.5) was even found in SPIRIT (The Stroke Prevention in Reversible Ischaemia Trial Study Group, 1997).

Specific issues
1 Some retrospective studies suggest that anticoagulation may be beneficial in specific circumstances: aortic atheroma (Dressler *et al.*, 1998), fusiform aneurysms of the basilar artery (Echiverri *et al.*, 1989) or arterial dissection. There are no consistent data relating to anticoagulation after cervical-artery dissection.
2 Oral anticoagulation should probably be avoided in elderly patients with leuko-araiosis (The Stroke Prevention in Reversible Ischaemia Trial Study Group, 1997).
3 It is unclear if patients with patent foramen ovale (PFO) benefit from oral anticoagulation. Patients without proven deep vein thrombosis or associated atrial septal aneurysm should probably be given aspirin. The roles of anticoagulation and closure of the PFO remain to be elucidated (Mas *et al.*, 2001).

RECOMMENDATIONS

1. Oral anticoagulation (INR 2.0–3.0) is indicated after ischaemic stroke associated with AF (Level I). Oral anticoagulation is not advisable in patients with co-morbid conditions such as falls, epilepsy, severe dementia, or gastro-intestinal bleedings.
2. Patients with prosthetic heart valves should receive long-term anticoagulation therapy with

a target INR between 2.5 and 3.5 or higher (Level II).

1. Patients with proven cardio-embolic stroke should be anticoagulated, if the risk of recurrence is high, with a target INR between 2.0 and 3.0 (Level III).

2. Anticoagulation should not be used after non-cardioembolic ischaemic stroke, except in some specific situations, such as aortic atheromas, fusiform aneurysms of the basilar artery or cervical artery dissection (Level IV).

they shift the autoregulation curve of the CBF towards normal values.

RECOMMENDATIONS

1. After stroke or TIA, blood pressure should be lowered, irrespective of its level, with a diuretic and/or an ACE inhibitor, subject to toleration of the treatment (Level I).

2. The effectiveness of other classes of BP lowering drugs has not yet been established by controlled trials.

Anti-hypertensive treatment

A meta-analysis from nine randomised controlled trials on antihypertensive drugs, in which a small number of stroke survivors had been included, led to an estimated RRR for stroke of 29% (95% CI: 5–47%) (The INDIANA Collaborators 1997). Indapamide (2.5 mg daily), a diuretic, reduces the risk of recurrent stroke by 29% (absolute reduction 2.9%) after 3 years in patients with high blood pressure and recent stroke or TIA (PATS collaborating group, 1995). The HOPE study showed an effective prevention of secondary ischaemic events by an ACE-inhibitor (ramipril) in high-risk patients including those who had already had a stroke (Yusuf et al., 2000), despite a modest reduction in blood pressure. The PROGRESS trial showed that patients who had had a stroke or TIA within 5 years, and received Perindopril (4 mg daily) plus Indapamide (2–2.5 mg daily), had a significant 43% reduction in the risk of recurrent stroke (PROGRESS collaborative group, 2001). This benefit was achieved regardless of blood pressure and type of stroke (PROGRESS collaborative group, 2001).

Specific issues

1. Although there is no convincing evidence, patients at risk of haemodynamic stroke as a consequence of occlusive or severe stenotic disease of the carotid or vertebro-basilar arteries, or who have cardiac failure, should not have their blood pressure lowered excessively.

2. ACE inhibitors may be considered in patients with haemodynamic brain compromise because

Cholesterol lowering therapy

A significant reduction in stroke risk is seen across all treatment groups (Di Mascio et al., 2000). Most of this effect was driven by trials involving patients with a prior vascular event using a statin, or where a reduction in total cholesterol levels of more than 10% was achieved. In secondary prevention, 57 patients would need to be treated with statins to prevent one stroke per year (Straus et al., 2002). The MRC/BHF Heart Protection study had a subgroup of 1820 patients with previous stroke or TIA and no previous coronary event: simvastatin (40 mg daily) reduced the risk of recurrent vascular events by 24% (Heart Protection Study Collaborative Group, 2002). The PROSPER trial showed that a similar reduction in the risk of coronary events was observed under pravastatin in older individuals, without significant effect on stroke or cognition after 3 years of follow-up (Sheperd et al., 2002). Gemfibrozil, a fibrate, can also reduce the risk of stroke (Rubins et al., 1999).

RECOMMENDATIONS

Patients with a history of ischaemic stroke or TIA should be considered for statin (Simvastatin) therapy (Level I).

Hormone replacement therapy (HRT)

In the Women's Oestrogen for Stroke Trial, a placebo-controlled randomised trial of oestrogen replacement therapy for the secondary prevention of ischaemic stroke, the risk of fatal stroke was higher (not significant), with oestrogens, and non-fatal strokes were associated with worse functional outcomes (Viscoli *et al.*, 2001).

RECOMMENDATIONS

There is no indication to use HRT for secondary stroke prevention in postmenopausal women (Level II).

Smoking

Smoking cessation leads to an early reduction in risk of both coronary events and stroke at any age (Kawachi *et al.*, 1993; Wannamethee *et al.*, 1995, *et al.* 1988).

RECOMMENDATIONS

All smokers should stop smoking, especially patients who have had stroke (Level IV).

Carotid endarterectomy

The NASCET (NASCET collaborators, 1991) and the ECST (European Carotid Surgery Trialists Collaborative Group, 1995) reported that surgery was efficacious for symptomatic patients with ipsilateral carotid stenosis greater than 70%. Although these trials used different methods of measurement, it is possible to predict the percentage of stenosis from one method to another, and there is little difference in their ability to predict ipsilateral stroke (Rothwell *et al.*, 2003). The NASCET analysis of surgery for symptomatic patients with less than 70% stenosis revealed an ARR of 6.5% and a RRR of 29% for patients with 50–69% stenosis allocated for surgery (Barnett *et al.*, 1998); the overall significance of carotid surgery in preventing ipsilateral stroke was marginal ($p = 0.045$) and the confidence intervals overlapped in the survival curves.

Specific issues
1. Elderly patients (>75 years) without organ failure or serious cardiac dysfunction benefit from CEA.

2. Women with symptomatic stenosis >70% should undergo CEA. Women with moderate stenosis should be treated medically.
3. Patients with few risk factors who present with amaurosis fugax only are better off with medical treatment. Patients with severe stenosis and high risk profile should be considered for CEA.
4. Patients with mild to moderate intracranial stenosis and severe extracranial stenosis are ideal candidates for CEA.
5. The benefit from CEA is lower for patients with lacunar stroke.
6. Patients with leuko-araiosis should be made aware of the increased operative risk.
7. Occlusion of the contralateral ICA is not a contraindication to CEA but carries a higher perioperative risk.
8. Continuation of aspirin is required until surgery, but heparin may be used in very severe stenosis.
9. The benefit from endarterectomy is marginal in patients with carotid near-occlusion.
10. All grading of stenoses should be according to NASCET-criteria.

RECOMMENDATIONS

1. Conventional angiography, or one or ideally more of the following investigations–ultrasonography, MRA, or CTA–may be used to identify and quantify carotid artery stenosis.
2. CEA is indicated for patients with stenosis of 70–99% without a severe neurological deficit with recent (<180 days) ischaemic events. This is valid only for centres with a perioperative complication rate (all strokes and death) of less than 6% (Level I).
3. CEA may be indicated for certain patients with stenosis of 50–69% without a severe neurological deficit. This is valid only for centres with a perioperative complication rate (all strokes and death) of less than 6%. The subgroup of patients most likely to benefit from surgery is males with recent hemispheric symptoms (Level III).
4. CEA is not recommended for patients with stenosis of less than 50% (Level I).

1. CEA should not be performed in centres not exhibiting low complication rates similar to those seen in NASCET or ECST (Level I).
2. Patients should remain on antithrombotic therapy before, during and after surgery (Level II).
3. Patients should be followed-up by the referring physician as well as the surgeon (Level IV).

Extracranial-intracranial anastomosis (EC-IC-Bypass)

Anastomosis between the superficial temporal and middle cerebral arteries is not beneficial in preventing stroke in patients with middle cerebral artery or internal carotid artery stenosis or occlusion (The EC/IC Bypass Study Group, 1985).

Carotid angioplasty and stenting

Angioplasty was compared with surgery in the Carotid and Vertebral Artery Trans-luminal Angioplasty Study, a randomised clinical trial (CAVATAS Investigators 2001): the 30-day death and stroke rate of carotid surgery was 9.9% and that of angioplasty 10.0%. We await the results of ongoing trials. The use of carotid angioplasty and stenting should be limited to well-designed, well-conducted, randomised studies.

RECOMMENDATIONS

1. Carotid PTA may be performed for patients with contraindications to CEA or with stenosis at surgically inaccessible sites (Level IV).
2. Carotid PTA and stenting may be indicated for patients with re-stenosis after initial CEA or stenosis following radiation (Level IV).
3. Patients should receive a combination of clopidogrel and aspirin immediately before, during and at least 1 month after stenting (Level IV).

Acute stroke management

There are five mainstays in the treatment of acute stroke.

1 Treatment of general conditions that need to be stabilised.

2 Specific therapy directed against particular aspects of stroke pathogenesis, either recanalisation of a vessel occlusion or prevention of mechanisms leading to neuronal death in the ischaemic brain (neuroprotection).

3 Prophylaxis and treatment of complications that may be either neurological (such as secondary haemorrhage, space-occupying oedema or seizures) or medical (such as aspiration, infections, decubital ulcers, deep venous thrombosis, or pulmonary embolism).

4 Early secondary prevention, which is aimed at reducing the incidence of early stroke recurrence.

5 Early rehabilitation.

Monitoring of vital neurological functions in the stroke unit or in a normal ward

In all stroke patients, the neurological status and vital functions (BP, pulse rate and temperature) should be continuously or regularly monitored. The neurological status is best monitored using validated neurological scales, such as the NIH Stroke Scale (Lyden *et al.*, 1994), the Scandinavian Stroke Scale (Lindstrom *et al.*, 1991) and the Glasgow Coma Scale (Teasdale and Jennet, 1976).

In selected cases with a past medical history of cardiac disease and/or arrhythmias and in case of unstable BP, on-line ECG monitoring is desirable. The electrodes for cardiac monitoring can also be used for respiratory monitoring, which are useful to detect respiration abnormalities during sleep (Iranzo *et al.*, 2002; Turkington *et al.*, 2002). When instrumental monitoring is not feasible, repeat ECG, clinical checks of respiratory function and blood pressure measurements with automatic inflatable sphygmomanometry should be performed. Pulse oxymetry is useful for continuous monitoring in stroke units. It provides relevant information on the patient's respiratory status. A central venous catheter and occasionally central venous pressure monitoring is needed in severe stroke patients treated in specialised wards. Via a central venous catheter, indirect information on intra-vascular volume, cardiac function, and compliance within the venous system can be achieved.

General stroke treatment

The term 'general treatment' refers to treatment strategies aimed at stabilising the critically ill patient to control systemic problems that may negatively influence stroke outcome and to provide an optimum physiological basis upon which specific therapeutic strategies may be applied. There is consensus that the management of general medical problems is the basis for stroke treatment (WHO Task Force, 1989; Brott and Reed, 1989; Adams et al., 1994; Hacke et al., 1995; European Ad Hoc Consensus Group, 1996). General management of stroke patients includes respiratory and cardiac care, fluid and metabolic management, BP control, and perhaps treatment of elevated intracranial pressure. In addition, treatment of seizures and prophylactic measures concerning DVT, pulmonary embolism, dysphagia, aspiration pneumonia, other infections, and decubital ulcer are part of the general treatment of the patients.

Most authors agree that adequate support of vital functions constitutes basic therapy. On the other hand, one has to keep in mind that even the proposed management of hypertension, hyperglycaemia or fever in stroke patients has never been tested prospectively.

Pulmonary function and airway protection

Normal respiratory function and adequate blood oxygenation are required for stroke management, being important for the preservation of metabolic function in the ischaemic penumbra. Although there is no convincing prospective clinical evidence that oxygen supply at low flow rates is useful in human brain infarction (Ronning and Guldvog, 1999), respiratory function has to be monitored to detect and treat hypoxia. This may be consequent to extensive brainstem or hemispheric infarction, large brain haemorrhage, sustained seizure activity, or to complications such as severe pneumonia particularly in patients at risk of aspiration, heart failure, pulmonary embolism, or exacerbation of chronic obstructive pulmonary disease. Ventilation may be particularly compromised during

sleep (Iranzo et al., 2002). Blood oxygenation is improved by the administration of 2–4 litres of O_2 per minute via a nasal tube, when indicated. In the event of a severely compromised respiratory pattern, severe hypoxaemia or hypercarbia, and in the unconscious patient (GCS ≤ 8) at high risk for aspiration, early intubation may be necessary. Prognosis of stroke patients undergoing intubation is not invariably bad (Grotta et al., 1995; Berrouschot et al., 2000) with some series reporting a 1-year survival rate of about one-third of the patients (Steiner et al., 1997). Of course, before intubation is performed, the general prognosis, coexisting life-threatening medical conditions and the presumed will of the patient and his family have to be taken into account.

Cardiac care

Cardiac arrhythmias secondary to stroke, particularly AF (Broderick et al., 1992; Vingerhoets et al., 1993), are not unusual, while heart failure, acute myocardial infarction (MI) or sudden death, (Bamford et al., 1990; Broderick et al., 1992) may complicate the clinical course. Significant ECG alterations in the ST segments and the T waves and QT prolongation mimicking myocardial ischaemia may appear in the acute phase (Norris, 1983), and cardiac enzymes may be elevated after stroke (Kaste et al., 1978; James et al., 2000). Most of the events are related to pre-existing coronary artery disease (Khechinashvili G, 2002) but there may also be coincidental MI, with cerebral ischaemia (Furlan, 1987). However, irrespective of previous cardiac disease, a correlation has been stressed between infarcts involving the insular cortex and cardiac complications (Oppenheimer et al., 1996).

Every stroke patient should have an initial ECG while indications on continuous ECG monitoring are reported above.

Optimizing cardiac output with maintenance of a high normal BP and a normal heart rate is the essential basis of stroke management. The central venous pressure should be maintained at approximately 8–10 cm H_2O, and its monitoring, although not frequently used in a normal ward, will give early warning of a volume deficiency or volume overload, which both have negative effects on cerebral perfusion. The intravascular volume must be kept stable. Among the inotropic agents, Dobutamine has the advantage of increasing cardiac output without substantially affecting either heart rate or BP. Dopamine may be particularly useful in patients with arterial hypotension or renal insufficiency. Increases in cardiac output may increase cerebral perfusion in areas that have lost their auto-regulative capacity after acute ischaemia. Restoration of normal cardiac rhythm using drugs, cardio-version, or pacemaker support should be performed in cooperation with internists or cardiologists, if necessary.

Blood pressure management

BP monitoring and treatment is a critical issue, as many patients with acute stroke have elevated BP (Leonardi-Bee et al., 2002). Some data would favour treatment (Hatashita et al., 1986; Davalos et al., 1990; Bowes et al., 1996; Fagan et al., 1998; Chamorro et al., 1998; Ahmed et al., 2001; Leonardi-Bee et al., 2002), but evidence opposing treatment is also available (Jorgensen et al., 1994; Ahmed et al., 2000; Leonardi-Bee et al., 2002). Cerebral blood flow autoregulation may be defective in an area of evolving infarction (Meyer et al., 1973). Eames et al. (2002) showed that flow in the ischaemic penumbra is passively dependent on the mean arterial pressure. Hence, abrupt drops in BP must be avoided if an adequate cerebral perfusion pressure is to be maintained. Moreover, blood pressure increase may be consequent to treatable conditions (Carlberg et al., 1991), and usually BP spontaneously decreases during the first days after stroke onset (Britton et al., 1986; Jansen et al., 1987; Oppenheimer and Hachinsky, 1992; Broderick et al., 1993; Harper et al., 1994).

A target systolic BP of 180 mm Hg and diastolic BP of 100–105 mm Hg is recommended in patients with prior hypertension. In other cases, lower blood pressure values are desirable (160–180/90–100 mm Hg). Obviously, extremely high BP levels are not acceptable. Systolic values over 220 mm Hg or diastolic values over 120 mm Hg (in some centres, especially in North America, thresholds of 240 systolic and 130 diastolic are accepted) constitute an indication for early but cautious drug treatment, avoiding a drastic or abrupt reduction in blood pressure (table 12.8) There are only few other indications for immediate anti-hypertensive therapy. Treatment may be appropriate in the setting of concomitant acute myocardial ischaemia (although extreme lowering of BP is deleterious for MI patients as well), cardiac insufficiency, acute renal failure or aortic arch dissection. In patients undergoing thrombolysis or heparin administration BP above 180 mmHg systolic should be avoided. In case the CT scan has shown a non-ischaemic cause of stroke, such as SAH, intracerebral haemorrhage or sub-dural haematoma, antihypertensive treatment may also be started.

The use of sublingual Nifedipine should be avoided because of the risk of abrupt reduction of blood pressure (Grossman et al., 1996), possible ischaemic steal (Graham, 1982; Power, 1993; Adams et al., 1994; Jorgensen et al., 1994; Ahmed et al., 2000) and overshoot hypertension. Oral Captopril (6.25–12.5 mg), may be used instead, but it has a short duration of action and can have an abrupt effect (table 12.9). In North America intravenous (i.v.) Labetalol (10 mg) is frequently recommended. Intravenous Urapidil is increasingly used in this situation. Finally, Sodium Nitroprusside is sometimes recommended despite possible major side-effects, such as reflex tachycardia and coronary artery ischaemia.

A low or normal-low BP at stroke onset is unusual (Leonardi-Bee et al., 2002) and may be consequent to a large infarct, or to cardiac failure or ischaemia, or sepsis. BP can be raised by adequate patient rehydration with crystalloid (saline) or, occasionally, colloid, solutions. Low cardiac output may need inotropic support.

Glucose metabolism

An increase of serum glucose level at hospital admission may be frequently found, due to previously known or unknown diabetes (Toni et al., 1992; Gray et al., 1987) and even in non-diabetic patients (van Kooten et al., 1993).

High glucose levels are harmful in stroke (Pulsinelli et al., 1983; Davalos et al., 1990;

Table 12.8 Characteristics of selected antihypertensive drugs that may be used in acute stroke (modified from Kaplan (1990) and Ringleb *et al.* (1998)).

	Dose	Onset, min	Duration, h	Adverse effects
Oral drugs				
Angiotensin-converting enzyme inhibitor				
Captopril	6–12.5 mg sl	15–30	4–6	decrease in CBF ortostatic hypotension
Parenteral drugs				
Central sympaticolytic				
Clonidine	0.2 mg initial then 0.1 mg/h up to 0.8 mg	5–15	6–8	profound hypotension caution if combined with diuretics
Vasodilators				
Nitroprusside	0.25–10 g/kg min^{-1}	1–5		nausea, vomiting muscle twitching, sweating, thiocyanate intoxication
Nitroglycerin	5–100 g/kg min^{-1}	2–5		tachycardia, headaches, vomiting
Dihydralazin	6.5–20 mg i.v. bolus 1.5–7.5 mg/h	1–2	1–2	tachycardia, headaches
β-Blocker				
Propranolol	1–10 mg i.v.	1–2	3–6	β-blocker side-effects (e.g. bronchospasm, decreased cardiac output, bradycardia)
α/β-Blocker				
Labetalol	20–80 mg i.v. bolus 2 mg/min i.v.	5–10	3–5	vomiting, postural infusion hypotension, nausea, dizziness
α-Blocker				
Urapidil	10–50 mg i.v. bolus 9–30 mg/h	2–5	3	no serious side-effects
Central sympatholytic				
Clonidine	0.075 mg s.c.	5–10	3–5	initial blood pressure increase, sedation
The use of oral calcium antagonists is strongly discouraged				

Toni *et al.*, 1994; Weir *et al.*, 1997; Capes *et al.*, 2001).

This is true not only for diabetic patients, whose metabolic derangement may be dramatically worsened in the acute stroke phase, but also for non-diabetic subjects (Weir *et al.*, 1997; Capes *et al.*, 2001). Hence, temporary insulin treatment may become necessary. A blood glucose level of 10 mmol/l or higher justifies immediate insulin titration. No glucose solution should be given to a stroke patient unless the patient's blood glucose Level Is known.

On the other hand, hypo-glycaemia can rarely mimic an acute ischaemic infarction (Huff, 2002) and should be treated by i.v. dextrose bolus or infusion of 10–20% glucose, preferably via a central venous line.

Body temperature

Experimentally hyperthermia increases infarct size (Fukuda *et al.*, 1999). Fever is frequent over the initial 48 h of stroke onset (Corbett *et al.*, 2000) and negatively influences clinical outcome (Reith *et al.*, 1996; Castillo *et al.*, 1999; Hajat *et al.*, 2000). On the other hand it has to be remembered that infection is a risk factor for stroke (Syrjanen *et al.*, 1988; Grau *et al.*, 1995), and that many patients develop an infection after stroke (Grau *et al.*, 1999; Georgilis *et al.*, 1999). Hence search of a possible infection is recommended to start tailored treatment, though empirical antibiotic, antimycotic or antiviral treatment is not recommended in immuno-competent patients.

Small randomised studies with high dose antipyretics provide contradictory data on the usefulness of this approach (Dippel *et al.*, 2001; Kasner *et al.*, 2002), but treating an elevated temperature in stroke patients is advisable. Although there are no prospective data, one may consider treating fever as early as the temperature reaches 37.5°C.

Fluid and electrolyte management

Stroke patients should have a balanced fluid and electrolyte status to avoid plasma volume contraction, which may influence brain perfusion and kidney function. Some degree of dehydration on admission is frequent and may be related to bad outcome (Bhalla A *et al.*, 2000). Virtually all acute stroke patients need i.v. fluid therapy, with a more or less positive balance according to level of dehydration. However, uncontrolled volume replacement may lead to cardiac failure and pulmonary oedema.

A slightly negative fluid balance is recommended in the presence of brain oedema. Hypotonic solutions (NaCl 0.45% or glucose 5%) are contraindicated due to the risk of brain oedema increase.

Serious electrolyte abnormalities are uncommon in patients with ischaemic stroke (Diringer *et al.*, 1992). However, electrolytes should be monitored daily and substituted accordingly. A peripheral venous access is usually sufficient for initial fluid management and blood sampling, while a central venous catheter is required in case of infusion of larger volumes of fluids or hyper-osmolal solutions.

RECOMMENDATIONS

Level IV recommendations:

1. Continuous cardiac monitoring is recommended in the first 48 h of stroke onset particularly in patients with:

   - previous known cardiac disease
   - history of arrhythmias
   - unstable blood pressure
   - clinical signs/symptoms of heart failure
   - abnormal baseline ECG
   - infarct involving the insular cortex.

2. Oxygenation monitoring with pulse oxymetry is recommended.
3. O$_2$ administration is recommended in case of hypoxemia
4. (blood gas analysis or O$_2$sat < 92% at pulse oxymetry).
5. Intubation is recommended in case of potentially reversible respiratory insufficiency.
6. Routine BP lowering is not recommended, except for extremely elevated values (>200–220 SBP or 120 DBP for ischaemic stroke, >180/105 for haemorrhagic stroke) confirmed by repeated measurements.
7. Immediate antihypertensive therapy for more moderate hypertension is recommended in case of stroke and heart failure, aortic dissection, acute myocardial infarction, acute renal failure, thrombolysis or i.v. heparin but should be applied cautiously.
8. Recommended target BP in patients with prior hypertension180/100–105 mmHg without prior hypertension: 160–180/90–100 mmHg under thrombolysis avoid SBP above 180 mmHg.
9. Recommended drugs for BP treatment:
   i.v. Labetalol or Urapidil
   i.v. Sodium Nitroprusside or Nitroglycerin
   oral Captopril.

10. Avoid Nifedipine and any drastic BP decrease. Avoid and treat hypotension particularly in unstable patients by administering adequate amounts of fluids (see further on) and, when required, volume expanders and/or catecholamines (Epinephrine 0.1–2 mg/h plus Dobutamine 5–50 mg/h).
11. Monitoring of serum glucose levels is recommended, particularly in known diabetic patients.
12. Glucose solutions are not recommended due to the detrimental effects of hyperglycaemia.
13. Treatment of serum glucose levels > 10 mMol/L with insulin titration is recommended.
14. Immediate correction of hypoglycaemia is recommended by i.v. dextrose bolus or infusion of 10–20% glucose.
15. Treatment of body temperature $\geq 37.5°C$ is recommended.
16. In case of fever the search of a possible infection (site and aetiology) is recommended to start tailored antibiotic treatment.
17. Antibiotic, anti-mycotic or anti-viral prophylaxis is not recommended in immuno-competent patients.
18. Monitoring and correction of electrolyte and fluid disturbances are recommended.
19. Hypo-tonic solutions (NaCl 0.45% or glucose 5%) are contraindicated due to the risk of brain oedema increase consequent to reduction of plasma osmolality.

Specific treatment

Thrombolytic therapy
iv-rtPA

Thrombolytic therapy with rtPA (0.9 mg/kg body weight) given within 3 h after stroke onset to patients with acute ischaemic stroke significantly improves outcome (The National Institute of Neurological Disorders and Stroke rtPA Stroke Study Group, NINDS, 1995), with a NNT of 7. Two European trials ECASS and ECASS II tested a 6-h time window and did not show statistically significant superiority of rtPA for the primary endpoints (Hacke *et al.*, 1995, 1998).

Eight trials have tested rtPA in 2889 patients. Overall, there was a significant reduction in the number of patients with a poor functional outcome (combined death or dependency) at the end of follow-up (OR 0.83, 95% CI 0.73–0.94). The subgroup of patients treated within 3 h showed a greater reduction in poor functional outcome with thrombolysis (OR 0.58, 95% CI 0.46–0.74) with no adverse effect on death (Hacke *et al.*, 1999; Wardlaw and Warlow, 1999; Wardlaw, 2001).

A pooled analysis of individual data of the 6 rtPA trials confirms that thrombolysis works at least until 4.5 h and potentially up to 6 h after stroke onset (Brott, 2002). Caution is advised before giving intravenous rtPA to persons with severe stroke (NIH stroke scale >25), or if the CT demonstrates extended early changes of a major infarction, such as sulcal effacement, mass effect and oedema.

Thrombolytic therapy should only be given if the diagnosis is established by a physician who has expertise in the diagnosis of stroke, and a CT of the brain is assessed by physicians who have expertise in reading this imaging study. Because the use of thrombolytic drugs carries the real risk of major bleeding, the risks and potential benefits of rtPA should be discussed whenever possible with the patient and family before treatment is initiated.

Intravenous administration of rtPA more than 3 h after stroke should be done only in an institutional protocol as experimental therapy or within a multicenter clinical trial. Continuous auditing of routine use of thrombolytic therapy is advisable. Safety monitoring of treatment (SITS-MOST) is a condition for approval of rtPA in the European Union.

Other thrombolytic approaches

Intravenous Streptokinase has been shown to be associated with an unacceptable risk of haemorrhage and haemorrhage-associated death (Donnan *et al.*, 1995; The Multicenter Acute Stroke Trial-Europe Study Group, 1996).

Intra-arterial thrombolytic therapy of occlusions of the proximal part of the middle cerebral artery, using pro-urokinase, has been shown to be significantly associated with better outcome in a randomised trial. This treatment is safe and efficacious in a 6-hour time window, but it requires super-selective angiography and is only available in selected centres (Furlan *et al.*, 1999). Intra-arterial treatment of acute basilar occlusion with urokinase or rtPA is frequently used in selected centres, but has not been subjected to a randomised trial (Hacke *et al.*, 1988; Brandt *et al.*, 1996).

De-fibrinogenating enzymes

Ancrod is a defibrinogenating enzyme that was shown to improve outcome after acute ischaemic stroke if given within 3 h after stroke onset and over 5 days (Sherman, for the STAT Writers Group, 1999). Recently, a European trial testing ancrod treatment in a 6-hour time window was terminated prematurely and did not confirm the US-findings.

RECOMMENDATIONS

1. Intravenous rtPA (0.9 mg/kg, maximum 90 mg), with 10% of the dose given as a bolus followed by an infusion lasting 60 min, is the recommended treatment within 3 h of onset of ischaemic stroke (Level I).

2. The benefit from the use of i.v. rtPA for acute ischaemic stroke beyond 3 h after onset of the symptoms is smaller, but present up to 4.5 h (Level I).

3. Intravenous rtPA is not recommended when the time of onset of stroke cannot be ascertained reliably; this includes persons whose strokes are recognised upon awakening (Level IV).

4. Intravenous administration of streptokinase is dangerous and not indicated for the management of persons with ischaemic stroke (Level I).

5. Data on the efficacy and safety of any other intravenously administered thrombolytic drugs are not available to provide a recommendation.

6. Intra-arterial treatment of acute middle cerebral artery occlusion in a 6-hour time window using pro-urokinase results in a significantly improved outcome (Level II).

7. Acute basilar occlusion may be treated with intra-arterial therapy in selected centres in an institutional protocol as experimental therapy or within a multicenter clinical trial (Level IV).

8. Ancrod cannot presently be recommended for use in acute ischaemic stroke outside the setting of clinical trials.

Aspirin

The results of two very large randomised, non-blinded intervention studies indicate that aspirin given within 48 h after stroke (IST, CAST) reduces mortality and rate of recurrent stroke minimally, but statistically significantly (International Stroke Trial Collaborative Group. 1997; Chinese Acute Stroke Trial, 1997), with a NNT of 111.

Early anticoagulation

Early anticoagulation with unfractionated heparin (UFH) has been used frequently in treatment after acute ischaemic stroke. Unfortunately, none of the early anticoagulation trials that have been performed in the past years selected full anticoagulant doses of UFH as the therapeutic option. Subcutaneous UFH at low- or moderate doses (International Stroke Trial Collaborative Group, 1997), Nadroparin (Kay *et al.*, 1995; Hommel *et al.*, 1998), Certoparin (Diener *et al.*; 2001), Tinzaparin (Bath *et al.*,2001), Dalteparin (Berge E *et al.*,2000) and i.v. Danaparoid (The TOAST Publication Committee, 1998) failed to show an overall benefit of treatment. While there was some kind of improvement in outcome or reduction in stroke recurrence rates, this was almost always counterbalanced by an increased number of haemorrhagic complications. In addition, most investigators believe that heparin is not a standard therapy for all stroke subtypes. Full-dose heparin may be used when there are selected indications such as cardiac sources with high risk of re-embolism, arterial dissection, or high grade arterial stenosis prior to surgery (table 12.10). Some investigators found greater functional recovery the sooner heparin was administered suggesting that in addition to its role in preventing early stroke recurrence, the agent also has therapeutic properties (Chamorro, 2001), including down-regulation of inflammatory markers (Chamorro *et al.*, 2002). Contra-indications for the treatment with heparin include large infarcts (e.g. more than 50% of MCA territory), uncontrollable arterial hypertension and advanced microvascular changes in the brain.

Haemodilution

Several large clinical trials of isovolaemic haemodilution failed to demonstrate a decline in mortality

Table 12.9 Suggested antihypertensive treatment in acute ischaemic stroke (modified from Brott *et al.*, 1994, and Ringleb *et al.*, 1998) (availability of substances may vary between countries).

1 Systolic BP 180–220 mm Hg and/or diastolic BP 105–140 mm Hg	Do not treat
2 Systolic BP $\geq$220 mm Hg and/or diastolic BP 120–140 mm Hg, on repeated measures	Captopril 6.25–12.5 mg p.o./i.m. Labetalol 5–20 mg i.v.[a] Urapidil 10–50 mg i.v., followed by 4–8 mg/h i.v[b] Clonidine 0.15–0.3 mg i.v. or s.c. Dihydralazine 5 mg i.v. plus metoprolol 10 mg
3 Diastolic BP $\geq$140	Nitroglycerin 5 mg i.v., followed by 1–4 mg/h i.v. Sodium nitroprusside 1–2 mg

[a] Avoid labetalol in patients with asthma, cardiac failure, severe conduction abnormalities and bradycardia.
[b] In patients with unstable conditions and rapidly fluctuating BP, alternating urapidil/labetalol and arterenol may be used.

Table 12.10 Remaining indications for heparin treatment after stroke.

- Stroke due to cardiac emboli with high risk of re-embolisation (artificial valves, atrial fibrillation, MI with mural thrombi, left atrial thrombosis)
- Coagulopathies such as protein C and S deficiency, APC-resistance
- Symptomatic dissection of extracranial arteries
- Symptomatic extra- and intracranial stenoses
  - Symptomatic internal carotid stenosis prior to operation
  - Crescendo TIAs or stroke in progression
- Sinus Venous Thrombosis

RECOMMENDATIONS

1 Aspirin (100–300 mg per day) may be given within 48 h after ischaemic stroke (Level I).
2 There is no recommendation for general use of heparin, low-molecular weight heparin or heparinoids after ischaemic stroke (Level I).
3 Full-dose heparin may be used when there are selected indications such as cardiac sources with high risk of re-embolism, arterial dissection, or high grade arterial stenosis prior to surgery (Level IV).
4 Haemodilution therapy is not presently recommended for the management of patient with acute ischaemic stroke (Level I).
5 Currently, there is no recommendation to treat stroke patients with neuroprotective substances (Level I).

or disability with treatment (Scandinavian Stroke Study Group, 1987; Italian Acute Stroke Study Group, 1988; The Haemodilution in Stroke Study Group, 1989; Strand, 1992). Hypervolaemic haemodilution has been examined in small randomised trials with conflicting results.

Neuroprotection

No neuroprotective trial has shown improved outcome after stroke on its predefined primary endpoint. Currently, there is no recommendation to treat patients with neuroprotective drugs after ischaemic stroke.

Prevention and treatment of complications

Acute stroke predisposes to medical complications (Davenport *et al.*, 1996; Langhorne *et al.*, 2000) such as pneumonia, urinary tract infections, malnutrition or volume depletion. Patients may also suffer from deep venous thrombosis and pulmonary embolism. Early supportive care and monitoring of physiological parameters may prevent such complications. This is best done in a dedicated stroke unit with experienced staff and early mobilisation. Immobility may lead to infections, contractions and decubital ulcers.

Aspiration and pneumonia

Bacterial pneumonia is one of the most important complications in stroke patients (Davenport *et al.*, 1996; Langhorne *et al.*, 2000; Weimar *et al.*, 2002), the majority being caused by aspiration (Horner *et al.* 1988). As aspiration may be detectable by video-fluoroscopy in as many as 50% of patients during the initial days after stroke onset, oral feeding should be withheld until the patient has demonstrated both intact swallowing with small amounts of water and intact coughing to command. Aspiration is frequently found, both in patients with reduced consciousness and in those with swallowing disturbances. Nasogastric tube (NGT) feeding is adequate for short-term enteral feeding, but a percutaneous enteral gastrostomy (PEG) should be inserted once it is clear that protracted enteral feeding will be required. As a rule of thumb, a PEG is indicated when abnormal swallowing is predicted for periods longer than one month.

NGT or PEG-feeding through avoidance of swallowing may be helpful in prevention of aspiration pneumonia. They do not completely reduce the risk, however, as reflux of liquid feed can itself promote aspiration. Other reasons for pneumonia include hypostasis, diminished cough and immobilisation. Frequent changes of the patient's position in bed and pulmonary physical therapy may prevent this type of pneumonia.

Urinary tract infection

Urinary tract infection is incidental in as many as 40% of patients dying from stroke (Silver *et al.*, 1984). Urinary retention is frequent in the early phase after stroke and will require insertion of a urine catheter or supra-pubic catheter. Otherwise, incontinent patients should be managed with a condom catheter or 'pad and pants'. The majority of hospital-acquired urinary tract infections are

associated with the use of indwelling catheters (Gerberding, 2002). In non-stroke patients suprapubic catheters are considered to carry lower risk of infection (Vandoni *et al.*, 1994), whereas intermittent catheterisation has not been shown to have a reduced risk. Once urinary infection is diagnosed, appropriate antibiotics should be chosen. To avoid bacterial resistance developing, prophylactic antibiotics are best avoided.

Pulmonary embolism and DVT

Pulmonary embolism is the cause of death in up to 25% of patients dying following ischaemic cerebral infarction. Nevertheless, the incidence of symptomatic PE and deep vein thrombosis is now <5%, presumably reflecting modern clinical practice and admission to a stroke unit. The risk of deep venous thrombosis and pulmonary embolism can be reduced by early hydration, and early mobilisation. Although graded compression stockings are effective in preventing venous thromboembolism in surgical patients, their efficacy after stroke is unproven. Whilst subcutaneous heparin or low molecular weight heparin reduce venous thromboembolism their effect is counterbalanced by an increase in haemorrhagic complications. Prophylaxis with subcutaneous low dose heparin (5000 i.u. twice daily) or low molecular weight heparines is reasonable in patients at particularly high risk of DVT or PE.

Decubital ulcer

Frequent turning of immobilised patients is useful for prevention of decubital ulcers. The skin of the incontinent patient must be kept dry. For patients at particularly high risk, an air- or fluid-filled mattress system should be used. If decubital ulcers do not respond to conservative therapy, antibiotic therapy may be justified for several days, preceding definitive surgical debridement.

Seizures

Partial (focal) or secondary generalised epileptic attacks may occur in the acute phase of ischaemic stroke. Post-stroke epilepsy may develop in 3–4% of cases (Olsen, 2001).

Standard i.v. and oral anti-epileptic drugs are in general used. There is no evidence that prophylactic anticonvulsive treatment is beneficial.

Agitation

Agitation and confusion are rarely caused by stroke, but are more frequently a symptom of other complications such as fever, volume depletion or infection. Adequate treatment of the underlying cause must precede any type of sedation or anti-psychotic treatment.

RECOMMENDATIONS

1 Low dose subcutaneous heparin or low molecular weight heparins should only be considered for patients at high risk of DVT or PE (Level II).

2 The incidence of venous thromboembolism may be reduced through early re-hydration and mobilisation, and graded compression stockings (Level IV).

3 Infections after stroke should be treated with appropriate antibiotics.

4 Aspiration pneumonia may not be prevented by naso-gastric feeding (Level IV).

5 Early mobilisation is helpful to prevent numerous complications after stroke including aspiration pneumonia, deep venous thrombosis and decubital ulcers (Level IV).

6 Administration of anti-convulsants to prevent recurrent seizures is strongly recommended (Level III).

7 Prophylactic administration of anticonvulsants to patients with recent stroke who have not had seizures is not recommended (Level IV).

Brain oedema and elevated intracranial pressure (ICP)

Ischaemic brain oedema occurs during the first 24–48 h after stroke onset and is the main reason for early (Toni *et al.*, 1995; Davalos *et al.*, 1999) and late (Davalos *et al.*, 1999) clinical deterioration. The most worrisome situation is that of younger patients with complete MCA infarction, in whom brain oedema and elevated ICP may lead to herniation within 2–4 days after onset of symptoms and to death in about 80% of cases with standard treatment (Rieke *et al.*, 1995; Hacke *et al.*, 1996; Steiner *et al.*, 2001).

Medical therapy

Basic management of elevated intracranial pressure following stroke includes head positioning at an elevation of up to 30°, avoidance of noxious stimuli, pain relief, appropriate oxygenation and normalising body temperature. If ICP monitoring is available, cerebral perfusion pressure should be kept >70 mm Hg (Unterberg *et al.*, 1997). Although strong evidence is lacking (Bereczki *et al.*, 2001; Righetti *et al.*, 2002), osmotherapy with 10% glycerol usually given intravenously (4×250 ml of 10% glycerol over 30–60 min) or i.v. mannitol, 25–50 g every 3–6 h is the first medical treatment to be used if clinical and/or radiological signs of space-occupying oedema occur. Hypertonic saline solutions given intravenously (5×100 ml Saline 3%) (Shackford *et al.*, 1992; Schwarz *et al.*, 1998, 2002), are probably similarly effective, though data available at present are not definitive (Qureshi *et al.*, 1998; Prough *et al.*, 1998). Hypotonic and glucose-containing solutions should be avoided as replacement fluids. Dexamethasone and cortico-steroids are not useful for brain oedema treatment after stroke (Qizilbash *et al.*, 2002). Short-acting barbiturates such as thiopental given as a bolus can quickly and significantly reduce ICP, but the effect is short-lived and may be exploited only to treat an acute crisis, for example, prior to operation. Barbiturate treatment requires ICP and EEG monitoring and careful monitoring of haemodynamic parameters, as a significant blood pressure drop may occur. ICP monitoring is also required when tris (hydroxy-methyl) aminomethane buffer solution is used after osmotherapy and barbiturate failure (Steiner *et al.*, 2001).

Volume loading by vasopressor induced hypertension may be attempted in case of severely compromised CPP, but haemodynamic monitoring and intensive care facilities are required (Kaste and Roine, in press).

Hypothermia

Hypothermia was shown to be neuroprotective after cardiac arrest (Bernard *et al.*, 2002; The HACA group, 2002). Mild hypothermia (i.e. brain temperature between 32 and 33°C) reduces the case fatality rate of patients with severe MCA infarcts, but causes a number of severe side-effects that may be encountered during therapy over several days. (Schwab *et al.*, 1998, 2001) The number of studied patients is still too small to draw any decisive conclusion, however this method is feasible and will be tested prospectively in randomised trials. One problem is recurrent ICP crisis, which was almost exclusively found during re-warming (Steiner *et al.*, 2001). Moreover, in a comparative trial hypothermia had more severe side-effects than decompressive surgery for malignant MCA infarction (Georgiadis *et al.*, 2002).

Decompressive surgery
Malignant MCA infarction The rationale of decompressive surgery is to allow expansion of the oedematous tissue to reduce ICP, to increase perfusion pressure, and to preserve cerebral blood flow by preventing further compression of the collateral vessels. In prospective case series, surgical, decompressive therapy in hemispheric space-occupying infarction lowered mortality from 80% down to 30% without increasing the rate of severely disabled survivors (Hacke and Schwab 1995; Rieke *et al.*, 1995; Mori 2001). Early decompressive surgery within the first 24 h after stroke onset can reduce mortality even more markedly (Schwab *et al.*, 1998). Prospective, multicenter study protocols have been recently developed and are underway.

Cerebellar infarction Ventriculostomy to reveal hydrocephalus and decompressive surgery is considered the treatment of choice of a space-occupying cerebellar infarction, although the scientific basis for this is no more solid than for hemispheric infarction. Comatose patients with space-occupying cerebellar infarctions have a mortality of about 80% if treated conservatively. This high mortality can be lowered down to less than 30% if decompressive surgery is performed (Heros, 1992; Rieke *et al.*, 1993). Like in space-occupying supratentorial infarction, the operation should be performed before signs of herniation are present.

The prognosis among survivors is very good, even if they were comatose when the operation was performed. It should be noted, however, that these are the results of open, small or medium-sized case series, one of them being prospective (Rieke *et al.*, 1993), the remainder being mostly retrospective. Data from a controlled, randomised trial are lacking.

RECOMMENDATIONS

1 Osmotherapy is recommended for patients whose condition is deteriorating secondary to increased intracranial pressure, including those with herniation syndromes (Level IV).
2 Ventriculostomy or surgical decompression and evacuation of large cerebellar infarctions that compress the brain stem is justified (Level III).
3 Surgical decompression and evacuation of a large hemispheric infarction can be a life-saving measure and survivors may have a residual neurological deficit that allows an independent life (Level III).

References

Abbott R, Yin Y, Reed D, Yano K (1986). Risk of stroke in male cigarette smokers. *N Eng J Med* **315**:717–720.
Aboderin I, Venables G, for the PAN European Consensus Meeting on Stroke Management (1996). Stroke management in Europe. *J Intern Med* **240**:173–180.
Adams HP Jr, Brott TG, Crowell RM, Furlan AJ, Gomez CR, Grotta J, Helgason CM, Marler JR, Woolson RF, Zivin JA, *et al.* (1994). Guidelines for the management of patients with acute ischaemic stroke. A statement for healthcare professionals from a special writing group of the Stroke Council, American Heart Association. *Stroke* **25**:1901–1914.
Ahmed N, Wahlgren G (2001). High initial blood pressure after acute stroke is associated with poor functional outcome. *J Intern Med* **249**:467–473.
Ahmed N, Nasman P, Wahlgren NG (2000). Effect of intravenous nimodipine on blood pressure and outcome after acute stroke. *Stroke* **31**:1250–1255.
Algra A, van Gijn J (1996). Aspirin at any dose above 30 mg offers only modest protection after cerebral ischaemia. *J Neurol Neurosurg Psychiatry* **60(2)**:197–199.
American Diabetes Association (2000). Aspirin treatment in diabetes. *Diabetes Care* **23**: S61–62.

Antithrombotic Trialists' Collaboration (2002). Collaborative meta-analysis of randomized trials of antiplatelet therapy for prevention of death, myocardial infarction, and stroke in high risk patients. *Br Med J* **324:**71–86.

Asplund K, Marke L-A, Terent A, Gustafsson C, Wester P (1993). Costs and gains in stroke prevention: European perspective. *Cerebrosvasc Dis* **3(Suppl):**34–42.

Baker WH, Howard VJ, Howard G, Toole JF, for the ACAS investigators (2000). Effect of contralateral occlusion on long-term efficacy of endarterectomy in the Asymptomatic Carotid Atherosclerosis Study (ACAS). *Stroke* **31:**2330–2334.

Bamford J, Dennis M, Sandercock P, Burn J, Warlow C (1990). The frequency, causes bad timing of death within 30 days of a first stroke. The Oxfordshire Community Stroke Project. *J Neurol Neurosurg Psychiatry* **53:**824–829.

Barber PA, Zhang J, Demchuk AM, Hill MD, Buchan AM (2001). Why are stroke patients excluded from TPA therapy? An analysis of patients eligibility. *Neurology* **56:**1015–1020.

Barnett HJ, Taylor DW, Eliasziw M, Fox AJ, Ferguson GG, Haynes RB, Rankin RN, Clagett GP, Hachinski VC, Sackett DL, Thorpe KE, Meldrum HE (1998). Benefit of endarterectomy in patients with symptomatic moderate or severe stenosis. *N Eng J Med* **339:**1415–1425.

Bath PM, Lindenstrom E, Boysen G, De Deyn P, Friis P, Leys D, Marttila R, Olsson J, O'Neill D, Orgogozo J, Ringelstein B, van der Sande J, Turpie AG (2001). Tinzaparin in acute ischaemic stroke (TAIST): a randomised aspirin-controlled trial. *Lancet* 358:702–710.

Becker K, Fruin M, Gooding T, Tirschwell D, Love P, Mankowski T (2001). Community-based education improves stroke knowledge. *Cerebrovasc Dis* **11:**34–43.

Benavente O, Moher D, Pham B (1998). Carotid endarterectomy for asymptomatic carotid stenosis: a meta-analysis. *Br Med J* **317:**1477–1480.

Bereczki D, Liu M, do Prado GF, Fekete I (2001). Mannitol for acute stroke. *Cochrane Database Syst Rev* **(1):**CD001153.

Berge E, Abdelnoor M, Nakstad PH, Sandset PM (2000). Low molecular-weight heparin versus aspirin in patients with acute ischaemic stroke and atrial fibrillation: a double-blind randomised study. HAEST Study Group. Heparin in Acute Embolic Stroke Trial. *Lancet* **355(9211):**1205–1210.

Bernabei R, Landi F, Gambassi G, *et al.* (1998). Randomised trial of impact of model of integrated care and case management for older people living in the community. *BMJ* **316:**1348–1351.

Bernard SA, Gray TW, Buist MD *et al.* (2002). Treatment of comatose survivors of out-of-hospital cardiac arrest with induced hypothermia. *NEJM* **346:**557–563.

Berrouschot J, Rossler A, Koster J, Schneider D (2000). Mechanical ventilation in patients with hemispheric ischemic stroke. *Crit Care Med* **28:**2956–2961.

Bhalla A, Sankaralingam S, Dundas R, Swaminathan R, Wolfe CD, Rudd AG (2000). Influence of raised plasma osmolality on clinical outcome after acute stroke. *Stroke* **31:**2043–2048.

Bhatt DL, Kapadia SR, Yadav JS, Topol EJ (2000). Update on clinical trials of antiplatelet therapy for cerebrovascular diseases. *Cerebrovasc Dis* **10(Suppl 5):**34–40.

Biller J, Feinberg W, Castaldo J, Whittemore A, Harbaugh R, Dempsey R, Caplan L, *et al.* (1998). Guidelines for carotid endarterectomy. A statement for healthcare professionals from a special writing group of the Stroke Council, American Heart Association. *Stroke* **97:**501– 509.

Bowes MP, Zivin JA, Thomas GR, Thibodeaux H, Fagan SC (1996). Acute hypertension, but not thrombolysis, increases the incidence and severity of hemorrhagic transformation following experimental stroke in rabbits. *Exp Neurol* **141:**40–46.

Brainin M, Steiner M (2003). Acute stroke units in Austria are being set up on a national level following evidence-based recommendations and structural quality criteria. *Cerebrovasc Dis* **15(Suppl 1):**29–32.

Brainin M, Kaste M, Czlonkowska A *et al.* for the European Federation of Neurological Societies Task Force on Acute Neurological Stroke Care (1997). The role of European neurology. *Eur J Neurol* **4:**435–441.

Brainin M, Olsen TS, Chamorro A *et al.* EUSI Executive Committee; EUSI Writing Committee (2004). Organization of stroke care: education, referral, emergency management and imaging, stroke units and rehabilitation. European Stroke Initiative. *Cerebrovasc Dis* **17(Suppl 2):**1–14.

Brainin M, Bornstein N, Boysen G, Demarin V for the EFNS Task Force on Acute Neurological Stroke Care (2000). Acute neurological stroke care in Europe: results of the European stroke care inventory. *Eur J Neurol* **7:**5–10.

Britton M, Carlsson A, de Faire U (1986). Blood pressure course in patients with acute stroke and matched controls. *Stroke* **17:**861–864.

Broderick JP, Phillips SJ, O'Fallon WM, Frye RL, Whisnant JP (1992). Relationship of cardiac disease to stroke occurrence, recurrence, and mortality. *Stroke* **23:**1250–1256.

Broderick J, Brott T, Barsan W, Clarke Haley E, Levy D, Marler J, Sheppard G, Blum C (1993). Blood pressure during the first inutes of focal cerebral ischaemia. *Ann Emerg Med* **22:**1438.

Brott T, Reed RL (1989). Intensive care for acute stroke in the community hospital setting. *Stroke* **20:**694–697.

Brott T, Fieschi C, Hacke W (1994). General therapy of acute ischemic stroke. in Hacke W, Hanley DF, Einhäupl K, Bleck Berlin TP (eds). *Neurocritical Care.* Heidelberg, Springer Verlag, 553–577.

Camerlingo M, Casto L, Censori B, Ferraro B, Gazzaniga G, Partziguian T, Signore M, Panagia C, Fascendini A, Cesana BM, Mamoli A (2001). Experience with a questionnaire administered by emergency medical service for pre-hospital identification of patients with acute stroke. *Neurol Sci* **22:**357–361.

Cannegieter S, Rosendaal F, Witzen A, Van Der Meer F, Vandenbroucke J, Briët E (1995). Optimal oral anticoagulation therapy in patients with mechanical heart valves. *N Eng J Med* **333:**11–17.

Capes SE, Hunt D, Malmberg K, Pathak P, Gerstein HC (2001). Stress hyperglycemia and prognosis of stroke in nondiabetic and diabetic patients:a systematic overview. *Stroke* **32:**2426–3223.

CAPRIE Steering Committee (1996). A randomised, blinded trial of clopidogrel versus aspirin in patients at risk of ischaemic events (CAPRIE). *Lancet* **348:**1329–1339.

Carlberg B, Asplund K, Hagg E (1991). Factors influencing admission blood pressure levels in patients with acute stroke. *Stroke* **22:**527–530.

Castillo J, Davalos A, Noya M (1999). Aggravation of acute ischemic stroke by hyperthermia is related to an excitotoxic mechanism. *Cerebrovasc Dis* **9:**22–27.

CAVATAS Investigators (2001). Endovascular versus surgical treatment in patients with carotid stenosis in the Carotid and Vertebral Artery Transluminal Angioplasty Study: a randomised trial. *Lancet* **357:**1729–1737.

Chambers BR, You RX, Donnan GA (2002). Carotid endarterectomy for asymptomatic carotid stenosis (Cochrane Review). *The Cochrane Library* Issue 4.

Chamorro A (2001). Immediate anticoagulation in acute focal brain ischemia revisited: gathering the evidence. *Stroke* **32:**577–578.

Chamorro A, Vila N, Ascaso C, Elices E, Schonewille W, Blanc R (1998). Blood pressure and functional recovery in acute ischemic stroke. *Stroke* **29:**1850–1853.

Chamorro A, Cervera A, Castillo J, Davalos A, Aponte JJ, Planas AM (2002). Unfractionated heparin is associated with a lower rise of serum vascular cell adhesion molecule-1 in acute ischemic stroke patients. *Neurosci Lett* **328:**229–232.

Colditz GA, Bonita R, Stampfer MJ, Willett WC, Rosner B, Speizer FE, Hennekens CH (1988). Cigarette smoking and risk of stroke in middle-aged women. *N Engl J Med* **318:**937–941.

Corbett D, Thornhill J (2000). Temperature modulation (hypothermic and hyperthermic conditions) and its influence on histological and behavioral outcomes following cerebral ischemia. *Brain Pathol* **10:**145–152.

Dahlof B, Devereux RB, Kjeldsen SE, Julius S, Beevers G, Faire U, Fyhrquist F, Ibsen H, Kristiansson K, Lederballe-Pedersen O, Lindholm LH, Nieminen MS, Omvik P, Oparil S, Wedel H (2002). Cardiovascular morbidity and mortality in the Losartan Intervention For Endpoint reduction in hypertension study (LIFE): a randomised trial against atenolol. *Lancet* **359:**995–1003.

Davalos A, Cendra E, Teruel J, Martinez M, Genis D (1990). Deteriorating ischemic stroke: risk factors and prognosis. *Neurology* **40:**1865–1869.

Davalos A, Toni D, Iweins F, Lesaffre E, Bastianello S, Castillo J (1999). Neurological deterioration in acute ischemic stroke: potential predictors and associated factors in the European cooperative acute stroke study (ECASS). *Stroke* **30:**2631–2636.

Davenport RJ, Dennis MS, Wellwood I, Warlow CP (1996). Complications after acute stroke. *Stroke* **27:**415–420.

de Gaetano G (2001). Low-dose aspirin and vitamin E in people at cardiovascular risk: a randomised trial in general practice. Collaborative Group of the Primary Prevention Project. *Lancet* **357:**89–95.

Derex L, Adeleine P, Nighoghossian N, Honnorat J, Trouillas P (2002). Factors influencing early admission in a French stroke unit. *Stroke* **33:**153–159.

Diener HC, Cunha L, Forbes C, Sivenius J, Smets P, Lowenthal A (1996). European Stroke Prevention Study. 2. Dipyridamole and acetylsalicylic acid in the secondary prevention of stroke. *J Neurol Sci* **143:**1–13.

Diener HC, Ringelstein EB, von Kummer R, Langohr HD, Bewermeyer H, Landgraf H, Hennerici M, Welzel D, Grave M, Brom J, Weidinger G (2001). Treatment of acute ischemic stroke with the low-molecular-weight heparin certoparin: results of the TOPAS trial. Therapy of Patients with Acute Stroke (TOPAS) Investigators. *Stroke* **32(1):**22–29.

Di Mascio R, Marchili R, Tognoni G (2000). Cholesterol reduction and stroke occurrence: an overview of randomized clinical trials. *Cerebrovascular Dis* **10:**85–92.

Dippel DW, van Breda EJ, van Gemert HM, van der Worp HB, Meijer RJ, Kappelle LJ, Koudstaal PJ (2001). Effect of paracetamol (acetaminophen) on body temperature in acute ischemic stroke: a double-blind, randomized phase II clinical trial. *Stroke* **32:**1607–1612.

Diringer MN (1992). Management of sodium abnormalities in patients with CNS disease. *Clin Neuropharmacol* **15**:427–447.

Dressler FA, Craig WR, Castello R, Labovitz AJ (1998). Mobile aortic atheroma and systemic emboli: efficacy of anticoagulation and influence of plaque morphology on recurrent stroke. *J Am Coll Cardiol* **31**:134–138.

Duncan PW (1997). Synthesis of intervention trials to improve motor recovery following stroke. *Top Stroke Rehabil* **3(4)**:1–20.

Eames PJ, Blake MJ, Dawson SL, Panerai RB, Potter JF (2002). Dynamic cerebral autoregulation and beat to beat blood pressure control are impaired in acute ischaemic stroke. *J Neurol Neurosurg Psychiatry* **72**:467–472.

Echiverri HC, Rubino FA, Gupta SR, Gujrati M (1989). Fusiform aneurysm of the vertebrobasilar arterial system. *Stroke* **20**:1741–1747.

ETDRS Investigators. Aspirin effects on mortality and morbidity in patients with diabetes mellitus (1992). Early Treatment Diabetic Retinopathy Study report 14. *JAMA* **268**:1292–1300.

European Carotid Surgery Trialists Collaborative Group (1995). Risk of stroke in the distribution of an asymptomatic carotid artery. *Lancet* **345**:209–212.

European Stroke Initiative (2000). European Stroke Initiative Recommendations for Stroke Management. *Cerebrovasc Dis* **10**:335–351.

Evenson KR, Rosamond WD, Morris DL (2001). Prehospital and in-hospital delays in acute stroke care. *Neuroepidemiology* **20**:65–76.

Executive Committee for the Asymptomatic Carotid Atherosclerosis Study (1995). Endarterectomy for asymptomatic carotid artery stenosis. *JAMA* **273**:1421–1428.

Fagan SC, Bowes MP, Lyden PD, Zivin JA (1998). Acute hypertension promotes hemorrhagic transformation in a rabbit embolic stroke model: effect of labetalol. *Exp Neurol* **150**:153–158.

Farrell B, Godwin J, Richards S, Warlow C (1991). The United Kingdom transient ischaemic attack (UK-TIA) aspirin trial: final results. *J Neurol Neurosurg Psychiatry* **54**:1044–1054.

Feinberg W, Albers G, Barnett H, Biller J, Caplan L, Carter L, *et al.* (1994). Guidelines for the management of transient ischemic attacks. From the ad hoc committee on guidelines for the management of transient ischemic attacks ofthe American Heart Association. *Circulation* **89**:2950–2965.

Ferro JM, Melo TP, Oliveira V, Crespo M, Canhão P, Pinto AN (1994). An analysis of the admission delay of acute stroke. *Cerebrovasc Dis* **4**:72–75.

Ferro JM, Pinto AN, Falcão I Rodrigues G, Ferreira J, Falcão F, Azevedo E, Canhão P, Melo TP, Rosas MJ, Oliveira V, Salgado AV (1998). Diagnosis of stroke by the nonneurologist. A validation study. *Stroke* **29**:1106–1109.

Fukuda H, Kitani M, Takahashi K (1999). Body temperature correlates with functional outcome and the lesion size of cerebral infarction. *Acta Neurol Scand* **100**:385–390.

Fuster V, Ryden LE, Asinger RW, Cannom DS, Crijns HJ, Frye RL, Halperin JL, Kay GN, Klein WW, Levy S, McNamara RL, Prystowsky EN, Wann LS, Wyse DG, Gibbons RJ, Antman EM, Alpert JS, Faxon DP, Fuster V, Gregoratos G, Hiratzka LF, Jacobs AK, Russell RO, Smith SC, Klein WW, Alonso-Garcia A, Blomstrom-Lundqvist C, De Backer G, Flather M, Hradec J, Oto A, Parkhomenko A, Silber S, Torbicki A (2001). ACC/AHA/ESC guidelines for the management of patients with atrial fibrillation: executive summary. A Report of the American College of Cardiology/ American Heart Association Task Force on Practice Guidelines and the European Society of Cardiology Committee for Practice Guidelines and Policy Conferences (Committee to Develop Guidelines for the Management of Patients with Atrial Fibrillation): developed in Collaboration with the North American Society of Pacing and Electrophysiology. *J Am Coll Cardiol* **38**:1231–1266.

Georgiadis D, Schwarz S, Aschoff A, Schwab S (2002). Hemicraniectomy and moderate hypothermia in patients with severe ischemic stroke. *Stroke* **33**:1584–1588.

Georgilis K, Plomaritoglou A, Dafni U, Bassiakos Y, Vemmos K (1999). Aetiology of fever in patients with acute stroke. *J Intern Med* **246**:203–209.

Gerberding JL (2002). Hospital-Onset Infections: A Patient Safety Issue. *Ann Int Med* **137**:665.

Goldstein LB, Adams R, Becker K, Furberg CD, Gorelick PB, Hademenos G, Hill M, Howard G, Howard VJ, Jacobs B, Levine SR, Mosca L, Sacco RL, Sherman DG, Wolf PA, del Zoppo GJ (2001). Primary prevention of ischemic stroke: A statement for healthcare professionals from the Stroke Council of the American Heart Association. *Stroke* **32**:280–299.

Grady D, Herrington D, Bittner V, Blumenthal R, Davidson M, Hlatky M, Hsia J, Hulley S, Herd A, Khan S, Newby LK, Waters D, Vittinghoff E, Wenger N (2002). Cardiovascular disease outcomes during 6.8 years of hormone therapy: Heart and Estrogen/progestin Replacement Study follow-up (HERS II). *JAMA* **288**:49–57.

Graham DI (1982). Ischemic brain damage following emergency blood pressure lowering in hypertensive patients. *Acta Med Scand* **678(Suppl):** 61–69.

Grau AJ, Buggle F, Schnitzler P, Spiel M, Lichy C, Hacke W (1999). Fever and infection early after ischemic stroke. *J Neurol Sci* **171:**115–120.

Gray CS, Taylor R, French JM, Alberti KG, Venables GS, James OF, Shaw DA, Cartlidge NE, Bates D (1987). The prognostic value of stress hyperglycaemia and previously unrecognized diabetes in acute stroke. *Diabet Med* **4:**237–240.

Grodstein F, Manson JE, Stampfer MJ (2001). Postmenopausal hormone use and secondary prevention of coronary events in the nurses' health study. A prospective, observational study. *Ann Intern Med* **135:**1–8.

Grossman E, Messerli FH, Grodzicki T, Kowey P (1996). Should a moratorium be placed on sublingual nifedipine capsules given for hypertensive emergencies and pseudoemergencies? *JAMA* **276:**1328–1331.

Hacke W, Kaste M, Bogousslavsky J *et al.*; European Stroke Initiative Executive Committee and the EUSI Writing Committee (2003). European Stroke Initiative Recommendations for Stroke Management–update 2003. *Cerebrovasc Dis* **16:**311–337.

Hacke W, Kaste M, Fieschi C, Toni D, Lesaffre E, *et al.* (1995). Intravenous thrombolysis with recombinant tissue plasminogen activator for acute hemispheric stroke. The European Cooperative Acute Stroke Study (ECASS). *JAMA* **274(13):**1017–1025.

Hacke W, Kaste M, Fieschi C, von Kummer R, Davalos A, Meier D, Larrue V, Bluhmki E, Davis S, Donnan G, Schneider D, Diez Tejedor E, Trouillas P (1998). Randomised double-blind placebo-controlled trial of thrombolytic therapy with intravenous alteplase in acute ischaemic stroke (ECASS II). Second European-Australasian Acute Stroke Study Investigators. *Lancet* **352:**1245–1251.

Hacke W, Schwab S, Horn M, Spranger M, DeGeorgia M, von Kummer R (1996). Malignant Middle Cerebral Artery Territory Infarction. *Arch Neurol* **53:**309–315.

Hacke W, Brott T, Caplan L, Meier D, Fieschi C, von Kummer R, Donnan G, Heiss WD, Wahlgren NG, Spranger M, Boysen F, Marler JR (1999). *Neurology* **537(Suppl 4):**3–14.

Hajat C, Hajat S, Sharma P (2000). Effects of poststroke pyrexia on stroke outcome: a meta-analysis of studies in patients. *Stroke* **31:**410–414.

Hankey GJ, Warlow CP (1999). Treatment and secondary prevention of stroke: evidence, costs, and effects on individuals and populations. *Lancet* **354:**1457–1463.

Hansson L, Zanchetti A, Carruthers S, Dahlof B, Elmfeldt D, Julius S, Menard J, Rahn KH, Wedel H, Westerling S (1998). Effects of intensive blood-pressure lowering and low-dose aspirin in patients with hypertension: principal results of the Hypertension Optimal Treatment (HOT) randomised trial. *Lancet* **351:**1755–1762.

Harper G, Castleden CM, Potter JF (1994). Factors affecting changes in blood pressure after acute stroke. *Stroke* **25(9):**1726–1729.

Harraf F, Sharma AK, Brown MM, Lees KR, Vass RI, Kalra L (2002). A multicentre observational study of presentation and early assessment of acute stroke. *BMJ* **325:**17.

Hart RG, Sherman DG, Easton JD, Cairns J (1998). Prevention of stroke in patients with nonvalvular atrial fibrillation. *Neurology* **51:**674–681.

Hart RG, Halperin JL, McBride R, Benavente O, Man-Son-Hing M, Kronmal RA (2000). Aspirin for the primary prevention of stroke and other major vascular events: meta-analysis and hypotheses. *Arch Neurol* **57:**326–332.

Hatashita S, Hoff JT, Ishii S (1986). Focal brain edema associated with acute arterial hypertension. *J Neurosurg* **64:**643–649.

He K, Rimm EB, Merchant A, Rosner BA, Stampfer MJ, Willett WC, Ascherio A (2002). Fish consumption and risk of stroke in men. *JAMA* **288:**3130–3136.

Heart Protection Study Collaborative Group (2000). MRC/BHF Heart Protection Study of cholesterol lowering with simvastatin in 20,536 high-risk individuals: a randomised placebo-controlled trial. *Lancet* **360:**7–22.

Hesse S (2001). Locomotor therapy in neurorehabilitation. *NeuroRehabilitation* **16:**133–139.

Hu FB, Willett WC (2002). Optimal diets for prevention of coronary heart disease. *JAMA* **288:**2569–2578.

Huff JS (2002). Stroke mimics and chameleon. Emerg Med Clin North Am 20:583–595.

Hughes RA, Barnes MP, Baron JC, Brainin M (2001). Guidance for the preparation of neurological management guidelines by EFNS scientific task forces. *Eur J Neurol* **6:**549–550.

Indredavik B, Bakke F, Solberg R, Rokseth R, Haaheim LL, Holme I (1991). Benefit of a stroke unit: a randomized controlled trial. *Stroke* **22:**1026–1031.

Indredavik B, Slordahl SA, Bakke F, Rokseth R, Haheim LL (1997). Stroke unit treatment: Long-term effects. *Stroke* **28:**1861–1866.

Inzitari D, Eliasziw M, Gates P, Sharpe BL, Chan RKT, Meldrum HE, Barnett HJM (2000). The causes and risk of stroke in patients with asymptomatic internal-carotid-artery stenosis. *N Engl J Med* **342:**1693–1700.

Iranzo A, Santamaría J, Berenguer J, Sánchez M, Chamorro A (2002). Prevalence and clinical importance of sleep apnea in the first night after cerebral infarction. Neurology 58:911–916.

James P, Ellis CJ, Whitlock RML., McNeil AR, Henley J, Anderson NE (2000). Relation between troponin T concentration and mortality in patients presenting with an acute stroke: observational study. *BMJ* **320:**1502.

Jansen PAF, Schulte BPM, Poels EFJ, Gribnau FWJ (1987). Course of blood pressure after cerebral infarction and transiemnt ischemic attack. *Clin Neurol Neurosurg* **89:**243–246.

Johansson BB (2000). Brain plasticity and stroke rehabilitation. The Willis lecture. *Stroke* **31:**223–230.

Jorgensen HS, Nakayama H, Raaschou HO, Olsen TS (1994). Effect of blood pressure and diabetes on stroke in progression. *Lancet* 16;344(8916):156–159.

Jorgensen H, Nakayama H, Raaschou H, Larsen K, Hübbe P, Olsen T (1995). The effect of a stroke unit: Reductions in mortality, discharge rate to nursing homne, length of hospital stay and cost. *Stroke* **26:**1176–1182.

Jørgensen HS, Kammersgaard LP, Houth J *et al.* (2000). Who benefits from treatment and rehabilitation in a stroke Unit? A community-based study. *Stroke* **31:**434–439.

Kawachi I, Colditz GA, Stampfer MJ, WC, Manson JE, Rosner B, Speizer FE, Hennekens CH (1993). Smoking cessation and decreased risk of stroke in women. *JAMA* **269:**232–236.

Kasner SE, Wein T, Piriyawat P, Villar-Cordova CE, Chalela JA, Krieger DW, Morgenstern LB, Kimmel SE, Grotta JC (2002). Acetaminophen for altering body temperature in acute stroke: a randomized clinical trial. *Stroke* **33:**130–134.

Kaste M, Palomaki H, Sarna S (1995). Where and how should elderly stroke patients be treated? A randomized trial. *Stroke* **26:**249–253.

Kaste M, Fogelholm R, Rissanen A (1998). Economic burden of stroke and the evaluation of new therapies. *Public Health* **112:**103–112.

Kaste M, Roine RO. General stroke management and stroke units. In: Grotta JC, Choi D, Mohr JP, Weir B, Wolf PA (Eds) Stroke: Physiology, Diagnosis and Management. Hartcourt Health Sciences Philadelphia. In press.

Khechinashvili G, Asplund K (2002). Electrocardiographic changes in patients with acute stroke: a systematic review. *Cerebrovasc Dis* **14:**67–76.

Klijn CJ, Hankey GJ; American Stroke Association and European Stroke Initiative. Management of acute ischaemic stroke: new guidelines from the American Stroke Association and European Stroke Initiative (2003). *Lancet Neurol* **2:**698–701.

Kothari R, Hall K, Brott T, Broderick J (1997). Early stroke recognition: developing and out-of-hospital NIH Stroke Scale. *Acad Emerg Med* **4:**986–990.

Kramer AM, Steiner JF, Schenkler RE *et al.* (1997). Outcomes and costs after hip fracture and stroke: a comparison of rehabilitation settings. *JAMA* **1277:**396–404.

Kwan J, Sandercock P (2003). In-hospital care pathways for stroke (Cochrane Review). In: *The Cochrane Library*, Issue 1 Oxford: Update Software.

Langhorne P, Stott DJ, Robertson L, MacDonald J, Jones L, McAlpine C, Dick F, Taylor GS, Murray G (2000). Medical complications after stroke: a multicenter study. *Stroke* **31:**1223–1229.

Langhorne P, Pollock A for the Stroke Unit Trialists' Collaboration (2002). What are the components of effective stroke unit care? *Age Ageing* **31:**365–371.

Lee IM, Hennekens CH, Berger K, Buring JE, Manson JE (1999). Exercise and risk of stroke in male physicians. *Stroke* **30:**1–6.

Leonardi-Bee J, Bath PMW, Philips SJ, Sandercock PAG, for the IST Collaborative Group (2002). Blood pressure and clinical outcomes in the International Stroke Trial. *Stroke* **33:**1315.

Leys D, Kwiecinski H, Bogousslavsky J *et al.*; EUSI Executive Committee; EUSI Writing Committee. Prevention. European Stroke Initiative (2004). *Cerebrovasc Dis* **17(Suppl 2):**15–29.

Lindstrom E, Boysen G, Christiansen LW, Nansen BR, Nielsen PW (1991). Reliability of Scandinavian neurological stroke scale. *Cerebrovascular Dis* **1:**103–107.

Lyden P, Brott T, Tilley B, Welch KM, Mascha EJ, Levine S, Haley EC, Grotta J, Marler J (1994). Improved reliability of the NIH Stroke Scale using video training. NINDS TPA Stroke Study Group. *Stroke* **25:**2220–2226.

Mas JL, Arquizan C, Lamy C, Zuber M, Cabanes L, Derumeaux G, Coste J (2001). Recurrent cerebrovascular events associated with patent foramen ovale, atrial sptal aneurysm, or both. *N Engl J Med* **345:**1740–1746.

Meade T (1998). Low dose warfarin and aspirin in preventing IHD. *Practitioner* **242:**799–803.

Meyer JS, Shimazu K, Fukuhuchi, Ohuchi T, Okamoto S, Koto A (1973). Impaired neurogenic cerebrovascular control and dysautoregulation after stroke. *Stroke* **4:**169.

Miltner WH, Bauder H, Sommer M, Dettmers C, Taub E (1999). Effects of constraint-induced movement therapy on patients with chronic motor deficits after stroke: a replication. *Stroke* **30:**586–592.

Mohr JP, Thompson JL, Lazar RM, Levin B, Sacco RL, Furie KL, Kistler JP, Albers GW, Pettigrew LC, Adams HP Jr, Jackson CM, Pullicino P (2001). A comparison of warfarin and aspirin for the prevention of recurrent ischemic stroke. *N Engl J Med* **345:**1444–1451.

Mori K, Aoki A, Yamamoto T, Maeda M (2001). Aggressive decompressive surgery in patients with massive hemispheric embolic cerebral infarction associated with severe brain swelling. *Acta Neurochir* **143:**483–492.

Neal B, MacMahon S, Chapman N (2000). Effects of ACE inhibitors, calcium antagonists, and other blood-pressure-lowering drugs: results of prospectively designed overviews of randomised trials. Blood Pressure Lowering Treatment Trialists' Collaboration. *Lancet* **356:**1955–1964.

North American Symptomatic Carotid Endarterectomy Trial Collaborators (1991). Beneficial effect of carotid endarterectomy in symptomatic patients with high-grade carotid stenosis. *N Eng J Med* **325:**445–453.

Odderson I, McKenna B (1993). A model for man agement of patients with stroke during the acute phase. Outcome and economic implica tions. *Stroke* **24:**1823–1827.

Olsen TS (2001). Post-stroke epilepsy. *Curr Atheroscler Rep* **3:**340–344.

Oppenheimer S, Hachinski V (1992). Complications of acute stroke. *Lancet* **339:**721–724.

Oppenheimer SM, Keden G, Martin WM (1996). Left-insular cortex lesions perturb cardiac autonomic tone in humans. *Clin Auton Res* **6:**131–140.

PATS Collaborating Group (1995). Post-stroke antihypertensive treatment study. A preliminary result. *Chin Med J* **108:**710–717.

Peto R, Gray R, Collins R, Wheatley K, Hennekens C, Jamrozik K, Warlow C, Hafner B, Thompson E, Norton S (1988). Randomised trial of prophylactic daily aspirin in British male doctors. *Br Med J* **296:**313–316.

Porteus GH, Corry MD, Smith WS (1999). Emergency medical services dispatcher identification of stroke and transient ischemic attack. *Prehosp Emerg Care* **3:**211–216.

Power WJ (1993). Acute hypertension after stroke: the scientific basis for treatment decisions. *Neurology* **43:**461–467.

PROGRESS Collaborative Group (2001). Randomised trial of a perindopril-based blood-pressure-lowering regimen among 6105 individuals with previous stroke or transient ischaemic attack. *Lancet* **358:**1033–1041.

Prospective Studies Collaboration (2002) Age-specific relevance of usual blood pressure to vascular mortality: a meta-analysis of individual data for one million adults in 61 prospective studies. *Lancet* **360:**1903–1991.

Prough DS, Zornow MH (1998). Hypertonic maintenance fluids for patients with cerebral edema: Does the evidence support a "phase II" trial? *Crit Care Med* **26:**421–422.

Qizilbash N, Lewington SL, Lopez-Arrieta JM (2002). Corticosteroids for acute ischaemic stroke. Cochrane Database Syst Rev (2):CD000064.

Qureshi AI, Suarez JI, Bhardwaj A, Mirski M, Schnitzer MS, Hanley DF, Ulatowski JA (1998). Use of hypertonic (3%) saline/acetate infusion in the treatment of cerebral edema: Effect on intracranial pressure and lateral displacement of the brain. *Crit Care Med* **26:**440–446.

Reynolds K, Lewis LB, Nolen JDL, Kinney GL, Sathya B, He J (2003). Alcohol consumption and risk of stroke. A meta-analysis. *JAMA* **289:**579–588.

Righetti E, Celani MG, Cantisani TA, Sterzi R, Boysen G, Ricci S (2002). Glycerol for acute stroke: a Cochrane systematic review. *J Neurol* **249:**445–451.

Ronning OM, Guldvog B (1999). Should stroke victims routinely receive supplemental oxygen? A quasi randomised controlled trial. *Stroke* **30:**2033–2037.

Rothwell PM, Eliasziv M, Gutnikov SA, Fox AJ, Taylor DW, Mayberg MR, Warlow CP, Barnett HJM (2003). Analysis of pooled data from the randomized controlled trials of endarterectomy for symptomatic carotid stenosis. *Lancet* **361:**107–116.

Roubin GS, New G, Iyer SS, Vitek JJ, Al-Mubarak N, Liu MW, Yadav J, Gomez C, Kuntz RE (2001). Immediate and late clinical outcomes of carotid artery stenting in patients with symptomatic and asymptomatic carotid artery stenosis: a 5-year prospective analysis. *Circulation* **103:**532–537.

Rubins HB, Robins SJ, Collins D, Fye CL, Anderson JW, Elam MB, Faas FH, Linares E, Schaefer EJ, Schectman G, Wilt TJ, Wittes J (1999). Gemfibrozil for the secondary prevention of coronary heart disease in men with low levels of high-density lipoprotein cholesterol. Veterans Affairs High-Density Lipoprotein Cholesterol Intervention Trial Study Group. *N Engl J Med* **341:**410–418.

Schellinger PD, Fiebach JB, Hacke W (2003). Imaging-based decision making in thrombolytic therapy for ischemic stroke- present state. *Stroke* **34:**575–583.

Schwab S, Schwarz S, Spranger M, Keller E, Bertram M, Hacke W (1998). Moderate hypothermia in the treatment of patients with severe middle cerebral artery infarction. *Stroke* **29:**2461–2466.

Schwab S, Georgiadis D, Berrouschot J, Schellinger PD, Graffangino C, Mayer SA (2001). Feasibility and safety of moderate hypothermia after massive hemispheric infarction. *Stroke* **32:**2033–2035.

Schwarz S, Schwab S, Bertram M, Aschoff A, Hacke W (1998). Effects of hypertonic saline hydroxyethyl starch solution and mannitol in patients with increased intracranial pressure after stroke. *Stroke* **29:**1550–1555.

Schwarz S, Georgiadis D, Aschoff A, Schwab S (2002). Effects of hypertonic (10%) saline in patients with raised intracranial pressure after stroke. *Stroke* **33:**136–140.

Shackford SR, Zhuang J, Schmoker J (1992). Intravenous fluid tonicity: effect on intracranial pressure, cerebral blood flow, and cerebral oxygen delivery in focal brain injury. *J Neurosurg* **76:**91–98.

Shepherd J, Blauw GJ, Murphy MB, Bollen EL, Buckley BM, Cobbe SM, Ford I, Gaw A, Hyland M, Jukema JW, Kamper AM, Macfarlane PW, Meinders AE, Norrie J, Packard CJ, Perry IJ, Stott DJ, Sweeney BJ, Twomey C, Westendorp RG, for the PROSPER (PROspective Study of Pravastatin in the Elderly at Risk) Study Group (2002). Pravastatin in elderly individuals at risk of vascular disease (PROSPER): a randomised controlled trial. *Lancet* **360:**1623–1630.

Shinton R, Beevers G (1989). Meta-analysis of relation between cigarette smoking and stroke. *Br Med J* **298:**789–794.

Sivenius J, Pyörälä K, Heinonen OP, Salonen J, Riekkinen P (1985). The significance of intensity of rehabilitation in the recovery of stroke. A controlled trial. *Stroke* **16:**928–931.

Staessen JA, Wang JG, Thijs L (2001). Cardiovascular protection and blood pressure reduction: a meta-analysis. *Lancet* **358:**1305–1315.

Steering Committee of the Physicians' Health Study Research Group (1989). Final report of the ongoing physicians health study. *N Eng J Med* **321:**129–135.

Stegmayr B, Vinogradova T, Malyutina S *et al.* (2000). Widening gap of stroke between East and West. *Stroke* **31:**2–8.

Steiner T, Ringleb P, Hacke W (2001). Treatment options for large hemispheric stroke. *Neurology* **57:**S61–S68.

Strand T, Asplund K, Eriksson S, Hagg E, Lithner F, Wester P (1985). A non-intensive stroke unit reduces functional disability and the need for long-term hospitalisation. *Stroke* **16(1):** 29–34.

Straus SE, Majumdar SR, McAlister FA (2002). New evidence for stroke prevention: Scientific review. *JAMA* **288:**1388–1395.

Stroke Unit Trialists' Collaboration (2002). Organised inpatient (stroke unit) care for stroke. The Cochrane Library 1, Oxford: Update Software.

Syrjanen J, Valtonen VV, Iivanainen M, Kaste M, Huttunen JK (1988). Preceding infection as an important risk factor for ischaemic brain infarction in young and middle aged patients. *Br Med J* (*Clin Res Ed*) **296:**1156–1160.

Taub E, Miller NE, Novack TA, *et al.* (1993). Technique to improve chronic motor deficit after stroke. *Arch Phys Med Rehabil* **74:**347–354.

Teasdale G, Jennett B (1976). Assessment and prognosis of coma after head injury. *Acta Neurochir* **34:**45–55.

The ALLHAT Officers and Coordinators for the ALLHAT Collaborative Research Group (2002). Major outcomes in moderately hypercholesterolaemic, hypertensive patients randomized to pravastatin vs usual care: The Antihypertensive and Lipid-Lowering Treatment to Prevent Heart Attack Trial (ALLHAT-LLT). *JAMA* **288:**2998–3007.

The Dutch TIA Trial Study Group (1991). A comparison of two doses of aspirin (30 mg vs. 283 mg a day) in patients after a transient ischaemic attack or minor ischaemic stroke. *N Engl J Med* **325:**1261–1266.

The EC/IC Bypass Study Group (1985). Failure of extracranial-intracranial arterial bypass to reduce the risk of ischaemic stroke. Results of an international randomised trial. *N Engl J Med* **313:**1191–2000.

The European Ad Hoc Consensus Group (1996). European strategies for early intervention in stroke. *Cerebrovasc Dis* **6:**315–324.

The European Ad Hoc Consensus Group (1997). Optimizing intensive care in stroke: A European perspective. A report of an Ad Hoc Consensus Group meeting. *Cerebrovasc Dis* **7:**113–128.

The European Atrial Fibrillation Study Group (1995). Optimal oral anticoagulation therapy with non-rheumatic atrial fibrillation and recent cerebral ischemia. *N Eng J Med* **333:**5–10.

The Hypothermia after Cardiac Arrest Study Group (2002). Mild therapeutic hypothermia to improve the neurologic outcome after cardiac arrest. *NEJM* **346:**549–556.

The INDIANA (Individual Data Analysis of Antihypertensive Intervention Trials) Project Collaborators (1997). Effect of antihypertensive treatment in patients having already suffered from stroke: gathering the evidence. *Stroke* **28:**2557–2562.

The Stroke Prevention in Reversible Ischaemia Trial Study Group (1997). A randomised trial of anticoagulants versus aspirin after cerebral ischemia of presumed arterial origin. *Ann Neurol* **42:**857–865.

Thomas SH, Kociszewski C, Schwamm LH, Wedel SK (2002). The evolving role of helicopter emergency medical services in the transfer of stroke patients to specialized centers. *Prehosp Emerg Care* **6:**210–204.

Thomassen L, Brainin M, Demarin V, Grond M, Toni D, Venables GS for the EFNS Task Force on Acute Neurological Stroke Care (in print). Acute stroke treatment in Europe: a questionnaire-based survey on behalf of the EFNS task force on acute neurological stroke care. *Europ J Neurol*

Toni D, Chamorro A, Kaste M, Lees K, Wahlgren NG, Hacke W; EUSI Executive Committee; EUSI Writing Committee (2004). Acute treatment of ischaemic stroke. European Stroke Initiative. *Cerebrovasc Dis* **17(Suppl 2)**:30–46.

Toni D, Sacchetti ML, Argentino C, Gentile M, Cavalletti C, Frontoni M, Fieschi C (1992). Does hyperglycaemia play a role on the outcome of acute ischaemic stroke patients? *J Neurol* **239**:382–386.

Toni D, De Michele M, Fiorelli M, Bastianello S, Camerlingo M, Sacchetti ML, Argentino C, Fieschi C (1994). Influence of hyperglycaemia on infarct size and clinical outcome of acute ischemic stroke patients with intracranial arterial occlusion. *J Neurol Sci* **123**:129–133.

Turkington PM, Bamford J, Wanklyn P, Elliott MW (2002). Prevalence and predictors of upper airway obstruction in the first 24 hours after acute stroke. *Stroke* **33**:2037–2042.

Turner RC, Cull CA, Frighi V, Holman RR (1999). Glycemic control with diet, sulfonylurea, metformin, or insulin in patients with type 2 diabetes mellitus: progressive requirement for multiple therapies (UKPDS 49). UK Prospective Diabetes Study (UKPDS) Group. *JAMA* **281**:2005–2012.

Vandoni RE, Lironi A, Tschantz P (1994). Bacteriuria during urinary tract catheterization: suprapubic versus urethral route: a prospective randomized trial. *Acta Chir Belg* **94**:12–16.

van Kooten F, Hoogerbrugge N, Naarding P, Koudstaal PJ (1993). Hyperglycemia in the acute phase of stroke is not caused by stress. *Stroke* **24**:1129–1132.

Vingerhoets F, Bogousslavsky J, Regli F, Van Melle G (1993). Atrial fibrillation after acute stroke. *Stroke* **24**:26–30.

Viscoli CM, Brass LM, Kernan WN, Sarrel PM, Suissa S, Horwitz RI (2001). A clinical trial of replacement-replacement therapy after ischemic stroke. *N Engl J Med* **345**:1243–1249.

Wade DT, Wood VA, Heller A, Maggs J, Langton-Hewer R (1987). Walking after stroke: measurement and recovery over the first 3 months. *Scand J Rehab Med* **19**:25–30.

Wannamethee SG, Shaper AG, Whincup PH, Walker M (1995). Smoking cessation and the risk of stroke in middle-aged men. *JAMA* **274**:155–160.

Wardlaw JM (2001). Overview of Cochrane thrombolysis meta-analysis. *Neurology* **57(5 Suppl 2)**:S69–76.

Weimar C, Roth MP, Zillessen G, Glahn J, Wimmer ML, Busse O, Haberl RL, Diener HC, German Stroke Date Bank Collaborators (2002). Complications following acute ischemic stroke. *Eur Neurol* **48**:133–140.

Weimar C, Glahn J, von Reutern GM, Kloth A, Busse O, Diener HC (2002). Treatment of ischemic stroke in 14 neurologic stroke units. An evaluation of the stroke databank of the German Stroke Aid Foundation. *Nervenarzt* **73**:342–348.

Wein TH, Staub L, Felberg R, Hickenbottom SL, Chan W, Grotta JC, Demchuck AM, Groff J, Bartholomew LK, Morgenstern LB (2000). Activation of emergency medical services for acute stroke in a nonurban population: the TLL Temple Foundation Stroke Project. *Stroke* **31**:1925–1928.

Weir CJ, Murray GD, Dyker AG, Lees KR (1997). Is hyperglycaemia an independent predictor of poor outcome after acute stroke? Results of a long-term follow up study. *BMJ* 3;**314**:1303–1306.

Werner C, Bardeleben A, Mauritz KH, Kirker S, Hesse S (2002). Treadmill training with partial body weight support and physiotherapy in stroke patients: a preliminary comparison. *Eur J Neurol* **9**:639–644.

Wester P, Radberg J, Lundgreen B, Peltonen M (1999). Factors associated with delayed admission to hospital and in-hospital delays in acute stroke and TIA. A prospective, multicenter study. *Stroke* **30**: 40–48.

West of Scotland Coronary Prevention Study Group (1998). Influence of pravastatin and plasma lipids on clinical events in the West of Scotland Coronary Prevention Study. *Circulation* **97**:1440–1445.

WHO Task Force on Stroke and Other Cerebrovascular Disorders: Recommendations on stroke prevention, diagnosis, and therapy (1989). Report of the WHO Task Force on Stroke and Other Cerebrovascular Disorders. *Stroke* **20**:1407–1431.

Wolf PA, D'Agostino RB, Kannel WB, Bonita R, Belanger AJ (1988). Cigarette smoking as a risk factor for stroke: the Framingham study. *JAMA* **259**:1025–1029.

Wolfe CDA, Giroud M, Kolomisnky-Rabas P *et al.* (2000). Variations in stroke incidence and survbvival in 3 areas of Europe. *Stroke* **31**:2074–2079.

Yoon SS, Byles J (2002). Preceptions in the general public and patients with stroke: a qualitative study. *BMJ* **324**:1065–1070.

Yusuf S, Sleight P, Pogue J, Bosch J, Davies R, Dagenais G (2000). Effects of an angiotensin-converting-enzyme inhibitor, ramipril, on cardiovascular events in high-risk patients. The Heart Outcome Prevention Evaluation Study Investigators. *New Engl J Med* **342**:145–153.

CHAPTER 13

Migraine

S. Evers,[a] J. Áfra,[b] A. Frese,[a] P.J. Goadsby,[c]
M. Linde,[d] A. May,[e] P.S. Sándor[f]

Abstract

Background Migraine is one of the most frequent disabling neurological conditions with a major impact on the patients' quality of life.

Objectives To give evidence-based or expert recommendations for the different drug treatment procedures of the different migraine syndromes based on a literature search and a consensus in an expert panel.

Methods All available medical reference systems were screened for all kinds of clinical studies on migraine with and without aura and on migraine-like syndromes. The findings in these studies were evaluated according to the recommendations of the EFNS resulting in Level A, B, or C recommendations and Good Practice Points.

For the acute treatment of migraine attacks, oral non-steroidal anti-inflammatory drugs (NSAIDs) and triptans are recommended. The administration should follow the concept of stratified treatment. Before intake of NSAIDs and triptans, oral metoclopramide or domperidon is recommended. In very severe attacks, intravenous acetylsalicylic acid or subcutaneous sumatriptan are drugs of first choice. A status migrainosus can probably be treated by steroids. For the prophylaxis of migraine, betablockers (propranolol and metoprolol), flunarizine, valproic acid and topiramate are drugs of first choice. Drugs of second choice for migraine prophylaxis are amitriptyline, naproxen, petasites and bisoprolol.

Objectives

These guidelines aim to give evidence-based recommendations for the drug treatment of migraine attacks and of migraine prophylaxis. The non-drug management (e.g. behavioural therapy) will not be included, although it is regarded as an important part of migraine treatment. Specific rare migraine syndromes will be considered as well as specific situations such as pregnancy and childhood. A brief clinical description of the headache disorders is included. The definitions follow the

[a]Department of Neurology, University of Münster, Germany; [b]National Institute of Neurosurgery, Budapest, Hungary; [c]Headache Group, Institute of Neurology, The National Hospital for Neurology and Neurosurgery, Queen Square, London, United Kingdom; [d]Cephalea Pain Center, Läkarhuset Södra vägen, Gothenburg, Sweden; [e]Department of Neurology, University of Hamburg, Germany; [f]Department of Neurology, University of Zurich, Switzerland.

diagnostic criteria of the International Headache Society (IHS).

Background

The second edition of the classification of the International Headache Society (IHS) provided a new subclassification of different migraine syndromes (Headache Classification Committee, 2004). The basic criteria for migraine attacks remained unchanged as compared to the first edition (except one semantic change). The different migraine syndromes with specific aura features, however, have been classified in a new system.

The purpose of this paper is to give evidence-based treatment recommendations for migraine attacks and for migraine prophylaxis. The recommendations are based on the scientific evidence from clinical trials and on the expert consensus by the respective task force of the European Federation of Neurological Societies (EFNS). The legal aspects of drug prescription and drug availability in the different European countries will not be considered. The definitions of the recommendation levels follow the EFNS criteria (Brainin et al., 2004).

Search strategy

A literature search was performed using the reference databases MedLine, Science Citation Index, and the Cochrane Library; the key words used were 'migraine' and 'aura' (last search in January 2005). All papers published in English, German, or French were considered when they described a controlled trial or a case series on the treatment of at least five patients. In addition, a review book (Olesen et al., 2000) and the German treatment recommendations for migraine (Diener et al., 2005b) were considered.

Method for reaching consensus

All authors performed an independent literature search. The first draft of the manuscript was written by the chairman of the task force. All other members of the task force read the first draft and discussed changes by email. A second draft was then written by the chairman that was again discussed by email. All recommendations had to be agreed to by all members of the task force unanimously. The background of the research strategy and of reaching consensus and the definitions of the recommendation levels used in this paper have been described in the EFNS recommendations (Brainin et al., 2004).

Clinical aspects

Migraine is an idiopathic headache disorder that is characterized by moderate to severe, often unilateral and pulsating headache attacks aggravated by physical activity and accompanied by vegetative symptoms such as nausea, vomiting, photophobia and phonophobia. The diagnostic criteria for migraine attacks and the migraine aura are given in table 13.1. The duration of the attacks is 4–72 h; at least five attacks must have occurred before the diagnosis can be established. Most of the patients suffer from migraine attacks without aura. However, there are several migraine syndromes with specific aura features and migraine syndromes with uncommon courses or complications. These syndromes have their own diagnostic criteria; the subclassification of these syndromes is given in table 13.2 (Headache Classification Committee,

Table 13.1 Diagnostic criteria of migraine of the IHS classification (2004).

A. At least five attacks fulfilling criteria B–D
B. Headache lasting 4–72 h (untreated or unsuccessfully treated)
C. Headache has at least two of the following characteristics:

   1. unilateral location
   2. pulsating quality
   3. moderate or severe pain intensity
   4. aggravation by or causing avoidance of routine physical activity (e.g. walking or climbing stairs)

D. During headache there is at least one of the following:

   1. nausea and/or vomiting
   2. photophobia and phonophobia

E. Not attributed to another disorder.

Table 13.2 Subclassification of migraine according to the IHS classification (2004).

1 Migraine without aura
2 Migraine with aura

   2.1 Typical aura with migraine headache
   2.2 Typical aura with non-migraine headache
   2.3 Typical aura without headache
   2.4 Familial hemiplegic migraine
   2.5 Sporadic hemiplegic migraine
   2.6 Basilar-type migraine

3 Childhood periodic syndromes that are commonly precursors of migraine

   3.1 Cyclical vomiting
   3.2 Abdominal migraine
   3.3 Benign paroxysmal vertigo of childhood

4 Retinal migraine
5 Complications of migraine

   5.1 Chronic migraine
   5.2 Status migrainosus
   5.3 Persistent aura without infarction
   5.4 Migrainous infarction
   5.5 Migraine-triggered seizure

6 Probable migraine

   6.1 Probable migraine without aura
   6.2 Probable migraine with aura
   6.3 Probable chronic migraine.

2004). The diagnostic criteria for these migraine syndromes have been published on the homepage of the IHS (www.i-h-s.org).

In children, migraine attacks can be shorter (even only 1 or 2 h) and the accompanying symptoms can be more prominent including syndromes such as abdominal migraine or periodic syndromes in childhood (Maytal, 1997; Lewis, 2004; Lewis *et al.*, 2004).

Epidemiology

Migraine is one of the most frequent headache disorders. About 6–8% of males and 12–14% of females suffer from migraine (Rasmussen *et al.*, 1991; Scher, 1998; Rasmussen, 2001; Lipton *et al.*, 2002). The life time prevalence of females might be even higher up to 25%. Before puberty, the prevalence of migraine is about 5%, both in boys and girls. The highest incidence of migraine attacks is in the age between 35 and 45 years with a female preponderance of 3 to 1. The median duration of untreated migraine attacks is 18 h, the median attack frequency is one per month.

Diagnosis

The diagnosis of migraine is based on the typical patient's history and a normal neurological examination. Apparative investigations, in particular brain imaging, is necessary if secondary headache is suspected (e.g. the headache characteristics are untypical), if the course of headache attacks changes, or if persistent neurological or psychopathological abnormalities are present (Quality Standards Subcommittee of the American Academy of Neurology, 1994). In particular, magnetic resonance imaging (MRI) (and not CT imaging with its inferior sensitivity to detect vascular abnormalities and lesions) of the brain in migraine is recommended when

- the neurological examination is not normal;
- typical migraine attacks occur for the first time after the age of 40;
- frequency or intensity of migraine attacks continuously increase;
- the accompanying symptoms of migraine attacks change;
- new psychiatric symptoms occur in relation to the attacks.

Drug treatment of migraine attacks

Several large randomized, placebo-controlled trials have been published to establish the best drugs for the acute management of migraine. In most of these trials, successful treatment of migraine attacks was defined as one or a combination of the following criteria:

- pain free after 2 h;
- improvement of headache from moderate or severe to mild or none after 2 h (Pilgrim, 1993);
- consistent efficacy in two out of three attacks;

- no headache recurrence and no further drug intake within 24 h after successful treatment (so-called sustained pain relief or pain free).

Analgesics

Drugs of first choice for mild or moderate migraine attacks are different analgesics. Evidence of efficacy in migraine treatment in at least one placebo-controlled study has been obtained for acetyl-salicylic acid (ASA) up to 1000 mg (Chabriat et al., 1994; Nebe et al., 1995; Tfelt-Hansen et al., 1995; Diener et al., 2004b), for ibuprofen 200–800 mg (Havanka-Kanniainen, 1989; Kloster et al., 1992; Nebe et al., 1995; Diener et al., 2004b), for diclofenac 50–100 mg (Karachalios et al., 1992; Dahlöf and Björkman, 1993; The Diclofenac-K/Sumatriptan Migraine Study Group, 1999), for phenazon 1000 mg (Göbel et al., 2004), for metamizol 1000 mg (Tulunay et al., 2004), tolfenamic acid 200 mg (Myllyla et al., 1998) and for paracetamol 1000 mg (Lipton et al., 2000). In addition, the fixed combination of ASA, parac-etamol and caffeine is effective in acute migraine treatment and is also more effective than the sin-gle substances or combinations without caffeine (Lipton et al., 1998; Diener et al., 2005a). Intra-venous ASA was more effective than subcutaneous ergotamine (Limmroth et al., 1999b); intravenous metamizol was superior to placebo in migraine without and with aura (Bigal et al., 2002). To prevent drug overuse headache, the intake of sim-ple analgesics should be restricted to 15 days per month and the intake of combined analgesics to 10 days per month. Coxibs are not recommended for acute migraine treatment because of the unde-termined cerebrovascular adverse events. Opioids are of only minor efficacy, no modern controlled trials are available for these substances. Table 13.3 presents an overview of analgesics with efficacy in acute migraine treatment.

Antiemetics

The use of antiemetics in acute migraine attacks is recommended to treat vegetative symptoms and because it is assumed that these drugs improve the resorption of analgesics (Ross-Lee et al., 1983; Waelkens, 1984; Schulman and Dermott, 2003).

However, prospective, placebo-controlled random-ized trials to prove this assumption are lacking. Metoclopramide also has a mild analgesic efficacy in migraine (Ellis et al., 1993). There is no evi-dence that the fixed combination of an antiemetic with an analgesic or with a triptan is more effec-tive than the analgesic or triptan alone. Metoclo-pramide 20 mg is recommended for adults and adolescents; in children domperidon 10 mg should be used because of the possible extrapyramidal side effects of metoclopramide. table 13.4 presents the antiemetics recommended for use in migraine attacks.

Ergot alkaloids

There are only very few randomised, placebo-controlled trials on the efficacy of ergot alka-loids in the acute migraine treatment; although these substances have been used for a very long time, very severe events have also been reported (Tfelt-Hansen et al., 2000). In comparative trials, triptans showed better efficacy than ergot alka-loids (The Multinational Oral Sumatriptan Cafer-got Comparative Study Group, 1991; Christie et al., 2002; Diener et al., 2002b). The advantage of ergot alkaloids in some patients is a longer half-life time and a lower recurrence rate. Therefore, these sub-stances should be restricted to patients with very long migraine attacks or with regular recurrence. The only compound with sufficient evidence of efficacy is ergotamine tartrate 2 mg (oral or sup-positories). Ergot alkaloids can induce drug overuse headache very fast and in very low doses (Evers et al., 1999b). Therefore, their use must be limited to 10 days per month. Major side effects are nausea, vomiting, paraesthesia and ergotism. Contraindi-cations are cardiovascular and cerebrovascular dis-eases, Raynaud's disease, arterial hypertension, renal failure, and pregnancy and lactation.

Triptans (5-HT$_{1B/1D}$-agonists)

The 5-HT$_{1B/1D}$ agonists sumatriptan, zolmitriptan, naratriptan, rizatriptan, almotriptan, eletriptan and frovatriptan (order in the year of marketing), the so-called triptans, are specific migraine medica-tions and should not be applied in other headache disorders except cluster headache. The different

Table 13.3 Analgesics with evidence of efficacy in at least one study on the acute treatment of migraine. The level of recommendation also considers side effects and consistency of the studies.

Substance	Dose (in mg)	Level of recommendation	Comment
Acetylsalicylic acid	1000 (oral)	A	Gastrointestinal side effects
(ASA)	1000 (i.v.)	A	Risk of bleeding
Ibuprofen	200–800	A	Side effects as for ASA
Naproxen	500–1000	A	Side effects as for ASA
Diclofenac	50–100	A	Including diclofenac-K
Paracetamol	1000 (oral)	A	Caution in liver and kidney
	1000 (supp.)	A	failure
ASA plus	250 (oral)	A	As for ASA and paracetamol plus
	200–250		paracetamol
Caffeine	50		
Metamizol	1000 (oral)	B	Risk of agranulocytosis
	1000 (i.v.)	B	Risk of hypotension
Phenazon	1000 (oral)	B	See paracetamol
Tolfenamic acid	200 (oral)	B	Side effects as for ASA

Table 13.4 Antiemetics recommended for the acute treatment of migraine attacks.

Substances	Dose	Level	Comment
Metoclopramide	10–20 mg(oral) 20 mg (suppository) 10 mg (intramuscular, intravenous, subcutaneous)	B	Side effect: dyskinesia; contraindicated in childhood and in pregnancy
Domperidon	20–30 mg (oral)	B	Side effects less severe than in metoclopramide; can be given to children

triptans for migraine therapy are presented in table 13.5. The efficacy of all triptans has been proven in large placebo-controlled trials the meta-analyses of which have been published (Ferrari *et al.*, 2001; Goadsby *et al.*, 2002). For sumatriptan (The Oral Sumatriptan and Aspirin plus Metoclopramide Comparative Study Group, 1992; Tfelt-Hansen, 1995) and zolmitriptan (Geraud *et al.*, 2002), comparative studies with ASA and metoclopramide exist. In these comparative studies, the triptans were not or only a little more effective than ASA. In about 60% of non-responders to NSAIDs, triptans are effective (Diamond *et al.*, 2004). Sumatriptan 6 mg subcutaneously is more effective than intravenous ASA 1000 mg s.c., but has more side effects (Diener *et al.*, 1999). Ergotaminetartrate was less effective in comparative studies with sumatriptan (The Multinational Oral Sumatriptan Cafergot Comparative Study Group, 1991) and with eletriptan (Diener *et al.*, 2002b). Triptans can be effective at any time during a migraine attack. However, there is evidence that the earlier triptans are taken the better is their efficacy (Burstein *et al.*, 2004; Dowson *et al.*, 2004). A strategy of strictly early intake can, however, lead to frequent drug treatment in certain patients. The use of triptans is restricted to maximum 10 days per month. Otherwise, the induction of a drug overuse headache

Table 13.5 Different triptans for the treatment of acute migraine attacks (order in the time of marketing). Not all doses or application forms are available in all European countries.

Substance	Dose	Level	Comment
Sumatriptan	25, 50, 100 mg (oral including rapid-release)	A	100 mg sumatriptan is reference to all triptans
	25 mg (suppository)	A	
	10, 20 mg (nasal spray)	A	
	6 mg (subcutaneous)	A	
Zolmitriptan	2.5, 5 mg (oral including disintegrating form)	A	
	2.5, 5 mg (nasal spray)	A	
Naratriptan	2.5 mg (oral)	A	less but longer efficacy than sumatriptan
Rizatriptan	10 mg (oral including wafer form)	A	5 mg when taking propranolol
Almotriptan	12.5 mg (oral)	A	probably less side effects than sumatriptan
Eletriptan	20, 40 mg (oral)	A	80 mg allowed if 40 mg not effective
Frovatriptan	2.5 mg (oral)	A	less but longer efficacy than sumatriptan

General side effects for all triptans: Chest symptoms, nausea, distal paraesthesia, fatigue.

General contraindications: Arterial hypertension (untreated), coronary heart disease, cerebrovascular disease, Raynaud's disease, pregnancy and lactation, age under 18 (except sumatriptan nasal spray) and age above 65, severe liver or kidney failure.

is possible for all triptans (Evers *et al.*, 1999b; Limmroth *et al.*, 1999a; Katsarava *et al.*, 2001). Therefore, in clinical practice, a reasonable trade-off has to be agreed on between early intake and a reasonable intake frequency.

One typical problem of attack treatment in migraine is headache recurrence. This is defined as a worsening of headache after a pain free state or mild pain has been achieved with a drug within 24 h (Ferrari, 1999). This problem is more eminent in triptans and NSAIDs than in ergotamine. About 15–40% (depending on the primary and the lasting efficacy of the drug) of the patients taking an oral triptan experience recurrence. A second dose of the triptan is effective in most cases (Ferrari *et al.*, 1994). If the first dose of a triptan is not effective, a second dose is useless.

After application of sumatriptan, severe adverse events have been reported such as myocardial infarction, cardiac arrhythmias and stroke. The incidence of these events was about 1 in 1,000,000 (O'Quinn *et al.*, 1999; Welch *et al.*, 2000). Reports of severe adverse events also exist for other triptans and for ergotamine tratrate. However, all of the reported patients had contraindications against triptans or the diagnosis of migraine was wrong. In population-based studies, no increased risk of vascular events could be detected for triptan users as compared to a healthy population (Velentgas *et al.*, 2004; Hall *et al.*, 2004). Thus, contraindications for the use of triptans are untreated arterial hypertension, coronary heart disease, Raynaud's disease, history of ischemic stroke, pregnancy, lactation, and severe liver or renal failure.

Due to safety aspects, triptans should not be taken during the aura although no specific severe adverse events have been reported. The best time for application is the very onset of headache. Furthermore, triptans are not efficacious when taken during the aura (Bates *et al.*, 1994; Olesen *et al.*, 2004).

Comparison of triptans

Triptans are a very homogenous group of acute migraine drugs with respect to efficacy, pharmacology and safety. However, some minor differences exist that will be discussed to give guidance on which triptan to use in an individual patient. It is important to notice that a triptan can be efficacious even if another (or more) triptan were not.

Subcutaneous sumatriptan has the fastest onset of efficacy of about 10 min (Tfelt-Hansen, 1993). Oral rizatriptan and eletriptan need about 30 min; oral sumatriptan, almotriptan and zolmitriptan need about 45–60 min (Ferrari *et al.*, 2001); a naratriptan and frovatriptan need up to 4 h for the onset of efficacy (Goadsby, 1997; McDavis, 1999). Zolmitriptan nasal spray has a shorter duration until efficacy than oral zolmitriptan (Charlesworth, 2003). There is no evidence that different oral formulations such as melting tablets, wafer forms, or rapid release forms (Dahlöf *et al.*, 2004) act earlier than others.

Pain relief after 2 h as the most important efficacy parameter is best in subcutaneous sumatripan with up to 80% responders (The Subcutaneous Sumatriptan International Study Group, 1991). Sumatriptan nasal spray has the same efficacy as oral sumatriptan 50 or 100 mg. Twenty-five milligram oral sumatriptan is less effective than the higher doses but has less side effects (Ferrari *et al.*, 2001). Sumatriptan suppositories are about as effective as oral sumatriptan 50 or 100 mg and should be given to patients who report vomiting (Becker *et al.*, 1995; Ryan *et al.*, 1997; Tepper *et al.*, 1998). Naratriptan and frovatriptan (2.5 mg) are less effective than sumatriptan 50 or 100 mg but have less side effects. The duration until the onset of efficacy is longer in these two triptans as compared to all others. Rizatriptan 10 mg is a little more effective than sumatriptan 100 mg. Oral zolmitriptan 2.5 or 5 mg, almotriptan 12.5 mg and eletriptan 40 mg show a similar efficacy and similar side effects (Goldstein *et al.*, 1998; Tfelt-Hansen *et al.*, 1998; Tfelt-Hansen and Ryan, 2000). Eletriptan 80 mg is the most effective oral triptan but also has the most side effects (Ferrari *et al.*, 2001).

Headache recurrence is a major problem in clinical practice. The recurrence rate is between 15 and 40%. The highest recurrence rate is observed after subcutaneous sumatriptan. Naratriptan and frovatriptan show the lowest recurrence rates. It might be that triptans with a longer half-life time have a lower recurrence rate (Geraud *et al.*, 2003). If migraine recurs after successful treatment with a triptan, a second dose of this triptan can be given. Another problem in clinical practice is inconsistency of efficacy. Therefore, efficacy only in two out of three attacks is regarded as good.

Migraine prophylaxis

Prophylactic drug treatment of migraine is possible with several drugs. Substances with good efficacy and tolerability and evidence of efficacy are betablockers, calcium channel blockers, antiepileptic drugs, NSAIDs, antidepressants and miscellaneous drugs. The use of all these drugs, however, is based on empirical data rather than on proven pathophysiological concepts. The decision to introduce a prophylactic treatment has to be discussed with the patient carefully. The efficacy of the drugs, their potential side effects, and their interactions with other drugs have to be considered in the individual patient. There is no commonly accepted indication for starting a prophylactic treatment. In the view of the Task Force, prophylactic drug treatment of migraine should be considered and discussed with the patient when

- the quality of life, business duties, or school attendance are severely impaired;
- frequency of attacks per month is two or higher;
- migraine attacks do not respond to acute drug treatment;
- frequent, very long, or uncomfortable auras occur.

A migraine prophylaxis is regarded as successful if the frequency of migraine attacks per month is decreased by at least 50% within 3 months. For therapy evaluation, a migraine diary is mandatory. In the following paragraphs, the placebo-controlled trials in migraine prophylaxis are summarized. The recommended drugs of first choice, according to the consensus of the Task

Table 13.6 Recommended substances (drugs of first choice) for the prophylactic drug treatment of migraine.

Substance	Daily dose	Level
Betablockers		
Metoprolol	50–200 mg	A
Propranolol	40–240 mg	A
Calcium channel blockers		
Flunarizine	5–10 mg	A
Antiepileptic drugs		
Valproic acid	500–1800 mg	A
Topiramate	25–100 mg	A

Table 13.7 Drugs of second choice for migraine prophylaxis (evidence of efficacy, but less effective or more side effects than drugs of table 13.6).

Substance	Daily Dose	Level
Amitriptyline	50–150 mg	B
Naproxen	2 × 250–500 mg	B
Petasites	2 × 75 mg	B
Bisoprolol	5–10 mg	B

Table 13.8 Drugs of third choice for migraine prophylaxis (only probable efficacy).

Substance	Daily Dose	Level
Acetylsalicylic acid	300 mg	C
Gabapentin	1200–1600 mg	C
Magnesium	24 mmol	C
Tanacetum parthenium	3 × 6.25 mg	C
Riboflavin	400 mg	C
Coenzyme Q10	300 mg	C
Candesartan	16 mg	C
Lisinopril	20 mg	C
Methysergide	4–12 mg	C

Force, are given in table 13.6. Tables 13.7 and 13.8 present drugs recommended as second or third choice when the drugs of table 13.6 are not effective, contraindicated, or when comorbidity of the patients suggests the respective drug of second or third choice (e.g. amitriptyline for migraine prophylaxis in depressed patients or in patients with sleep disturbances or with tension-type headache).

Betablockers

Betablockers are clearly effective in migraine prophylaxis and very well studied in a lot of placebo-controlled, randomized trials. The best evidence has been obtained for the selective betablocker metoprolol (Kangasniemi and Hedman, 1984; Olsson et al., 1984; Steiner et al., 1988; Sorensen et al., 1991; Wörz et al., 1991) and for the non-selective betablocker propranolol (Diamond and Medina, 1976; Kangasniemi and Hedman, 1984; Olsson et al., 1984; Tfelt-Hansen et al., 1984; Nadel-mann et al., 1986; Havanka-Kanniainen et al., 1988; Ludin, 1989; Holroyd et al., 1991; Gawel et al., 1992). Also, bisoprolol (Wörz et al., 1991; van de Ven et al., 1997), timolol (Tfelt-Hansen et al., 1984; Stellar et al., 1984), and atenolol (Johannsson et al., 1987) might be effective but evidence is less convincing compared to propranolol and metoprolol.

Calcium channel blockers

The 'non-specific' calcium channel blocker flunarizine has been shown to be effective in migraine prophylaxis in several studies (Louis, 1981; Diamond and Schenbaum, 1983; Amery et al., 1985; Bono et al., 1985; Centonze et al., 1985; Nappi et al., 1987; Freitag et al., 1991; Sorensen et al., 1991; Gawel et al., 1992; Bassi et al., 1992; Diamond and Freitag, 1993; Balkan et al., 1994). The dose is 5–10 mg; female patients seem to benefit from lower doses than male patients (Diener et al., 2002a). Another 'non-specific' calcium channel blocker, cyclandelate, has also been studied but with conflicting results (Nappi et al., 1987; Gerber et al., 1995; Diener et al., 1996; Siniatchkin et al., 1998; Diener et al., 2001). As the better designed studies were negative, cyclandelate cannot be recommended.

Antiepileptic drugs

Valproic acid in a dose of at least 600 mg (Kaniecki, 1997; Klapper, 1997; Silberstein et al., 2000b; Freitag et al., 2002) and topiramte in a dose between 25 and 100 mg (Brandes *et al.*, 2004a; Diener *et al.*, 2004a; Mei *et al.*, 2004; Silberstein *et al.*, 2004b) are the two antiepileptic drugs with evidence of efficacy in more than one placebo-controlled trial. The efficacy rates are comparable to those of metoprolol, propranolol and flunarizine. Other antiepilpetic drugs studied in migraine prophylaxis are lamotrigine and gabapentin. Lamotrigine did not reduce the frequency of migraine attacks but is probably effective in reducing the frequency of migraine auras (Steiner *et al.*, 1997; Lampl *et al.*, 1999). Gabapentin showed a significant efficacy in one placebo-controlled trial in doses between 1200 and 1600 mg (Mathew *et al.*, 2001).

NSAIDs

In some comparative trials, ASA was equivalent to or worse than a comparator (which had shown efficacy in other trials) but never achieved a better efficacy than placebo in direct comparison. However, in two large cohort trials, ASA 200–300 mg reduced the frequency of migraine attacks (Peto *et al.*, 1988; Buring *et al.*, 1990). Naproxen 1000 mg was better than placebo in three controlled trials (Ziegler and Ellis, 1985; Welch *et al.*, 1985; Bellavance and Meloche, 1990). Also tolfenamic acid showed efficacy in two placebo-controlled trials (Mikkelsen and Falk, 1982; Mikkelsen *et al.*, 1986). Other NSAIDs studied were ketoprofen, mefenamic acid, indobufen, flurbiprofen and rofecoxib (Evers and Mylecharane, 2005). However, all studies for the latter substances were small and had no sufficient design.

Antidepressants

The only antidepressant with consistent efficacy in migraine prophylaxis is amitriptyline in doses between 10 and 150 mg. It has been studied in four older placebo-controlled trials, all with positive results (Gomersall and Stuart, 1973; Couch and Hassanein, 1979; Ziegler *et al.* 1987; Ziegler *et al.*, 1993). As the studies with amitriptyline were small and showed central side effects, this drug is recommended only with Level B. For femoxetine, two small positive placebo-controlled trials have been published (Zeeberg *et al.*, 1981; Orholm *et al.*,

1986). Fluoxetine in doses between 10 and 40 mg was effective in three (Adly *et al.*, 1992; Steiner *et al.*, 1998; d'Amato *et al.*, 1999) and not effective in one placebo-controlled trial (Saper *et al.*, 1994).

Other antidepressants not effective in placebo-controlled trials were clomipramine and sertraline; for several further antidepressants, only open or not placebo-controlled trials are available (Evers and Mylecharane, 2005).

Miscellaneous drugs

The antihypertensive drugs lisinopril (Schrader *et al.*, 2001) and candesartan (Tronvik *et al.*, 2002) showed efficacy in migraine prophylaxis in one placebo-controlled trial each. However, these results have to be confirmed before the drugs can definitely be recommended. The same is true for high-dose riboflavin (400 mg) and coenzyme Q10 which have shown efficacy in one placebo-controlled trial each (Schoenen *et al.*, 1998; Sándor *et al.*, 2005). For oral magnesium, conflicting studies (one positive, one negative) have been published (Pfaffenrath *et al.*, 1996; Peikert *et al.*, 1996). A herbal drug with evidence of efficacy is butterbur root extract (Petasites hybridus). This has been shown for a remedy with 75 mg in two placebo-controlled trials (Diener *et al.*, 2004c; Lipton *et al.*, 2004). Another herbal remedy, feverfew (Tanacetum parthenium), has been studied in several placebo-controlled trials with conflicting results. The most recent and best-designed study showed negative results (Pfaffenrath *et al.*, 2002), and a Cochrane review resulted in a negative meta-analysis of all controlled studies on tanacetum (Pittler and Ernst, 2004). However, as there exist positive placebo-controlled trials, Tanacetum can be tried as a third-line drug.

In older studies, clonidin, pizotifen and methysergide have shown efficacy in migraine prophylaxis. The more recent and better designed studies on clonidine, however, did not confirm any efficacy (for review see Evers and Mylecharane, 2005). Methysergide, which is clearly effective, can be recommended for short-term use only (maximum 6 months per treatment period) because of potentially severe side effects (Silberstein, 1998); it can be re-established after a wash-out period of 4–6 weeks.

Pizotifen is not recommended because the efficacy is not better than in the substances mentioned above and the side effects (dizziness, weight gain) are classified as very severe by the task force and limit the use too much (Mylecharane, 1991). Ergot alkaloids have also been used in migraine prophylaxis. The evidence for dihydroergotamine is weak as several studies reported both positive and negative results (for review see Evers and Mylecharane, 2005). Dihydroergocryptine has also shown efficacy in one small placebo-controlled study (Canonico et al., 1989).

Botulinum toxin was studied in four published placebo-controlled trials (Silberstein et al., 2000a; Brin et al., 2000; Evers et al., 2004; Dodick et al., 2005). Only one study showed an efficacy for the low-dose (but not the high-dose) treatment with botulinum toxin (Silberstein et al., 2000a). In another study, only the subgroup of chronic migraine patients without further prophylactic treatment showed benefit from botulinum toxin A (Dodick et al., 2005). However, this was not the primary endpoint of the study.

Finally, those substances with negative modern randomized, placebo-controlled, double-blind trials and which are not mentioned above are listed as follows: no efficacy at all in migraine prophylaxis has been shown for homoeopathic remedies (Whitmarsh et al., 1997; Walach et al., 1997; Straumsheim et al., 2000); for the antagonist of the cysteinyl-leukotriene receptor antagonist montelukast (Brandes et al., 2004b); for acetazolamide 500 mg per day (Vahedi et al., 2002); and for the neurokinin-1 receptor antagonist lanepitant (Goldstein et al., 2001).

Specific situations

Menstrual migraine

In the recent 2nd edition of IHS diagnostic criteria, the entity of menstrual migraine is to be found in the appendix (and not the main criteria), reflecting a certain degree of uncertainty about the best criteria. Nevertheless, different drug regimes have been studied to treat this condition of quite some importance in clinical practice. On the one hand, acute migraine treatment with triptans has been

studied showing the same efficacy of triptans in menstrual migraine attacks as compared to non-menstrual migraine attacks. On the other hand, short-term prophylaxis of menstrual migraine has also been studied.

Naproxen sodium (550 mg twice daily) has been shown to reduce pain including headache in the premenstrual syndrome (Facchinetti et al., 1989). Its specific effects on menstrual migraine (550 mg twice daily) have also been evaluated (Sargent et al., 1985; Sances et al., 1990; Szekely et al., 1989). In one trial (Sargent et al., 1985), patients reported fewer and less severe headaches during the week before menstruation than patients treated with placebo, but only severity was significantly reduced. In the other two placebo-controlled trials, naproxen sodium, given 1 week before and 1 week after the start of menstruation, resulted in fewer perimenstrual headaches; in one study, severity was not reduced (Szekely et al., 1989), but in the other both severity and analgesic requirements were decreased (Sances et al., 1990). Even triptans have been used as short-term prophylaxis of menstrual migraine. For naratriptan (2×1 mg per day for 5 days starting 2 days prior to the expected onset of menses) and for frovatriptan (2×2.5 mg given for 6 days perimenstrually), superiority over placebo has been shown (Newman et al., 2001; Silberstein et al., 2004a).

Another prophylactic treatment regime of menstrual migraine is oestrogen replacement therapy. The best evidence, although not as effective as betablockers or other first line prophylactic drugs, has been achieved for transdermal estradiol (not less than 100 μg given for 6 days perimenstrually as a gel or a patch) (De Lignieres et al., 1986; Dennerstein et al., 1988; Smits et al., 1994; Pradalier et al., 1994).

Migraine in pregnancy

There are no specific clinical trials evaluating drug treatment of migraine during pregnancy, most of the migraine drugs are contraindicated. Fortunately, most of the pregnant migraineurs experience less or even no migraine attacks. If migraine occurs during pregnancy, only paracetamol is allowed during the whole period. NSAIDs can be given in the second trimester. These recommendations are based on the advices of the regulatory authorities in most European countries. There might be differences in some respect between different countries (in particular, NDAIDs might be allowed in the first trimester).

Triptans and ergot alkaloids are contraindicated. For sumatriptan, a large pregnancy register has been established with no reports of any adverse events or complications during pregnancy that might be attributed to sumatriptan (Olesen *et al.*, 2000; Källen and Lygner, 2001; Fox *et al.*, 2002). For migraine prophylaxis, only magnesium and metoprolol are recommended during pregnancy (Recommendation Level B).

Migraine in children and adolescents

The only analgesics with evidence of efficacy for acute migraine treatment in children and adolescents are ibuprofen 10 mg per kg body weight and paracetamol 15 mg per kg body weight (Evers *et al.*, 2001). The only antiemetic licensed for use in children up to 12 years is domperidon. Sumatriptan nasal spray 5–20 mg is the only triptan with positive placebo-controlled trials in acute migraine treatment of children and adolescents (Überall and Wenzel, 1999; Winner *et al.*, 2000; Ahonen *et al.*, 2004), the recommended dose for adolescents from the age of 12 is 10 mg. Oral triptans did not show significant efficacy in placebo-controlled childhood and adolescents studies (Hämäläinen *et al.*, 1997; Evers, 1999a; Winner *et al.*, 2002). This was in particular due to high placebo responses of about 50% in this age group. In post-hoc analyses, however, 2.5–5 mg zolmitriptan were effective in adolescents from the age of 12 to 17 (Solomon *et al.*, 1997; Tepper *et al.* 1999). Ergot alkaloids should not be used in children and adolescents. Also children and adolescents can develop drug-induced headache due to analgesic, ergotamine or triptan overuse.

For migraine prophylaxis, flunarizine 10 mg and propranolol 40–80 mg per day showed the best evidence of efficacy in children and adolescents (Evers, 1999a; Lewis *et al.*, 2004). Other drugs have not been studied or did not show efficacy in appropriate studies.

Conflicts of interest

The present guidelines were developed without external financial support. The authors report the following financial supports:

Stefan Evers: Salary by the government of the State Northrhine-Westphalia; honoraries and research grants by Almirall, AstraZeneca, Berlin Chemie, Boehringer, GlaxoSmithKline, Ipsen Pharma, Janssen Cilag, MSD, Pfizer, Novartis, Pharm Allergan, Pierre Fabre

Judit Áfra: Salary by the Hungarian Ministry of Health; honoraries by GlaxoSmithKline

Achim Frese: Salary by the government of the State Northrhine-Westphalia; no honoraries

Peter J. Goadsby: Salary by the University College of London; honoraries by Almirall, AstraZeneca, GlaxoSmithKline, MSD, Pfizer, Medtronic

Mattias Linde: Salary by the Swedish government; honoraries by AstraZeneca, GlaxoSmithKline, MSD, Nycomed, Pfizer

Arne May: Salary by the University Hospital of Hamburg; honoraries by Almirall, AstraZeneca, Bayer Vital, Berlin Chemie, GlaxoSmithKline, Janssen Cilag, MSD, Pfizer

Peter S. Sándor: Salary by the University Hospital of Zurich; honoraries by AstraZeneca, GlaxoSmithKline, Janssen Cilag, Pfizer, Pharm Allergan.

References

Adly C, Straumanis J, Chesson A (1992). Fluoxetine prophylaxis of migraine. *Headache* **32:** 101–104.

Ahonen K, Hämäläinen M, Rantala H, Hoppu K (2004). Nasal sumatriptan is effective in treatment of migraine attacks in children: A randomized trial. *Neurology* **62:**883–887.

Amery WK, Caers LI, Aerts TJL (1985). Flunarizine, a calcium entry blocker in migraine prophylaxis. *Headache* **25:**249–254.

Balkan S, Aktekin B, Önal Z (1994). Efficacy of flunarizine in the prophylactic treatment of migraine. *Gazi Medical J* **5:**81–84.

Bassi P, Brunati L, Rapuzzi B, Alberti E, Mangoni A (1992). Low dose flunarizine in the prophylaxis of migraine. *Headache* **32:**390–392.

Bates D, Ashford E, Dawson R, Ensink FB, Gilhus NE, Olesen J, Pilgrim AJ, Shevlin P (1994). Subcutaneous sumatriptan during the migraine aura. *Neurology* **44:**1587–1592.

Becker WJ, on behalf of the Study Group (1995). A placebo-controlled, dose-defining study of sumatriptan nasal spray in the acute treatment of migraine. *Cephalalgia* **15(Suppl 14):** 271–276.

Bellavance AJ, Meloche JP (1990). A comparative study of naproxen sodium, pizotyline and placebo in migraine prophylaxis. *Headache* **30:**710–715.

Bigal ME, Bordini CA, Tepper SJ, Speciali JG (2002). Intravenous dipyrone in the acute treatment of migraine without aura and migraine with aura: a randomized, double blind, placebo controlled study. *Headache* **42:**862–871.

Bono G, Manzoni GC, Martucci N, Baldrati A, Farina S, Cassabgi F, De Carolis P, Nappi G (1985). Flunarizine in common migraine: Italian cooperative trial. II. Long-term follow-up. *Cephalalgia* **5(Suppl 2):**155–158.

Brainin M, Barnes M, Baron JC, Gilhus NE, Hughes R, Selmaj K, Waldemar G (2004). Guidance for the preparation of neurological management guidelines by EFNS scientific task forces – revised recommendations 2004. *Eur J Neurol* **11:**577–581.

Brandes J, Saper J, Diamond M, Couch JR, Lewis DW, Schmitt J, Neto W, Schwabe S, Jacobs D; MIGR-002 Study Group (2004a). Topiramate for migraine prevention: a randomized controlled trial. *JAMA* **291:**965–973.

Brandes JL, Visser WH, Farmer MV, Schuhl AL, Malbecq W, Vrijens F, Lines CR, Reines SA; Protocol 125 study group (2004b). Montelukast for migraine prophylaxis: a randomized, double-blind, placebo-controlled study. *Headache* **44:**581–586.

Brin MF, Swope DM, O'Brian C, Abbasi S, Pogoda JM (2000). Botox? for migraine: double-blind, placebo-controlled, region-specific evaluation. *Cephalalgia* **20:**421–422.

Buring JE, Peto R, Hennekens CH (1990). Lowdose aspirin for migraine prophylaxis. *JAMA* **264:**1711–1713.

Burstein R, Collins B, Jakubowski M (2004). Defeating migraine pain with triptans: a race against the development of cutaneous allodynia. *Ann Neurol* **55:** 19–26.

Canonico PL, Scapagnini U, Genazzani E, Zanotti A (1989). Dihydroergokryptine (DEK) in the prophylaxis of common migraine: doubleblind clinical study vs placebo. *Cephalalgia* **9(Suppl 10):**446–447.

Centonze V, Tesauro P, Magrone D, Vino M, Macinagrossa G, Campanozzi F, Altomare E, Attolini E, Albano O (1985). Efficacy and tolerability of flunarizine in the prophylaxis of migraine. *Cephalalgia* **5(Suppl 2):**163–168.

Chabriat H, Joire JE, Danchot J, Grippon P, Bousser MG (1994). Combined oral lysine acetylsalicylate and metoclopramide in the acute treatment of migraine: a multicentre double-blind placebo-controlled study. *Cephalalgia* **14:**297–300.

Christie S, Göbel H, Mateos V, Allen C, Vrijens F, Shivaprakash M (2003); Rizatriptan-Ergotamine/Caffeine Preference Study Group. Crossover comparison of efficacy and preference for rizatriptan 10 mg versus ergotamine/caffeine in migraine. *Eur Neurol* **49:**20–29.

Couch JR, Hassanein RS (1979). Amitriptyline in migraine prophylaxis. *Arch Neurol* **36:**695–699.

d'Amato CC, Pizza V, Marmolo T, Giordano E, Alfano V, Nasta A (1999). Fluoxetine for migraine prophylaxis: a double-blind trial. *Headache* **39:**716–719.

Dahlöf C, Björkman R. Diclofenac-K (50 and 100 mg) and placebo in the acute treatment of migraine (1993). *Cephalalgia* **13:**117–123.

Dahlöf C, Cady R, Poole AC (2004). Speed of onset and efficacy of sumatriptan fast-disintegrating/rapid release tablets: results of two replicate randomised, placebo-controlled studies. *Headache Care* **1:**277–280.

De Lignieres B, Mauvais-Javis P, Mas JML, Mas JL, Touboul PJ, Bousser MG (1986). Prevention of menstrual migraine by percutaneous oestradiol. *BMJ* **293:**1540.

Dennerstein L, Morse C, Burrows G, Oats J, Brown J, Smith M (1988). Menstrual migraine: a double blind trial of percutaneous oestradiol. *Gynecol Endocrinol* **2:**113–120.

Diamond S, Medina JL (1976). Double blind study of propranolol for migraine prophylaxis. *Headache* **16:**24–27.

Diamond S, Schenbaum H (1983). Flunarizine, a calcium channel blocker, in the prophylactic treatment of migraine. *Headache* **23:**39–42.

Diamond S, Freitag FG (1993). A double blind trial of flunarizine in migraine prophylaxis. *Headache Quart* **4:**169–172.

Diamond M, Hettiarachchi J, Hilliard B, Sands G, Nett R (2004). Effectiveness of eletriptan in acute migraine: primary care for Excedrin nonresponders. *Headache* **44:**209–216.

Diener HC, Föh M, Iaccarino C, Wessely P, Isler H, Strenge H, Fischer M, Wedekind W, Taneri Z (1996). Cyclandelate in the prophylaxis of migraine: A randomized, parallel, double-blind study in comparison with placebo and propranolol. *Cephalalgia* **16:**441–447.

Diener HC, for the ASASUMAMIG Study Group (1999). Efficacy and safety of intravenous acetylsalicylic acid lysinate compared to subcutaneous sumatriptan and parenteral placebo in the acute treatment of migraine.

A double-blind, double-dummy, randomized, multi-center, parallel group study. *Cephalalgia* **19**:581–588.

Diener H, Krupp P, Schmitt T, Steitz G, Milde K, Freytag S; On behalf of the Study Group (2001). Cyclandelate in the prophylaxis of migraine: a placebo-controlled study. *Cephalalgia* **21**:66–70.

Diener H, Matias-Guiu J, Hartung E, Pfaffenrath V, Ludin HP, Nappi G, De Beukelaar F (2002a). Efficacy and tolerability in migraine prophylaxis of flunarizine in reduced doses: a comparison with propranolol 160 mg daily. *Cephalalgia* **22**:209–221.

Diener HC, Reches A, Pascual J, Pascual J, Pitei D, Steiner TJ; Eletriptan and Cafergot Comparative Study Group (2002b). Efficacy, tolerability and safety of oral eletriptan and ergotamine plus caffeine (Cafergot) in the acute treatment of migraine: a multicentre, randomised, double-blind, placebo-controlled comparison. *Europ Neurol* **47**:99–107.

Diener H, Tfelt-Hansen P, Dahlöf C, Lainez MJ, Sandrini G, Wang SJ, Neto W, Vijapurkar U, Doyle A, Jacobs D; MIGR-003 Study Group (2004a). Topiramate in migraine prophylaxis: results from a placebo-controlled trial with propranolol as an active control. *J Neurol* **251**:943–950.

Diener HC, Bussone G, de Liano H, Eikermann A, Englert R, Floeter T, Gallai V, Gobel H, Hartung E, Jimenez MD, Lange R, Manzoni GC, Mueller-Schwefe G, Nappi G, Pinessi L, Prat J, Puca FM, Titus F, Voelker M; EMSASI Study Group (2004b). Placebo-controlled comparison of effervescent acetylsalicylic acid, sumatriptan and ibuprofen in the treatment of migraine attacks. *Cephalalgia* **24**:947–954.

Diener HC, Rahlfs VW, Danesch U (2004c). The first placebo-controlled trial of a special butterbur root extract for the prevention of migraine: reanalysis of efficacy criteria. *Eur Neurol* **51**:89–97.

Diener H, Pfaffenrath V, Pageler L (2005a). The fixed combination of acetylsalicylic acid, paracetamol and caffeine is more effective than single substances and dual combination for the treatment of headache: a multi-centre, randomized, double-blind, single-dose, placebo-controlled parallel group study. *Cephalalgia* 25 (in press).

Diener HC (Hrsg) (2005b). Therapie der Migräneattacke und Migräneprophylaxe. Leitlinie der Deutschen Gesellschaft für Neurologie und der Deutschen Migräne- und Kopfschmerzgesellschaft. (in press).

Dodick DW, Mauskop A, Elkind AH, DeGryse R, Brin MF, Silberstein SD; BOTOX CDH Study Group (2005). Botulinum toxin type A for the prophylaxis of chronic daily headache: subgroup analysis of patients not receiving other prophylactic medications: a randomized double-blind, placebo-controlled study. *Headache* **45**:315–324.

Dowson A, Massiou H, Lainez J, Cabarrocas X (2004). Almotriptan improves response rates when treatment is within 1 hour of migraine onset. *Headache* **44**:318–322.

Ellis GL, Delaney J, DeHart DA, Owens A (1993). The efficacy of metoclopramide in the treatment of migraine headache. *Ann Emerg Med* **22**:191–195.

Evers S (1999a). Drug treatment of migraine in children. A comparative review. *Paediatr Drugs* **1**:7–18.

Evers S, Gralow I, Bauer B, Suhr B, Buchheister A, Husstedt IW, Ringelstein EB (1999b). Sumatriptan and ergotamine overuse and drug-induced headache: a clinicoepidmiologic study. *Clin Neuropharmacol* **22**:201–206.

Evers S, Pothmann, R, Überall M, Naumann E, Gerber WD (2001). Therapie idiopathischer Kopfschmerzen im Kindesalter. *Nervenheilkunde* **20**:306–315.

Evers S, Vollmer-Haase J, Schwaag S, Rahmann A, Husstedt IW, Frese A (2004). Botulinum toxin A in the prophylactic treatment of migraine - a randomized, double-blind, placebo-controlled study. *Cephalalgia* **24**:838–843.

Evers S, Mylecharane E (2005). Nonsteroidal antiinflammatory and miscellaneous drugs in migraine prophylaxis. In: Olesen J, Goadsby PJ, Ramadan N, Tfelt-Hansen P, Welch KMA. *The Headaches*, 3rd edition. Lippincott, Philadelphia (in press).

Facchinetti F, Fioroni L, Sances G, Romano G, Nappi G, Genazzani AR (1989). Naproxen sodium in the treatment of premenstrual symptoms: a placebo-controlled study. *Gynecol Obstet Invest* **28**:205–208.

Ferrari MD (1999). How to assess and compare drugs in the management of migraine: success rates in terms of response and recurrence. *Cephalalgia* **19(Suppl 23)**:2–8.

Ferrari MD, James MH, Bates D, Pilgrim A, Ashford E, Anderson BA, Nappi G (1994). Oral sumatriptan: effect of a second dose, and incidence and treatment of headache recurrences. *Cephalalgia* **14**:330–338.

Ferrari MD, Roon KI, Lipton RB, Goadsby PJ (2001). Oral triptans (serotonin 5-HT$_{1B/1D}$ agonists) in acute migraine treatment: a meta-analysis of 53 trials. *Lancet* **358**:1668–1675.

Fox AW, Chambers CD, Anderson PO, Diamond ML, Spierings EL (2002). Evidence-based assessment of pregnancy outcome after sumatriptan exposure. *Headache* **42**:8–15.

Freitag FG, Diamond S, Diamond M (1991). A placebo controlled trial of flunarizine in migraine prophylaxis. *Cephalalgia* **11(Suppl 11)**:157–158.

Freitag F, Collins S, Carlson H, Goldstein J, Saper J, Silberstein S, Mathew N, Winner PK, Deaton R, Sommerville K; Depakote ER Migraine Study Group (2002). A randomized trial of divalproex sodium extended-release tablets in migraine prophylaxis. *Neurology* **58**:1652–1659.

Gawel MJ, Kreeft J, Nelson RF, Simard D, Arnott WS (1992). Comparison of the efficacy and safety of flunarizine to propranolol in the prophylaxis of migraine. *Can J Neurol Sci* **19**:340–345.

Geraud G, Compagnon A, Rossi A (2002). Zolmitriptan versus a combination of acetylsalicylic acid and metoclopramide in the acute oral treatment of migraine: a double-blind, randomised, three-attack study. *Eur Neurol* **47**:88–98.

Geraud G, Keywood C, Senard JM (2003). Migraine headache recurrence: relationship to clinical, pharmacological, and pharmacokinetic properties of triptans. *Headache* **43**:376–388.

Gerber WD, Schellenberg R, Thom M, Haufe C, Bolsche F, Wedekind W, Niederberger U, Soyka D (1995). Cyclandelate versus propranolol in the prophylaxis of migraine - a double-blind placebo-controlled study. *Funct Neurol* **10**:27–35.

Goadsby PJ (1997). Role of naratriptan in clinical practice. *Cephalalgia* **17**:472–473.

Goadsby PB, Lipton RB, Ferrai MD (2002). Migraine: current understanding and management. *N Engl J Med* **346**:257–270.

Göbel H, Heinze A, Niederberger U, Witt T, Zumbroich V (2004). Efficacy of phenazone in the treatment of acute migraine attacks: a double-blind, placebo-controlled, randomized study. *Cephalalgia* **24**:888–893.

Goldstein J, Ryan R, Jiang K, Getson A, Norman B, Block GA, Lines C (1998). Crossover comparison of rizatriptan 5 mg and 10 mg versus sumatriptan 25 and 50 mg in migraine. *Headache* **38**:737–747.

Goldstein DJ, Offen WW, Klein EG, Phebus LA, Hipskind P, Johnson KW, Ryan RE Jr (2001). Lanepitant, an NK-1 antagonist, in migraine prevention. *Cephalalgia* **21**:102–106.

Gomersall JD, Stuart A (1973). Amitriptyline in migraine prophylaxis: changes in pattern of attacks during a controlled clinical trial. *J Neurol Neurosurg Psychiatry* **36**:684–690.

Hall G, Brown M, Mo J, MacRae KD (2004). Triptans in migraine: the risks of stroke, cardiovascular disease, and death in practice. *Neurology* **62**:563–568.

Hämäläinen ML, Hoppu K, Santavuori P (1997). Sumatriptan for migraine attacks in children: A randomized placebo-controlled study. Do children with migraine attacks respond to oral sumatriptan differently from adults? *Neurology* **48**:1100–1103.

Havanka-Kanniainen H, Hokkanen E, Myllylä VV (1988). Long acting propranolol in the prophylaxis of migraine. Comparison of the daily doses of 80 mg and 160 mg. *Headache* **28**:607–611.

Havanka-Kanniainen H (1989). Treatment of acute migraine attack: ibuprofen and placebo compared. *Headache* **29**:507–509.

Headache Classification Committee of the International Headache Society (2004). The international classification of headache disorders, 2nd edition. *Cephalalgia* **24(Suppl 1)**:1–160.

Holroyd KA, Penzien DB, Cordingley GE (1991). Propranolol in the management of recurrent migraine: a meta-analytic review. *Headache* **31**:333–340.

Johannsson V, Nilsson LR, Widelius T, Javerfalk T, Hellman P, Akesson JA, Olerud B, Gustafsson CL, Raak A, Sandahl G (1987). Atenolol in migraine prophylaxis a double-blind cross-over multicentre study. *Headache* **27**:372–374.

Källen B, Lygner PE (2001). Delivery outcome in women who used drugs for migraine during pregnancy with special reference to sumatriptan. *Headache* **41**:351–356.

Kangasniemi P, Hedman C (1984). Metoprolol and propranolol in the prophylactic treatment of classical and common migraine. A double-blind study. *Cephalalgia* **4**:91–96.

Kaniecki RG (1997). A comparison of divalproex with propranolol and placebo for the prophylaxis of migraine without aura. *Arch Neurol* **54**:1141–1145.

Karachalios GN, Fotiadou A, Chrisikos N, Karabetsos A, Kehagioglou K (1992). Treatment of acute migraine attack with diclofenac sodium: A double-blind study. *Headache* **32**:98–100.

Katsarava Z, Fritsche G, Muessig M, Diener HC, Limmroth V (2001). Clinical features of withdrawal headache following overuse of triptans and other headache drugs. *Neurology* **57**:1694–1698.

Klapper J, on behalf of the Divalproex Sodium in Migraine Prophylaxis Study Group (1997). Divalproex sodium in migraine prophylaxis: a dose-controlled study. *Cephalalgia* **17**:103–108.

Kloster R, Nestvold K, Vilming ST (1992). A double-blind study of ibuprofen versus placebo in the treatment of acute migraine attacks. *Cephalalgia* **12**:169–171.

Lampl C, Buzath A, Klinger D, Neumann K (1999). Lamotrigine in the prophylactic treatment of migraine aura - a pilot study. *Cephalalgia* **19**:58–63.

Lewis DW (2004). Toward the definition of childhood migraine. *Curr Opin Pediatr* **16**:628–636.

Lewis D, Ashwal S, Hershey A, Hirtz D, Yonker M, Silberstein S; American Academy of Neurology Quality Standards Subcommittee; Practice Committee of the Child Neurology Society (2004). Practice parameter: pharmacological treatment of migraine headache in children and adolescents: report of the American Academy of Neurology Quality Standards Subcommittee and the Practice Committee of the Child Neurology Society. *Neurology* **63:**2215–2224.

Limmroth V, Kazarawa S, Fritsche G, Diener HC (1999a). Headache after frequent use of new serotonin agonists zolmitriptan and naratriptan. *Lancet* **353:**378.

Limmroth V, May A, Diener HC (1999b). Lysineacetylsalicylic acid in acute migraine attacks. *Eur Neurol* **41:**88–93.

Lipton RB, Stewart WF, Ryan RE, Saper J, Silberstein S, Sheftell F (1998). Efficacy and safety of acetaminophen, aspirin, and caffeine in alleviating migraine headache pain – Three double-blind, randomized, placebo-controlled trials. *Arch Neurol* **55:**210–217.

Lipton RB, Baggish JS, Stewart WF, Codispoti JR, Fu M (2000). Efficacy and safety of acetaminophen in the treatment of migraine: results of a randomized, double-blind, placebo-controlled, population-based study. *Arch Intern Med* **160:**3486–3492.

Lipton R, Scher A, Kolodner K, Liberman J, Steiner TJ, Stewart WF (2002). Migraine in the United States: epidemiology and patterns of health care use. *Neurology* **58:**885–894.

Lipton RB, Göbel H, Einhäupl KM, Wilks K, Mauskop A (2004). Petasites hybridus root (butterbur) is an effective preventive treatment for migraine. *Neurology* **63:**2240–2244.

Louis P (1981). A double-blind placebo-controlled prophylactic study of flunarizine in migraine. *Headache* **21:**235–239.

Ludin H-P (1989). Flunarizine and propranolol in the treatment of migraine. *Headache* **29:**218–223.

Mathew NT, Rapoport A, Saper J, Magnus L, Klapper J, Ramadan N, Stacey B, Tepper S (2001). Efficacy of gabapentin in migraine prophylaxis. *Headache* **41:**119–128.

Maytal J, Young M, Shechter A, Lipton RB (1997). Pediatric migraine and the International Headache Society (IHS) criteria. *Neurology* **48:**602–607.

Mei D, Capuano A, Vollono C, Evangelista M, Ferraro D, Tonali P, Di Trapani G (2004). Topiramate in migraine prophylaxis: a randomised double-blind versus placebo study. *Neurol Sci* **25:**245–250.

Mikkelsen BM, Falk JV (1982). Prophylactic treatment of migraine with tolfenamic acid: a comparative doubleblind crossover study between tolfenamic acid and placebo. *Acta Neurol Scand* **66:**105–111.

Mikkelsen B, Pedersen KK, Christiansen LV (1986). Prophylactic treatment of migraine with tolfenamic acid, propranolol and placebo. *Acta Neurol Scand* **73:**423–427.

Mylecharane EJ (1991). 5-HT2 receptor antagonists and migraine therapy. *J Neurol* **238(Suppl 1):**S45–52.

Myllyla VV, Havanka H, Herrala L, Kangasniemi P, Rautakorpi I, Turkka J, Vapaatalo H, Eskerod O (1998). Tolfenamic acid rapid release versus sumatriptan in the acute treatment of migraine: comparable effect in a double-blind, randomized, controlled, parallel-group study. *Headache* **38:**201–207.

Nadelmann JW, Stevens J, Saper JR (1986). Propranolol in the prophylaxis of migraine. *Headache* **26:**175–182.

Nappi G, Sandrini G, Savoini G, Cavallini A, de Rysky C, Micieli G (1987). Comparative efficacy of cyclandelate versus flunarizine in the prophylactic treatment of migraine. *Drugs* **33(Suppl 2):**103–109.

Nebe J, Heier M, Diener HC (1995). Low-dose ibuprofen in self-medication of mild to moderate headache: a comparison with acetylsalicylic acid and placebo. *Cephalalgia* **15:**531–535.

Newman L, Mannix LK, Landy S, Silberstein S, Lipton RB, Putnam DG, Watson C, Jobsis M, Batenhorst A, O'Quinn S (2001). Naratriptan as short-term prophylaxis in menstrually associated migraine: a randomised, double-blind, placebo-controlled study. *Headache* **41:**248–256.

Olesen C, Steffensen FH, Sorensen HT, Nielsen GL, Olsen J (2000). Pregnancy outcome following prescription for sumatriptan. *Headache* **40:**20–24.

Olesen J, Diener HC, Schoenen J, Hettiarachchi J (2004). No effect of eletriptan administration during the aura phase of migraine. *Europ J Neurol* **11:**671–677.

Olsson JE, Behring HC, Forssman B *et al.* (1984). Metoprolol and propranolol in migraine prophylaxis: a double-blind multicenter study. *Acta Neurol Scand* **70:**160–168.

O'Quinn S, Davis RL, Guttermann DL *et al.* (1999). Prospective large-scale study of the tolerability of subcutaneous sumatriptan injection for the acute treatment of migraine. *Cephalalgia* **19:**223–231.

Orholm M, Honoré PF, Zeeberg I (1986). A randomized general practice groupcomparative study of femoxetine and placebo in the prophylaxis of migraine. *Acta Neurol Scand* **74:**235–239.

Peikert A, Wilimzig C, Köhne-Volland R (1996). Prophylaxis of migraine with oral magnesium: results from a prospective, multi-center, placebo-controlled and double-blind randomized study. *Cephalalgia* **16**:257–263.

Peto R, Gray R, Collins R, Wheatly K, Hennekens C, Jamrozik K (1988). Randomised trial of prophylactic daily aspirin in male british doctors. *BMJ* **296**:313–316.

Pfaffenrath V, Wessely P, Meyer C, Isler HR, Evers S, Grotemeyer KH, Taneri Z, Soyka D, Gobel H, Fischer M (1996). Magnesium in the prophylaxis of migraine - a double-blind, placebo-controlled study. *Cephalalgia* **16**:436–440.

Pfaffenrath V, Diener HC, Fischer M, Friede M, Henneicke-von Zepelin HH; Investigators (2002). The efficacy and safety of Tanacetum parthenium (feverfew) in migraineprophylaxis – a double-blind, multicentre, randomized placebo-controlled dose-response study. *Cephalalgia* **22**:523–532.

Pilgrim AJ (1993). The methods used in clinical trials of sumatriptan in migraine. *Headache* **33**:280–293.

Pittler MH, Ernst E (2004). Feverfew for preventing migraine. *Cochrane Database Syst Rev* **(1):**CD002286.

Pradalier A, Vincent D, Beaulieu PH, Baudesson G, Launay J-M (1994). Correlation between estradiol plasma Level and therapeutic effect on menstrual migraine. Proc 10th Migraine Trust Symp, pp. 129–132.

Quality Standards Subcommittee of the American Academy of Neurology (1994). Practice parameter: the utility of neuroimaging in the evaluation of headache in patients with normal neurologic examinations. *Neurology* **44**:1353–1354.

Rasmussen BK (2001). Epidemiology of headache. *Cephalalgia* **21**:774–777.

Rasmussen BK, Jensen R, Schroll M, Olesen J (1991). Epidemiology of headache in a general population - a prevalence study. *J Clin Epidemiol* **44**:1147–1157.

Ross-Lee LM, Eadie MJ, Heazlewood V, Bochner F, Tyrer JH (1983). Aspirin pharmacokinetics in migraine. The effect of metoclopramide. *Eur J Clin Pharmacol* **24**:777–785.

Ryan R, Elkind A, Baker CC, Mullican W, DeBussey S, Asgharnejad M (1997). Sumatriptan nasal spray for the acute treatment of migraine. *Neurology* **49**:1225–1230.

Sances G, Martignoni E, Fioroni L, Blandini F, Facchinetti F, Nappi G (1990). Naproxen sodium in menstrual migraine prophylaxis: a double-blind placebo controlled study. *Headache* **30**:705–709.

Sandor PS, di Clemente L, Coppola G, Saenger U, Fumal A, Magis D, Seidel L, Agosti RM, Schoenen J (2005). Efficacy of coenzyme Q10 in migraine prophylaxis: a randomised controlled trial. *Neurology* **64**:713–715.

Saper JR, Silberstein SD, Lake AE, Winters ME (1994). Doubleblind trial of fluoxetine: chronic daily headache and migraine. *Headache* **34**:497–502.

Sargent J, Solbach P, Damasio H, Baumel B, Corbett J, Eisner L, Jessen B, Kudrow L, Mathew N, Medina J (1985). A comparison of naproxen sodium to propranolol hydrochloride and a placebo control for the prophylaxis of migraine headache. *Headache* **25**: 320–324.

Scher A, Stewart WF, Liberman J, Lipton RB (1998). Prevalence of frequent headache in a population sample. *Headache* **38**:497–506.

Schoenen J, Jacquy J, Lenaerts M (1998). Effectiveness of high-dose riboflavin in migraine prophylaxis - A randomized controlled trial. *Neurology* **50**:466–470.

Schrader H, Stovner LJ, Helde G, Sand T, Bovim G (2001). Prophylactic treatment of migraine with angiotensin converting enzyme inhibitor (lisinopril): randomised, placebo-controlled, crossover trial. *BMJ* **322**:19–22.

Schulman E, Dermott K (2003). Sumatriptan plus metoclopramide in triptan-nonresponsive migraineurs. *Headache* **43**:729–733.

Silberstein SD (1998). Methysergide. *Cephalalgia* **18**:421–435.

Silberstein S, Mathew N, Saper J, Jenkins S (2000a). Botulinum toxin type A as a migraine preventive treatment. *Headache* **40**:445–450.

Silberstein SD, Collins SD, Carlson H (2000b). Safety and efficacy of once-daily, extended-release divalproex sodium monotherapy for the prophylaxis of migraine headaches. *Cephalalgia* **20**:269.

Silberstein SD, Elkind AH, Schreiber C, Keywood C (2004a). A randomized trial of frovatriptan for the intermittent prevention of menstrual migraine. *Neurology* **63**:261–269.

Silberstein SD, Neto W, Schmitt J, Jacobs D (2004b). Topiramate in migraine prevention: results of a large controlled trial. *Arch Neurol* **61**:490–495.

Siniatchkin M, Gerber WD, Vein A (1998). Clinical efficacy and central mechanisms of cyclandelate in migraine: a double-blind placebo-controlled study. *Funct Neurol* **13**:47–56.

Smits MG, van den Meer YG, Pfeil JPJM, Rijnierse JJMM, Vos AJM (1994). Perimenstrual migraine: effect of Estraderm®TTS and the value of contingent negative variation and exteroceptive temporalis muscle suppression test. *Headache* **34**:103–106.

Solomon GD, Cady RK, Klapper JA, Earl NL, Saper JR, Ramadan NM (1997). Clinical efficacy and tolerability of 2.5 mg zolmitriptan for the acute treatment of migraine. *Neurology* **49**:1219–1225.

Sorensen PS, Larsen BH, Rasmussen MJK, Kinge E, Iversen H, Alslev T, Nohr P, Pedersen KK, Schroder P, Lademann A (1991). Flunarizine versus metoprolol in migraine prophylaxis: a double-blind, randomized parallel group study of efficacy and tolerability. *Headache* **31**:650–657.

Steiner TJ, Joseph R, Hedman C, Rose FC (1988). Metoprolol in the prophylaxis of migraine: parallel group comparison with placebo and dose-ranging follow-up. *Headache* **28**:15–23.

Steiner TJ, Findley LJ, Yuen AWC (1997). Lamotrigine versus placebo in the prophylaxis of migraine with and without aura. *Cephalalgia* **17**:109–112.

Steiner TJ, Ahmed F, Findley LJ, MacGregor EA, Wilkinson M (1998). S-fluoxetine in the prophylaxis of migraine: a phase II double-blind randomized placebo-controlled study. *Cephalalgia* **18**:283–286.

Stellar S, Ahrens SP, Meibohm AR, Reines SA (1984). Migraine prevention with timolol. A double-blind crossover study. *JAMA* **252**:2576–2580.

Straumsheim P, Borchgrevink C, Mowinckel P, Kierulf H, Hafslund O (2000). Homeopathic treatment of migraine: a double blind, placebo controlled trial of 68 patients. *Br Homeopath J* **89**:4–7.

Szekely B, Merryman S, Croft H, Post G (1989). Prophylactic effects of naproxen sodium on perimenstrual headache: a double-blind, placebo-controlled study. *Cephalalgia* **9(Suppl 10)**:452–453.

Tepper SJ, Cochran A, Hobbs S, Woessner M (1998). Sumatriptan suppositories for the acute treatment of migraine. *Int J Clin Pract* **52**:31–35.

Tepper SJ, Donnan GA, Dowson AJ, Bomhof MA, Elkind A, Meloche J, Fletcher PE, Millson DS (1999). A long-term study to maximise migraine relief with zolmitriptan. *Curr Med Res Opin* **15**:254–271.

Tfelt-Hansen P, Standnes B, Kangasniemi P, Hakkarainen H, Olesen J (1984). Timolol vs. propranolol vs. placebo in common migraine prophylaxis: a double-blind multicenter trial. *Acta Neurol Scand* **69**:1–8.

Tfelt-Hansen P, Henry P, Mulder LJ, Scheldewaert RG, Schoenen J, Chazot G (1995). The effectiveness of combined oral lysine acetylsalicylate and metoclopramide compared with oral sumatriptan for migraine. *Lancet* **346**:923–926.

Tfelt-Hansen P, Teall J, Rodriguez F, Giacovazzo M, Paz J, Malbecq W, Block GA, Reines SA, Visser WH (1998). Oral rizatriptan versus oral sumatriptan: a direct comparative study in the acute treatment of migraine. *Headache* **38**:748–755.

Tfelt-Hansen P, Ryan RE (2000). Oral therapy for migraine: comparisons between rizatriptan and sumatriptan. A review of four randomized, double-blind clinical trials. *Neurology* **55(Suppl 2)**:S19–S24.

Tfelt-Hansen P, Saxena PR, Dahlöf C, Pascual J, Lainez M, Henry P, Diener H, Schoenen J, Ferrari MD, Goadsby PJ (2000). Ergotamine in the acute treatment of migraine. A review and European consensus. *Brain* **123**:9–18.

The Diclofenac-K/Sumatriptan Migraine Study Group (1999). Acute treatment of migraine attacks: efficacy and safety of a nonsteroidal antiinflammatory drug, diclofenac-potassium, in comparison to oral sumatriptan and placebo. *Cephalalgia* **19**:232–240.

The Multinational Oral Sumatriptan Cafergot Comparative Study Group (1991). A randomized, double-blind comparison of sumatriptan and Cafergot in the acute treatment of migraine. *Eur Neurol* **31**:314–322.

The Oral Sumatriptan and Aspirin plus Metoclopramide Comparative Study Group (1992). A study to compare oral sumatriptan with oral aspirin plus oral metoclopramide in the acute treatment of migraine. *Eur Neurol* **32**:177–184.

The Subcutaneous Sumatriptan International Study Group (1991). Treatment of migraine attacks with sumatriptan. *N Engl J Med* **325**:316–321.

Tronvik E, Stovner LJ, Helde G, Sand T, Bovim G (2002). Prophylactic treatment of migraine with an angiotensin II receptor blocker. A randomized controlled trial. *JAMA* **289**:65–69.

Tulunay FC, Ergun H, Gulmez SE, Ozbenli T, Ozmenoglu M, Boz C, Erdemoglu AK, Varlikbas A, Goksan B, Inan L (2004). The efficacy and safety of dipyrone (Novalgin) tablets in the treatment of acute migraine attacks: a double-blind, cross-over, randomized, placebo-controlled, multi-center study. *Funct Neurol* **19**:197–202.

Überall MA, Wenzel D (1999). Intranasal sumatriptan for the acute treatment of migraine in children. *Neurology* **52**:1507–1510.

Vahedi K, Taupin P, Djomby R, El-Amrani M, Lutz G, Filipetti V, Landais P, Massiou H, Bousser MG; DIAMIG investigators (2002). Efficacy and tolerability of acetazolamide in migraine prophylaxis: a randomised placebo-controlled trial. *J Neurol* **249**:206–211.

van de Ven LLM, Franke CL, Koehler PJ (1997). Prophylactic treatment of migraine with bisoprolol: a placebo-controlled study. *Cephalalgia* **17**:596–599.

Velentgas P, Cole JA, Mo J, Sikes CR, Walker AM (2004). Severe vascular events in migraine patients. *Headache* **44**:642–651.

Waelkens J (1984). Dopamine blockade with domperidone: bridge between prophylactic and abortive treatment of migraine? A dose-finding study. *Cephalalgia* **4**:85–90.

Walach H, Haeusler W, Lowes T, Mussbach D, Schamell U, Springer W, Stritzl G, Gaus W, Haag G (1997). Classical homeopathic treatment of chronic headaches. *Cephalalgia* **17:**119–126.

Welch KMA, Ellis DJ, Keenan PA (1985). Successful migraine prophylaxis with naproxen sodium. *Neurology* **35:**1304–1310.

Welch KMA, Mathew NT, Stone P, Rosamond W, Saiers J, Gutterman D (2000). Tolerability of sumatriptan: clinical trials and post-marketing experience. *Cephalalgia* **20:**687–695.

Whitmarsh TE, Coleston-Shields DM, Steiner TJ (1997). Double-blind randomized placebo-controlled study of homoeopathic prophylaxis of migraine. *Cephalalgia* **17:**600–604.

Winner P, Rothner AD, Saper J, Nett R, Asgharnejad M, Laurenza A, Austin R, Peykamian M (2000). A randomized, double-blind, placebo-controlled study of sumatriptan nasal spray in the treatment of acute migraine in adolescents. *Pediatrics* **106:**989–997.

Winner P, Lewis D, Visser H, Jiang K, Ahrens S, Evans JK; Rizatriptan Adolescent Study Group (2002). Rizatriptan 5 mg for the acute treatment of migraine in adolescents: a randomized, double-blind, placebo-controlled study. *Headache* **42:**49–55.

Wörz R, Reinhardt-Benmalek B, Grotemeyer KH (1991). Bisoprolol and metoprolol in the prophylactic treatment of migraine with and without aura - a randomized double-blind cross-over multicenter study. *Cephalalgia* **11(Suppl 11):**152–153.

Zeeberg I, Orholm M, Nielsen JD, Honore PLF, Larsen JJV (1981). Femoxetine in the prophylaxis of migraine - a randomised comparison with placebo. *Acta Neurol Scand* **64:**452–459.

Ziegler DK, Ellis DJ (1985). Naproxen in prophylaxis of migraine. *Arch Neurol* **42:**582–584.

Ziegler DK, Hurwitz A, Hassanein RS Kodanaz HA, Preskorn SH, Mason J (1987). Migraine prophylaxis. A comparison of propranolol and amitriptyline. *Arch Neurol* **44:**486–489.

Ziegler DK, Hurwitz A, Preskorn S, Hassanein R, Seim J (1993). Propranolol and amitriptyline in prophylaxis of migraine: pharmacokinetic and therapeutic effects. *Arch Neurol* **50:**825–830.

CHAPTER 14

Cluster headache

S. Evers,[a] J. Áfra,[b] A. Frese,[a] P.J. Goadsby,[c]
M. Linde,[d] A. May,[e] P.S. Sándor[f]

Abstract

Background: Cluster headache and other trigemino-autonomic headache disorders (paroxysmal hemicrania, SUNCT syndrome) are rare but very disabling conditions with a major impact on the patients' quality of life.

Objectives: To give evidence-based or expert treatment recommendations for these headache disorders based on a literature search and a consensus in an expert panel.

Methods: All available medical reference systems were screened for all kinds of studies on cluster headache, paroxysmal hemicrania and SUNCT syndrome. The findings in these studies were evaluated according to the recommendations of the EFNS resulting in Level A, B, or C recommendations and Good Practice Points.

Recommendations: For the acute treatment of cluster headache attacks, oxygen (100%) with a flow of at least 7 l/min over 15 min and 6 mg subcutaneous sumatriptan are drugs of first choice. As second choice, 20 mg sumatriptan nasal spray is recommended. Prophylaxis of cluster headache should be performed with verapamil in a daily dose of at least 240 mg (maximum dose depends on efficacy or tolerability). Although no class I or II trials are available, steroids are clearly effective in cluster headache. Therefore, the use of at least 100 mg oral up to 500 mg i.v. per day methylprednisone (or equivalent corticosteroid) over 5 days (then tapering down) is recommended. Methysergide, lithium and topiramate are recommended as alternative drugs of second choice. Surgical procedures, although in part promising, require further scientific evaluation before they can be recommended. For paroxysmal hemicranias, only indomethacin in a daily dose of up to 200 mg is the drug of first (and only) choice. For treatment of SUNCT syndrome, no drug has shown consistent efficacy. Based on case reports, oral lamotrigine, gabapentin, and topiramate and intravenous phenytoin and lidocaine are recommended.

Objectives

These guidelines aim to give evidence-based recommendations for the treatment of cluster

[a]Department of Neurology, University of Münster, Germany; [b]National Institute of Neurosurgery, Budapest, Hungary; [c]Headache Group, Institute of Neurology, The National Hospital for Neurology and Neurosurgery, Queen Square, London, United Kingdom; [d]Cephalea Pain Center, Läkarhuset Södra vägen, Gothenburg, Sweden; [e]Department of Neurology, University of Hamburg, Germany; [f]Department of Neurology, University of Zurich, Switzerland.

headache attacks, for the prophylaxis of cluster headache, for the treatment of paroxysmal hemicranias and for the treatment of SUNCT syndrome. A brief clinical description of the headache disorders is included. The definition of the headache disorders follows the diagnostic criteria of the International Headache Society (IHS).

Background

The second edition of the classification of the International Headache Society (IHS) provided a new primary headache grouping named the trigemino-autonomic cephalgias (TAC) (Headache Classification Committee, 2004). All these headache syndromes have two features in common: relatively short-lasting, unilateral, severe headache attacks and typical accompanying cranial autonomic symptoms (although the latter are not obligatory). These autonomic symptoms occur on the side of headache and comprise lacrimation, conjunctival injection, rhinorrhea, miosis and ptosis. The following syndromes belong to the TAC:

- episodic and chronic cluster headache
- episodic and chronic paroxysmal hemicrania
- SUNCT-syndrome (short-lasting unilateral neuralgiform headache attacks with conjunctival injection and tearing).

These syndromes differ in duration, frequency and rhythmicity of the attacks, and in the intensity of pain and autonomic symptoms. The pathophysiology of TAC has been in the focus of intensive research for several years (Sjaastad, 1992; Goadsby, 1999; May, 2003).

The purpose of this paper is to give evidence-based treatment recommendations for the different TAC. The recommendations are based on the scientific evidence from clinical trials and on the expert consensus by this European Federation of Neurological Societies (EFNS) task force. The legal aspects of drug prescription and drug availability in the different European countries will not be considered. The definitions of the recommendation levels follow the EFNS criteria (Brainin *et al.*, 2004).

Search strategy

A literature search was performed using the reference databases MedLine, Science Citation Index and the Cochrane Library; the key words used were 'cluster headache', 'paroxysmal hemicrania', 'SUNCT', 'treatment' and 'trial' (last search in January 2005). All papers published in English, German or French were considered when they described a controlled trial or a case series on the treatment of at least five patients (or less in paroxysmal hemicrania or SUNCT syndrome). In addition, a review book (Olesen *et al.*, 2000) and the German treatment recommendations for cluster headache (May *et al.*, 2004) were considered.

Method for reaching consensus

All authors performed an independent literature search. The first draft of the manuscript was written by the chairman of the task force. All other members of the task force read the first draft and discussed changes by email. A second draft was then written by the chairman that was again discussed by email. All recommendations had to be agreed to by all members of the task force unanimously. The background of the research strategy and of reaching consensus and the definitions of the recommendation levels used in this paper have been described in the EFNS recommendations (Brainin *et al.*, 2004).

Clinical syndromes

The diagnosis of a headache belonging to the TAC is based on the patient's history and on neurological examination. Electrophysiological and laboratory examinations including examination of the CSF are not helpful. For the first diagnosis and in the case of an abnormal neurological examination, a cranial magnetic resonance imaging (MRI) or a computerised tomography (CT) scan should be performed to exclude abnormalities of the brain. Particularly in older patients, mass lesions or malformations in the midline have been described to be associated with symptomatic cluster headache.

Table 14.1 Diagnostic criteria of cluster headache.

A. At least five attacks fulfilling criteria B–D
B. Severe or very severe unilateral orbital, supraorbital and/or temporal pain lasting 15–180 min if untreated
C. Headache is accompanied by at least one of the following:

  1. ipsilateral conjunctival injection and/or lacrimation
  2. ipsilateral nasal congestion and/or rhinorrhea
  3. ipsilateral eyelid oedema
  4. ipsilateral forehead and facial sweating
  5. ipsilateral miosis and/or ptosis
  6. sense of restlessness or agitation

D. Attacks have a frequency from one every other day to 8 per day
E. Not attributed to another disorder.

Episodic and chronic cluster headache (IHS 3.1)

The diagnostic criteria of cluster headache are presented in table 14.1. Cluster headache is defined as a paroxysmal, strongly unilateral, very severe headache, typically with a retro-orbital maximum of pain. The occurrence of cranial autonomic symptoms such as Horner's syndrome, lacrimation and rhinorrhea ipsilateral, and simultaneous to the pain is obligatory (but can be replaced by restlessness/agitation). The attacks occur up to eight times a day, sometimes with a nocturnal preponderance, and last between 15 and 180 min, rarely several hours. The episodic form of cluster headache occurs in 80% of patients with bouts lasting between 7 and 365 days separated by pain-free remission periods longer than 1 month. Sometimes, asymptomatic periods lasting even years can be observed. If the cluster attacks occur for longer than 1 year without remission periods or with remission periods lasting less than 1 month, the diagnosis is chronic cluster headache. This is the case in 15–20% of patients. The two forms do not necessarily evolve from one another. Often, the attacks start at the same time of day or night, frequently about 1–2 h after falling asleep (mostly during the first REM period in the sleep) or in the early morning. Cluster headache is regarded as a biorhythmic disorder because the attacks often occur with a strong periodicity and because the cluster bouts regularly occur during spring and autumn. Furthermore, changes of the diurnal release of hormones involved in biorhythmicity have been detected. The lifetime prevalence of cluster headache is between 0.06% (Tonon *et al.*, 2002) and 0.4% (Sjaastad and Bakketeig, 2003) with a male to female ratio between 2.5:1 and 7.1:1 (Bahra *et al.*, 2002). In recent years, the number of female patients who report cluster headache has increased (Ekbom *et al.*, 2002; Manzoni, 1998). It is not clear if this is a genuine change or simply increased recognition. A genetic background for cluster headache has not been described but is likely (Russell, 2004). Cluster headache can be seen in children and is just as devastating in that age group. There is a familial occurrence in 2–7%. On average, the headache starts at the age of 28–30 years (but can start at any age). After 15 years, 80% of the cluster headache patients still have attacks (Bahra *et al.*, 2002).

Episodic and chronic paroxysmal hemicrania (IHS 3.2)

Paroxysmal hemicrania was first described in 1974 in its chronic form (Sjaastad and Dale, 1974; for a recent review see Dodick, 2004). The paroxysmal headache attacks, the character and localization of pain and the autonomic symptoms are very similar to those observed in cluster headache. In contrast to cluster headache, the attacks are shorter (2–30 min) and more frequent (more than five attacks per day). The autonomic symptoms are often less severe than in cluster headache. The diagnostic criteria of paroxysmal hemicrania are given in table 14.2. Some patients report that their attacks can be triggered by irritation of the neck, in particular in the cervical segments C2 and C3. As for cluster headache, there is an episodic and a chronic form of paroxysmal hemicrania. The criteria for this differentiation are the same as in cluster headache (see above). The most important criterion for the diagnosis of paroxysmal hemicrania is the complete response to indomethacin. Within 1 week (often within 3 days) after the initiation of indomethacin at an adequate dose, the attacks disappear, and this effect is maintained long term. The prevalence is very low, but the exact figures

Table 14.2 Diagnostic criteria of paroxysmal hemicrania.

A. At least 20 attacks fulfilling criteria B–D
B. Attacks of severe unilateral orbital, supraorbital or temporal pain lasting 2–30 min
C. Headache is accompanied by at least one of the following:

    1. ipisilateral conjunctival injection and/or lacrimation
    2. ipsilateral nasal congestion and/or rhinorrhea
    3. ipsilateral eyelid oedema
    4. ipsilateral forehead and facial sweating
    5. ipsilateral miosis and/or ptosis

D. Attacks have a frequency above 5 per day for more than half the time, although periods with lower frequency may occur
E. Attacks are prevented completely by therapeutic doses of indomethacin
F. Not attributed to another disorder.

Table 14.3 Diagnostic criteria of SUNCT syndrome.

A. At least five attacks fulfilling criteria B–D
B. Attacks of unilateral orbital, supraorbital or temporal stabbing or pulsating pain lasting 5–240 s
C. Pain is accompanied by ipsilateral conjunctival injection and lacrimation
D. Attacks occur with a frequency from 3 to 200 per day
E. Not attributed to another disorder.

are not known. It is estimated that paroxysmal hemicranias comprise about 3–6% of all TAC. The headache usually starts between the age of 20 and 40 years, although children as young as 3 years old with clear indomethacin responses have been described. In contrast to cluster headache, the male to female ratio is 1:3.

SUNCT syndrome (IHS 3.3)

The name of this syndrome (short-lasting unilateral neuralgiform headache attacks with conjunctival injection and tearing) describes its typical clinical features. It was first described in 1989 (Sjaastad et al., 1989; for review see Matharu et al., 2003b). The diagnostic criteria are given in table 14.3. SUNCT syndrome is characterized by very short (5–240 s) attacks with neuralgiform pain quality and severe intensity. The attacks occur at a frequency of on average 60 per day (3–200 per day), are strictly unilateral (periorbital), and are often triggered by touching, speaking or chewing. When triggerable there is no refractory period of triggering attacks. The autonomic symptoms are mostly restricted to lacrimation and conjunctival injection. Distinct episodic and chronic forms of SUNCT syndrome are yet to be recognized in formal classifications, but both types occur. The most

important differential diagnosis is classical trigeminal neuralgia. In trigeminal neuralgia, unlike as in SUNCT syndrome, autonomic symptoms are not prominent and triggered attacks have a clear refractory period. The SUNCT syndrome is uncommon and its true frequency is completely unclear. The male to female ratio is 1:4. The diagnosis of SUNCT syndrome follows the same algorithm as described for cluster headache.

Treatment of cluster headache

The treatment of cluster headache is based on empirical data rather than on a pathophysiological concept of this disorder (May and Leone, 2003; May, 2003). Drug treatment can be divided into acute attack abortion and prophylaxis (Matharu et al., 2003a; May et al., 2004). Non-drug treatment is ineffective in nearly all patients. It has, however, to be considered that drug treatment in cluster headache shows a placebo rate similar to that observed in migraine treatment (Nilsson Remahl et al., 2003) (table 14.4).

Attack treatment

Inhalation of pure (100%) oxygen with a flow of at least 7 l/min (sometimes more than 10 l/min) is effective in abortion of cluster headache attacks (Horton, 1956; Kudrow, 1981; Fogan, 1985). The inhalation should be for 20 min in a sitting, upright position with a face mask. There are no contraindications known for the use of oxygen. It is safe and without side effects. About 60% of all cluster headache patients respond to this treatment with a significant pain reduction within 30 min (Ekbom, 1995; Gallagher et al., 1996).

Table 14.4 Treatment recommendations for cluster headache, paroxysmal hemicrania and SUNCT syndrome. For exact doses see text.

	Cluster headache	Paroxysmal hemicrania	SUNCT syndrome
Attack treatment	Oxygen inhalation (A) Sumatriptan 6 mg s.c. (A) Sumatriptan 20 mg nasal (A) Zolmitriptan 10 mg oral (B) Lidocaine nasal (B) Zolmitriptan 5 mg oral (B) Octreotide (B)	None	None
Prophylactic treatment	Verapamil (A) Steroids (A) Lithium (B) Methysergide (B) Topiramate (B) Valproic acid (C) Ergotamine tartrate (B) Melatonin (C) Baclofen (C)	Indomethacin (A) Verapamil (C) NSAIDs (C)	Lamotrigine (C)

A denotes effective; B denotes probably effective; C denotes possibly effective.

In double-blind, placebo-controlled trials, the 5-HT1$_{B/D}$ agonist sumatriptan injected subcutaneously is effective in about 75% of all cluster headache patients (i.e. pain free within 20 min) (The Sumatriptan Study Group, 1991; Ekbom *et al.*, 1993). It is safe and without side effects in most of the patients even after frequent use (Ekbom *et al.*, 1995; Göbel *et al.*, 1998). Contraindications are cardio- and cerebrovascular disorders and untreated arterial hypertension. The most unpleasant side effects are chest pain and distal paresthesia. In open prospective observational studies (Krabbe, 1989; Gregor *et al.*, 2004), even 3 mg of subcutaneous sumatriptan is effective in the majority of patients. In recent open and double-blind, placebo-controlled trials, sumatriptan nasal spray 20 mg (Schuh-Hofer *et al.*, 2002; van Vliet *et al.*, 2003) and oral zolmitriptan 10 mg (Bahra *et al.*, 2000) were also effective within 30 min. In the latter study, only patients with episodic cluster headache responded and even 5 mg oral zolmitriptan was effective in a part of efficacy parameters.

Oral ergotamine has been used in the treatment of cluster headache attacks since more than 50 years (Horton *et al.*, 1948; Kunkle *et al.*, 1952; Friedman and Mikropoulos, 1958) and is effective when given very early in the attack. It was then recommended for the acute cluster headache attack treatment as an aerosol spray (Speed, 1960; fGraham *et al.*, 1960; Duvoisin *et al.*, 1961; Ekbom *et al.*, 1983). However, more recent trials are missing. The intranasal application of dihydroergotamine in cluster headache attacks was not superior to placebo in a single trial (Andersson and Jespersen, 1986). Very recently, the intravenous application of 1 mg of dihydroergotamine over 3 days has been shown to be effective in the abortion of severe cluster attacks in an open retrospective trial (Magnoux and Zlotnik, 2004).

For short-term prophylaxis, ergotamine has also been studied. Ergotamine suppositories need a long time until the onset of efficacy. They have been proposed in a dose of 2 mg for short term prophylaxis, given in the evening to prevent cluster headache attacks in the night (Horton, 1952). Also, regular intramuscular or subcutaneous injections of ergotamine tartrate 0.25–0.5 mg have been found to be successful in the prevention of nightly attacks (Schiller, 1960; Symonds, 1956).

The nasal installation of lidocaine (1 ml with a concentration of 4–10%; the head should be reclined by 45° and rotated to the affected side by 30°–40°) is effective in at least one third of the patients (Kitrelle *et al.*, 1985; Markley, 2003; Mills and Scoggin, 1997; Robbins, 1995; Costa *et al.*, 2000). The use of lidocaine evolved from early observations that cocaine is effective in aborting cluster headache attacks. This has been supported in a recent open, but not controlled trial with 10% intranasal cocaine (Costa *et al.*, 2000).

Very recently, 100 µg of subcutaneous octreotide has been shown to be effective in the treatment of acute cluster headache attacks in a double-blind, placebo-controlled trial (Matharu *et al.*, 2004a) confirming previous observations on the efficacy of parenteral somatostatin in cluster headache.

Prophylactic drug treatment

Verapamil in a daily dose of 240–960 mg has been established as the drug of first choice in the prophylaxis of episodic and chronic cluster headache (Matharu *et al.*, 2003; May *et al.*, 2004), although only few sufficient double-blind, placebo-controlled trials are available. Controlled trials compared verapamil and lithium with placebo showing an efficacy of both the substances with a more rapid action of verapamil (Bussone *et al.*, 1990) or compared verapamil (360 mg) with placebo showing the superiority of verapamil (Leone *et al.*, 2000). In some cases, a daily dose of more than 720 mg can be necessary (Gabai and Spierings, 1989). Regular ECG controls are required to control for increase in cardiac conduction time. Sometimes, echocardiography can be necessary due to the negative inotropic effects of verapamil. Side effects of verapamil are bradycardia, oedema, constipation, gastrointestinal discomfort, gingival hyperplasia and dull headache. There is no evidence for the optimal way of dosing verapamil. An increase of 80 mg every 3 days is recommended. The full efficacy of verapamil can be expected within 2–3 weeks. As verapamil is usually well tolerated, it is also the drug of first choice for continuous treatment in chronic cluster headache. In the first 2 weeks of verapamil administration, corticosteroids are also administered by some clinicians.

In two small open studies nimodipine was also effective (Meyer *et al.*, 1985; de Carolis *et al.*, 1987).

There are no sufficient randomised, placebo-controlled trials for the use of corticosteroids in cluster headache. Several open studies and case series have been published and reviewed by Ekbom (2000). All reported efficacy of corticosteroids given in different regimes (30 mg prednisone and higher; 2 × 4 mg dexamethasone per day). By expert consensus, steroids are recommended for short-term over 2–3 weeks when rapid control of attacks is desired. However, some patients are attack-free only under steroids and rarely is continuous administration of steroids necessary. There is no evidence upon which to use corticosteroids, although their high morbidity suggests caution, short-courses, and avoidance in chronic cluster headache. For the beginning of corticosteroid treatment, prednisone 60–100 mg given once a day for at least 5 days is recommended, to be decreased by 10 mg every daily. At high dose, about 70–80% of all cluster headache patients respond to steroids. Intravenous and oral application of steroids can successfully be combined (Mir *et al.*, 2003). In the experience of the Task Force, 500 mg of methylprednisone given intravenously for up to 5 days can be even more effective.

Lithium (given as lithium carbonate) has been studied in cluster headache prophylaxis in a daily dose between 600 and 1,500 mg in more than twenty open trials reviewed by Ekbom (1981). An improvement in chronic cluster headache was reported to be as high as 78% (63% in episodic cluster headache). A recent placebo-controlled trial, however, did not show any efficacy of lithium in episodic cluster headache (Steiner *et al.*, 1997). In a comparative, double-blind crossover study, lithium and verapamil showed similar efficacy with a more rapid improvement and better tolerability for verapamil (Bussone *et al.*, 1990). Lithium should be monitored by the plasma level which should be between 0.3 and 1.2 mmol/l (Manzoni *et al.*, 1983). Regular control of liver, renal and thyroid function and of electrolytes is required. Major side effects are hypothyroidosis, tremor and renal dysfunction. Lithium is commonly used in cluster headache. This is, however, based on very small and open studies with the evidence being somewhat more convincing in chronic cluster headache. Therefore, lithium is recommended in particular for chronic cluster headache and only when other drugs are ineffective or contraindicated.

The anti-iserotonergic drug pizotifen (3 mg per day) has been shown to be effective in cluster headache prophylaxis in a single-blind, placebo-controlled older trial (Ekbom, 1969). However, its use is limited by side effects such as tiredness and weight gain.

Methysergide has been recommended as a prophylactic drug in episodic cluster headache (Ekbom, 2000; May *et al.*, 2004). However, no placebo-controlled, double-blind studies are available. The efficacy rates reported in open studies were reviewed by Ekbom and Solomon (2000). The number of patients with a benefit of methysergide ranged between 20 and 73%; it was more effective in episodic cluster headache. The doses applied in the open studies varied from 4 mg to 16 mg. In the experience of the Task Force, methysergide can be given in a daily dose of up to 12 mg (starting with 1 mg per day). As there is a small but important incidence of pulmonary and retroperitoneal fibrosis, the continuous use of methysergide is limited to a maximum of 6 months.

Valproic acid has been studied in two open trials with acceptable results (Gallagher *et al.*, 2002; Hering and Kuritzky, 1989) and in one controlled study in which it did not differentiate from placebo (El Amrani *et al.*, 2002). The objective evidence, and our experience, is that valproic acid is generally ineffective in cluster headache but can be tried as the drug of third choice in a daily dose between 5 and 20 mg per kg body weight.

Open studies suggest that topiramate is effective in the prophylaxis of cluster headache (Förderreuther *et al.*, 2002; Rozen, 2001; McGeeney, 2003). The recommended dose is at least 100 mg per day, the starting dose should be 25 mg. The main side effects are cognitive disturbances, paresthesias and weight loss. It is contraindicated in nephrolithiasis.

The pre-emptive use of 5-HT$1_{B/D}$ agonists (triptans) in cluster headache remains controversial. Hundred milligram of oral sumatriptan given tid

was not effective in preventing cluster headache attacks in a placebo-controlled trial (Monstad *et al.*, 1995). In open trials, 40 mg eletriptan per day (Zebenholzer *et al.*, 2004) or 2.5–5 mg naratriptan per day (Mulder and Spierings, 2002) reduced the number of cluster headache attacks.

For the ipsilateral intranasal application of capsaicin, two open (Sicuteri *et al.*, 1989; Fusco *et al.*, 1994) and one double-blind, placebo-controlled (Marks *et al.*, 1993) trials have been published showing an efficacy in about two-third of the patients after repeated application. Intranasal application of civamide showed a modest efficacy in a recent double-blind, placebo-controlled study (Saper *et al.*, 2002). Although such studies are claimed to be blinded, this is a major design issue given the irritating nature of the nasally applied treatment.

Oral melatonin, 10 mg, was effective in a single double-blind, placebo-controlled study (Leone *et al.*, 1996). In cluster headache refractory to other medication, however, melatonin used open-label did not produce any additional efficacy (Pringsheim *et al.*, 2002).

There is very weak evidence from a small open study for the efficacy of baclofen, 15–30 mg, (Hering-Hanit and Gadoth, 2000), and no sufficient evidence for the efficacy of botulinum toxin (Evers, 2004) and of transdermal clonidine (Leone *et al.*, 1997) in the prophylactic treatment of cluster headache. In our experience these approaches offer nothing useful to patients with cluster headache.

Hyperbaric oxygen inhalation was suggested to be effective as a prophylaxis in an open trial (di Sabato *et al.*, 1993). However, a more recent placebo-controlled, double-blind trial could not confirm that hyperbaric oxygen is effective in preventing cluster headache attacks (Nilsson Remahl *et al.*, 2002).

There is no evidence for the superiority of combined prophylactic drug treatment in cluster headache, although this question has not been systematically studied.

Interventional and surgical treatment

It has been observed that greater occipital nerve blockade resulted in a significant reduction of cluster headache attacks in about two-third of the patients (Anthony, 1985; Peres *et al.*, 2002). This finding confirmed previous observations but needs to be replicated in controlled trials. Also, suboccipital injection of long-acting steroids was shown to be effective in the prophylaxis of cluster headache in a double-blind, placebo-controlled trial (Ambrosini *et al.*, 2003).

If all drugs are ineffective, contraindicated, or not tolerated and a secondary cluster headache has been excluded, surgical treatment can be discussed. Surgical procedures should be approached with great caution because no reliable long-term observational data is available and because some procedures can induce trigeminal neuralgia or anaesthesia dolorosa (Ekbom, 2000). Unlike in trigeminal neuralgia, surgical treatment of cluster headache is not a causal therapy and continuation of cluster headache after the procedure is observed regularly. Different methods have been suggested to prevent cluster headache: application of glycerrhol or local anaesthetics into the cisterna trigeminalis of the Gasserian ganglion (Ekbom *et al.*, 1987); radio frequency rhizotomy or gamma knife treatment of the Gasserian ganglion (Taha and Tew, 1995) or of the trigeminal nerve (Ford *et al.*, 1998); microvascular decompression (Lovely *et al.*, 1998); resection or blockade of the N. petrosus superficialis (Onofrio and Campbell, 1986) or of the ganglion sphenopalatinum (Sanders and Zuurmond, 1997). However, there are also case reports on different surgical procedures (Matharu and Goadsby, 2002; Black and Dodick, 2002; Jarrar *et al.*, 2003) and one prospective study on gamma knife treatment (Donnet *et al.*, 2005) showing inefficacy of surgical treatment in TACs.

Given that trigeminal destructive procedures have a certain morbidity and that the nerve root section has a well-described morbidity, the Task Force sees these procedures as supplanted by neuromodulatory procedures. Very recently, deep brain stimulation of the posterior inferior hypothalamus has been shown to be effective in the majority of a sample of patients with intractable cluster headache (Franzini *et al.*, 2003; Leone *et al.*, 2001; Schoenen *et al.*, 2005). Recommendations for the selection of patients for these procedure

have been published recently (Leone *et al.*, 2004).

RECOMMENDATIONS

Level A. As first choice, acute attacks of cluster headache should be treated with the inhalation of 100% oxygen with at least 7 l/min over 15 min (class II trials) or with the subcutaneous injection of 6 mg sumatriptan (class I trials). As second choice, sumatriptan 20 mg nasal spray can be used (class I trial with minor efficacy or more side effects).

Prophylaxis of cluster headache should be first tried with verapamil in a daily dose of at least 240 mg (maximum dose depends on efficacy or tolerability, ECG controls are obligatory with increasing doses). Although no class I or II trials are available, steroids are clearly effective in cluster headache. Therefore, the use of at least 100 mg oral up to 500 mg i.v. per day methylprednisone (or equivalent corticosteroid) over 5 days (then tapering down) is recommended.

Level B. Intranasal lidocaine (4%) and subcutaneous octreotide (100 μg) can be tried in acute cluster headache attacks if Level A medication is ineffective or contraindicated. Oral zolmitriptan 5–10 mg is effective in some patients (class I trial but high dose produces many side effects and limits practical use).

Methysergide and lithium are drugs of second choice if verapamil is ineffective or contraindicated. Corticosteroids can be used for short courses where bouts are short or to help establish another medicine. Topiramate is promising but only open trials exist at this point. Melatonin is useful in some patients. Except for lithium, the maximum dose depends on efficacy and tolerability. Ergotamine tratrate is recommended in short-term prophylaxis (class III studies). In spite of positive class II studies, pizotifen and intranasal capsaicin should not be used because of side effects.

Level C. Baclofen 15–30 mg and valproic acid showed possible efficacy and can be tried as drugs of third choice. Surgical procedures are not indicated in most of the patients with cluster headache. Patients with intractable chronic cluster headache should be referred to centres with expertise in both destructive and neuromodulatory procedures to be offered all reasonable alternatives before a definitive procedure is conducted. This recommendation is regarded as a Good Practice Point.

Treatment of paroxysmal hemicrania

By definition, indomethacin in a daily dose of up to 200 mg is completely effective (Antonaci and Sjaastad, 1989; Sjaastad et al. 1995; Evers and Husstedt, 1996). For the same reason, no placebo-controlled trials exist. Indomethacin should be administered in three or more doses per day because of its short half-life time of 4 h. Many patients need a high dose of indomethacin only in the first weeks of treatment, then a lower dose can be tried. Very rarely, doses higher than 200 mg per day are required. The major contraindication is a gastrointestinal disorder. Gastrointestinal discomfort and bleeding are the major side effects. Therefore, a protone pump inhibitor should be given in addition. For diagnostic and rapid therapeutic purposes, the so-called indo-test has been suggested (Antonaci et al., 1998). Intramuscular indomethacin 50 mg should result in freedom of attacks within 30 min.

There is no drug of similar efficacy as indomethacin for the treatment of paroxysmal hemicrania. However, open studies (class IV) suggest a moderate efficacy of alternative drugs if indomethacin is not tolerated. The best evidence in these open studies has been observed for verapamil (Shabbir and McAbee, 1994; Evers and Husstedt, 1996). Fewer positive reports have been published for acetazolamide (Warner et al., 1994) and the NSAIDs piroxicam (Sjaastad and Antonaci, 1995) and acetylsalicylic acid (Sjaastad and Dale, 1974; Evers and Husstedt, 1996). Subcutaneous sumatriptan is ineffective (Dahlöf, 1993). Anaesthetic blockades of pericranial nerves (Antonaci

et al. 1997) are said to be ineffective although one of us has seen excellent response to greater occipital nerve blockade.

In summary, proxysmal hemicrania is to be treated with indomethacin up to 200 mg (Recommendation Level A). Alternatively, verapamil and other NSAIDs can be tried (Recommendation Level C).

Treatment of SUNCT syndrome

There is no consistently effective treatment known for SUNCT syndrome including high doses of indomethacin and anaesthetic blockades (Pareja et al., 1995). No controlled trials have been published, and the rareness of the syndrome makes this a difficult task. However, some case reports have been published with individual efficacy of some drugs. Because of the extreme burden caused by this disorder, all reasonable treatment options should be tried.

Among all drugs tried in SUNCT syndrome (Gutierrez-Garcia, 2002), lamotrigine was most efficacious in the published case reports (with however the majority of patients not responding to this drug) (D'Andrea et al., 2001; Malik et al., 2002; Chakravarty and Mukherjee, 2003). Other treatment options include gabapentin (Hunt et al., 2002; Porta-Etessam et al., 2002), topiramate (Rossi et al., 2003), intravenous lidocaine (Matharu et al., 2004b), and intravenous phenytoin (Schwaag et al., 2003). In part, these drugs were applied in combination.

In summary, no recommendation can be given for the treatment of SUNCT syndrome. Treatment with lamotrigine (at least 100 mg) is considered a Good Practice Point.

Conflicts of interest
The present guidelines were developed without external financial support. The authors report the following financial supports:

Stefan Evers: Salary by the government of the State Northrhine-Westphalia; honoraries and research grants by Almirall, AstraZeneca, Berlin Chemie, Boehringer, GlaxoSmithKline, Ipsen Pharma, Janssen Cilag, MSD, Pfizer, Novartis, Pharm Allergan, Pierre Fabre

Judit Áfra: Salary by the Hungarian Ministry of Health; honoraries by GlaxoSmithKline

Achim Frese: Salary by the government of the State Northrhine-Westphalia; no honoraries

Peter J. Goadsby: Salary by the University College of London; honoraries by Almirall, AstraZeneca, GlaxoSmithKline, MSD, Pfizer, Medtronic

Mattias Linde: Salary by the Swedish government; honoraries by AstraZeneca, GlaxoSmith-Kline, MSD, Nycomed, Pfizer

Arne May: Salary by the University Hospital of Hamburg; honoraries by Almirall, AstraZeneca, Bayer Vital, Berlin Chemie, GlaxoSmithKline, Janssen Cilag, MSD, Pfizer

Peter S. Sándor: Salary by the University Hospital of Zurich; honoraries by AstraZeneca, Glaxo-SmithKline, Janssen Cilag, Pfizer, Pharm Allergan

References

Ambrosini A, Vandenheede M, Rossi P, Aloj F, Sauli E, Buzzi MG, Pierelli F, Schoenen J (2003). Suboccipital (GON) injection with long-acting steroids in cluster headache: a double-blind placebo-controlled study. *Cephalalgia* **23:**734.

Andersson PG, Jespersen LT (1986). Dihydroergotamine nasal spray in the treatment of attacks of cluster headache. *Cephalalgia* **6:**51–54.

Anthony M (1985). Arrest of attacks of cluster headache by local steroid injection of the occipital nerve. In: Rose C (Ed). *Migraine.* Basel, Karger, pp. 169–173.

Antonaci F, Sjaastad O (1989). Chronic paroxysmal hemicrania(CPH): a review of its clinical manifestations. *Headache* **29:**648–656.

Antonaci F, Pareja JA, Caminero AB, Sjaastad O (1997). Chronic paroxysmal hemicrania and hemicrania continua: anaesthetic blockades of pericranial nerves. *Funct Neurol* **12:**11–15.

Antonaci F, Pareja JA, Caminero AB, Sjaastad O (1998). Chronic paroxysmal hemicrania and hemicrania continua. Parenteral indomethacin: the 'indotest'. *Headache* **38:**122–128.

Bahra A, Gawel MJ, Hardebo JE, Millson D, Breen SA, Goadsby PJ (2000). Oral zolmitriptan is effective in the acute treatment of cluster headache. *Neurology* **54:**1832–1839.

Bahra A, May A, Goadsby PJ (2002). Cluster headache: A prospective clinical study with diagnostic implications. *Neurology* **58:**354–361.

Black DF, Dodick DW (2002). Two cases of medically and surgically intractable SUNCT: a reason for caution and an argument for a central mechanism. *Cephalalgia* **22:**201–204.

Brainin M, Barnes M, Baron JC, Gilhus NE, Hughes R, Selmaj K, Waldemar G (2004). Guidance for the preparation of neurological management guidelines by EFNS scientific task forces – revised recommendations 2004. *Eur J Neurol* **11:**577–581.

Bussone G, Leone M, Peccarisi C, Micieli G, Granella F, Magri M, Manzoni GC, Nappi G (1990). Double blind comparison of lithium and verapamil in cluster headache prophylaxis. *Headache* **30:**411–417.

Chakravarty A, Mukherjee A (2003). SUNCT syndrome responsive to lamotrigine: documentation of the first Indian case. *Cephalalgia* **23:**474–475.

Costa A, Pucci E, Antonaci F, Sances G, Granella F, Broich G, Nappi G (2000). The effect of intranasal cocaine and lidocaine on nitroglycerin-induced attacks in cluster headache. *Cephalalgia* **20:**85–91.

Dahlöf C (1993). Subcutaneous sumatriptan does not abort attacks of chronic paroxysmal hemicrania (CPH). *Headache* **33:**201–202.

D'Andrea G, Granella F, Ghiotto N, Nappi G (2001). Lamotrigine in the treatment of SUNCT syndrome. *Neurology* **57:**1723–1725.

De Carolis P, Baldrati A, Agati R, De Capoa D, D'Alessandro R, Sacquegna T (1987). Nimodipine in episodic cluster headache: results and methodological considerations. *Headache* **27:**397–399.

Di Sabato F, Fusco BM, Pelaia P, Giacovazzo M (1993). Hyperbaric oxygen therapy in cluster headache. *Pain* **52:**243–245.

Dodick DW (2004). Indomethacin-responsive headache syndromes. *Curr Pain Headache Rep* **8:**19–26.

Donnet A, Valade D, Regis J (2005). Gamma knife treatment for refractory cluster headache: prospective open trial. *J Neurol Neurosurg Psychiatry* **76:**218–221.

Duvoisin RC, Parker GW, Kenoyer WL (1961). The cluster headache. *Arch Intern Med* **108:**711–716.

Ekbom K (1969). Prophylactic treatment of cluster headache with a new serotonin antagonist, BC 105. *Acta Neurol Scand* **45:**601–610.

Ekbom K (1981). Lithium for cluster headache: review of the literature and preliminary results of long-term treatment. *Headache* **21:**132–139.

Ekbom K, Krabbe AE, Paalzow G, Paalzow L, Tfelt-Hansen P, Waldenlind E (1983). Optimal routes of administration of ergotamine tartrate in cluster headache patients. A pharmacokinetic study. *Cephalalgia* **3**:15–20.

Ekbom K, Lindgren L, Nilsson BY, Hardebo JE, Waldenlind E (1987). Retro-Gasserian glycerol injection in the treatment of chronic cluster headache. *Cephalalgia* **7**:21–27.

Ekbom K, Monstad I, Prusinski A, Cole JA, Pilgrim AJ, Noronha D (1993). Subcutaneous sumatriptan in the acute treatment of cluster headache: a dose comparison study. The Sumatriptan Cluster Headache Study Group. *Acta Neurol Scand* **88**:63–69.

Ekbom K (1995). Treatment of cluster headache: clinical trials, design and results. *Cephalalgia* **15**:33–36.

Ekbom K, Krabbe A, Micieli G, Prusinski A, Cole JA, Pilgrim AJ, Noronha D (1995). Cluster headache attacks treated for up to three months with subcutaneous sumatriptan (6 mg). Sumatriptan Cluster Headache Long-term Study Group. *Cephalalgia* **15**:230–236.

Ekbom K, Solomon S (2000). Management of cluster headache. In: Olesen J, Tfelt-Hansen P, Welch KMA (Eds). *The Headaches*. Philadelphia, Lippincott, pp. 731–740.

Ekbom K, Svensson DA, Traff H, Waldenlind E (2002). Age at onset and sex ratio in cluster headache: observations over three decades. *Cephalalgia* **22**:94–100.

El Amrani M, Massiou H, Bousser MG (2002). A negative trial of sodium valproate in cluster headache: methodological issues. *Cephalalgia* **22**:205–208.

Evers S, Husstedt IW (1996). Alternatives in drug treatment of chronic paroxysmal hemicrania. *Headache* **36**:429–432.

Evers S (2004). Botulinum toxin and the management of chronic headaches. *Curr Opin Otolaryngol Head Neck Surg* **12**:197–203.

Fogan L (1985). Treatment of cluster headache. A double-blind comparison of oxygen v air inhalation. *Arch Neurol* **42**:362–363.

Ford RG, Ford KT, Swaid S, Young P, Jennelle R (1998). Gamma knife treatment of refractory cluster headache. *Headache* **38**:3–9.

Förderreuther S, Mayer M, Straube A (2002). Treatment of cluster headache with topiramate: effects and side-effects in five patients. *Cephalalgia* **22**:186–189.

Franzini A, Ferroli P, Leone M, Broggi G (2003). Stimulation of the posterior hypothalamus for treatment of chronic intractable cluster headaches: first reported series. *Neurosurgery* **52**:1095–1101.

Friedman AP, Mikropoulos HE (1958). Cluster headaches. *Neurology* **8**:653–663.

Fusco BM, Marabini S, Maggi CA, Fiore G, Geppetti P (1994). Preventative effect of repeated nasal applications of capsaicin in cluster headache. *Pain* **59**:321–325.

Gabai IJ, Spierings EL (1989). Prophylactic treatment of cluster headache with verapamil. *Headache* **29**:167–168.

Gallagher RM, Mueller L, Ciervo CA (1996). Analgesic use in cluster headache. *Headache* **36**:105–107.

Gallagher RM, Mueller LL, Freitag FG (2002). Divalproex sodium in the treatment of migraine and cluster headaches. *J Am Osteopath Assoc* **102**:92–94.

Goadsby PJ (1999). Short-lasting primary headaches: focus on trigeminal automatic cephalgias and indomethacin-sensitive headaches. Curr Opin Neurol **12**:273–277.

Göbel H, Lindner V, Heinze A, Ribbat M, Peuschl G (1998). Acute therapy for cluster headache with sumatriptan: findings of a one-year long-term study. *Neurology* **51**:908–911.

Graham JR, Malvea BP, Gramm HF (1960). Aerosol ergotamine tartrate for migraine and Horton's syndrome. *New Engl J Med* **263**:802–804.

Gregor N, Schlesiger C, Kraemer C, Akova-Öztürk E, Husstedt IW, Evers S (2004). Wirksamkeit von subkutanem Sumatriptan in verschiedenen Dosierungen und reinem Sauerstoff zur akuten Behandlung des Clusterkopfschmerzes – eine Patientenbefragung. *Schmerz* **18(Suppl 1)**:S65.

Gutierrez-Garcia JM (2002). SUNCT syndrome responsive to lamotrigine. *Headache* **42**:823–825.

Headache Classification Committee of the International Headache Society (2004). The international classification of headache disorders, 2nd edition. *Cephalalgia* **24(Suppl 1)**:1–160.

Hering R, Kuritzky A (1989). Sodium valproate in the treatment of cluster headache: an open clinical trial. *Cephalalgia* **9**:195–198.

Hering-Hanit R, Gadoth N (2000). Baclofen in cluster headache. *Headache* **40**:48–51.

Horton BT, Ryan R, Reynolds JL (1948). Clinical observations of the use of E.C. 110, a new agent for the treatment of headache. *Mayo Clin Proc* **23**:104–108.

Horton BT (1952). Histaminic cephalgia. *Lancet* ii: 92–98.

Horton BT (1956). Histaminic cephalgia: differential diagnosis and treatment. *Mayo Clin Proc* **31**:325–333.

Hunt CH, Dodick DW, Bosch EP (2002). SUNCT responsive to gabapentin. *Headache* **42**: 525–526.

Jarrar RG, Black DF, Dodick DW, Davis DH (2003). Outcome of trigeminal nerve section in the treatment of chronic cluster headache. *Neurology* **60**:1360–1362.

Kittrelle JP, Grouse DS, Seybold ME (1985). Cluster headache. Local anesthetic abortive agents. *Arch Neurol* **42**:496–498.

Krabbe A (1989). Early clinical epxerience with GR43175 in acute cluster headache attacks. *Cephalalgia* **9(Suppl 10)**:404–405.

Kudrow L (1981). Response of cluster headache to oxygen inhalation. *Headache* **21**:1–4.

Kunkle EC, Pfeiffer JB, Wilhoit WM, Hamrick LW (1952). Recurrent brief attacks in cluster pattern. *Trans Am Neurol Assoc* **77**:240–243.

Leone M, D'Amico D, Moschiano F, Fraschini F, Bussone G (1996). Melatonin versus placebo in the prophylaxis of cluster headache: a double-blind pilot study with parallel groups. *Cephalalgia* **16**:494–496.

Leone M, Attanasio A, Grazzi L, Libro G, D'Amico D, Moschiano F, Bussone G (1997). Transdermal clonidine in the prophylaxis of episodic cluster headache: an open study. *Headache* **37**:559–560.

Leone M, D'Amico D, Frediani F, Moschiano F, Grazzi L, Attanasio A, Bussone G (2000). Verapamil in the prophylaxis of episodic cluster headache: a double-blind study versus placebo. *Neurology* **54**:1382–1385.

Leone M, Franzini A, Bussone G (2001). Stereotactic stimulation of posterior hypothalamic gray matter in a patient with intractable cluster headache. *N Engl J Med* **345**:1428–1429.

Leone M, May A, Franzini A, Broggi G, Dodick D, Rapoport A, Goadsby PJ, Schoenen J, Bonavita V, Bussone G (2004). Deep brain stimulation for intractable chronic cluster headache: proposals for patient selection. *Cephalalgia* **24**:934–937.

Lovely TJ, Kotsiakis X, Jannetta PJ (1998). The surgical management of chronic cluster headache. *Headache* **38**:590–594.

Magnoux E, Zlotnik G (2004). Outpatient intravenous dihydroergotamine for refractory cluster headache. Headache **44**:249–255.

Malik K, Rizvi S, Vaillancourt PD (2002). The SUNCT syndrome: successfully treated with lamotrigine. *Pain Med* **3**:167–168.

Manzoni GC, Bono C, Lanfranchi M, Micieli G, Terzano MG, Nappi G (1983). Lithium carbonate in cluster headache: assessment of its short- and long-term therapeutic efficacy. *Cephalalgia* **3**:109–114.

Manzoni GC (1998). Gender ratio of cluster headache over the years: a possible role of changes in lifestyle. *Cephalalgia* **18**:138–142.

Markley HG (2003). Topical agents in the treatment of cluster headache. *Curr Pain Headache Rep* **7**:139–143.

Marks DR, Rapoport A, Padla D *et al.* (1993). A double-blind, placebo-controlled trial of intranasal capsaicin for cluster headache. *Cephalalgia* **13**:114–116.

Matharu MS, Goadsby PJ (2002). Persistence of attacks of cluster headache after trigeminal nerve root section. *Brain* **125**:976–984.

Matharu MS, Boes CJ, Goadsby PJ (2003a). Management of trigeminal autonomic cephalgias and hemicrania continua. *Drugs* **63**:1637–1677.

Matharu MS, Cohen AS, Boes CJ, Goadsby PJ (2003b). Short-lasting unilateral neuralgiform headache with conjunctival injection and tearing syndrome: a review. *Curr Pain Headache Rep* **7**:308–318.

Matharu MS, Levy MJ, Meeran K, Goadsby PJ (2004a). Subcutaneous octreotide in cluster headache: randomized placebo-controlled double-blind crossover study. *Ann Neurol* **56**:488–494.

Matharu MS, Cohen AS, Goadsby PJ (2004b). SUNCT syndrome responsive to intravenous lidocaine. *Cephalalgia* **24**:985–992.

May A (2003). Headaches with (ipsilateral) autonomic symptoms. *J Neurol* **250**:1273–1278.

May A, Leone M (2003). Update on cluster headache. *Curr Opin Neurol* **16**:333–340.

May A, Evers S, Straube A, Pfaffenrath V, Diener HC (2004). Therapie und Prophylaxe von Clusterkopfschmerzen und anderen trigemino-autonomen Kopfschmerzen. *Nervenheilkunde* **23**:478–490.

McGeeney BE (2003). Topiramate in the treatment of cluster headache. *Curr Pain Headache Rep* **7**:135–138.

Meyer JS, Nance M, Walker M, Zetusky WJ, Dowell RE (1985). Migraine and cluster headache treatment with calcium antagonists supports a vascular pathogenesis. *Headache* **25**: 358–367.

Mills TM, Scoggin JA (1997). Intranasal lidocaine for migraine and cluster headaches. *Ann Pharmacother* **31**:914–915.

Mir P, Alberca R, Navarro A, Montes E, Martinez E, Franco E, Cayuela A, Lozano P (2003). Prophylactic treatment of episodic cluster headache with intravenous bolus of methylprednisolone. *Neurol Sci* **24**:318–324.

Monstad I, Krabbe A, Micieli G, Prusiniki A, Cole J, Pilgrim A, Shevlin P (1995). Preemptive oral treatment with sumatriptan during a cluster period. *Headache* **35**:607–613.

Mulder LJ, Spierings EL (2002). Naratriptan in the preventive treatment of cluster headache. *Cephalalgia* **22**:815–817.

Nilsson Remahl AI, Ansjon R, Lind F, Waldenlind E (2002). Hyperbaric oxygen treatment of active cluster headache: a double-blind placebo-controlled crossover study. *Cephalalgia* **22:**730–739.

Nilsson Remahl AI, Laudon Meyer E, Cordonnier C, Goadsby PJ (2003). Placebo response in cluster headache trials: a review. *Cephalalgia* **23:**504–510.

Olesen J, Tfelt-Hansen P, Welch KMA (Eds) (2000). *The Headaches*. Philadelphia, Lippincott.

Onofrio BM, Campbell JK (1986). Surgical treatment of chronic cluster headache. *Mayo Clin Proc* **61:**537–544.

Pareja JA, Kruszewski P, Sjaastad O (1995). SUNCT syndrome: trials of drugs and anaesthetic blockades. *Headache* **35:**138–142.

Peres MF, Stiles MA, Siow HC, Rozen TD, Young WB, Silberstein SD (2002). Greater occipital nerve blockade for cluster headache. *Cephalalgia* **22:**520–522.

Porta-Etessam J, Benito-Leon J, Martinez-Salio A, Berbel A (2002). Gabapentin in the treatment of SUNCT syndrome. *Headache* **42:**523–524.

Pringsheim T, Magnoux E, Dobson CF, Hamel E, Aube M (2002). Melatonin as adjunctive therapy in the prophylaxis of cluster headache: a pilot study. *Headache* **42:**787–792.

Robbins L (1995). Intranasal lidocaine for cluster headache. *Headache* **35:**83–84.

Rossi P, Cesarino F, Faroni J, Malpezzi MG, Sandrini G, Nappi G (2003). SUNCT syndrome successfully treated with topiramate: case reports. *Cephalalgia* **23:**998–1000.

Rozen TD (2001). Antiepileptic drugs in the management of cluster headache and trigeminal neuralgia. *Headache* **41(Suppl 1):** 25–33.

Russell MB (2004). Epidemiology and genetics of cluster headache. *Lancet Neurol* **3:**279–283.

Sanders M, Zuurmond WW (1997). Efficacy of sphenopalatine ganglion blockade in 66 patients suffering from cluster headache: a 12- to 70-month follow-up evaluation. *J Neurosurg* **87:**876–880.

Saper JR, Klapper J, Mathew NT, Rapoport A, Phillips SB, Bernstein JE (2002). Intranasal civamide for the treatment of episodic cluster headaches. *Arch Neurol* **59:**990–994.

Schiller F (1960). Prophylatcic and other treatment for histaminic, cluster, or limited variant migraine. *JAMA* **173:**1907–1911.

Schoenen J, Di Clemente L, Vandenheede M, Fumal A, De Pasqua V, Mouchamps M, Remacle JM, de Noordhout AM (2005). Hypothalamic stimulation in chronic cluster headache: a pilot study of efficacy and mode of action. *Brain* **28:**940–947.

Schuh-Hofer S, Reuter U, Kinze S, Einhaupl KM, Arnold G (2002). Treatment of acute cluster headache with 20 mg sumatriptan nasal spray - an open pilot study. *J Neurol* **249:**94–99.

Schwaag S, Frese A, Husstedt IW, Evers S (2003). SUNCT syndrome: the first German case series. *Cephalalgia* **23:**398–400.

Shabbir N, McAbee G (1994). Adolescent chronic paroxysmal hemicrania responsive to verapamil monotherapy. *Headache* **34:**209–210.

Sicuteri F, Fusco BM, Marabini S, Campagnolo V, Maggi CA, Gepetti C, Fanciullacci M (1989). Beneficial effect of capsaicin application to the nasal mucosa in cluster headache. *Clin J Pain* **5:**49–53.

Sjaastad O (1992). Cluster Headache Syndrome. London, WB Saunders.

Sjaastad O, Antonaci F (1995). A piroxciam derivative partly effective in chronic paroxysmal hemicrania and hemicrania continua. *Headache* **35:**549–550.

Sjaastad O, Bakketeig LS (2003). Cluster headache prevalence. Vaga study of headache epidemiology. *Cephalalgia*. **23:**528–533.

Sjaastd O, Dale I (1974). Evidence for a new (?) treatable headache entity. *Headache* **14:**105–108.

Sjaastad O, Saunte C, Salvesen R, Fredriksen TA, Seim A, Roe OD, Fostad K, Lobben OP, Zhao JM (1989). Short-lasting, unilateral neuralgiform headache attacks with conjunctival injection, tearing, sweating, and rhinorrhea. *Cephalalgia* **19:**147–156.

Sjaastad O, Stovner LJ, Stolt Nielsen A, Antonaci F, Fredriksen TA (1995). CPH and hemicrania continua: requirements of high indomethacin dosages - an ominous sign? *Headache* **35:**363–367.

Speed WG (1960). Ergotamine tartrate inhalation: a new approach for the management of recurrent vascular headaches. *Am J Med Sci* **240:**327–331.

Steiner TJ, Hering R, Couturier EGM, Davies PTG, Whitmarsh TE (1956). Double-blind placebo-controlled trial of lithium in episodic cluster headache. *Cephalalgia* **17:**673–675.

Symonds C (1956). A particular variety of headache. *Brain* **79:**217–232.

Taha JM, Tew JM Jr (1995). Long-term results of radiofrequency rhizotomy in the treatment of cluster headache. *Headache* **35:**193–196.

The Sumatriptan Cluster Headache Study Group (1991). Treatment of acute cluster headache with sumatriptan. *N Engl J Med* **325:**322–326.

Tonon C, Guttmann S, Volpini M, Naccarato S, Cortelli P, D'Alessandro R (2002). Prevalence and incidence of cluster headache in the Republic of San Marino. *Neurology* **58:**1407–1409.

Van Vliet JA, Bahra A, Martin V, Ramadan N, Aurora SK, Mathew NT, Ferrari MD, Goadsby PJ (2003). Intranasal sumatriptan in cluster headache: randomized placebo-controlled double-blind study. *Neurology* **60:**630–633.

Warner JS, Wamil AW, McLean MJ (1994). Acetazolamide for the treatment of chronic paroxysmal hemicrania. *Headache* **34:**597–599.

Zebenholzer K, Wober C, Vigl M, Wessely P (2004). Eletriptan for the short-term prophylaxis of cluster headache. *Headache* **44:**361–364.

CHAPTER 15

Dystonia

A. Albanese,[a] M.P. Barnes,[b] K.P. Bhatia,[c]
E. Fernandez-Alvarez,[d] G. Filippini,[a] T. Gasser,[e]
J.K. Krauss,[f] A. Newton,[g] I. Rektor,[h]
M. Savoiardo,[a] J. Valls-Solè[i]

Abstract

Objectives To review the literature on primary dystonia and dystonia plus and to provide evidence-based recommendations.

Background Primary dystonia and dystonia plus are chronic and often disabling conditions with a widespread spectrum mainly in young people.

Search strategy Computerised MEDLINE and EMBASE literature reviews (1966–1967 February 2005) were conducted. The Cochrane Library was searched for relevant citations.

Results on diagnosis Diagnosis and classification of dystonia are highly relevant for providing appropriate management and prognostic information, and genetic counselling. Expert observation is suggested. DYT-1 gene testing in conjunction with genetic counselling is recommended for patients with primary dystonia with onset before the age of 30 and in those with an affected relative with early onset. Positive genetic testing for dystonia (e.g. DYT-1) is not sufficient to diagnose dystonia. Individuals with myoclonus should be tested for the epsilon-sarcoglycan gene (DYT-11). A levodopa trial is warranted in every patient with early onset dystonia without an alternative diagnosis. Brain imaging is not routinely required when there is a confident diagnosis of primary dystonia in adult patients, whereas it is necessary in the paediatric population.

Results on treatment Botulinum toxin (BoNT) type A (or type B if there is resistance to type A) can be regarded as first line treatment for primary cranial (excluding oromandibular) or cervical dystonia and can be effective in writing dystonia. Actual evidence is lacking on direct comparison of the clinical efficacy and safety of BoNT-A vs. BoNT-B. Pallidal deep brain stimulation (DBS) is

[a]Istituto Nazionale Neurologico Carlo Besta, Milan, Italy; [b]Hunters Moor Regional Rehabilitation Centre, Newcastle Upon Tyne, United Kingdom; [c]Institute of Neurology, University College London, Queen Square, London, United Kingdom; [d]Neuropediatric Department, Hospital San Joan de Dieu, Barcelona, Spain; [e]Department of Neurodegenerative Diseases, Hertie-Institute for Clinical Brain Research, University of Tübingen, Germany; [f]Department of Neurosurgery, Medical University of Hanover, MHH, Hanover, Germany; [g]European Dystonia Federation, Brussels, Belgium; [h]First Department of Neurology, Masaryk University, St. Anne's Teaching Hospital, Brno, Czech Republic; [i]Neurology Department, Hospital Clínic, Barcelona, Spain.

considered a good option, particularly for generalised or cervical dystonia, after medication or BoNT has failed to provide adequate improvement. Selective peripheral denervation is a safe procedure that is indicated exclusively in cervical dystonia. Intrathecal baclofen can be indicated in patients where secondary dystonia is combined with spasticity. The absolute and comparative efficacy and tolerability of drugs in dystonia, including anticholinergic and antidopaminergic drugs, is poorly documented and no evidence-based recommendations can be made to guide prescribing.

Objectives

The objective of the task force was to review the literature on diagnosis and treatment of primary dystonia and dystonia plus to provide evidence-based recommendations for diagnosis and treatment.

Background

Dystonia is characterised by sustained muscle contractions, frequently causing repetitive twisting movements or abnormal postures (Fahn *et al.*, 1987, 1998). Although it is thought to be rare, it is possibly underdiagnosed or misdiagnosed due to the lack of specific clinical criteria. A recent study evaluated the ability among neurologists with different expertise in movement disorders to recognise adult onset focal dystonia and found relevant disagreement, particularly among examiners with lesser expertise (Logroscino *et al.*, 2003).

The prevalence of dystonia is difficult to ascertain. On the basis of the best available prevalence estimates, primary dystonia may be 11.1 per 100 000 or early-onset cases in Ashkenazi Jews from New York area, 60 per 100 000 or late-onset cases in Northern England, and 300 per 100 000 for late-onset cases in the Italian population over the age of 50 (Defazio *et al.*, 2004).

Primary dystonia and dystonia plus are chronic and often disabling conditions with a widespread spectrum mainly in young people. Areas of specific concern include differential diagnosis with other movement disorders, aetiological diagnosis, drug treatment, surgical interventions and genetic counselling.

Search strategy

Computerised MEDLINE and EMBASE searches (1966–February 2005) were conducted using a combination of text words and MeSH terms 'dystonia', 'blepharospasm', 'torticollis', 'writer's cramp', 'Meige syndrome', 'dysphonia' and 'sensitivity and specificity' or 'diagnosis', and 'clinical trial' or 'random allocation' or 'therapeutic use' limited to human studies. The Cochrane Library and the reference lists of all known primary and review articles were searched for relevant citations. No language restrictions were applied. Studies of diagnosis, diagnostic test, and various treatments for patients suffering from dystonia were considered and rated as Level A to C according to the recommendations for European Federation of Neurological Societies (EFNS) scientific task forces (Brainin *et al.*, 2004). Where only class IV evidence was available but consensus could be achieved we have proposed Good Practice Points.

Method for reaching consensus

The results of the literature searches were circulated by e-mail to the task force members for comments. The task force chairman prepared a first draft of the manuscript based on the results of the literature review, data synthesis and comments from the task force members. The draft and the recommendations were discussed during a conference held in Milan on 11–12 February 2005, until consensus was reached within the task force.

Results

Diagnosis

Literature search on the diagnosis of dystonia identified no existing guidelines or systematic reviews. Two consensus agreements (Fahn *et al.*, 1987; Deuschl *et al.*, 1998), two reports of workshops or taskforces (Hallett and Daroff, 1996; Sanger *et al.*, 2003), 69 primary studies on clinically based diagnosis and 292 primary studies on the diagnostic accuracy of different laboratory tests were found. Dealing with primary clinical studies, there were 6 cohort studies, 23 case-control studies, 3 cross-sectional and 37 clinical series.

Table 15.1 Classification of dystonia based on three axes.

By cause (aetiology)

- Primary (or idiopathic): dystonia is the only clinical sign and there is no identifiable exogenous cause or other inherited or degenerative disease. Example: DYT-1 dystonia.
- Dystonia plus: dystonia is a prominent sign, but is associated with another movement disorder. There is no evidence of neurodegeneration. Example: Myoclonus-dystonia (DYT-11).
- Heredo-degenerative: dystonia is a prominent sign, among other neurological features, of a heredo-degenerative disorder. Example: Wilson's disease.
- Secondary: dystonia is a symptom of an identified neurological condition, such as a focal brain lesion, exposure to drugs or chemicals. Examples: dystonia due to a brain tumour, off-period dystonia in Parkinson's disease.
- Paroxysmal: dystonia occurs in brief episodes with normalcy in between. These disorders are classified as idiopathic (often familial although sporadic cases also occur) and symptomatic due to a variety of causes. Three main forms are known depending on the triggering factor. In paroxysmal kinesigenic dyskinesia (PKD; DYT-9) attacks are induced by sudden movement; in paroxysmal exercise induced dystonia (PED) by exercise such as walking or swimming, and in the non-kinesigenic form (PNKD; DYT-8) by alcohol, coffee, tea, etc. A complicated familial form with PNKD and spasticity (DYT-10) has also been described.

By age at onset

- Early onset (variably defined as ≤20–30 years): usually starts in a leg or arm and frequently progresses to involve other
- limbs and the trunk.
- Late onset: usually starts in the neck (including the larynx), the cranial muscles or one arm. Tends to remain localised with restricted progression to adjacent muscles.

By distribution

- Focal: single body region (e.g. writer's cramp, blepharospasm)
- Segmental: contiguous body regions (e.g. cranial and cervical, cervical and upper limb)

Dystonia

- Multifocal: non-contiguous body regions (e.g. upper and lower limb, cranial and upper limb)
- Generalised: both legs and at least one other body region (usually one or both arms)
- Hemidystonia: half of the body (usually secondary to a structural lesion in the contralateral basal ganglia)

Classification

The classification of dystonia is based on three axes: (a) aetiology, (b) age at onset of symptoms, and (c) distribution of body regions affected (table 15.1). The aetiological axis discriminates primary (idiopathic) dystonia, in which dystonia is the only clinical sign without any identifiable exogenous cause or other inherited or degenerative disease, from non-primary forms in which dystonia is usually just one of several clinical signs. Dystonia plus is characterised by dystonia in combination with other movement disorders, for example, myoclonus or parkinsonism. Paroxysmal dystonia is characterised by brief episodes of dystonia with normalcy in between. Primary dystonia and dystonia plus, whether sporadic or familial, are thought to be of genetic origin in most cases.

The clinical features of dystonia encompass a combination of dystonic movements and postures to create a sustained postural twisting (torsion dystonia). Dystonic postures can precede the occurrence of dystonic movements and in rare cases can persist without the occurrence of dystonic movements (called 'fixed dystonia') (Albanese, 2003). Dystonia has some specific features that can be recognised by clinical examination. The speed of contractions of dystonic movements may be slow or rapid, but at the peak of movement, it is sustained. Contractions almost always have a consistent directional or posture-assuming character. Dystonia is commonly aggravated during voluntary movement and may only be present with specific voluntary actions (called 'task-specific dystonia') (Bressman, 2000), or may be temporarily alleviated by specific voluntary tasks, called *gestes antagonistes*, also known as 'sensory tricks' (Gomez-Wong *et al.*, 1998; Greene and Bressman, 1998). Overflow to other body parts, while activating the affected region, is often seen. Dystonia manifesting as tremor may precede clear abnormal posturing.

Two articles have addressed the possibility of identifying clinical features to distinguish between primary and non-primary forms (Tan and Jankovic, 2000; Svetel *et al.*, 2004;). The committee has evaluated that the evidence provided by these studies (both Level IV) does not allow the use of their criteria as indicators for aetiological classification.

> ## GOOD PRACTICE POINTS
>
> 1. Diagnosis and classification of dystonia are highly relevant for providing appropriate management, prognostic information, genetic counselling and treatment (Good Practice Point).
> 2. Based on the lack of specific diagnostic tests, expert observation is recommended. Referral to a movement disorders expert increases the diagnostic accuracy (Logroscino *et al.*, 2003) (Good Practice Point).
> 3. Neurological examination alone allows the clinical identification of primary dystonia and dystonia plus, but not the distinction among different aetiological forms of heredo-degenerative and secondary dystonias (Good Practice Point).

Use of genetic test in diagnosis and counselling

Only one gene (DYT-1) has been identified for primary dystonias (Ozelius *et al.*, 1989). DYT-1 dystonia typically presents in childhood and usually starts in a limb, gradually progressing to a generalised form. However, many exceptions to

this typical presentation have been reported. Other phenotypes of primary dystonia that have been described are: DYT-2, DYT-4, DYT-6, DYT-7 and DYT-13 (de Carvalho and Ozelius, 2002).

Phenotype–genotype correlations have been assessed in DYT-1 dystonia, where one class II study has been published (Bressman *et al.*, 2002). DYT-1 testing had a specificity of up to 100% in dystonia patients with positive family history consistently showing twisting or directional movements and postures. This has led to the recommendation that only patients with such features be considered for genetic studies (Bentivoglio *et al.*, 2002; Bressman *et al.*, 2002); however, this evidence was obtained from American Ashkenazi Jews and does not necessarily apply to the Western European population (Valente *et al.*, 1998). In patients with primary torsion dystonia, age at onset below 30 years, the site of onset in a limb and a positive family history are the three crucial predictors of the diagnostic accuracy of DYT-1 genetic testing (Valente *et al.*, 1998; Klein *et al.*, 1999; Bressman *et al.*, 2000) (class III evidence). Asymptomatic carriers of DYT-1 genetic mutations have been described; the penetrance of DYT-1 dystonia is considered to be around 30%. Four dystonia plus syndromes have been characterised.

The most common form of dopa-responsive dystonia is linked to the DYT-5 gene (GCH1; GTP-cyclohydrolase I). This is a treatable and often misdiagnosed disease for which efforts should be made to warrant a correct diagnosis. The classical phenotype comprises childhood-onset dystonia, sometimes with additional parkinsonism and sustained response to low doses of levodopa, and diurnal fluctuations, with patients being less affected in the morning and more in the evening (Segawa *et al.*, 1976). However, several atypical presentations and several private mutations have been reported (Bandmann and Wood, 2002) (see the database cured by N. Blau and B. Thöny: http://www.bh4.org/biomdb1.html). If genetic testing of the GCH1-gene is negative, parkin mutations should be considered, as the two disorders are sometimes difficult to distinguish (Tassin *et al.*, 2000). There is no evidence for supporting guidelines for genetic testing. It has been proposed to make a diagnostic therapeutic trial with levodopa (Robinson *et al.*, 1999) (class IV) or to perform ancillary diagnostic tests. Phenylalanine loading tests and CSF pterin and dopamine metabolite studies may be useful diagnostic complements (Hyland *et al.*, 1997,1999; Bandmann *et al.*, 2003;), but there is no clear evidence regarding their predictive value. Hence, the recommendation still remains that every patient with early onset dystonia without an alternative diagnosis should have a trial with levodopa.

Myoclonus dystonia is characterised by onset in childhood; the initial symptoms usually consist of lightning jerks and dystonia mostly affecting the neck and the upper limbs, with a prevalent proximal involvement and slow progression (Asmus and Gasser, 2004). Myoclonus and dystonia are strikingly alleviated by the ingestion of alcohol in many but not all patients (Vidailhet *et al.*, 2001). When the phenotype is typical and inheritance is dominant more than 50% of patients will have mutations of the epsilon-sarcoglycan gene (DYT-11) (Klein *et al.*, 2000; Leung *et al.*, 2001; Asmus *et al.*, 2002; Valente *et al.*, 2005).

The DYT-12 gene (mutated gene: ATP1A3) is affected in rapid-onset dystonia-parkinsonism, an extremely rare disease with onset in childhood or early adulthood in which patients develop dystonia, bradykinesia, postural instability, dysarthria and dysphagia over a period ranging from several hours to weeks (Dobyns *et al.*, 1993).

A gene for the paroxysmal non-kinesigenic (PNKD) form of dystonia (DYT-8) has been identified. This condition is characterised by episodes of choreo-dystonia lasting many hours and is induced by coffee, tea, alcohol and fatigue (Demirkiran and Jankovic, 1995). Sporadic and more frequently familial cases with an autosomal dominant inheritance have been described (Bhatia, 2001). Mutations in the myofibrillogenesis regulator 1 (MR-1) gene have been found to cause PNKD in all families with the typical PNKD phenotype (Lee *et al.*, 2004; Rainier *et al.*, 2004; Chen *et al.*, 2005).

RECOMMENDATIONS

1. Diagnostic DYT-1 testing in conjunction with genetic counselling is recommended for patients with primary dystonia with onset before the age of 30 (Klein *et al.*, 1999) (Level B).

2. Diagnostic DYT-1 testing in patients with onset after the age of 30 may also be warranted in those having an affected relative with early onset (Klein *et al.*, 1999; Bressman *et al.*, 2000) (Level B).

3. Diagnostic DYT-1 testing is not recommended in patients with onset of symptoms after the age of 30 who either have focal cranial-cervical dystonia or have no affected relative with early onset dystonia (Klein *et al.*, 1999; Bressman *et al.*, 2000) (Level B).

4. Diagnostic DYT-1 testing is not recommended in asymptomatic individuals, including those under the age of 18, who are relatives of familial dystonia patients. Positive genetic testing for dystonia (e.g. DYT-1) is not sufficient to make a diagnosis of dystonia unless clinical features indicate dystonia (Anon. 1995; Klein *et al.*, 1999) (Level B).

5. A diagnostic levodopa trial is warranted in every patient with early onset dystonia without an alternative diagnosis (Robinson *et al.*, 1999) (Good Practice Point).

6. Individuals with myoclonus affecting the arms or neck, particularly if positive for autosomal dominant inheritance, should be tested for the DYT-11 gene (Valente *et al.*, 2005) (Good Practice Point).

7. Diagnostic testing for the PNKD gene (DYT-8) is not widely available but this may become possible in the near future (Good Practice Point).

Use of neurophysiology in the diagnosis and classification of dystonia

Various neurophysiological techniques can document functional abnormalities in patients with dystonia and assist in differential diagnosis, evaluation of the pathophysiology and directing treatment with botulinum toxin injections.

Studies with surface electromyography show co-contraction between muscles with antagonistic functions, overflow of activity to muscles not intended to move, and disordered configuration of the triphasic pattern for ballistic movements (Rothwell *et al.*, 1983; Hughes and McLellan, 1985; Cohen and Hallett, 1988; van der *et al.*, 1989; Deuschl *et al.*, 1992). Studies of brainstem and spinal reflexes demonstrate an enhanced excitability of brainstem or spinal interneurones that is either limited to the affected area or spreads to adjacent areas in focal dystonia (Berardelli *et al.*, 1985; Rothwell *et al.*, 1988; Tolosa *et al.*, 1988; Nakashima *et al.*, 1989; Panizza *et al.*, 1989;). Studies performed with cortical transcranial magnetic stimulation (TMS) have shown depressed intracortical inhibition, decreased duration of the silent period, and abnormally enhanced recruitment of the motor evoked potential with increasing stimulus intensity and degree of muscle contraction (Ridding *et al.*, 1995; Ikoma *et al.*, 1996; Chen *et al.*, 1997).

Abnormalities of a number of neurophysiological tests of cortical excitability have been reported in symptomatic and non-symptomatic DYT-1 carriers; in contrast, abnormalities of spinal excitability were found only in symptomatic patients. All neurophysiological studies of dystonia are class IV studies, being done in case-control conditions, but not blinded.

GOOD PRACTICE POINTS

Neurophysiological tests are not routinely recommended for the diagnosis or classification of dystonia; however, the observation of abnormalities typical of dystonia is an additional diagnostic tool in cases where the clinical features are considered insufficient to the diagnosis (Hughes and McLellan, 1985; Deuschl *et al.*, 1992) (Good Practice Point).

Use of brain imaging in the diagnosis of dystonia

Most authors agree that conventional or structural magnetic resonance imaging (MRI) studies in primary dystonia are normal. Indeed, a normal MRI study is usually considered a prerequisite to state that a patient's dystonia is primary. Only one conventional MRI class IV study (Schneider *et al.*, 1994) showed T2 bilateral abnormalities in the lentiform nucleus in primary cervical dystonia. However, the abnormalities were only detected on calculated T2 values; no obvious signal changes could be recognized on visual inspection of T2-weighted images. Structural changes in the lentiform nuclei, predominantly in the contralateral pallidum in patients with adult-onset primary focal dystonia, have been suggested by the increased echogenicity of these structures on transcranial sonography (class IV) (Becker and Berg, 2001).

Interesting prospects to understanding the pathophysiological mechanisms of primary and secondary dystonia are offered by functional MRI studies. Class IV studies conducted in series of patients with blepharospasm (Schmidt *et al.*, 2003), writer's cramp (Preibisch *et al.*, 2001; Oga *et al.*, 2002) or other focal dystonia of the arm (Butterworth *et al.*, 2003) demonstrated that several deep structures and cortical areas may be activated in primary dystonia, depending on the different modalities of examination. Recent class IV voxel-based morphometry studies demonstrated an increase in grey matter density or volume in various areas, including cerebellum, basal ganglia, and primary somatosensory cortex (Draganski *et al.*, 2003; Garraux *et al.*, 2004). The increase in grey matter volume might represent plastic changes secondary to overuse, but different interpretations have been considered.

Positron emission tomography studies with different tracers have provided information about areas of abnormal metabolism in different types of dystonia and in different conditions (e.g. during active involuntary movement or during sleep), providing insight on the role of cerebellar and subcortical structures versus cortical areas in the pathophysiology of dystonia (all class IV studies) (Hutchinson *et al.*, 2000; Asanuma *et al.*, 2005). At present, a practical approach to differentiate patients with dystonia plus syndromes from patients with parkinsonism and secondary dystonia is to obtain a single photon emission computerized tomography study with ligands for dopamine transporter; this is readily available and less expensive than positron emission tomography. Patients with dopa-responsive dystonia have normal studies, whereas patients with early-onset Parkinson's disease show reduction of striatal ligand uptake (class IV) (Marshall and Grosset, 2003).

GOOD PRACTICE POINTS

1. Structural brain imaging is not routinely required when there is a confident diagnosis of primary dystonia in adult patients, because a normal study is expected in primary dystonia (Rutledge *et al.*, 1988) (Good Practice Point).
2. Structural brain imaging is necessary for screening of secondary forms of dystonia, particularly in the paediatric population due to the more widespread spectrum of dystonia at this age (Meunier *et al.*, 2003) (Good Practice Point).
3. MRI is preferable to CT, except when brain calcifications are suspected (Good Practice Point).
4. There is no evidence that more sophisticated imaging techniques (e.g., voxel-based morphometry, diffusion weighted imaging (DWI), fMRI) are currently of any value in either the diagnosis or the classification of dystonia (Good Practice Point).

Treatment

Botulinum toxins

Botulinum toxin (BoNT) treatment was recommended for blepharospasm, adductor spasmodic dysphonia, jaw-closing oromandibular dystonia and cervical dystonia by the National Institutes of Health consensus statement .(Anon. 1990).

BoNT treatment for cervical dystonia was analysed in four Cochrane reviews. The first review evaluated BoNT-A therapy and included results from thirteen randomised, placebo-controlled trials. They were short-term studies (6–16 weeks) of BoNT-A enrolling 680 patients overall. All trials reported a benefit of a single injection cycle of BoNT-A for cervical dystonia, but did not provide controlled evidence of the long-term effects of repeated BoNT-A injections. Enriched trials (using patients previously treated with BoNT-A),

suggested that further injections maintained efficacy in most patients. The most frequently reported treatment-related adverse events were dysphagia, neck weakness, local pain at injection site, and sore throat/dry mouth. Most of the adverse events in patients receiving BoNT-A were mild or moderate; no serious adverse events or laboratory abnormalities were associated with the use of BoNT-A (Costa *et al.*, 2005d).

The second review evaluated BoNT-B and included three short-term (16 weeks) studies enrolling 308 participants. All were multicentre and conducted in the United States. All patients included had previously received BoNT-A. A single injection of BoNT-B improved cervical dystonia (Costa *et al.*, 2005c). A similar conclusion was reached in a different review, which included the same three trials (Figgitt and Noble, 2002).

The third review compared BoNT-A versus BoNT-B, but no preliminary results were yet available from two ongoing trials (Costa *et al.*, 2005a). Evidence is currently lacking on direct comparison of the clinical efficacy and safety of BoNT-A vs. BoNT-B.

The fourth review analysed BoNT-A versus anticholinergics and found only one randomised trial comparing BoNT-A versus trihexyphenidyl in 66 patients with cervical dystonia. The results favoured BoNT-A (Costa *et al.*, 2005e).

One Cochrane review analysed BoNT-A efficacy in blepharospasm, but the authors concluded that there were no high quality randomised controlled studies to support the use of BoNT-A for blepharospasm (Costa *et al.*, 2005b). A narrative review of 55 open control studies conducted on 4340 patients in 28 countries reported a success rate of approximately 90% (American Academy of Ophthalmology, 1989).

One Cochrane review analysed BoNT-A for laryngeal dystonia. Only one randomised study was included in this review and no conclusion was drawn about the effectiveness of BoNT for all types of spasmodic dysphonia (Watts *et al.*, 2004).

The efficacy of BoNT-A treatment for writing dystonia has been reviewed by a recent meta-analysis (Balash and Giladi, 2004). Two trials provided class III data suggesting the efficacy of BoNT-A in this condition.

An open randomised class II study compared the costs and effectiveness of a trained outreach nurse practitioner giving injections of botulinum toxin with the standard procedure carried out by medical practitioners within the clinic. The patients had spasmodic torticollis, blepharospasm, or other segmental dystonia, hemidystonia, or generalised dystonia. The study found that the outreach nurse service was as effective and safe as the standard clinic-based service, and the patients preferred it. Although the costs to the National Health System were slightly higher in the nurse practitioner group, the overall costs for society were lower than in the clinic-based service (Whitaker *et al.*, 2001).

RECOMMENDATIONS

1. BoNT-A (or type B if there is resistance to type A) can be regarded as first line treatment for primary cranial (excluding oromandibular) or cervical dystonia (American Academy of Ophthalmology, 1989; Costa *et al.*, 2005b) (Level A).
2. Due to the large number of patients who require BoNT injections, the burden of performing treatment could be shared with properly trained nurse specialists, except in complex dystonia or where electromyography (EMG) guidance is required (Whitaker *et al.*, 2001) (Level B).
3. BoNT-A may be considered in patients with writing dystonia (Balash and Giladi, 2004) (Level C).

Other treatments

One systematic review is available on other types of symptomatic treatment (Balash and Giladi, 2004).

Anticholinergic drugs

Two small class III crossover studies have investigated if trihexyphenidyl treatment was superior to placebo for childhood onset primary or secondary dystonias (Burke and Fahn, 1983; Burke *et al.*, 1986). These studies showed benefit during a follow-up period of 9 months (Burke *et al.*, 1986) and after a mean follow up of 2.4 years (Burke and Fahn, 1983). In contrast, a class III crossover study on cranial adult-onset dystonia (Nutt *et al.*, 1984) did not reveal differences between centrally acting anticholinergics, peripheral anticholinergics, and placebo in patients with cranial dystonia. A retrospective class IV study on adult-onset dystonia (Lang *et al.*, 1982) found no consistent benefit from anticholinergics in patients with adult-onset focal dystonia and concluded that only a minority of patients with cranial dystonia respond to anticholinergics.

GOOD PRACTICE POINTS

The absolute and comparative efficacy and tolerability of anticholinergic agents in dystonia is poorly documented in children and there is no proof of efficacy in adults; therefore, no recommendations can be made to guide prescribing (Good Practice Point).

Antiepileptic drugs

Two double blind randomised crossover studies of oral gamma-vinyl GABA (six patients) and valproate (five patients) were considered not representative, due to the small sample size (class IV) (Carella *et al.*, 1986; Snoek *et al.*, 1987). All other available studies are only case-series evaluating the effects of benzodiazepines or carbamazepine in dystonia.

GOOD PRACTICE POINTS

There is lack of evidence to give recommendations for this type of treatment (Good Practice Point).

Anti-dopaminergic drugs

No controlled trials were available on the effects of this type of treatment. Class IV studies reported symptomatic relief with classic neuroleptics like haloperidol or pimozide (Lang, 1988; Balash and Giladi, 2004).

Tetrabenazine was effective in one double-blind randomised crossover study that was considered class IV due to the small sample size (Jankovic, 1982). The positive effect of this treatment was confirmed in a large class IV series of patients with different types of movement disorders, including dystonia, followed up retrospectively for a mean duration of 6.6 years (Jankovic and Beach, 1997). All other available studies are also of class IV, thus insufficient to prove the effect of tetrabenazine.

Two class IV studies evaluated the effects of risperidone in patients with different forms of dystonia and did not provide sufficient evidence of efficacy. One class IV study on tiapride and three studies on clozapine did not provide evidence of efficacy.

> ## GOOD PRACTICE POINTS
> There is lack of evidence to give recommendations for this type of treatment (Good Practice Point).

Dopaminergic drugs

Levodopa is the treatment of choice for dopa-responsive dystonia. There are no evidence-based data to support the use of levodopa or dopamine agonists in other primary dystonias. Patients with dopa-responsive dystonia typically experience marked long-term benefit with low doses of levodopa. The optimal dose differs among patients; while some respond magnificently to small doses, others require higher doses.

A class IV trial performed on a small sample of dopa-responsive dystonia patients showed no differences in the short- and long-duration responses (Nutt and Nygaard, 2001). Many uncontrolled studies reported improvement of parkinsonism and dystonia with variable doses of levodopa, from 100 mg daily (Gherpelli *et al.*, 1995) to 750 mg daily (Rajput *et al.*, 1994). In a case series of 20 patients clinical benefit was observed at a mean dose of 343.8 mg daily for patients with dyskinesias, and 189.1 mg daily for patients without dyskinesias; in addition, there was an inverse correlation between the daily dose of levodopa and duration of treatment (Hwang *et al.*, 2001).

> ## GOOD PRACTICE POINTS
> Following a positive diagnostic trial with levodopa, chronic treatment with levodopa should be initiated and adjusted according to the clinical response (Hwang *et al.*, 2001) (Good Practice Point).

Other drugs

A class I study on the acute effect of nabilone (a cannabinoid receptor agonist) did not show efficacy (Fox *et al.*, 2002). Only class IV evidence is available regarding alcohol, lidocaine, diphenhydramine, L-tryptophan, tizanidine or oestrogens.

Neurosurgical procedures

The available studies were classified according to the following categories: deep brain stimulation; selective peripheral denervation/myectomy; intrathecal baclofen; radiofrequency lesions; rare, uncommon or obsolete procedures.

Deep brain stimulation (DBS)

Long-term electrical stimulation of the globus pallidus internus (GPi) or the thalamus has been applied in patients with various features of dystonia, mainly those who do not achieve adequate benefit with medical treatment. At this time, the consensus is that patients with primary (familial or sporadic) generalised or segmental dystonia and patients with complex cervical dystonia are the best candidates for pallidal DBS (Krauss *et al.*, 2004). Several other manifestations are currently being explored. DBS has received approval from the Food and Drug Administration in the United States in the form of an humanitarian device exemption and has received the CE-mark for dystonia in Europe.

All studies published thus far are class IV, with the exception of a recent class III study on primary generalised dystonia (Vidailhet *et al.*, 2005).

It has been observed that the improvement of dystonia following DBS implants follows a specific sequence. While dystonic movements (including phasic, myoclonic and tremulous features) may improve immediately or within hours or days after surgery, dystonic postures (i.e. tonic features) generally have a delayed improvement over weeks or months (Yianni et al., 2003; Coubes et al., 2004; Krause et al., 2004; Vidailhet et al., 2005).

Primary versus secondary dystonia. The postoperative improvement of patients with primary dystonia who receive GPi implants is within a range of 40–90% using standard dystonia rating scales. The improvement of patients with secondary dystonia is much less pronounced (Eltahawy et al., 2004; Krauss et al., 2004).

Targets other than the pallidum. The GPi is currently considered the target of choice in primary dystonia; however, the ventrolateral thalamus has been considered by some a suitable target for secondary dystonia by some. Other targets (e.g. the subthalamic nucleus) have also been considered for primary dystonia. Due to the paucity of data, no conclusions can be made at this time and no recommendations can be given.

Generalised dystonia. The most beneficial results with pallidal DBS were reported in children with DYT-1 dystonia with improvement in the range of 40–90% (Coubes et al., 2000). However, also adult patients with non-DYT-1 primary generalised dystonia can achieve equivalent benefit (Yianni et al., 2003; Coubes et al., 2004; Krause et al., 2004). A class III French multicentre study investigated the effect of bilateral pallidal DBS in primary generalised dystonia including blinded assessment of clinical outcome (Vidailhet et al., 2005). The mean percentage of improvement of the Burke–Fahn–Marsden rating scale after pallidal DBS in primary generalised dystonia in this study was on average 54%, and the mean improvement of disability was on average 44%.

Cervical dystonia. Pallidal DBS has been primarily used in patients who were thought not to be ideal candidates for peripheral denervation, including those with head tremor and myoclonus, marked phasic dystonic movements, sagittal and lateral shift, antecollis, and combined complex forms of cervical dystonia. Postoperative benefit in these patients most often was evaluated with the Toronto Western Spasmodic Torticollis Rating Scale. At 1–2 year follow-up, the improvement in severity score ranged between 50 and 70%, the disability score improved between 60 and 70%, and the pain score between 50 and 60% (Level C) (Krauss et al., 1999; Parkin et al., 2001; Eltahawy et al., 2004).

Chronic stimulation uses both higher pulse width and voltage than in PD, which results in much higher energy consumption and earlier battery depletion. Batteries must be replaced every 2 years or even more often. Sudden battery depletion may induce acute recurrence of dystonia, sometimes resulting in a medical emergency. Three safety aspects have to be considered: surgery-related complications, stimulation-induced side effects and hardware-related problems.

GOOD PRACTICE POINTS

Pallidal DBS is considered a good option, particularly for generalized or cervical dystonia, after medication or BoNT have failed to provide adequate improvement. While it can be considered second-line treatment in patients with generalized dystonia, this is not the case in cervical dystonia as there are other surgical options available (see below). This procedure requires a specialised expertise, and is not without side effects (Eltahawy et al., 2004; Vidailhet et al., 2005) (Good Practice Point).

Selective peripheral denervation and myectomy

The National Institute for Clinical Excellence of the United Kingdom has produced a guideline for selective peripheral denervation in cervical dystonia which was issued in August 2004 (The National Institute for Clinical Excellence, 2004). Selective peripheral denervation should not be confused with intradural rhizotomy, which has a high incidence of complications; it is indicated in patients with cervical dystonia who do not achieve adequate response with medical treatment or repeated botulinum toxin injections. It is indicated in non-responders to botulinum toxin injections. Additional myectomy may be carried out if necessary. Patients with prominent (phasic or myoclonic) dystonic movements or with dystonic head tremor are not good candidates for this procedure.

In some patients, selective peripheral denervation can also be an alternative to botulinum toxin injections. Overall, about one to two-thirds of patients achieve useful long-term improvement. This proportion has been higher, up to 90%, in some studies (Bertrand, 1993); however it is unclear how follow-up was performed in these studies. Denervation of C2 invariably involves numbness in the territory of the greater occipital nerve in the early postoperative period. Patients should be informed about the invariable procedure-related numbness; neuropathic pain can develop rarely. Swallowing difficulties have been noted in some studies. In about 1–2% of patients the procedure causes weakness in non-dystonic muscles, in particular in the trapezius. Re-innervation can occur and the patient may require further surgery.

RECOMMENDATIONS

Selective peripheral denervation is a safe procedure with infrequent and minimal side effects that is indicated exclusively in cervical dystonia. This procedure requires specialised expertise (The National Institute for Clinical Excellence, 2004) (Level C).

Intrathecal baclofen

Intrathecal baclofen has been used in patients with severe generalised dystonia; in particular, patients who have concomitant severe spasticity may benefit from this therapeutic option. The number of publications has decreased as the use of DBS for dystonia has become more prevalent. All the available evidence on outcome is Class IV and furthermore no standardized dystonia scales have been used; thus results are difficult to compare. Controlled studies have only been performed on the screening procedure to select candidates for long-term treatment. There is no evidence to set the procedure in perspective with other treatments.

Overall, the results from different centres are variable.

The surgical risk is low, but the method is burdened by medication-related side effects, infections and long-term hardware-related problems. Intrathecal baclofen for treatment of dystonia requires frequent pump refills and follow-up visits.

GOOD PRACTICE POINTS

There is insufficient evidence to use this treatment in primary dystonia; the procedure can be indicated in patients where secondary dystonia is combined with spasticity (Albright *et al.*, 2001) (Good Practice Point).

Radiofrequency lesions

Until recently, unilateral or bilateral stereotactic radiofrequency ablations of the thalamus or the pallidum were the preferred surgical methods to treat patients with severe and otherwise refractory dystonia. Most of the available literature suffers from methodological flaws and there is little data available to compare the benefits achieved with thalamotomy as opposed to pallidotomy (Ondo *et al.*, 2001; Loher *et al.*, 2004). In a retrospective series of 32 patients with primary and secondary dystonias, it was found that patients with primary dystonia who underwent pallidotomy demonstrated significantly better long-term outcomes than did patients who underwent thalamotomy (Yoshor *et al.*, 2001). Patients with secondary dystonia experienced more modest improvement after either procedure, with little or no difference in outcome between the two procedures.

GOOD PRACTICE POINTS

Radiofrequency ablations are currently discouraged for bilateral surgery because of the relatively high risk of side effects (Good Practice Point). The focus of treatment has currently shifted to DBS because of its lower risk for bilateral procedures.

Rare, uncommon or obsolete procedures

Intradural anterior cervical rhizotomy was the most common operation for cervical dystonia before the advent of peripheral denervation (Hamby, 1970; Friedman *et al.*, 1993). Several variations of this procedure have been developed. As the 'standard procedure' was rather non-selective and resulted in high complication rates, modified techniques aimed to denervate the dystonic muscles and to preserve normal activity. Both the reported results and the complication rates in different series were highly variable (Colbassani, Jr. and Wood, 1986). Side effects included dysphagia, weakness of the neck, cerebrospinal fluid fistulas and infection. Weak or unstable neck has been estimated to occur in about 40% of patients after bilateral rhizotomy, and transient dysphagia in about 30% of patients.

Microvascular decompression of the spinal accessory nerve for treatment of cervical dystonia has been used in analogy to the therapeutic benefit of this procedure in other cranial neuropathies such as hemifacial spasm (Jho and Jannetta, 1995). Pathophysiological concepts do not support microvascular decompression as a valid treatment option for cervical dystonia, and data on outcome are very limited.

GOOD PRACTICE POINTS

1. Intradural rhizotomy has been replaced by selective ramisectomy and peripheral denervation or myotomy. These procedures are no longer recommended.
2. Microvascular decompression is not recommended for treatment of cervical dystonia.

Acknowledgement

The authors wish to thank Dr. Antonio E. Elia, who performed literature searches and preparatory work.

References

1991 Clinical use of botulinum toxin. *Arch Neurol* **48:**1294–298.

1995 Points to consider: ethical, legal, and psychosocial implications of genetic testing in children and adolescents. American Society of Human Genetics Board of Directors, American College of Medical Genetics Board of Directors. *Am J Hum Genet* **57:**1233–1241.

Albanese A (2003). The clinical expression of primary dystonia. *J Neurol* **250:**1145–1151.

Albright AL, Barry MJ, Shafton DH, Ferson SS (2001). Intrathecal baclofen for generalized dystonia. *Develop Med Child Neurol* **43:**652–657.

American Academy of Ophthalmology (1989). Botulinum toxin therapy of eye muscle disorders. Safety and effectiveness. *Ophthalmology* **96(2):**37–41.

Asanuma K, Ma Y, Huang C, Carbon-Correll M, Edwards C, Raymond D, Bressman SB, Moeller J R, Eidelberg D (2005). The metabolic pathology of dopa-responsive dystonia. *Ann Neurol* **57:**596–600.

Asmus F, Gasser T (2004). Inherited myoclonus-dystonia. *Adv Neurol* **94:**113–119.

Asmus F, Zimprich A, Tezenas du MS, Kabus C, Deuschl G, Kupsch A, Ziemann U, Castro M, Kuhn AA, Strom TM, Vidailhet M, Bhatia KP, Durr A, Wood NW, Brice A, Gasser T (2002). Myoclonus-dystonia syndrome: epsilon-sarcoglycan mutations and phenotype. *Ann Neurol* **52:**489–492.

Balash Y, Giladi N (2004). Efficacy of pharmacological treatment of dystonia: evidence-based review including meta-analysis of the effect of botulinum toxin and other cure options. *European J Neurol* **11:**361–370.

Bandmann O, Wood NW (2002). Dopa-responsive dystonia. The story so far. *Neuropediatrics* **33:**1–5.

Bandmann O, Goertz M, Zschocke J, Deuschl G, Jost W, Hefter H, Muller U, Zofel P, Hoffmann G, Oertel W (2003). The phenylalanine loading test in the differential diagnosis of dystonia. *Neurology* **60:**700–702.

Becker G, Berg D (2001). Neuroimaging in basal ganglia disorders: perspectives for transcranial ultrasound. *Mov Disord* **16:**23–32.

Bentivoglio AR, Loi M, Valente EM, Ialongo T, Tonali P, Albanese A (2002). Phenotypic variability of DYT1-PTD: Does the clinical spectrum include psychogenic dystonia? *Mov Disord* **17:**1058–1063.

Berardelli A, Rothwell JC, Day BL, Marsden CD (1985). Pathophysiology of blepharospasm and oromandibular dystonia. *Brain* **108:**593–608.

Bertrand CM (1993). Selective peripheral denervation for spasmodic torticollis: surgical technique, results, and observations in 260 cases. *Surg Neurol* **40:**96–103.

Bhatia KP (2001). Familial (idiopathic) paroxysmal dyskinesias: an update. *Semin Neurol* **21:** 69–74.

Brainin M, Barnes M, Baron JC, Gilhus NE, Hughes R, Selmaj K, Waldemar G (2004). Guidance for the preparation of neurological management guidelines by EFNS scientific task forces–revised recommendations 2004. *Euro J Neurol* **11:**577–581.

Bressman SB (2000). Dystonia update. *Clin Neuropharmacol* **23:**239–251.

Bressman SB, Sabatti C, Raymond D, de Leon D, Klein C, Kramer PL, Brin MF, Fahn S, Breakefield X, Ozelius LJ, Risch NJ (2000). The DYT1 phenotype and guidelines for diagnostic testing. *Neurology* **54:**1746–1752.

Bressman SB, Raymond D, Wendt K, Saunders-Pullman R, de Leon D, Fahn S, Ozelius L, Risch N (2002). Diagnostic criteria for dystonia in DYT1 families. *Neurology* **59:**1780–1782.

Burke RE, Fahn S (1983). Double-blind evaluation of trihexyphenidyl in dystonia. *Adv Neurol* **37:**189–192.

Burke RE, Fahn S, Marsden CD (1986). Torsion dystonia: a double blind, prospective trial of high-dosage trihexyphenidil. *Neurology* **36:**160–164.

Butterworth S, Francis S, Kelly E, McGlone F, Bowtell R, Sawle GV (2003). Abnormal cortical sensory activation in dystonia: an fMRI study. *Mov Disord* **18:**673–682.

Carella F, Girotti F, Scigliano G, Caraceni T, Joder-Ohlenbusch AM, Schechter PJ (1986). Double-blind study of oral gamma-vinyl GABA in the treatment of dystonia. *Neurology* **36:**98–100.

Chen R, Wassermann EM, Canos M, Hallett M (1997). Impaired inhibition in writer's cramp during vountary muscle activation. *Neurology* **49:**1054–1059.

Chen DH, Matsushita M, Rainier S, Meaney B, Tisch L, Feleke A, Wolff J, Lipe H, Fink J, Bird T D, Raskind WH (2005). Presence of alanine-to-valine substitutions in myofibrillogenesis regulator 1 in paroxysmal nonkinesigenic dyskinesia: confirmation in 2 kindreds. *Arch Neurol* **62:**597–600.

Cohen LG, Hallett M (1988). Hand cramps: clinical features and electromyographic patterns in a focal dystonia. *Neurology* **38:**1005–1012.

Colbassani HJ Jr, Wood JH (1986). Management of spasmodic torticollis. *Surg Neurol* **25:** 153–158.

Costa J, Borges A, Espirito-Santo C, Ferreira J, Coelho M, Moore P, Sampaio C (2005a). Botulinum toxin type A versus botulinum toxin type B for cervical dystonia. *Cochrane Database Syst Rev* CD004314.

Costa J, Espirito-Santo C, Borges A, Ferreira J, Coelho M, Moore P, Sampaio C (2005b). Botulinum toxin type A therapy for blepharospasm. *Cochrane Database Syst Rev* CD004900.

Costa J, Espirito-Santo C, Borges A, Ferreira J, Coelho M, Moore P, Sampaio C (2005c). Botulinum toxin type B for cervical dystonia. *Cochrane Database Syst Rev* CD004315.

Costa J, Espirito-Santo C, Borges A, Ferreira J, Coelho M, Moore P, Sampaio C (2005d). Botulinum toxin type A therapy for cervical dystonia. *Cochrane Database Syst Rev* CD003633.

Costa J, Espirito-Santo C, Borges A, Ferreira J, Coelho M, Sampaio C (2005e). Botulinum toxin type A versus anticholinergics for cervical dystonia. *Cochrane Database Syst Rev* CD004312.

Coubes P, Roubertie A, Vayssiere N, Hemm S, Echenne B (2000). Treatment of DYT1-generalised dystonia by stimulation of the internal globus pallidus. *Lancet* **355:**2220–2221.

Coubes P, Cif L, El Fertit H, Hemm S, Vayssiere N, Serrat S, Picot MC, Tuffery S, Claustres M, Echenne B, Frerebeau P (2004). Electrical stimulation of the globus pallidus internus in patients with primary generalized dystonia: long-term results. *J Neurosurg* **101:**189–194.

de Carvalho PM, Ozelius LJ (2002). Classification and genetics of dystonia. *Lancet Neurol* **1:**316–325.

Defazio G, Abbruzzese G, Livrea P, Berardelli A (2004). Epidemiology of primary dystonia. *Lancet Neurol* **3:**673–678.

Demirkiran M, Jankovic J (1995). Paroxysmal dyskinesias: clinical features and classification. *Ann Neurol* **38:**571–579.

Deuschl G, Heinen F, Kleedorfer B, Wagner M, Lucking CH, Poewe W (1992). Clinical and polymyographic investigation of spasmodic torticollis. *J Neurol* **239:**9–15.

Deuschl G, Bain P, Brin M (1998). Consensus statement of the Movement Disorder Society on Tremor. Ad Hoc Scientific Committee. *Mov Disord* **13(3):**2–23.

Dobyns WB, Ozelius LJ, Kramer PL, Brashear A, Farlow MR, Perry TR, Walsh LE, Kasarskis EJ, Butler IJ, Breakefield XO (1993). Rapid-onset dystonia-parkinsonism. *Neurology* **43:**2596–2602.

Draganski B, Thun-Hohenstein C, Bogdahn U, Winkler J, May A (2003). "Motor circuit" gray matter changes in idiopathic cervical dystonia. *Neurology* **61:**1228–1231.

Eltahawy HA, Saint-Cyr J, Poon YY, Moro E, Lang AE, Lozano AM (2004). Pallidal deep brain stimulation in cervical dystonia: clinical outcome in four cases. *Canad J Neurol Sci* **31:**328–332.

Fahn S, Marsden CD, Calne DB (1987). Classification and investigation of dystonia, In *Movement disorders 2*, C. D. Marsden S. Fahn, eds., Butterworths, London, pp. 332–358.

Fahn S, Bressman S, Marsden CD (1998). Classification of dystonia. *Adv Neurol* **78:**1–10.

Figgitt DP, Noble S (2002). Botulinum toxin B: a review of its therapeutic potential in the management of cervical dystonia. *Drugs* **62:**705–722.

Fox SH, Kellett M, Moore AP, Crossman AR, Brotchie JM (2002). Randomised, double-blind, placebo-controlled trial to assess the potential of cannabinoid receptor stimulation in the treatment of dystonia. *Mov Disord* **17:**145–149.

Friedman AH, Nashold BS, Sharp R, Caputi F, Arruda J (1993). "Treatment of spasmodic torticollis with intradural selective rhizotomies," *J Neurosurg* **78:**46–53.

Garraux G, Bauer A, Hanakawa T, Wu T, Kansaku K, Hallett M (2004). Changes in brain anatomy in focal hand dystonia. *Ann Neurol* **55:**736–739.

Gherpelli JL, Nagae LM, Diament A (1995). DOPA-sensitive progressive dystonia of childhood with diurnal fluctuations of symptoms: a case report. *Arquivos de Neuro-Psiquiatria* **53:** 298–301.

Gomez-Wong E, Marti MJ, Cossu G, Fabregat N, Tolosa ES, Valls-Sole J (1998). The 'geste antagonistique' induces transient modulation of the blink reflex in human patients with blepharospasm. *Neurosci Lett* **251:**125–128.

Greene PE, Bressman S (1998). Exteroceptive and interoceptive stimuli in dystonia. *Mov Disord* **13:**549–551.

Hallett M, Daroff RB (1996). Blepharospasm: report of a workshop. *Neurology* **46:**1213–1218.

Hamby WB (1970). Schiffer S:Spasmodic torticollis; results after cervical rhizotomy in 80 cases. *Clin Neurosurg* **17:**28–37.

Hughes M, McLellan DL (1985). Increased co-activation of the upper limb muscles in writer's cramp. *J Neurol Neurosurg Psych* **48:**782–787.

Hutchinson M, Nakamura T, Moeller JR, Antonini A, Belakhlef A, Dhawan V, Eidelberg D (2000). The metabolic topography of essential blepharospasm: a focal dystonia with general implications. *Neurology* **55:**673–677.

Hwang WJ, Calne DB, Tsui JK, Fuente-Fernandez R (2001). The long-term response to levodopa in dopa-responsive dystonia. *Parkinsonism Relat Disord* **8:**1–5.

Hyland K, Fryburg JS, Wilson WG, Bebin EM, Arnold LA, Gunasekera RS, Jacobson RD, Rost-Ruffner E, Trugman JM (1997). Oral phenylalanine loading in dopa-responsive dystonia: a possible diagnostic test. *Neurology* **48:**1290–1297.

Hyland K, Nygaard TG, Trugman JM, Swoboda KJ, Arnold LA, Sparagana SP (1999). Oral phenylalanine loading profiles in symptomatic and asymptomatic gene carriers with dopa-responsive dystonia due to dominantly inherited GTP cyclohydrolase deficiency. *J Inherit Metab Dis* **22:**213–215.

Ikoma K, Samii A, Mercuri B, Wassermann EM, Hallett M (1996). Abnormal cortical motor excitability in dystonia. *Neurology* **46:**1371–1376.

Jankovic J (1982). Treatment of hyperkinetic movement disorders with tetrabenazine: a double-blind crossover study. *Ann Neurol* **11:**41–47.

Jankovic J, Beach J (1997). Long-term effects of tetrabenazine in hyperkinetic movement disorders. *Neurology* **48:**358–362.

Jho HD, Jannetta PJ (1995). Microvascular decompression for spasmodic torticollis. *Acta Neurochirurgica* **134:**21–26.

Klein C, Friedman J, Bressman S, Vieregge P, Brin MF, Pramstaller PP, de Leon D, Hagenah J, Sieberer M, Fleet C, Kiely R, Xin W, Breakefield XO, Ozelius LJ, Sims KB (1999). Genetic testing for early-onset torsion dystonia (DYT1): introduction of a simple screening method, experiences from testing of a large patient cohort, and ethical aspects. *Genet Test* **3:**323–328.

Klein C, Schilling K, Saunders-Pullman RJ, Garrels J, Breakefield XO, Brin MF, deLeon D, Doheny D, Fahn S, Fink JS, Forsgren L, Friedman J, Frucht S, Harris J, Holmgren G, Kis B, Kurlan R, Kyllerman M, Lang AE, Leung J, Raymond D, Robishaw JD, Sanner G, Schwinger E, Tabamo RE, Tagliati M (2000). A major locus for myoclonus-dystonia maps to chromosome 7q in eight families. *Amer J Hum Genet* **67:**1314–1319.

Krause M, Fogel W, Kloss M, Rasche D, Volkmann J, Tronnier V (2004). Pallidal stimulation for dystonia. *Neurosurgery* **55:**1361–1370.

Krauss JK, Pohle T, Weber S, Ozdoba C, Burgunder JM (1999). Bilateral stimulation of globus pallidus internus for treatment of cervical dystonia. *Lancet* **354:**837–838.

Krauss JK, Yianni J, Loher TJ, Aziz TZ (2004). Deep brain stimulation for dystonia. *J Clin Neurophysiol* **21:**18–30.

Lang AE (1988). Dopamine agonists and antagonists in the treatment of idiopathic dystonia. *Adv Neurol* **50:**561–570.

Lang AE, Sheehy MP, Marsden CD (1982). Anticholinergics in adult-onset focal dystonia. *Canad J Neurol Sci* **9:**313–319.

Lee HY, Xu Y, Huang Y, Ahn AH, Auburger GW, Pandolfo M, Kwiecinski H, Grimes DA, Lang AE, Nielsen JE, Averyanov Y, Servidei S, Friedman A, Van BP, Abramowicz MJ, Bruno MK, Sorensen BF, Tang L, Fu YH, Ptacek LJ (2004). The gene for paroxysmal non-kinesigenic dyskinesia encodes an enzyme in a stress response pathway. *Hum Mol Genet* **13:** 3161–3170.

Leung JC, Klein C, Friedman J, Vieregge P, Jacobs H, Doheny D, Kamm C, deLeon D, Pramstaller PP,

Penney JB, Eisengart M, Jankovic J, Gasser T, Bressman SB, Corey DP, Kramer P, Brin MF, Ozelius LJ, Breakefield XO (2001). Novel mutation in the TOR1A (DYT1) gene in atypical early onset dystonia and polymorphisms in dystonia and early onset parkinsonism. *Neurogenetics* **3:**133–143.

Logroscino G, Livrea P, Anaclerio D, Aniello MS, Benedetto G, Cazzato G, Giampietro L, Manobianca G, Marra M, Martino D, Pannarale P, Pulimeno R, Santamato V, Defazio G (2003). Agreement among neurologists on the clinical diagnosis of dystonia at different body sites. *J Neurol Neurosurg Psych* **74:**348–350.

Loher TJ, Pohle T, Krauss JK (2004). Functional stereotactic surgery for treatment of cervical dystonia: review of the experience from the lesional era. *Stereotac Funct Neurosurg* **82:**1–13.

Marshall V, Grosset D (2003). Role of dopamine transporter imaging in routine clinical practice. *Mov Disord* **18:**1415–1423.

Meunier S, Lehericy S, Garnero L, Vidailhet M (2003). Dystonia: lessons from brain mapping. *Neuroscientist* **9:**76–81.

Nakashima K, Rothwell JC, Day BL, Thompson PD, Shannon K, Marsden CD (1989). Reciprocal inhibition between forearm muscles in patients with writer's cramp and other occupational cramps, symptomatic hemidystonia and hemiparesis due to stroke. *Brain* **112:**681–697.

Nutt JG, Hammerstad JP, deGarmo P, Carter J (1984). Cranial dystonia: double-blind crossover study of anticholinergics. *Neurology* **34:**215–217.

Nutt JG, Nygaard TG (2001). Response to levodopa treatment in dopa-responsive dystonia. *Arch Neurol* **58(6):**905–910.

Oga T, Honda M, Toma K, Murase N, Okada T, Hanakawa T, Sawamoto N, Nagamine T, Konishi J, Fukuyama H, Kaji R, Shibasaki H (2002). Abnormal cortical mechanisms of voluntary muscle relaxation in patients with writer's cramp: an fMRI study. *Brain* **125:**895–903.

Ondo WG, Desaloms M, Krauss JK, Jankovic J, Grossman RG (2001). Pallidotomy and thalamotomy for dystonia In *Surgery for Parkinson's Disease and Movement Disorders*, J. K. Krauss, J. Jankovic, R. G. Grossman, eds., Lippincott, Philadelphia, pp. 299–306.

Ozelius L, Kramer PL, Moskowitz CB, Kwiatkowski DJ, Brin MF, Bressman SB, Schuback DE, Falk CT, Risch N, de Leon D, Burke RE, Haines J, Gusella JF, Fahn S, Breakefield XO (1989). Human gene for torsion dystonia located on chromosome 9q32-q34. *Neuron* **2:**1427–1434.

Panizza ME, Hallett M, Nilsson J (1989). Reciprocal inhibition in patients with hand cramps. *Neurology* **39:**85–89.

Parkin S, Aziz T, Gregory R, Bain P (2001). Bilateral internal globus pallidus stimulation for the treatment of spasmodic torticollis. *Move Disord* **16:**489–493.

Preibisch C, Berg D, Hofmann E, Solymosi L, Naumann M (2001). Cerebral activation patterns in patients with writer's cramp: a functional magnetic resonance imaging study. *J Neurol* **248:**10–17.

Rainier S, Thomas D, Tokarz D, Ming L, Bui M, Plein E, Zhao X, Lemons R, Albin R, Delaney C, Alvarado D, Fink JK (2004). Myofibrillogenesis regulator 1 gene mutations cause paroxysmal dystonic choreoathetosis. *Arch Neurol* **61:**1025–1029.

Rajput AH, Gibb WR, Zhong XH, Shannak KS, Kish S, Chang LG, Hornykiewicz O (1994). Dopa-responsive dystonia: pathological and biochemical observations in a case. *Ann Neurol* **35(4):**396–402.

Ridding MC, Sheean G, Rothwell JC, Inzelberg R, Kujirai T (1995). Changes in the balance between motor cortical excitation and inhibition in focal, task specific dystonia. *J Neurol Neurosurg Psych* **59:**493–498.

Robinson R, McCarthy GT, Bandmann O, Dobbie M, Surtees R, Wood NW (1999). GTP cyclohydrolase deficiency; intrafamilial variation in clinical phenotype, including levodopa responsiveness. *J Neurol Neurosurg Psych* **66:**86–89.

Rothwell JC, Obeso JA, Marsden CD (1983). Pathophysiology of dystonias In *Motor Control Mechanisms in Health and Disease*, J. E. Desmedt, ed., Raven, New York, pp. 851–863.

Rothwell JC, Day BL, Obeso JA, Berardelli A, Marsden CD (1988). Reciprocal inhibition between muscles of the human forearm in normal subjects and in patients with idiopathic torsion dystonia. *Adv Neurol* **50:**133–140.

Rutledge JN, Hilal SK, Silver AJ, Defendini R, Fahn S (1988). Magnetic resonance imaging of dystonic states. *Adv Neurol* **50:**265–275.

Sanger TD, Delgado MR, Gaebler-Spira D, Hallett M, Mink JW (2003). Classification and definition of disorders causing hypertonia in childhood. *Pediatrics* **111:**e89–e97.

Schmidt KE, Linden DE, Goebel R, Zanella FE, Lanfermann H, Zubcov AA (2003). Striatal activation during blepharospasm revealed by fMRI. *Neurology* **60:**1738–1743.

Schneider S, Feifel E, Ott D, Schumacher M, Lucking CH, Deuschl G (1994). Prolonged MRI T2 times of the lentiform nucleus in idiopathic spasmodic torticollis. *Neurology* **44:**846–850.

Segawa M, Hosaka A, Miyagawa F, Nomura Y, Imai H (1976). Hereditary progressive dystonia with marked diurnal fluctuation. *Adv Neurol* **14:**215–233.

Snoek JW, van Weerden TW, Teelken AW, van den BW, Lakke JP (1987). Meige syndrome: double-blind crossover study of sodium valproate. *J Neurol Neurosurg Psych* **50:**1522–1525.

Svetel M, Ivanovic N, Marinkovic J, Jovic J, Dragasevic N, Kostic VS (2004). Characteristics of dystonic movements in primary and symptomatic dystonias. *J Neurol Neurosurg Psych* **75:**329–330.

Tan EK, Jankovic J (2000). Tardive and idiopathic oromandibular dystonia: a clinical comparison. *J Neurol Neurosurg Psych* **68:**186–190.

Tassin J, Durr A, Bonnet AM, Gil R, Vidailhet M, Lucking CB, Goas JY, Durif F, Abada M, Echenne B, Motte J, Lagueny A, Lacomblez L, Jedynak P, Bartholome B, Agid Y, Brice A (2000). Levodopa-responsive dystonia. GTP cyclohydrolase I or parkin mutations? *Brain* **123:**1112–1121.

The National Institute for Clinical Excellence. Selective peripheral denervation of cervical dystonia (2004). http://www.nice.org.uk

Tolosa E, Montserrat L, Bayes A (1988). Blink reflex studies in focal dystonias: enhanced excitability of brainstem interneurons in cranial dystonia and spasmodic torticollis. *Mov Disord* **3:**61–69.

Valente EM, Warner TT, Jarman PR, Mathen D, Fletcher NA, Marsden CD, Bhatia KP, Wood N W (1998). The role of DYT1 in primary torsion dystonia in Europe. *Brain* **121:** 2335–2339.

Valente EM, Edwards MJ, Mir P, Digiorgio A, Salvi S, Davis M, Russo N, Bozi M, Kim HT, Pennisi G, Quinn N, Dallapiccola B, Bhatia KP (2005). The epsilon-sarcoglycan gene in myoclonic syndromes. *Neurology* **64:**737–739.

van der KW, Berardelli A, Rothwell JC, Thompson PD, Day BL, Marsden CD (1989). Rapid elbow movements in patients with torsion dystonia. *J Neurol Neurosurg Psych* **52:**1043–1049.

Vidailhet M, Tassin J, Durif F, Nivelon-Chevallier A, Agid Y, Brice A, Durr A (2001). A major locus for several phenotypes of myoclonus–dystonia on chromosome 7q. *Neurology* **56:** 1213–1216.

Vidailhet M, Vercueil L, Houeto JL, Krystkowiak P, Benabid AL, Cornu P, Lagrange C, Tezenas du MS, Dormont D, Grand S, Blond S, Detante O, Pillon B, Ardouin C, Agid Y, Destee A, Pollak P (2005). Bilateral deep-brain stimulation of the globus pallidus in primary generalized dystonia. *New England J Med* **352:**459–467.

Watts CC, Whurr R, Nye C (2004). Botulinum toxin injections for the treatment of spasmodic dysphonia. *Cochrane Database Syst Rev* p. CD004327.

Whitaker J, Butler A, Semlyen JK, Barnes MP (2001). Botulinum toxin for people with dystonia treated by an outreach nurse practitioner: a comparative study between a home and a clinic treatment service. *Arch Phys Med Rehabil* **82:**480–484.

Yianni J, Bain P, Giladi N, Auca M, Gregory R, Joint C, Nandi D, Stein J, Scott R, Aziz T (2003). Globus pallidus internus deep brain stimulation for dystonic conditions: a prospective audit. *Mov Disord* **18:**436–442.

Yoshor D, Hamilton WJ, Ondo W, Jankovic J, Grossman RG (2001). Comparison of thalamotomy and pallidotomy for the treatment of dystonia. *Neurosurgery* **48:**818–824.

CHAPTER 16

Mild traumatic brain injury

P.E. Vos,[a] Yuri Alekseenko,[b] L. Battistin,[c]
G. Birbamer,[d] F. Gerstenbrand,[d] A. Potapov,[e]
T. Prevec,[f] Ch.A. Stepan,[g] P. Traubner,[h]
A. Twijnstra,[i] L. Vecsei,[j] K. von Wild[k]

Abstract

Background The incidence of traumatic brain injury (TBI) is high, varying between 229 and 1967 per 100 000, with the highest incidence occurring in men, aged 15–24 years. Approximately 90–95% of all TBIs are considered mild. Intracranial complications of mild traumatic brain injury (MTBI) are infrequent but potentially life-threatening, and may require neurosurgical intervention in a minority of cases (0.2–3.1%). Hence, a true health management problem exists because of the need to exclude the small chance of a life-threatening complication in large numbers of individual patients.

Objective To construct from the literature acceptable evidence-based guidelines for initial management with respect to ancillary investigations, hospital admission, observation, and follow-up after MTBI.

Methods Systematic review.

Results A systematic review of the literature revealed risk factors with sufficient sensitivity to predict the presence of intracranial complications (evidence Level I–IV) including Glasgow Coma Scale Score at the time of hospital admission, presence of persistent anterograde amnesia, retrograde amnesia longer than 30 min, trauma above the clavicles including facial or cranial soft tissue injury and clinical signs of skull fracture (skull base- or depressed skull fracture), severe headache, nausea, vomiting (≥2 times), focal neurological deficit, cranial nerve deficit, motor deficit, dysphasia, seizure, age, coagulation disorders, high-energy accident (dangerous mechanism of injury) and intoxication with alcohol/drugs.

Conclusion The guidelines in this paper present evidence for the importance of careful neurological

[a]Department of Neurology, Radboud University Nijmegen Medical Centre; [b]Department of Neurology and Neurosurgery, Vitebsk Medical University, Vitebsk, Belarus; [c]Clinica Neurologica I, Padova, Italy; [d]Ludwig Boltzmann Institute for Restorative Neurology and Neuromodulation, Vienna, Austria; [e]Institute of Neurosurgery, Russian Academy of Medical Sciences, Moscow, Russia; [f]University Institute of Clinical neurophysiology, University Medical Centre, Ljubljana, Slovenia; [g]Neurological Hospital Rosenhügel, Vienna, Austria; [h]Department of Neurology, Comenius University School of Medicine, Bratislava, Slovak Republic; [i]Department of Neurology, University Medical Centre Maastricht, The Netherlands; [j]Department of Neurology, Szent-Györgyi University Hospital, Szeged, Hungary; [k]Medical Faculty Westphalien University Münster and of functional neurorehabilitation and re-engineering of brain and spinal cord lesions at the International Neuroscience Institute INI Hanover, Germany.

examination, assessment of trauma history, recognition of risk factors and use of CT to detect all intracranial complications after MTBI.

Background

Trauma of the head can cause brain injury (Denny-Brown and Russell, 1941; Frowein and Firsching, 1990) and is a common cause of morbidity and mortality (Kraus *et al.*, 1996). After mild traumatic brain injury (MTBI), that is, patients with a hospital admission Glasgow Coma Score (GCS) of 13–15) (Teasdale and Jennett, 1974), mortality, almost exclusively caused by intracranial haemorrhage, is very low (between 0.04 and 0.29%) (Klauber *et al.*, 1989; af Geijerstam and Britton, 2003). The International Classification of Diseases (ICD-10) classifies acute traumatic brain injury (TBI) as S-02, S-04, S-06, S-07, S-09 in combination with dizziness or vomiting, retrograde or anterograde amnesia, impaired consciousness, skull fracture, and/or focal neurological impairment (Bellner *et al.*, 2003). As the incidence of TBI is high, varying between 229 and 1967 per 100 000, with the highest incidence occurring in men, aged 15–24 years (Jennet, 1996; Kraus *et al.*, 1996; von Wild and Wenzlaff, 2005) and 90–95% of all TBIs are considered mild, formal evidence-based clinical decision rules are warranted (Haydel *et al.*, 2000; Meerhoff *et al.*, 2000; Stiell *et al.*, 2001). There are practically no Class I and II data on TBI management in the literature. These guidelines try to provide a set of rules aimed at early recognition of symptoms and signs known to increase the risk of development of an intracranial haemorrhage after MTBI (Krau *et al.*, 1996; Jennet, 1996; Stiell *et al.*, 2001).

Search strategy

The Task Force systematically searched the English literature in the medline, EMBASE, Cochrane database (1966–2005) using the key words 'minor head injury', 'mild head injury', 'mild traumatic brain injury', 'traumatic brain injury', 'guidelines' and 'management'. Additional articles were identified from the bibliographies of the articles retrieved (including those in the German language), and from textbooks. Articles were included if they contained data on the classification system used (i.e. admission GCS 13–15) and outcome data (CT abnormalities, need for neurosurgical intervention, mortality) or management. Articles judged to be of historical value were also included. Initially, 540 articles were retrieved. Articles were reviewed by one author (PEV). For the purpose of this report, a total of 109 papers were finally included. Additional information can be found on the European Federation of Neurological Societies (EFNS) website. Where appropriate, a classification of evidence level (EL) was given for interventions, diagnostic tests, and grades of recommendation for management according to the neurological management guidelines of the EFNS (Brainin *et al.*, 2004). Where there was a lack of evidence but consensus was clear we have stated our opinion as Good Practice Points (GPP).

Mechanisms of traumatic brain injury

Focal impact or contact injuries may cause closed and open skull fractures, extradural haematoma, subdural haematoma, cortical contusion, rupture of the dura mater with CSF leakage and/or prolaps of brain tissue. Direct collisional forces acting on the skull might compress the underlying tissue structures (coup) or of tissue remote from the site of the impact (contre-coup) (Pudenz and Shelden, 1946; Sellier, 1963).

Impact to the head *per se* is not mandatory to evoke brain dysfunction or brain damage. Except for skull fracture and extradural haematoma, all types of brain injury can be produced by (angular) acceleration of the head without impact, provided that there is a period of loss of consciousness (Gennarelli *et al.*, 1982; Birbamer *et al.*, 1994). Shear forces generated in the brain upon sudden rotation may cause damage to axons and blood vessels (Houlbourn, 1943; Gennarelli, 1983; Grcevic, 1988; Gerstenbrand and Stepan, 2001). Controversy exists whether diffuse brain dysfunction can occur in MTBI without there being structural damage (Trotter, 1924; Spatz, 1936).

Classification of mild traumatic brain injury

Many terms exist to describe and define MTBI (Frowein and Firsching, 1990; Williams *et al.*, 1990; Evans, 1992; Pople *et al.*, 1993; Birbamer *et al.*, 1994; Stein and Spettell, 1995; Teasdale, 1995; Culotta *et al.*, 1996; Gomez *et al.*, 1996; Saab *et al.*, 1996; Arienta *et al.*, 1997; Ingebrigsten, *et al.*, 2000; Gerstenbrand and Stepan, 2001; von Wild and Terwey, 2001; Stepan *et al.*, 2001). Here, a classification for MTBI is proposed based on admission GCS, trauma history (i.e., the duration of loss of consciousness [LOC] and post-traumatic amnesia [PTA]), age, neurological signs and symptoms), and risk factors for intracranial complications. Several sub-classifications are recognized to facilitate initial management decisions (Recommendation Level B) (table 16.1, figure 16.1).

RECOMMENDATIONS

MTBI is defined as the consequence of blunt (non-penetrating) impact with sudden acceleration, deceleration, or rotation of the head (ICD-10 codes: S-02, S-04, S-06, S-07, S-09) with a GCS score of 13–15 at the time of hospital admission (table 16.1).

Admission GCS

The risk of intracranial complications and the need for neurosurgical interventions are inversely related to the admission GCS (Gomez *et al.*, 1996; Culotta *et al.*, 1996). Reported rates depend on the definition of neurosurgical intervention and vary between 0.6 and 13% in patients with an admission GCS of 15 to 25–37.5% in patients with an admission GCS of 13 (Teasdale *et al.*, 1990; Stein and Ross, 1992; Stein *et al.*, 1995; Gomez *et al.*, 1996; Culotta *et al.*, 1996; Dunham *et al.*, 1996; Haydel *et al.*, 2000; Steill *et al.*, 2001; af Geijerstam and Britton, 2003). A meta-analysis in patients with a GCS=15 found a complication rate (CI), defined as neurosurgical procedure, medical treatment of brain oedema, start of intracranial pressure monitoring or transfer to intensive care,

Table 16.1 Classification of traumatic brain injury.

Classification	Admission Glasgow Coma Scale Score (GCS) and clinical characteristics modified from the Dutch, Scandinavian and American classification systems (Maas *et al.*, 1997; Stein and Spettell, 1995; Ingebrigsten *et al.*, 2000; Twijnstra *et al.*, 2001)
Mild	GCS = 13–15
Category	
0	GCS = 15 No LOC, no PTA = head injury, no TBI No risk factors
1	GCS = 15 LOC < 30 min, PTA < 1 h No risk factors
2	GCS = 15 and risk factors present*
3	GCS = 13–14 With or without risk factors present*
Moderate	GCS = 9–12
Severe	GCS ≤ 8
Critical	GCS = 3–4, with loss of pupillary reactions and absent or decerebrate motor reactions

Abbreviations: TBI, traumatic brain injury; GCS, Glasgow Coma Scale; LOC, loss of consciousness; PTA, post-traumatic amnesia.
*Risk factors are shown in table 16.2.

of 0.9 (0.6–1.2)% (5). The time between the accident and hospital admission can influence the GCS (Jennett, 1996; Haydel *et al.*, 2000; Stiell *et al.*, 2001). The GCS is also the most frequently used scoring tool in children; however, it is less appropriate for very young children whose motor and verbal skills are not yet fully developed, and for this reason alternative scales have been developed (Reilly *et al.*, 1988; Simpson *et al.*, 1991; Durham *et al.*, 2000).

Duration of loss of consciousness

Verification of whether LOC has occurred and assessment of the duration of LOC are essential because LOC increases the risk of intracranial complications (EL = Class III) (Teasdale *et al.*, 1990; Stein and Spettell, 1995; Gomez *et al.*, 1996).

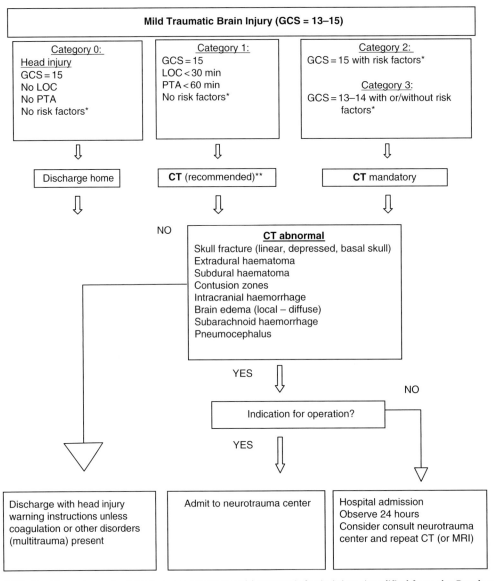

Figure 16.1. Decision scheme for initial management in mild traumatic brain injury (modified from the Dutch and Scandinavian guidelines) (Ingebrigtsen et al., 2000; Twijnstra et al., 2001)
GCS, Glasgow Coma Scale; LOC, loss of consciousness; PTA, post-traumatic amnesia; TBI, traumatic brain injury; CT, computed tomography; MRI, magnetic resonance imaging. *Risk factors are shown in table 16.2. **If CT availability is limited, conventional skull radiography can be performed but the sensitivity and specificity for intracranial abnormalities is unacceptably low.

Compatible with a diagnosis of MTBI are LOC duration times of 5–30 min (Rimel et al., 1981; Williams et al., 1990; Evans, 1992; Hahn and McLone, 1993; Mild Traumatic Brain Injury Committee, 1993; Gomez et al., 1996; Jennett, 1996; Haydel et al., 2000; Ingebrigsten et al., 2000). Although LOC increases the risk of intracranial complications, long-term outcome is not necessarily adversely affected by a short period of LOC. In children, a 100% good outcome was found if LOC was less than 15 min (Hahn and McLeone, 1993) (EL = II). Also, the number of post-traumatic subjective complaints, neurocognitive performance, and pre-existing emotional risk factors does not correlate with the duration of LOC (EL = II) (Ruff and Jurica, 1999). A duration of altered consciousness of less than 15–30 min can be considered as mild (EL = IV) (Jennett, 1996).

RECOMMENDATIONS

A duration of LOC of 30 minutes maximum is considered compatible with MTBI (Level B).

PTA

Post-traumatic (or anterograde) amnesia is the period of inability to lay down continuous memories (amnesic for ongoing events) and is often characterised by confusion (Levin et al., 1979; Tate et al., 2000). A distinction is usually made between disorientation and amnesia because the two do not always disappear at the same time (Tate et al., 2000). Retrograde amnesia is the loss of memory for the period before the accident.

Failure to reach GCS 15 within 2 h post injury and deficits in short-term memory increase the risk of intracranial complications (table 16.2) (Haydel et al., 2000; Stiell et al., 2001). Retrograde amnesia >30 min increases the risk for neurological intervention (Stiell et al., 2001).

RECOMMENDATIONS

If the duration of LOC is maximally 30 min and PTA is less than 1 h, outcome is considered good (mortality 0.1%) especially in the absence of risk factors (Level B).

Of note is that the presence of PTA is synonymous with a GCS of 14 in patients with an otherwise normal GCS score.

Risk factors

Several symptoms, signs and risk factors associated with an increased risk of intracranial injury have been identified (EL = I-III) (See table 16.2 for overview) (Masters et al., 1987; Chan et al., 1990; Arienta et al., 1997; Haydel et al., 2000; Stiell et al., 2001).

RECOMMENDATIONS

Recognition of risk factors is important and such factors should be included in a classification system to further assess the risk of immediate complications (intracranial haemorrhage) (Level B).

Complications
Intracranial abnormalities

Post-traumatic intracerebral complications can be divided into: (1) Intracranial (mass) lesions, that is, abnormalities that (often) need neurosurgical intervention (extracerebral haematoma, depressed skull fracture, growing skull fracture, secondary haemorrhagic contusion, subdural effusions, malignant brain oedema with diffuse brain swelling). (2) Intracranial lesions that are treated conservatively (contusion zones, brain oedema, diffuse axonal injury, small haemorrhages, traumatic subarachnoid haemorrhage, pneumocephalus) (Teasdale et al., 1990; Lloyd et al., 1997; Ingebrigsten et al., 2000).

Computerised Tomography (CT) is very sensitive in the detection of extracerebral haematoma and other intracranial abnormalities and is the gold standard in imaging acute TBI, although no formal CT classification for MTBI exists. The incidence of intracranial abnormalities varies with the definitions used, the clinical inclusion criteria, and the radiography method used (Stein et al., 1995; Culotta et al., 1996). Normal CT findings may predict the absence of late disease progression. The negative predictive value of a normal CT for neurosurgical intervention was 100% in a study involving 2032 patients and 99.7% in a study of 2124 patients (EL = Class II) (Dunham et al., 1996; Livingston et al., 2000).

Table 16.2 Risk factors for intracranial complications after MTBI.

Reference	Risk factor	Level of evidence	N	Follow up	% CT	Endpoint
	Glasgow Coma Scale Score					
Stiell *et al.*, 2001	GCS < 15 at 2 h after injury	II	3121	14 day telephone interview	67	[1]Neurosurgery, CT
	Continued post-traumatic amnesia*					
Haydel *et al.*, 2000	Persistent anterograde amnesia	I	1429	Discharge	100	CT
	Retrograde amnesia longer than 30 min					
Stiell *et al.*, 2001	Amnesia before impact	II	3121	14 day telephone interview	67	[1]Neurosurgery, CT
	Trauma above the clavicles including clinical signs of skull fracture					
	(skull base- or depressed skull fracture)					
Haydel *et al.*, 2000	Any external evidence of injury including contusions, abrasions, lacerations, deformities, and signs of facial or skull fracture	I	1429	Discharge	100	CT
Borczuk 1995	Cranial or facial injury	III	1448	—	100	CT
Madden *et al.*, 1995	Facial injury- signs of basilar skull fracture, depressed skull fracture	II	813	—	100	CT
Miller *et al.*, 1997	Signs of depressed skull fracture	I	2143	Discharge	100	[2]Neurosurgery, CT
Jeret *et al.*, 1993	Signs of basilar skull fracture	II	712	Discharge	100	[3]Neurosurgery, CT
Stiell *et al.*, 2001	Signs of basal skull fracture or depressed skull fracture	II	3121	14 day telephone interview	67	[1]Neurosurgery, CT
Dunham *et al.*, 1996	Cranial soft tissue injury	II	2252	?	91.3	CT
	Headache					
Haydel *et al.*, 2000	Any	I	1429	Discharge	100	CT
Miller *et al.*, 1997	Severe headache	I	2143	Discharge	100	[2]Neurosurgery, CT
	Nausea					
Miller *et al.*, 1997	n.d.	I	2143	Discharge	100	[2]Neurosurgery, CT
	Vomiting					
Miller *et al.*, 1997	n.d	I	2143	Discharge	100	[2]Neurosurgery, CT
Haydel *et al.*, 2000	Any	I	1429	Discharge	100	CT
Stiell *et al.*, 2001	≥ 2 times	II	3121	14 day telephone interview	67	[1]Neurosurgery, CT
	Focal neurological deficit					
Gomez *et al.*, 1996	Cranial nerve deficit, motor deficit, dysphasia	III	2484	—	7.5	[4]Neurosurgery, CT
	Seizure					
Haydel *et al.*, 2000	Suspected or witnessed seizure after the event	I	1429	Discharge	100	CT

Table 16.2 Contd.

Reference	Risk factor	Level of evidence	N	Follow up	% CT	Endpoint
	Age					
Masters et al., 1987	<2 years	IV	7035	National Health Statistics	?	Intracranial injury
Haydel et al., 2000	>60 years	I	1429	Discharge	100	CT
Stiell et al., 2001	>65 years	II	3121	14 day telephone interview	67	[1]Neurosurgery, CT
Gomez et al., 1996	Linear	IV	2484	—	7.5	[4]Neurosurgery, CT
	Coagulation disorders					
Fabbri et al., 2004	Warfarin	III	501	instructions	100	CT
Li et al., 2001	Warfarin	IV	144	—	100	CT
	High-energy accident**					
Stiell et al., 2001	Dangerous mechanism of injury	II	3121	14 day telephone interview	67	[1]Neurosurgery, CT
Jeret et al., 1993	Pedestrian hit by car or victim of assault	II	712	Discharge	100	[3]Neurosurgery, CT
	Intoxication with alcohol/drugs					
Haydel et al., 2000	Alcohol or drugs	I	1429	Discharge	100	CT

*Continued post-traumatic amnesia may be interpreted as a GCS verbal reaction of 4 and hence be defined as GCS <15.
**According to Advanced Trauma Life Support principles, a high-energy (vehicle) accident is defined as initial speed >64 km/h, major auto-deformity, intrusion into passenger compartment >30 cm, extrication time from vehicle >20 min, falls >6 m, roll over, auto–pedestrian accidents, or motor cycle crash >32 km/h or with separation of rider and bike (American College of Surgeons, 1997; Bartlett et al., 1998). Neurosurgery defined as: [1]death within 7 days, craniotomy, elevation of skull fracture, intracranial pressure monitoring or intubation for head injury; [2]craniotomy, or placing of monitoring bolt; [3]death or craniotomy; [4]craniotomy, elevation of depressed skull fracture, ICP monitoring.

> ## RECOMMENDATIONS
>
> CT is the gold standard for the detection of intracranial abnormalities (Level B). The term post-traumatic intracranial complication includes all extracerebral, and intracerebral abnormalities in relation to head trauma that can be visualized on CT and that are likely to be the result of the head trauma (Level C).

Neurosurgical intervention

Absolute indications for emergency decompressive neurosurgical intervention are signs and symptoms of an existing or rapidly developing intracranial mass lesion including deterioration of consciousness, functional motor impairment and brain stem compression signs. Intracranial haemorrhage (extradural or subdural) often needing quick neurosurgical intervention occurs in 0.2–3.1 % (Stein and Ross, 1992; Shackford et al., 1992; Borczuk, 1995; Culotta et al., 1996; Dunham et al., 1996; Hsiang et al., 1997; Haydel et al., 2000; Steill et al., 2001; af Geijerstam and Britton, 2003).

The mortality of MTBI, after systemic (multiple) injuries are excluded, is very low and is almost exclusively caused by the late or missed diagnosis of deterioration in patients with an intracranial haemorrhage (specifically an extradural haematoma) (EL = II-III) (Mendelow et al., 1979; Klauber et al., 1989; Shackford et al., 1992; Culotta et al., 1996; Dunham et al., 1996; Gomez et al., 1996; Jennett, 1996; Mendelow and Bartlett, 1998; Servadei et al., 2001; Stiell et al., 2001). The prognosis of extradural haematoma is good, especially when it is detected early in fully conscious patients and surgery is performed as soon as possible (Paterniti et al., 1994; Servadei et al., 1995; Servadei, 1997). However, when rapid neurological deterioration occurs or when patients are already in coma, mortality rises sharply with the delay between deterioration and surgery (EL = III) (Mendelow et al., 1979; Seelig et al., 1984; Servadei, 1997).

Growing skull fractures are rare (frequency 0.05–0.6%). It is most likely to occur in children younger than 6 years old, when a dural tear beneath a skull fracture is present. Neurosurgical treatment is mandatory when systolic–diastolic pulsations result in widening of the fracture margins and interposition of leptomeninges or brain tissue into the fracture. It is mentioned here as a long-term complication that occurs if early diagnosis and intervention are deferred.

RECOMMENDATIONS

The primary goal of initial management in MTBI is to identify the patients at risk of intracranial abnormalities and especially those that may need neurosurgical intervention. Use of a clinical decision scheme based on risk factors may facilitate this process (Level B) (see figure 16.1).

The extracerebral haemorrhage (extradural haematoma) is potentially the most threatening complication after MTBI (Level B). An extradural haematoma can be easily identified with CT, which should be carried out urgently (Level B).

Seizures

Patients with MTBI have only a slightly increased risk of developing post-traumatic seizures including early post-traumatic seizures (= a seizure occurring in the first week) (Schierhout and Roberts, 1997;

Annegers et al., 1998). Prophylactic antiepileptic treatment is not warranted. A systematic review of randomised controlled trials including 2036 patients showed that prophylactic antiepileptic treatment did not reduce mortality, neurological disability, or late seizures (EL = I) (Schierhout and Roberts, 1998). If recurrent seizures occur, treatment is probably necessary and alternative explanations (i.e. delayed haematoma, Wernicke-Korsakoff syndrome, alcohol withdrawal or electrolyte disturbances) should be taken into account.

RECOMMENDATIONS

Prophylactic antiepileptic treatment is not indicated (Level A).

Skull base fracture

A skull base or temporal bone fracture or open fracture increases the risk of cerebrospinal fluid (CSF) leakage and CSF fistula formation (Dagi et al., 1983; Brodie, 1997; Brodie and Thompson, 1997). The reported incidence of CSF leakage after basal skull fracture varies from approximately 10 to 20%, and the incidence of bacterial meningitis from 2 to 50% (Leech and Paterson, 1973; Dagi et al., 1983; Helling et al., 1988; Marion, 1991; Brodie, 1997; Brodie and Thompson, 1997). The role of antibiotic prophylaxis in open or basilar skull fractures remains controversial; the conclusions of two recent meta-analysis on the prophylactic use of antibiotics were contradictory (Demetriades et al., 1992; Working Party of the British Society for Antimicrobial Chemotherapy, 1994; Brodie, 1997; Villalobos, 1998).

RECOMMENDATIONS

There is insufficient proof for prophylactic antibiotic treatment against meningitis in patients with clinical signs of a skull base fracture (Level C).

Patients on anticoagulation

No randomised clinical trials exist on the discontinuation of anticoagulation therapy after head injury. The scarce available literature shows conflicting results. Post hoc analysis of a large Italian cohort with mild head injury showed increased odds of coagulopathy for intracranial abnormalities as shown with CT (Fabbri *et al.*, 2004). Retrospective studies concluded that elderly patients on warfarin may have an increased risk for intracranial haemorrhage as well as equal morbidity and mortality after head injury (Kennedy *et al.*, 2000; Karni *et al.*, 2001).

The question what to do in a patient under anticoagulation for a cardiovascular cause and with an intracranial haematoma is hence not easy to answer. The indications for antiocoagulation and the underlying cardiovascular disease should be reviewed. A retrospective study in 39 patients with intracranial haemorrhage and mechanical heart valves without previous evidence of systemic embolization revealed that discontinuation of warfarin therapy for 1 to 2 weeks had a low probability of embolic events (Wijdicks *et al.*, 1998). It is uncertain however if these findings are applicable to head injury patients on anticoagulation therapy.

GOOD PRACTICE POINTS

All patients with head injury should be questioned about the use of anticoagulation therapy (Level C). All patients with head injury on anticoagulation therapy should have their international normalized ratio (INR) checked and the indication for anticoagulation reviewed (Level C). These patients should be admitted for neurological observation (Level C) (Saab *et al.*, 1996). If CT demonstrates an intracranial haematoma, the INR should be corrected immediately. (Over-) anticoagulation can be best corrected with fresh frozen plasma and vitamin K. If spontaneous coagulation disorders or additional injuries with bleeding exist consultation of a coagulation specialist should be sought (Good Practice Point).

Ancillary investigations

Skull radiography versus CT

The diagnostic value of plain skull radiography(Masters *et al.*, 1987; Teasdale *et al.*, 1990; Mendelow *et al.* 1983; Borczuk 1995; Mendelow and Bartlett 1998; Nee *et al.* 1999) is now considered insufficient to demonstrate intracranial complications (Masters *et al.*, 1987; Teasdale *et al.*, 1990). Mendelow *et al.* (1983), Borczuk (1995), Mendelow and Bartlett (1998) and Nee *et al.* (1999). showed that sSkull radiography is of little value in the initial assessment of MTBI (EL = I) (Hofman *et al.*, 2000). A meta-analysis of 13 studies, in which at least 50a CT of the brain, showed that the estimated sensitivity of radiographic evidence of skull fracture for a diagnosis of intracranial haemorrhage was only 0.38 with a corresponding specificity of 0.95 (EL = 1) (Hofman *et al.*, 2000).

RECOMMENDATIONS

Skull radiography is of insufficient value in the detection of intracranial abnormalities in patients with MTBI (Level A).

Clinical decision rules for CT

Two large prospective studies investigated a clinical decision rule for use of CT to demonstrate the need for neurosurgical intervention or clinically important brain injury after MTBI (Haydel *et al.*, 2000; Stiell *et al.*, 2001). In a North-American prospective study involving 1429 patients with minor head injury (defined as LOC and an admission GCS of 15), seven predictors (headache, vomiting, seizure, PTA, trauma above the clavicles, drug or alcohol intoxication, or age over 60 years) were retrieved after Chi-square analysis and determination of likelihood ratios for each criterion. This model showed 100% (95% CI: 95–100%) sensitivity for intracranial complications.

In a Canadian prospective multicentre study involving 3121 patients with minor head injury (defined as blunt trauma with LOC and/or amnesia or disorientation and initial ED GCS = 13–15),

250 patients (8%) had clinically important brain injury and 31(1%) required neurosurgical intervention. Five high-risk factors (failure to reach GCS of 15 within 2 h, suspected open skull fracture, any signs of basal skull fracture, vomiting >2 episodes, or age >65 years) were derived which had 100% sensitivity (95% CI: 92–100%) for predicting the need for neurosurgical intervention (Stiell *et al.*, 2001). Interestingly, this would lead to a CT ordering proportion of 32%. In addition, two medium-risk factors (amnesia before impact >30 min and dangerous mechanism of injury) were 98.4% sensitive (95% CI 96–99%) and 49.6% specific for predicting clinically important brain damage. This would lead to a CT ordering proportion of 54%. Both studies concluded that in patients with MTBI the use of CT can be safely limited to those who have certain clinical findings (Haydel *et al.*, 2000; Stiell *et al.*, 2001). However the generalisability of existing guidelines has been questioned. In an independent sample of 1101 patients, the reliability (detection of intracranial abnormalities) of 11 existing guidelines was lower than described in the original studies (Ibanez *et al.*, 2004).

RECOMMENDATIONS

CT is a gold standard for the detection of life-threatening (and other intracranial) abnormalities after MTBI and is recommended in those with documented LOC and/or PTA and is considered mandatory in all patients with certain clinical findings (GCS = 13–14, or GCS = 15 in the presence of risk factors) (Level B).

Clinical decisions for MRI

Cerebral MRI is not routinely used in TBI. The relationship between intracranial abnormalities on MRI and outcome is not entirely clear, and more research is needed (Voller *et al.*, 2001). When early MRI (within 21 days from the injury) and late MRI (between 5 and 18 months) findings were compared in patients with mild, moderate or severe TBI, measures of neuropsychological outcome correlated with late MRI findings only (Wilson *et al.*, 1988).

RECOMMENDATIONS

MRI may be of value for the detection of structural brain damage in patients without CT abnormalities, and especially in those with long-term complaints (Level B).

PET and SPECT-examination

Positron emission tomography (PET) and technetium ^{99m}-hexa-methylpropyleneamineoxime SPECT may show abnormalities in the acute and chronic stages when CT or MRI and neurological examination do not show damage (Ichise *et al.*, 1994; Jacobs *et al.*, 1994; Ruff *et al.*, 1994). Normal SPECT findings within 1–4 weeks after mild and moderate TBI predicted good outcome after 1 year, with a negative predictive value of 97% (Jacobs *et al.*, 1994). The specificity of abnormal findings, however, has been questioned (Alexander, 1998). Similar patterns of hypometabolism in the frontopolar and lateral temporal cortices and the basal ganglia have been reported among patients with depression but no injury (Mayberg, 1994; Dolan *et al.*, 1994).

RECOMMENDATIONS

No recommendations for the use of PET or SPECT in the initial phase after MTBI can be given at present.

Biochemical markers of traumatic brain injury

Brain-specific proteins, in particular S100β and neuron-specific enolase, may be released into the circulation after TBI. Serum levels of S100β are higher in patients with intracranial pathology and correlate with clinical outcome and the severity of primary and secondary brain damage (EL = II)

(Raabe *et al.*, 1999; Romner *et al.*, 2000). Unde-tectable or normal serum levels of S100β are predic-tive of normal intracranial findings on CT, and thus S100β could be used to select patients for CT after MTBI (Class II) (Romner *et al.*, 2000; Biberthaler *et al.*, 2004). These results have to be confirmed in large prospective studies. Although this finding has already been questioned: normal serum S100β levels may be present after epidural haematoma (Unden *et al.*, 2005). In the future, this may be of relevance in the medical–legal context to prove that the acute symptoms and signs and/or the long-term disability or neuropsychological impair-ments after MTBI are indeed a consequence of structural brain damage or of psychological stress in reaction to the event, alcohol intoxication, pre-existent disorders, systemic injury, or other causes (see also Romner *et al.*, 2000).

RECOMMENDATIONS

The study of biochemical markers of MTBI is of considerable interest (especially the negative pre-dictive value of normal serum concentrations for the absence of intracranial abnormalities), but at present no recommendations can be given and more research is needed (Level B).

Initial patient management

According to the Advanced Trauma Life Sup-port (ATLS) guidelines, any patient with trauma should be evaluated for surgical trauma (EL = III) (American College of Surgeons, 1997). Proper triage includes assessing the airways, breathing, and circulation, and the cervical spine. A neurolog-ical examination is obligatory and should include level of consciousness, presence of anterograde or retrograde amnesia and disorientation, higher cog-nitive functions, presence of focal neurological deficit (asymmetrical motor reactions or reflexes, unilateral paresis or cranial nerve deficit), pupillary responses, blood pressure, and pulse rate (Valadka and Narayan, 1996; Ingebrigsten *et al.*, 2000; Tate *et al.*, 2000). In addition, the presence of frontal lobe signs, cerebellar symptoms, or sensory deficits should be actively investigated.

GOOD PRACTICE POINTS

Following acute TBI all patients should undergo urgent neurological examination, in addition to a surgical examination. Furthermore, accurate history taking (including medication), preferably with information being obtained from a witness of the accident or personnel involved in first-aid procedures outside the hospital, is important to ascertain the circumstances (mechanism of injury) under which the accident took place and to assess the duration of LOC and amnesia (Good Practice Point).

An algorithm for the initial management of MTBI is given in figure 16.1.

RECOMMENDATIONS

Hospitals should have a protocol for resuscitation and triage of patients with MTBI (Level C). Cat-egory 2 and 3 patients should be admitted to a neurotrauma centre. All children with MTBI should be seen by a paediatrician or a child neurolo-gist (Level C). CT is recommended for category 1 patients and is mandatory for all category 2 and 3 patients (see figure 16.1) (Level B)*. If CT find-ings are normal, adult category 1 patients can be discharged and head injury warning instruc-tions should be given to the patient and family members. Compliance is greater if both verbal and written instructions are given (EL = III) (de Louw *et al.*, 1994; Valadka and Narayan, 1996; Ingebrig-sten *et al.*, 2000). A repeat CT should be considered if the admission CT findings were abnormal or if risk factors are present (table 16.2) (Level C).

  *Note: If CT availability is limited, conventional skull radiography can be performed but because of low sensitivity and specificity for intracranial abnor-malities it is insufficient for patient management.

Clinical observation

Another issue is the necessity for and duration of neurological observation after MTBI. Patients in category 1 can be discharged to home with head injury warning instructions if CT findings are normal (Appendix available on the web site of the EFNS: http://www.efns.org/) (Warren and Kissoon, 1989; Ward *et al.*, 1992; Valadka and Narayan, 1996). Patients in category 2 or 3 should preferably be admitted to the hospital for observation, although the necessity of this can be questioned in some patients in category 2 (e.g. patients older then 60 years of age who are not on anticoagulation therapy). Most guidelines recommend an observation period of minimally 12–24 h (Masters *et al.*, 1987; Bartlett *et al.*, 1998; American Academy of Pediatrics, 1999; Ingebrigsten *et al.*, 2000; Twijnstra *et al.*, 2001). The main goal of clinical observation is to detect, at an early stage, the development of extradural or subdural haematoma or diffuse cerebral oedema. A secondary goal is to determine the duration of PTA.

An extradural haematoma usually develops within 6 h, and thus the initial CT may be false negative when performed very early (within 1 h) (Frowein *et al.*, 1989; Smith and Miller 1991; Servadei *et al.*, 1995). Repeated neurological observation (see above) is therefore obligatory for the timely detection of clinical deterioration and other neurological deficits (such as sensory deficits, frontal lobe signs, cerebellar symptoms, etc.).

RECOMMENDATIONS

A complete neurological examination is mandatory after admission and should include assessment of the GCS. Repeat neurological examination should be carried out, its frequency being dependent on the clinical condition of the patient. The patient should be examined every 30 min and if no complications or deterioration occurs, every 1–2 h. The use of a neurological checklist may be helpful to document the neurological condition and its course. If deterioration occurs, possible intracranial causes should be evaluated with (repeated) CT (Level C).

Rules for bed rest

No randomised trials exist on the value and duration of bed rest and on the duration of sick leave after MTBI. A survey among various European hospitals showed major differences in management with regard to the ordering (and duration) of bed rest, home observation, sick leave, and follow-up examination (de Kruijk *et al.*, 2001). When patients were randomised for complete bed rest (for a period of 6 days) versus no bedrest no treatment effect was found on the number of post traumatic complaints and quality of life 6 months after the trauma (de Kruijk *et al.*, 2002). Graded resumption of activities after discharge and follow-up may beneficially influence the recovery process (EL = IV) (Alexander, 1995; Kibby and Long, 1997; Ingebrigsten *et al.*, 1998).

RECOMMENDATIONS

No recommendations can be given for the need for or duration of bed rest. Early graded resumption of activities (including return to work) is probably the best strategy (Level B).

Follow-up

It has been shown that regular specialised outpatient follow-up visits are effective in reducing social morbidity and the severity of symptoms after MTBI (Wade *et al.*, 1998). In a large randomised controlled trial, patients with a PTA shorter than 7 days who received specialist intervention had significantly less social disability and fewer post-concussion symptoms 6 months after injury than those who did not receive the service (EL = II) (Wade *et al.*, 1998).

RECOMMENDATIONS

It is recommended that all patients in MTBI category 3 who have been admitted to hospital should be seen at least once in the outpatient clinic in the first 2 weeks after discharge (Level C) (Wade *et al.*, 1998). Patients who are discharged immediately with head injury instructions should contact their general practitioners, who can decide to refer the patient to the neurologist if complaints persist (Level C).

Conclusions

The guidelines presented in this paper stress the importance of careful neurological examination, assessment of trauma history and extensive use of CT. Moreover, the use of a clinical decision rule for CT and hospital admission after MTBI may increase the use of CT compared with other existing protocols.

CT is the preferred imaging method for MTBI even though MRI is more sensitive. As MRI becomes more widely available, it may have a greater role in the evaluation of more subtle intracranial abnormalities in patients with MTBI (Haydel *et al.*, 2000; Voller *et al.*, 2001).

Conflicts of interest

The authors declare that they have no conflict of interest regarding this Chapter.

References

af Geijerstam JL, Britton M (2003). Mild head injury - mortality and complication rate: meta-analysis of findings in a systematic literature review. *Acta Neurochir* **145(10)**:843–850.

Alexander MP (1995). Mild traumatic brain injury: pathophysiology, natural history, and clinical management. *Neurology* **45(7)**:1253–1260.

Alexander MP (1998). In the pursuit of proof of brain damage after whiplash injury. *Neurology* **51(2)**: 336–340.

American Academy of Pediatrics (1999). The management of minor closed head injury in children. Committee on Quality Improvement, American Academy of Pediatrics. Commission on Clinical Policies and Research, American Academy of Family Physicians. *Pediatrics* **104(6)**:1407–1415.

American College of Surgeons (1997). *Advanced Trauma Life Support for Doctors*. 6th ed. Chicago.

Annegers JF, Hauser WA, Coan SP, Rocca WA (1998). A population-based study of seizures after traumatic brain injuries. *New Engl J Med* **338(1)**:20–24.

Arienta C, Caroli M, Balbi S (1997). Management of head-injured patients in the emergency department: a practical protocol. *Surg Neurol* **48(3)**:213–219.

Bartlett J, Kett-White R, Mendelow AD, Miller JD, Pickard J, Teasdale G (1998). Recommendations from the Society of British Neurological Surgeons. *Br J Neurosurg* **12(4)**:349–352.

Bellner J, Jensen SM, Lexell J, Romner B (2003). Diagnostic criteria and the use of ICD-10 codes to define and classify minor head injury. *J Neurol Neurosurg Psychiatry* **74(3)**:351–352.

Biberthaler P, Mussack T, Kanz KG (2004). Identification of high-risk patients after minor craniocerebral trauma. Measurement of nerve tissue protein S 100. *Unfallchirurg* **107(3)**:197–202.

Birbamer G, Gerstenbrand F, Aichner F *et al.* (1994). Imaging of inner cerebral trauma. *Acta Neurol (Napoli)* **16(3)**:114–120.

Borczuk P (1995). Predictors of intracranial injury in patients with mild head trauma. *Ann Emerg Med* **25(6)**:731–736.

Brainin M, Barnes M, Baron JC *et al.* (2004). Guidance for the preparation of neurological management guidelines by EFNS scientific task forces–revised recommendations 2004. *Eur J Neurol* **11(9)**:577–581.

Brodie HA (1997). Prophylactic antibiotics for posttraumatic cerebrospinal fluid fistulae. A meta-analysis. *Arch Otolaryngol Head Neck Surg* **123(7)**:749–752.

Brodie HA, Thompson TC (1997). Management of complications from 820 temporal bone fractures. *Am J Otol* **18(2)**:188–197.

Chan KH, Yue CP, Mann KS (1990). The risk of intracranial complications in pediatric head injury. Results of multivariate analysis. *Childs Nerv Syst* **6(1)**:27–29.

Culotta VP, Sementilli ME, Gerold K, Watts CC (1996). Clinicopathological heterogeneity in the classification of mild head injury. *Neurosurgery* **38(2)**:245–250.

Dagi TF, Meyer FB, Poletti CA (1983). The incidence and prevention of meningitis after basilar skull fracture. *Am J Emerg Med* **1(3)**:295–298.

de Kruijk JR, Twijnstra A, Meerhoff S, Leffers P (2001). Management of mild traumatic brain injury: lack of consensus in Europe. *Brain Injury* **15(2)**: 117–123.

de Kruijk JR, Leffers P, Meerhoff S, Rutten J, Twijnstra A (2002). Effectiveness of bed rest after mild traumatic brain injury: a randomised trial of no versus six days of bed rest. *J Neurol Neurosurg Psychiatry* **73(2)**: 167–172.

de Louw A, Twijnstra A, Leffers P (1994). Lack of uniformity and low compliance concerning wake-up advice following head trauma. *Ned Tijdschr Geneeskd* **138(44):**2197–2199.

Demetriades D, Charalambides D, Lakhoo M, Pantanowitz D (1992). Role of prophylactic antibiotics in open and basilar fractures of the skull: a randomized study. *Injury* **23(6):**377–380.

Denny-Brown D, Russell WR (1941). Experimental cerebral concussion. **Brain 64:**93–163.

Dolan RJ, Bench CJ, Brown RG, Scott LC, Frackowiak RS (1994). Neuropsychological dysfunction in depression: the relationship to regional cerebral blood flow. *Psychol Med* **24(4):**849–857.

Dunham CM, Coates S, Cooper C (1996). Compelling evidence for discretionary brain computed tomographic imaging in those patients with mild cognitive impairment after blunt trauma. *J Trauma* **41(4):** 679–686.

Durham SR, Clancy RR, Leuthardt E *et al.* (2000). CHOP Infant Coma Scale ("Infant Face Scale"): a novel coma scale for children less than two years of age. *J Neurotrauma* **17(9):**729–737.

Evans RW (1992). The postconcussion syndrome and the sequelae of mild head injury. *Neurol Clin* **10(4):**815–847.

Fabbri A, Vandelli A, Servadei F, Marchesini G (2004). Coagulopathy and NICE recommendations for patients with mild head injury. *J Neurol Neurosurg Psychiatry* **75(12):**1787–1788.

Frowein RA, Schiltz F, Stammler U (1989). Early post-traumatic intracranial hematoma. *Neurosurg Rev* **12(Suppl 1):**184–187.

Frowein RA, Firsching R (1990). *Classification of Head Injury. Handbook of Clinical Neurology.* Elsevier Science Publishers, pp. 101–122.

Gennarelli TA, Thibault LE, Adams JH, Graham DI, Thompson CJ, Marcincin RP (1982). Diffuse axonal injury and traumatic coma in the primate. *Ann Neurol* **12(6):**564–574.

Gennarelli TA (1983). Head injury in man and experimental animals: clinical aspects. *Acta Neurochir Suppl (Wien)* **32:**1–13.

Gerstenbrand F, Stepan CH (2001). Mild traumatic brain injury. *Brain Injury* **15(2):**95–97.

Gomez PA, Lobato RD, Ortega JM, De La Cruz J (1996). Mild head injury: differences in prognosis among patients with a Glasgow Coma Scale score of 13 to 15 and analysis of factors associated with abnormal CT findings. *Br J Neurosurg* **10(5):**453–460.

Grcevic N (1988). The concept of inner cerebral trauma. *Scand J Rehabil Med Suppl* **17:**25–31.

Hahn YS, McLone DG (1993). Risk factors in the outcome of children with minor head injury. *Pediatr Neurosurg* **19(3):**135–142.

Haydel MJ, Preston CA, Mills TJ, Luber S, Blaudeau E, DeBlieux PM (2000). Indications for computed tomography in patients with minor head injury. *New Engl J Med* **343(2):**100–105.

Helling TS, Evans LL, Fowler DL, Hays LV, Kennedy FR (1988). Infectious complications in patients with severe head injury. *J Trauma* **28(11):**1575–1577.

Hofman PA, Nelemans P, Kemerink GJ, Wilmink JT (2000). Value of radiological diagnosis of skull fracture in the management of mild head injury: meta-analysis. *J Neurol Neurosurg Psychiatry* **68(4):**416–422.

Houlbourn AHS (1943). Mechanics of head injuries. *Lancet* **1:**438–441.

Hsiang JN, Yeung T, Yu AL, Poon WS (1997). High-risk mild head injury. *J Neurosurg* **87(2):**234–238.

Ibanez J, Arikan F, Pedraza S *et al.* (2004). Reliability of clinical guidelines in the detection of patients at risk following mild head injury: results of a prospective study. *J Neurosurg* **100(5):**825–834.

Ichise M, Chung DG, Wang P, Wortzman G, Gray BG, Franks W (1994). Technetium-99m-HMPAO SPECT, CT and MRI in the evaluation of patients with chronic traumatic brain injury: a correlation with neuropsychological performance. *J Nucl Med* **35(2):**217–226.

Ingebrigtsen T, Waterloo K, Marup Jensen S, Attner E, Romner B (1998). Quantification of post-concussion symptoms 3 months after minor head injury in 100 consecutive patients. *J Neurol* **245(9):**609–612.

Ingebrigtsen T, Romner B, Kock-Jensen C (2000). Scandinavian guidelines for initial management of minimal, mild, and moderate head injuries.The Scandinavian Neurotrauma Committee. *J Trauma* **48(4):**760–766.

Jacobs A, Put E, Ingels M, Bossuyt A (1994). Prospective evaluation of technetium-99m-HMPAO SPECT in mild and moderate traumatic brain injury. *J Nucl Med* **35(6):**942–947.

Jennett B (1996). Epidemiology of head injury. *J Neurol Neurosurg Psychiatry* **60(4):**362–369.

Jeret JS, Mandell M, Anziska B *et al.* (1993). Clinical predictors of abnormality disclosed by computed tomography after mild head trauma. *Neurosurgery* **32(1):** 9–15.

Karni A, Holtzman R, Bass T *et al.* (2001). Traumatic head injury in the anticoagulated elderly patient: a lethal combination. *Am Surg* **67(11):**1098–1100.

Kennedy DM, Cipolle MD, Pasquale MD, Wasser T (2000). Impact of preinjury warfarin use in elderly trauma patients. *J Trauma* **48(3):**451–453.

Kibby MY, Long CJ (1997). Effective treatment of minor head injury and understanding its neurological consequences. *Appl Neuropsych* **4:**34–42.

Klauber MR, Marshall LF, Luerssen TG, Frankowski R, Tabaddor K, Eisenberg HM (1989). Determinants of head injury mortality: importance of the low risk patient [see comments]. *Neurosurgery* **24(1):** 31–36.

Kraus JF, McArthur DL, Silverman TA, Jayaraman M (1996). Epidemiology of brain injury. In: Narayan RK, Wilberger JE, Jr., Povlishock JT (eds). *Neurotrauma*. New York: McGraw-Hill pp. 13–30.

Leech PJ, Paterson A (1973). Conservative and operative management for cerebrospinal-fluid leakage after closed head injury. *Lancet* **1(7811):**1013–1016.

Levin HS, O'Donnell VM, Grossman RG (1979). The Galveston Orientation and Amnesia Test. A practical scale to assess cognition after head injury. *J Nerv Ment Dis* **167(11):**675–684.

Li J, Brown J, Levine M (2001). Mild head injury, anticoagulants, and risk of intracranial injury. *Lancet* **357(9258):**771–772.

Livingston DH, Lavery RF, Passannante MR *et al.* (2000). Emergency department discharge of patients with a negative cranial computed tomography scan after minimal head injury. *Ann Surg* **232(1):**126–132.

Lloyd DA, Carty H, Patterson M, Butcher CK, Roe D (1997). Predictive value of skull radiography for intracranial injury in children with blunt head injury. *Lancet* **349(9055):**821–824.

Maas AI, Dearden M, Teasdale GM *et al.* (1997). EBIC-guidelines for management of severe head injury in adults. European Brain Injury Consortium. *Acta Neurochir* **139(4):**286–294.

Madden C, Witzke DB, Sanders AB, Valente J, Fritz M (1995). High-yield selection criteria for cranial computed-tomography after acute trauma. *Academic Emergency Medicine* **2(4):**248–253.

Marion DW (1991). Complications of head injury and their therapy. *Neurosurg Clin N Am* **2(2):**411–424.

Masters SJ, McClean PM, Arcarese JS *et al.* (1987). Skull x-ray examinations after head trauma. Recommendations by a multidisciplinary panel and validation study. *N Engl J Med* **316(2):**84–91.

Mayberg HS (1994). Frontal lobe dysfunction in secondary depression. *J Neuropsychiatry Clin Neurosci* **6(4):**428–442.

Meerhoff SR, de Kruijk JR, Rutten J, Leffers P, Twijnstra A (2000). De incidentie van traumatisch schedel-of hersenletsel in het adherentie gebied van het Academisch Ziekenhuis Maastricht in 1997. *Ned Tijdschr Geneeskd* **144(40):**1915–1918.

Mendelow AD, Bartlett J (1998). Recommendations from the society of British neurological surgeons. *Br J Neurosurg* **12:**349–352.

Mendelow AD, Karmi MZ, Paul KS, Fuller GA, Gillingham FJ (1979). Extradural haematoma: effect of delayed treatment. *Br Med J* **1(6173):**1240–1242.

Mendelow AD, Teasdale GM, Jennett B, Bryden J, Hessett C, Murray G (1983). Risks of intracranial haematoma in head injured adults. *Br Med J Clin Res Ed* **287(6400):**1173–1176.

Mild Traumatic Brain Injury Committee (1993). Definition of mild traumatic brain injury. *J Head Trauma Rehabil* **8(3):**86–87.

Miller EC, Holmes JF, Derlet RW (1997). Utilizing clinical factors to reduce head CT scan ordering for minor head trauma patients. *J Emerg Med* **15(4):**453–457.

Nee PA, Hadfield JM, Yates DW, Faragher EB (1999). Significance of vomiting after head injury. *J Neurol Neurosurg Psychiatry* **66(4):**470–473.

Paterniti S, Fiore P, Macri E *et al.* (1994). Extradural haematoma. Report of 37 consecutive cases with survival. *Acta Neurochir* **131(3–4):**207–210.

Pople IK, Stranjalis G, Nelson R (1993). Anticoagulant-related intracranial haemorrhage. *Br J Hosp Med* **49(6):**428–429.

Pudenz RH, Shelden CH (1946). The lucite calvarium- A method for direct observation of the brain. *J Neurosurg* **3:**487–505.

Raabe A, Grolms C, Sorge O, Zimmermann M, Seifert V (1999). Serum S-100B protein in severe head injury. *Neurosurgery* **45(3):**477–483.

Reilly PL, Simpson DA, Sprod R, Thomas L (1988). Assessing the conscious level in infants and young children: a paediatric version of the Glasgow Coma Scale. *Childs Nerv Syst* **4(1):**30–33.

Rimel RW, Giordani B, Barth JT, Boll TJ, Jane JA (1981). Disability caused by minor head injury. *Neurosurgery* **9(3):**221–228.

Romner B, Ingebrigtsen T, Kongstad P, Borgesen SE (2000). Traumatic brain damage: serum S-100 protein measurements related to neuroradiological findings. *J Neurotrauma* **17(8):**641–647.

Ruff RM, Jurica P (1999). In search of a unified definition for mild traumatic brain injury. *Brain Injury* **13(12):**943–952.

Ruff RM, Crouch JA, Troster AI *et al.* (1994). Selected cases of poor outcome following a minor brain trauma: comparing neuropsychological and positron emission tomography assessment. *Brain Injury* **8(4):**297–308.

Saab M, Gray A, Hodgkinson D, Irfan M (1996). Warfarin and the apparent minor head injury. *J Accid Emerg Med* **13(3):**208–209.

Seelig JM, Marshall LF, Toutant SM *et al.* (1984). Traumatic acute epidural hematoma: unrecognized high lethality in comatose patients. *Neurosurgery* **15(5):** 617–620.

Schierhout G, Roberts I (1997). The Cochrane Brain and Spinal Cord Injury Group. *J Neurol Neurosurg Psychiatry* **63(1):**1–3.

Schierhout G, Roberts I (1998). Prophylactic antiepileptic agents after head injury: a systematic review. *J Neurol Neurosurg Psychiatry* **64(1):**108–112.

Sellier K, Unterharnscheidt F (1963). *Hefte zur Unfallheilkunde; Mechanik und pathomorfologie der hirnschaden nach stumpfer gewalteinwirkung auf den schadel.* Berlin: Springer Verlag.

Servadei F (1997). Prognostic factors in severely head injured adult patients with epidural haematoma's. *Acta Neurochir* **139(4):**273–278.

Servadei F, Vergoni G, Staffa G *et al.* (1995). Extradural haematomas: how many deaths can be avoided? Protocol for early detection of haematoma in minor head injuries. *Acta Neurochir* **133(1–2):**50–55.

Servadei F, Teasdale G, Merry G (2001). Defining acute mild head injury in adults: a proposal based on prognostic factors, diagnosis, and management. *J Neurotrauma* **18(7):**657–664.

Shackford SR, Wald SL, Ross SE *et al.* (1992). The clinical utility of computed tomographic scanning and neurologic examination in the management of patients with minor head injuries. *J Trauma* **33(3):** 385–394.

Simpson DA, Cockington RA, Hanieh A, Raftos J, Reilly PL (1991). Head injuries in infants and young children: the value of the Paediatric Coma Scale. Review of literature and report on a study. *Childs Nerv Syst* **7(4):**183–190.

Smith HK, Miller JD (1991). The danger of an ultra-early computed tomographic scan in a patient with an evolving acute epidural hematoma. *Neurosurgery* **29(2):**258–260.

Spatz H (1936). Pathology der gedeckten Hirnverletzung unter besonderer Berucksichtigung der Rindenkontusion. Zeitschrift fur die gesamte *Neurologie und Psychiatrie* **78:**615–616.

Stein SC, Ross SE (1992). Mild head injury: a plea for routine early CT scanning. *J Trauma* **33(1):**11–13.

Stein SC, Spettell C (1995). The Head Injury Severity Scale (HISS): a practical classification of closed-head injury. *Brain Injury* **9(5):**437–444.

Stepan CH, Binder H, Gerstenbrand F (2001). Terminology of mild traumatic brain injury, results of a survey in Austria 2000. World Congres on Traumatic Brain Injury (Torino, 2001), p. 209.

Stiell IG, Wells GA, Vandemheen K *et al.* (2001). The Canadian CT Head Rule for patients with minor head injury. *Lancet* **357(9266):**1391–1396.

Tate RL, Pfaff A, Jurjevic L (2000). Resolution of disorientation and amnesia during post-traumatic amnesia. *J Neurol Neurosurg Psychiatry* **68(2):**178–185.

Teasdale GM (1995). Head injury. *J Neurol Neurosurg Psychiatry* **58(5):**526–539.

Teasdale GM, Jennett B (1974). Assessment of coma and impaired consciousness. A practical scale. *Lancet* **2(872):**81–84.

Teasdale GM, Murray G, Anderson E *et al.* (1990). Risks of acute traumatic intracranial haematoma in children and adults: implications for managing head injuries. *BMJ* **300(6721):**363–367.

Trotter W (1924). Annual Oration on certain minor head injuries of the brain. *Lancet* **1:**935–939.

Twijnstra A, Brouwer OF, Keyser A *et al.* (2001). Richtlijnen voor de diagnostiek en behandeling van patienten met licht schedel-hersenletsel. Commissie Kwaliteitsbevordering van de Nederlandse Vereniging voor Neurologie 1–26.

Unden J, Bellner J, Astrand R, Romner B (2005). Serum S100β levels in patients with epidural haematomas. *Br J Neurosurg* **19:**43–45.

Valadka AB, Narayan RK (1996). Emergency room management of the head-injured patient. In: Narayan RK, Wilberger JE, Povlishock JT, editors. *Neurotrauma.* New York: McGraw-Hill, pp. 119–135.

Villalobos T, Arango C, Kubilis P, Rathore M (1998). Antibiotic prophylaxis after basilar skull fractures: a meta-analysis. *Clin Infect Dis* **27(2):**364–369.

Voller B, Auff E, Schnider P, Aichner F (2001). To do or not to do? Magnetic resonance imaging in mild traumatic brain injury. *Brain Injury* **15(2):**107–115.

von Wild KRH, Terwey S (2001). Diagnostic confusion in mild traumatic brain injury (MTBI). Lessons from clinical practice and EFNS–inquiry. European Federation of Neurological Societies. *Brain Injury* **15(3):** 273–277.

von Wild KRH, Wenzlaff P (2005). Quality management in traumatic brain injury (TBI). Lessons from the prospective study in 6800 patients after acute TBI in respect of neurorehabilitation. *Acta Neurochir Suppl* **93:**15–25.

Wade DT, King NS, Wenden FJ, Crawford S, Caldwell FE (1998). Routine follow up after head injury: a second randomised controlled trial. *J Neurol Neurosurg Psychiatry* **65(2):**177–183.

Ward AB, Boughey AM, Aung TS, Barrett K (1992). Use of head injury instruction cards in accident centres. *Arch Emerg Med* **9(3):**314–316.

Warren D, Kissoon N (1989). Usefulness of head injury instruction forms in home observation of mild head injuries. *Pediatr Emerg Care* **5(2):**83–85.

Wijdicks EF, Schievink WI, Brown RD, Mullany CJ (1998). The dilemma of discontinuation of anticoagulation therapy for patients with intracranial hemorrhage and mechanical heart valves. *Neurosurgery* **42(4):**769–773.

Williams DH, Levin HS, Eisenberg HM (1990). Mild head injury classification. *Neurosurgery* **27(3):**422–428.

Wilson JT, Wiedmann KD, Hadley DM, Condon B, Teasdale GM, Brooks DN (1988). Early and late magnetic resonance imaging and neuropsychological outcome after head injury. *J Neurol Neurosurg Psychiatry* **51(3):**391–396.

Working Party of the British Society for Antimicrobial Chemotherapy (1994). Infection in Neurosurgery. Antimicrobial prophylaxis in neurosurgery and after head injury. *Lancet* **344(8936):** 1547–1551.

CHAPTER 17

Early (uncomplicated) Parkinson's disease*

M. Horstink (EFNS),[a] E. Tolosa (MDS-ES),[b]
U. Bonuccelli,[c] G. Deuschl,[d] A. Friedman,[e]
P. Kanovsky,[f] J.P. Larsen,[g] A. Lees,[h] W. Oertel,[i]
W. Poewe,[j] O. Rascol,[k] C. Sampaio[l]

Abstract

Objective To provide evidence-based recommendations for the management of early (uncomplicated) Parkinson's disease (PD), based on a review of the literature. Uncomplicated PD refers to patients suffering from the classical motor syndrome of PD only, without treatment-induced motor complications and without neuropsychiatric or autonomic problems.

Methods MEDLINE, Cochrane Library and INAHTA database literature searches were conducted. National guidelines were requested from all EFNS societies. Non-European guidelines were searched for using MEDLINE.

Results Part I of the guidelines deals with prevention of disease progression, symptomatic treatment of motor features (Parkinsonism), and prevention of motor and neuropsychiatric complications of therapy. For each topic, a list of therapeutic interventions is provided, including classification of evidence. Following this, recommendations for management are given, alongside ratings of efficacy. Classifications of evidence and ratings of efficacy are made according to EFNS guidance. In cases where there is insufficient scientific evidence, a consensus statement ('Good Practice Point') is made.

Background

In the initial stages of disease, levodopa is the most effective therapy for improving motor symptoms in Parkinson's disease (PD). However, long-term treatment is accompanied by the development of fluctuations in motor performance, dyskinesias,

---

*Review of the therapeutic management of Parkinson's disease. Report of a joint task force of the European Federation of Neurological Societies (EFNS) and the Movement Disorder Society-European Section (MDS-ES).

[a]Department of Neurology, Radboud University Medical Centre, Nijmegen, The Netherlands; [b]Neurology Service, Hospital Clínic, Universitat de Barcelona, Spain; [c]Department of Neurosciences, University of Pisa, Italy; [d]Dept of Neurology, Christian-Albrechts-University Kiel, Germany; [e]Department of Neurology, Medical University of Warsaw, Poland; [f]Department of

Neurology, Palacky University, Olomouc, Czech Republic; [g]Department of Neurology, Stavanger University Hospital, Norway; [h]Reta Lila Weston Institute of Neurological Studies, London, UK; [i]Philipps-University of Marburg, Centre of Nervous Diseases, Marburg, Germany; [j]Department of Neurology, Innsbruck Medical University, Austria; [k]Clinical Investigation Centre, Departments of Clinical Pharmacology and Neurosciences, University Hospital, Toulouse, France; [l]Laboratório de Farmacologia Clinica e Terapeutica e Instituto de Medicina Molecular, Faculdade de Medicina de Lisboa, Portugal.

and neuropsychiatric complications. Furthermore, as PD progresses, patients develop features that do not respond well to levodopa therapy, such as freezing episodes, autonomic dysfunction, falling, and dementia, and symptoms related to the administration of other drugs. The increasingly diverse possibilities in the therapy of PD, and the many side effects and complications of therapy, require reliable standards for patient care that are based on current scientific knowledge.

This document provides these scientifically supported treatment recommendations. If the level of available evidence is less than Level C, or if scientific evidence is lacking, best practice is recommended ('Good Practice Point'), based on the experience of the guidelines development group.

Methods

The authors were invited by EFNS and MDS-ES to prepare an evidence-based review.

Search strategy

Searches were made in MEDLINE, the full database of the Cochrane Library, and the International Network of Agencies for Health Technology Assessment (INAHTA), up to the first complete draft in May 2005. During the following discussions, relevant articles were added up to January 2006. The databases were also searched for existing guidelines and management reports, and requests were made to EFNS societies for their National Guidelines. Reference lists from (review) articles and other reports were also checked.

Method for reaching consensus

Classification of scientific evidence and the rating of recommendations are made according to the EFNS guidance (Brainin *et al.*, 2004). This report focuses on the highest levels of evidence available and, when only class IV evidence is available, or there is no scientific evidence, a Good Practice Point is given.

After a first meeting, held to discuss the principal format and methodology, six members of the task force provided a first draft of the report, which was commented on by all members via e-mail and through discussion at four EFNS and MDS congress

meetings, until consensus was reached (informative consensus approach). At a final meeting in September 2005, the six primary authors finalised the text for approval by all members of the task force.

For recommendations concerning drug dosage, method and route of administration and contraindications the reader is referred to the local formulary or manufacturer's instruction, except when provided within the guidelines' recommendation itself.

Interventions for the management of early (uncomplicated) Parkinson's disease

This section discusses drug classes used in the pharmacological treatment of PD. Following this, there is consideration of the non-pharmacological interventions in early (uncomplicated) PD.

Neuroprotection

To date, no adequate clinical trial has provided definite evidence for pharmacological neuroprotection. While many agents appear to be promising based on laboratory studies, selecting clinical endpoints for clinical trials that are not confounded by symptomatic effects of the study intervention has been difficult. As matters stand at present, neuroprotective trials of riluzole (class II: Jankovic and Hunter, 2002), coenzyme Q10 (CoQ) (class II: Shults *et al.*, 2002), and glial-derived neurotrophic factor (GDNF) (class II: Nutt *et al.*, 2003) do not support the use of any of these drugs for neuroprotection in routine practice. Although a meta-analysis of seven observational studies suggests that dietary intake of vitamin E protects against PD (class III: Etminan *et al.*, 2005), vitamin E did not have a neuroprotective effect in patients with PD (class I: Parkinson Study Group, 1989).

The sections below describe the neuroprotective use of drugs primarily known for their symptomatic effect.

MAO-B inhibitors

Studies in early PD (class I and II: Tetrud and Langston, 1989; Parkinson Study Group, 1989; Myllyla *et al.*, 1992; Olanow *et al.*, 1995;

Palhagen *et al.*, 1998) show that selegiline postpones the need for dopaminergic treatment by >6 months, indicating a delay in disability progression. However, the initial advantages of selegiline were not sustained (Parkinson Study Group, 1996). Furthermore, evidence is insufficient to make a conclusion on the neuroprotective, as opposed to the symptomatic, effect of selegiline in PD. Rasagiline had been shown to have symptomatic effect in the Trial of Rasagiline Mesylate (TVP-1012) in Early Mononotherapy for Parkinson's Disease Outpatients (TEMPO) study (Parkinson Study Group, 2002a). However, these patients were followed thereafter in a so-called late-start design, showing that patients treated with rasagiline for 12 months showed less functional decline than subjects whose treatment was delayed for 6 months, suggesting that a neuroprotective effect could be present (Parkinson Study Group, 2004a).

Levodopa

The only available placebo-controlled study of levodopa in relation to neuroprotection is inconclusive about any neuroprotective, as opposed to symptomatic, effect (class I: Parkinson Study Group, 2004b). Mortality studies suggest improved survival with levodopa therapy (class III: Rajput, 2001; review: Clarke, 1995).

Dopamine agonists

Class I randomised, controlled trials with bromocriptine, pramipexole and ropinirole produced no convincing evidence of neuroprotection (Olanow *et al.*, 1995; Parkinson Study Group, 2002b; Whone *et al.*, 2003).

Starting treatment of PD patients with bromocriptine, rather than with levodopa, is not effective in improving mortality (class II: Lees *et al.*, 2001; Montastruc *et al.*, 2001).

Anticholinergics, amantadine, COMT inhibitors

For these medications, either clinical studies are not available, or the agents are unable to prevent the progression of PD.

Symptomatic pharmacotherapy of parkinsonism

Anticholinergics

Mechanism of action

Anticholinergics are believed to act by correcting the disequilibrium between striatal dopamine and acetylcholine activity. Some anticholinergics, for example, benzotropine, can also block dopamine uptake in central dopaminergic neurons. The anticholinergics used to treat PD specifically block muscarinic receptors.

Symptomatic treatment of parkinsonism (monotherapy)

Three class II trials found anticholinergic monotherapy more effective than placebo in improving motor function in PD [bornaprine (Iivainen, 1974), benzhexol (Parkes *et al.*, 1974; Cooper *et al.*, 1992)]. Biperiden is as effective as apomorphine in patients with parkinsonian tremor (Class III: Schrag *et al.*, 1999). However, data conflict over whether anticholinergic drugs have a better effect on tremor than on other outcome measures. These results are consistent with reviews concluding that anticholinergics have only a small effect on PD symptoms, and that evidence for a special effect on tremor is inconclusive ('Management of Parkinson's disease', 2002; Katzenschlager *et al.*, 2002).

Adjunctive therapy of parkinsonism

Class II studies of trihexyphenidyl (Martin *et al.*, 1974), benzotropine (Tourtellotte *et al.*, 1982) and bornaprine (Cantello *et al.*, 1986) in levodopa-treated patients, and two reviews, indicate that adjunctive anticholinergics have only a minor effect on PD symptoms in patients on levodopa therapy, and that the tremor-specific data is inconclusive ('Management of Parkinson's disease', 2002; Katzenschlager *et al.*, 2002).

Prevention of motor complications

No studies available.

Symptomatic treatment of non-motor problems

Because of the risk of side effects (see below), centrally acting anticholinergics are usually not advised for the therapy of non-motor, that is, autonomic, dysfunctions.

Safety
The clinical use of anticholinergics has been limited by their side-effect profiles and contraindications. The most commonly reported side effects are blurred vision, urinary retention, nausea, constipation (rarely leading to paralytic ileus), and dry mouth. The incidence of reduced sweating, particularly in those patients on neuroleptics, can lead to fatal heat stroke. Anticholinergics are contraindicated in patients with narrow-angle glaucoma, tachycardia, hypertrophy of the prostate, gastrointestinal obstruction and megacolon.

Impaired mental function (mainly immediate memory and memory acquisition) is a well-documented central side effect that resolves after drug withdrawal (class IV: van Herwaarden *et al.*, 1993). Therefore, if dementia is present, the use of anticholinergics is contraindicated.

The abrupt withdrawal of anticholinergics may lead to a rebound effect with marked deterioration of parkinsonism. Consequently, anticholinergics should be discontinued gradually and with caution (Hughes *et al.*, 1971; Horrocks *et al.*, 1973).

Amantadine
Mechanism of action
Amantadine's mechanism of action remains unclear. A blockade of NMDA glutamate receptors and an anticholinergic effect are proposed, whereas other evidence suggests an amphetamine-like action to release presynaptic dopamine stores.

Symptomatic treatment of parkinsonism (monotherapy)
Class II studies (Cox *et al.*, 1973; Parkes *et al.*, 1974; Butzer *et al.*, 1975; Fahn and Isgreen, 1975) and reviews ('Management of Parkinson's disease', 2002; Crosby *et al.*, 2003a) show that amantadine induces symptomatic improvement.

Adjunctive therapy of parkinsonism
The addition of amantadine to anticholinergic agents is superior to placebo, with the improvement more pronounced in severely affected patients (class II: Appleton *et al.*, 1970; Jorgensen *et al.*, 1971).

Over 9 weeks, amantadine was beneficial as an adjunctive treatment to levodopa (class II: Savery, 1971), with a more noticeable improvement in patients on low levodopa doses (class II: Fehling, 1973). Together with the results of low class evidence studies (reviews: 'Management of Parkinson's disease', 2002; Crosby *et al.*, 2003a), data suggest that amantadine is probably effective as adjunct therapy, with an unproven long-term duration of effect.

Prevention of motor complications
No studies available.

Symptomatic treatment of non-motor problems
Not applicable.

Safety
Side effects are generally mild, most frequently including dizziness, anxiety, impaired coordination and insomnia (>5%), nausea and vomiting (5–10%), and headache, nightmares, ataxia, confusion/agitation, drowsiness, constipation/diarrhoea, anorexia, xerostomia, and livedo reticularis (<5%). Less common side effects include psychosis, abnormal thinking, amnesia, slurred speech, hyperkinesia, hypertension, urinary retention, decreased libido, dyspnoea, rash, and orthostatic hypotension (during chronic administration) ('Management of Parkinson's disease', 2002).

MAO-B inhibitors
Mechanism of action
Selegiline and rasagiline inhibit the action of monoamine oxidase isoenzyme type B (MAO-B). MAO-B prevents the breakdown of dopamine, producing greater dopamine availability. Mechanisms besides MAO-B inhibition may also contribute to the clinical effects (Olanow and Riederer, 1996). Unlike selegiline, rasagiline is not metabolised to amphetamine, and has no sympathomimetic activity.

Symptomatic treatment of parkinsonism (monotherapy)

Five of six studies with a typical follow-up period of 3–12 months (class I and II: Parkinson Study Group, 1989; Teravainen, 1990; Myllyla *et al.*, 1992; Allain *et al.*, 1993; Mally *et al.*, 1995; Palhagen *et al.*, 1998), and a meta-analysis (Ives *et al.*, 2004), demonstrated a small symptomatic effect of selegiline monotherapy (class I). One study of rasagiline also showed significant improvements on the PD Quality of Life questionnaire and although there was no difference in Unified PD Rating Scale (UPDRS) versus baseline at 6 months, there was a significant improvement versus placebo on UPDRS at 6 months (class I: Parkinson Study Group, 2002b).

Adjunctive therapy of parkinsonism

In clinical studies (class I: Przuntek and Kuhn, 1987; Sivertsen *et al.*, 1989; Nappi *et al.*, 1991; Lees, 1995; Larsen and Boas, 1997) and a meta-analysis (Ives *et al.*, 2004), investigating the addition of selegiline to other antiparkinsonian therapies (mainly levodopa), no consistent beneficial effect was demonstrated on the core symptoms of PD in non-fluctuating patients. Rasagiline has not been studied in this context.

Prevention of motor complications

Selegiline has shown no effect in preventing motor fluctuations including wearing-off, ON–OFF fluctuations and dyskinesia (class I: Larsen *et al.*, 1999; class II: PD Research Group in the UK, 1993; Shoulson *et al.*, 2002). Rasagiline has not been studied in this context.

Symptomatic treatment of non-motor problems

A class II study detected no effect of selegiline on depression in PD (Lees *et al.*, 1977). MAO-B inhibitors have not been investigated for the treatment of other non-motor problems.

Safety

As with any dopaminergic drug, MAO-B inhibitors can induce a variety of dopaminergic adverse reactions. At the daily doses currently recommended, the risk of tyramine-induced hypertension (the 'cheese effect') is low (Heinonen and Myllyla, 1998).

Concerns that the selegiline/levodopa combination increased mortality rates (Ben-Shlomo *et al.*, 1998) have been allayed (Olanow *et al.*, 1998).

COMT inhibitors

Mechanism of action

Catechol-O-methyltransferase (COMT) inhibitors reduce the metabolism of levodopa, extending its plasma half-life and prolonging the action of each levodopa dose. Therapeutic doses of entacapone only act peripherally and do not alter cerebral COMT activity.

Symptomatic treatment of parkinsonism (monotherapy)

Not applicable (COMT inhibitors should always be given with levodopa).

Adjunctive therapy of parkinsonism

There are four published studies (class I and II) where the issue of efficacy in non-fluctuating patients is addressed. Two of these tested tolcapone (Waters *et al.*, 1997; Dupont *et al.*, 1997), and the other two examined entacapone (Myllyla *et al.*, 2001; Brooks *et al.*, 2003). All trials showed a small benefit in the control of the symptoms of parkinsonism, mostly reflected in UPDRS part II (activities of daily living), but the results were not consistent across all endpoints.

Prevention of motor complications

No studies available.

Symptomatic treatment of non-motor problems

No studies available.

Safety

COMT inhibitors increase levodopa bioavailability, so they can increase the incidence of dopaminergic adverse reactions, including nausea, and cardiovascular and neuropsychiatric complications. Diarrhoea and urine discoloration are the most frequently reported non-dopaminergic adverse reactions.

Tolcapone can elevate liver transaminases, and fatal cases of liver injury are reported. The European Agency for the Evaluation of Medicinal Products (EMEA) lifted the suspension of tolcapone for use in patients on levodopa who fail to respond to other COMT inhibitors, but imposed strict safety restrictions (EMEA, 2004). Tolcapone can only be prescribed by physicians experienced in the management of advanced PD, with a recommended daily dose of 100 mg three times daily. Patients must have fortnightly blood tests for liver function in the first year, at four-weekly intervals for the next 6 months and, subsequently, every 8 weeks. Patients with abnormal liver function or a history of neuroleptic malignant syndrome, rhabdomyolysis or hyperthermia have to be excluded. The combination with selective MAO-B inhibitors (selegiline) is allowed if the dose of MAO-B inhibitor does not exceed the recommended dose.

Levodopa
a. Standard levodopa formulation
Mechanism of action
Levodopa exerts its symptomatic benefits through conversion to dopamine, and is routinely administered in combination with a decarboxylase inhibitor (carbidopa, benserazide) to prevent its peripheral conversion to dopamine and the resultant nausea and vomiting.

Symptomatic treatment of parkinsonism (monotherapy)
The efficacy of levodopa is firmly established from over 30 years of use in clinical practice ('Management of Parkinson's disease', 2002; Levine *et al.*, 2003). A recent class I trial confirmed a dose-dependent significant reduction in UPDRS scores with levodopa versus placebo (Parkinson Study Group, 2004b).

In terms of symptomatic effects, levodopa proved to be better than the dopamine agonists. Levodopa was better than bromocriptine, at least during the first year (class II: Lees *et al.*, 2001), and a Cochrane review found comparable effects of bromocriptine and levodopa on impairment and disability (Ramaker and van Hilten, 2000).

Levodopa's symptomatic effect also proved better than ropinirole (class I: Whone *et al.*, 2003), pramipexole (class I: Parkinson Study Group, 2004c), pergolide (class III: Kulisevsky *et al.*, 1998), lisuride (class III: Rinne, 1989), and cabergoline (class I: Rinne *et al.*, 1997). The results of these individual studies are confirmed by systematic reviews showing that levodopa monotherapy produced better UPDRS scores than cabergoline, pramipexole, and ropinirole ('Management of Parkinson's disease', 2002; Levine *et al.*, 2003), and bromocriptine, lisuride, and pergolide (Levine *et al.*, 2003).

Adjunctive therapy of parkinsonism
Supplementation of levodopa to other antiparkinsonian medications in stable PD is common clinical practice to improve symptomatic control (class IV).

Prevention of motor complications (risk reduction)
The prevention of motor complications (i.e. fluctuations and dyskinesia) by levodopa seems contradictory because these complications are actually caused by levodopa. Usually, levodopa is started three times daily, which offers symptomatic control throughout the day, but after several months or years of chronic treatment, motor complications may arise (see safety section, below). However, by carefully shortening the dose interval in order to compensate for shortening of the duration of effect of each levodopa dose (wearing-off), and by reducing the dose of each levodopa intake to reduce the magnitude of the effect (peak dose dyskinesia), the clinical emergence of these motor problems can be postponed.

Symptomatic treatment of non-motor problems
Whether or not levodopa improves mood in PD is a matter of debate (Marsh and Markham, 1973; Maricle *et al.*, 1995; Morrison *et al.*, 2004), as is the influence of levodopa on cognition (reviews: Nieoullon, 2002; Pillon *et al.*, 2003; Bosboom *et al.*, 2004). Off-period psychiatric symptoms (anxiety, panic attacks, depression) and other non-motor symptoms (drenching sweats, pain, fatigue, and akathisia) may be alleviated by modifying the treatment schedule of levodopa (class IV: Nissenbaum

et al., 1987; Raudino, 2001; Olanow *et al.*, 2001; Witjas *et al.*, 2002).

Safety

Most studies in animal models and humans failed to show accelerated dopaminergic neuronal loss with long-term levodopa therapy at usual clinical doses (reviews: 'Management of Parkinson's disease', 2002; Katzenschlager and Lees, 2002; Olanow *et al.*, 2004). A meta-analysis reported no treatment-related deaths or life-threatening events (Levine *et al.*, 2003). Peripheral side effects include gastrointestinal and cardiovascular dysfunction (reviews: Olanow *et al.*, 2001; 'Management of Parkinson's disease', 2002; Levine *et al.*, 2003; Jankovic, 2005; Adler, 2005).

Central adverse effects include levodopa motor problems such as fluctuations, dyskinesia and dystonia, and psychiatric side effects such as confusion, hallucinations and sleep disorders (reviews: Olanow *et al.*, 2001; Levine *et al.*, 2003; Jankovic, 2005). A meta-analysis found ~40% likelihood of motor fluctuations and dyskinesias after 4–6 years of levodopa therapy (Ahlskog and Muenter, 2001). Risk factors are younger age, longer disease duration, and levodopa (Poewe *et al.*, 1986; Kostic *et al.*, 1991; Blanchet *et al.*, 1996; Grandas *et al.*, 1999; Denny and Behari, 1999; Parkinson Study Group, 2004b; Kumar *et al.*, 2005; reviews: Olanow *et al.*, 2001; Levine *et al.*, 2003; Jankovic, 2005). In individual studies, the percentage of fluctuations and dyskinesia may range from 10–60% of patients at 5 years, and up to 80–90% in later years (Olanow *et al.*, 2001; Levine *et al.*, 2003). Neuropsychiatric complications occur in less than 5% of *de novo* patients on levodopa monotherapy (reviews: Olanow *et al.*, 2001; Levine *et al.*, 2003).

b. Controlled-release levodopa formulations

Mechanism of action

Levodopa has a short half-life, which eventually results in short-duration responses with a wearing-off (end-of-dose) effect. Controlled-release (CR) formulations aim to prolong the effect of a single dose of levodopa, and reduce the number of daily doses.

Symptomatic treatment of parkinsonism (monotherapy)

Standard and CR levodopa maintain a similar level of control in *de novo* PD after 5 years (class I: Koller *et al.*, 1999), and also in more advanced PD with a duration of about 10 years and without motor fluctuations (class I: Goetz *et al.*, 1988).

Prevention of motor complications

CR levodopa has no significant preventive effect on the incidence of motor fluctuations or dyskinesia, as compared with standard levodopa (class I: Dupont *et al.*, 1996; Block *et al.*, 1997; Koller *et al.*, 1999).

Dopamine agonists

Mechanism of action

Of the nine dopamine agonists presently marketed for the treatment of PD, five are ergot derivatives (bromocriptine, cabergoline, dihydroergocryptine, lisuride and pergolide) and four are non-ergot derivatives (apomorphine, piribedil, pramipexole and ropinirole).

It is generally accepted that the shared D_2-like receptor agonistic activity produces the symptomatic antiparkinsonian effect. This D_2 effect also explains peripheral (gastrointestinal – nausea and vomiting), cardiovascular (orthostatic hypotension), and neuropsychiatric (somnolence, psychosis, and hallucinations) side effects. In addition, dopamine agonists have other properties (e.g. anti-apoptotic effect) that have prompted their testing as putative neuroprotective agents.

Apart from apomorphine, which can only be used via the subcutaneous route (penject and pumps) (Katzenschlager *et al.*, 2005), all dopamine agonists are used orally. A transdermal patch of a new non-ergot dopamine agonist, rotigotine, is currently under development for the treatment of PD (Parkinson Study Group, 2003).

Symptomatic treatment of parkinsonism (monotherapy)

Agonists versus placebo Dihydroergocryptine (Bergamasco *et al.*, 2000), pergolide (Barone *et al.*, 1999), pramipexole (Shannon *et al.*, 1997), and ropinirole (Adler *et al.*, 1997), are effective in early

PD (class I). Bromocriptine and cabergoline are probably effective as monotherapy in early PD (class II and III: Riopelle, 1987; Montastruc *et al.*, 1994; Rinne *et al.*, 1997, 1998). Lisuride (Rinne, 1989) and piribedil (Rondot and Ziegler, 1992) are possibly effective (class IV).

Agonists versus levodopa Levodopa is more efficacious than any orally active dopamine agonist monotherapy (see section on levodopa). The proportion of patients able to remain on agonist monotherapy falls progressively over time to <20% after 5 years of treatment [class I: bromocriptine (Montastruc *et al.*, 1994; PD Research Group in the UK, 1993), cabergoline (Rinne *et al.*, 1998), pramipexole (Parkinson Study Group, 2000), and ropinirole (Rascol *et al.*, 2000)]. For this reason, after a few years of treatment, most patients who start on an agonist will receive levodopa as a replacement or adjunct treatment to keep control of motor parkinsonian signs. Over the last decade, a commonly tested strategy has been to start with an agonist and to add levodopa later if worsening of symptoms can not be controlled with the agonist alone. However, previously, it was common practice to combine an agonist like bromocriptine or lisuride with levodopa within the first months of treatment ('early combination strategy') [class II: bromocriptine (Przuntek *et al.*, 1996) and lisuride (Allain *et al.*, 2000)]. There are no studies assessing whether one strategy is better than the other.

Agonists versus agonists From the limited data available [class II: bromocriptine versus ropinirole (Korczyn *et al.*, 1998,1999); class III: bromocriptine versus pergolide (Mizuno *et al.*, 1995)], the clinical relevance of the reported difference between agonists, if any, remains questionable.

Agonists versus other antiparkinsonian medications There are no published head-to-head comparisons between agonist monotherapy and any other antiparkinsonian medication in early PD. Changes in UPDRS scores reported for most agonists are usually larger than those reported with MAO-B inhibitors, suggesting a greater symptomatic effect with the agonists.

Adjunctive therapy of parkinsonism
Agonists versus placebo Based on class I evidence, most agonists have been shown to be effective in improving the cardinal motor signs of parkinsonism in patients already treated with levodopa. This is true for apomorphine (Dewey *et al.*, 2001), bromocriptine (Guttman, 1997; Mizuno *et al.*, 2003), cabergoline (Hutton *et al.*, 1996), pergolide (Olanow *et al.*, 1994), piribedil (Ziegler *et al.*, 2003), and pramipexole (Pinter *et al.*, 1999; Pogarell *et al.*, 2002; Moller *et al.*, 2005). The available evidence is less convincing (class II) for dihydroergocryptine (Martignoni *et al.*, 1991), lisuride (Allain *et al.*, 2000), and ropinirole (Lieberman *et al.*, 1998).

Agonists versus agonists Several class I and II studies have compared the symptomatic effect of two different dopamine agonists on parkinsonism when given as adjunct to levodopa – with bromocriptine as the reference comparator. Such data cannot have a strong impact on clinical practice because of methodological problems in the reported studies [cabergoline (Inzelberg *et al.*, 1996), lisuride (Le Witt *et al.*, 1982; Laihinen *et al.*, 1992), pergolide (Le Witt *et al.*, 1983; Mizuno *et al.*, 1995; Pezzoli *et al.*, 1995; Boas *et al.*, 1996), pramipexole (Mizuno *et al.*, 2003), and ropinirole (Brunt *et al.*, 2002)]. Switching from one agonist to another for reasons of efficacy or safety is sometimes considered in clinical practice. Most of the available data are based on open-label class IV trials with an overnight switch (Goetz *et al.*, 1989,1999; Canesi *et al.*, 1999; Gimenez-Roldan *et al.*, 2001; Hanna *et al.*, 2001; Reichmann *et al.*, 2003; Linazasoro *et al.*, 2004; Grosset *et al.*, 2004). An empirical conversion chart of dose equivalence is usually proposed, with 10 mg bromocriptine = 1 mg pergolide = 1 mg pramipexole = 2 mg cabergoline = 5 mg ropinirole.

Agonists versus other antiparkinsonian medications Bromocriptine (Tolcapone Study Group, 1999) and pergolide (Koller *et al.*, 2001) have been compared with the COMT inhibitor tolcapone (class II), and no significant difference was reported in terms of efficacy on parkinsonian cardinal signs.

Prevention of motor complications
Agonists versus levodopa Class I randomised, controlled trials demonstrate how early use of an agonist can reduce the incidence of motor complications versus levodopa [cabergoline (Rinne *et al.*, 1998), pramipexole (Parkinson Study Group, 2000), and ropinirole (Rascol *et al.*, 2000; Whone *et al.*, 2003)]. Similar conclusions were reported with bromocriptine (class II: PD Research Group in the UK, 1993; Hely *et al.*, 1994; Montastruc *et al.*, 1994), and pergolide (class II: Oertel *et al.*, 2005). Conflicting results have been reported with lisuride (Rinne, 1989; Allain *et al.*, 2000).

Agonists versus agonists There is no available indication that one agonist might be more efficacious than another in preventing or delaying 'time to motor complications'. The only published class II comparison (ropinirole versus bromocriptine: Korczyn *et al.*, 1999) did not show any difference in dyskinesia incidence at 3 years.

Agonists versus other antiparkinsonian medications No studies available.

Symptomatic treatment of non-motor problems
There is no indication that symptoms such as anxiety, sleep disturbance or pain are responsive to dopamine agonists. It is conceivable that such symptoms, if partly 'dopa-responsive' and occurring or worsening during OFF episodes, might be improved by dopamine agonists, as with any dopaminergic medication, but no convincing data are available. Conversely, dysautonomic parkinsonian symptoms, like orthostatic hypotension, are aggravated by dopaminergic medication, including agonists, probably through sympatholytic mechanisms (see also the management recommendations section on neuropsychiatric complications in Part II of the guidelines).

Safety
Dopamine agonists and all other active dopamine-mimetic medications share a common safety profile reflecting dopamine stimulation. Accordingly, side effects such as nausea, vomiting, orthostatic hypotension, confusion, psychosis, and somnolence may occur with administration of any of these agents. Peripheral leg oedema is also commonly observed with most agonists.

Hallucinations and somnolence are more frequent with some agonists than with levodopa (class I: Etminan *et al.*, 2001; Avorn *et al.*, 2005). There is no convincing evidence that any agonist is better tolerated than bromocriptine. However, the rare but severe risk of pleuropulmonary/retroperitoneal fibrosis is greater with ergot agonists than with non-ergot agonists. The same is probably true for valvular heart disorders, although pergolide has been the most frequently reported drug at the present time (Van Camp *et al.*, 2004). For this reason, pergolide is presently only used as a second-line alternative option, when other agonists have not provided an adequate response.

Occupational, physical and speech therapy
Mechanism of action
Occupational therapy, physical therapy and speech therapy, are designed to teach patients how to cope with emotional problems, disabilities and handicaps.

Prevention of disease progression
Higher levels of physical activity may lower the risk of PD in men (class IV: Sasco *et al.*, 1992; Tsai *et al.*, 2002; Chen *et al.*, 2005).

Symptomatic treatment of parkinsonism (monotherapy)
No studies available.

Adjunctive therapy of parkinsonism
Most studies of physical therapy, speech therapy, and rehabilitation programmes in PD report improvements in at least one outcome measure. However, it is often difficult to interpret the clinical importance of these improvements, and long-term effects remain unclear.

Some class II–III studies suggest that physical therapy, especially exercise, improves parkinsonian motor impairments or disabilities (Gauthier *et al.*, 1987; Formisano *et al.*, 1992; Comella *et al.*, 1994; Dam *et al.*, 1996; Schenkman *et al.*, 1998; Baatile *et al.*, 2000; Hirsch *et al.*, 2003; Ellis *et al.*, 2005). Several review articles also highlight the positive effects of physiotherapy (de Goede *et al.*, 2001; Health Council of the Netherlands, 2003; Levine *et al.*, 2003; Gage and Storey, 2004), although others have found insufficient evidence to support or refute its efficacy in PD (Deane *et al.*, 2001a,b, 2002; 'Management of Parkinson's disease', 2002; Levine *et al.*, 2003). Practice and specific training strategies have been shown to improve motor performance (class III: Platz *et al.*, 1998; Soliveri *et al.*, 1992).

Sensory cue strategies such as walking sticks and auditory pacing can improve gait and reduce freezing in some patients (class III–IV: Dietz *et al.*, 1990; Thaut *et al.*, 1996; McIntosh *et al.*, 1997; Lewis *et al.*, 2000; Marchese *et al.*, 2000; Suteerawattananon *et al.*, 2004; Rochester *et al.*, 2005; review: Rubinstein *et al.*, 2002), but may reduce walking speed and be ineffective against ON-freezing in others (class III: Kompoliti *et al.*, 2000; Cubo *et al.*, 2004).

The effect of non-pharmacological therapies on falls has been evaluated in elderly people, but no class I–III study specifically evaluates the effect in PD patients. In elderly people, health/environmental risk factor intervention, muscle strengthening and balance retraining, home hazard modification, and withdrawal of psychotropic medication, are all likely to be effective (class III–IV: Gillespie *et al.*, 2003; Bloem *et al.*, 2003).

Three reviews found insufficient evidence for the efficacy of speech and language therapy for dysarthria (Deane *et al.*, 2001c; 'Management of Parkinson's disease', 2002; Pinto *et al.*, 2004). Ramig *et al.* (1996, 2001) showed that Lee Silverman Voice Therapy (LSVT) improves vocal intensity and phonation. Pitch Limiting Voice Treatment (PLVT) produces the same increase in loudness, but limits an increase in vocal pitch and prevents a strained voicing (class IV: de Swart *et al.*, 2003). No scientific evidence supports or refutes the efficacy of non-pharmacological swallowing therapy for dysphagia in PD (Deane *et al.*, 2001d; Deane *et al.*, 2002).

Prevention of motor complications

No qualified studies in these areas.

Symptomatic treatment of non-motor problems

Not specifically addressed by class I–III studies. The Good Practice Point is to adhere to the usual management rules in general practice.

Safety

Practice suggests that these therapies are safe.

RECOMMENDATIONS

Conclusion for patient care

Physical therapy, especially exercise and cueing strategies, is probably effective (Level B). Speech therapy is possibly effective (Level C). However, the long-term benefits of these therapies remain to be proven. The studies discussed above and the conclusion address physical and speech therapy as adjunctive therapy in PD. No recommendation can be made regarding the effect of physiotherapy as monotherapy in early PD.

Early untreated patients

The optimal time frame for onset of therapy has not been clearly defined. Once parkinsonian signs start to have an impact on the patient's life, initiation of treatment is recommended. For each patient, the choice between the numerous effective drugs available is based on a subtle combination of subjective and objective factors. These factors include considerations related to the drug (efficacy for symptomatic control of parkinsonism/prevention of motor complications, safety, practicality, costs, etc.), to the patient (symptoms, age, needs, expectations, experience, co-morbidity, socio-economic level, etc.), and to his/her environment (drug availability according to national markets in the European Union, variability in economic and health insurance systems, etc.). However, based on the available level of evidence alone, two main issues are usually considered when initiating a symptomatic therapy for early PD: the symptomatic control of parkinsonism, and the prevention of motor complications (see table 17.1).

Currently, there is no uniform proposal across Europe on initiating symptomatic medication for PD.

continued

Options include starting treatment with:

- *MAO-B inhibitor*, like selegiline or rasagiline (Level A). The symptomatic effect is more modest than that of levodopa and (probably) dopamine agonists, but they are easy to administer (one dose, once daily, no titration).
- *amantadine or an anticholinergic* (Level B). The impact on symptoms is smaller than that of levodopa. Anticholinergics are poorly tolerated in the elderly and their use is mainly restricted to young patients.
- *levodopa*, the most effective symptomatic antiparkinsonian drug (Level A). After a few years of treatment, levodopa is frequently associated with the development of motor complications. As older patients are more sensitive to neuropsychiatric adverse reactions and are less prone to developing motor complications, the early use of levodopa is recommended in the older population (Good Practice Point). The early use of controlled-release levodopa formulations is not effective in the prevention of motor complications (Level A).
- *orally active dopamine agonist*. Pramipexole and ropinirole are effective as monotherapy in early PD, with a lower risk of motor complications than levodopa (Level A). Older drugs like bromocriptine are supported by lower class evidence, giving a Level B recommendation. However, there is no convincing evidence that they are less effective in managing patients with early PD. The benefit of agonists in preventing motor complications (Level A, with data up to 5 years only) must be balanced with the smaller effect on symptoms and the greater incidence of hallucinations, somnolence, and leg oedema, as compared with levodopa. Patients must be informed of these risks, for example, excessive daytime somnolence is especially relevant to drivers. Younger patients are more prone to developing levodopa-induced motor complications, and therefore initial treatment with an agonist can be recommended in this population (Good Practice Point). Ergot derivatives such as pergolide, bromocriptine, and cabergoline are not recommended as first-line medication

because of the risk of fibrotic reactions. Subcutaneous apomorphine is not appropriate at this stage of the disease. The early combination of low doses of a dopamine agonist with low doses of levodopa is another option, although the benefits of such a combination have not been properly documented.
- *rehabilitation*. Due to the lack of evidence of the efficacy of physical therapy and speech therapy at this stage of the disease, a recommendation cannot be made.

Adjustment of initial monotherapy in patients without motor complications
Patients not on dopaminergic therapy

If a patient has started on an MAO-B inhibitor, anticholinergic, amantadine, or a combination of these drugs, a stage will come when, because of worsening motor symptoms, there is a requirement for:

- *addition of levodopa or a dopamine agonist* (Good Practice Point). Just like in *de novo* patients, at this stage, the choice between levodopa and an agonist again mainly depends on the impact of improving motor disability (better with levodopa) compared with the risk of motor complications (less with agonists) and neuropsychiatric complications (greater with agonists). In addition, there is the effect of age upon the occurrence of motor complications (more frequent in younger patients), and neuropsychiatric complications (more frequent in older and cognitively impaired patients). In general, dopaminergic therapy could be started with agonists in younger patients, whereas levodopa may be preferred in older patients (Good Practice Point, see previous section).

Patients on dopaminergic therapy

Once receiving therapy with a dopamine agonist or levodopa, adjustments of these drugs will also become necessary over time because of worsening motor symptoms.

Table 17.1 Recommendations for the treatment of early PD.

Therapeutic interventions	Recommendation level	
	Symptomatic control of parkinsonism	Prevention of motor complications
Levodopa	Effective (Level A)	Not applicable
Levodopa CR	Effective (Level A)	Ineffective (Level A)
Apomorphine	Not used[a]	Not used[a]
Bromocriptine[b]	Effective (Level B)	Effective (Level B)
Cabergoline[b]	Effective (Level B)	Effective (Level A)
Dihydroergocryptine[b]	Effective (Level A)	No recommendation[c]
Lisuride[b]	Effective (Level B)	Effective (Level C)
Pergolide[b]	Effective (Level A)	Effective (Level B)
Piribedil	Effective (Level C)	No recommendation[c]
Pramipexole	Effective (Level A)	Effective (Level A)
Ropinirole	Effective (Level A)	Effective (Level A)
Selegiline	Effective (Level A)	Ineffective (Level A)
Rasagiline	Effective (Level A)	No recommendation[c]
Entacapone[d]	No recommendation[c]	No recommendation[c]
Tolcapone[d]	No recommendation[c]	No recommendation[c]
Amantadine	Effective (Level B)	No recommendation[c]
Anticholinergics	Effective (Level B)	No recommendation[c]
Rehabilitation	No recommendation[c]	No recommendation[c]
Surgery	Not used	Not used

[a]Subcutaneous apomorphine is not used in early PD.
[b]Pergolide, bromocriptine, cabergoline and, precautionarily, other ergot derivates, cannot be recommended as a first-line treatment for early PD because of the risk of valvular heart disorder (Rascol *et al.*, 2004a,b).
[c]No recommendation can be made due to insufficient data.
[d]As COMT inhibitors, entacapone and tolcapone should always be given with levodopa. Due to hepatic toxicity, tolcapone is not recommended in early PD.

RECOMMENDATIONS

If on dopamine agonist therapy:
- *increase the dopamine agonist dose* (Good Practice Point). However, even when the dopamine agonist dose is increased over time, it cannot control parkinsonian symptoms for more than about 3–5 years of follow-up in most patients.
- *switch between dopamine agonists* (Level C).
- *add levodopa* (Good Practice Point).

If on levodopa:
- *increase the levodopa dose* (Good Practice Point).
- *add a dopamine agonist* (Good Practice Point), although the efficacy of adding an agonist has been insufficiently evaluated.

Patients with persistent, or emerging disabling, tremor

If a significant tremor persists despite usual therapy with dopaminergic agents or amantadine, the following treatment options exist for tremor at rest.

RECOMMENDATIONS

- *anticholinergics* (Good Practice Point: possibly useful, although no full consensus could be made). Cave: anticholinergic side effects, particularly cognitive dysfunction in older patients. See section on anticholinergics.

continued

- *clozapine* (Level B: Bonuccelli *et al.*, 1997; Friedman *et al.*, 1997; Parkinson Study Group, 1999). Due to safety concerns (see Part II of the guidelines on the treatment of psychosis), clozapine is not advised for routine use, but it is considered as an experimental approach for exceptionally disabled patients requiring specialised monitoring (Good Practice Point).
- *beta-blockers (propanolol)*. Beta-blockers can be effective in both resting and postural tremor (Level C: Marsden *et al.*, 1974; Foster *et al.*, 1984; Koller and Herbster, 1987; Henderson *et al.*, 1994). However, due to methodological problems, a Cochrane review found it impossible to determine whether beta-blocker therapy is effective for tremor in PD (Crosby *et al.*, 2003b). Further studies are needed to judge the efficacy of beta-blockers in the treatment of tremor in PD (no recommendation can be made).
- *consider deep brain stimulation.* Usually subthalamic nucleus stimulation, rarely thalamic stimulation (Good Practice Point, see Part II of the guidelines).

Conflicts of interest

M Horstink has not received any departmental research grants or honoraria since starting this guidelines project.

E Tolosa has received honoraria for research funding and consultancy from Novartis, Boehringer Ingelheim, Teva, Medtronic, Schwarz and Servier.

U Bonuccelli has acted as scientific advisor for, or obtained speaker honoraria from, Novartis, Boehringer Ingelheim, Pfizer, Chiesi, Schwarz and GlaxoSmithKline. During the past 2 years he has received departmental grants and performed clinical studies for GlaxoSmithKline, Novartis, Teva, Chiesi, Boehringer, Schwarz and Eisai.

G Deuschl has acted as scientific advisor for, or obtained speaker honoraria from, Orina, Novartis, Boehringer Ingelheim, and Medtronic, during the past 2 years.

JP Larsen has received honoraria and research support from Orion Pharma and Pfizer, and has acted as a consultant for Lundbeck.

A Lees has received honoraria for lectures from Novartis, Orion, Valeant, Britannia, GE-Amersham, Servier, Teva, GlaxoSmithKline, Boehringer Ingelheim and Lundbeck.

W Oertel has received honoraria for research funding and consultancy from Novartis, Boehringer Ingelheim, Schwarz, Medtronic, Teva, Orion, GlaxoSmithKline, Pfizer and Solvay.

W Poewe has received honoraria for lecturing and advisory board membership from Novartis, GlaxoSmithKline, Teva, Boehringer Ingelheim, Schwarz and Orion.

O Rascol has received honoraria for research funding and/or consultancy from GlaxoSmithKline, Novartis, Boehringer Ingelheim, Eli Lilly, Teva, Lundbeck, Schwarz and Servier.

C Sampaio has received departmental research grants from Novartis Portugal. Her department has also charged consultancy fees to Servier and Lundbeck, and she has received honoraria for lectures from Boehringer Ingelheim.

A Friedman and P Kanovsky have nothing to declare.

Disclosure statement

The opinions and views expressed in the paper are those of the authors and not necessarily those of the MDS or its Scientific Issues Committee (SIC).

Acknowledgments

The authors thank Prof Niall Quinn for his constructive criticism and comments on this manuscript. The authors thank Juliet George for helping with the preparation of the text and Karen Henley for secretarial assistance during earlier meetings. They also acknowledge the significant contribution of Dr Yaroslau Compte to the sections on dysautonomia, amantadine and anticholinergics.

Funding sources supporting the work: Financial support from MDS-ES, EFNS and Stichting De Regenboog (the Netherlands).

References
Adler CH (2005). Nonmotor complications in Parkinson's disease. *Mov Disord* **20(Suppl 11):**S23–S29.

Adler CH, Sethi KD, Hauser RA *et al.* for the Ropinirole Study Group (1997). Ropinirole for the treatment of early Parkinson's disease. *Neurology* **49:**393–399.

Ahlskog JE, Muenter MD (2001). Frequency of levodopa-related dyskinesias and motor fluctuations as estimated from the cumulative literature. *Mov Disord* **16:** 448–458.

Allain H, Pollak P, Neukirch HC (1993). Symptomatic effect of selegiline in de novo Parkinsonian patients. The French Selegiline Multicenter Trial. *Mov Disord* **8(Suppl 1):**S36–S40.

Allain H, Destée A, Petit H *et al.* (2000). Five-year follow-up of early lisuride and levodopa combination therapy versus levodopa monotherapy in de novo Parkinson's disease. The French Lisuride Study Group. *Eur Neurol* **44:**22–30.

Appleton DB, Eadie MJ, Sutherland JM (1970). Amantadine hydrochloride in the treatment of parkinsonism. A controlled study. *Med J Aust* **2:**626–629.

Avorn J, Schneeweiss S, Sudarsky LR, Benner J, Kiyota Y, Levin R, Glynn RJ (2005). Sudden uncontrollable somnolence and medication use in Parkinson disease. *Arch Neurol* **62:**1242–1248.

Baatile J, Langbein WE, Weaver F, Maloney C, Jost MB (2000). Effect of exercise on perceived quality of life of individuals with Parkinson's disease. *J Rehabil Res Dev* **37:**529–534.

Barone P, Bravi D, Bermejo-Pareja F *et al.* and the Pergolide Monotherapy Study Group (1999). Pergolide monotherapy in the treatment of early PD. A randomized controlled study. *Neurology* **53:**573–579.

Ben-Shlomo Y, Churchyard A, Head J, Hurwitz B, Overstall P, Ockelford J, Lees AJ (1998). Investigation by Parkinson's Disease Research Group of United Kingdom into excess mortality seen with combined levodopa and selegiline treatment in patients with early, mild Parkinson's disease: further results of randomised trial and confidential inquiry. *BMJ* **316:**1191–1196.

Bergamasco B, Frattola L, Muratorio A, Piccoli F, Mailland F, Parnetti L (2000). Alpha-dihydroergocryptine in the treatment of de novo parkinsonian patients: results of a multicentre, randomized, double-blind, placebo-controlled study. *Acta Neurol Scand* **101:**372–380.

Blanchet PJ, Allard P, Gregoire L, Tardif F, Bedard PJ (1996). Risk factors for peak dose dyskinesia in 100 levodopa-treated parkinsonian patients. *Can J Neurol Sci* **23:**189–193.

Block G, Liss C, Reines S, Irr J, Nibbelink D (1997). Comparison of immediate-release and controlled release carbidopa/levodopa in Parkinson's disease. A multicenter 5-year study. The CR First Study Group. *Eur Neurol* **37:**23–27.

Bloem BR, Steijns JA, Smits-Engelsman BC (2003). An update on falls. *Curr Opin Neurol* **16:**15–26.

Boas J, Worm-Petersen J, Dupont E, Mikkelsen B, Wermuth L (1996). The levodopa dose-sparing capacity of pergolide compared with that of bromocriptine in an open-label, cross-over study. *Eur J Neurol* **3:**44–49.

Bonuccelli U, Ceravolo R, Salvetti S, D'Avino C, Del Dotto P, Rossi G, Murri L (1997). Clozapine in Parkinson's disease tremor. Effects of acute and chronic administration. *Neurology* **49:**1587–1590.

Bosboom JL, Stoffers D, Wolters EC (2004). Cognitive dysfunction and dementia in Parkinson's disease. *J Neural Transm* **111:**1303–1315.

Brainin M, Barnes M, Baron JC, Gilhus NE, Hughes R, Selmaj K, Waldemar G (2004). Guidance for the preparation of neurological management guidelines by EFNS scientific task forces – revised recommendations 2004. *Eur J Neurol* **11:**577–581.

Brooks DJ, Sagar H; UK-Irish Entacapone Study Group (2003). Entacapone is beneficial in both fluctuating and non-fluctuating patients with Parkinson's disease: a randomised, placebo controlled, double blind, six month study. *J Neurol Neurosurg Psychiatry* **74:**1071–1079.

Brunt ER, Brooks DJ, Korczyn AD, Montastruc JL, Stocchi F; 043 study group (2002). A six-month multicentre, double-blind, bromocriptine-controlled study of the safety and efficacy of ropinirole in the treatment of patients with Parkinson's disease not optimally controlled by L-dopa. *J Neural Transm* **109:**489–502.

Butzer JF, Silver DE, Sans AL (1975). Amantadine in Parkinson's disease. A double-blind, placebo-controlled, crossover study with long-term follow-up. *Neurology* **25:**603–606.

Canesi M, Antonini A, Mariani CB, Tesei S, Zecchinelli AL, Barichella M, Pezzoli G (1999). An overnight switch to ropinirole therapy in patients with Parkinson's disease. Short communication. *J Neural Transm* **106:**925–929.

Cantello R, Riccio A, Gilli M *et al.* (1986). Bornaprine vs placebo in Parkinson disease: double-blind controlled cross-over trial in 30 patients. *Ital J Neurol Sci* **7:**139–143.

Chen H, Zhang SM, Schwarzschild MA, Hernan MA, Ascherio A (2005). Physical activity and the risk of Parkinson disease. *Neurology* **64:**664–669.

Clarke CE (1995). Does levodopa therapy delay death in Parkinson's disease? A review of the evidence. *Mov Disord* **10:**250–256.

Comella CL, Stebbins GT, Brown-Toms N, Goetz CG (1994). Physical therapy and Parkinson's disease: a controlled clinical trial. *Neurology* **44:**376–378.

Cooper JA, Sagar HJ, Doherty SM, Jordan N, Tidswell P, Sullivan EV (1992). Different effects of dopaminergic and anticholinergic therapies on cognitive and motor function in Parkinson's disease. *Brain* **115:** 1701–1725.

Cox B, Danta G, Schnieden H, Yuill GM (1973). Interactions of levodopa and amantadine in patients with parkinsonism. *J Neurol Neurosurg Psychiatry* **36:**354–361.

Crosby NJ, Deane KH, Clarke CE (2003a). Amantadine for dyskinesia in Parkinson's disease. *Cochrane Database Syst Rev* **2:**CD003467.

Crosby NJ, Deane KHO, Clarke CE (2003b). Beta-blocker therapy for tremor in Parkinson's disease. *Cochrane Database Syst Rev* **1:**CD003361. [This ref will need an a/b designation]

Cubo E, Leurgans S, Goetz CG (2004). Short-term and practice effects of metronome pacing in Parkinson's disease patients with gait freezing while in the 'on' state: randomized single blind evaluation. *Parkinsonism Relat Disord* **10:**507–510.

Dam M, Tonin P, Casson S, Bracco F, Piron L, Pizzolato G, Battistin L (1996). Effects of conventional and sensory-enhanced physiotherapy on disability of Parkinson's disease patients. *Adv Neurol* **69:**551–555.

de Goede CJ, Keus SH, Kwakkel G, Wagenaar RC (2001). The effects of physical therapy in Parkinson's disease: a research synthesis. *Arch Phys Med Rehabil* **82:**509–515.

de Swart BJ, Willemse SC, Maassen BA, Horstink MW (2003). Improvement of voicing in patients with Parkinson's disease by speech therapy. *Neurology* **60:**498–500.

Deane KHO, Jones D, Ellis-Hill C, Clarke CE, Playford ED, Ben-Shlomo Y (2001a). Physiotherapy for Parkinson's disease: a comparison of techniques. *Cochrane Database Syst Rev* **1:**CD002815.

Deane KHO, Jones D, Playford ED, Ben-Shlomo Y, Clarke CE (2001b). Physiotherapy versus placebo or no intervention in Parkinson's disease. *Cochrane Database Syst Rev* **3:**CD002817.

Deane KHO, Whurr R, Playford ED, Ben-Shlomo Y, Clarke CE (2001c). Speech and language therapy versus placebo or no intervention for dysarthria in Parkinson's disease. *Cochrane Database Syst Rev* **2:**CD002812.

Deane KHO, Whurr R, Clarke CE, Playford ED, Ben-Shlomo Y (2001d). Non-pharmacological therapies for dysphagia in Parkinson's disease. *Cochrane Database Syst Rev* **1:**CD002816.

Deane KH, Ellis-Hill C, Jones D, Whurr R, Ben-Shlomo Y, Playford ED, Clarke CE (2002). Systematic review of paramedical therapies for Parkinson's disease. *Mov Disord* **17:**984–991.

Denny AP, Behari M (1999). Motor fluctuations in Parkinson's disease. *J Neurol Sci* **165:**18–23.

Dewey RB Jr, Hutton JT, LeWitt PA, Factor SA (2001). A randomized, double-blind, placebo-controlled trial on subcutaneously injected apomorphine for parkinsonian off-state events. *Arch Neurol* **58:**1385–1392.

Dietz MA, Stebbins GT, Goetz CG (1990). Evaluation of a modified inverted walking stick as a treatment for parkinsonian freezing episodes. *Mov Disord* **5:**243–247.

Dupont E, Andersen A, Boas J *et al.* (1996). Sustained-release Madopar HBS compared with standard Madopar in the long-term treatment of de novo parkinsonian patients. *Acta Neurol Scand* **93:**14–20.

Dupont E, Burgunder JM, Findley LJ, Olsson JE, Dorflinger E (1997). Tolcapone added to levodopa in stable parkinsonian patients: a double-blind placebo-controlled study. Tolcapone in Parkinson's Disease Study Group II (TIPS II). *Mov Disord* **12:**928–934.

Ellis T, de Goede CJ, Feldman RG, Wolters EC, Kwakkel G, Wagenaar RC (2005). Efficacy of a physical therapy program in patients with Parkinson's disease: a randomized controlled trial. *Arch Phys Med Rehabil* **86:**626–632.

Etminan M, Samii A, Takkouche B, Rochon P (2001). Increased risk of somnolence with the new dopamine agonists in patients with Parkinson's disease. A meta-analysis of randomised controlled trials. *Drug Saf* **24:**863–868.

Etminan M, Gill SS, Samii A (2005). Intake of vitamin E, vitamin C, and carotenoids and the risk of Parkinson's disease: a meta-analysis. *Lancet Neurol* **4:**362–365.

European Agency for the Evaluation of Medicinal Products (EMEA) (2004). EMEA public statement on the lifting of the suspension of the marketing authorisation for tolcapone (Tasmar). London, 29 April 2004 (http://www.emea.eu.int/pdfs/human/press/pus/1185404en.pdf, date accessed 10 January 2006).

Fahn S, Isgreen WP (1975). Long-term evaluation of amantadine and levodopa combination by double-blind crossover analyses. *Neurology* **25:**695–700.

Fehling C (1973). The effect of adding amantadine to optimum levodopa dosage in Parkinson's syndrome. *Acta Neurol Scand* **49:**245–251.

Formisano R, Pratesi L, Modarelli FT, Bonifati V, Meco G (1992). Rehabilitation and Parkinson's disease. *Scand J Rehabil Med* **24:**157–160.

Foster NL, Newman RP, LeWitt PA, Gillespie MM, Larsen TA, Chase TN (1984). Peripheral beta-adrenergic blockade treatment of parkinsonian tremor. *Ann Neurol* **16:**505–508.

Friedman JH, Koller WC, Lannon MC, Busenbark K, Swanson-Hyland E, Smith D (1997). Benztropine versus clozapine for the treatment of tremor in Parkinson's disease. *Neurology* **48:**1077–1081.

Gage H, Storey L (2004). Rehabilitation for Parkinson's disease: a systematic review of available evidence. *Clin Rehabil* **18:**463–482.

Gauthier L, Dalziel S, Gauthier S (1987). The benefits of group occupational therapy for patients with Parkinson's disease. *Am J Occup Ther* **41:**360–365.

Gillespie LD, Gillespie WJ, Robertson MC, Lamb SE, Cumming RG, Rowe BH (2003). Interventions for preventing falls in elderly people. *Cochrane Database Syst Rev* **4:**CD000340.

Gimenez-Roldan S, Esteban EM, Mateo D (2001). Switching from bromocriptine to ropinirole in patients with advanced Parkinson's disease: open label pilot responses to three different dose-ratios. *Clin Neuropharmacol* **24:**346–351.

Goetz CG, Tanner CM, Shannon KM, Carroll VS, Klawans HL, Carvey PM, Gilley D (1988). Controlled-release carbidopa/levodopa (CR4-Sinemet) in Parkinson's disease patients with and without motor fluctuations. *Neurology* **38:**1143–1146.

Goetz CG, Shannon KM, Tanner CM, Carroll VS, Klawans HL (1989). Agonist substitution in advanced Parkinson's disease. *Neurology* **39:**1121–1122.

Goetz CG, Blasucci L, Stebbins GT (1999). Switching dopamine agonists in advanced Parkinson's disease: is rapid titration preferable to slow? *Neurology* **52:**1227–1229.

Grandas F, Galiano ML, Tabernero C (1999). Risk factors for levodopa-induced dyskinesias in Parkinson's disease. *J Neurol* **246:**1127–1133.

Grosset K, Needleman F, Macphee G, Grosset D (2004). Switching from ergot to nonergot dopamine agonists in Parkinson's disease: a clinical series and five-drug dose conversion table. *Mov Disord* **19:**1370–1374.

Guttman M (1997). Double-blind randomized, placebo controlled study to compare safety, tolerance and efficacy of pramipexole and bromocriptine in advanced Parkinson's disease. International Pramipexole-Bromocriptine Study Group. *Neurology* **49:**1060–1065.

Hanna PA, Ratkos L, Ondo WG, Jankovic J (2001). Switching from pergolide to pramipexole in patients with Parkinson's disease. *J Neural Transm* **108:**63–70.

Health Council of the Netherlands (2003). Therapeutic exercise. *Den Haag, Netherlands* **2003/22:**108.

Heinonen EH, Myllyla V (1998). Safety of selegiline (deprenyl) in the treatment of Parkinson's disease. *Drug Saf* **19:**11–22.

Hely MA, Morris JGL, Reid WGJ (1994). The Sydney multicentre study of Parkinson's disease: a randomized, prospective five year study comparing low dose bromocriptine with low dose levodopa-carbidopa. *J Neurol Neurosurg Psychiatry* **57:**903–910.

Henderson JM, Yiannikas C, Morris JG, Einstein R, Jackson D, Byth K (1994). Postural tremor of Parkinson's disease. *Clin Neuropharmacol* **17:**277–285.

Hirsch MA, Toole T, Maitland CG, Rider RA (2003). The effects of balance training and high-intensity resistance training on persons with idiopathic Parkinson's disease. *Arch Phys Med Rehabil* **84:**1109–1117.

Horrocks PM, Vicary DJ, Rees JE, Parkes JD, Marsden CD (1973). Anticholinergic withdrawal and benzhexol treatment in Parkinson's disease. *J Neurol Neurosurg Psychiatry* **36:**936–941.

Hughes RC, Polgar JG, Weightman D, Walton JN (1971). Levodopa in Parkinsonism: the effects of withdrawal of anticholinergic drugs. *Br Med J* **2:**487–491.

Hutton JT, Koller WC, Ahlskog JE *et al.* (1996). Multicenter, placebo-controlled trial of cabergoline taken once daily in the treatment of Parkinson's disease. *Neurology* **46:**1062–1065.

Iivanainen M (1974). KR 339 in the treatment of Parkinsonian tremor. *Acta Neurol Scand* **50:**469–470.

Inzelberg R, Nisipeanu P, Rabey JM *et al.* (1996). Double-blind comparison of cabergoline and bromocriptine in Parkinson's disease patients with motor fluctuations. *Neurology* **47:**785–788.

Ives NJ, Stowe RL, Marro J *et al.* (2004). Monoamine oxidase type B inhibitors in early Parkinson's disease: meta-analysis of 17 randomised trials involving 3525 patients. *BMJ* **329:**593.

Jankovic J (2005). Motor fluctuations and dyskinesias in Parkinson's disease: Clinical manifestations. *Mov Disord* **20(Suppl 11):**S11–S16.

Jankovic J, Hunter C (2002). A double-blind, placebo-controlled and longitudinal study of riluzole in early Parkinson's disease. *Parkinsonism Relat Disord* **8:**271–276.

Jorgensen PB, Bergin JD, Haas L *et al.* (1971). Controlled trial of amantadine hydrochloride in Parkinson's disease. *N Z Med J* **73:**263–267.

Katzenschlager R, Lees AJ (2002). Treatment of Parkinson's disease: levodopa as the first choice. *J Neurol* **249(Suppl 2):**II19–II24.

Katzenschlager R, Sampaio C, Costa J, Lees A (2002). Anticholinergics for symptomatic management of Parkinson's disease. *Cochrane Database Syst Rev* **3:**CD003735.

Katzenschlager R, Hughes A, Evans A *et al.* (2005). Continuous subcutaneous apomorphine therapy improves dyskinesias in Parkinson's disease: a prospective study using single-dose challenges. *Mov Disord* **20:**151–157.

Koller WC, Herbster G (1987). Adjuvant therapy of parkinsonian tremor. *Arch Neurol* **44:**921–923.

Koller WC, Hutton JT, Tolosa E, Capilldeo R (1999). Immediate-release and controlled-release carbidopa/levodopa in PD: a 5-year randomized multicenter study. Carbidopa/Levodopa Study Group. *Neurology* **53:**1012–1019.

Koller W, Lees A, Doder M, Hely M; Tolcapone/Pergolide Study Group (2001). Randomised trial of tolcapone versus pergolide as add-on to levodopa therapy in Parkinson's disease patients with motor fluctuations. *Mov Disord* **16:**858–866.

Kompoliti K, Goetz CG, Leurgans S, Morrissey M, Siegel IM (2000). "On" freezing in Parkinson's disease: resistance to visual cue walking devices. *Mov Disord* **15:**309–312.

Korczyn AD, Brooks DJ, Brunt ER, Poewe WH, Rascol O, Stocchi F (1998). Ropinirole versus bromocriptine in the treatment of early Parkinson's disease: a 6-month interim report of a 3-year study. 053 Study Group. *Mov Disord* **13:**46–51.

Korczyn AD, Brunt ER, Larsen JP, Nagy Z, Poewe WH, Ruggieri S (1999). A 3-year randomized trial of ropinirole and bromocriptine in early Parkinson's disease. The 053 Study Group. *Neurology* **53:**364–370.

Kostic V, Przedborski S, Flaster E, Sternic N (1991). Early development of levodopa-induced dyskinesias and response fluctuations in young-onset Parkinson's disease. *Neurology* **41:**202–205.

Kulisevsky J, Lopez-Villegas D, Garcia-Sanchez C, Barbanoj M, Gironell A, Pascual-Sedano B (1998). A six-month study of pergolide and levodopa in de novo Parkinson's disease patients. *Clin Neuropharmacol* **21:**358–362.

Kumar N, Van Gerpen JA, Bower JH, Ahlskog JE (2005). Levodopa-dyskinesia incidence by age of Parkinson's disease onset. *Mov Disord* **20:**342–344.

Laihinen A, Rinne UK, Suchy I (1992). Comparison of lisuride and bromocriptine in the treatment of advanced Parkinson's disease. *Acta Neurol Scand* **86:**593–595.

Larsen JP, Boas J (1997). The effects of early selegiline therapy on long-term levodopa treatment and parkinsonian disability: an interim analysis of a Norwegian–Danish 5-year study. Norwegian-Danish Study Group. *Mov Disord* **12:**175–182.

Larsen JP, Boas J, Erdal JE (1999). Does selegiline modify the progression of early Parkinson's disease? Results from a five-year study. The Norwegian-Danish Study Group. *Eur J Neurol* **6:**539–547.

Le Witt PA, Gopinathan G, Ward CD *et al.* (1982). Lisuride versus bromocriptine treatment in Parkinson disease: a double-blind study. *Neurology* **32:**69–72.

Le Witt PA, Ward CD, Larsen TA *et al.* (1983). Comparison of pergolide and bromocriptine therapy in parkinsonism. *Neurology* **33:**1009–1014.

Lees AJ (1995). Comparison of therapeutic effects and mortality data of levodopa and levodopa combined with selegiline in patients with early, mild Parkinson's disease. Parkinson's Disease Research Group of the United Kingdom. *BMJ* **311:**1602–1607.

Lees AJ, Shaw KM, Kohout LJ, Stern GM (1977). Deprenyl in Parkinson's disease. *Lancet* **15:**791–795.

Lees AJ, Katzenschlager R, Head J, Ben-Shlomo Y (2001). Ten-year follow-up of three different initial treatments in de-novo PD. A randomized trial. *Neurology* **57:**1687–1694.

Levine CB, Fahrbach KR, Siderowf AD, Estok RP, Ludensky VM, Ross SD (2003). Diagnosis and treatment of Parkinson's disease: a systematic review of the literature. *Evid Rep Technol Assess* **57:**1–306.

Lewis GN, Byblow WD, Walt SE (2000). Stride length regulation in Parkinson's disease: the use of extrinsic, visual cues. *Brain* **123:**2077–2090.

Lieberman A, Olanow CW, Sethi K, Swanson P, Waters CH, Fahn S, Hurtig H, Yahr M (1998). A multicenter trial of ropinirole as adjunct treatment for Parkinson's disease. Ropinirole Study Group. *Neurology* **51:**1057–1062.

Linazasoro G; Spanish Dopamine Agonists Study Group (2004). Conversion from dopamine agonists to pramipexole. An open-label trial in 227 patients with advanced Parkinson's disease. *J Neurol* **251:**335–339.

Mally J, Kovacs AB, Stone TW (1995). Delayed development of symptomatic improvement by (–)-deprenyl in Parkinson's disease. *J Neurol Sci* **134:**143–145.

Management of Parkinson's disease: an evidence-based review (2002). *Mov Disord* **17:**S1–S166.

Marchese R, Diverio M, Zucchi F, Lentino C, Abbruzzese G (2000). The role of sensory cues in the rehabilitation of parkinsonian patients: a comparison of two physical therapy protocols. *Mov Disord* **15:**879–883.

Maricle RA, Nutt JG, Carter JH (1995). Mood and anxiety fluctuation in Parkinson's disease associated with levodopa infusion: preliminary findings. *Mov Disord* **10:**329–332.

Marsden CD, Parkes JD, Rees JE (1974). Propranolol in Parkinson's disease. *Lancet* **2:**410.

Marsh GG, Markham CH (1973). Does levodopa alter depression and psychopathology in Parkinsonism patients? *J Neurol Neurosurg Psychiatry* **36:**925–935.

Martignoni E, Pacchetti C, Sibilla L, Bruggi P, Pedevilla M, Nappi G (1991). Dihydroergocryptine in the treatment of Parkinson's disease: a six month's double-blind clinical trial. *Clin Neuropharmacol* **14:**78–83.

Martin WE, Loewenson RB, Resch JA, Baker AB (1974). A controlled study comparing trihexyphenidyl hydrochloride plus levodopa with placebo plus levodopa in patients with Parkinson's disease. *Neurology* **24:**912–919.

McIntosh GC, Brown SH, Rice RR, Thaut MH (1997). Rhythmic auditory-motor facilitation of gait patterns in patients with Parkinson's disease. *J Neurol Neurosurg Psychiatry* **62:**22–26.

Mizuno Y, Kondo T, Narabayashi H (1995). Pergolide in the treatment of Parkinson's disease. *Neurology* **45(Suppl 31):**S13–S21.

Mizuno Y, Yanagisawa N, Kuno S, Yamamoto M, Hasegawa K, Origasa H, Kowa H; Japanese Pramipexole Study Group (2003). Randomized double-blind study of pramipexole with placebo and bromocriptine in advanced Parkinson's disease. *Mov Disord* **18:**1149–1156.

Moller JC, Oertel WH, Koster J, Pezzoli G, Provinciali L (2005). Long-term efficacy and safety of pramipexole in advanced Parkinson's disease: results from a European multicenter trial. *Mov Disord* **20:**602–610.

Montastruc JL, Rascol O, Senard JM, Rascol A (1994). A randomized controlled study comparing bromocriptine to which levodopa was later added, with levodopa alone in previously untreated patients with Parkinson's disease: a five year follow-up. *J Neurol Neurosurg Psychiatry* **57:**1034–1038.

Montastruc JL, Desboeuf K, Lapeyre-Mestre M, Senard JM, Rascol O, Brefel-Courbon C (2001). Long-term mortality results on the randomized controlled study comparing bromocriptine to which levodopa was later added with levodopa alone in previously untreated patients with Parkinson's disease. *Mov Disord* **16:**511–514.

Morrison CE, Borod JC, Brin MF, Halbig TD, Olanow CW (2004). Effects of levodopa on cognitive functioning in moderate-to-severe Parkinson's disease (MSPD). *J Neural Transm* **111:**1333–1341.

Myllyla VV, Sotaniemi KA, Vuorinen JA, Heinonen EH (1992). Selegiline as initial treatment in de novo parkinsonian patients. *Neurology* **42:**339–343.

Myllyla VV, Kultalahti ER, Haapaniemi H, Leinonen M; FILOMEN Study Group (2001). Twelve-month safety of entacapone in patients with Parkinson's disease. *Eur J Neurol* **8:**53–60.

Nappi G, Martignoni E, Horowski R, Pacchetti C, Rainer E, Bruggi P, Runge I (1991). Lisuride plus selegiline in the treatment of early Parkinson's disease. *Acta Neurol Scand* **83:**407–410.

Nieoullon A (2002). Dopamine and the regulation of cognition and attention. *Prog Neurobiol* **67:**53–83.

Nissenbaum H, Quinn NP, Brown RG, Toone B, Gotham AM, Marsden CD (1987). Mood swings associated with the 'on-off' phenomenon in Parkinson's disease. *Psychol Med* **17:**899–904.

Nutt JG, Burchiel KJ, Comella CL, Jankovic J, Lang AE, Laws ER Jr *et al.* (2003). Randomized, double-blind trial of glial cell line-derived neurotrophic factor (GDNF) in PD. *Neurology* **60:**69–73.

Oertel WH, Wolters E, Sampaio C *et al.* (2005). Pergolide versus levodopa monotherapy in early Parkinson's disease patients: the PELMOPET study. *Mov Disord.* Published online 6 Oct, DOI: 10.1002/mds.20724.

Olanow CW, Riederer P (1996). Selegiline and neuroprotection in Parkinson's disease. *Neurology* **47C(Suppl 3):**51.

Olanow CW, Fahn S, Muenter M *et al.* (1994). A multicenter double-bind placebo-controlled trial of pergolide as an adjunct to Sinemet in Parkinson's disease. *Mov Disord* **9:**40–47.

Olanow CW, Hauser RA, Gauger L *et al.* (1995). The effect of deprenyl and levodopa on the progression of Parkinson's disease. *Ann Neurol* **38:**771–777.

Olanow CW, Myllyla VV, Sotaniemi KA *et al.* (1998). Effect of selegiline on mortality in patients with Parkinson's disease: a meta-analysis. *Neurology* **51:**825–830.

Olanow CW, Watts RL, Koller WC (2001). An algorithm (decision tree) for the management of Parkinson's disease (2001): treatment guidelines. *Neurology* **56(Suppl 5):**S1-S88.

Olanow CW, Agid Y, Mizuno Y *et al.* (2004). Levodopa in the treatment of Parkinson's disease: current controversies. *Mov Disord* **19:**997–1005.

Palhagen S, Heinonen EH, Hagglund J *et al.* (1998). Selegiline delays the onset of disability in de novo parkinsonian patients. Swedish Parkinson Study Group. *Neurology* **51:**520–525.

Parkes JD, Baxter RC, Marsden CD, Rees J (1974). Comparative trial of benzhexol, amantadine, and levodopa in the treatment of Parkinson's disease. *J Neurol Neurosurg Psychiatry* **37:**422–426.

Parkinson Study Group (1989). Effect of deprenyl on the progression of disability in early Parkinson's disease. *N Engl J Med* **321:**1364–1371.

Parkinson Study Group (1996). Impact of deprenyl and tocopherol treatment on Parkinson's disease in DATATOP patients requiring levodopa. *Ann Neurol* **39:**37–45.

Parkinson Study Group (1999). Low-dose clozapine for the treatment of drug-induced psychosis in Parkinson's disease. The Parkinson Study Group. *N Engl J Med* **340:**757–763.

Parkinson Study Group (2000). Pramipexole vs levodopa as initial treatment for Parkinson disease: a randomized controlled trial. *JAMA* **284**:1931–1938.

Parkinson Study Group (2002a). A controlled trial of rasagiline in early Parkinson disease. The TEMPO study. *Arch Neurol* **59**:1937–1943.

Parkinson Study Group (2002b). Dopamine transporter brain imaging to assess the effects of pramipexole vs levodopa on Parkinson disease progression. *JAMA* **287**:1653–1661.

Parkinson Study Group (2003). A controlled trial of rotigotine monotherapy in early Parkinson's disease. *Arch Neurol* **60**:1721–1728.

Parkinson Study Group (2004a). A controlled, randomized, delayed-start study of rasagiline in early Parkinson disease. *Arch Neurol* **61**:561–566.

Parkinson Study Group (2004b). Levodopa and the progression of Parkinson's disease. *N Engl J Med* **351**:2498–2508.

Parkinson Study Group (2004c). Pramipexole vs levodopa as initial treatment for Parkinson disease: a 4-year randomized controlled trial. *Arch Neurol* **61**:1044–1053.

Parkinson's Disease Research Group in the United Kingdom (1993). Comparisons of therapeutic effects of levodopa, levodopa and selegiline, and bromocriptine in patients with early, mild Parkinson's disease: three year interim report. *BMJ* **307**:469–472.

Pezzoli G, Martignoni E, Pacchetti C *et al.* (1995). A cross-over, controlled study comparing pergolide with bromocriptine as an adjunct to levodopa for the treatment of Parkinson's disease. *Neurology* **45(Suppl 3)**:S22–S27.

Pillon B, Czernecki V, Dubois B (2003). Dopamine and cognitive function. *Curr Opin Neurol* **16(Suppl 2)**:S17–S22.

Pinter MM, Pogarell O, Oertel WH (1999). Efficacy, safety, and tolerance of the non-ergoline dopamine agonist pramipexole in the treatment of advanced Parkinson's disease: a double-blind, placebo controlled, randomized, multicentre study. *J Neurol Neurosurg Psychiatry* **66**:436–441.

Pinto S, Ozsancak C, Tripoliti E, Thobois S, Limousin-Dowsey P, Auzou P (2004). Dysarthria in Parkinson's disease. *Lancet Neurol* **3**:547–556.

Platz T, Brown RG, Marsden CD (1998). Training improves the speed of aimed movements in Parkinson's disease. *Brain* **121**:505–514.

Poewe WH, Lees AJ, Stern GM (1986). Low-dose L-dopa therapy in Parkinson's disease: a 6-year follow-up study. *Neurology* **36**:1528–1530.

Pogarell O, Gasser T, van Hilten JJ, Spieker S, Pollentier S, Meier D, Oertel WH (2002). Pramipexole in patients with Parkinson's disease and marked drug resistant tremor: a randomized, double-blind, placebo-controlled multicentre trial. *J Neurol Neurosurg Psychiatry* **72**:713–720.

Przuntek H, Kuhn W (1987). The effect of R-(-)-deprenyl in de novo Parkinson patients on combination therapy with levodopa and decarboxylase inhibitor. *J Neural Transm Suppl* **25**:97–104.

Przuntek H, Welzel D, Gerlach M *et al.* (1996). Early institution of bromocriptine in Parkinson's disease inhibits the emergence of levodopa-associated motor side effects. Long-term results of the PRADO study. *J Neural Transm* **103**:699–715.

Rajput AH (2001). Levodopa prolongs life expectancy and is non-toxic to substantia nigra. *Parkinsonism Relat Disord* **8**:95–100.

Ramaker C, van Hilten JJ (2000). Bromocriptine versus levodopa in early Parkinson's disease. *Cochrane Database Syst Rev* **2**:CD002258.

Ramig LO, Countryman S, O'Brien C, Hoehn M, Thompson L (1996).Intensive speech treatment for patients with Parkinson's disease: short-and long-term comparison of two techniques. *Neurology* **47**:1496–1504.

Ramig LO, Sapir S, Fox C, Countryman S (2001). Changes in vocal loudness following intensive voice treatment (LSVT) in individuals with Parkinson's disease: a comparison with untreated patients and normal age-matched controls. *Mov Disord* **16**:79–83.

Rascol O, Brooks DJ, Korczyn AD, De Deyn PP, Clarke CE, Lang AE (2000). A five-year study of the incidence of dyskinesia in patients with early Parkinson's disease who were treated with ropinirole or levodopa. 056 Study Group. *N Engl J Med* **342**:1484–1491.

Rascol O, Pathak A, Bagheri H, Montastruc J-L (2004a). New concerns about old drugs: valvular heart disease on ergot derivative dopamine agonists as an exemplary situation of pharmacovigilance. *Mov Disord* **19**:611–613.

Rascol O, Pathak A, Bagheri H, Montastruc J-L (2004b). Dopaminagonists and fibrotic valvular heart disease: further considerations. *Mov Disord* **19**:1524–1525.

Raudino F (2001). Non motor off in Parkinson's disease. *Acta Neurol Scand* **104**:312–315.

Reichmann H, Herting B, Miller A, Sommer U (2003). Switching and combining dopamine agonists. *J Neural Transm* **110**:1393–1400.

Rinne UK (1989). Lisuride, a dopamine agonist in the treatment of early Parkinson's disease. *Neurology* **39**:336–339.

Rinne UK, Bracco F, Chouza C *et al.* (1997). Cabergoline in the treatment of early Parkinson's disease: results of the first year of treatment in a double-blind comparison of cabergoline and levodopa. The PKDS009 Collaborative Study Group. *Neurology* **48**:363–368.

Rinne UK, Bracco F, Chouza C, Dupont E, Gershanik O, Marti Masso JF, Montastruc JL, Marsden CD (1998). Early treatment of Parkinson's disease with cabergoline delays the onset of motor complications. The PKDS009 Study Group. *Drugs* **55(Suppl 1)**:23–30.

Riopelle RJ (1987). Bromocriptine and the clinical spectrum of Parkinson's disease. *Can J Neurol Sci* **14**:455–459.

Rochester L, Hetherington V, Jones D, Nieuwboer A, Willems AM, Kwakkel G, Van WE (2005). The effect of external rhythmic cues (auditory and visual) on walking during a functional task in homes of people with Parkinson's disease. *Arch Phys Med Rehabil* **86**:999–1006.

Rondot P, Ziegler M (1992). Activity and acceptability of piribedil in Parkinson's disease: a multicentre study. *J Neurol* **239(Suppl 1)**:28–34.

Rubinstein TC, Giladi N, Hausdorff JM (2002). The power of cueing to circumvent dopamine deficits: a review of physical therapy treatment of gait disturbances in Parkinson's disease. *Mov Disord* **17**:1148–1160.

Sasco AJ, Paffenbarger RS, Gendre I, Wing AL (1992). The role of physical exercise in the occurrence of Parkinson's disease. *Arch Neurol* **49**:360–365.

Savery F (1971). Amantadine and a fixed combination of levodopa and carbidopa in the treatment of Parkinson's disease. *Dis Nerv Syst* **38**:605–608.

Schenkman M, Cutson TM, Kuchibhatla M, Chandler J, Pieper CF, Ray L, Laub KC (1998). Exercise to improve spinal flexibility and function for people with Parkinson's disease: a randomized, controlled trial. *J Am Geriatr Soc* **46**:1207–1216.

Schrag A, Schelosky L, Scholz U, Poewe W (1999). Reduction of parkinsonian signs in patients with Parkinson's disease by dopaminergic versus anticholinergic single-dose challenges. *Mov Disord* **14**:252–255.

Shannon KM, Bennett JP, Friedman JH (1997). Efficacy of pramipexole, a novel dopamine agonist, as monotherapy in mild to moderate Parkinson's disease. The Pramipexole Study Group. *Neurology* **49**:724–728.

Shoulson I, Oakes D, Fahn S *et al.*; Parkinson Study Group (2002). Impact of sustained deprenyl (selegiline) in levodopa-treated Parkinson's disease: a randomized placebo-controlled extension of the deprenyl and toco-pherol antioxidative therapy of parkinsonism trial. *Ann Neurol* **51**:604–612.

Shults CW, Oakes D, Kieburtz K, Beal MF, Haas R, Plumb S *et al.* (2002). Effects of coenzyme Q10 in early Parkinson disease: evidence of slowing of the functional decline. *Arch Neurol* **59**:1541–1550.

Sivertsen B, Dupont E, Mikkelsen B, Mogensen P, Rasmussen C, Boesen F, Heinonen E (1989). Selegiline and levodopa in early or moderately advanced Parkinson's disease: a double-blind controlled short- and long-term study. *Acta Neurol Scand Suppl* **126**:147–152.

Soliveri P, Brown RG, Jahanshahi M, Marsden CD (1992). Effect of practice on performance of a skilled motor task in patients with Parkinson's disease. *J Neurol Neurosurg Psychiatry* **55**:454–460.

Suteerawattananon M, Morris GS, Etnyre BR, Jankovic J, Protas EJ (2004). Effects of visual and auditory cues on gait in individuals with Parkinson's disease. *J Neurol Sci* **219**:63–69.

Teravainen H (1990). Selegiline in Parkinson's disease. *Acta Neurol Scand* **81**:333–336.

Tetrud JW, Langston JW (1989). The effect of deprenyl (selegiline) on the natural history of Parkinson's disease. *Science* **245**:519–522.

Thaut MH, McIntosh GC, Rice RR, Miller RA, Rathbun J, Brault JM (1996). Rhythmic auditory stimulation in gait training for Parkinson's disease patients. *Mov Disord* **11**:193–200.

Tolcapone Study Group (1999). Efficacy and tolerability of tolcapone compared with bromocriptine in levodopa-treated parkinsonian patients. *Mov Disord* **14**:38–44.

Tourtellotte WW, Potvin AR, Syndulko K *et al.* (1982). Parkinson's disease: Cogentin with Sinemet, a better response. *Prog Neuropsychopharmacol Biol Psychiatry* **6**:51–55.

Tsai CH, Lo SK, See LC *et al.* (2002). Environmental risk factors of young onset Parkinson's disease: a case-control study. *Clin Neurol Neurosurg* **104**:328–333.

Van Camp G, Flamez A, Cosyns B *et al.* (2004). Treatment of Parkinson's disease with pergolide and relation to restrictive valvular heart disease. *Lancet* **363**:1179–1183.

van Herwaarden G, Berger HJ, Horstink MW (1993). Short-term memory in Parkinson's disease after withdrawal of long-term anticholinergic therapy. *Clin Neuropharmacol* **16**:438–443.

Waters CH, Kurth M, Bailey P, Shulman LM, LeWitt P, Dorflinger E, Deptula D, Pedder S (1997). Tolcapone in stable Parkinson's disease: efficacy and safety of long-term treatment. The Tolcapone Stable Study Group. *Neurology* **49**:665–671.

Whone AL, Watts RL, Stoess AJ *et al.* (2003). Slower progression of Parkinson's disease with ropinirole versus levodopa: the REAL-PET study. *Ann Neurol* **54:**93–101.

Witjas T, Kaphan E, Azulay JP *et al.* (2002). Nonmotor fluctuations in Parkinson's disease: frequent and disabling. *Neurology* **59:**408–413.

Ziegler M, Castro-Caldas A, Del Signore S, Rascol O (2003). Efficacy of piribedil as early combination to levodopa in patients with stable Parkinson's disease: a 6-month, randomized placebo-controlled study. *Mov Disord* **18:**418–425.

CHAPTER 18

Late (complicated) Parkinson's disease*

M. Horstink (EFNS),[a] E. Tolosa (MDS-ES),[b]
U. Bonuccelli,[c] G. Deuschl,[d] A. Friedman,[e]
P. Kanovsky,[f] J.P. Larsen,[g] A. Lees,[h] W. Oertel,[i]
W. Poewe,[j] O. Rascol,[k] C. Sampaio[l]

Abstract

Objective To provide evidence-based recommendations for the management of late (complicated) Parkinson's disease (PD), based on a review of the literature. Complicated PD refers to patients suffering from the classical motor syndrome of PD along with other motor or non-motor complications, either disease-related (e.g. freezing) or treatment-related (e,g. dyskinesias or hallucinations).

Methods MEDLINE, Cochrane Library and INAHTA database literature searches were conducted. National guidelines were requested from all EFNS societies. Non-European guidelines were searched for using MEDLINE.

Results Part II of the guidelines deals with treatment of motor and neuropsychiatric complications and autonomic disturbances. For each topic, a list of therapeutic interventions is provided, including classification of evidence. Following this, recommendations for management are given, alongside ratings of efficacy. Classifications of evidence and ratings of efficacy are made according to EFNS guidance. In cases where there is insufficient scientific evidence, a consensus statement ('Good Practice Point') is made.

Methods

For background, search strategy and method for reaching consensus, see Part I of these guidelines.

Patients with advanced Parkinson's disease (PD) may suffer from any combination of motor and non-motor problems. Doctors and patients must make choices and decide which therapeutic strategies should prevail for each particular instance.

*Review of the therapeutic management of Parkinson's disease. Report of a joint task force of the European Federation of Neurological Societies (EFNS) and the Movement Disorder Society-European Section (MDS-ES)

[a]Department of Neurology, Radboud University Medical Centre, Nijmegen, The Netherlands; [b]Neurology Service, Hospital Clínic, Universitat de Barcelona, Spain;[c]Department of Neurosciences, University of Pisa, Italy; [d]Department of Neurology, Christian-Albrechts-University Kiel, Germany; [e]Department of Neurology, Medical University of Warsaw, Poland; [f]Department of Neurology, Palacky University, Olomouc, Czech Republic; [g]Department of Neurology, Stavanger University Hospital, Norway; [h]Reta Lila Weston Institute of Neurological Studies, London, United Kingdom; [i]Philipps-University of Marburg, Centre of Nervous Diseases, Marburg, Germany; [j]Department of Neurology, Innsbruck Medical University, Austria; [k]Clinical Investigation Centre, Departments of Clinical Pharmacology and Neurosciences, University Hospital, Toulouse, France;[l]Laboratório de Farmacologia Clinica e Terapeutica e Instituto de Medicina Molecular, Faculdade de Medicina de Lisboa, Portugal.

Interventions for the symptomatic control of motor complications

Motor complications are divided into motor fluctuations and dyskinesia. With advancing PD, patients may begin to fluctuate in motor performance, that is, they experience a wearing-off (end-of-dose) effect because the motor improvement after a dose of levodopa becomes reduced in duration and parkinsonism reappears. However, wearing-off can also manifest in symptoms such as depression, anxiety, akathisia, unpleasant sensations, and excessive sweating. Besides fluctuations, dyskinesias may occur, which are involuntary movements in response to levodopa and/or dopamine agonist intake. Most dyskinesias emerge at peak-dose levels and are typically choreiform, but may involve dystonia or myoclonus. A minority of patients may experience diphasic dyskinesia, in which they exhibit dyskinesia at the beginning of turning ON and/or at the beginning of turning OFF, but have different and less severe or absent dyskinesias at the time of peak levodopa effect. Eventually, patients may begin to experience rapid and unpredictable fluctuations between ON and OFF periods, known as the ON–OFF phenomenon.

The diagnosis and therapeutic management of motor complications depends on detecting the type of movement involved and the time of day when they occur in relation to the timing of levodopa and the resulting ON–OFF cycle. Diaries may be helpful in assessing this course over time. It must be noted that many patients prefer being ON with dyskinesia rather than OFF without dyskinesia.

Pharmacological interventions

Mechanisms of action: if not mentioned, see Part I of the guidelines.

Amantadine

Using patient diaries, one study found that the duration of daily OFF time decreased significantly (class I: Verhagen Metman et al., 1998), whereas a second study found no significant differences in ON or OFF duration (class I: Luginger et al., 2000).

During 3 weeks of steady-state infusion with amantadine, dyskinesia was reduced by 60%, with a similar effect observed at 1-year follow-up (class I: Verhagen Metman et al., 1998,1999). In patients on chronic levodopa, oral amantadine significantly reduced the dyskinetic effect of an orally administered acute levodopa/decarboxylase inhibitor challenge of 1.5 times their usual dose (class I: Snow et al., 2000). Similar results were found by Luginger et al. (2000) (class I). However, the antidyskinetic effect of oral amantadine may only last for 3–8 months, according to one study (class I: Thomas et al., 2004), in which, several subjects experienced a rebound in dyskinesia severity after discontinuation.

MAO-B inhibitors

Short-duration studies (<3 months) showed no consistent effect of selegiline in the reduction of OFF time, although an improvement in PD symptoms was observed (class I and II: Lees et al., 1977; Lieberman et al., 1987; Golbe et al., 1988). Zydis selegiline, which dissolves on contact with saliva, reduces daily OFF time when used as adjunctive therapy with levodopa (class I: Waters et al., 2004).

Rasagiline produced a significant reduction in OFF time in patients on levodopa [class I: rasagiline 1 mg, -0.78 hour/day (Rascol et al., 2005) and -0.94 hour/day (Parkinson Study Group, 2005)]. In the study by Rascol et al., rasagiline achieved a similar magnitude of effect to the active comparator, entacapone, which reduced OFF time by 0.80 hour/day (class I: Rascol et al., 2005).

Selegiline might increase or provoke dyskinesia in levodopa-treated patients, but this was not the primary outcome measure in the studies referred to (class I: Lees et al., 1977; Shoulson et al., 2002). Golbe et al. noted that dyskinesia abated after levodopa was reduced (class I: Golbe et al., 1988). Rasagiline increased dyskinesia in one study (Parkinson Study Group, 2005), whereas it had no significant impact in another (Rascol et al., 2005). The reason for this difference remains unknown, as levodopa dose adjustment was allowed equally in both trials.

COMT inhibitors

Due to their mechanism of action, COMT inhibitors should always be given with levodopa.

Class I studies demonstrated that tolcapone was efficacious in reducing OFF time (Rajput *et al.*, 1997; Kurth *et al.*, 1997; Baas *et al.*, 1997; Adler *et al.*, 1998). The effect size of tolcapone and dopamine agonists (bromocriptine, pergolide) may be similar (class II: Agid *et al.*, 1997; Tolcapone Study Group, 1999; Koller *et al.*, 2001), but these studies lacked the power to be fully conclusive (Deane *et al.*, 2004a). The overall conclusion from four studies of entacapone was a reduction in OFF time of 41 min/day (95% CI: 13 min, 1 hour 8 min) as compared with placebo (class I: Deane *et al.*, 2004b). Entacapone reduces mean daily OFF time in levodopa-treated patients by a similar extent to rasagiline (class I: Rascol *et al.*, 2005).

In the trials quoted above, dyskinesias were more frequent with entacapone groups than with placebo. In the majority of the trials, entacapone produced an improvement in Unified PD Rating Scale (UPDRS) motor scores.

Levodopa

It is common practice to lower the individual doses of levodopa in cases of peak-dose dyskinesia, whereas the dose interval is shortened in wearing-off ('Management of Parkinson's disease', 2002; Levine *et al.*, 2003).

To lower the occurrence of delayed ON, no ON, or reduced symptomatic effect due to gastrointestinal absorption failure, methods are being developed to improve levodopa absorption. Fluctuations and wearing-off could be reduced by methods providing more constant gastrointestinal delivery (reviews: 'Management of Parkinson's disease', 2002; Nyholm and Aquilonius, 2004).

Controlled-release (CR) levodopa formulations
Controlled-release (CR) levodopa has been shown to have a significant beneficial effect on daily ON time in a minority of studies, but the improvement is often only minor and transient. No class I study shows long-lasting (>6 months) daily improvement of >1 hour ON, or a reduction in hours with dyskinesia as measured by diaries, although some studies found an improvement using 1–4 ratings similar to the UPDRS-Complications scale (Ahlskog *et al.*, 1988; Jankovic *et al.*, 1989; Lieberman *et al.*, 1990; 'Management of Parkinson's disease', 2002).

Alternative levodopa formulations and delivery routes
In fluctuating PD, oral dispersible levodopa/benserazide significantly shortened time to peak plasma levels compared with the standard formulation (class III: Contin *et al.*, 1999).

Continuous duodenal infusions of levodopa/carbidopa resulted in statistically significant increases in ON time (class III: Kurth *et al.*, 1993). Continuous intraduodenal infusion of levodopa/carbidopa enteral gel resulted in a significant improvement in motor function during ON time, accompanied by a significant decrease in OFF time, and no increase in dyskinesia. Median total UPDRS score also decreased (class III: Nyholm *et al.*, 2005).

Dopamine agonists

Several dopamine agonists have been shown to reduce the duration of OFF episodes. There is class I evidence for pergolide (Olanow *et al.*, 1994), pramipexole (Guttman, 1997; Mizuno *et al.*, 2003), ropinirole (Rascol *et al.*, 1996; Lieberman *et al.*, 1998), and for apomorphine as intermittent subcutaneous injection (class I: Ostergaard *et al.*, 1995; Dewey *et al.*, 2001) or continuous infusion (class IV: Manson *et al.*, 2002). There is class II evidence for bromocriptine (Hoehn and Elton, 1985; Toyokura *et al.*, 1985; Guttman, 1997) and cabergoline (Hutton *et al.*, 1996), and class IV evidence for other agonists such as lisuride or piribedil ('Management of Parkinson's disease', 2002).

The available comparative class II–III trials showed no major differences between bromocriptine and other agonists such as cabergoline (Inzelberg *et al.*, 1996), lisuride (Laihinen *et al.*, 1992), pergolide (Mizuno *et al.*, 1995), and pramipexole (Guttman, 1997). The same was true when comparing bromocriptine (Tolcapone Study Group, 1999) and pergolide (Koller *et al.*, 2001), to the COMT inhibitor tolcapone (class II).

When levodopa-treated patients with advanced PD receive an agonist to reduce OFF episodes, dyskinesia may occur or, if already present, worsen. In clinical practice, when an agonist is given as adjunct in patients with dyskinesias, the levodopa dose is usually reduced to minimise this problem.

Dopamine agonists can deliver more continuous dopamine stimulation than levodopa, due to their longer plasma elimination half-life. Therefore, high doses of dopamine agonists might allow a reduction in levodopa daily dose and, consequently, lessen the duration and severity of levodopa-induced dyskinesias. There are only a few open-label reports to support this practice (class IV), involving small cohorts of patients with continuous subcutaneous infusions of apomorphine (Colzi et al., 1998; Stocchi et al., 2001; Kanovsky et al., 2002; Katzenschlager et al., 2005) or oral administration of high doses of pergolide (Facca and Sanchez-Ramos, 1996) or ropinirole (Cristina et al., 2003).

Functional neurosurgery

Pallidotomy and deep brain stimulation (DBS) are discussed in detail here, as they are the only surgical treatments frequently used to treat PD symptoms. Other treatments are covered only briefly and the reader is referred to special reviews (Deuschl et al., 2002).

All surgical interventions for PD involve lesioning or stimulating nuclei or fibre connections of the basal ganglia loop (direct or indirect loop) (Alexander et al., 1990). Lesioning of these nuclei destroys the circuit, and continuous electrical stimulation is likely to reversibly block the neuronal activity in the loop.

Pallidotomy

This section focuses on unilateral pallidotomy. Bilateral pallidotomy is only rarely performed and there are insufficient studies to allow a conclusion on the safety of the technique.

Adjunctive therapy of parkinsonism
Unilateral pallidotomy has been tested in prospective studies with control groups receiving best medical treatment or subthalamic nucleus (STN) stimulation (class II: de Bie et al., 1999,;002; Vitek et al., 2003; Esselink et al., 2004) and was found to be efficacious for the treatment of PD.

Symptomatic control of motor complications
The improvement of dyskinesia on the body side contralateral to pallidotomy is usually 50–80% (class III: Baron et al., 1996; Hariz and De Salles

1997; Kumar et al., 1998; de Bie et al., 1999, 2001; Kondziolka et al., 1999; ;sselink et al., 2004).

Safety
Side effects with unilateral pallidotomy are generally limited, but the potential for severe complications due to haemorrhage or peri-operative complications is common to all stereotactic procedures. Symptomatic infarction was found in 3.9% of patients, and the mortality rate was 1.2%. Speech problems were found in 11.1% of patients and facial paresis in 8.4% (reviews: Hariz and De Salles 1997; de Bie et al., 2002). Neuropsychological functioning is usually unaffected (Green et al., 2002; Gironell et al., 2003), but frontal lobe functions and depression may show a modest deterioration (class III: Perrine et al., 1998; Trepanier et al., 1998). Visual field defects were common in earlier series, but have decreased to <5% with modification of the surgical technique (Biousse et al., 1998).

Deep brain stimulation (DBS)

Stimulation of the STN (reviews: Levine et al., 2003; Volkmann et al., 2004; Verhagen Metman and O'Leary, 2005; Lang et al., 2006; Rezai et al., 2006; Deuschl et al., 2006) has become the most frequently applied surgical procedure for PD (at least in Europe), because treating neurologists and neurosurgeons consider it more efficient than pallidal stimulation. However, this is not scientifically proven.

Stimulation of the posteroventral pallidum
Adjunctive therapy of parkinsonism Pallidal DBS may improve the symptoms of advanced PD, as assessed by the UPDRS-Motor score, by 33% for study periods of up to 6 and 12 months (class II: DBS Study Group, 2001). Over time, deterioration occurs in some patients who are subsequently successfully reoperated on, with implantation of electrodes into the STN (class III: Volkmann et al., 2004).

Symptomatic control of motor complications One of the most consistent effects of DBS upon the pallidum is the reduction of dyskinesias and the reduction of OFF time. In class II and III studies, the reduction in OFF time was shown to be 35–60% (DBS Study Group, 2001; Volkmann *et al.*, 2004). The few long-term observations available show no loss of effect on dyskinesias (Lang *et al.*, 2006).

Symptomatic control of non-motor problems Under stimulation, there is a mild but significant improvement in mood (Ardouin *et al.*, 1999), but the symptomatic control of non-motor complications has not been primarily studied.

Safety The general surgical risks for pallidal stimulation are the same as for STN DBS (see next section). However, stimulation-specific side effects are less frequent. The incidence and severity of the neuropsychological and psychiatric effects of this technique are understudied (Vingerhoets *et al.*, 1999; Fields and Troster 2000; Trepanier *et al.*, 2000; Troster *et al.*, 2002; Volkmann *et al.*, 2004). A recent review found neuropsychiatric complications in 2.7% of patients, speech and swallowing disturbances in 2.6%, sensory disturbances in 0.9%, and oculomotor disturbances in 1.8% of patients (Lang *et al.*, 2006).

Stimulation of the subthalamic nucleus
Adjunctive therapy of parkinsonism in patients with dyskinesia The UPDRS-Motor score improved by 56% for subthalamic nucleus (STN) stimulation, compared with 33% for pallidal stimulation (class III: DBS Study Group, 2001). This is consistent with a meta-analysis of 20 studies, showing an average improvement of 53% (Volkmann *et al.*, 2004). Smaller controlled studies found similar results (Katayama *et al.*, 2001; Ostergaard *et al.*, 2002; Esselink *et al.*, 2004). At the same time, the levodopa equivalence dosage could be reduced by 50–60%. UPDRS-Motor scores during stimulation were clearly improved after 1 year, but had deteriorated slightly 5 years after the operation (class III: Krack *et al.*, 2003).

Symptomatic control of motor complications A class III study found a 61% reduction in OFF time (DBS Study Group, 2001), and dyskinesias have been reduced by 59–75% (DBS Study Group, 2001; Kleiner-Fisman *et al.*, 2006). Thus, STN stimulation is as effective in reducing dyskinesia as pallidotomy or pallidal stimulation. A 5-year study showed an ongoing improvement of dyskinesia (class III: Krack *et al.*, 2003).

Symptomatic control of non-motor problems Depression scores improve at 6 and 12 months after the operation (Romito *et al.*, 2002a; Daniele *et al.*, 2003; Krack *et al.*, 2003; Herzog *et al.*, 2003a). However, there is insufficient evidence to assume a consistent positive or negative effect of STN stimulation on mood or neuropsychological functions. See also safety section, below.

Safety In general, reviews (Levine *et al.*, 2003; Kleiner-Fisman *et al.*, 2006) and those studies referred to below show that adverse effects of DBS may occur in about 50% of patients, but are permanent in about 20% only. However, the severity of adverse events seldom warrants suspension of DBS. The occurrence of *adverse effects related to the procedure*, that is, acute confusion, intracerebral bleeding, stroke and seizures, or *to device dysfunction*, that is, infection or stimulator repositioning, causing permanent severe morbidity or death, reaches up to about 4% (review: Kleiner-Fisman *et al.*, 2006).

However, *most adverse effects are related to the treatment* (either stimulatory or stimulatory in combination with pharmacological). Neuropsychological tests were not worsened or showed only slight deterioration in various areas of cognition (Burchiel *et al.*, 1999; Morrison *et al.*, 2000; Saint-Cyr *et al.*, 2000; Alegret *et al.*, 2001; Dujardin *et al.*, 2001; Berney *et al.*, 2002; Daniele *et al.*, 2003; Gironell *et al.*, 2003; Funkiewiez *et al.*, 2004). Older patients or patients with moderate cognitive impairment prior to surgery may be at greater risk of cognitive deterioration (Saint-Cyr *et al.*, 2000; Trepanier *et al.*, 2000; Alegret *et al.*, 2001; Dujardin *et al.*, 2001; Kleiner-Fisman *et al.*, 2003). Apathy, hypomania, psychosis, depression, anxiety, and emotional liability occur in up to 10% of patients (Houeto *et al.*, 2002; Krack *et al.*, 2003; Volkmann *et al.*, 2004; Funkiewiez *et al.*, 2004; Rodriguez-Oroz *et al.*, 2005), although many of these might instead be caused by a reduction in dopaminergic therapy.

Suicide has been reported in up to about 4% of patients with DBS (Romito *et al.*, 2002b; Daniele *et al.*, 2003; Krack *et al.*, 2003; Herzog *et al.*, 2003b; Burkhard *et al.*, 2004). Weight gain is reported in 13% of patients, speech and swallowing disturbances in 7.1%, sensory disturbances in 0.4%, and oculomotor disturbances (apraxia of eyelid opening) in 1.5% (Deuschl *et al.*, 2006). However, a number of these stimulation-associated side effects can be corrected. Gait disorder, speech and swallowing difficulties, and disequilibrium are probably not related to the stimulation itself (Krack *et al.*, 2003; Rodriguez-Oroz *et al.*, 2005), but could in part result from disease progression or a reduction in levodopa dose.

Surgical treatments that are rarely used in the treatment of PD

Thalamotomy

Thalamotomy has been performed in patients with tremor insufficiently controlled by oral medications. It improves tremor, and rigidity is also reduced in 70% of patients, but it has no consistent effect on akinesia (class IV: Speelman *et al.*, 2002). Unilateral thalamotomy, as assessed in historical case series, has a permanent morbidity rate of 4–47%, and bilateral thalamotomy is associated with a 30% chance of developing serious dysarthria (Tasker, 1998).

Stimulation of the thalamus

Stimulation of the thalamus is frequently used for the treatment of tremors, especially essential tremor (Koller *et al.*, 1999; Limousin *et al.*, 1999). Stimulation of the thalamus improves tremor (and rigidity) in PD, but not akinesia (Koller *et al.*, 1997; Limousin *et al.*, 1999), and is therefore rarely employed. Thalamotomy and stimulation of the thalamus were found to be equally efficient, but DBS had fewer side effects (class I: Schuurman *et al.*, 2000).

Lesioning of the subthalamic nucleus

Lesioning of the STN has only been used in experimental protocols in small patient series with a high incidence of persistent dyskinesias (class III: Alvarez *et al.*, 2001; Alvarez *et al.*, 2005). Therefore,

presently, this technique is not recommended if STN DBS is an available option.

Foetal mesencephalic grafts

Two class I studies found that the symptoms of parkinsonism were not improved by foetal mesencephalic grafts, and some patients developed serious dyskinesias (Freed *et al.*, 2001; Olanow *et al.*, 2003). However, in the study by Freed *et al.*, the younger group, but not the older, showed an improvement of UPDRS-Motor OFF scores of 34%, and of Schwab and England OFF scores of 31%, while sham surgery patients did not improve. Subsequent analysis showed that it was not the patient's age, but the preoperative response to levodopa that predicted the magnitude of neurological change after transplant. Some patients in open studies (class IV) have also shown major improvement (Lopez-Lozano *et al.*, 1997; Brundin *et al.*, 2000; Schumacher *et al.*, 2000). Therefore, although transplantation of mesencephalic cells has, at the moment, to be considered ineffective as routine treatment for PD (Level A), further investigation is probably warranted.

RECOMMENDATIONS

Symptomatic control of motor complications

Motor fluctuations

Wearing-off

- *Adjust levodopa dosing.* In an early phase, when motor fluctuations are just becoming apparent, adjustments in the frequency of levodopa dosing during the day, tending to achieve 4–6 daily doses, might attenuate the wearing-off (Good Practice Point).
- *Switch from standard levodopa to CR formulation.* CR formulations of levodopa can also improve wearing-off (Level C).
- *Add COMT inhibitors or MAO-B inhibitors.* No recommendations can be made on which treatment should be chosen first – on average, all reduce OFF time by about 1–1.5 h/day. The only published direct comparison (Level A) showed

no difference between entacapone and rasagi-line. Tolcapone is potentially hepatotoxic, and is only recommended in patients failing on all other available medications (see Part I of the guidelines). Rasagiline should not be added to selegiline (Level C) because of cardiovascular safety issues.

- *Add dopamine agonists.* Oral dopamine ago-nists are efficacious in reducing OFF time in patients experiencing wearing-off. Currently, no dopamine agonist has proven better than another, but switching from one agonist to another can be helpful in some patients (Level B/C). Pergolide and other ergot agonists are reserved for second-line treatment, due to their association with valvulopathy.
- *Add amantadine or an anticholinergic.* In patients with disabling recurrent OFF symptoms that fail to improve further with the above mentioned strategies, the addition of an anticholinergic (in younger patients), or amantadine, may improve symptoms in some cases (Good Practice Point).

Most patients will eventually receive a combi-nation of several of these treatments because a single treatment fails to provide adequate control of fluctuations. There is insufficient evidence on the combination of more than two strategies, and the choice of drugs is mainly based on safety, toler-ability and ease of use. All the above options may provoke or increase dyskinesias, but usually this can be managed by decreasing the levodopa dose.

Note: reduction or redistribution of total daily dietary proteins may reduce wearing-off effects in some patients. Restricting protein intake to one meal a day may facilitate better motor responses to levodopa following other daily meals during the day. A more practical approach could be to take lev-odopa on an empty stomach about 1 h before, or at least 1 h after, each meal (class IV: Bracco *et al.*, 1991; Karstaedt and Pincus JH, 1992).

If oral therapy fails, the following strategies can be recommended.

- Deep brain stimulation of the STN (Level B).
- Subcutaneous apomorphine as penject (Level A) or pump (Level C).

- Alternative delivery routes or alternative formu-lations of levodopa:
  - oral dispersible levodopa might be useful for delayed ON (Level C).
  - levodopa/carbidopa enteric gel administered through percutaneous gastrostomy (PEG) can also be considered to stabilise patients with refractory motor fluctuations (Level B).

Unpredictable ON–OFF

In the large studies of wearing-off, patients with unpredictable ON–OFF were either not included or constituted <5% of the total population. There-fore, insufficient evidence exists to conclude whether the results that are valid for wearing-off are also valid for unpredictable ON–OFF. There are only a few small studies specifically including patients suffering from unpredictable ON–OFF, although studies evaluating continuous dopaminergic stimulation also include patients suffering concomitantly from wearing-off and unpredictable ON–OFF. The same is true for con-comitant dyskinesia, which frequently occurs dur-ing the ON phase of ON–OFF. Thus, there is insufficient evidence to conclude on specific strate-gies for ON–OFF, although the strategies described for dyskinesia and for wearing-off should be con-sidered for unpredictable ON–OFF (Good Practice Point).

RECOMMENDATIONS

Unpredictable ON–OFF can have several compo-nents, one of which is delayed ON and, for which, oral dispersible levodopa formulations could have some value (Level C).

Note: by shortening the interval between lev-odopa doses to prevent wearing-off, the relation between the moment of intake of each dose and the subsequent motor effect can become difficult to disclose, especially when inadequate absorption also occurs. The resulting pattern of fluctuation and dyskinesia may falsely suggest unpredictable ON–OFF. In such patients, the actual mecha-nism of wearing-off and peak-dose dyskinesia may reappear by increasing the levodopa intake interval to about 4 h. However, in some patients, the benefit may wane after weeks or months.

RECOMMENDATIONS

Dyskinesias
Peak-dose dyskinesia
- *Add amantadine* (Level A) – most studies use 200–400 mg/day. The benefit may last <8 months. The use of other antiglutaminergic drugs is investigational.
- *Reduce individual levodopa dose size*, at the risk of increasing OFF time. The latter can be compensated for by increasing the number of daily doses of levodopa or increasing the doses of a dopamine agonist (Level C).
- *Discontinue or reduce dose of MAO-B inhibitors or COMT inhibitors* (Good Practice Point), at the risk of worsening wearing-off.
- *Add atypical antipsychotics*, clozapine (Level A: Pierelli *et al.*, 1998; Durif *et al.*, 2004), with doses ranging between 12.5 and 75 mg/day up to 200 mg/day, or quetiapine (Level C: Morgante *et al.*, 2004; Katzenschlager *et al.*, 2004). However, clozapine is associated with potential serious adverse events (agranulocytosis and myocarditis), which limits its use (Good Practice Point).
- *Deep brain stimulation of the STN*, which allows reduction of dopaminergic treatment (Level B).
- *Apomorphine continuous subcutaneous infusion*, which allows reduction of levodopa therapy (Level C).

Biphasic dyskinesia

Biphasic dyskinesias can be very difficult to treat, and have not been the subject of specific and adequate class I–III studies. Usually, the strategies described for peak-dose dyskinesias can also be considered for biphasic dyskinesia (Good Practice Point). Another option is increasing the size and frequency of levodopa dose, at the risk of inducing or increasing peak-dose dyskinesia. This latter strategy can be helpful, generally transiently, in those cases without peak-dose dyskinesia, or where

they are considered less disabling than the biphasic type. A further option could be larger, less frequent doses, to give a more predictable response, which would better enable patients to plan daily activities (Good Practice Point).

RECOMMENDATIONS

Off-period and early morning dystonias
- *Usual strategies for wearing-off* can be applied in cases of off-period dystonia (Good Practice Point).
- *Additional doses of levodopa or dopamine agonist therapy at night* may be effective for the control of dystonia appearing during the night or early in the morning (Good Practice Point).
- *Deep brain stimulation of the STN* (Level B).
- *Botulinum toxin* can be employed in both off-period and early morning dystonia (Good Practice Point).

Freezing

Freezing, particularly freezing of gait, often occurs during the OFF phase, and less frequently in both OFF and ON. The latter scenario often does not respond to dopaminergic strategies.

Options for OFF freezing are the same as those described for wearing-off. In addition, the use of visual or auditory cues is empirically useful for facilitating the start of the motor act once freezing has occurred (Level C).

In ON freezing, trying a reduction in dopaminergic therapy is recommended, although this may result in worsening of wearing-off.

Interventions and recommendations for the symptomatic control of non-motor problems

Neuropsychiatric complications

Dementia

Dementia is a late feature of PD, found in about 30–40% of patients (Marttila and Rinne, 1976; Mayeux *et al.*, 1992; Aarsland *et al.*, 1996; Bosboom *et al.*, 2004; Schrag, 2004), with reported frequencies up to 78.2% (Aarsland *et al.*, 2003a). Besides abnormalities in monoaminergic functions, another neurochemical brain change associated with dementia in PD is cortical cholinergic denervation (Reviews: Zgaljardic *et al.*, 2004; Bosboom *et al.*, 2004).

Interventions for the treatment of dementia in PD
Several drugs, particularly anticholinergics, can impair cognitive function and considering discontinuation of such drugs is recommended. Another possible intervention is therapy with cholinesterase inhibitors (see below).

Cholinesterase inhibitors Several reports on cognitive dysfunction in patients with dementia in PD have claimed beneficial treatment effects with donepezil (class II: Aarsland *et al.*, 2002; Leroi *et al.*, 2004), rivastigmine (class I: Emre *et al.*, 2004), galantamine (class IV: Aarsland *et al.*, 2003b), and tacrine (class IV: Hutchinson and Fazzini, 1996; Werber and Rabey, 2001). However, it must be noted that the cognitive improvements are only modest, while tremor worsened in some patients, although UPDRS scores did not change (Emre *et al.*, 2004). Besides tremor, nausea and vomiting can also result in discontinuation of therapy in a minority of patients.

RECOMMENDATIONS

Treatment of dementia in PD

- *Discontinue potential aggravators.* Anticholinergics (Level B), amantadine (Level C), tricyclic antidepressants (Level C), tolterodine and oxybutynin (Level C), and benzodiazepines (Level C).
- *Add cholinesterase inhibitors.* Rivastigmine (Level A), donepezil (Level C), galantamine (Level C). Given the hepatotoxicity of tacrine, its use is not recommended (Good Practice Point).

Psychosis

Psychosis is one of the most disabling non-motor complications of PD. Visual hallucinations have been observed in up to 40% of patients with advanced disease in hospital-based series (Fenelon *et al.*, 2000).

Interventions for the treatment of psychosis in PD
Due to the prominent role of dopaminergic treatment-induced psychosis in PD, interventions are primarily based on reduction or withdrawal of the offending drugs, complemented by adjunct treatment with atypical antipsychotics, if necessary. However, infection and metabolic disorders can provoke psychosis and, in such cases, the underlying disorder should be treated.

Atypical antipsychotics
Clozapine The efficacy of clozapine was documented in two 4-week trials (class I: Parkinson Study Group, 1999; French CPSG, 1999). There was no worsening of UPDRS-Motor scores, and one study (Parkinson Study Group, 1999) found significant improvement of tremor in patients receiving clozapine versus placebo. In an open-label extension of one of these studies, efficacy was maintained over an additional 12 weeks (Factor *et al.*, 2001). Leucopenia is a rare (0.38%) but serious adverse event with clozapine (Honigfeld *et al.*, 1998). Consistently reported side effects (even with low-dose clozapine) include sedation, dizziness, increased drooling, orthostatic hypotension, and weight gain.

Olanzapine In two class I studies, olanzapine failed to show antipsychotic efficacy (Ondo *et al.*, 2002; Breier *et al.*, 2002). Both studies also found significant motor worsening with olanzapine, as did Goetz *et al.* (2000) (class I). Olanzapine is associated with unacceptable worsening of PD, and is no longer recommended because of the risk of cerebrovascular events in the elderly (Bullock, 2005). However, a relationship between olanzapine and stroke has been denied by others (Herrmann and Lanctot, 2005).

Quetiapine A recent trial found no significant improvement in psychosis rating with quetiapine versus placebo (class I: Ondo *et al.*, 2005). This study contradicts previous encouraging results from several class III studies (Fernandez *et al.*, 1999,

2002, 2003; Dewey and O'Suilleabhain, 2000; Brandstadter and Oertel, 2002; Reddy *et al.*, 2002; Juncos *et al.*, 2004), and a study by Morgante *et al.* (2004) (class II), which found no difference between quetiapine and clozapine.

Risperidone Risperidone improves hallucinations and psychosis in PD (class IV: Mohr *et al.*, 2000; Ellis *et al.*, 2000; Leopold, 2000; Meco *et al.*, 1994). However, motor worsening was observed in most of these reports and, therefore, risperidone is not recommended in patients with PD (Friedman and Factor, 2000).

Cholinesterase inhibitors
Rivastigmine (class III: Reading *et al.*, 2001; Bullock and Cameron, 2002) and donepezil (class IV: Fabbrini *et al.*, 2002; Bergmann and Lerner, 2002) have been reported to improve psychosis in PD patients. In a study of dementia in PD, rivastigmine improved hallucinations (class III, since hallucination was analysed post hoc in this trial: Emre *et al.*, 2004). Motor worsening was reported in two cases in one study only. A small minority of patients discontinued therapy because of increased tremor, nausea or vomiting.

RECOMMENDATIONS

Treatment of psychosis in PD

- *Control triggering factors* (Good Practice Point). Treat infection and metabolic disorders, rectify fluid/electrolyte balance, treat sleep disorder.
- *Reduce polypharmacy* (Good Practice Point). Reduce/stop anticholinergic antidepressants, reduce/stop anxiolytics/sedatives.
- *Reduce antiparkinsonian drugs* (Good Practice Point). Stop anticholinergics, stop amantadine, reduce/stop dopamine agonists, reduce/stop MAO-B and COMT inhibitors, finally, reduce levodopa. Stopping antiparkinsonian drugs can be at the cost of worsening motor symptoms.
- *Add atypical antipsychotics.* Clozapine (Level A) – although it can be associated with serious haematological adverse events, requiring monitoring. There is insufficient data on quetiapine,

but it is possibly useful (Good Practice Point). Quetiapine is thought to be relatively safe and does not require blood monitoring. Olanzapine (Level A) and risperidone (Level C) are not recommended (harmful).
- *Typical antipsychotics* (e.g. phenothiazines, butyrophenones) should not be used because they worsen parkinsonism.
- *Add cholinesterase inhibitors.* Rivastigmine (Level B), donepezil (Level C).

Depression

Depression is one of the most common non-motor symptoms of PD and, overall, available studies suggest that it may be found in about 40% of patients (Cummings, 1992; Burn, 2002). Depressive episodes and panic attacks may occur before the onset of overt motor symptoms (Santamaria *et al.*, 1986; Gonera *et al.*, 1997) and, in established PD, depression is a major determinant of quality of life (Findley, 1999; Schrag *et al.*, 2000).

There is consensus that PD-specific neurobiological changes also play a key role (Hornykiewicz, 1982; Mayeux *et al.*, 1984; Zgaljardic *et al.*, 2004).

Interventions for the treatment of depression in PD
Despite its clinical importance, pharmacological interventions to treat PD-associated depression have been poorly studied.

Levodopa There are no studies on the effects of chronic levodopa treatment on depressive symptoms in PD.

Dopamine agonists There have been early anecdotal claims of antidepressant effects of the dopamine agonists, initially related to bromocriptine (class IV: Agid *et al.*, 1986). In addition, a small study has compared the antidepressive efficacy of standard doses of pergolide and pramipexole as adjunct therapy. After 8 months, both treatments were associated with significant improvements in depression scores (class III: Rektorová *et al.*, 2003).

MAO inhibitors In a study of the effects of selegiline on motor fluctuations, Lees *et al.* (1977) (class II) failed to detect any significant changes in depression score in a subgroup analysis. However, depression was not the primary target of this trial.

In another study, after 6 weeks of therapy, Hamilton Depression rating scale (HAM-D) scores showed significantly greater improvement in patients receiving combined MAO-A (moclobemide 600 mg/day) plus MAO-B (selegiline 10 mg/day) inhibition, as compared with treatment with moclobemide alone (class III: Steur and Ballering, 1997). However, this study was confounded by motor improvement in the combined treatment group.

Tricyclic antidepressants This class of agents with among other things an anticholinergic effect is an established treatment modality in major depression. The only randomised placebo-controlled study dates back more than 20 years and is related to nortryptiline (titrated from 25 mg/day to a maximum of 150 mg/day) (class II: Andersen *et al.*, 1980), which showed a significant improvement over placebo, on a depression rating scale designed by the author. Recent evidence-based reviews ('Management of Parkinson's disease', 2002; Ghazi-Noori *et al.*, 2003) found little evidence supporting the use of tricyclic antidepressants in PD.

Selective serotonin reuptake inhibitors Although the use of Selective serotonin reuptake inhibitors (SSRIs) in PD-associated depression has been reported as beneficial in numerous small, open-label studies covering a variety of agents (fluoxetine, sertraline, paroxetine; class II–IV: see Weintraub *et al.*, 2005 for review), to date only one small double-blind placebo-controlled study of sertraline has assessed this approach. No statistically significant differences in the change of Montgomery Åsberg Depression Rating Scale (MADRS) scores was detected between treatment arms (class II: Leentjens *et al.*, 2003).

The two largest uncontrolled trials of SSRIs in the treatment of depression in PD investigated the use of paroxetine in 33 and 65 patients over a period of 3–6 months (class III: Ceravolo *et al.*, 2000; Tesei *et al.*, 2000). In both studies, paroxetine was titrated to 20 mg/day and produced statistically significant improvements over baseline in HAM-D rating scores. There were no changes in UPDRS-Motor scores in either study but, in the Ceravolo study, one patient reported worsening of tremor and, in the Tesei study, there were two (3%) withdrawals related to worsened OFF time or tremor. Avila *et al.* (2003) (class II) compared nefazodone with fluoxetine. Significant improvements in BDI scores were observed with both treatments. However, according to a recent review, large effect sizes have been seen with both active and placebo treatment in PD, but there is no difference between the two groups (Weintraub *et al.*, 2005).

When added to dopaminergic therapy, SSRIs have the potential to induce a 'serotonin syndrome', which is a rare but serious adverse event.

'New' antidepressants Reboxetine (class III: Lemke, 2002) and venlafaxine (class III: Bayulkem and Torun, 2002) have been reported beneficial in PD-associated depression. However, these studies have been small, and of short duration.

Non-pharmacological interventions A recent review identified 21 articles, covering a total of 71 patients with PD receiving electroconvulsive therapy (ECT) to treat concomitant depression ('Management of Parkinson's disease', 2002). These data are insufficient to conclude on the efficacy and safety of ECT to treat depression in PD.

Two double-blind studies have assessed repetitive transcranial magnetic stimulation (rTMS) in PD depression. There was no difference between sham and effective stimulation with respect to depression and PD measures (class I: Okabe *et al.*, 2003). A class I study (Fregni *et al.*, 2004) found rTMS as effective as fluoxetine in improving depression at week 2 – an effect maintained to week 8. However, interpretation of this study is hampered by lack of a placebo.

Autonomic dysfunction

Autonomic dysfunction is a common complication of PD. However, it may also occur as a side effect of standard medical therapy in PD. A significant minority of parkinsonian patients experience very severe and disabling autonomic impairment.

Orthostatic hypotension

Interventions for the treatment of orthostatic hypotension in PD

Midodrine Midodrine is a peripheral alpha-adrenergic agonist, without cardiac effect. Two class II studies of midodrine that included PD and other causes of neurogenic orthostatic hypotension revealed a significant increase in standing blood pressure (Jankovic *et al.*, 1993; Low *et al.*, 1997). Supine hypertension was found in up to 4% of patients (Low *et al.*, 1997).

Fludrocortisone Fludrocortisone (also called fluorohydrocortisone) enhances sodium reabsorption and potassium excretion in the kidney. The rise in blood pressure is assumed to be due to an increase in blood volume and cardiac output. Only one study (class IV) evaluated PD patients and showed an increase in systolic pressure upon standing, as well as disappearance of orthostatic symptoms (Hoehn, 1975). Hypertension, hypokalaemia, and ankle oedema (Riley, 2000) are the main side effects. Other studies find fludrocortisone effective in various other causes of orthostatic hypotension.

Dihydroergotamine, etilefrine hydrochloride, indomethacin, yohimbine, L-DOPS (L-threo-3,4-dihydroxyphenylserine), and EPO (erythropoietin) Insufficient evidence is available in PD and in other disorders causing neurogenic orthostatic hypotension.

Urinary disturbance

Interventions for the treatment of urinary incontinence in PD

Peripherally acting anticholinergics Drugs with anticholinergic effects (oxybutynin, amytriptyline), antispasmodic agents (propiverine, tolterodine), and alpha-1 agonists (prazosin and derived drugs) have not been specifically evaluated in PD ('Management of Parkinson's disease', 2002).

Intranasal desmopressin spray Intranasal desmopressin spray showed a good response in PD patients with nocturia (class IV: Suchowersky *et al.*, 1995).

RECOMMENDATIONS

Treatment of urinary incontinence in PD

- *General measures for treating urinary urgency and incontinence.* Avoid coffee before bedtime, limit water ingestion before bedtime, etc.
- *Add peripherally acting anticholinergic drugs* (Good Practice Point).
- *Add intranasal desmopressin spray* for nocturnal polyuria (insufficient evidence, no recommendation can be made).

Gastrointestinal motility problems

Constipation and reduced gastric motility are common problems in PD. Anorexia, nausea and vomiting frequently occur as side effects of dopamine agonist therapy.

Interventions for the treatment of gastrointestinal motility problems in PD
Cisapride has been withdrawn from the market in several European countries due to its association with cardiac arrhythmias and death (Tooley *et al.*, 1999).

Domperidone Domperidone blocks peripheral dopamine receptors, thus increasing gastric emptying. It reduces dopaminergic drug-related gastrointestinal symptoms in patients with PD (class II–IV: Agid *et al.*, 1979; Quinn *et al.*, 1981; Day and Pruitt, 1989; Soykan *et al.*, 1997).

Metoclopramide Metoclopramide also blocks peripheral dopamine receptors. However, in contrast to domperidone, it crosses the blood–brain barrier and reduces nausea and vomiting (Quinn *et al.*, 1981) by blocking dopamine receptors in the area postrema. However, it can also increase parkinsonism (Bateman *et al.*, 1985; Miller and Jankovic,

1989; Ganzini *et al.*, 1993), which is considered an unacceptable risk in patients with PD.

RECOMMENDATIONS

Treatment of gastrointestinal motility problems in PD

- *Apply general measures for treating constipation.* Diet, laxatives, etc.
- *Reduce or discontinue drugs with anticholinergic activity* (Good Practice Point).
- *Add domperidone* (Level B).

Erectile dysfunction

Interventions for the treatment of erectile dysfunction in PD

Sildenafil On the basis of trials using validated questionnaires, sildenafil was found to be efficacious in the treatment of erectile dysfunction (class I: Hussain *et al.*, 2001; class IV: Zesiewicz *et al.*, 2000; Raffaele *et al.*, 2002). Side effects of this drug include a group of mild and transitory adverse reactions (headache, transient visual effects, flushing) and, occasionally, severe reactions (hypotension, priapism, cardiac arrest).

Alprostadil Insufficient evidence.

Dopamine agonists Apomorphine, administered 30 min before sexual activity, may improve erectile function (class IV: O'Sullivan and Hughes, 1998). Nausea, headache, yawning and orthostatic hypotension are the most common side effects of apomorphine. Pergolide may improve sexual function in younger male patients (class IV: Pohanka *et al.*, 2004).

RECOMMENDATIONS

Treatment of erectile dysfunction in PD

- *Add sildenafil* (Level A).
- *Add dopamine agonists.* Apomorphine and pergolide (insufficient evidence, no recommendation can be made).

Conflicts of interest

M Horstink has not received any departmental research grants or honoraria since starting this guidelines project.

E Tolosa has received honoraria for research funding and consultancy from Novartis, Boehringer Ingelheim, Teva, Medtronic, Schwarz and Servier.

U Bonuccelli has acted as scientific advisor for, or obtained speaker honoraria from, Novartis, Boehringer Ingelheim, Pfizer, Chiesi, Schwarz and GlaxoSmithKline. During the past 2 years he has received departmental grants and performed clinical studies for GlaxoSmithKline, Novartis, Teva, Chiesi, Boehringer, Schwarz and Eisai.

G Deuschl has acted as scientific advisor for, or obtained speaker honoraria from, Orina, Novartis, Boehringer Ingelheim and Medtronic, during the past 2 years.

JP Larsen has received honoraria and research support from Orion Pharma and Pfizer, and has acted as a consultant for Lundbeck.

A Lees has received honoraria for lectures from Novartis, Orion, Valeant, Britannia, GE-Amersham, Servier, Teva, GlaxoSmithKline, Boehringer Ingelheim and Lundbeck.

W Oertel has received honoraria for research funding and consultancy from Novartis, Boehringer Ingelheim, Schwarz, Medtronic, Teva, Orion, GlaxoSmithKline, Pfizer and Solvay.

W Poewe has received honoraria for lecturing and advisory board membership from Novartis, GlaxoSmithKline, Teva, Boehringer Ingelheim, Schwarz and Orion.

O Rascol has received honoraria for research funding and/or consultancy from GlaxoSmithKline, Novartis, Boehringer Ingelheim, Eli Lilly, Teva, Lundbeck, Schwarz and Servier.

C Sampaio has received departmental research grants from Novartis Portugal. Her department has also charged consultancy fees to Servier and Lundbeck, and she has received honoraria for lectures from Boehringer Ingelheim.

A Friedman and P Kanovsky have nothing to declare.

Disclosure statement

The opinions and views expressed in the paper are those of the authors and not necessarily those of the MDS or its Scientific Issues Committee (SIC).

Acknowledgments

The authors thank Prof Niall Quinn for his constructive criticism and comments on this manuscript. The authors thank Juliet George for helping with the preparation of the text and Karen Henley for secretarial assistance during earlier meetings. They also acknowledge the significant contribution of Dr Yaroslau Compte to the sections on dysautonomia, amantadine and anticholinergics.

Funding sources supporting the work: Financial support from MDS-ES, EFNS and Stichting De Regenboog (the Netherlands).

References

Aarsland D, Tandberg E, Larsen JP, Cummings JL (1996). Frequency of dementia in Parkinson's disease. *Arch Neurol* **53:**538–542.

Aarsland D, Laake K, Larsen JP, Janvin C (2002). Donepezil for cognitive impairment in Parkinson's disease: a randomised controlled study. *J Neurol Neurosurg Psychiatry* **72:**708–712.

Aarsland D, Andersen K, Larsen JP, Lolk A, Kragh-Sorensen P (2003a). Prevalence and characteristics of dementia in Parkinson disease: an 8-year prospective study. *Arch Neurol* **60:**387–392.

Aarsland D, Hutchinson M, Larsen JP (2003b). Cognitive, psychiatric and motor response to galantamine in Parkinson's disease with dementia. *Int J Geriatr Psychiatry* **18:**937–941.

Adler CH, Singer C, O'Brien C (1998). Randomized, placebo-controlled study of tolcapone in patients with fluctuating Parkinson disease treated with levodopa-carbidopa. Tolcapone Fluctuator Study Group III. *Arch Neurol* **55:**1089–1095.

Agid Y, Pollak P, Bonnet AM, Signoret JL, Lhermitte F (1979). Bromocriptine associated with a peripheral dopamine blocking agent in treatment of Parkinson's disease. *Lancet* **1:** 570–572.

Agid Y, Ruberg M, Dubois B *et al.* (1986). Parkinson's disease and dementia. *Clin Neuropharmacol* **9(Suppl 2):**22–36.

Agid Y, Destee A, Durif F, Montastruc J-L, Pollak P (1997). Tolcapone, bromocriptine, and Parkinson's disease. French Tolcapone Study Group. *Lancet* **350:**712–713.

Ahlskog JE, Muenter MD, McManis PG, Bell GN, Bailey PA (1988). Controlled-release Sinemet (CR-4): a double-blind crossover study in patients with fluctuating Parkinson's disease. *Mayo Clin Proc* **63:** 876–886.

Alegret M, Junque C, Valldeoriola F, Vendrell P, Pilleri M, Rumia J, Tolosa E (2001). Effects of bilateral subthalamic stimulation on cognitive function in Parkinson disease. *Arch Neurol* **58:**1223–1227.

Alexander GE, Crutcher MD, DeLong MR (1990). Basal ganglia-thalamocortical circuits: parallel substrates for motor, oculomotor, "prefrontal" and "limbic" functions. *Prog Brain Res* **85:**119–146.

Alvarez L, Macias R, Guridi J *et al.* (2001). Dorsal subthalamotomy for Parkinson's disease. *Mov Disord* **16:**72–78.

Alvarez L, Macias R, Lopez G *et al.* (2005). Bilateral subthalamotomy in Parkinson's disease: initial and long-term response. *Brain* **128:**570–583.

Andersen J, Aabro E, Gulmann N, Hjelmsted A, Pedersen HE (1980). Antidepressive treatment in Parkinson's disease: a controlled trial of the effect of nortriptyline in patients with Parkinson's disease treated with L-dopa. *Acta Neurol Scand* **62:** 210–219.

Ardouin C, Pillon B, Peiffer E *et al.* (1999). Bilateral subthalamic or pallidal stimulation for Parkinson's disease affects neither memory nor executive functions: a consecutive series of 62 patients. *Ann Neurol* **46:**217–223.

Avila A, Cardona X, Martin-Baranera M, Maho P, Sastre F, Bello J (2003). Does nefazodone improve both depression and Parkinson disease? A pilot randomized trial. *J Clin Psychopharmacol* **23:**509–513.

Baas H, Beiske AG, Ghika J, Jackson M, Oertel WH, Poewe W, Ransmayr G (1997). Catechol-O-methyltransferase inhibition with tolcapone reduces the "wearing off" phenomenon and levodopa requirements in fluctuating parkinsonian patients. *J Neurol Neurosurg Psychiatry* **63:**421–428.

Baron MS, Vitek JL, Bakay RA *et al.* (1996). Treatment of advanced Parkinson's disease by posterior GPi pallidotomy: 1-year results of a pilot study. *Ann Neurol* **40:**355–366.

Bateman DN, Rawlins MD, Simpson JM (1985). Extrapyramidal reactions with metoclopramide. *Br Med J* **291:**930–932.

Bayulkem K, Torun F (2002). Therapeutic efficiency of venlafaxin in depressive patients with Parkinson's disease. *Mov Disord* **17(Suppl 5):**P204.

Bergmann J, Lerner V (2002). Successful use of donepezil for the treatment of psychotic symptoms in patients with Parkinson's disease. *Clin Neuropharmacol* **25:**107–110.

Berney A, Vingerhoets F, Perrin A *et al.* (2002). Effect on mood of subthalamic DBS for Parkinson's disease: a consecutive series of 24 patients. *Neurology* **59:**1427–1429.

Biousse V, Newman NJ, Carroll C *et al.* (1998). Visual fields in patients with posterior GPi pallidotomy. *Neurology* **50:**258–265.

Bosboom JL, Stoffers D, Wolters EC (2004). Cognitive dysfunction and dementia in Parkinson's disease. *J Neural Transm* **111:**1303–1315.

Bracco F, Malesani R, Saladini M, Battistin L (1991). Protein redistribution diet and antiparkinsonian response to levodopa. *Eur Neurol* **31:**68–71.

Brandstadter D, Oertel WH (2002). Treatment of drug-induced psychosis with quetiapine and clozapine in Parkinson's disease. *Neurology* **58:**160–161.

Breier A, Sutton VK, Feldman PD, Kadam DL, Ferchland I, Wright P, Friedman JH (2002). Olanzapine in the treatment of dopaminetic-induced psychosis in patients with Parkinson's disease. *Biol Psychiatry* **52:**438–445.

Brundin P, Pogarell O, Hagell P *et al.* (2000). Bilateral caudate and putamen grafts of embryonic mesencephalic tissue treated with lazaroids in Parkinson's disease. *Brain* **123:**1380–1390.

Bullock R (2005). Treatment of behavioural and psychiatric symptoms in dementia: implications of recent safety warnings. *Curr Med Res Opin* **21:**1–10.

Bullock R, Cameron A (2002). Rivastigmine for the treatment of dementia and visual hallucinations associated with Parkinson's disease: a case series. *Curr Med Res Opin* **18:**258–264.

Burchiel KJ, Anderson VC, Favre J, Hammerstad JP (1999). Comparison of pallidal and subthalamic nucleus deep brain stimulation for advanced Parkinson's disease: results of a randomized, blinded pilot study. *Neurosurgery* **45:**1375–1384.

Burkhard PR, Vingerhoets FJ, Berney A, Bogousslavsky J, Villemure JG, Ghika J (2004). Suicide after successful deep brain stimulation for movement disorders. *Neurology* **63:**2170–2172.

Burn DJ (2002). Beyond the iron mask: towards better recognition and treatment of depression associated with Parkinson's disease. *Mov Disord* **17:**445–454.

Ceravolo R, Nuti A, Piccinni A *et al.* (2000). Paroxetine in Parkinson's disease: effects on motor and depressive symptoms. *Neurology* **55:**1216–1218.

Colzi A, Turner K, Lees AJ (1998). Continuous subcutaneous waking day apomorphine in the long term treatment of levodopa induced interdose dyskinesias in Parkinson's disease. *J Neurol Neurosurg Psychiatry* **64:**573–576.

Contin M, Riva R, Martinelli P, Cortelli P, Albani F, Baruzzi A (1999). Concentration-effect relationship of levodopa-benserazide dispersible formulation versus standard form in the treatment of complicated motor response fluctuations in Parkinson's disease. *Clin Neuropharmacol* **22**:351–355.

Cristina S, Zangaglia R, Mancini F, Martignoni E, Nappi G, Pacchetti C (2003). High-dose ropinirole in advanced Parkinson's disease with severe dyskinesias. *Clin Neuropharmacol* **26**:146–150.

Cummings JL (1992). Depression and Parkinson's disease: a review. *Am J Psychiatry* **149**:443–454.

Daniele A, Albanese A, Contarino MF *et al.* (2003). Cognitive and behavioural effects of chronic stimulation of the subthalamic nucleus in patients with Parkinson's disease. *J Neurol Neurosurg Psychiatry* **74**:175–182.

Day JP, Pruitt RE (1989). Diabetic gastroparesis in a patient with Parkinson's disease: effective treatment with domperidone. *Am J Gastroenterol* **84**:837–838.

de Bie RM, de Haan RJ, Nijssen PC *et al.* (1999). Unilateral pallidotomy in Parkinson's disease: a randomised, single-blind, multicentre trial. *Lancet* **354**:1665–1669.

de Bie RM, Schuurman PR, Bosch DA, de Haan RJ, Schmand B, Speelman JD (2001). Outcome of unilateral pallidotomy in advanced Parkinson's disease: cohort study of 32 patients. *J Neurol Neurosurg Psychiatry* **71**:375–382.

de Bie RM, de Haan RJ, Schuurman PR, Esselink RA, Bosch DA, Speelman JD (2002). Morbidity and mortality following pallidotomy in Parkinson's disease: a systematic review. *Neurology* **58**:1008–1012.

Deane KHO, Spieker S, Clarke CE (2004a). Catechol-O-methyltransferase inhibitors versus active comparators for levodopa-induced complications in Parkinson's disease. *Cochrane Database Syst Rev* **4**:CD004553.

Deane KHO, Spieker S, Clarke CE (2004b). Catechol-O-methyltransferase inhibitors for levodopa-induced complications in Parkinson's disease. *Cochrane Database Syst Rev* **4**:CD004554.

Deep Brain Stimulation for Parkinson's Disease Study Group (2001). Deep-brain stimulation of the subthalamic nucleus or the pars interna of the globus pallidus in Parkinson's disease. *N Engl J Med* **345**:956–963.

Deuschl G, Volkmann J, Krack P (2002). Deep brain stimulation for movement disorders. *Mov Disord* **17**:S1.

Deuschl G, Herzog J, Kleiner-Fisman G *et al.* (2006). Deep brain stimulation: postoperative issues. *Mov Disord*, in press.

Dewey RB Jr, O'Suilleabhain PE (2000). Treatment of drug-induced psychosis with quetiapine and clozapine in Parkinson's disease. *Neurology* **55**:1753–1754.

Dewey RB Jr, Hutton JT, LeWitt PA, Factor SA (2001). A randomized, double-blind, placebo-controlled trial

on subcutaneously injected apomorphine for parkinsonian off-state events. *Arch Neurol* **58**:1385–1392.

Dujardin K, Defebvre L, Krystkowiak P, Blond S, Destee A (2001). Influence of chronic bilateral stimulation of the subthalamic nucleus on cognitive function in Parkinson's disease. *J Neurol* **248**:603–611.

Durif F, Debilly B, Galitzky M (2004). Clozapine improves dyskinesias in Parkinson disease: a double-blind, placebo-controlled study. *Neurology* **62**:381–388.

Ellis T, Cudkowicz ME, Sexton PM, Growdon JH (2000). Clozapine and risperidone treatment of psychosis in Parkinson's disease. *J Neuropsychiatry Clin Neurosci* **12**:364–369.

Emre M, Aarsland D, Albanese A *et al.* (2004). Rivastigmine in Parkinson's disease patients with dementia: a randomized, double-blind, placebo-controlled study. *N Engl J Med* **351**:2509–2518.

Esselink RA, de Bie RM, de Haan RJ *et al.* (2004). Unilateral pallidotomy versus bilateral subthalamic nucleus stimulation in PD: a randomized trial. *Neurology* **62**:201–207.

Fabbrini G, Barbanti P, Aurilia C, Pauletti C, Lenzi GL, Meco G (2002). Donepezil in the treatment of hallucinations and delusions in Parkinson's disease. *Neurol Sci* **23**:41–43.

Facca A, Sanchez-Ramos J (1996). High-dose pergolide monotherapy in the treatment of severe levodopa-induced dyskinesias. *Mov Disord* **11**:327–329.

Factor SA, Friedman JH, Lannon MC, Oakes D, Bourgeois K; Parkinson Study Group (2001). Clozapine for the treatment of drug-induced psychosis in Parkinson's disease: results of the 12 week open label extension in the PSYCLOPS trial. *Mov Disord* **16**:135–139.

Fenelon G, Mahieux F, Huon R, Ziegler M (2000). Hallucinations in Parkinson's disease. Prevalence, phenomenology and risk factors. *Brain* **123**:733–745.

Fernandez H, Friedman J, Jacques C, Rosenfeld M (1999). Quetiapine for the treatment of drug-induced psychosis in Parkinson's disease. *Mov Disord* **14**:484–487.

Fernandez H, Trieschmann ME, Burke MA, Friedmann JH (2002). Quetiapine for psychosis in Parkinson's disease versus dementia with Lewy bodies. *J Clin Psychiatry* **63**:513–515.

Fernandez HH, Trieschmann ME, Burke MA, Jacques C, Friedman JH (2003). Long-term outcome of quetiapine use for psychosis among Parkinsonian patients. *Mov Disord* **18**:510–514.

Fields JA, Troster AI (2000). Cognitive outcomes after deep brain stimulation for Parkinson's disease: a review of initial studies and recommendations for future research. *Brain Cogn* **42**:268–293.

Findley LJ (1999). Quality of life in Pakinson's disease. *Int J Clin Pract* **53**:404–405.

Freed CR, Greene PE, Breeze RE *et al.* (2001). Transplantation of embryonic dopamine neurons for severe Parkinson's disease. *N Engl J Med* **344**:710–719.

Fregni F, Santos CM, Myczkowski ML *et al.* (2004). Repetitive transcranial magnetic stimulation is as effective as fluoxetine in the treatment of depression in patients with Parkinson's disease. *J Neurol Neurosurg Psychiatry* **75**:1171–1174.

French Clozapine Parkinson Study Group (1999). Clozapine in drug-induced psychosis in Parkinson's disease. *Lancet* **353**:2041.

Friedman JH, Factor SA (2000). Atypical antipsychotics in the treatment of drug-induced psychosis in Parkinson's disease. *Mov Disord* **15**:201–211.

Funkiewiez A, Ardouin C, Caputo E *et al.* (2004). Long term effects of bilateral subthalamic nucleus stimulation on cognitive function, mood, and behaviour in Parkinson's disease. *J Neurol Neurosurg Psychiatry* **75**:834–839.

Ganzini L, Casey DE, Hoffman WF, McCall AL (1993). The prevalence of metoclopramide-induced tardive dyskinesia and acute extrapyramidal movement disorders. *Arch Int Med* **153**:1469–1475.

Ghazi-Noori S, Chung TH, Deane KHO, Rickards H, Clarke CE (2003). Therapies for depression in Parkinson's disease. *Cochrane Database Syst Rev* **2**:CD003465.

Gironell A, Kulisevsky J, Rami L, Fortuny N, Garcia-Sanchez C, Pascual-Sedano B (2003). Effects of pallidotomy and bilateral subthalamic stimulation on cognitive function in Parkinson disease. A controlled comparative study. *J Neurol* **250**:917–923.

Goetz C, Blasucci L, Leurgans S, Pappert E (2000). Olanzapine and clozapine: comparative effects on motor function in hallucinating PD patients. *Neurology* **55**:748–749.

Golbe LI, Lieberman AN, Muenter MD *et al.* (1988). Deprenyl in the treatment of symptom fluctuations in advanced Parkinson's disease. *Clin Neuropharmacol* **11**:45–55.

Gonera EG, van't Hof M, Berger HJC, van Weel C, Horstink MWIM (1997). Prodromal symptoms in Parkinson's disease. *Mov Disord* **12**:871–876.

Green J, McDonald WM, Vitek JL *et al.* (2002). Neuropsychological and psychiatric sequelae of pallidotomy for PD: clinical trial findings. *Neurology* **58**:858–865.

Guttman M (1997). Double-blind randomized, placebo controlled study to compare safety, tolerance and efficacy of pramipezole and bromocriptine in advanced Parkinson's disease. International Pramipexole-Bromocriptine Study Group. *Neurology* **49**:1060–1065.

Hariz MI, De Salles AA (1997). The side-effects and complications of posteroventral pallidotomy. *Acta Neurochir Suppl* **68**:42–48.

Herrmann N, Lanctot KL (2005). Do atypical antipsychotics cause stroke? *CNS Drugs* **19**:91–103.

Herzog J, Volkmann J, Krack P *et al.* (2003a). Two-year follow-up of subthalamic deep brain stimulation in Parkinson's disease. *Mov Disord* **18**:1332–1337.

Herzog J, Reiff J, Krack P, Witt K, Schrader B, Muller D, Deuschl G (2003b). Manic episode with psychotic symptoms induced by subthalamic nucleus stimulation in a patient with Parkinson's disease. *Mov Disord* **18**:1382–1384.

Hoehn MM (1975). Levodopa induced postural hypotension. Treatment with fludrocortisone. *Arch Neurol* **32**:50–51.

Hoehn MMM, Elton RL (1985). Low dosages of bromocriptine added to levodopa in Parkinson's disease. *Neurology* **35**:199–206.

Honigfeld G, Arellano F, Sethi J, Bianchini A, Schein J (1998). Reducing clozapine-related morbidity and mortality: 5 years of experience with the Clozaril National Registry. *J Clin Psychiatry* **59**:3–7.

Hornykiewicz O (1982). Imbalance of brain monoamines and clinical disorders. *Prog Brain Res* **55**:419–429.

Houeto JL, Mesnage V, Mallet L *et al.* (2002). Behavioural disorders, Parkinson's disease and subthalamic stimulation. *J Neurol Neurosurg Psychiatry* **72**:701–707.

Hussain IF, Brady CM, Swinn MJ, Mathias CJ, Fowler CJ (2001). Treatment of erectile dysfunction with sildenafil citrate in parkinsonism due to Parkinson's disease and multiple system atrophy with observations on orthostatic hypotension. *J Neurol Neurosurg Psychiatry* **71**:371–374.

Hutchinson M, Fazzini E (1996). Cholinesterase inhibition in Parkinson's disease. J Neurol *Neurosurg Psychiatry* **61**:324–325.

Hutton JT, Koller WC, Ahlskog JE *et al.* (1996). Multicenter, placebo-controlled trial of cabergoline taken once daily in the treatment of Parkinson's disease. *Neurology* **46**:1062–1065.

Inzelberg R, Nisipeanu P, Rabey JM *et al.* (1996). Double-blind comparison of cabergoline and bromocriptine in Parkinson's disease patients with motor fluctuations. *Neurology* **47**:785–788.

Jankovic J, Schwartz K, Vander LC (1989). Comparison of Sinemet CR4 and standard Sinemet: double blind and long-term open trial in parkinsonian patients with fluctuations. *Mov Disord* **4**:303–309.

Jankovic J, Gilden JL, Hiner BC *et al.* (1993). Neurogenic orthostatic hypotension: a double-blind placebo-controlled study with midodrine. *Am J Med* **95**:38–48.

Juncos JL, Roberts VJ, Evatt ML *et al.* (2004). Quetiapine improves psychotic symptoms and cognition in Parkinson's disease. *Mov Disord* **19**:29–35.

Kanovsky P, Kubova D, Bares M, Hortova H, Streitova H, Rektor I, Znojil V (2002). Levodopa-induced dyskinesias and continuous subcutaneous infusions of apomorphine: results of a two-year, prospective follow-up. *Mov Disord* **17**:188–191.

Karstaedt PJ, Pincus JH (1992). Protein redistribution diet remains effective in patients with fluctuating parkinsonism. *Arch Neurol* **49**:149–151.

Katayama Y, Kasai M, Oshima H, Fukaya C, Yamamoto T, Ogawa K, Mizutani T (2001). Subthalamic nucleus stimulation for Parkinson disease: benefits observed in levodopa-intolerant patients. *J Neurosurg* **95**:213–221.

Katzenschlager R, Manson AJ, Evans A, Watt H, Lees AJ (2004). Low dose quetiapine for drug induced dyskinesias in Parkinson's disease: a double blind cross over study. *J Neurol Neurosurg Psychiatry* **75**:295–297.

Katzenschlager R, Hughes A, Evans A *et al.* (2005). Continuous subcutaneous apomorphine therapy improves dyskinesias in Parkinson's disease: a prospective study using single-dose challenges. *Mov Disord* **20**:151–157.

Kleiner-Fisman G, Fisman DN, Sime E, Saint-Cyr JA, Lozano AM, Lang AE (2003). Long-term follow up of bilateral deep brain stimulation of the subthalamic nucleus in patients with advanced Parkinson disease. *J Neurosurg* **99**:489–495.

Kleiner-Fisman G, Herzog J, Fisman D *et al.* (2006). Subthalamic nucleus deep brain stimulation: summary and meta-analysis of outcomes. *Mov Disord*, in press.

Koller W, Pahwa R, Busenbark K *et al.* (1997). High-frequency unilateral thalamic stimulation in the treatment of essential and parkinsonian tremor. *Ann Neurol* **42**:292–299.

Koller WC, Lyons KE, Wilkinson SB, Pahwa R (1999). Efficacy of unilateral deep brain stimulation of the VIM nucleus of the thalamus for essential head tremor. *Mov Disord* **14**:847–850.

Koller W, Lees A, Doder M, Hely M; Tolcapone/Pergolide Study Group (2001). Randomised trial of tolcapone versus pergolide as add-on to levodopa therapy in Parkinson's disease patients with motor fluctuations. *Mov Disord* **16**:858–866.

Kondziolka D, Bonaroti E, Baser S, Brandt F, Kim YS, Lunsford LD (1999). Outcomes after stereotactically guided pallidotomy for advanced Parkinson's disease. *J Neurosurg* **90**:197–202.

Krack P, Batir A, Van Blercom N *et al.* (2003). Five-year follow-up of bilateral stimulation of the subthalamic nucleus in advanced Parkinson's disease. *N Engl J Med* **349**:1925–1934.

Kumar R, Lozano AM, Montgomery E, Lang AE (1998). Pallidotomy and deep brain stimulation of the pallidum and subthalamic nucleus in advanced Parkinson's disease. *Mov Disord* **13**:73–82.

Kurth MC, Tetrud JW, Tanner CM, Irwin I, Stebbins GT, Goetz CG, Langston JW (1993). Double-blind, placebo-controlled, crossover study of duodenal infusion of levodopa/carbidopa in Parkinson's disease patients with 'on-off' fluctuations. *Neurology* **43**:1698–1703.

Kurth MC, Adler CH, Hilaire MS *et al.* (1997). Tolcapone improves motor function and reduces levodopa requirement in patients with Parkinson's disease experiencing motor fluctuations: a multicenter, double-blind, randomized, placebo-controlled trial. Tolcapone Fluctuator Study Group I. *Neurology* **48**:81–87.

Laihinen A, Rinne UK, Suchy I (1992). Comparison of lisuride and bromocriptine in the treatment of advanced Parkinson's disease. *Acta Neurol Scand* **86**:593–595.

Lang AE, Houeto J-L, Krack P *et al.* (2006). Deep brain stimulation: preoperative issues. *Mov Disord*, in press.

Leentjens AF, Vreeling FW, Luijeckx GJ, Verhey FR (2003). SSRIs in the treatment of depression in Parkinson's disease. *Int J Geriatr Psychiatry* **18**:552–554.

Lees AJ, Shaw KM, Kohout LJ, Stern GM (1977). Deprenyl in Parkinson's disease. *Lancet* **15**:791–795.

Lemke MR (2002). Effect of reboxetine on depression in Parkinson's disease patients. *J Clin Psychiatry* **63**:300–304.

Leopold NA (2000). Risperidone treatment of drug-related psychosis in patients with parkinsonism. *Mov Disord* **15**:301–304.

Leroi I, Brandt J, Reich SG, Lyketsos CG, Grill S, Thompson R, Marsh L (2004). Randomized placebo-controlled trial of donepezil in cognitive impairment in Parkinson's disease. *Int J Geriatr Psychiatry* **19**:1–8.

Levine CB, Fahrbach KR, Siderowf AD, Estok RP, Ludensky VM, Ross SD (2003). Diagnosis and treatment of Parkinson's disease: a systematic review of the literature. *Evid Rep Technol Assess* **57**:1–306.

Lieberman AN, Gopinathan G, Neophytides A, Foo SH (1987). Deprenyl versus placebo in Parkinson disease: a double-blind study. *N Y State J Med* **87**:646–649.

Lieberman A, Gopinathan G, Miller E, Neophytides A, Baumann G, Chin L (1990). Randomized double-blind cross-over study of Sinemet-controlled release (CR4 50/200) versus Sinemet 25/100 in Parkinson's disease. *Eur Neurol* **30**:75–78.

Lieberman A, Olanow CW, Sethi K, Swanson P, Waters CH, Fahn S, Hurtig H, Yahr M(1998). A multicenter trial of ropinirole as adjunct treatment for Parkinson's disease. Ropinirole Study Group. *Neurology* **51:**1057–1062.

Limousin P, Speelman JD, Gielen F, Janssens M (1999). Multicentre European study of thalamic stimulation in parkinsonian and essential tremor. *J Neurol Neurosurg Psychiatry* **66:**289–296.

Lopez-Lozano JJ, Bravo G, Brera B, Millan I, Dargallo J, Salmean J, Uria J, Insausti J (1997). Long-term improvement in patients with severe Parkinson's disease after implantation of fetal ventral mesencephalic tissue in a cavity of the caudate nucleus: 5-year follow up in 10 patients. Clinica Puerta de Hierro Neural Transplantation Group. *J Neurosurg* **86:**931–942.

Low PA, Gilden FL, Freeman R, Sheng KN, McElligott MA (1997). Efficacy of midodrine vs placebo in neuogenic orthostatic hypotension. A randomized double-blind multicenter study. Midodrine study group. *JAMA* **277:**1046–1051.

Luginger E, Wenning GK, Bosch S, Poewe W (2000). Beneficial effects of amantadine on levodopa-induced dyskinesias in Parkinson's disease. *Mov Disord* **15:**873–878.

Management of Parkinson's disease: an evidence-based review (2002). *Mov Disord* **17:**S1–S166.

Manson AJ, Turner K, Lees AJ (2002). Apomorphine monotherapy in the treatment of refractory motor complications of Parkinson's disease: long-term follow-up study of 64 patients. *Mov Disord* **17:**1235–1241.

Marttila RJ, Rinne UK (1976). Epidemiology of Parkinson's disease in Finland. *Acta Neurol Scand* **53:**81–102.

Mayeux R, Stern Y, Cote L, Williams JBW (1984). Altered serotonin metabolism in depressed patients with Parkinson's disease. *Neurology* **34:**642–646.

Mayeux R, Denaro J, Hemenegildo N, Marder K, Tang MX, Cote LJ, Stern Y (1992). A population-based investigation of Parkinson's disease with and without dementia. Relationship to age and gender. *Arch Neurol* **49:**492–497.

Meco G, Alessandria A, Bonifati V, Giustini P (1994). Risperidone for hallucinations in levodopa-treated Parkinson's disease patients. *Lancet* **343:**1370–1371.

Miller LG, Jankovic J (1989). Metoclopramide-induced movement disorders. Clinical findings with a review of the literature. *Arch Intern Med* **149:**2486–2492.

Mizuno Y, Kondo T, Narabayashi H (1995). Pergolide in the treatment of Parkinson's disease. *Neurology* **45(Suppl 31):**S13–S21.

Mizuno Y, Yanagisawa N, Kuno S, Yamamoto M, Hasegawa K, Origasa H, Kowa H; Japanese Pramipexole Study Group (2003). Randomized double-blind study of pramipexole with placebo and bromocriptine in advanced Parkinson's disease. *Mov Disord* **18:**1149–1156.

Mohr E, Mendis T, Hildebrand K, De Deyn PP (2000). Risperidone in the treatment of dopamine-induced psychosis in Parkinson's disease: an open pilot trial. *Mov Disord* **15:**1230–1237.

Morgante L, Epifanio A, Spina E *et al.* (2004). Quetiapine and clozapine in parkinsonian patients with dopaminergic psychosis. *Clin Neuropharmacol* **27:**153–156.

Morrison CE, Borod JC, Brin MF, Raskin SA, Germano IM, Weisz DJ, Olanow CW (2000). A program for neuropsychological investigation of deep brain stimulation (PNIDBS) in movement disorder patients: development, feasibility, and preliminary data. *Neuropsychiatry Neuropsychol Behav Neurol* **13:**204–219.

Nyholm D, Aquilonius SM (2004). Levodopa infusion therapy in Parkinson disease: state of the art in 2004. *Clin Neuropharmacol* **27:**245–256.

Nyholm D, Nilsson Remahl AI, Dizdar N *et al.* (2005). Duodenal levodopa infusion monotherapy vs oral polypharmacy in advanced Parkinson disease. *Neurology* **64:**216–223.

O'Sullivan JD, Hughes AJ (1998). Apomorphine-induced penile erections in Parkinson's disease. *Mov Disord* **13:**536–539.

Okabe S, Ugawa Y, Kanazawa I; Effectiveness of rTMS on Parkinson's Disease Study Group (2003). 0.2-Hz repetitive transcranial magnetic stimulation has no add-on effects as compared to a realistic sham stimulation in Parkinson's disease. *Mov Disord* **18:**382–388.

Olanow CW, Fahn S, Muenter M *et al.* (1994). A multicenter double-blind placebo-controlled trial of pergolide as an adjunct to Sinemet in Parkinson's disease. *Mov Disord* **9:**40–47.

Olanow CW, Goetz CG, Kordower JH *et al.* (2003). A double-blind controlled trial of bilateral fetal nigral transplantation in Parkinson's disease. *Ann Neurol* **54:**403–414.

Ondo W, Levy J, Vuong K, Hunter C, Jankovic J (2002). Olanzapine treatment for dopaminergic-induced hallucinations. *Mov Disord* **17:**1031–1035.

Ondo WG, Tintner R, Voung KD, Lai D, Ringholz G (2005). Double-blind, placebo-controlled, unforced titration parallel trial of quetiapine for dopaminergic-induced hallucinations in Parkinson's disease. *Mov Disord* **20:**958–963.

Ostergaard L, Werdelin L, Odin P (1995). Pen injected apomorphine against off phenomena in late Parkinson's disease: a double blind, placebo controlled study. *J Neurol Neurosurg Psychiatry* **58:**681–687.

Ostergaard K, Sunde N, Dupont E (2002). Effects of bilateral stimulation of the subthalamic nucleus in patients with severe Parkinson's disease and motor fluctuations. *Mov Disord* **17**:693–700.

Parkinson Study Group (1999). Low-dose clozapine for the treatment of drug-induced psychosis in Parkinson's disease. *N Engl J Med* **340**:757–763.

Parkinson Study Group (2005). A randomized placebo-controlled trial of rasagiline in levodopa-treated patients with Parkinson disease and motor fluctuations. The PRESTO study. *Arch Neurol* **62**:241–248.

Perrine K, Dogali M, Fazzini E *et al.* (1998). Cognitive functioning after pallidotomy for refractory Parkinson's disease. *J Neurol Neurosurg Psychiatry* **65**:150–154.

Pierelli F, Adipietro A, Soldati G, Fattapposta F, Pozzessere G, Scoppetta C (1998). Low dosage clozapine effects on L-dopa induced dyskinesias in parkinsonian patients. *Acta Neurol Scand* **97**:295–299.

Pohanka M, Kanovsky P, Bares M, Pulkrabek J, Rektor I (2004). Pergolide mesylate can improve sexual dysfunction in patients with Parkinson's disease: the results of an open, prospective, 6-month follow-up. *Eur J Neurol* **11**:483–488.

Quinn N, Illas A, Lhermitte F, Agid Y (1981). Bromocriptine and domperidone in the treatment of Parkinson's disease. *Neurology* **31**:662–667.

Raffaele R, Vecchio I, Giammusso B, Morgia G, Brunetto MB, Rampello L (2002). Efficacy and safety of fixed-dose oral sildenafil in the treatment of sexual dysfunction in depressed patients with idiopathic Parkinson's disease. *European Urology* **41**:382–386.

Rajput AH, Martin W, Saint-Hilaire MH, Dorflinger E, Pedder S (1997). Tolcapone improves motor function in parkinsonian patients with the "wearing-off" phenomenon: a double-blind, placebo-controlled, multicenter trial. *Neurology* **49**:1066–1071.

Rascol O, Lees AJ, Senard JM, Pirtosek Z, Montastruc JL, Fuell D (1996). Ropinirole in the treatment of levodopa-induced motor fluctuations in patents with Parkinson's disease. *Clin Neuropharmacol* **19**:234–245.

Rascol O, Brooks DJ, Melamed E, Oertel W, Poewe W, Stocchi F, Tolosa E; LARGO study group. (2005). Rasagiline as an adjunct to levodopa in patients with Parkinson's disease and motor fluctuations (LARGO, Lasting effect in Adjunct therapy with Rasagiline Given Once daily, study): a randomised, double-blind, parallel-group trial. *Lancet* **365**:947–954.

Reading P, Luce A, McKeith I (2001). Rivastigmine in the treatment of parkinsonian psychosis and cognitive impairment. *Mov Disord* **16**:1171–1174.

Reddy S, Factor SA, Molho ES, Feustel PJ (2002). The effect of quetiapine on psychosis and motor function in parkinsonian patients with and without dementia. *Mov Disord* **17**:676–681.

Rektorová I, Rektor I, Bares M *et al.* (2003). Pramipexole and pergolide in the treatment of depression in Parkinson's disease: a national multicentre prospective randomized study. *Eur J Neurol* **10**:399–406.

Rezai AR, Kopell BH, Gross R, Vitek J, Sharan A, Limousin P, Benabid AL (2006). Deep brain stimulation for Parkinson's disease: surgical issues. *Mov Disord*, in press.

Riley DE (2000). Orthostatic hypotension in multiple system atrophy. *Curr Treat Options Neurol* **2**:225–230.

Rodriguez-Oroz MC, Obeso JA, Lang AE *et al.* (2005). Bilateral deep brain stimulation in Parkinson's disease: a multicentre study with 4 years follow-up. *Brain* **128**:2240–2249.

Romito LM, Scerrati M, Contarino MF, Bentivoglio AR, Tonali P, Albanese A (2002a). Long-term follow up of subthalamic nucleus stimulation in Parkinson's disease. *Neurology* **58**:1546–1550.

Romito LM, Raja M, Daniele A *et al.* (2002b). Transient mania with hypersexuality after surgery for high frequency stimulation of the subthalamic nucleus in Parkinson's disease. *Mov Disord* **17**:1371–1374.

Saint-Cyr JA, Trepanier LL, Kumar R, Lozano AM, Lang AE (2000). Neuropsychological consequences of chronic bilateral stimulation of the subthalamic nucleus in Parkinson's disease. *Brain* **123**:2091–2108.

Santamaria J, Tolosa E, Valles A (1986). Parkinson's disease with depression: a possible subgroup of idiopathic parkinsonism. *Neurology* **36**:1130–1133.

Schrag A, Jahanshahi M, Quinn N (2000). What contributes to quality of life in patients with Parkinson's disease? *J Neurol Neurosurg Psychiatry* **69**:308–312.

Schrag A (2004). Psychiatric aspects of Parkinson's disease – an update. *J Neurol* **251**:795–804.

Schumacher JM, Ellias SA, Palmer EP *et al.* (2000). Transplantation of embryonic porcine mesencephalic tissue in patients with PD. *Neurology* **54**:1042–1050.

Schuurman PR, Bosch DA, Bossuyt PM *et al.* (2000). A comparison of continuous thalamic stimulation and thalamotomy for suppression of severe tremor. *N Engl J Med* **342**:461–468.

Shoulson I, Oakes D, Fahn S *et al.*; Parkinson Study Group (2002). Impact of sustained deprenyl (selegiline) in levodopa-treated Parkinson's disease: a randomized placebo-controlled extension of the deprenyl and tocopherol antioxidative therapy of parkinsonism trial. *Ann Neurol* **51**:604–612.

Snow BJ, Macdonald L, Mcauley D, Wallis W (2000). The effect of amantadine on levodopa-induced dyskinesias in Parkinson's disease: a double-blind, placebo-controlled study. *Clin Neuropharmacol* **23:**82–85.

Soykan I, Sarosiek I, Shifflett J, Wooten GF, McCallum RW (1997). Effect of chronic oral domperidone therapy on gastrointestinal symptoms and gastric emptying in patients with Parkinson's disease. *Mov Disord* **12:**952–957.

Speelman JD, Schuurman R, de Bie RM, Esselink RA, Bosch DA (2002). Stereotactic neurosurgery for tremor. *Mov Disord* **17(Suppl 3):**S84–S88.

Steur EN, Ballering LA (1997). Moclobemide and selegeline in the treatment of depression in Parkinson's disease. *J Neurol Neurosurg Psychiatry* **63:**547.

Stocchi F, Vacca L, De Pandis MF, Barbato L, Valente M, Ruggieri S (2001). Subcutaneous continuous apomorphine infusion in fluctuating patients with Parkinson's disease: long-term results. *Neurol Sci* **22:**93–94.

Suchowersky O, Furtado S, Rohs G (1995). Beneficial effect of intranasal desmopressin for nocturnal polyuria in Parkinson's disease. *Mov Disord* **10:**337–340.

Tasker RR (1998). Deep brain stimulation is preferable to thalamotomy for tremor suppression. *Surg Neurol* **49:**145–154.

Tesei S, Antonini A, Canesi M, Zecchinelli A, Mariani CB, Pezzoli G (2000). Tolerability of paroxetine in Parkinson's disease: a prospective study. *Mov Disord* **15:**986–989.

Thomas A, Iacono D, Luciano AL, Armellino K, Di Iorio A, Onofrj M (2004). Duration of amantadine benefit on dyskinesia of severe Parkinson's disease. *J Neurol Neurosurg Psychiatry* **75:**141–143.

Tolcapone Study Group (1999). Efficacy and tolerability of tolcapone compared with bromocriptine in levodopa-treated parkinsonian patients. *Mov Disord* **14:**38–44.

Tooley PJ, Vervaet P, Wager E (1999). Cardiac arrhythmias reported during treatment with cisapride. *Pharmacoepidemiol Drug Saf* **8:**57–58.

Toyokura Y, Mizuno Y, Kase M *et al.* (1985). Effects of bromocriptine on parkinsonism. A nation-wide collaborative double-blind study. *Acta Neurol Scand* **72:**157–170.

Trepanier LL, Saint-Cyr JA, Lozano AM, Lang AE (1998). Neuropsychological consequences of posteroventral pallidotomy for the treatment of Parkinson's disease. *Neurology* **51:**207–215.

Trepanier LL, Kumar R, Lozano AM, Lang AE, Saint-Cyr JA (2000). Neuropsychological outcome of GPi pallidotomy and GPi or STN deep brain stimulation in Parkinson's disease. *Brain Cogn* **42:**324–347.

Troster AI, Woods SP, Fields JA, Hanisch C, Beatty WW (2002). Declines in switching underlie verbal fluency changes after unilateral pallidal surgery in Parkinson's disease. *Brain Cogn* **50:**207–217.

Verhagen Metman L, O'Leary ST (2005). Role of surgery in the treatment of motor complications. *Mov Disord* **20(Suppl 11):**S45–S56.

Verhagen Metman L, Del Dotto P, van den Munckhof P, Fang J, Mouradian MM, Chase TN (1998). Amantadine as treatment for dyskinesias and motor fluctuations in Parkinson's disease. *Neurology* **50:**1323–1326.

Verhagen Metman L, Del Dotto P, LePoole K, Konitsiotis S, Fang J, Chase TN (1999). Amantadine for levodopa-induced dyskinesias. A 1-year follow-up. *Arch Neurol* **56:**1383–1386.

Vingerhoets G, van der Linden C, Lannoo E, Vandewalle V, Caemaert J, Wolters M, Van den Abbeele D (1999). Cognitive outcome after unilateral pallidal stimulation in Parkinson's disease. *J Neurol Neurosurg Psychiatry* **66:**297–304.

Vitek JL, Bakay RA, Freeman A *et al.* (2003). Randomized trial of pallidotomy versus medical therapy for Parkinson's disease. *Ann Neurol* **53:**558–569.

Volkmann J, Allert N, Voges J, Sturm V, Schnitzler A, Freund HJ (2004). Long-term results of bilateral pallidal stimulation in Parkinson's disease. *Ann Neurol* **55:**871–875.

Waters CH, Sethi KD, Hauser RA, Molho E, Bertoni JM; Zydis Selegiline Study Group (2004). Zydis selegiline reduces off time in Parkinson's disease patients with motor fluctuations: a 3-month, randomized, placebo-controlled study. *Mov Disord* **19:**426–432.

Weintraub D, Morales KH, Moberg PJ *et al.* (2005). Antidepressant studies in Parkinson's disease: a review and meta-analysis. *Mov Disord* **20:**1161–1169.

Werber E, Rabey J (2001). The beneficial effect of cholinesterase inhibitors on patients suffering from Parkinson's disease and dementia. *J Neural Transm* **108:**1319–1325.

Zesiewicz TA, Helal M, Hauser RA (2000). Sildenafil citrate (Viagra) for the treatment of erectile dysfunction in men with Parkinson's disease. *Mov Disord* **15:**305–308.

Zgaljardic DJ, Foldi NS, Borod JC (2004). Cognitive and behavioral dysfunction in Parkinson's disease: neurochemical and clinicopathological contributions. *J Neural Transm* **111:**1287–1301.

CHAPTER 19

Alzheimer's disease and other disorders associated with dementia

G. Waldemar,[a] B. Dubois,[b] M. Emre,[c] J. Georges,[d]
I.G. McKeith,[e] M. Rossor,[f] P. Scheltens,[g]
P. Tariska,[h] B. Winblad[i]

Abstract

Background and objectives The aim of this international guideline on dementia was to present a peer-reviewed evidence-based statement for the guidance of practice for clinical neurologists, geriatricians, psychiatrists, and other specialist physicians responsible for the care of patients with dementia. It covers major aspects of diagnostic evaluation and treatment, with particular emphasis on the type of patient often referred to the specialist physician. The main focus is Alzheimer's disease, but many of the recommendations apply to dementia disorders in general.

Methods The task force working group considered and classified evidence from original research reports, meta-analysis, and systematic reviews, published before January 2006. The evidence was classified and consensus recommendations graded according to the European Federation of Neurological Societies (EFNS) guidance. Where there was a lack of evidence, but clear consensus, Good Practice Points were provided.

Results The recommendations for clinical diagnosis, blood tests, neuroimaging, EEG, CSF analysis, genetic testing, tissue biopsy, disclosure of diagnosis, treatment of Alzheimer's disease, and counselling and support for caregivers were all revised as compared with the previous EFNS guideline. New recommendations were added for the treatment of vascular dementia, Parkinson's disease dementia, and dementia with Lewy Bodies, for monitoring treatment, for treatment of behavioural and psychological symptoms in dementia and for legal issues.

Conclusion The specialist physician plays an important role together with primary care physicians in the multidisciplinary dementia teams that have been established throughout Europe. This

[a]Memory Disorders Research Group, Department of Neurology, Rigshospitalet, Copenhagen University Hospital, Denmark; [b]Department of Neurology and Dementia Research Center, Hopital de la Salpetriere, Paris, France; [c]Department of Neurology, Istanbul Faculty of Medicine, Istanbul University, Turkey; [d]Alzheimer Europe, Luxembourg; [e]Institute for Ageing and Health, Newcastle General Hospital, Newcastle upon Tyne, United Kingdom; [f]Dementia Research Centre, Institute of Neurology, University College London, Queen Square, London United Kingdom; [g]Department of Neurology and Alzheimer Center, VU University Medical Center, Amsterdam, The Netherlands; [h]National Institute of Psychiatry & Neurology, Budapest, Hungary; [i]Department of Geriatric Medicine, Karolinska University Hospital, Huddinge, Sweden.

guideline may contribute to the definition of the role of the specialist physician in providing dementia health care.

Introduction

Dementia afflicts at least five million people in Europe (Andlin-Sobocki *et al.*, 2005) and is associated with significant physical, social and psychiatric disability in the patients and with significant burden and distress in family caregivers. Furthermore, Alzheimer's disease (AD) and other dementia disorders rank second in Western Europe when comparing the burden of brain diseases by the loss of disability adjusted life years (Olesen and Leonardi, 2003). The total health care costs in Europe related to dementia amount to at least 55 billion € per year, not including indirect costs and costs in young patients with dementia (Andlin-Sobocki *et al.*, 2005; Jönsson and Berr, 2005), and the majority of the costs are spent on institutional care.

Despite the fact that there is significant evidence for the benefits of early diagnostic evaluation, treatment and social support, the rate of diagnosis and treatment in people with dementia varies considerably in Europe (Waldemar *et al.*, 2006). General practitioners play a major role in the identification, diagnosis and management of patients with dementia. In many places multidisciplinary teams have been established to facilitate the management of the complex needs of patients and caregivers during the course of the dementia disease. The neurologist and other specialist physicians play a major role in these teams and clinics together with other professionals with special training in dementia.

In 2003, a task force was set up to develop a revision of the EFNS guideline on dementia published in 2000 (Waldemar *et al.*, 2000), with the aim to provide peer-reviewed evidence-based guidance for clinical neurologists, geriatricians, old age psychiatrists and other specialist physicians responsible for the care of patients with dementia. This guideline addresses major issues in the diagnosis and management of AD and other disorders with dementia. Since the previous guideline was published in 2000

significant evidence has accumulated, and new methods have become available for diagnosis and treatment.

The task force panel, appointed by the Scientific Committee of the EFNS, included neurologists, and representatives from geriatrics and old age psychiatry, with clinical and research expertise in dementia, and a representative from the patient organisation, Alzheimer Europe. The guideline applies to patients with suspected or diagnosed dementia, and covers aspects of diagnostic evaluation, as well as treatment, with particular emphasis on the type of patient often referred to the specialist. It does not, however, include treatment of mild cognitive impairment (MCI). The main focus of the guideline is AD, but there are many other conditions, although lower in prevalence, which require specific assessment and treatment, and many of the recommendations apply to dementia disorders in general. The guideline represents the minimum desirable standards for the guidance of practice, but does not include an analysis of cost-effectiveness of the recommended diagnostic and treatment interventions.

The evidence for this guideline was collected from Cochrane Library reviews, other published meta-analyses and systematic reviews, other evidence-based management guidelines in dementia, including the practice parameters from the American Academy of Neurology (AAN) (Petersen *et al.*, 2001; Knopman *et al.*, 2001; Doody *et al.*, 2001), and original scientific papers published in peer-reviewed journals before January 2006. For each topic, the evidence was sought in MEDLINE according to predefined search protocols. The scientific evidence for diagnostic investigations and treatments were evaluated according to pre-specified levels of certainty (class I, II, III and IV), and the recommendations were graded according to the strength of evidence (Level A, B or C), using the definitions given in the EFNS guidance (Brainin *et al.*, 2004). In addressing important clinical questions, for which no evidence was available, the task force group recommended 'Good Practice Points' based on the experience and consensus of the task force group. Consensus was reached by circulating drafts of the manuscript to the task force members and by discussion of the classification of evidence and recommendations at four task force meetings during 2004 and 2005.

This guideline may not be appropriate in all circumstances, and decisions to apply the recommendations must be made in the light of the clinical presentation of the individual patient and of available resources.

Diagnostic evaluation

Clinical diagnosis

With the remarkable exception of autosomal dominant causes of dementia, there is no specific biological marker for degenerative dementias. Therefore, in the absence of neuropathological confirmation, the aetiological diagnosis of a dementia syndrome can only be made in terms of probability. The clinical diagnosis should rely on criteria that have been proposed to increase the reliability and accuracy of the diagnosis. The accuracy of these diagnostic criteria varies as a function of the dementia. For AD, both the *Diagnostic and Statistical Manual,* 3rd edition, revised (DSM-IIIR) (American Psychiatric Association, 1993) and the National Institute of Neurologic, Communicative Disorders and Stroke-Alzheimer's Disease and Related Disorders Association (NINCDS-ADRDA) (McKhann *et al.*, 1984) criteria achieved a good sensitivity (up to 100%, average 81% across studies), but a low specificity (average across studies 70%) for 'probable' AD, based on class I–II studies with post-mortem confirmation (Knopman *et al.*, 2001). For dementia with Lewy bodies (DLB), the Consortium for DLB diagnostic criteria from 1996 (McKeith *et al.*, 1996) showed rather low sensitivities in class I and II studies (Knopman *et al.*, 2001). For fronto-temporal dementia (FTD) (Neary *et al.*, 1998; McKhann *et al.*, 2001), advances in the understanding of the underlying pathophysiology and genetic mechanisms have indicated that the clinical syndromes are associated with several different neuropathological abnormalities, although generally, specific sets of pathological findings have not been associated with specific clinical syndromes. For vascular dementia (VaD), the National Institute of Neurologic Disorders and Stroke and the Association Internationale pour la Recherche et l'Enseignement en Neuroscience (NINDS-AIREN) diagnostic criteria (Roman *et al.*, 1993) achieved a low sensitivity (43%), but a good specificity (95%) in the only published class I study (Holmes *et al.*, 1999). Mixed pathologies and the prevalent findings of vascular lesions in all patients with dementia add to the complexity of the diagnosis of vascular dementia.

Medical history

Clinical history is a cornerstone of medical practice and serves to focus the examination and investigations. The history should include the cognitive domains affected, the mode of onset, the pattern of progression and the impact on activities of daily living (ADL). Past medical history, current co-morbidities, family history and educational history are important. Due both to the presence of cognitive deficit and to the possibility of anosognosia it is important to obtain a history from an independent informant. Several class I to II studies have confirmed the value of informant-based instruments, such as the Informant Questionnaire on Cognitive Decline in the Elderly (IQCODE) and the Blessed Roth Dementia Scale (BRDS) in the detection of dementia (Jorm and Jacomb, 1989; Fuh *et al.*, 1995; Jorm 1997; Lam *et al.*, 1997; MacKinnon and Mulligan, 1998; MacKinnon *et al.*, 2003).

RECOMMENDATIONS

Medical history The clinical history should be supplemented by an independent informant where available (Level A).

Neurological and physical examination

The neurological examination in early AD is unremarkable apart from the cognitive impairment. However, for many of the other dementing disorders, for example DLB and prion diseases, the presence of additional neurological features, such as an extra pyramidal syndrome or myoclonus, is a key component of the diagnostic criteria. Moreover, many of the disorders in which dementia is part of a broader range of neurological dysfunction (the dementia plus syndromes) or in which abnormalities on physical examination such as organomegaly occur, the examination is critical in the diagnostic process. Furthermore, the general physical examination may reveal relevant co-morbidities. Whilst no formal studies have addressed the issue of the added value of a neurological and physical examination this is an important part of the differential diagnosis of dementia.

RECOMMENDATIONS

Neurological and physical examination A general neurological and physical examination should be performed on all patients presenting with dementia (Good Practice Point).

Assessment of Cognitive Functions

Assessment of cognitive function is important for several reasons: (1) the diagnosis of dementia mainly relies on the evidence of cognitive deficits (episodic memory, instrumental and executive functions); (2) most of aetiologies of dementia (e.g. AD, FTD, DLB) can be identified by the nature of their cognitive and behavioural changes; (3) as specialist physicians increasingly see patients at early stages of the disease, it is now important to be able to identify the specific degenerative disorders at a prodromal phase before the symptoms reach the threshold of dementia. Accordingly, an evaluation of cognitive function by a physician and by a clinical neuropsychologist is required for the management of patients with a prodromal, mild or moderate stage of dementia, whereas it is less essential for severely demented patients. The battery should investigate the following domains:

Global cognitive functions. The mini-mental state examination (MMSE) of Folstein *et al.* (1975) may help in the detection of cognitive impairment (I), and its sensitivity increases, if a decline of the score over time is taken into account. The 7-minute screen and the clinical dementia rating (CDR) (score = 1) demonstrate a specificity of 96%

and 94% with sensitivity of 92% for the diagnosis of dementia (Juva *et al.*, 1995 (II); Solomon *et al.*, 1998 (IV)) and can be useful for the detection of dementia. These two tests can be used as screening instruments for assessing general intellectual functioning. The Mattis dementia rating scale (Mattis, 1976) takes a longer time and tests in addition several areas related to executive functions. It is therefore more appropriate for the assessment and follow up of FTD and fronto-subcortical dementias.

Memory function. Memory has to be systematically assessed. Episodic long-term memory impairment is required to fulfil the diagnosis criteria for dementia. Word recall, such as the Rey auditory verbal learning test (RAVLT), can distinguish between patients with AD and those without dementia (I) (Incalzi *et al.*, 1995). However, an effective encoding of information should be controlled to exclude the influence of depression, anxiety and other emotional states to cognitive problems. Semantic cueing may also help in separating retrieval for storage deficits (Pillon *et al.*, 1996). For that reason, the memory impairment scale (MIS) (sensitivity of 60% and specificity of 96% for identification of dementia; Buschke *et al.*, 1999) and the '5 word' test (sensitivity of 91% and specificity of 87% for the identification of AD; Dubois *et al.*, 2002) are short and simple memory tests that can be useful for a first-line screening tool for medical practitioners. Semantic memory should also be assessed (category fluency test, pictures naming task, word and picture definition), as deficits may be observed in AD and be prominent in semantic dementia (SD) (Hodges *et al.*, 1992).

Executive functions. Executive dysfunctions are observed in several dementia conditions. This impairment results in decreased verbal fluency with speech reduction, verbal stereotypes and echolalia; perseverations of mental set; retrieval deficits; attentional disorders; concrete thinking and in some cases disinhibition, impaired adaptation, and uncontrolled behaviours. These deficits are currently assessed by the Wisconsin card sorting test (Nelson, 1976), the trail making test (Reitan, 1958), the Stroop test (Stroop, 1935), the verbal fluency tests (Benton, 1968), and the digit ordering test (Cooper *et al.*, 1992), which trigger the cognitive processes needed for executive functions. In some dementias, executive dysfunction is only an epiphenomenon, part of a more diffuse and global picture. By contrast, it can be a prominent feature and essential for the diagnosis of other dementias, such as FTD (Bozeat *et al.*, 2000) and progressive supranuclear palsy (PSP) (Pillon *et al.*, 1996).

Instrumental functions. Language (comprehension and expression), reading and writing, praxis (execution and recognition), visuospatial and visuoconstructive abilities can also be more or less affected according to the type of dementia disorder. These cognitive domains, often referred to as instrumental functions, are particularly impaired in diseases with prominent cortical involvement such as AD and DLB and may be the initial domain of dysfunction in lobar atrophy (progressive aphasia syndromes, progressive apraxia, corticobasal degeneration (CBD) or posterior cortical atrophy).

RECOMMENDATIONS

Assessment of cognitive functions Cognitive assessment is central to the diagnosis and management of dementias and should be performed in all patients (Level A). Quantitative neuropsychological testing, ideally performed by someone trained in neuropsychology, should be considered in patients with questionable, prodromal, mild, or moderate dementia (Level C). The specialist physician should include a global cognitive measure and in addition more detailed testing of the main cognitive domains including memory, executive functions and instrumental functions (Level C).

Assessment of behavioural and psychological symptoms

Various terms including 'behavioural and psychological symptoms of dementia' (BPSD), 'neuropsychiatric features', and 'non-cognitive symptoms', are used to describe a range of symptoms that are common in dementia and which contribute substantially to patient distress and caregiver burden (McKeith and Cummings, 2005). They are frequently a major factor leading to the prescription of psychotropic medications and to nursing home placement (Finkel and Burns, 2000) (III). Their presence may contribute to the process of differential diagnosis, for example, visual hallucinations are a prominent feature of DLB (McKeith *et al.*, 1996) (II), whereas disinhibition and lack of personal concern are characteristic of FTD (Neary and Snowden, 1996) (II). Their temporal course also varies, for example, apathy, depression and anxiety tend to occur early in the course of AD with delusions, hallucinations and agitation appearing in the middle to late stages. BPSD may be worsened or caused by somatic co-morbidity. Patients with psychosis experience a more rapid cognitive decline than those without, and neuropsychiatric features may predict an increased rate of conversion to dementia in patients diagnosed with MCI (Hwang and Cummings, 2004) (II).

The accurate identification of BPSD is essential both for diagnosis and management of patients with dementia, but often such symptoms may not be disclosed by patients or caregivers, until they are intolerable or they precipitate a crisis (Gustavson and Cummings, 2004). Earlier detection can be achieved by routine and repeated enquiry. Several rating instruments have been designed for this purpose, enquiring not only about the presence or absence of different symptoms but also about their frequency, severity and impact upon the caregiver. They usually rely upon the report of an informant who should have regular contact with the patient. Repeated use of such scales can also be useful in monitoring the effects of treatment interventions. Suitable scales include the neuropsychiatric inventory (NPI) (Cummings *et al.*, 1994), BEHAVE-AD (Reisberg *et al.*, 1987) and the Manchester and Oxford Universities scale for the psychopathological assessment of dementia (MOUSEPAD) (Allen *et al.*,1996).

The most common neuropsychiatric feature of AD is apathy (72%), followed by aggression/agitation (60%), anxiety (48%) and depression (48%) (Mega *et al.*, 1996) (II).

Apathy and *inertia* may occur independently of depressed mood and may be particularly frustrating for carers, especially in the early stages. *Agitation* and *aggression* may be very persistent and frequent causes of requests for institutionalisation. *Anxiety* may manifest physically with tension, insomnia, palpitations and shortness of breath and also with excessive worrying and fearfulness particularly if separated from the spouse or carer. *Depressed mood* should be assessed independently of weight loss, appetite changes, sleep disturbances and retardation that may occur as features of the dementia. Core psychological manifestations of depression such as sadness, thoughts of worthlessness and hopelessness, and statements about death and suicide should be enquired about. *Delusions* are common in dementia, usually of theft, intruders or imposters, often rather vaguely expressed and transient. They are typically based in forgetfulness and misinterpretation. Hallucinations, misidentifications and illusions in dementia are usually visual, particularly in DLB, but perceptual disturbances can also be auditory, olfactory or tactile. They are more common in those with impaired vision and hearing. *Purposeless activities* such as pacing and rummaging are characteristic of AD, while compulsions and stereotyped behaviours are more common in FTD as are *disinhibition and euphoria* exhibited as impulsivity, hyperorality, socially inappropriate behaviour and emotional lability. *Sleep disturbances* may be secondary to other psychiatric features, may be associated with daytime drowsiness and are particularly burdensome to carers who are also likely to be kept awake. Rapid eye movement (REM) sleep behaviour disorder is characteristic of DLB (Boeve *et al.*, 2001) (II).

RECOMMENDATIONS

Assessment of behavioural and psychological symptoms Assessment of behavioural and psychological symptoms of dementia is essential for both diagnosis and management, and should be performed in all patients (Level A). Symptoms should be actively enquired about from the patient and a closely involved carer using appropriate rating scales (Good Practice Point). Co-morbidity should always be considered as a possible cause (Level C).

Assessment of activities of daily living

Decline in every day functional abilities is a major component of the dementia syndrome. It has a great influence on the quantity and quality of care and its level is extremely important for the caregiver. Assessment of function in daily life is part of diagnostic process and allows clinicians to evaluate the need for personal and institutional care. Different scales are used to objectively measure these abilities. These are based mainly on the interview with the patient and his/her caregiver. Two classic fields measured are basic, or general (such as eating, dressing etc.) and instrumental activities (such as the use of devices, shopping). Frequently used scales include the Alzheimer disease cooperative study (ADCS) ADL Scale (Galasko *et al.*, 1997), functional activities questionnaire (FAQ) (Pfeffer *et al.*, 1982); the progressive deterioration scale (PDS) (DeJong *et al.*, 1989), and the disability assessment for dementia (DAD) (Gelinas *et al.*, 1999).

RECOMMENDATIONS

Assessment of activities of daily living Impairment of activities of daily living due to cognitive impairment is an essential part of the criteria for dementia and should be assessed in the diagnostic evaluation (Level A). A semi-structured interview from the caregiver is the most practical way to obtain relevant information, and a panel of validated scales are available (Good Practice Point).

Assessment of co-morbidity

Co-morbidities are frequent, particularly in elderly patients (IV), and may rapidly worsen the cognitive and functional status of the patient. There is a strong association between medical co-morbidity and cognitive status in AD (IV), and optimal management of medical illnesses may offer potential to improve cognition (Doraiswamy *et al.*, 2002). Depression, cardiovascular disease, infections, adverse effects of drugs, delirium, falls, incontinence, and anorexia are frequently observed co-morbidities or complications. Some of the co-morbid conditions that were identified in a large post-mortem study of patients with dementia would have affected the clinical management of the patient, had they been known ante mortem (IV) (Fu *et al.*, 2004).

RECOMMENDATIONS

Assessment of co-morbidity   Assessment of co-morbidity is important in the evaluation of the patient with dementia, and should be performed not only at the time of diagnosis, but throughout the course of the disease, with particular attention to episodes of sudden worsening of cognitive or behavioural symptoms (Good Practice Point).

Blood tests

Laboratory screening with blood tests is recognised as an important integral part of the general screening of a patient presenting with cognitive disturbances. The aims of blood tests include (1) to identify co-morbidity and/or complications; (2) to reveal potential risk factors; (3) to explore the background of frequently associated confusional states, and (4) more rarely to identify the primary cause of dementia. Cognitive disturbances may be associated with a wide range of metabolic, infectious, and toxic conditions, which should be identified and treated. For most of these conditions, there is no specific evidence from randomised controlled trials that treatment will reverse cognitive symptoms. Yet, the specialist physician is often dealing with patients with confusional states, rapid progression or atypical presentation, in whom blood tests may be of diagnostic value.

RECOMMENDATIONS

Blood tests   The following blood tests are generally proposed as mandatory tests for all patients at first evaluation, both as a potential cause of cognitive impairment or as co-morbidity: blood sedimentation rate, complete blood cell count, electrolytes, calcium, glucose, renal and liver function tests, and thyroid stimulating hormone. More extensive tests will often be required, e.g. vitamin B12 and serological tests for syphilis, HIV, and Borrelia, in individual cases (Good Practice Point).

Neuroimaging

Traditionally, imaging was considered important solely as a means of excluding treatable causes of dementia. These conditions account for a small proportion of all causes of dementia with far more common causes being AD, VaD, DLB and FTD (Ott *et al.*, 1995). Neuroimaging is now the most important ancillary investigation in the work-up of dementia to aid in differential diagnosis and management decisions.

CT

CT is mostly used to exclude other illnesses that are potentially amenable to (surgical) treatment, for example, tumours, haematomata and hydrocephalus. The yield of such a procedure has been debated but probably lies somewhere between 1% and 10% and may even be lower (Hejl *et al.*, 2002; Clarfield, 2003) (II). Farina *et al.* performed CT in 513 patients referred to a memory clinic of whom 362 were found demented (Farina *et al.*, 1999) (II). In 26 of them (7.2%) a potential reversible cause of dementia was detected. However, in none of the cases did CT reveal findings that had not been discovered clinically. Foster *et al.* carried out a systematic review on the use of CT scanning in dementia (Foster *et al.*, 1999). Comparing costs and outcome they concluded that scanning each patient under 65 years and treating only subdural haematomas would be the most cost-effective approach. Recently, Condefer *et al.* (2004) showed that in a memory clinic setting, routine CT impacted on diagnosis in 12% of cases and on management in 11% (II), mainly because of the identification of vascular changes. Because Gifford *et al.* (2000) showed that there is considerable uncertainty in the evidence underlying clinical prediction rules to identify which patients with dementia should undergo neuroimaging and application of these rules may miss patients with potentially reversible causes of dementia, it is generally felt that a structural imaging investigation in the evaluation of a patient suspected of dementia should be performed routinely.

Magnetic Resonance Imaging

Magnetic resonance imaging (MRI) may be used for the same reason as CT but has the ability to increase specificity to an already quite high sensitivity of the clinical diagnosis.

Hippocampal atrophy in AD

Hippocampal atrophy is an early and specific marker of the AD process (de Leon *et al.*, 1989, 1997; Jack *et al.*, 1992; Killiany *et al.*, 1993; De Carli *et al.*, 1995) (II–IV). This structure has been measured using a variety of tracing techniques and anatomical boundaries. Some studies have employed linear or visual measurements (Scheltens *et al.*, 1992, 1995, 1997; de Leon *et al.*, 1996; O'Brien *et al.*, 1997; Frisoni *et al.*, 2002). Because of their supposedly (but debatable) greater accuracy and reliability, other studies have used volumetric measures of medial temporal lobe structures. Comparative studies have found good correlations between these assessment techniques (Desmond *et al.*, 1994; Wahlund *et al.*, 2000). Several studies used a qualitative method that involves a visual rating scale, usually a four- or five-point scale ranging from absent to severe atrophy (Scheltens *et al.*, 1992; Erkinjuntti *et al.*, 1993). Frisoni *et al.* used a compound score of linear measurements that included the temporal horn (Frisoni *et al.*, 1996). Pucci *et al.* found the best discriminating parameter to be just the height of the left hippocampus (Pucci *et al.*, 1998). In a novel approach Frisoni and co-workers used the radial width of the temporal horn of the lateral ventricle on axial MR scans as measured with a calliper on paper printouts (Frisoni *et al.*, 2002). Visual assessment is considerably less time consuming than volumetry and easily applicable in clinical practice (Wahlund *et al.*, 1999). The down-side may be a larger interrater variability (Scheltens *et al.*, 1995). The overall sensitivity and specificity figures for detection of mild to moderate AD vs controls were 85% and 88% in a meta-analysis (Scheltens *et al.*, 2002), and the accuracy of hippocampal atrophy in mild AD ranged from 67% to 100% in a systematic review (Chetelat *et al.*, 2003) (I–II).

Fronto-temporal lobar degeneration

Asymmetric, predominantly left sided peri-sylvian atrophy characterises progressive non-fluent aphasia and asymmetric anterior temporal lobe atrophy

is diagnostic of SD. In both conditions, with time, atrophy becomes more widespread but usually remains asymmetric. The pattern of atrophy may be more useful than atrophy of single regions in the differential diagnosis of FTD vs AD (II) (Galton *et al.*, 2001; Chan *et al.*, 2001; Varma *et al.*, 2002; Boccardi *et al.*, 2003).

Vascular Dementia

In the most often used NINDS-AIREN international work group criteria for VaD brain imaging is thought to be essential for the diagnosis, and without it VaD will be 'possible' at best (Roman *et al.*, 1993). In addition, the criteria specify which vascular territories are 'relevant' for VaD. These include large vessel strokes, such as bilateral infarcts in the anterior or posterior cerebral artery areas, in the association areas, or in the watershed regions. Using operational guidelines on how to classify radiological features as fitting into the NINDS-AIREN criteria, inter-observer reliability of the diagnosis went up significantly from 40% to 60% (vanStraaten *et al.*, 2003) (II).

Identifying vascular disease in dementia

Like AD, the prevalence of cerebrovascular disease (CVD), both symptomatic and asymptomatic, increases dramatically with age, and pathological studies often find concomitant cerebral infarction in patients with definite AD (Snowdon *et al.*, 1997). Even small, concurrent infarctions significantly increase the likelihood of expressed dementia, suggesting a synergistic effect. Given that concurrent CVD may be amenable to targeted interventions potentially ameliorating disease progression, brain imaging may prove important to the clinical care of the demented patient with coexisting CVD. Preliminary evidence from anti-hypertensive treatment trials of older individuals supports this notion, although further prospective clinical trials involving brain imaging are necessary.

Miscellaneous

In addition to the above specific imaging signs may include: bilateral caudate atrophy in Huntington's disease, hyperintense signal in the putamen in sporadic Creutzfeldt Jakob Disease (CJD) and hyperintense signal change in the pulvinar in new variant CJD (Schroter *et al.*, 2000) (II). Diffusion-weighted MRI shows (the earliest) focal changes in CJD not yet apparent on FLAIR images, and may widely involve the cortex (Collie *et al.*, 2001) (II). Corticobasal degeneration shows a typical MRI pattern, with striking, asymmetric parietal (peri-Rolandic) and frontal atrophy, sparing medial temporal regions (Kitagaki *et al.*, 2000) (II). Normal pressure hydrocephalus (NPH) is a questionable disease entity, and it may be difficult to decide whether such a patient would benefit from a shunting procedure. Strict adherence to clinical and MRI criteria is important, with additional information from a positive – but not a negative – cerebrospinal fluid (CSF) tap and the occurrence of B-waves (Vanneste, 2000) (II). These MRI criteria include widened ventricles with normal sulci and without white matter pathology. In DLB MRI has been reported to show medial temporal lobe atrophy in a lower frequency than in AD, and therefore the *absence* of medial temporal lobe atrophy may be suggestive of a diagnosis of DLB (Barber *et al.*, 1999) (II).

SPECT and PET

SPECT and PET are often used as a part of the work-up especially in memory clinics and as a complement to structural imaging in difficult differential diagnostic questions. Here again, the quest should be to increase specificity to augment clinical diagnostic criteria and structural imaging. The most often applied functional imaging studies include regional blood flow measurements performed with SPECT (^{99m}Tc-HMPAO or ^{133}Xe) and measurement of glucose metabolism performed with ^{18}F-FDG-PET. A reduction in blood flow or glucose metabolism in parieto-temporal areas is the most commonly described diagnostic criterion for AD. In a recent meta-analysis, functional imaging studies with SPECT in which AD was contrasted against control subjects yielded pooled weighted sensitivities ranging from 65% to 71%, with specificity of 79% (Dougall *et al.*, 2004). Very few SPECT studies have adequately addressed the comparison between AD and other dementias. The few that did provided a pooled weighted

sensitivity and specificity for AD vs FTD of 71% and 78%, respectively, and for AD vs VaD of 71% and 75%, respectively (Dougall *et al.*, 2004). In a recent meta-analysis, the summary sensitivity of PET in diagnosing AD vs control subjects was 86%, and the summary specificity was 86% (Patwardhan *et al.*, 2004). The majority of SPECT and PET studies were class II, although many did not have blinded evaluation of imaging results (IV). The fact that all positive likelihood ratios were <5, indicates that cerebral blood flow assessed with SPECT or glucose metabolism assessed with PET moderately improves the diagnostic certainty either when AD is contrasted against controls or against other dementias (Jagust *et al.*, 2002). Interestingly, there is no difference in diagnostic value between regional cerebral blood flow assessed with SPECT and glucose metabolism assessed with PET. Furthermore, very few studies addressed the additional value of functional imaging over structural imaging. On the other hand, an international consortium of investigators argued that, although FDG-PET had moderate specificity (73–78%) for the diagnosis of AD both for clinical and pathological diagnosis, due to its high sensitivity, a negative (i.e. normal) PET strongly favours a normal outcome at follow-up (Silverman *et al.*, 2001).

There have been studies suggesting that SPECT using the presynaptic dopamine transporter ligand ^{123}I-FP-CIT (DAT-SPECT) can distinguish DLB from AD and normal aging. Low striatal dopamine transporter activity is seen in idiopathic Parkinson's disease (PD), DLB, and PSP, but not in AD (II–III) (Walker *et al.*, 2002; O'Brien *et al.*, 2004; Tolosa *et al.*, 2006). The positive outcome has led the consensus committee on the diagnosis of DLB to include it in the most recent version of its guidelines (McKeith *et al.*, 2005).

RECOMMENDATIONS

Neuroimaging Structural imaging should be used in the evaluation of every patient suspected of dementia: Non-contrast CT can be used to identify surgically treatable lesions and vascular disease (Level A). To increase specificity, MRI (with a protocol including T1, T2 and FLAIR sequences) should be used (Level A). SPECT and PET may be useful in those cases where diagnostic uncertainty remains after clinical and structural imaging work up, and should not be used as the only imaging measure (Level B).

Electroencephalography (EEG)

EEG is widely available, non-invasive and suitable for repeated recording. Generalised slowing of background rhythm is a feature of AD and DLB. The EEG may be entirely normal in advanced frontal lobe degeneration although abnormalities are relatively common in the overall group of FTD (Chan et al., 2004). There is an overall relationship between the severity of dementia and abnormalities on the EEG in AD and DLB. There have been many studies demonstrating the ability of the EEG to distinguish clinically diagnosed AD from controls with a sensitivity that is comparable to other techniques such as neuroimaging (Claus et al., 1998, 1999; Jelic et al., 1999, 2000). However, there is a paucity of studies that explore the differential diagnosis of the dementia and which have neuropathological confirmation. Robinson et al. reported a series of neuropathologically confirmed AD (86 patients) and mixed and VaD (17 patients) with blinded assessment of the EEG (II) (Robinson et al., 1994). Abnormalities on the EEG were frequent in uncomplicated AD with a sensitivity of 87%. Importantly, a normal EEG had a negative predictive value of 82% with respect to a diagnosis of AD. There have been few studies exploring the added value of the EEG over and above a full clinical and neuroimaging assessment. Claus et al. investigated the added value of the EEG in a study of 49 control subjects with and without minimal cognitive impairment and 86 probable AD patients (II) (Claus et al., 1999). The maximum diagnostic gain of 38% for an abnormal EEG was found when the prior probability was low at 30–40%. If there was a high pre-test probability of 80–90% then the diagnostic gain of an abnormal EEG was much lower, between 7 and 14%.

In some specific dementia conditions, the EEG has a higher diagnostic contribution. Periodic sharp wave complexes are part of the clinical criteria for the diagnosis of CJD, particularly the sporadic variety. Zerr et al. reported on 805 patients with neuropathologically confirmed CJD disease in whom the EEG was available (I) (Zerr et al., 2000). The presence of periodic sharp wave complexes provided 66% sensitivity and 74% specificity, comparable to the smaller series of Steinhoff et al. (I) (1996). The appearance of periodic sharp wave complexes is however variable and can disappear during the course of the disease making repeated EEG measurements valuable.

Transient epileptic amnesia due to focal temporal lobe seizure activity can masquerade as AD (Zeman et al., 1998; Høgh et al., 2002). The EEG may be diagnostic in this situation.

RECOMMENDATIONS

EEG The EEG may be a useful adjunct, and should be included in the diagnostic work up of patients suspected of having Creutzfeldt–Jakob disease or transient epileptic amnesia (Level B).

CSF analysis

Examination of CSF (with routine cell count, protein, glucose, and protein electrophoresis) is mandatory when inflammatory disease, vasculitis or demyelination is suspected, and in cases of dementia with early onset, rapid decline, marked fluctuations, or extensive white matter changes on MRI or CT. A vast body of literature has emerged investigating the added value of 'specific' biomarkers in CSF such as amyloid β (1-42) (Aβ42), total tau (tau), phospho-tau and the 14-3-3 protein. Aβ42 is decreased in the CSF of AD patients possibly as a result of the deposition of fibrillar Aβ42 in senile plaques. Tau is increased in CSF of AD patients, as a reflection of the release of tau in CSF with neuronal loss. Phospho-tau derives from tangle deposition. The presence of the 14-3-3 protein in CSF is a measure for (acute) neuronal loss and brain damage and is associated with CJD.

AD vs Controls

Aβ42 is decreased and tau increased in CSF of AD patients compared to non-demented controls, patients with depression, and patients with memory complaints on the basis of alcohol abuse (Sunderland *et al.*, 2003; Blennow *et al.*, 2003a, b). The pooled sensitivity and specificity for Aβ42 in AD vs controls from 13 studies was 86% and 90%. For tau the sensitivity was 81% and the specificity 90%, pooled from 36 studies (II–III) (Blennow *et al.*, 2003a). A recent meta-analysis showed considerable differences in absolute concentrations of Aβ42 and tau between laboratories, even when the same test kit was used (Sjögren *et al.*, 2001). Using the combination of both markers for AD versus controls, a high sensitivity (85–94%) and specificity (83–100%) can be reached (II) (Verbeek *et al.*, 2003). In patients with early onset AD compared to controls, a sensitivity of 81% with specificity of 100% was found (III) (Schoonenboom *et al.*, 2004). As the reference test, the clinical diagnosis is usually used, sometimes also with a follow-up period in which the diagnosis did not change (Schoonenboom *et al.*, 2004; Pijnenburg *et al.*, 2004). Only two studies had neuropathological validation of the diagnosis (Tapiola *et al.*, 2000; Clark *et al.*, 2003). In these studies the same high sensitivity and specificity for the distinction of AD from controls was found (I). One study investigated and found an association between the number of senile plaques and concentration of Aβ42 in CSF (Strozyk *et al.*, 2003).

AD vs other dementias

A decreased CSF-Aβ42 is being found in FTD (Riemenschneider *et al.*, 2002; Schoonenboom *et al.*, 2004;), DLB (Kanemaru *et al.*, 2000), VaD (Hulstaert *et al.*, 1999; Nagga *et al.*, 2002), and CJD (Van Everbroeck *et al.*, 1999) when compared to controls (for AD vs FTD: specificity 59–81% (I) (Riemenschneider *et al.*, 2002; Schoonenboom *et al.*, 2004; Pijnenburg *et al.*, 2004); for AD vs VaD: specificity 71% (II) (Kapaki *et al.*, 2003). Tau is increased in many other dementias such as FTD (II) (Green *et al.*, 1999; Fabre *et al.*, 2001; Riemenschneider *et al.*, 2002; Schoonenboom *et al.*, 2004) and CJD (I) (Otto *et al.*, 2002). In VaD conflicting results have been reported; specificity varied between 14% and-83% (II–III) (Blennow *et al.*, 1995; Andreasen *et al.*, 1998; Kapaki *et al.*,

2003) compared to AD. In FTD specificity varied from 26% to 75% (II–III) (Riemenschneider *et al.*, 2002; Schoonenboom *et al.*, 2004; Pijnenburg *et al.*, 2004). In DLB tau is usually normal (II) (Kanemaru *et al.*, 2000). The combination of Aβ42 and total tau increases specificity and the negative predictive value (II): AD vs total group other dementias: 58–85% (Verbeek *et al.*, 2003); AD vs FTD: 85% (Riemenschneider *et al.*, 2002); AD vs DLB and VaD specificity 67% and 48%, respectively, with a negative predictive value of 95% (I) (Andreasen *et al.*, 2001).

AD compared to an age matched FTD group yielded good sensitivity (72%), and high specificity (89%) and a very low negative likelihood ratio (-LR =0.03) (Schoonenboom *et al.*, 2004). In general, for studies in which phospho tau was added, specificity was even higher (II–III) (Blennow *et al.*, 2003).

CJD

In CJD very high tau levels have been reported, higher than in AD, yielding a high sensitivity and specificity, 93% and 90–100% (I) (Kapaki *et al.*, 2001; Otto *et al.*, 2002). Assessment of the 14-3-3 protein in the sporadic form of CJD has a sensitivity of 90–100% and a specificity of 84–96% (I–II) (Zerr *et al.*, 1998, 2000; Lemstra *et al.*, 2000; Otto *et al.*; 2002; Van Everbroeck *et al.*, 2003). False positive results are found in cerebral infarcts, encephalitis, tumours and rapidly progressive AD (I–II) (Zerr *et al.*, 1998; Poser *et al.*, 1999; Lemstra *et al.*, 2000). When the clinical suspicion of CJD is high, the combination of EEG (Poser *et al.*, 1999), MRI, and 14-3-3-assessment has the maximum accuracy (I–II) (Lemstra *et al.*, 2001).

RECOMMENDATIONS

CSF CSF analysis with routine cell count, protein, glucose and protein electrophoresis is recommended in patients with a clinical suspicion of certain diseases and in patients with atypical clinical presentations (Good Practice Point). CSF total tau, phospo-tau, and Ab42 can be used as an adjunct in cases of diagnostic doubt (Level B).

For the identification of CJD in cases with rapidly progressive dementia, assessment of the 14-3-3 protein is recommended (Level B).

Genetic testing

Many degenerative dementias can occur as autosomal dominant disorders with similar phenotypes to sporadic disease apart from an earlier age at onset. The prevalence of autosomal dominant disease varies from less than 1% in AD to nearly 50% in some series of FTD. Three causative genes have been identified in familial AD, the amyloid precursor protein (APP) gene and the presenilin 1 and 2 genes. Tau mutations are found in some cases of familial FTD and mutations in the prion protein gene in familial CJD. There is an increasing range of rarer genes, especially in the dementia plus syndromes. The yield of mutation screening in unselected populations is low, for example, no tau mutations were found in a large series of clinically diagnosed non Alzheimer dementias (Houlden et al., 1999). However, with an appropriate phenotype an autosomal dominant family history gene testing for known mutations can provide a specific diagnosis. This should only be undertaken in specialist centres with appropriate consent and counselling. The identification of a known pathogenic mutation in an affected family member can permit pre-symptomatic testing, and the Huntington's disease protocol for predictive testing and counselling should be followed (Harper et al., 1990). Autopsy diagnosis in familial dementias can be valuable for establishing the significance of gene sequence variation in a family for subsequent diagnosis and counselling.

A variety of risk genes have been identified and the most carefully studied has been the Apolipoprotein (Apo) E4 polymorphism. The addition of Apo E testing increased the positive predictive value of a diagnosis of AD from 90 to only 94% in a neuropathologically confirmed series (Mayeux et al., 1998). In those patients with a clinical diagnosis of non-Alzheimer dementia the absence of an Apo E4 ε4 allele increased the negative predictive value from 64% to 72%.

RECOMMENDATIONS

Genetic testing Screening for known pathogenic mutations can be undertaken in patients with appropriate phenotype or a family history of an autosomal dominant dementia. This should only be undertaken in specialist centres with appropriate counselling of the patient and family caregivers, and with consent (Good Practice Point).

Presymptomatic testing may be performed in adults where there is a clear family history, and when there is a known mutation in an affected individual to ensure that a negative result is clinically significant. It is recommended that the Huntington's disease protocol is followed (Good Practice Point).

Routine Apo E genotyping is not recommended (Level B).

Other investigations

Additional investigations may provide critical information in the differential diagnosis of dementia, for example, metabolic studies from fibroblast cultures, white cell enzyme assays, urinary aminoacids, and the like. Moreover, extensive imaging may provide diagnostic information in paraneoplastic syndromes. Biopsies of specific tissues can also be invaluable, for example, liver biopsy in Wilson's disease and skin and muscle biopsies in conditions such as cerebral autosomal dominant arteriopathy with subcortical infarcts and leucoencephalopathy (CADASIL) (100% specificity and 45% sensitivity) (Markus et al., 2002), Lafora body disease and mitochondrial cytopathies. Tonsillar biopsy can demonstrate the presence of prion protein in variant CJD.

Cerebral biopsy can provide a specific histological diagnosis but should only be undertaken where a treatable disorder is considered, such as cerebral vasculitis. In general, a non-dominant frontal or temporal pole full thickness biopsy to include leptomeninges and white matter should be performed. In many cases, prion disease cannot be excluded from the differential diagnosis and either disposable craniotomy instruments should be used or the instruments should be quarantined until a specific diagnosis has been made.

> **RECOMMENDATIONS**
>
> *Tissue biopsy* Tissue biopsy can provide a specific diagnosis some rare dementias. This should only be undertaken in specialist centres in carefully selected cases (Good Practice Point).

Disclosure of diagnosis

Of particular interest to specialist physicians are laws pertaining to the disclosure of diagnosis to the person him/herself rather than his/her family. Most European countries have not established the right to a diagnosis into an absolute right without any possible exceptions and most legislations allow doctors to refrain from disclosing a diagnosis, if this is considered to be in the 'best interests' of the person or if such disclosure could cause 'serious harm' to the physical or mental health of the patient (Alzheimer Europe, 2000). Nevertheless, a growing consensus (Alzheimer Europe, 2001) has emerged in favour of disclosing a diagnosis to the person at a time when the person is capable of understanding this. It has been shown that such disclosure relieves the anxiety of uncertainty and maximises individual autonomy and choice by providing information necessary for decision making and advance planning (IV) (Fearnley *et al.*, 1997), including the decision to give informed consent to research projects and autopsy.

> **RECOMMENDATIONS**
>
> *Disclosure of diagnosis* Disclosure of diagnosis should be done tactfully and should be accompanied by information about the consequences and the progression of the disease, as well as useful contacts such as the local or national Alzheimer's association. In countries where this is possible physicians may also wish to encourage patients to draw up advance directives containing future treatment and care preferences (Good Practice Point).

Management of Alzheimer's disease and other disorders associated with dementia

To address the complex needs of the patient with dementia and the caregiver during the course of a dementia disorder the specialist physicians should collaborate with other health care professionals with special training in dementia. The specialist physician should schedule regular follow-up visits, the purposes of which include: (1) to assess cognitive, emotional, and behavioural symptoms together with the functional status; (2) to evaluate treatment indications and to monitor pharmacological and non-pharmacological treatment effects; (3) to ensure identification and appropriate treatment of concomitant conditions and of complications of the primary dementia disorder; (4) to assess caregiver burden and needs; (5) to assess sources of care and support; (6) to provide continuous advice and guidance to patient and caregiver on health and psychological issues, safety measures, driving, and legal and financial matters; and (7) to administer appropriate patient and caregiver interventions. The primary caregiver, when available, should accompany the patient with dementia at follow-up visits and investigations.

In this guideline the main emphasis is on recommendations for pharmacological treatment, and many important aspects of the care for patients with dementia, for example, living arrangements, cognitive rehabilitation, nursing care and end-of-life issues are not covered. For pharmacological treatment, this review is confined to dementia (not MCI) and to drugs that have been clinically tested in dementia and which are available on the market, although they may not be registered for dementia worldwide. Negative results were also included, if published, whereas experimental substances were not covered. It must be emphasised that the class of evidence does not necessarily reflect the effect size and the potential clinical relevance thereof, which were taken into consideration in making recommendations.

Treatment of Alzheimer's disease
Cholinesterase inhibitors

Cholinesterase inhibitors (ChEIs) represent the first class of drugs approved for the specific symptomatic treatment of AD. Following the introduction of tacrine, the first ChEI to be approved, donepezil, rivastigmine and galantamine became available. There are multiple randomised, placebo-controlled, large-scale clinical trials with these substances establishing efficacy on cognitive functions, overall evaluation, and ADL in patients with mild to moderate AD, with modest effect sizes (Rogers *et al.*, 1996,1998; Rösler *et al.*, 1999; Raskind *et al.*, 2000; Tariot *et al.*, 2000; Brodaty *et al.*, 2005) (I). The ChEIs are generally well tolerated, although gastrointestinal adverse effects such as nausea, diarrhoea, and vomiting are the most common adverse effects, and may lead to discontinuation of treatment in some patients. The use of ChEIs in mild to moderate AD has also been subject to systematic reviews and meta-analyses, and their efficacy was confirmed (Birks *et al.*, 2000; Birks and Harvey, 2006; Loy and Schneider, 2006). Likewise, practice parameters such as those provided by AAN, recommend that ChEIs should be considered in patients with mild to moderate AD (Doody *et al.*, 2001). Although their appraisal report is currently being revised, the National Institute for Clinical Excellence (NICE) in the UK in their health technology appraisal from 2001 recommended that ChEIs should be considered in mild to moderate AD (NICE, 2001).

With regard to duration of efficacy the longest lasting placebo-controlled studies with continuous treatment were with donepezil, performed over 1 year. These studies revealed that efficacy, in terms of difference from placebo-treated patients, was maintained for at least 1 year and there was a 38% reduction in the risk of functional decline compared to placebo (Winblad *et al.*, 2001; Mohs *et al.*, 2001) (I). A recent placebo-controlled study over 3 years, in which multiple withdrawal phases were involved, revealed that cognitive scores and functionality were significantly better with donepezil over 2 years, but the differences were small and did not translate into benefits in primary outcome measures defined as institutionalisation or progression of disability over 3 years (AD 2000 Collaborative Group, 2004) (II). There have been extensions of placebo-controlled studies with follow-up up to 5 years, where historical data or model-based predictions for non-treatment were used as a control.

These studies suggest a slower progression of symptoms in treated patients. Lack of control in these studies and bias due to dropouts, however, limit their conclusions (Rogers *et al.*, 2000; Pirttala *et al.*, 2004; Winblad *et al.*, 2006) (III).

The initial assessments of efficacy of ChEI were focused on cognitive functions, scales of global change and ADL. Subsequently, small beneficial effects of ChEI on behavioural symptoms of AD were also shown (Tariot *et al.*, 2000; Feldman *et al.*, 2001; Trinh *et al.* 2003) (I). With regard to disease stage, placebo-controlled randomised trials with donepezil confirmed efficacy in patients with early, mild AD as well as those with moderate to moderately severe AD (Feldman *et al.*, 2001; Seltzer *et al.*, 2004) (I). There has been only one large randomised controlled double-blind study with direct comparison of the efficacy of cholinesterase inhibitors: A comparison of rivastigmine with donepezil in a large, randomised controlled trial over 2 years revealed that the efficacy was comparable in the primary outcome measure, some of the secondary efficacy measures favoured rivastigmine, and tolerability was better with donepezil (Bullock *et al.*, 2005) (II). There is some evidence from open-label studies that patients who do not tolerate or do not seem to benefit from one AChE-I may tolerate or draw benefit from the other (III) (Auriacombe *et al.*, 2002; Bartorelli *et al.*, 2005). Several attempts were made to quantify the clinical usefulness of ChEIs, which are not considered to be disease modifying (Livingston and Katona, 2000; Clegg *et al.*, 2001; Trinh *et al.*, 2003). A meta-analysis on the cost-effectiveness of ChEIs concluded that on the basis of the current evidence the implications of the use of donepezil, rivastigmine or galantamine to treat patients with AD are unclear (Clegg *et al.*, 2001). A meta-analysis of 29 controlled studies with ChEIs revealed a modest beneficial impact on neuropsychiatric and functional outcomes, but there seemed to be no difference between the different drugs in this regard (Trinh *et al.*, 2003) (I).

Memantine

Memantine, a non-competitive *N*-Methyl-D-Aspartate (NMDA) receptor antagonist, represents the second class of drugs approved for the specific symptomatic treatment of AD. The compound blocks the chronic hyper-activation of NMDA receptors that is thought to contribute to the symptomatology and pathogenesis of AD. A number of large-scale, randomised placebo-controlled trials with memantine were reported in patients with dementia.

Two studies were performed in patients with moderate-to-severe AD (I) (Reisberg et al., 2003; Tariot et al., 2004); one of them in patients on stable treatment with donepezil (Tariot et al., 2004). Another randomised placebo-controlled study was performed in a mixed population of severe AD and severe VaD patients (Winblad and Poritis, 1999) (I). To date, no studies in mild AD have been published in peer-reviewed journals.

Recently, the available data were reviewed in a Cochrane meta-analysis, and the authors concluded from the published data that memantine at 6 months caused a clinically noticeable reduction in deterioration in patients with moderate to severe Alzheimer's disease (I) (Areosa SA et al., 2005). This was supported by less functional and cognitive deterioration (I). Memantine was well tolerated when given alone, and also in the study where it was combined with donepezil (I) (Tariot et al., 2004), and patients taking memantine appeared to be less likely to develop agitation. Whether memantine has any effect in mild to moderate AD is unknown (Areosa SA et al., 2005).

With the exception of Winblad and Poritis (1999), where no performance-based cognitive assessment was performed, all of these studies showed statistically significant superiority in the cognitive performance of memantine treatment of the patients over placebo using the severe impairment battery (SIB) (I). In the study of Winblad and Poritis, statistically significant effects were demonstrated in functional and global assessments (I). One of the trials in moderate-to-severe AD included a pharmaco-economic questionnaire and demonstrated a reduction in caregiver time and in total societal costs (Wimo et al., 2003). In the study by Tariot et al. (2004), memantine showed positive effects on the behavioural disturbances, as assessed by the NPI (I).

Other drugs and interventions

There are several other treatment measures that have been suggested for the treatment of AD, including gingko biloba, non-steroidal anti-inflammatory drugs (NSAIDs), oestrogens and statins. Three randomised, controlled trials with the gingko biloba extract Egb 761 were reported in AD. All of these studies involved mixed patient populations including those with AD, multi-infarct dementia, and in one study also patients with MCI, and the duration of treatment was up to 1 year. In two studies some parameters measuring cognition and behaviour improved significantly (Kanowski et al., 1996; Le Bars et al., 1997), although assessment methods in one and analysis of results in the other were not standard (II); in the third study there were no significant differences between gingko biloba and placebo (II) (van Dongen et al., 2003). A meta-analysis of all published data in patients with dementia concluded that although overall there is promising evidence of improvement in cognition and function, the three more modern trials showed inconsistent results, and there is a need for a large trial using modern methodology (Birks et al., 2002) (I).

Anti-oxidants such as vitamin E have been studied to see if they can delay progression in patients with AD. In a large randomised, placebo-controlled study (Sano et al., 1997) in patients with moderate AD, vitamin E (given at the dose of 1000 IU, twice a day over 2 years) was found to significantly delay the time to a composite outcome of primary measures, indicative of clinical worsening, and fewer patients receiving vitamin E were institutionalised as compared to those receiving placebo (I). An attempted meta-analysis of randomised, controlled studies with vitamin E, which could find only the above-mentioned study, concluded that there is insufficient evidence for the efficacy of vitamin E in the treatment of AD, but there is sufficient evidence of possible benefit to justify further studies (I) (Tabet et al., 2004). Furthermore, a large meta-analysis of studies with vitamin E has shown that high-dosage (> or = 400 IU/d) vitamin E supplements may increase all cause mortality (I) (Miller et al., 2004).

Chronic exposure to non-steroidal anti-inflammatory drugs was suggested to be protective against AD in a retrospective analysis of epidemiological data (McGeer *et al.*, 1996). In prospective studies, however, only indomethacin was suggested to stabilise cognition in a 6-month trial with a high dropout rate (I) (Rogers *et al.*, 1993; Scharf *et al.*, 1999; Aisen *et al.*, 2000; Van Gool *et al.*, 2001; Aisen *et al.*, 2003). Similarly, in a recent large, randomised, double-blind, placebo-controlled trial the cyclo-oxygenase-2 inhibitor rofecoxib, administered for 1 year, was not found to be effective in slowing the progression of AD (Reines *et al.*, 2004) (I).

Statins used for the treatment of hypercholesterolaemia were found to decrease the prevalence of AD in two studies with retrospective or cross-sectional analysis (Jick *et al.*, 2000; Wolozin *et al.*, 2000). This effect was found to be independent of indication bias (healthier cohort effect), but confined to those below the age of 80 (Rockwood *et al.*, 2002), and appeared to be modified by the presence of certain chronic medical conditions, in that the reduced risk of AD was observed among those with diseases such as hypertension and ischemic heart disease (Zamrini *et al.*, 2004). Pravastatin showed no significant effect on cognitive function or disability (Shepherd *et al.*, 2002); atorvastatin showed significant effect on cognitive function at 6 months, but not at 12 months (III) (Sparks *et al.*, 2005). A meta-analysis of available data concluded that there is no good evidence to recommend statins for reducing the risk of AD (Scott and Laake, 2003) (II).

In retrospective or cross-sectional analyses postmenopausal use of oestrogens has been suggested to provide symptomatic benefits or reduce the risk of AD. Prospective, randomised, placebo-controlled studies, however, failed to demonstrate symptomatic beneficial effects of oestrogens, given up to 1 year, in women with mild to moderate AD, with or without hysterectomy (III) (Wang *et al.*, 2000; Henderson *et al.*, 2000; Mulnard *et al.*, 2000). Although treatment with oestrogen elevated blood oestradiol and oestrone levels, there was no association between hormone levels and cognitive functioning after 1 year of treatment (Thal *et al.*, 2003). A meta-analysis concluded that oestrogen replacement therapy is not indicated for cognitive improvement or maintenance for

women with AD (I) (Hogervorst *et al.*, 2002). Likewise, the results of the large, prospective, placebo-controlled 'Women's Health Initiative Memory Study' revealed that the use of oestrogen plus progestin in post-menopausal women, after a mean follow-up time of 4 years, was associated with a significantly increased risk of dementia (Shumaker *et al.*, 2003) (I).

Meta-analyses for several other drugs including selegiline (Birks and Flicker, 2003), nicergoline (Fioravanti and Flicker, 2001), nimodipine (Lopez-Arrieta, 2002) and piracetam (Flicker and Grimley Evans, 2004) concluded that there was not sufficient evidence to recommend their use in AD (II).

RECOMMENDATIONS

Treatment of Alzheimer's disease In patients with AD, treatment with ChEIs (donepezil, galantamine, or rivastigmine) should be considered at the time of diagnosis, taking into account expected therapeutic benefits and potential safety issues (Level A). Realistic expectations for treatment effects and potential side effects should be discussed with the patient and caregivers (Good Practice Point).

In patients with moderate to severe AD, treatment with memantine can be considered, alone or in combination with a ChEI, taking into account expected therapeutic benefits and potential safety issues (Level A). Realistic expectations for treatment effects and potential side effects should be discussed with the patient and caregivers (Good Practice Point).

Currently, there is insufficient evidence to consider the use of gingko biloba, anti-inflammatory drugs, nootropics, selegiline, oestrogens, vitamin E or statins in the treatment or prevention of AD (Level A–C).

Treatment of vascular dementia
Cholinesterase inhibitors

After it became apparent that VaD is also associated with cholinergic deficits, ChEIs were investigated in patients with VaD. Along with patients with dementia due to pure or predominant CVD, vascular pathology can also co-exist with AD pathology, constituting mixed dementia. There have been two large, randomised, placebo-controlled studies with donepezil in patients with possible or probable VaD and one large, randomised, placebo-controlled study with galantamine in patients with VaD or AD combined with CVD. In the two donepezil studies there was a significant improvement in the two main outcome parameters (cognitive functions and overall scales); ADL was significantly improved in one and showed a trend for improvement in the second study at the end of treatment period (Black *et al.*, 2003; Wilkinson *et al.*, 2003) (I). Results with galantamine were similar: patients on active drug had significant improvement on both primary end-points as well as in ADL and behavioural scales, as compared to placebo (I) (Erkinjuntti *et al.*, 2002). Although the study was not powered to detect changes in the two diagnostic sub-groups (i.e. probable VaD and AD with CVD) the cognitive and overall scales showed significant improvement in AD with CVD group whereas the differences as compared to placebo were not significant in the probable VaD sub-group (Erkinjuntti *et al.*, 2002). An open label 6-month extension of this study suggested that the benefits may be maintained up to 1 year (III) (Erkinjutti *et al.*, 2003). A Cochrane meta-analysis concluded that there are some weak indications that galantamine is useful in dementia secondary to vascular damage, but it was associated with higher rates of adverse events and withdrawal (I) (Craig and Birks, 2006). From existing trial data (III–IV), most of which are from open studies or post-hoc analyses, there is some evidence of benefit of rivastigmine in vascular cognitive impairment, but larger placebo-controlled double blind RCTs are needed (Craig and Birks, 2004). A meta-analysis of the two studies with donepezil concluded that the evidence indicates that donepezil is well tolerated and can improve cognitive symptoms and functional ability in patients with vascular cognitive impairment (Malouf and Birks, 2004) (I).

Memantine

Two randomised placebo-controlled 6-month studies are available in patients suffering from mild-to-moderate VaD (Wilcock *et al.*, 2002; Orgogozo *et al.*, 2002), using 20 mg/d memantine. These studies included close to 900 patients and were designed according to modern standards, using the ADAS-Cog and a clinical global rating of change as primary efficacy endpoints. They were summarised by the recent Cochrane meta-analysis (Areosa SA *et al.*, 2005): in the two studies memantine improved cognition and behaviour, but this was not supported by clinical global measures (I). Memantine was well tolerated (I). In a subgroup analysis of these studies (Möbius and Stöffler, 2003), the cognitive benefit seemed to be more pronounced in the subgroup of patients with small vessel disease, which is more closely linked to AD (III). In addition, a number of short-term studies in less well-defined dementia populations have been published and were also reviewed in the Cochrane database, including studies in patients with VaD, and with dementia of unspecified type. In summary, there were beneficial effects on cognition (Ditzler, 1991), ADL (Ditzler, 1991), behaviour and global scales (Ditzler, 1991; Görtelmeyer, 1992) and in global impression of change (Ditzler, 1991; Görtelmeyer, 1992) (III–IV). The meta-analysis concluded that patients with mild to moderate vascular dementia receiving memantine had less cognitive deterioration at 28 weeks, but the effects were not clinically discernible. The drug was well tolerated in general and the incidence of adverse effects was low (Areosa SA *et al.*, 2005).

Anti-aggregants and other drugs

There has been one small study with aspirin in patients with VaD. In this study, where the control group was no-treatment, patients treated with aspirin had a better outcome on a cognitive scale by the third year and also a significant improvement in cerebral perfusion in the first 2 years (Meyer *et al.*, 1989) (III). A meta-analysis of available data revealed that, despite its widespread use, there is still no evidence that aspirin is effective in treating patients with a diagnosis of VaD (Rands *et al.*, 2004). In a systematic review of clinical studies with pentoxifylline in VaD, four studies were identified fulfilling the criteria (being randomised, double-blind, and placebo-controlled), which revealed a trend towards improved cognitive function, but no statistically significant differences versus placebo (Sha and Callahan, 2003)

(I). When the calcium channel blocker nimodipine was tested in patients with 'multi-infarct dementia' in a large, randomised placebo-controlled study, there were no significant benefits from nimodipine treatment over placebo in cognitive, functional and global assessments (Pantoni *et al.*, 2000) (I). Furthermore, in a recent randomised placebo-controlled trial in patients with subcortical vascular dementia there was no significant effect of nimodipine on the primary outcome measure, a global clinical assessment scale (Pantoni *et al.*, 2005). Studies with gingko biloba are mentioned above.

RECOMMENDATIONS

Treatment of vascular dementia ChEIs (currently evidence exists for donepezil) may be considered in patients fulfilling diagnostic criteria for VaD of mild to moderate severity (Level B). Realistic expectations for treatment effects and potential side effects should be discussed with the patient and caregivers (Good Practice Point). In the presence of severe focal neurological deficits, the accuracy of diagnosis and expected therapeutic benefits should be carefully considered based on the presumed contribution of sensory-motor impairment versus cognitive deficits to the overall disability of the patient (Good Practice Point).

There is insufficient evidence to consider the use of memantine in patients with vascular dementia (Level B).

There is insufficient evidence to support the use of aspirin, gingko biloba, calcium antagonists or pentoxifylline in the treatment of VaD (Level A–C).

Optimum management of vascular risk factors, including anti-platelet drugs, should be ensured, not only in vascular dementia, but also in patients with other dementias or co-morbid vascular disease (Good Practice Point).

Treatment of Parkinson disease dementia (PD-D) and Dementia with Lewy bodies (DLB)

There are substantial cholinergic deficits both in PD-D and DLB, and ChEIs have been tested in both these indications. In total there have been fourteen studies with four compounds (tacrine, donepezil, rivastigmine and galantamine) describing the use of ChEIs in patients with PD-D. All of these studies were small (all including less than 30 patients), three of them were placebo-controlled, eight were open studies and two case series. Improvement in cognition and neuropsychiatric symptoms, notably hallucinations, were described in the majority of these studies, worsening of parkinsonism was infrequent, and was mostly related to tremor (Aarsland *et al.*, 2004; Ravina *et al.*, 2004). A recent, large, placebo-controlled study with rivastigmine revealed that there was a statistically significant improvement in favour of rivastigmine in both primary endpoints with modest effect sizes (ADAS-cog for cognitive functions and ADCS Clinical Global Impression of Change (CGIC) for CGIC overall evaluation) as well as on all secondary measures. Adverse event profile was comparable to that seen in patients with AD, nausea and vomiting being the most frequent adverse events. In the rivastigmine group 10% of patients reported subjective worsening of tremor, and 1.7% discontinued treatment for this reason. There were, however, no significant differences between rivastigmine and placebo in objectively measured motor scores (Emre *et al.*, 2004) (I).

There have been eight studies reporting the use of ChEIs in DLB, involving tacrine, donepezil and rivastigmine. One of these studies was placebo-controlled, three were controlled, but not-randomised and others were case series. All studies but one reported improvement in cognitive functions, and half of them reported improvement in neuropsychiatric symptoms, commonly apathy and hallucinations; worsening of parkinsonism was rare (Aarsland *et al.*, 2004). In the large, prospective, randomised, placebo-controlled study, rivastigmine was found to be significantly better than placebo for one of the two main outcome parameters, cognitive speed score. There was also more improvement in the rivastigmine group for the other parameter, neuropsychiatric symptom score, in the last observation carried forward (LOCF) and observed case analyses, but not in the intention to treat (ITT) population. A responder analysis showed significantly greater reductions in NPI score in all three groups. Rivastigmine did not cause worsening of motor symptoms (McKeith *et al.*, 2000) (I).

The efficacy of memantine has not been formally assessed in DLB. The very limited case report literature available suggests that about two thirds of DLB patients can tolerate memantine, but the symptomatic effects are variable A significant minority experience worsening of agitation, paranoid delusions, and visual hallucinations when exposed to memantine (Sabbagh *et al.*, 2005; Ridha *et al.*, 2005) (IV).

RECOMMENDATIONS

Treatment of Parkinson disease dementia and Dementia with Lewy Bodies Treatment with ChEIs (currently evidence exists for rivastigmine) can be considered in patients with PD-D or DLB (Level A), taking into account expected therapeutic benefits and potential safety issues. Realistic expectations for treatment effects and potential side effects should be discussed with the patient and caregivers (Good Practice Point).

There is insufficient evidence for the use of memantine in PD-D or DLB (Level C) and it may be associated with worsening of agitation and psychosis.

Monitoring treatment with ChEIs and memantine in patients with dementia disorders

Monitoring treatment with ChEIs and memantine must be guided by the adverse event profiles and the clinical condition of the patient. Monitoring should include regular assessments of compliance, efficacy (cognitive functions, ADL, and behavioural symptoms), and side effects. In patients with known cardiac disease or significant cardoivascular risk factors a baseline ECG may be heplful for future monitoring purposes. There is no evidence from appropriately designed studies that can guide the clinician in determining when to stop treatment.

RECOMMENDATIONS

Monitoring of treatment with ChEIs and memantine Efficacy and side effects should be regularly monitored during treatment (Good Practice Point). In case of rapid worsening or an apparent loss of efficacy discontinuation of treatment may be considered on a trial basis. Such patients should be closely monitored to assess withdrawal effects or worsening in which case the treatment should be re-started (Level C).

Treatment of other dementia disorders

There have been no large, randomised, controlled studies in other types of degenerative dementias such as FTD, PSP or CBD. In a small open and another small randomised, double-blind, placebo-controlled cross-over study, donepezil was not found to be effective in patients with PSP: there were at best modest effects on cognition but deleterious effects on ADL and mobility (Fabbrini *et al.*, 2001; Litvan *et al.*, 2001) (III). Selective serotonin reuptake inhibitors, particularly paroxetine, were used in two open and one small placebo-controlled cross-over study in patients with FTD. While the open studies suggested some benefits, especially with regard to behaviour, the placebo-controlled study suggested no benefits, rather a deterioration of cognitive functions (Swartz *et al.*, 1997; Moretti *et al.*, 2003; Deakin *et al.*, 2004) (III).

RECOMMENDATIONS

Treatment of other dementia disorders There are no drugs available for the specific treatment of other degenerative dementias such as FTD, PSP and CBD (Level C). A number of pathological conditions and systemic or central nervous system disorders can be associated with dementia. Their specific treatment must be based on the underlying aetiology (Good Practice Point).

Treatment of behavioural and psychological symptoms in dementia

It is the behavioural and psychological symptoms of dementia that contribute most to patient distress and carer burden and which frequently need treatment, sometimes urgently (McKeith and Cummings, 2005). The sudden onset or worsening of symptoms such as hallucinations, insomnia, anxiety, agitation or aggression may be indicative of a superadded delirium, as may apathy or apparent depression. A physical re-evaluation should therefore always be the first stage of managing BPSD, paying close attention to recent changes in medications, signs of infection or systemic toxicity and evidence for parallel decline in cognitive function (Gustavson and Cummings, 2004) (II). Drugs with potential to worsen confusion and psychosis, e.g. anticholinergics, are contra-indicated and should be avoided. Pre-intervention measures of behavioural disturbance or psychiatric symptoms should ideally be established using an appropriate rating scale to help assess treatment effects. Psychosocial interventions may be classified as cognition-orientated, behaviour-orientated, emotion-orientated and stimulation-orientated. There is limited randomised controlled trial evidence about their specific effects upon BPSD, and they tend to be applied in an individualised way or to group settings such as care homes. Education, information and support groups for patients and carers are helpful and should be offered by a skilled multidisciplinary team. Environmental manipulations can be important. A non-confrontational approach to dealing with delusions, wandering, agitation and aggression may be difficult for lone carers to maintain at home and there may be considerable value in providing day and respite care. Locked doors may reduce concerns about wandering although may increase patients' attempts to escape from their surroundings. Specific behavioural interventions may help reduce incontinence (Doody et al., 2001) (I), and good sleep hygiene may reduce insomnia.

The pharmacological management of BPSD is particularly problematic as very few placebo-controlled randomised controlled trials have been conducted (McKeith and Cummings, 2005). A target symptom approach, for example, a focus upon the reduction of agitation or psychosis, is preferable to attempting to reduce BPSD generally. Such fine distinctions may not always however be easy to apply in clinical practice.

There has been recent interest in the potential role of ChEIs for managing BPSD, for example, rivastigmine reduced apathy, anxiety, hallucinations, delusions and irritability in DLB (McKeith et al., 2000) (I) and galantamine reduced the emergence of neuropsychiatric features in mild to moderately impaired AD patients (Loy and Schneider, 2006) (I). ChEIs are increasingly being used for BPSD in AD and other dementias. Although they may impact on BPSD they may also need to be used in combination with other agents. The mainstay of pharmacological management of the symptom cluster agitation, delusions, hallucinations and irritability has been with neuroleptic agents such as haloperidol (Lonergan et al., 2002) and more recently with atypical antipsychotics, usually prescribed at a third to half the young adult dose. There is little consistent evidence that these drugs significantly modify unwanted behaviours other than aggression (O'Brien and Ballard, 1999; Ballard and Waite, 2006), and there is often a considerable side effect cost with sedation, weight gain, extrapyramidal features and falls. There are recent reports that atypical antipsychotic medication may be associated with an increased risk of cerebrovascular events and mortality in elderly patients with dementia (UK Committee on Safety of Medicines, 2004; Schneider et al., 2005; Carson et al., 2006; Ballard and Waite, 2006). However, a retrospective cohort study suggested that conventional antipsychotic medications are at least as likely as atypical agents to increase the risk of death among elderly persons (Wang et al., 2005), and more information is required to help clinicians make judgements about risk-benefits in individual patients (McKeith and Cummings, 2005). In DLB, severe neuroleptic sensitivity reactions are associated with a two- to threefold increased mortality, and antipsychotics should only be used with great caution (McKeith et al., 1992) (II). Thus, in all elderly patients with dementia, conventional as well as atypical antipsychotics should be used with caution and only after careful estimation of risk-benefits. Patients and caregivers should be informed about the expected therapeutic benefits and risks, and the treatment must be reviewed at close intervals. Carbamazepine (Olin et al., 2001) and valproic acid (Lonergan et al., 2002) have both been used to treat agitation in dementia, but with inconsistent effects (II).

The principles of treatment of depression in dementia are probably similar to that in non-demented people of the same age, although adequately conducted trials are lacking for most agents (Bains *et al.*, 2004). Selective serotonin reuptake inhibitors (SSRIs) and other newer antidepressants are less likely to induce confusion and the anticholinergic effects typically seen with tricyclics. Emotional lability and compulsive behaviours have been reported to improve with SSRIs in FTD, and they may have similar effects in other dementias (McKeith and Cummings, 2005) (II).

RECOMMENDATIONS

Treatment of Behavioural and Psychological Symptoms in Dementia (BPSD) Clinicians treating patients with dementia should be aware of the importance of treating behavioural and psychiatric symptoms and the potential benefits for patient and carer (Good Practice Point). Somatic co-morbidity should be considered as the cause of the symptoms (Level C). Non-pharmacological and then pharmacological interventions for BPSD may both be effective and should be applied in a targeted symptom approach. The short, medium and long term benefits and adverse effects of such interventions should be regularly reviewed (Level C). Antipsychotics, conventional as well as atypical, may be associated with significant side effects and should be used with caution (Level A).

Counselling and support for caregivers

In patients with mild to moderate dementia, the assistance of a caregiver is necessary for many complex ADL, for instance travelling, financial matters, dressing, planning, and communication with family and friends. With the progression of the disease, increasing amounts of time must be spent on supervision. In patients with moderate to severe dementia caregivers often provide full time assistance with basic ADL, dealing with incontinence, bathing, feeding, and transfer or use of a wheelchair or walker. The majority of AD caregivers provide high levels of care, and at the same

time they are burdened by the loss of their spouse or good friend. Caregivers are twice as likely to report physical strain and high levels of emotional stress as a direct result of caregiving responsibilities. They are more likely to report family conflicts, to spend less time with other family members, and to give up vacations, hobbies, and other personal activities. Caring for someone with dementia may also cause a high level of financial strain. Interventions developed to offer support for caregivers to patients living at home include: counselling, training and education programmes, homecare/health care teams, respite care, information-technology based support. Many small quantitative or qualitative studies on the effectiveness of formal interventions seeking to support carers and alleviate the burden of caring have been published. Two meta-analyses (Brodaty *et al.*, 2003; Sørensen *et al.*, 2002) and one systematic review (Pusey and Richards, 2001) on the effect of caregiver intervention have been published. In general, there is evidence from a few class II randomised trials to support the view that carers to patients with moderate to severe dementia benefit from structured support initiatives that may reduce depressive symptoms (Mittelmann *et al.*, 1993, 1995). There is a lack of appropriately designed randomised controlled studies, particularly in mild dementia (Thompson *et al.*, 2004). As a dementia diagnosis is often established early in the course of the disease, intervention programmes should also include support, counselling, and education activities for the patient, but there are no appropriately designed quantitative studies that have addressed the outcome of supportive interventions directed towards the patient with mild dementia.

RECOMMENDATIONS

Counselling and support for caregivers A dementia diagnosis mandates an inquiry to the community for available public health care support programs (Good Practice Point). Specialist physicians should assess caregiver distress and needs at regular intervals throughout the course of the disease (Level C). Caregivers should be offered support and counselling (Level B). This includes information about patient organisations (Good Practice Point).

Legal issues

Dementia involves a gradual loss of cognitive and physical capacities and thereby affects memory, decision-making and the ability to communicate one's wishes to others. For these reasons, a person with dementia may be unable to consent to treatment, take part in research or be involved in decisions relating to his or her care. In everyday life, problems may arise if the person with dementia wants to continue driving, make a will or carry out financial transactions. In many cases, it may be necessary to appoint a guardian or tutor (Alzheimer Europe, 2000).

In almost all countries specialist physicians play an important role in the assessment of mental capacity or incapacity, as they may be required to: make an assessment of capacity prior to medical treatment, provide a medical certificate at a lawyer's request as to a particular capacity unrelated to medical treatment, witness or otherwise certify a legal document signed by someone, or give an opinion as to a particular legal capacity that is relevant to court proceedings (British Medical Association, 1995).

Although assessing a person's capacity does not require a high degree of legal knowledge, the doctor should understand the relevant legal terms in broad terms as the doctor's role is to provide information on which an assessment of the person's capacity can be based (British Medical Association, 1995).

RECOMMENDATIONS

Legal issues Specialist physicians responsible for the care of patients with dementia should be aware of national legislations relating to assessment of capacity, consent to treatment and research, disclosure of diagnosis, and advance directives (Good Practice Point).

A diagnosis of dementia is not synonymous with mental incapacity, as a determination of capacity should always involve a 'functional' analysis: does the person possess the skills and abilities to perform a specific act in its specific context? (Good Practice Point).

Driving

At the time of diagnosis, a patient's driving skills should also be assessed and discussed, as advice about driving is an essential part of the management of dementia (Johansson and Lundberg, 1997) and because patients with AD who continue to drive are at an increased risk for crashes (Hunt *et al.*, 1997) (I). In particular, drivers with mild AD (CDR 1) pose a significant traffic safety problem (Dubinsky *et al.*, 2000). There is, however, considerable variability across Europe with respect to the national driving regulations for patients suffering from disorders associated with dementia, the role of specialist physicians in the assessment of driving capabilities, and the confidentiality of medical data with regard to third parties, such as national driving licence authorities (White and O'Neill, 2000).

RECOMMENDATIONS

Driving Assessment of driving ability should be done after diagnosis and be guided by current cognitive function, and by a history of accidents or errors whilst driving. Particular attention should be paid to visuo-spatial, visuo-perceptual, praxis and frontal lobe functions together with attention. Advice either to allow driving, but to review after an interval, to cease driving, or to refer for retesting should be given (Level A). This decision must accord with the national regulations of which the specialist physician must be aware (Good Practice Point).

Conclusion

The assessment, interpretation, and treatment of symptoms, disability, needs, and caregiver stress during the course of AD and other dementia disorders require the contribution of many different professional skills. Ideally, the appropriate care and management of patients with dementia requires a multidisciplinary and multi-agency approach. Neurologists should be involved together with old age psychiatrists and geriatricians in the development and leadership of multidisciplinary teams responsible for clinical practice and research in dementia. This review contributes to the definition of standards of care in dementia by providing evidence for important aspects of the diagnosis and management of dementia.

Conflicts of interest

Potential conflicts of interest: Gunhild Waldemar, Bruno Dubois, Murat Emre, Ian McKeith, Philip Sheltens, Peter Tariska, and Bengt Winblad have received speaker's and/or consultancy honoraria from Janssen-Cilag, Lundbeck, Mertz, Novartis, and/or Pfizer. Jean Georges: none declared. For the conception and writing of this guideline no honoraria or any other compensations were received by any of the authors. The development of the guideline was supported by a task force grant from the EFNS.

Acknowledgments

This guideline task force was supported by a task force grant from the EFNS

References

Aarsland D, Mosimann UP, McKeith IG (2004). Role of cholinesterase inhibitors in Parkinson's disease and dementia with Lewy bodies. *J Geriatr Psychiatry Neurol* **17:**164–171.

AD 2000 Collaborative Group. Long-term donepezil treatment in 565 patients with Alzheimer's disease (AD 2000): randomized double-blind trial (2004). *Lancet* **363:**2105–2115.

Aisen PS, Davis KL, Berg JD *et al.* (2000). A randomized controlled trial of prednisone in Alzheimer's disease. Alzheimer's Disease Cooperative Study. *Neurology* **54:**588–593.

Aisen PS, Schafer KA, Grundman M *et al.* (2003). Alzheimer's Disease Cooperative Study. Effects of rofecoxib or naproxen vs placebo on Alzheimer disease progression: a randomized controlled trial. *JAMA* **289:**2819–2826.

Allen NH, Gordon S, Hope T, Burns A (1996). Manchester and Oxford Universities Scale for the Psychopathological Assessment of Dementia (MOUSEPAD). *Br J Psychiatry* **169:**293–307.

Alzheimer Europe (2000). Lawnet – Final report. http://www. alzheimer-europe.org (accessed February 24, 2006).

Alzheimer Europe (2001). Recommendations on how to improve the legal rights and protection of adults with incapacity due to dementia. http://www.alzheimer-europe.org (accessed February 24, 2006).

American Psychiatric Association (APA) (1993). *Diagnostic and Statistical Manual of Mental Disorders*. DSM-IV, 4th edition. Washington, D.C.: American Psychiatric Association.

Andreasen N, Vanmechelen E, Van de Voorde A *et al.* (1998). Cerebrospinal fluid tau protein as a biochemical marker for Alzheimer's disease: a community based follow up study. *J Neurol Neurosurg Psychiatry* **64:**298–305.

Andreasen N, Minthon L, Davidsson P *et al.* (2001). Evaluation of CSF-tau and CSF-Aβ42 as diagnostic markers for Alzheimer disease in clinical practice. *Arch Neurol* **58:**373–379.

Andlin-Sobocki P, Jönsson B, Wittchen H-U, Olesen J (2005). Cost of disorders of the brain in Europe *Euro J Dement* **12(Suppl 1):**1–27.

Areosa Sastre A, Sherriff F, McShane R (2005). Memantine for dementia. *The Cochrane Database of Systematic Reviews*, Issue 3. Art. No.: CD003154. DOI: 10.1002/14651858.CD003154.pub4.

Auriacombe S, Pere J-J, Loria-Kanza Y *et al.* (2002). Efficacy and safety of rivastigmine in patients with Alzheimer's disease who failed to benefit from treatment with donepezil. *Curr Med Res Opin* **18:**129–138.

Bains J, Birks JS, Dening TD (2002). Antidepressants for treating depression in dementia. *The Cochrane Database of Systematic Reviews*, Issue 4. Art. No.: CD003944. DOI: 10.1002/14651858.CD003944.

Ballard C, Waite J (2006). The effectiveness of atypical antipsychotics for the treatment of aggression and psychosis in Alzheimer's disease. *The Cochrane Database of Systematic Reviews*, Issue 1. Art. No.: CD003476. DOI: 10.1002/14651858.CD003476.pub2.

Barber R, Gholkar A, Scheltens P, Ballard C, McKeith IG, O'Brien JT (1999). Medial temporal lobe atrophy on MRI in dementia with Lewy bodies. *Neurology* **52:**1153–1158.

Bartorelli L, Giraldi C, Saccardo M *et al.* (2005). Effects of switching from and AChEI to a dual AChE-BuChE inhibitor in patients with Alzheimer's disease. *Curr Med Res Opin* **21:**1809–1818.

Benton AL (1968). Differential behavioral effects in frontal lobe disease. *Neuropsychologia* **6:** 53–60.

Birks J, Flicker L (2003). Selegiline for Alzheimer's disease. *The Cochrane Database of Systematic Reviews*, Issue 1. Art. No.: CD000442. DOI: 10.1002/14651858.CD000442.

Birks J, Grimley Evans J, Iakovidou V, Tsolaki M (2000). Rivastigmine for Alzheimer's disease. *The Cochrane Database of Systematic Reviews*, Issue 4. Art. No.: CD001191. DOI: 10.1002/14651858.CD001191.

Birks J, Grimley Evans J (2002). Ginkgo Biloba for cognitive impairment and dementia. *The Cochrane Database of Systematic Reviews* 2002, Issue 4. Art. No.: CD003120. DOI: 10.1002/14651858.CD003120.

Birks J, Harvey RJ (2006). Donepezil for dementia due to Alzheimer's disease. *The Cochrane Database of Systematic Reviews* 2006, Issue 1. Art. No.: CD001190. DOI: 10.1002/14651858.CD001190.pub2.

Black S, Roman GC, Geldmacher DS *et al.* (2003). Efficacy and tolerability of donepezil in vascular dementia: positive results of a 24-week, multicenter, international, randomized, placebo-controlled clinical trial. *Stroke* **34**:2323–2330.

Blennow K, Hampel H (2003a). Cerebrospinal fluid markers for incipient Alzheimer's disease. *Lancet Neurol* **2**:605–613.

Blennow K, Vanmechelen E (2003b). CSF markers for pathogenic processes in Alzheimer's disease: diagnostic implications and use in clinical neurochemistry. *Brain Res Bull* **61**:235–242.

Blennow K, Wallin A, Ågren H *et al.* (1995). Tau protein in cerebrospinal fluid: a biochemical marker for axonal degeneration in Alzheimer's disease? *Mol Chem Neuropathol* **26**:231–245.

Boccardi M, Laakso MP, Bresciani L *et al.* (2003). The MRI pattern of frontal and temporal brain atrophy in fronto-temporal dementia. *Neurobiol Aging* **24**:95–103.

Boeve, B, Silber, M, Ferman, T *et al.* (2001). Association of REM sleep behavior disorder and neurodegenerative disease may reflect an underlying synucleinopathy. *Mov Disord* **16**:622–630.

Bozeat S, Gregory CA, Ralph MA, Hodges JR (2000). Which neuropsychiatric and behavioural features distinguish frontal and temporal variants of frontotemporal dementia from Alzheimer's disease? *J Neurol Neurosurg Psychiatry* **69**:178–186.

Brainin M, Barnes M, Gilhus NE, Selmaj K, Waldemar G (2004). Guidance for the preparation of neurological management guidelines by EFNS scientific task forces - revised recommendations. *Euro J Neurol* **11**:577–581.

British Medical Association (1995). *Assessment of Mental capacity: Guidance for doctors and lawyers. A report of the British Medical Association and The Law Society.* Plymouth: Latimer Trend and Company Ltd, 1995.

Brodaty H, Green A, Koschera A (2003). Meta-Analysis of Psychosocial Interventions for Caregivers of People with Dementia. *J Am Geriatr Soc* **51**:657–664.

Brodaty H, Cory-Bloom J, Potocnik FC, Tryen L, Gold M, Damaraju CR (2005). Galantamine prolonged-release formulation in the treatment of mild to moderate Alzheimer's disease. *Dement Geriatr Cognit Disord* **20**:120–132.

Bullock R, Touchon J, Bergman H *et al.* (2005). Rivastigmine and donepezil treatment in moderate to moderately-severe Alzheimer's disease over a 2-year period. *Curr Med Res Opin* **21**:1317–1327.

Buschke H, Kuslansky G, Katz M *et al.* (1999). Screening for dementia with the Memory impairment Screen. *Neurology* **52**:231–238.

Carson S, McDonagh MS, Peterson K *et al.* (2006). A systematic review of the efficacy and safety of atypical antipsychotics in patients with psychological and behavioral symptoms of dementia. *J Am Geriatr Assoc* **54**:354–361.

Chan D, Fox NC, Jenkins R, Scahill RI, Crum WR, Rossor MN (2001). Rates of global and regional cerebral atrophy in AD and frontotemporal dementia. *Neurology* **57**:1756–1763..

Chan D, Walters RJ, Sampson EL, Schott JM, Smith SJ, Rossor MN (2004). EEG abnormalities in frontotemporal lobar degeneration. *Neurology* **62**:1628–1630.

Chetelat G, Baron JC (2003). Early diagnosis of Alzheimer's disease: Contribution of structural neuroimaging. *Neuroimage* **18**:525–541.

Clarfield AM (2003). The decreasing prevalence of reversible dementias: an updated meta-analysis. *Arch Int Med* **163**:2219–2229.

Clark CM, Sharon X, Chittams J *et al.* (2003). Cerebrospinal fluid Tau and β-Amyloid. How well do these biomarkers reflect autopsy-confirmed dementia diagnoses? *Arch Neurol* **60**:1696–1702.

Claus JJ, Kwa VIH, Teunisse S *et al.* (1998). Slowing on quantitative spectral EEG is a marker for rate of subsequent cognitive and functional decline in early Alzheimer disease. *Alzheimer's Dis Associated Disord* **12**:167–174.

Claus JJ, Strijers RL, Jonkman EJ *et al.* (1999). The diagnostic value of electroencephalography in mild senile Alzheimer's Disease. *Clin Neurophysiol* **110**:825–832.

Clegg A, Bryant J, Nicholson T *et al.* (2001) Clinical and cost-effectiveness of donepezil, rivastigmine and galantamine for Alzheimer's disease: a rapid and systematic review. *Health Technol Assess* **5**:1–137.

Collie DA SR, Zeidler M, Colchester AC, Knight R, Will RG (2001). MRI of Creutzfeldt-Jakob disease: imaging features and recommended MRI protocol. *Clin Radiol* **56**:726–739.

Condefer KA, Haworth J, Wilcock GK (2004). Clinical utility of computed tomography in the assessment of dementia: e memory clinic study. *Int J Geriatr Psychiatry* **19:**414–421.

Cooper JA, Sagar HJ, Doherty SM, Jordan N, Tidswell P, Sullivan EV (1992). Different effects of dopaminergic and antticholinergic therapies on cognitive and motor function in Parkinson's disease. A follow-up study of untreated patients. *Brain* **115:**1701–1725.

Craig D, Birks J (2004). Rivastigmine for vascular cognitive impairment. *Cochrane Database of Systematic Reviews*, Issue 2. Art. No.: CD004744. DOI: 10.1002/14651858.CD004744.pub2.

Craig D, Birks J (2006). Galantamine for vascular cognitive impairment. *The Cochrane Database of Systematic Reviews*, Issue 1. Art. No.: CD004746. DOI: 10.1002/14651858.CD004746.pub2.

Cummings JL, Mega M, Gray K, Rosenberg-Thompson S, Carusi DA, Gornbein J (1994). The Neuropsychiatric Inventory: comprehensive assessment of psychopathology in dementia. *Neurology* **44:**2308–2314.

de Leon MJ, George AE, Stylopoulos LA, Smith G, Miller DC (1989). Early marker for Alzheimer's disease: the atrophic hippocampus. *Lancet* **2(8664):**672–673.

de Leon MJ, Convit A, George AE *et al.* (1996). In vivo structural studies of the hippocampus in normal aging and in incipient Alzheimer's disease. *Ann N Y Acad Sci* **777:**1–13.

de Leon MJ, Convit A, DeSanti S *et al.* (1997). Contribution of structural neuroimaging to the early diagnosis of Alzheimer's disease. *Int Psychogeriatr* **9(Suppl 1):**183–190.

Deakin JB, Rahman S, Nestor PJ, Hodges JR, Sahakian BJ (2004). Paroxetine does not improve symptoms and impairs cognition in frontotemporal dementia: a double-blind randomized controlled trial. *Psychopharmacology (Berl)* **172:**400–408.

DeCarli C, Murphy DG, McIntosh AR, Teichberg D, Schapiro MB, Horwitz B (1995). Discriminant analysis of MRI measures as a method to determine the presence of dementia of the Alzheimer type. *Psychiatry Res* **57:**119–130.

DeJong R, Osterlund OW, Roy GW (1989). Measurement of quality of life changes in patients with Alzheimer's disease. *Clin Ther* **11:**545–554.

Desmond PM, O'Brien JT, Tress BM *et al.* (1994). Volumetric and visual assessment of the mesial temporal structures in Alzheimer's disease. *Aust N Z J Med* **24:**547–553.

Ditzler K (1991). Efficacy and tolerability of memantine in patients with dementia syndrome. A double-blind, placebo controlled trial. *Arzneimittelforschung* **41:**773–780.

Doody RC, Stevens JC, Beck RN *et al.* (2001). Practice parameter: Management of dementia (an evidence-based review). Report of the quality standards sub-committee of the Amerian Academy of Neurology. *Neurology* **56:**1154–1166.

Doraiswamy M, Leon J, Cummings JL, Martin D, Neumann PJ (2002). Prevalence and impact of medical comorbidity in Alzheimer's disease. *J Gerontol A Biol Sci Med Sci* **57:**M1 73–77.

Dougall NJ, Bruggink S, Ebmeier KP (2004). Systematic review of the diagnostic accuracy of 99mTc-HMPAO-SPECT in dementia. *Am J Geriatr Psychiatry* **12:**554–570.

Dubinsky RM, Stein AC, Lyons K (2000). Practice parameter: Risk of driving and Alzheimer's disease (an evidence-based review): Report of the Quality Standards Subcommittee of the American Academy of Neurology. *Neurology* **54:**2205–2211.

Dubois B, Touchon J, Portet F, Ousset PJ, Vellas B, Michel B (2002). [The '5 words' test: a simple and sensitive test for the diagnosis of Alzheimer's disease]. *Presse Médicale* **31:**1696–1699.

Emre M, Aarsland D, Albanese A *et al.* (2004). Rivastigmine for dementia associated with Parkinson's disease. *N Engl J Med* **351:**2509–2518.

Erkinjuntti T, Lee DH, Gao F *et al.* (1993). Temporal lobe atrophy on magnetic resonance imaging in the diagnosis of early Alzheimer's disease. *Arch Neurol* **50:**305–310.

Erkinjuntti T, Kurz A, Gauthier S, Bullock R, Lilienfeld S, Damaraju CV (2002). Efficacy of galantamine in probable vascular dementia and Alzheimer's disease combined with cerebrovascular disease: a randomised trial. *Lancet* **359:**1283–1290.

Erkinjuntti T, Kurz A, Small GW, Bullock R, Lilienfeld S, Damaraju CV; GAL-INT-6 Study Group (2003). An open-label extension trial of galantamine in patients with probable vascular dementia and mixed dementia. *Clin Ther* **25:**1765–1782.

Fabbrini G, Barbanti P, Bonifati V *et al.* (2001). Donepezil in the treatment of progressive supranuclear palsy. *Acta Neurol Scand* **103:**123–125.

Fabre SF, Forsell C, Viitanen M *et al.* (2001). Clinic-based cases with frontotemporal dementia show increased cerebrospinal fluid tau and high apolipoprotein E epsilon 4 frequency, but no tau gene mutations. *Exp Neurol* **168:**413–418.

Farina E, Pomati S, Mariani C (1999). Observations on dementias with possibly reversible symptoms. *Aging (Milano)* **11:**323–328.

Fearnley K, McLennan J., Weaks D (1999). *The Right to Know – Sharing the Diagnosis of Dementia*. Edinburgh: Alzheimer Scotland – Action on dementia.

Feldman H, Gauthier S, Hecker J, Vellas B, Subbiah P, Whalen E; Donepezil MSAD Study Investigators Group (2001). A 24-week, randomized, double-blind study of donepezil in moderate to severe Alzheimer's disease. *Neurology* **57**:613–620.

Finkel S, Burns A (2000). Introduction. In: Ames D, O'Brien J (eds.). Behavioral and Psychological Symptoms of Dementia (BPSD): A Clinical and Research Update. *Internat Psychogeriatr* **12(Suppl 13)**:9–12.

Fioravanti M, Flicker L (2001). Nicergoline for dementia and other age associated forms of cognitive impairment. *The Cochrane Database of Systematic Reviews*, Issue 4. Art. No.: CD003159. DOI: 10.1002/14651858.CD003159.

Flicker L, Grimley Evans J (2004). Piracetam for dementia or cognitive impairment. *The Cochrane Database of Systematic Reviews*, Issue 1. Art. No.: CD001011. DOI: 10.1002/14651858.CD001011.

Folstein MF, Folstein SE, McHugh PR (1995). Mini-Mental State. A practical method for grading the cognitive state of patients for the clinician. *J Psychiatric Res* **12**:189–198.

Foster GR, Scott DA, Payne S (1999). The use of CT scanning in dementia. *A systematic review. Internat J Technol Assess Health Care* **15**:406–423.

Frisoni GB, Weiss C, Geroldi C, Bianchetti A, Trabucchi M (1996). Linear measures of atrophy in mild Alzheimer's disease. *Am J Neuroradiol* **17**:913–923.

Frisoni GB, Geroldi C, Beltramello A *et al.* (2002). Radial width of the temporal horn: a sensitive measure in Alzheimer disease. *Am J Neuroradiol* **23**:35–47.

Fu C, Chute DJ, Farag ES, Garakian J, Cummings JL, Vinters HV (2004). Comorbidity in dementia: an autopsy study. *Arch Pathol Lab Med* **128**:32–38.

Fuh JL, Teng EL, Lin KN *et al.* (1995). The Informant Questionnaire on Cognitive Decline in the Elderly (IQCODE) as a screening tool for dementia for a predominantly illiterate Chinese population. *Neurology* **45**:92–96.

Galasko D, Bennett D, Sano M *et al.*, and the Alzheimer's Disease Cooperative Study (1997). An Inventory to assess activities of daily living for clinical trials in Alzheimer's disease. *Alzheimer's Dis Assoc Disord* **11(Suppl 2)**:S33–S39.

Galton CJ, Gomez-Anson B, Antoun N *et al.* (2001). Temporal lobe rating scale: application to Alzheimer's disease and frontotemporal dementia. *J Neurol Neurosurg Psychiatry* **70**:165–173.

Gelinas I, Gauthier L, McIntyre M, Gauthier S (1999). Development of a functional measure for persons with Alzheimer's disease: The disability assessment for dementia. *Am J Occup Ther* **53**:471–481.

Gifford DR, Holloway RG, Vickrey BG (2000). Systematic review of clinical prediction rules for neuroimaging in the evaluation of dementia. *Arch Intern Med* **160**:2855–2862.

Görtelmeyer R, Erbler H (1992). Memantine in the treatment of mild to moderate dementia syndrome. A double-blind placebo-controlled study. *Arzneimittel-Forschung* **42**:904–913.

Green AJE, Harvey RJ, Thompson EJ, Rossor MN (1999). Increased tau in the cerebrospinal fluid of patients with frontotemporal dementia and Alzheimer's disease. *Neurosci Lett* **259**:133–135.

Gustavson AR, Cummings JL (2004). Assessment and Treatment of Neuropsychiatric Symptoms in Alzheimer's disease. In: Richter RW, Richter ZR, eds Alzheimer's Disease. *A Physician's Guide to Practical Management.* New Jersey: Humana Press, pp. 371–385.

Harper PS, Morris MJ, Tyler A (1990). Genetic testing for Huntington's disease. *BMJ* **300**:1089–1090.

Hejl AM, Høgh P, Waldemar G (2002). Potentially reversible conditions in 1000 consecutive memory clinic patients. *J Neurol Neurosurg Psychiatry* **73**:390–394.

Henderson VW, Paganini-Hill A, Miller BL *et al.* (2000). Estrogen for Alzheimer's disease in women: randomized, double-blind, placebo-controlled trial. *Neurology* **54**:295–301.

Hodges JR, Patterson K, Oxbury S, Funnell E (1992). Semantic dementia. Progressive fluent aphasia with temporal lobe atrophy. *Brain* **115**:1783–1806.

Hogervorst E, Yaffe K, Richards M, Huppert F (2002). Hormone replacement therapy to maintain cognitive function in women with dementia. *The Cochrane Database of Systematic Reviews*, Issue 3. Art. No.: CD003799. DOI: 10.1002/14651858.CD003799.

Høgh P, Smith SJ, Scahill RI *et al.* (2002). Epilepsy presenting as AD: Neuroimaging, electroclinical features, and response to treatment. *Neurology* **58**:298–301.

Holmes C, Cairns N, Lantos P *et al.* (1999). Validity of current clinical criteria for Alzheimer's disease, vascular dementia and dementia with Lewy bodies. *Br J Psychiatry* **174**:45–50.

Houlden H, Baker M, Adamson J *et al.* (1999). Frequency of tau mutations in three series of non-Alzheimer's degenerative dementia. *Ann Neurol* **46**:243–248.

Hulstaert F, Blennow K, Ivanoiu A *et al.* (1999). Improved discrimination of AD patients using beta amyloid 1-42 and tau levels in CSF. *Neurology* **52**:1555–1562.

Hunt LA, Murphy CF, Carr D, Duchek JM, Buckles V, Morris JC (1997). Reliability of the Washington University Road Test: A performance-based assessment for drivers with dementia of the Alzheimer type. *Arch Neurol* **54**:707–712.

Hwang TJ, Cummings JL (2004). Neuropsychiatric symptoms of mild cognitive impairment. In: Gauthier S, Scheltens Ph, Cummings JL, eds. *Alzheimer's Disease and Related Disorders Annual 2004*. London: Martin Dunitz, pp. 71–80.

Incalzi RA, Capparella O, Gemma A, Marra C, Carbonin P (1995). Effects of aging and of Alzheimer's disease on verbal memory. *J Clin Experiment Neuropsychol* **17**:580–589.

Jack CR, Jr., Petersen RC, O'Brien PC, Tangalos EG (1992). MR-based hippocampal volumetry in the diagnosis of Alzheimer's disease. *Neurology* **42**:183–188.

Jagust W, Chui H, Lee A-Y (2002). Functional imaging in dementia. In: Quizilbash N., Schneider LS, Chui H, Tariot P, *et al.*, eds. *Evidence-based dementia practice* Oxford, UK: Blackwell, pp. 162–169.

Jelic V, Wahlund L-O, Almkvist O *et al.* (1999). Diagnostic accuracies of quantitative EEG and PET in mild Alzheimer's disease. *Alzheimer's Reports* **2**:291–298.

Jelic V, Johansson S-E, Almkvist O, *et al.* (2000). Quantitative EEG in mild cognitive impairment: longitudinal changes and possible prediction of Alzheimer's disease. *Neurobiolology of Aging* **21**:533–540.

Jick H, Zornberg GL, Jick SS, Seshadri S, Drachman DA (2000). Statins and the risk of dementia. *Lancet* **356**:1627–1631.

Johannson K, Lundberg C (1997). The 1994 International Consensus Conference on Dementia and Driving: a brief report. Swedish National Road Administration. *Alzheimer's Dis Assoc Disord* **11(Suppl 1)**:62–69.

Jönsson L, Berr C (2005). Cost of dementia in Europe. *Euro J Neurol* **12(Suppl 1)**:50–53.

Jorm AF (1997). Methods of screening for dementia: a meta-analysis of studies comparing an informant questionnaire with a brief cognitive test. *Alzheimer's Dis Assoc Disord* **11**:158–162.

Jorm AF, Jacomb PA (1989). The Informant Questionnaire on Cognitive Decline in the Elderly (IQCODE): sociodemographic correlates, reliability, validity and some norms. *Psychol Med* **19**:1015–1022.

Juva K, Sulkava R, Erkinjutti K, Ylikoski R, Valvanne J, Tilvis R (1995). Usefulness of the clinical Dementia Rating scale in screening for dementia. *Int Psychogeriatr* **7**:17–24.

Kanemaru K, Kameda N, Yamanouchi H (2000). Decreased CSF amyloid beta42 and normal tau levels in dementia with Lewy bodies. *Neurology* **54**:1875–1876.

Kanowski S, Herrmann WM, Stephan K, Wierich W, Horr R (1996). Proof of efficacy of the ginkgo biloba special extract EGb 761 in outpatients suffering from mild to moderate primary degenerative dementia of the Alzheimer type or multi-infarct dementia. *Pharmacopsychiatry* **29**:47–56.

Kapaki E, Kilidireas K, Paraskevas GP, Michalopoulou M, Patsouris E (2001). Highly increased CSF tau protein and decreased beta-amyloid (1-42) in sporadic CJD: a discrimation from Alzheimer's disease? *J Neurol Neurosurg Psychiatry* **71**:401–403.

Kapaki E, Paraskevas GP, Zalonis I, Zournas C (2003). CSF tau protein and β-amyloid (1-42) in Alzheimer's disease diagnosis: discrimination from normal aging and other dementias in the Greek population. *Euro J Neurol* **10**:119–128.

Killiany RJ, Moss MB, Albert MS, Sandor T, Tieman J, Jolesz F (1993). Temporal lobe regions on magnetic resonance imaging identify patients with early Alzheimer's disease. *Arch Neurol* **50**:949–954.

Kitagaki H, Hirono N, Ishii K, Mori E (2000). Corticobasal degeneration: evaluation of cortical atrophy by means of hemispheric surface display generated with MR images. *Radiology* **216**:31–38.

Knopman DS, DeKosky ST, Cummings JL *et al.* (2001). Practice parameter: Diagnosis of dementia (an evidence-based review). Report of the quality standards subcommittee of the Amerian Academy of Neurology. *Neurology* **56**:1143–1153.

Lam LC, Chiu HF, Li SW *et al.* (1997). Screening for dementia: a preliminary study on the validity of the Chinese version of the Blessed-Roth Dementia Scale. *Int Psychogeriatr* **9**:39–46.

Le Bars PL, Katz MM, Berman N, Itil TM, Freedman AM, Schatzberg AF (1997). A placebo-controlled, double-blind, randomized trial of an extract of Ginkgo biloba for dementia. North American EGb Study Group. *JAMA* **278**:1327–1332.

Lemstra AW, van Meegen MT, Vreyling JP *et al.* (2000). 14-3-3 testing in diagnosing Creutzfeldt-Jakob disease: a prospective study in 112 patients. *Neurology* **55**:514–516.

Lemstra AW, van Meegen M, Baas F, van Gool WA (2001). [Clinical algorithm for cerebrospinal fluid test of 14-3-3 protein in diagnosis of Creutzfeldt-Jacob disease]. *Ned Tijdschr Geneeskd* **145**:1467–1471.

Livingston G, Katona C (2000). How useful are cholinesterase inhibitors in the treatment of Alzheimer's disease? A number needed to treat analysis. *Int J Geriatr Psychiatry* **15**:203–207.

Litvan I, Phipps M, Pharr VL, Hallett M, Grafman J, Salazar A (2001). Randomized placebo-controlled trial of donepezil in patients with progressive supranuclear palsy. *Neurology* **57**:467–473.

Lonergan E, Luxenberg J, Colford J, Birks J (2002). Haloperidol for agitation in dementia. *The Cochrane Database of Systematic Reviews* Issue 2. Art. No.: CD002852. DOI: 10.1002/14651858.CD002852.

Lonergan ET, Luxenberg J (2004). Valproate preparations for agitation in dementia. *The Cochrane Database of Systematic Reviews*, Issue 2. Art. No.: CD003945. DOI: 10.1002/14651858.CD003945.pub2.

López-Arrieta, Birks J (2002). Nimodipine for primary degenerative, mixed and vascular dementia. *The Cochrane Database of Systematic Reviews*, Issue 3. Art. No.: CD000147. DOI: 10.1002/14651858.CD000147.

Loy C, Schneider L (2006). Galantamine for Alzheimer's disease and mild cognitive impairment. *The Cochrane Database of Systematic Reviews*, Issue 1. Art. No.: CD001747. DOI: 10.1002/14651858.CD001747.pub3.

Mackinnon A, Mulligan R (1998). Combining cognitive testing and informant report to increase accuracy in screening for dementia. *Am J Psychiatry* **155:**1529–1535.

Mackinnon A, Khalilian A, Jorm AF, Korten AE, Christensen H, Mulligan R (2003). Improving screening accuracy for dementia in a community sample by augmenting cognitive testing with informant report. *J Clin Epidemiol* **56:**358–366.

Malouf R, Birks J (2004). Donepezil for vascular cognitive impairment. *The Cochrane Database of Systematic Reviews*, Issue 1. Art. No.: CD004395. DOI: 10.1002/14651858.CD004395.pub2.

Markus HS, Martin RJ, Simpson MA *et al.* (2002). Diagnostic strategies in CADASIL. *Neurology* **59:**1134–1138.

Mattis S (1976). Mental status examination for organic mental syndrome in the elderly patient. In: Bellack L, Karusu TB eds. *Geriatric Psychiatry: a Handbook for Psychiatrist and Primary Care Physicians* New York: Grune & Straton, pp. 77–121.

Mayeux R, Saunders AM, Shea S *et al.* (1998). Utility of the apolipoprotein E genotype in the diagnosis of Alzheimer's disease. Alzheimer's Disease Centres Consortium on Apolipoprotein E and Alzheimer's Disease. *N Engl J Med* **338:**506–511.

McGeer PL, Schulzer M, McGeer EG (1996). Arthritis and anti-inflammatory agents as possible protective factors for Alzheimer's disease: a review of 17 epidemiologic studies. *Neurology* **47:**425–432.

McKhann G, Drachman D, Folstein M, Katzman R, Price D, Stadlan EM (1984). Clinial diagnosis of Alzheimer's disease: Report of the NINCDS-ADRDA Work Group under the auspices of Department of Health and Human Services Task Force on Alzheimer's Disease. *Neurology* **34:**939–944.

McKhann GM, Albert MS, Grossman M, Miller B, Dickson D, Trojanowski JQ (2001). Clinical and Pathological Diagnosis of Frontotemporal Dementia: Report of the Work Group on Frontotemporal Dementia and Pick's Disease. *Arch Neurol* **58:**1803–1809.

McKeith IG, Cummings J (2005). Behavioural changes and psychological symptoms in dementia disorders. *Lancet Neurology* **4:**735–742.

McKeith IG, Fairbairn AF, Perry RH, Thompson P, Perry EK (1992). Neuroleptic sensitivity in patients with senile dementia of Lewy body type. *BMJ* **305:**673–678.

McKeith IG, Galasko D, Kosaka K *et al.* (1996). Consensus guidelines for the clinical and pathological diagnosis of dementia with Lewy bodies (DLB): Report of the consortium on DLB international workshop. *Neurology* **47:**1113–1124.

McKeith IG, Grace JB, Walker Z, Byrne EJ, Wilkinson D, Stevens T, Perry EK (2000). Rivastigmine in the treatment of dementia with Lewy bodies: Preliminary findings from an open trial. *Int J Geriatr Psychiatry* **15:**387–392.

McKeith IG, Dickson D, Emre M *et al.* (2005). Dementia with Lewy Bodies: Diagnosis and Management: Third Report of the DLB Consortium. *Neurology* **65:**1863–1872.

Mega MS, Cummings JL, Fiorello T, Gornbein J (1996). The spectrum of behavioral changes in Alzheimer's disease. *Neurology* **46:**130–135.

Meyer JS, Chowdhury MH, Xu G, Li YS, Quach M (2002). Donepezil treatment of vascular dementia. *Ann N Y Acad Sci* **977:**482–486.

Miller ER 3rd, Pastor-Barriuso R, Dalal D, Riemersma RA, Appel LJ, Guallar E (2005). Meta-analysis: high-dosage vitamin E supplementation may increase all-cause mortality. *Ann Intern Med* **142:**37–46.

Mittelmann MS, Ferris SH, Steinberg G *et al.* (1993). An Intervention That Delays Institutionalization of Alzheimer's Disease Patients: Treatment of Spouse-Caregivers. *Gerontologist* **33:**730–740.

Mittelmann MS, Ferris SH, Shulman E, Steinberg G, Ambinder A, Mackell JA, Cohen J (1995). A Comprehensive Support Program: Effect on Depression in Spouse-Caregivers of AD Patients. *Gerontologist* **35:**792–803.

Möbius HJ, Stöffler A (2002). New approaches to clinical trials in vascular dementia: memantine in small vessel disease. *Cerebrovasc Dis* **13(Suppl 2):**61–66.

Mohs RC, Doody RS, Morris JC *et al.* (2001). A 1-year, placebo-controlled preservation of function survival study of donepezil in AD patients. *Neurology* **57:**481–488.

Moretti R, Torre P, Antonello RM, Cazzato G, Bava A (2003). Frontotemporal dementia: paroxetine as a possible treatment of behavior symptoms. A randomized, controlled, open 14-month study. *Euro Neurol* **49**:13–19.

Mulnard RA, Cotman CW, Kawas C *et al.* (2000). Estrogen replacement therapy for treatment of mild to moderate Alzheimer disease: a randomized controlled trial. Alzheimer's Disease Cooperative Study. *JAMA* **283**:1007–1015.

Nagga K, Gottfries J, Blennow K, Marcusson J (2002). Cerebrospinal fluid phospho-tau, total tau and beta-amyloid(1-42) in the differentiation between Alzheimer's disease and vascular dementia. *Demen Geriatr Cognit Disord* **14**:183–190.

Neary D, Snowden JS (1996). Clinical features of frontotemporal dementia. In: Pasquier F, Lebert F, Scheltens Ph, eds *Frontotemporal Dementia Current Issues in Neurodegeneration* Vol 8. Dordrecht: ICG Publications, pp. 31–47.

Neary D, Snowden JS, Gustafson L *et al.* (1998). Frontotemporal lobar degeneration: a consensus on clinical diagnostic criteria. *Neurology* **51**:1546–1554.

Nelson HE (1976). Modified card sorting test sensitive to frontal lobe defects. *Cortex* **12**:313–324.

NICE. Alzheimer's disease - donepezil, rivastigmine and galantamine. NICE Tehnology Appraisal Guidance-No 19. 2001 www.nice.org.uk (accessed February 24, 2006).

O'Brien JT, Ames D, Schweitzer I, Chiu E, Tress B (1997). Temporal lobe magnetic resonance imaging can differentiate Alzheimer's disease from normal ageing, depression, vascular dementia and other causes of cognitive impairment. *Psychol Med* **27**:1267–1275.

O'Brien JT, Ballard CG (1999). Treating behavioural and psychological signs in Alzheimer's disease (editorial) *BMJ* **319**:138–139.

O'Brien JT, Colloby S, Fenwick J *et al.* (2004). Dopamine transporter loss visualized with FP-CIT SPECT in the differential diagnosis of dementia with Lewy bodies. *Arch Neurol* **61**:919–925.

Olesen J, Leonardi M (2003). The burden of brain diseases in Europe. *Euro J Neurol* **10**:471–477.

Olin JT, Fox LS, Pawluczyk S, Taggart NA, Schneider LS (2001). A pilot randomized trial of carbamazepine for behavioral symptoms in treatment-resistant outpatients with Alzheimer disease. *Am J Geriatr Psychiatry* **9**:400–405.

Orgogozo JM, Rigaud AS, Stöffler A, Möbius HJ, Forette F (2002). Efficacy and safety of memantine in patients with mild to moderate vascular dementia: a randomized, placebo-controlled trial (MMM 300). *Stroke* **33**:1834–1839.

Ott A, Breteler MM, van Harskamp F *et al.* (1995). Prevalence of Alzheimer's disease and vascular dementia: association with education. The Rotterdam study. *BMJ* **310**:970–973.

Otto M, Wiltfang J, Cepek L *et al.* (2002). Tau protein and 14-3-3 protein in the differential diagnosis of Creutzfeldt-Jakob disease. *Neurology* **58**:192–197.

Pantoni L, Bianchi C, Beneke M, Inzitari D, Wallin A, Erkinjuntti T (2000). The Scandinavian Multi-Infarct Dementia Trial: a double-blind, placebo-controlled trial on nimodipine in multi-infarct dementia. *J Neurol Sci* **175**:116–123.

Pantoni L, del Ser T, Soglian AG *et al.* (2005). Efficacy and safety of nimodipine in subcortical vascular dementia: a randomized placebo-controlled trial. *Stroke* **36**:619–624.

Patwardhan MB, McCrory DC, Marchar DB, Sams GP, Rutschmann OT (2004). Alzheimer Disease: Operating Characteristics of PET: A Meta-Analysis. *Radiology* **231**:73–80.

Petersen RC, Stevens JC, Ganguli M, Tangalos EG, Cummings JL, DeKosky ST (2001). Practice parameter: Early detection of dementia: Mild cognitive impairment (an evidence-based review). Report of the quality standards subcommittee of the Amerian Academy of Neurology. *Neurology* **56**:1133–1142.

Pfeffer RI, Kurosaki TT, Harrah CH *et al.* (1982). Measurement of functional activities in older adults in the community. *J Gerontol* **37**:323–329.

Pijnenburg YAL, Schoonenboom NSM, Rosso SM *et al.* (2004). CSF tau and Aβ42 are not useful in the diagnosis of frontotemporal lobar degeneration. *Neurology* **62**:1649.

Pillon B, Dubois B, Agid Y (1996). Testing cognition may contribute to the diagnosis of movement disorders. *Neurology* **46**:329–333.

Pirttala T, Wilcock G, Truyen L, Damaraju CV (2004). Long-term efficacy and safety of galantamine in patients with mild-to-moderate Alzheimer's disease: multicenter trial. *Euro J Neurol* **11**:734–741.

Poser S, Mollenhauer B, Krauss A *et al.* (1999). How to improve the clinical diagnosis of Creutzfeldt Jakob Disease. *Brain* **122**:2345–2351.

Pucci E BN, Regnicolo L, Nolfe G, Signorino M, Salvolini U, Angeleri F (1998). Hippocampus and parahippocampal gyrus linear measurements based on magnetic resonance in Alzheimer's disease. *Euro J Neurol* **39**:16–25.

Pusey H, Richards R (2001). A systematic review of the effectiveness of psychosocial interventions for carers of people with dementia. *Aging Ment Health* **5:**107–119.

Rands G, Orrel M, Spector A, Williams P (2000). Aspirin for vascular dementia. *The Cochrane Database of Systematic Reviews*, Issue 4. Art. No.: CD001296. DOI: 10.1002/14651858.CD001296.

Raskind MA, Peskind ER, Wessel T, Yuan W (2000). Galantamine in AD: A 6-month randomized, placebo-controlled trial with a 6-month extension. The Galantamine USA-1 Study Group. *Neurology* **54:**2261–2268.

Ravina B, Putt M, Siderowf A *et al.* (2005). Donepezil for dementia in Parkinson's disease: a randomized double blind placebo controlled crossover study. *J Neurol Neurosurg Psychiatry* **76:**903–904.

Reines SA, Block GA, Morris JC *et al.* (2004). Rofecoxib: no effect on Alzheimer's disease in a 1-year, randomized, blinded, controlled study. *Neurology* **62:**66–71.

Reisberg B, Borenstein J, Salob SP, Ferris SH, Franssen E, Georgotas A (1987). Behavioral symptoms in Alzheimer's disease: phenomenology and treatment. *J Clin Psychiatry* **48(Supp 9):**9–15.

Reisberg B, Doody R, Stoffler A, Schmitt F, Ferris S, Mobius HJ; Memantine Study Group (2003). Memantine in moderate-to-severe Alzheimer's disease. *N Engl J Med* **348:**1333–1341.

Reitan RM (1958). Validity of the Trail Making Test as an indication of organic brain damage. *Percept Mot Skills* **8:**271–276.

Ridha BH, Josephs KA, Rossor MN (2005). Delusions and hallucinations in dementia with Lewy bodies: Worsening with memantine. *Neurology* **65:**481–482.

Riemenschneider M, Wagenpfeil S, Diehl J *et al.* (2002). Tau and Abeta42 protein in CSF of patients with frontotemporal degeneration. *Neurology* **58:**1622–1628.

Robinson DJ, Merskey H, Blume WT, Fry R, Williamson PC, Hachinski VC (1994). Electroencephalography as an aid in the exclusion of Alzheimer's disease. *Arch Neurol* **51:**280–284.

Rockwood K, Kirkland S, Hogan DB *et al.* (2002). Use of lipid-lowering agents, indication bias, and the risk of dementia in community-dwelling elderly people. *Arch Neurol* **59:**223–227.

Rogers SL, Friedhoff LT (1996). The efficacy and safety of donepezil in patients with Alzheimer's disease: results of a US Multicentre, Randomized, Double-Blind, Placebo-Controlled Trial. The Donepezil Study Group. *Dementia* **7:**293–303.

Rogers J, Kirby LC, Hempelman SR *et al.* (1993). Clinical trial of indomethacin in Alzheimer's disease. *Neurology* **43:**1609–1611.

Rogers SL, Doody RS, Mohs RC, Friedhoff LT (1998). Donepezil improves cognition and global function in Alzheimer disease: a 15-week, double-blind, placebo-controlled study. *Arch Intern Med* **158:**1021–1031.

Rogers S, Doody RS, Pratt RD, Ieni JR (2000). Long-term efficacy and safety of donepezil in the treatment of Alzheimer's disease: final analysis of a US multicentre open-label study. *European Neuropsychopharmacology* **10:**195–203.

Roman GC, Tatemichi TK, Erkinjuntti T *et al.* (1993). Vascular dementia: diagnostic criteria for research studies. Report of the NINDS-AIREN International Workshop. *Neurology* **43:**250–260.

Rosler M, Anand R, Cicin-Sain A *et al.* (1999). Efficacy and safety of rivastigmine in patients with Alzheimer's disease: international randomised controlled trial. *BMJ* **318:**633–638.

Sabbagh M, Hake A, Ahmed S, Farlow M (2005). The use of memantine in dementia with Lewy bodies. *J Alzheimer's Dis* **7:**285–289.

Sano M, Ernesto C, Thomas RG *et al.* (1997). A controlled trial of selegiline, alpha-tocopherol, or both as treatment for Alzheimer's disease. The Alzheimer's Disease Cooperative Study. *N Engl J Med* **336:**1216–1222.

Scharf S, Mander A, Ugoni A, Vajda F, Christophidis N (1999). A double-blind, placebo-controlled trial of diclofenac/misoprostol in Alzheimer's disease. *Neurology* **53:**197–201.

Scheltens P, Leys D, Barkhof F *et al.* (1992). Atrophy of medial temporal lobes on MRI in "probable" Alzheimer's disease and normal ageing: diagnostic value and neuropsychological correlates. *J Neurol Neurosurg Psychiatry* **55:**967–972.

Scheltens P, Launer LJ, Barkhof F, Weinstein HC, van Gool WA (1995). Visual assessment of medial temporal lobe atrophy on magnetic resonance imaging: interobserver reliability. *J Neurol* **242:**557–560.

Scheltens P, Launer LJ, Barkhof F, Weinstein HC, Jonker C (1997). The diagnostic value of magnetic resonance imaging and technetium 99m-HMPAO single-photon-emission computed tomography for the diagnosis of Alzheimer disease in a community-dwelling elderly population. *Alzheimers Dis Assoc Disord* **11:**63–70.

Scheltens P, Fox N, Barkhof F, De Carli C (2002). Structural magnetic resonance imaging in the practical assessment of dementia: beyond exclusion. *Lancet Neurol* **1:**13–21.

Schneider LS, Dagerman KS, Insel P (2005). Risk of death with atypical antipsychotic drug treatment for dementia: meta-analysis of randomized placebo-controlled trials. *JAMA* **294:**1934–1943.

Schoonenboom SNM, Pijnenburg YAL, Mulder C et al. (2004). Amyloid β 1-42 and phosphorylated tau in CSF as markers for early ones et al. zheimer's disease. Neurology **62**:1580–1584.

Schroter A ZI, Henkel K, Tschampa HJ, Finkenstaedt M, Poser S (2000). Magnetic Resonance Imaging in the clinical diagnosis of Creutzfeldt-Jakob disease. Arch Neurol **57**:1751–1757.

Scott HD, Laake K (2001). Statins for the prevention of Alzheimer's disease. The Cochrane Database of Systematic Reviews, Issue 3. Art. No.: CD003160. DOI: 10.1002/14651858.CD003160.

Seltzer B, Zolnouni B, Nunez M et al. Donepezil "402" study group (2004). Efficacy of donepezil in early-stage Alzheimer disease: a randomized placebo-controlled trial. Arch Neurol **61**:1852–1856.

Sha MC, Callahan CM (2003). The efficacy of pentoxifylline in the treatment of vascular dementia: a systematic review. Alzheimer's Dis Assoc Disord **17**:46–54.

Shepherd J, Blauw GJ, Murphy MB et al. (2002). PROspective Study of Pravastatin in the Elderly at Risk. Pravastatin in elderly individuals at risk of vascular disease (PROSPER): a randomised controlled trial. Lancet **360**:1623–1630.

Shumaker SA, Legault C, Rapp SR et al. (2003). Estrogen plus progestin and the incidence of dementia and mild cognitive impairment in postmenopausal women: the Women's Health Initiative Memory Study: a randomized controlled trial. JAMA **289**:2651–2662.

Silverman DH, Small GW, Chang CY et al. (2001). Positron emission tomography in evaluation of dementia: Regional brain metabolism and long-term outcome. JAMA **286**:2120–2127.

Sjögren M, Vanderstichele H, Ågren H et al. (2001). Tau and Aβ42 in cerebrospinal fluid from healthy adults 21–93 years of age: establishment of reference values. Clin Chem **47**:1776–1781.

Snowdon DA GL, Mortimer JA, Riley KP, Greiner PA, Markesberry WR (1997). Brain infarction and the clinical expression of Alzheimer disease. JAMA **277**:813–817.

Solomon PR, Hirschoff A, Kelly B et al. (1998). A 7-minute neurocognitive screening battery highly sensitive to Alzheimer's disease. Arch Neurol **55**:349–355.

Sörensen S, Pinquart M, Dr Habil, Duberstein P (2002). How Effective Are Interventions With Caregivers? An Updated Meta-Analysis. Gerontologist **42**:356–372.

Sparks DL, Sabbagh MN, Connor DJ et al. (2005). Atorvastatin therapy lowers circulating cholesterol but not free radical activity in advance of identifiable clinical benefit in the treatment of mild-to-moderate AD. Curr Alzheimer Res **2**:343–353.

Steinhoff BJ, Racker S, Herrendorf G, Poser S, Grosche S, Zerr I, Kretzschmar H, Weber T (1996). Accuracy and reliability of periodic sharp wave complexes in Creutzfeldt-Jakob disease. Arch Neurol **53**:162–166.

Stroop JR (1935). Studies of interference in serial verbal reactions. J Exp Psychol **18**:643–662.

Strozyk D, Blennow K, White LR, Launer LJ (2003). CSF Aβ42 levels correlate with amyloid-neuropathology in a population-based autopsy study. Neurology **60**:652–656.

Sunderland T, Linker G, Mirza N et al. (2003). Decreased β-Amyloid 1-42 and increased tau levels in cerebrospinal fluid of patients with Alzheimer's disease. JAMA **289**:2094–2103.

Swartz JR, Miller BL, Lesser IM, Darby AL (1997). Frontotemporal dementia: treatment response to serotonin selective reuptake inhibitors. J Clin Psychiatry **58**:212–216.

Tabet N, Birks J, Grimley Evans J, Orrel M, Spector A (2000). Vitamin E for Alzheimer's disease. The Cochrane Database of Systematic Reviews, Issue 4. Art. No.: CD002854. DOI: 10.1002/14651858.CD002854.

Tapiola T, Pirttila T, Mehta PD, Alafuzofff I, Lehtovirta M, Soininen H (2000). Relationship between apoE genotype and CSF beta-amyloid (1-42) and tau in patients with probable and definite Alzheimer's disease. Neurobiol Aging **21**:735–740.

Tariot PN, Solomon PR, Morris JC, Kershaw P, Lilienfeld S, Ding C (2000). A 5-month, randomized, placebo-controlled trial of galantamine in AD. The Galantamine USA-10 Study Group. Neurology **54**:2269–2276.

Tariot PN, Farlow MR, Grossberg GT, Graham SM, McDonald S, Gergel I (2004). Memantine treatment in patients with moderate to severe Alzheimer disease already receiving donepezil: a randomized controlled trial. JAMA **291**:317–324.

Thal LJ, Thomas RG, Mulnard R, Sano M, Grundman M, Schneider L (2003). Estrogen levels do not correlate with improvement in cognition. Arch Neurol **60**:209–212.

Thompson CA, Spilsbury K, Barnes C (2003). Information and support interventions for carers of people with dementia. (Protocol) The Cochrane Database of Systematic Reviews, Issue 4. Art. No.: CD004513. DOI: 10.1002/14651858.CD004513.

Tolosa E, Wenning G, Poewe W (2006). The diagnosis of Parkinson's disease. Lancet Neurol **5**:75–86.

Trinh NH, Hoblyn J., Mohanty S, Yaffe K (2003). Efficacy of cholinesterase inhibitors in the treatment of neuropsychiatric symptoms and functional impairment in Alzheimer disease: a meta-analysis. JAMA **289**:210–216.

UK Committee on Safety of Medicines (2004). New advice issued on risperidone and olanapine. http://www.mhra.gov.uk (accessed February 24, 2006).

van Dongen M, van Rossum E, Kessels A, Sielhorst H, Knipschild P (2003). Ginkgo for elderly people with dementia and age-associated memory impairment: a randomized clinical trial. *J Clin Epidemiol* **56:**367–376.

van Everbroeck B, Green AJ, Pals P, Martin JJ, Cras P (1999). Decreased Levels of Amyloid-beta 1-42 in Cerebrospinal Fluid of Creutzfeldt-Jakob Disease Patients. *J Alzheimers Dis* **1:**419–424.

van Everbroeck B, Quoilin S, Boons J, Martin JJ, Cras P (2003). A prospective study of CSF markers in 250 patients with possible Creutzfeldt-Jakob disease. *J Neurol Neurosurg Psychiatry* **74:**1210–1214.

Van Gool WA, Weinstein HC, Scheltens P, Walstra GJ (2001). Effect of hydroxychloroquine on progression of dementia in early Alzheimer's disease: an 18-month randomised, double-blind, placebo-controlled study. *Lancet* **358:**455–460.

van Straaten EC, Scheltens P, Knol DL, van Buchem MA, *et al.* (2003). Operational definitions for the NINDS-AIREN criteria for vascular dementia: an interobserver study. *Stroke* **34:**1907–1912.

Vanneste JA (2000). Diagnosis and management of normal-pressure hydrocephalus. *J Neurol* **247:**5–14.

Varma AR, Adams W, Lloyd JJ, Carson KJ, Snowden JS, Testa HJ, Jackson A, Neary D (2002). Diagnostic patterns of regional atrophy on MRI and regional cerebral blood flow change on SPECT in young onset patients with Alzheimer's disease, frontotemporal dementia and vascular dementia. *Acta Neurol Scand* **105:**261–269.

Verbeek MM, De Jong D, Kremer HPH (2003). Brain-specific proteins in cerebrospinal fluid for the diagnosis of neurodegenerative diseases. *Ann Clin Biochem* **40:**25–40.

Wahlund LO, Julin P, Lindqvist J, Scheltens P (1999). Visual assessment of medical temporal lobe atrophy in demented and healthy control subjects: correlation with volumetry. *Psychiatry Res* **90:**193–199.

Wahlund LO, Julin P, Johansson SE, Scheltens P (2000). Visual rating and volumetry of the medial temporal lobe on magnetic resonance imaging in dementia: a comparative study. *J Neurol Neurosurg Psychiatry* **69:**630–635.

Waldemar G, Dubois B, Emre M, Scheltens P, Tariska P, Rossor M (2000). Diagnosis and management of Alzheimer's disease and related disorders: The role of neurologists in Europe. *Euro J Neurol* **7:**133–144.

Waldemar G, Phungh KTT, Burns A, Georges J, Hansen FR, Iliffe S, Marking C, Olde-Rikkert M, Selmes J, Stoppe G, Sartorius N (2006). Access to diagnostic evaluation and treatment for dementia in Europe. *Int J Geriatr Psychiatry (in press).*

Walker Z, Costa DC, Walker RWH, Shaw K, Gacinovic S, Stevens T, *et al.* (2002). Differentiation of dementia with Lewy bodies from Alzheimer's disease using a dopaminergic presynaptic ligand. *J Neurol Neurosurg Psychiatry* **73:**134–140.

Wang PN, Liao SQ, Liu RS *et al.* (2000). Effects of estrogen on cognition, mood, and cerebral blood flow in AD: a controlled study. *Neurology* **54:**2061–2066.

Wang PS, Schneeweiss S, Avorn J *et al.* (2005). Risk of death in elderly users of conventional vs. atypical antipsychotic medications. *N Engl J Med* **353:**2335–2341.

White S, O'Neill D (2000). Health and relicensing policies for older drivers in the European Union. *Gerontology* **46:**146–152.

Wilcock G, Möbius HJ, Stöffler A (2002). A double-blind, placebo-controlled multicentre study of memantine in mild to moderate vascular dementia (MMM500). *Int Clin Psychopharmacol* **17:**297–305.

Wilkinson D, Doody R, Helme R *et al.* (2003). Donepezil in vascular dementia: a randomized, placebo-controlled study. *Neurology* **61:**479–486.

Wimo A, Winblad B, Stöffler A, Wirth Y, Möbius HJ (2003). Resource utilisation and cost analysis of memantine in patients with moderate to severe Alzheimer's disease. *Pharmacoeconomics* **21:**327–340.

Winblad B, Poritis N (1999). Memantine in severe dementia: results of the M-Best Study (Benefit and efficacy in severely demented patients during treatment with memantine). *Int J Geriatr Psychiatry* **14:**135–146.

Winblad B, Engedal K, Soininen H *et al.* (2001). A 1-year, randomized, placebo-controlled study of donepezil in patients with mild to moderate AD. *Neurology* **57:**489–495.

Winblad B, Wimo A, Engedal K, Soininen H, Verhey F, Waldemar G, Wetterholm A-L, Haglund A, Zhang R, Schindler R and the Donepezil Nordic Study Group (2006). 3-year study of donepezil therapy in Alzheimer's disease: Effects of early and continuous therapy. *Dementia and Geriatric Cognitive Impairment* **21:**353–361.

Wolozin B, Kellman W, Ruosseau P, Celesia GG, Siegel G (2000). Decreased prevalence of Alzheimer disease associated with 3-hydroxy-3-methyglutaryl coenzyme A reductase inhibitors. *Arch Neurol* **57:**1439–1443.

Zamrini E, McGwin G, Roseman JM (2004). Association between statin use and Alzheimer's disease. *Neuroepidemiology* **23:**94–98.

Zeman AZ, Boniface SJ, Hodges JR (1998). Transient epileptic amnesia: a description of the clinical and neuropsychological features in 10 cases and a review of the literature. *J Neurol Neurosurg Psychiatry* **64:**435–443.

Zerr I, Bodemer M, Gefeller O *et al.* (1998). Detection of 14-3-3 protein in the cerebrospinal supports the diagnosis of Creutzfeldt Jakob disease. *Ann Neurol* **43:**32–40.

Zerr I, Pocchiari M, Collins S *et al.* (2000). Analysis of EEG and CSF 14-3-3 proteins as aids to the diagnosis of Creutzfeldt-Jakob disease. *Neurology* **55:**811–815.

CHAPTER 20

Amyotrophic lateral sclerosis

P.M. Andersen,[a] G.D. Borasio,[b] R. Dengler,[c]
O. Hardiman,[d] K. Kollewe,[c] P.N. Leigh,[e]
P.-F. Pradat,[f] V. Silani,[g] B. Tomik[h]

Abstract

Background Despite being one of the most dev-astating diseases known, there is little evidence for diagnosing and managing patients with amy-otrophic lateral sclerosis (ALS). Although specific therapy is lacking, correct early diagnosis and introduction of symptomatic and specific therapy can have a profound influence on the care and quality of life of the patient and may increase sur-vival time. This document addresses the optimal clinical approach to ALS.

Methods The final literature search was performed in the spring of 2005. Consensus recommenda-tions are given graded according to the EFNS guid-ance regulations. Where there was lack of evidence but consensus was clear we have stated our opinion as Good Practice Points.

People affected with possible ALS should be examined as soon as possible by an experienced neurologist. Early diagnosis should be pursued and a number of investigations should be per-formed with high priority. The patient should be informed of the diagnosis by a consultant with a good knowledge of the patient and the disease. Fol-lowing diagnosis, the patient and relatives should receive regular support from a multidisciplinary care team. Medication with riluzole should be ini-tiated as early as possible. Percutaneous endocopic gastrostomy (PEG) is associated with improved nutrition and should be inserted early. The oper-ation is hazardous in patients with vital capacity (VC) < 50%. Non-invasive positive pressure ven-tilation improves survival and quality of life but is underused. Maintaining the patient's ability to communicate is essential. During the entire course of the disease, every effort should be made to maintain patient autonomy. Advance directives for palliative end of life care are important and should be fully discussed early with the patient and rel-atives respecting the patient's social and cultural background.

[a]Department of Neurology, Umeå University Hospital, Sweden; [b]Interdisciplinary Center for Palliative Medicine and Department of Neurology, Munich University Hospital – Grosshadern, Munich, Germany; [c]Department of Neurology, Medizinische Hochschule Hannover, Hannover, Germany; [d]Department of Neurology, Beaumont Hospital, Dublin, Ireland; [e]Department of Neurology, Institute of Psychiatry and Guy's, King's and St Thomas's School of Medicine, Institute of Psychiatry, King's College, London UK; [f]Fédération des Maladies du Système Nerveux, Hôpital de la Salpêtrière, Paris, France; [g]Department of Neurology and Laboratory of Neuroscience, "Dino Ferrari" Center – University of Milan Medical School, Milano, Italy; [h]Department of Neurology, Institute of Neurology, Collegium Medicum, Jagiellonian University, Krakow, Poland.

European Journal of Neurology 2005, 12:921–938

Introduction

Amyotrophic lateral sclerosis (ALS, also known as MND, SLA) is a fatal syndrome characterized by the onset of symptoms and signs of degeneration of primarily the upper (UMN) and lower (LMN) motor neurons, leading to progressive weakness of the bulbar, limb, thoracic and abdominal muscles. Other brain functions, including oculomotor and sphincter functions, are relatively spared, though these may be involved in some cases. Cognitive dysfunction is seen in 20–50%, and 3–5% develop dementia that is usually of the frontotemporal type (Abrahams *et al.*, 1996). Death due to respiratory failure follows on average 2–4 years after onset, but a small group may survive for a decade or more (Forsgren *et al.*, 1983). The mean age of onset is 47–52 years in familial cases (FALS) and 58–63 years in sporadic (SALS) cases (Haverkamp *et al.*, 1995). The life-time risk of developing ALS is about 1:1000 ($\approx$ half the risk of getting MS), with male sex, increasing age and hereditary disposition being the main risk factors (Bobowick and Brody, 1973). When diagnosing and managing a patient with ALS it is important to recognize that ALS is a heterogeneous syndrome that overlaps with a number of other conditions (figure 20.1) (Ince *et al.*, 1998; Brugman *et al.*, 2005). This systematic review comprises of an objective appraisal of the evidence in regard to the diagnosis and clinical management of patients with ALS. The primary aim has been to establish evidence-based and patient and carer-centred guidelines, with secondary aims of identifying areas where further research is needed.

Methods

Two investigators screened potentially relevant citations independently. We searched the Cochrane Central Register of Controlled Trials (CENTRAL) (The Cochrane Library to date); MEDLINE-OVID (January 1966 to date); MEDLINE-ProQuest; MEDLINE-EIFL; EMBASE-OVID (January 1990 to date); Science Citation Index (ISI); The National Research Register; Oxford Centre for Evidenced-based Medicine; American Speech Language Hearing Association (ASHA); the world Federation of Neurology ALS Page of reviews of published

research; the Oxford Textbook of Palliative Medicine, and the UK Department of Health National Research Register (http://www.update-software.com/National/nrr-frame.html). We also searched national neurological databases (e.g. www.alsa.org, alsod.org) and personal collections of references and reference lists of articles. There were no constraints based on language or publication status. Any difference at any stage of the review was resolved by discussion.

Results

Ten central issues in the management of ALS were addressed by the Task Force. The following is an abbreviated report; the full report with all tables, figures and references is available at www.efns.org. Tables and figures referred to *in oblique* are only listed on www.efns.org. The guidelines were prepared following the European Federation of Neurological Societies (EFNS) criteria (Brainin *et al.*, 2004) and the level of evidence and grade of recommendation are expressed in accordance with this reference. Where there was lack of evidence but consensus was clear we have stated our opinion as Good Practice Points.

Diagnosing ALS/MND

Diagnosing ALS is usually considered straightforward if the patient has been ill for some time and has generalized symptoms (table 20.1) (Li *et al.*, 1986). Diagnosing the disease *early* in the disease when the patient has only limited focal symptoms from one or two regions (bulbar, upper limb, truncal, lower limb) may be difficult and depends on the presence of signs in other affected regions and a number of investigations (Wilbourn, 1998; Meininger, 1999). The mean time from onset of symptoms to confirmation of diagnosis of ALS is 13–18 months (Chio, 1999). Delays may arise from a complex referral pathway, and early symptoms are often intermittent and nonspecific and may be denied or go unrecognized by the patient. However, three studies have shown that the longest delay occurs after the patient actually has seen the neurologist (Chio, 1999). There are four cogent reasons for making the diagnosis as early as possible:

For psychological reasons, as the progressive loss of motor symptoms causes anxiety and discomfort,

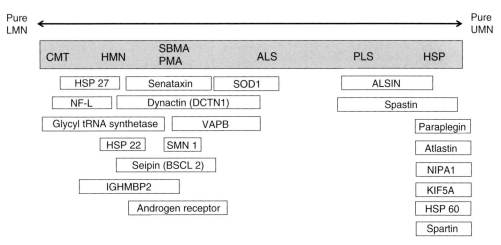

Figure 20.1. Shematic illustration of the relationship between ALS and some other motor neuron syndromes and motor neuronopathies.

On the far left are syndromes affecting lower motor neurons (LMN) and/or the peripheral motor axons, on the right syndromes affecting the upper motor neurons and/or the corticospinal and corticobulbar tract systems. The approximate clinical spectrum associated with mutations in some genes is shown below the bar. At present, 44 genes have been associated with motor neuron disease or neuronopathy. CMT, Charcot-Marie-Tooth's; HMN, distal hereditary motor neuronopathies; SBMA, Spino-bulbar muscular atropy; PMA, progressive spinal muscular atrophies; PLS, primary lateral sclerosis syndrome; HSP, hereditary spastic paraplegias.

Table 20.1 Diagnostic criteria for ALS.

The diagnosis of ALS requires the presence of: (positive criteria)
    LMN signs (including EMG features in clinically unaffected muscles)
    UMN signs
    Progression of symptoms and signs

The diagnosis of ALS requires the absence of: (diagnosis by exclusion)
    Sensory signs
    Sphincter disturbances
    Visual disturbances
    Autonomic features
    Basalganglia dysfunction
    Alzheimer-type dementia
    ALS 'mimic' syndromes (table 20.3)

The diagnosis of ALS is supported by:
    Fasciculations in one or more regions
    Neurogenic changes in EMG
    Normal motor and sensory nerve conduction
    Absence of conduction block

---

impairing the patient's social and professional life; *for ethical reasons*, so that the patient can better plan the remaining part of her or his life; *for economic reasons*, as many patients go on a tour of the health care system undergoing series of (expensive) unnecessary tests; *for neurological reasons* to be able to initiate neuroprotective medication before too many neuronal cells become dysfunctional and lost. Though no hard evidence exists on the kinetics of cell loss in ALS, it is reasonable to assume that the earlier medication is started the greater the neuroprotective effect will be (Bromberg, 1999). Studies in experimental animal models and humans with SOD1 gene mutations indicate that loss of motor neurons is preceded by a period of cellular dysfunction (Aggarwal and Nicholson, 2002). Both in humans and animal models the life-prolonging effect of riluzole is greater the earlier medication is initiated. Also, early administration of medication can have a profound positive psychological effect on the patient and carers.

The objective is to present guidelines for making the correct diagnosis *and* doing this as early as possible. As no single investigation is specific for the diagnosis, making the diagnosis should be based on symptoms, a thorough clinical examination, electrodiagnostic studies, neuroimaging and laboratory studies (tables 20.1 and 20.2) (Lima *et al.*, 2003). Great care should be taken to rule out diseases that can masquerade as ALS (*Supplementary*

Table 20.2 Diagnosing ALS/MND: recommended investigations.

Clinical chemistry	Test class	Evidence	Recommended mandatory tests	Recommended additional tests in selected cases
Blood	Erythrocyte sedimentation rate	IV	x	
	C-reactive protein (CRP)	IV	x	
	Haematological screen	IV	x	
	ASAT, ALAT, LDH	IV	x	
	TSH, FT4, FT3 hormone assays	IV	x	
	Vitamins B12 and folate	IV	x	
	Serum protein electrophoresis	IV	x	
	Serum immunoelectrophoresis	IV	x	
	Creatine kinase (CK)	IV	x	
	Creatinine	IV	x	
	Electrolytes (Na^+,K^+,Cl^+,$Ca2^+$,PO4)	IV	x	
	Glucose	IV	x	
	Angiotensin converting enzyme (ACE)	IV		x
	Lactate	IV		x
	Hexoaminidase A and B assay	IV		x
	Ganglioside GM-1 antibodies	IV		x
	Anti-Hu, anti-MAG	IV		x
	RA, ANA, anti-DNA	IV		x
	Anti-AChR, anti-MUSK antibodies	IV		x
	Serology (Borrelia, virus including HIV)	IV		x
	DNA analysis (for details see figure 20.1)	IV		x
CSF	Cell count	IV		x
	Cytology	IV		x
	Total protein concentration	IV		x
	Glucose, lactate	IV		x
	Protein electrophoresis including IgG index	IV		x
	Serology (Borrelia, virus)	IV		x
	Ganglioside antibodies	IV		x
Urine	Cadmium	IV		x
	Lead (24-h secretion)	IV		x
	Mercury	IV		x
	Manganese	IV		x
	Urine immunoelectrophoresis	IV		x
Neurophysiology	EMG	III	x	
	Nerve conduction velocity	III	x	
	MEP	IV		x
Radiology	MRI/CAT (head/cervical, thoracic, lumbar)	IV	x	
	Chest X-ray	IV	x	
	Mammography	IV		x
Biopsy	Muscle	III		x
	Nerve	IV		x
	Bone marrow	IV		x
	Lymph node	IV		x

table 1 online at the European Journal of Neurology, www.blackwellpublishing.com; see Anderson *et al.* 2005) (Evangelista *et al.*, 1996; Traynor *et al.*, 2000). In specialist practice, 5–8% of apparent ALS cases have an alternative diagnosis, which may be treatable in about half the cases (Belsh and Schiffman, 1990; Davenport *et al.*, 1996; Traynor *et al.*, 2000). Evolution of atypical symptoms or failure of the patient to show progress are the most important 'red flags' suggesting that the diagnosis may be wrong (Traynor *et al.*, 2000). The revised El Escorial criteria are research diagnostic criteria for clinical trials (table 20.3, adapted from Brooks *et al.*, 2000). The criteria are too restrictive for use in routine clinical practice and are not suitable if the objective is to establish the diagnosis as early as possible (Ross *et al.*, 1998). In practice, we do not recommend that patients are told they have 'definite, probable or possible' ALS. The clinician must decide, on the balance of probability, whether or not the patient has ALS, even in the absence of unequivocal UMN and LMN signs (Leigh *et al.*, 2003).

GOOD PRACTICE POINTS

1. The diagnosis should be pursued as early as possible. Patients in whom ALS is suspected should be referred with high priority to an experienced neurologist.
2. All suspected new cases should undergo prompt detailed clinical and paraclinical examinations (tables 20.1 and 20.2).
3. In some cases, additional investigations may be needed (table 20.2).
4. Repetition of the investigations may be needed if the initial series of tests do not result in a diagnosis.
5. Review of the diagnosis is advisable if there is no evidence of progression or if the patient develops atypical features (table 20.1).

Breaking the news: communicating the diagnosis

Telling the patient and the family that the diagnosis is ALS is a daunting task for the physician. If not performed appropriately, the effect can be devastating, leaving the patient with a sense of abandonment and destroying the patient–physician relationship (Lind *et al.*, 1989). Studies of other fatal illnesses (Damian and Tattersall, 1991; Doyle, 1996; Davies and Hopkins, 1997) clearly demonstrated the advantages of utilizing specific techniques (table 20.4). Surveys in ALS patients and caregivers have demonstrated that the way the diagnosis is communicated is less than satisfactory in half of the cases (Borasio *et al.*, 1998; McCluskey *et al.*, 2004). Better performance on all attributes of effective communication as well as greater time spent discussing the diagnosis was correlated with higher patient/caregiver satisfaction (McCluskey *et al.*, 2004). A survey in ALS centres has shown that physicians in 44 % of centres usually spend 30 min or less discussing the diagnosis (Borasio *et al.*, 2001a). Callous delivery of the diagnosis may affect the psychological adjustment to bereavement (Ackerman and Oliver, 1997).

GOOD PRACTICE POINTS

1. The diagnosis should be communicated by a consultant with a good knowledge of the patient.
2. The physician should start the consultation by asking what the patient already knows or suspects.
3. Respect the cultural and social background of the patient by asking whether the patient wishes to receive information or prefers that the information be communicated to a family member.
4. The physician should give the diagnosis to the patient and discuss its implications in a step-wise fashion, checking repeatedly if the patient understands what is said, and reacting appropriately to the verbal and non-verbal cues of the patient.
5. The diagnosis should always be given in person and never by mail or telephone, with enough time available (at least 45–60 minutes) on the part of the physician.
6. Provide printed materials about the disease, about support and advocacy organizations, and about informative websites on the internet.

continued

Table 20.3 Revised El Escorial research diagnostic criteria for ALS (summary).

Clinically definite ALS
UMN and LMN signs in three regions

Clinically definite ALS – laboratory supported
UMN and/or LMN signs in one region *and* the patient is a carrier of a pathogenic gene mutation
MN and LMN signs in two regions with some UMN signs rostral to the LMN signs

Clinically probable ALS – laboratory supported
UMN signs in one or more regions *and* LMN signs defined by EMG in at least two regions

Clinically possible ALS
UMN and LMN signs in one region, or
UMN signs in at least two regions, or
UMN and LMN signs in two regions with no UMN signs rostral to LMN signs

---

Optionally, a letter or audiotape summarizing what the physician has discussed can be very helpful for the patients and family.

7. Assure the patient that he or her and their family will not be on their own ('abandoned') but will be supported by a professional ALS-care team (where available) and with regular follow-up visits to a neurologist. Make arrangements for a close follow-up visit before the end of the consultation, ideally within 2–4 weeks (or sooner if appropriate).

8. Avoid the following: withholding the diagnosis, providing insufficient information, delivering information callously, or taking away or not providing hope. Remember to switch off mobile phones and pagers, and put up 'Do not disturb' signs.

Multi-disciplinary care in the management of ALS

Specialist multidisciplinary (MD) clinics provide secondary or tertiary services to patients with ALS. These clinics comprise a wide range of health care professionals with expertise in ALS. Ideally, such clinics provide both diagnostic and management services, and facilitate continuity of care by close liaising with the primary care physician and community-based services (Chio *et al.*, 2001; Howard and Orrell, 2002; Leigh *et al.*, 2003, Traynor *et al.*, 2003). The emphasis of

care should be on patient autonomy and choice. Patients who attend specialist MD clinics tend to be younger and to have had symptoms for longer than those who do not (Lee *et al.*, 1995; Traynor *et al.*, 2003). Comparison between clinic-based cohorts and population-based cohorts of patients have confirmed a referral bias (Lee *et al.*, 1995, Traynor *et al.*, 2003). However, an independent survival benefit has been identified in two studies, which is independent of other prognostic factors including age, disease duration, bulbar onset disease and rate of progression (Traynor *et al.*, 2003; Chio *et al.*, 2004). Importantly, patients attending a MD clinic have fewer hospital admissions and shorter durations of stay than those who attend general clinics (Chio *et al.*, 2004). Increased use of non-invasive ventilation, attention to nutrition and earlier referral to palliative referral services are likely to contribute to the increased survival of those attending MD clinics (Traynor *et al.*, 2003; Leigh *et al.*, 2003).

GOOD PRACTICE POINTS

1. Multi-disciplinary care should be available for people affected by ALS as attendance at a MD clinic improves care, and may extend survival.

2. The following specialists should be part of or be readily available to the MD team: A consultant in neurology, pulmonologist, gastroenterologist, rehabilitation medicine physician, social counsellor, occupational therapist, speech

Table 20.4 How should a physician tell the patient that they have ALS (Modified from Miller *et al.*, 1999).

Task	Recommendations
Location Structure	Quiet, comfortable, and private. In person, face-to-face. Convenient time (at least 45–60 min). Enough time to ensure no rushing or interruptions. Make eye contact and sit close to patient.
Participants	Know the patient *before* the meeting including family, emotional and social situation, case history, and all relevant test results. Have all the facts at hand. Have patient's support network present (relatives). Have a clinical nurse specialist or equivalent present or available.
What is said	Find out what the patient already knows about the condition. Ascertain how much the patient wants to know about ALS and tailor your information accordingly. Give a warning comment that bad news is coming. The whole truth may need to come by instalments. Use the correct ALS-term, not 'wear and tear of the motor nerves'. Explain the anatomy of the disease (make a simple drawing). If the patient indicates that they want to know the course of the disease, be honest about the likely progression and prognosis but give a broad time frame, and recognise the limitations of any predictions. There is no cure, symptoms tend to steadily worsen, and prognosis is highly variable. Some patients survive five or ten or more years. Acknowledge and explore patient's reaction and allow for emotional expression. Summarize the discussion verbally, in writing, and/or audiotape. Allow plenty of time for questions.
Reassurance	Acknowledge that this is devastating news but discuss reasons for hope such as research, drug trials and the variability of the disease. Explain that the complications of ALS are treatable. Reassure that every attempt will be made to maintain the patient's function and that the patient's treatment decisions will be respected. Reassure that the patient will continue to be cared for and will not be abandoned. Inform about patient support groups (offer contact details and leaflets). Inform about neuroprotective treatment (i.e. riluzole) and ongoing research. Discuss opportunities to participate in research treatment protocols (if available). Acknowledge willingness to get a second opinion if the patient wishes.
How it is said	Emotional manner: warmth, caring, empathy, respect. Be honest, sympathetic but not sentimental. Give news at person's pace; allow the patient to dictate what he or she is told.
Language	Simple and careful word choice, yet direct; no euphemisms or medical jargon.

therapist, specialized nurse, physical therapist, dietician, psychologist, dentist.

3. Schedule clinical visits every 2–3 months and more frequently if needed. This is particularly often the case in the first half year following diagnosis, and in late stages of the disease. Patients with very slowly progressing disease can be seen once or twice a year.

4. It is important that between visits the patient support team maintains regular contact with the patient and relatives (e.g. by phone, letter or email).

5. Ideally, from the outset the patient should be followed by a single named neurologist working in close liaison with the patient's primary care physician (family general practitioner).

6. Effective channels of communication and co-ordination are essential between the hospital-based MD-team, the primary care team, the palliative care team and community services.

Neuroprotective treatment

At present, only riluzole, a presumed glutamate-release antagonist, has been shown to slow the course of ALS in two class I studies (Bensimon *et al.*, 1994; Lacomblez *et al.*, 1996; Cochrane review by Miller *et al.*, 2002). Patients with early disease (i.e. with suspected or possible ALS according to the El Escorial Criteria) were not included. Oral administration of 100 mg riluzole daily prolonged survival by about 3 months after 18 months of treatment. There was a clear dose effect. The drug is safe with few serious side effects. Guidelines for monitoring have been published (www.nice.org.uk/search.aspx?search-mode=simple&ss=ALS). Although patients with progressive muscular atrophy (PMA) or primary lateral sclerosis (PLS) were not included in the riluzole trials, pathological and genetic studies show that some PMA and PLS cases fall within the ALS-syndrome (figure 20.1) (Andersen *et al.*, 2003; Brugman *et al.*, 2005). Riluzole may have little effect in late stage ALS and it is not clear if and when treatment should be terminated. A large number of other drugs have been tested in ALS alas with negative results (table 20.5).

GOOD PRACTICE POINTS

1. ALS patients should be offered treatment with riluzole 50 mg twice daily. (Class I A).
2. Patients treated with riluzole should be monitored regularly for safety. (Class I A).
3. Treatment should be initiated as early as possible after the patient has been informed of the diagnosis.
4. Treatment with riluzole should be considered in PMA and PLS patients who have a first degree relative with ALS.
5. Patients with sporadic PMA, sporadic PLS or hereditary spastic paraplegias (HSP) should as a rule not be treated with riluzole.
6. Irrespective of familial disposition, all patients with a symptomatic motor neuron disease and carrying a SOD1 gene mutation should be offered treatment with riluzole.

Symptomatic treatment

Symptomatic treatment aims to improve the quality of life of patients and caregivers. Symptoms should be treated as they become prominent and incapacitating in individual patients.

Sialorrhea

Sialorrhea (drooling or excessive salivation) is a socially disabling symptom. It results from impaired handling of saliva rather than from over-production. Sialorrhea is treatable. Most evidence, however, comes from studies in other conditions. Amitriptyline is commonly used with reasonable efficacy at low cost (Forshew and Bromberg, 2003). Oral doses of not more than 25–50 mg twice to three times a day are usually sufficient.

Atropine drops can be administered sublingually. A Class IV study in seven patients with Parkinson's disease demonstrated statistically significant decline in saliva production (Hyson *et al.*, 2002). For ALS patients, 0.25–0.75 mg three times a day is recommended empirically (Leigh *et al.*, 2003). Glycopyrrolate (in nebulized or i.v. form) has been shown to be effective in patients with cerebral palsy or developmental disabilities in a

Table 20.5 Summary of the most important controlled therapeutic studies in ALS.

Completed trials
N-Acetylcysteine*
Brain-derived neurotrophic factor (BDNF)*
Branched-chain amino acids*
Celecoxib*
Ciliary neurotrophic factor (CNTF)* (two trials)
Creatine* (three trials)
Cyclosporin*
Dextromethorphan*
Gabapentin*
Glial-derived neurotrophic factor (GDNF)*
Indinavir*
Interferon beta-1a*
Insulin-like growth factor (IGF-1)*
Lamotrigine* (two trials)
Lymphoid irradiation*
Nimodipine*
ONO-2506*
Pentoxifylline*
Riluzole
Selegiline*
TCH-346*
Topiramate*
Verapamil*
Vitamin E* (two trials)
Xaliproden*

Ongoing phase II/III trials (summer of 2006)
Arimoclomol
Ceftriaxone
IGF-1 polypeptide
Minocycline

Phase III trials being planned or considered
AEOL 10150
Celastrol
Coenzyme Q10
Copaxone
IGF-1 – viral delivery
Memantine
NAALADase inhibitors
Nimesulide
Scriptaid
Sodium Phenylbutyrate
Talampanel
Tamoxifen
Thalidomide
Trehalose

---

*No therapeutic benefit was observed.

Class I study (Mier *et al.*, 2000), but no studies in ALS are known. Hyoscine (scopolamine) can be given orally or applied as a dermal patch. Two Class IV studies (Talmi *et al.*,1989 and 1990) showed a reduction of salivary flow with transdermal scopolamine (1.5 mg every three days). Patients with severe drooling may need two patches.

Benzotropine demonstrated in a Class I study in developmentally disabled patients a decrease in drooling up to 70% (Camp-Bruno *et al.*, 1989). An alternative to anticholinergic drugs is botulinum toxin: in a Class IV study in ALS-patients, Giess *et al.*, 2000 showed a reduction of sialorrhea by injections of botulinum toxin type A into the salivary glands. The effect faded in several months, and repeated injections were necessary. Studies with similar results have been carried out in patients with other neurological disorders (Porta *et al.*, 2001; Dogu *et al.*, 2004). However, serious side effects have been reported (Tan *et al.*, 2001; Winterholler *et al.*, 2001). There are no studies using botulinum toxin type B. Another alternative is radiological interventions. Three Class IV studies in ALS patients showed satisfactory results in the treatment of drooling with external radiation of the parotid and submandibular glands (Andersen *et al.*, 2001; Harriman *et al.*, 2001; Stalpers and Moser, 2002). Low dosage palliative radiation in a single fraction of 7–8 Gy to the parotid glands is a simple, fast, safe and inexpensive procedure to reduce drooling in ALS patients.

Surgical interventions, such as transtympanic neurectomy, parotid duct ligation and relocation and submandibular gland excision, showed effective long-term results in children with drooling (Burton 1991; Hockstein *et al.*, 2004). Case reports suggest less efficacy in ALS patients with reports of increased secretions of thick mucus production and side effects like recurrent jaw dislocation and inflammation (Winterholler *et al.*, 2001).

GOOD PRACTICE POINTS

1. Treat sialorrhea in ALS with oral or transdermal hyoscine, atropine drops, glycopyrrolate or amitriptyline.

continued

2. Provide a portable mechanical home suction device.
3. Botulinum toxin injections into the parotid glands can be tried but insufficient data are available yet to appraise safety and long-term efficacy, and this intervention is judged as still experimental.
4. Irradiation of the salivary glands may be tried when pharmacological treatment fails.
5. Surgical interventions are not recommended.

anticholinergic bronchodilator or a mucolytic or furosemide in combination.
5. The use of a mechanical insufflator-exsufflator may be helpful, particularly in the setting of an acute respiratory infection.
6. Cricopharyngeal myotomy may be helpful in the rare cases with frequent episodes with cricopharyngeal spasm and severe bronchial secretions.

Bronchial secretions

Clearing tenacious secretions can be difficult for the patient with respiratory insufficiency causing much distress to the patient. The mucosa of the nasal cavity, larynx, trachea, bronchial airways and lungs contribute a constant flow of serous and particularly mucoid fluids. Stimulation of cholinergic receptors produces thin serous secretions whereas stimulation of β adrenergic receptors produces thick protein- and mucus-rich secretions. A portable home suction device is useful for clearing the upper airways (and excess saliva in the mouth). However, secretions in the lower airways can be difficult to reach. Medication with mucolytics like guaifenesin or N-acetylcysteine, a β-receptor antagonist (such as metoprolol or propranolol) and an anticholinergic bronchodilator like ipratropium and theophylline or even furosemide can be of value, but no controlled studies in ALS exist (Newall et al., 1996). Mechanical cough assisting devices (insufflator-exsufflator) via a face mask were very effective in ALS patients in uncontrolled trials (Hanayama et al., 1997; Sancho et al., 2004).

GOOD PRACTICE POINTS

1. Teach the patient and carers the technique of assisting expiratory movements using a manual assisted cough (can also be performed by a physical therapist).
2. Provide a portable home suction device and a room humidifier.
3. Consider using a mucolytic like N-acetyl-cysteine, 200–400 mg three times daily.
4. If these measures are insufficient, try a nebulizer with saline and a β-receptor antagonist and an

Pseudobulbar emotional lability

Pseudobulbar signs such as pathological weeping, laughing or yawning can be socially disabling. Emotional lability occurs in at least 50% of ALS patients and can be seen in patients without bulbar motor signs (Gallagher, 1989). Occasionally, the emotional outbursts are more troubling for the relatives and nursing staff than the patient, and treatment may not be necessary. A randomised controlled trial of a combination of dextrometorphan and quinidine showed this to be effective in improving emotional lability and quality of life (Brooks et al., 2004). Side effects were experienced by 89% of patients and 24% discontinued treatment during the trial's 4-week duration. Fluvoxamine (Iannaccone et al., 1996), amitriptyline, citalopram and even dopamine and lithium have been tested with good effect in other neurological diseases (Schiffer et al.,1985; Andersen et al.,1993). There appears to be no advantage for a particular medication so the emphasis should be on tolerability, safety and cost.

GOOD PRACTICE POINTS

1. Inform the patient and relatives that the emotional lability is not a sign of a mood disorder but is due to an organic lesion in the brain (Poeck, 1996).
2. Only troublesome emotional lability should be treated. If treatment is deemed necessary, an antidepressant such as amitriptyline, fluvoxamine, citalopram is usually sufficient.
3. A combination of dextrometorphan and quinidine has been shown to be effective in a Class I A study but further experience on the long-term side effects and tolerability are needed.

Cramps

Cramps may be an early and troublesome symptom in ALS, in particular before falling asleep. Class I studies in patients with non-ALS leg cramps with quinine sulfate and vitamin E (Conolly *et al.*, 1992; Diener *et al.*, 2002) showed a positive effect only for quinine. Empirically, massage, physical exercise (in the evening), hydrotherapy, Mg^{2+}, carbamazepine, diazepam, phenytoin, verapamil, gabapentin can alleviate muscle cramps.

GOOD PRACTICE POINTS

1. Treat cramps in ALS with physiotherapy, physical exercise and hydrotherapy.
2. If necessary, treat cramps in ALS with quinine sulfate.
3. Mg^{2+}, carbamazepine, phenytoin, verapamil, gabapentin are alternatives.

Spasticity

Spasticity can be a troublesome symptom in patients with ALS. Physical therapy is vital and helped in reducing spasticity in a Class IIB study (Drory *et al.*, 2001). Modalities such as hydrotherapy, heat, cold, ultrasound, electrical stimulation, and in rare cases surgery can be used, though no controlled studies in ALS exist. In a Class III study of 20 patients with spinal cord injury, the use of hydrotherapy in heated pools three times per week produced a significant decrease in spasm severity and reduction of oral baclofen medication (Kesiktas *et al.*, 2004). Cryotherapy of the facial muscles reduced spasticity to facilitate dental care in 24 patients with cerebral palsy (dos Santos and de Oliveira, 2004). Oral baclofen (up to 80 mg daily) revealed no significant effect in spasticity in ALS in one small study (Norris *et al.*, 1979). Intrathecal baclofen in two ALS-patients with intractable spasticity was more effective than oral medication and greatly improved the patient's quality of life (Marquardt and Seifert, 2002). Other drugs have not been tested formally in ALS, but in clinical practice gabapentin (900–2400 mg daily), tizanidine (6–24 mg daily), memantine (10–60 mg daily), dantrolene (25–100 mg daily) and diazepam (10–30 mg daily) have been used with effect. Botulinum toxin A has successfully been used to treat trismus and stridor in case reports (Winterholler *et al.*, 2002).

GOOD PRACTICE POINTS

1. Physical therapy should be available regularly when there is significant spasticity.
2. Hydrotherapy with exercises in heated pools with 32–34°C warm water, and cryotherapy should be considered.
3. Antispastic drugs such as baclofen and tizanidine may be tried.

Depression, anxiety and insomnia

Depression occurs frequently at all stages of ALS as well as insomnia (Dengler, 1999). Anxiety can become marked when respiratory insufficiency occurs. The four mostly used antidepressants in ALS are amitriptyline, sertraline, fluoxetine and paroxetine. Amitriptyline has the best therapeutic effect and the lowest costs. For insomnia in ALS, amitriptyline and zolpidem are the most commonly used medications (Forshew and Bromberg, 2003). There are no systematic studies on anxiolytics in ALS, but oral diazepam or sub-lingual lorazepam are useful.

GOOD PRACTICE POINTS

1. Treat depression in ALS with an appropriate antidepressant (e.g. amitriptyline or an SSRI).
2. Treat insomnia with amitriptyline or appropriate hypnotics (e.g. zolpidem, diphenhydramine).
3. Treat anxiety with bupropion or benzodiazepines such as diazepam tablets or suppositories, temesta tablets 0.5 mg 2–3 times daily, or lorazepam sublingually.

Pain

Pain occurs frequently in ALS. Some familial ALS syndromes include pain of the neuralgic type. Treatment is unspecific and should follow accepted principles. Opioids can be used, following the 1990-WHO analgesic ladder guidelines, when nonnarcotics fail (Miller, 2001). Begin with simple anagelsics such as paracetamol, followed by weak

Table 20.6 Frequency of FALS in some epidemiological studies.

Study area	% FALS	n	Year	Reference
Germany	13.5	251	1959	Haberlandt (1959)
Central Finland	11.6	36	1983	Murros, Fogelholm (1983)
USA	9.5	1200	1995	Haverkamp et al. (1995)
Belgium	8.6	140	2000	Thijs et al. (2000)
Nova Scotia, Canada	5.8	52	1974	Murray et al. (1974)
Wärmland, Sweden	5.6	89	1984	Gunnarsson, Palm (1984)
England	5.0	580	1988	Li et al. (1988)
USA	4.9	668	1978	Rosen AD (1978)
Northern Sweden	4.7	128	1983	Forsgren et al. (1983)
Sardinia, Italy	4.4	182	1983	Giagheddu et al. (1983)
Jutland, Denmark	2.7	186	1989	Højer-Pedersen et al. (1989)
Hong Kong	1.2	84	1996	Fong et al. (1996)
Finland	0.8	255	1977	Jokelainen (1977)

opioids such as tramadol, followed by strong opioids such as morphine or ketobemidon. Liberal use of opioids may be appropriate when non-narcotics fail and have the secondary advantages of alleviating dyspnea and anxiety. However, constipation may become a problem.

GOOD PRACTICE POINTS

Treat pain in ALS following accepted guidelines.

Venous thrombosis

Patients with leg paralysis have an increased risk of venous thrombosis.

GOOD PRACTICE POINTS

Physiotherapy, limb elevation, compression stockings can be used. Prophylactic treatment with anti-coagulants is not recommended.

Genetic testing and counselling

In different populations, the frequency of familial ALS (FALS) is reportedly 5–10% of all ALS cases (table 20.6) but may be underestimated for a number of reasons (*Supplementary table 2 online*). At present four genes have been found to cause ALS (figures 20.1 and 20.2), SOD1, VAPB, SETX and

ALSIN. At present mutations in the latter three genes appear to be very rare and analysis is only performed in a scientific setting.

Since 1993 some 128 mutations have been found in the SOD1 gene with five different modes of inheritance (figure 20.2) (www.ALSOD.org; Andersen et al., 2003). The most frequent mutation is the D90A which in most European countries is inherited as a recessive trait with a characteristic slowly progressing phenotype (Andersen et al., 1996). Twelve to twenty-three per cent of diagnosed FALS and 2–7% of apparently SALS patients carry a SOD1 mutation (table 20.7). It must be emphasized that diminished disease penetrance is not infrequent and that SOD1 mutations can be found in cases of apparent SALS (*Supplementary tables 3 and 4 online*) (Jones et al., 1995). A DNA-SOD1 diagnostic test speeds up the diagnostic process and can be of help in patients with atypical features (Andersen et al., 2003) as well as providing some prognostic information (*Supplementary tables 5 and 6*) (Andersen et al., 1996). Presymptomatic (predictive) genetic testing should only be performed in first degree adult blood relatives of patients with a known SOD1 gene mutation. Testing should only be performed on a strictly volunteer basis as outlined (*Supplementary table 7 online*) (Gasser et al., 2001). Special consideration should be taken before presymptomatic testing is performed in FALS families where the

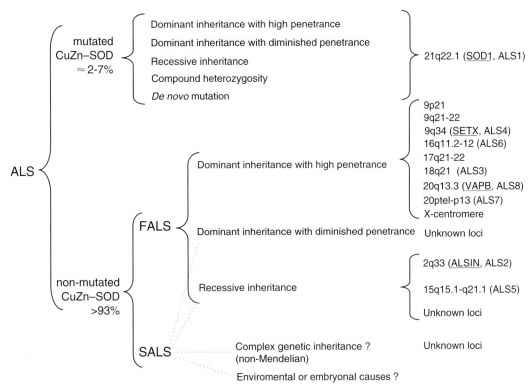

Figure 20.2. The different patterns of inheritance and genetic loci found in ALS. It is important to remember that reduced disease penetrance has been recognized in many families with ALS. Some cases diagnosed as SALS are in fact FALS with very low disease penetrance, recessive inheritance or oligogenic inheritance in a complicated pattern not always understood.

mutation is associated with reduced disease penetrance (*Supplementary table 3 online*) or with a variable prognosis (*Supplementary table 5 online*).

GOOD PRACTICE POINTS

1. Clinical DNA analysis for SOD1 gene mutation should only be performed in cases with a known familial history of ALS or in SALS cases with the characteristic phenotype of the D90A mutation.
2. Clinical DNA analysis for SOD1 gene mutations should *not* be performed in cases with SALS with a typical classical ALS-phenotype.
3. Before blood is drawn for DNA analysis, the patient should receive genetic counselling. Give the patient time for consideration. DNA analysis should not be performed without the patient's consent.

4. Presymptomatic genetic testing should *only* be performed in first degree adult blood relatives of patients with a known SOD1 gene mutation. Testing should only be performed on a strictly volunteer basis as outlined (*Supplementary table 7 online*).
5. Results of DNA analysis performed on patients and their relatives as part of a research project should not be used in clinical practice or disclosed to the unaffected relative. Also, the results should be kept in a separate file, not in the patient's medical chart.

Non-invasive and invasive ventilation in ALS Patients

Respiratory insufficiency in ALS patients is caused mainly by respiratory muscle or bulbar weakness

Table 20.7 Frequency of CuZn-SOD mutations in ALS.

In SALS

7.3% (3/41) in Italy	(Corrado L. *et al.*, personal communication June 2005)
7% (4/56) in Scotland	(Jones CT et al., *J Med Genet* 1995;32:290–292)
6% (3/48) in Italy	(Gellera C et al., ALS & other MNDs 2001;2(suppl 1):543–546)
4% (14/355) in Scandinavia	(Andersen PM et al., *Brain* 1997;10:1723–1737)
3% (5/175) in the UK	(Shaw CE et al., *Ann Neurol* 1998;43:390–394)
3% (5/155) in England	(Jackson M et al., *Ann Neurol* 1997;42:803–807)
1.2% (1/87) in Spain	(García-Redondo A et al., *Muscle & Nerve* 2002;26:274–278)
0% (0/225) in Italy	(Battistini S et al., *J Neurol* 2005;252:782–788)

In FALS

23.5% (12/51) in Scandinavia	(Andersen PM et al., *Brain* 1997;10:1723–1737)
23.5% (68/290) in the USA	(Cudkowicz ME et al., *Ann Neurol* 1997;2:210–221)
21% (8/38) in the UK	(Shaw CE et al., *Ann Neurol* 1998;43:390–394)
19.7% (14/71) in the UK	(Orrell R et al., *Neurology* 1997;48:746–751)
18% (2/11) in Spain	(García-Redondo A et al., *Muscle & Nerve* 2002;26:274–278)
18% (7/39) in Italy	(Battistini S et al., *J Neurol* 2005;252:782–788)
14.3% (10/70) in France	(Boukaftane Y et al., *Can J Neurol Sci* 1998;25:192–196)
12% (9/75) in Germany	(Niemann S et al., *JNNP* 2004;75:1186–1188)

Without classification to hereditary disposition

7.2% (148/2045) in North America	(Andersen PM et al., ALS & Other MNDs 2003;4:62–73).

Table 20.8 Symptoms and signs of respiratory insufficiency in ALS (modified from Leigh *et al.*, 2003).

Symptoms	Signs
Dyspnoea on exertion or talking	Tachypnea
Ortopnoea	Use of auxillary respiratory muscles
Frequent nocturnal awakenings	Paradoxical movement of abdomen
Excessive day-time sleepiness	Decreased chest movement
Daytime fatigue	Weak cough
Difficulty clearing secretions	Sweating
Morning headache	Tachycardia
Nocturia	Weight loss
Depression	Confusion, hallucinations, dizziness
Poor appetite	Papilloedema (rare)
Poor concentration and/or memory	Syncope
	Mouth dryness

and can be aggravated by aspiration and bronchopneumonia (Howard and Orrell, 2002). Some patients present with thoracic paresis and respiratory insufficiency (table 20.8). Vital capacity (VC) is the most widely available test of respiratory muscle function and should be measured regularly in parallel with assessments of symptoms suggestive of respiratory insufficiency (Leigh *et al.*, 2003). Sniff nasal pressure (SNP) may be a more accurate predictor of respiratory failure than VC, but neither VC nor SNP are sensitive predictors of respiratory failure in patients with severe bulbar involvement (Lyall *et al.*, 2001). Nocturnal oximetry can detect nocturnal hypoventilation and can be done at home. Blood exchange abnormalities ($\uparrow$ PCO_2) are generally a late finding. Non-invasive positive-pressure ventilation (NIV) and invasive mechanical ventilation via tracheostomy

Table 20.9 Proposed criteria for NIV (modified from Leigh *et al.*, 2003).

---

1. Symptoms related to respiratory muscle weakness. At least one of the following:

   (a) Dyspnoea
   (b) Orthopnoea
   (c) Disturbed sleep not due to pain
   (d) Morning headache
   (e) Poor concentration
   (f) Loss of appetite
   (g) Excessive daytime sleepiness (ESS > 9)

2. Signs of respiratory muscle weakness (FVC <80% or SNP < 40 cm H_2O)

3. Evidence of either:

   (a) Significant nocturnal desaturation on overnight oximetry, or
   (b) Morning blood-gas $pCO2$ > 6.5 Kpa.

ESS, Epworth Sleepiness Score.

(TV) are used to alleviate respiratory symptoms, improve quality of life and prolong survival. There is no clear evidence regarding timing and criteria of use of NIV and TV in ALS patients (table 20.9). The use of mechanical ventilation varies between countries with cross-cultural and ethical differences (Miller *et al.*, 1999; Bourke and Gibson, 2004). The patient's advance directives and a clear plan for management of respiratory failure should be established before respiratory failure occurs (Miller *et al.*, 1999; Leigh *et al.*, 2003; Bourke and Gibson, 2004). The choice of ventilation will depend on hypoventilation symptoms and upper airway obstruction symptoms, bronchial secretions and factors such as availability, cost, patient preference and care.

NIV has become the preferred initial therapy to alleviate respiratory symptoms in ALS patients and should be considered before TV (Miller *et al.*, 1999; Annane *et al.*, 2000; Leigh *et al.*, 2003; Bourke and Gibson, 2004). It is usually initially used for intermittent nocturnal support to alleviate symptoms of nocturnal hypoventilation (table 20.8). Observational studies suggest that NIV improves survival and quality of life (Bourke *et al.*, 2003). Secretion management is a major factor in the success of NIV (Leigh *et al.*, 2003), (see section on bronchial secretions). As respiratory muscle

strength declines, daytime NIV usually becomes necessary and patients may become dependent on non-stop ventilation. Patients who cannot use NIV should be informed about the terminal phase, TV, hospice referral and palliative care. Patients with flaccid paresis of the facial muscles may have difficulty using NIV, but the method should be offered to patients with predominating UMN bulbar paresis and little atrophy.

TV may be proposed when NIV treatment is not effective due to progression of the disease or when the patient cannot cooperate with NIV because of loss of bulbar tone and difficulty clearing secretions (Figure 20.3) (Miller *et al.*, 1999). TV can prolong survival for many years, can be acceptable for some patients and caregivers and in these cases can improve patients' quality of life, although some patients become unable to communicate in a state of locked-in (Leigh *et al.*, 2003). However, home TV is costly and has a significant emotional and social impact on patients and caregivers (Cazzolli and Oppenheimer, 1996; Miller *et al.*, 1999). The advantages and drawbacks of TV are summarized in table 20.10. A difficult issue is when to terminate ventilatory support. Parenteral diamorphine, a benzodiazepine and an antiemetic are used when the patient decides that ventilatory support should be withdrawn (Miller *et al.*, 1999). For symptomatic treatment of dyspnea with opioids and oxygen, the class of evidence is IA in cancer and chronic obstructive pulmonary disease (Jennings *et al.*, 2002; Bruera *et al.*, 2003), but no controlled studies in ALS exist.

GOOD PRACTICE POINTS

1. Symptoms or signs of respiratory insufficiency (including symptoms of nocturnal hypoventilation) should be checked at each visit.
2. VC is the most available and practical test for the monitoring of respiratory function on a regular basis. If possible, VC should be measured both standing/sitting and lying.
3. SNP may be used for monitoring of inspiratory muscle strength, particularly in some bulbar patients who cannot perform VC accurately.

continued

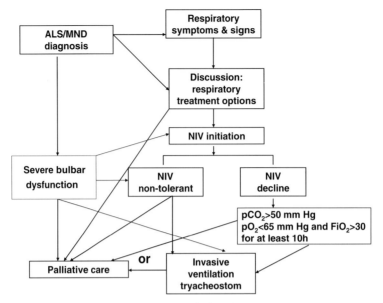

Figure 20.3. Flowchart for the management of respiratory dysfunction in ALS.

4. Nocturnal oximetry, available at home, is recommended in patients with symptoms of nocturnal hypoventilation.

5. Symptoms or signs of respiratory insufficiency should initiate discussions with the patient and the caregivers about all treatment options such as NIV, TV and the terminal phase. Early discussions are needed to allow advance planning and directives. The patient should be informed about the temporary nature of NIV (which is primarily directed towards improving quality of life rather than prolonging it (as opposed to TV)). Care should adapt to the changing needs of patients and carers over the course of the disease.

6. NIV should be considered before TV in patients with symptoms of respiratory insufficiency.

7. TV can prolong survival for many months and can improve patient's quality of life, but it has a major impact upon carers, and must be undertaken only after a thorough discussion of the pro's and con's with the patient and carers.

8. Unplanned (emergency) TV should be avoided at all costs through early discussion of end of life issues, palliative care and advance directives.

9. Oxygen therapy alone should be avoided as it may exacerbate CO_2 retention and mouth dryness.

10. Medical treatment of intermittent dyspnea:

   – short dyspneic bouts: relieve anxiety and give lorazepam 0.5–2.5 mg sublingually
   – longer phases of dyspnea (>30 min): give morphine.

11. Medical treatment of chronic dyspnea: start with morphine 2.5 mg orally 4–6 times daily. For severe dyspnea give morphine s.c. or i.v. infusion. Start with 0.5 mg/h and titrate.

Enteral nutrition in ALS patients

Initial management of dysphagia in patients with ALS is based on dietary counselling, modification of food and fluid consistency (blending food, adding thickeners to liquids), prescription of high protein and caloric supplements and education of the patient and carers in feeding and swallowing techniques such as supraglottic swallowing and postural changes (Miller *et al.*, 1999; Desport *et al.*, 2000; Heffernan *et al.*, 2004). Flexing the neck forward on swallowing to protect the airway

Table 20.10 The advantages and drawbacks of invasive ventilation tracheostomy.

1. Advantages

   (a) preventing aspiration
   (b) more secure ventilator – patients interface
   (c) ability to provide higher ventilator pressures

2. Drawbacks

   (a) more secretions generating
   (b) impairing swallowing risk
   (c) increasing aspiration
   (d) increasing risk of infections
   (e) tracheoesophageal fistula
   (f) tracheal stenosis or tracheomalacia
   (g) costs
   (h) 24 h nursing care

(chin tuck manoeuvre) may be helpful. Some patients having difficulty swallowing tap water can drink carbonated fluids or ice-cold fluids. Empirically, this is in particular the case for patients with predominantly spastic dysphagia. Sufficient oral fluid intake is important also to improve articulation, to maintain good oral hygiene and reduce the risk of constipation. As dysphagia progresses, these measures become insufficient and tube feeding is needed. Three procedures obviate the need for major surgery and general anaesthesia: Percutaneous endocopic gastrostomy (PEG), percutaneous radiologic gastrostomy (PRG or RIG, radiologically inserted gastrostomy) and nasogastric tube (NGT) feeding.

PEG is the standard procedure for enteral nutrition in ALS and is wildly available (Desport *et al.*, 2000; Heffernan *et al.*, 2004). PEG improves nutrition, but there is no convincing evidence that PEG prevents aspiration or improves quality of life or survival (Miller *et al.*, 1999; Heffernan *et al.*, 2004). The procedure requires mild sedation and is therefore more hazardous in patients with respiratory impairment and at an advanced stage of the disease (Miller *et al.*, 1999; Desport *et al.*, 2000; Heffernan *et al.*, 2004). Non-invasive ventilation during the PEG procedure may be feasible in ALS patients with respiratory impairment (Heffernan *et al.*, 2004). The timing of PEG is mainly based on symptoms, nutritional status and respiratory function (Miller *et al.*, 1999; Heffernan *et al.*, 2004). To minimize risks, evidence suggests that PEG should be performed before VC falls below 50% of the predicted level (Mathus-Vliegen LM *et al.*, 1994).

PRG is a new alternative to PEG in ALS patients (Heffernan *et al.*, 2004; Chio *et al.*, 2004; Shaw *et al.*, 2004). A major advantage of PRG is that it does not require sedation and therefore is suitable in patients with respiratory impairment or in poor general condition. The success rate of the PRG procedure has also been shown to be higher than PEG (Thornton *et al.*, 2002; Chio *et al.*, 2004). However, this procedure is not yet widely available and is less well documented than PEG.

NGT is a minor and non-invasive procedure that can be used with all patients but presents numerous disadvantages that limit its use (Scott and Austin, 1994; Heffernan *et al.*, 2004). NGT increases oropharyngeal secretions and is associated with nasopharyngeal discomfort, pain or even ulceration.

GOOD PRACTICE POINTS

1. Bulbar dysfunction and nutritional status, including at least weight, should be checked at each visit.
2. The patient and spouse should be referred to a dietician as soon as dysphagia appears. A speech and language therapist can give valuable advice on swallowing techniques.
3. The timing of PEG/PRG is based on an individual approach taking into account bulbar symptoms, malnutrition (weight loss > 10 %), respiratory function and the patient's general condition. Thus, early operation is highly recommended.
4. When PEG is indicated, patient and carers should be informed: (a) of the benefits and risks of the procedure; (b) that it is possible to continue to take food orally as long as it is possible; (c) that deferring PEG to a late disease stage may increase the risk of the procedure.
5. PRG is a suitable alternative to PEG. This procedure can be used as the procedure of choice or when the PEG is deemed hazardous.

continued

6. Tubes with relatively large diameters (e.g. 18–22 Charriere) are recommended for both PEG and PRG to prevent tube obstruction.
7. Prophylactic medication with antibiotics on the day of the operation may reduce the risk of infections.
8. NGT may be used for short-term feeding and when PEG or PRG is not suitable.

GOOD PRACTICE POINTS

1. Regular assessment (i.e. every 3–6 months) of communication by a trained SLT is recommended.
2. The use of appropriate communication support systems (ranging from pointing boards with figures or words, to computerised speech synthesisers) should be provided as required.

Communication in ALS patients

Most commonly communication difficulties in ALS result from progressive dysarthria, with language functions remaining largely intact. However, changes of language function may occur, especially in patients with cognitive impairment of the frontal type. This is shown by reduced verbal output (in rare cases leading to mutism), reduced spelling ability, word finding difficulty and auditory comprehension of more complex input (Bak and Hodges, 2004). In others, the deficits are subtle and only exposed on formal testing (Cobble, 1998). Language impairment can have a deleterious effect on the quality of life of the patients and carers, and can make the clinical management of the patient difficult (Cobble, 1998; Murphy, 2004).

Communication should be routinely assessed by a speech and language therapist (SLT). The goal of management of communication difficulties in ALS patients is to optimize the effectiveness of communication for as long as possible and to concentrate not only on the disabled person, but on personal partner-to-partner communication as well. When dysarthria progresses the use of an augmentive and alternative communication (AAC) system is needed. An ACC system substantially improves the quality of life. Prosthetic treatments (palatal lift and/or palatal augmentation prosthesis) can be useful in reduction of hypernasality and improvement of articulation. For ventilated patients eye-pointing or eye-gaze augmentive high-tech communication devices are useful. Brain-computer-interfaces, EEG & EP (SCP) methods, thought translation devices can be used as the new communication channels.

Palliative and end-of-life care

A palliative care approach should be incorporated into the care plan for patients and carers from the time of diagnosis (Borasio et al., 2001b, Class III recommendation). Early referral to a specialist palliative care team is often appropriate. Palliative care based in the community or through hospice contacts (e.g. home care teams) can proceed in partnership with clinic-based neurological multidisciplinary care. The aim of palliative care is to maximise quality of life of patients and families by relieving symptoms, providing emotional, psychological and spiritual support as needed, removing obstacles to a peaceful death, and supporting the family in bereavement (Oliver et al., 2000). Various other aspects of terminal care have been covered in several sections in this chapter.

GOOD PRACTICE POINTS

1. Whenever possible, offer input from a palliative care team early in the course of the disease.
2. Initiate discussions on end-of-life decisions whenever the patient asks – or 'opens the door' – for end-of-life information and/or interventions.
3. Discuss the options for respiratory support and end-of-life issues if the patient has dyspnea, other symptoms of hypoventilation (table 20.8), or a forced vital capacity <50%.
4. Inform the patient of the legal situation regarding advance directives and naming of a health care proxy. Offer assistance in formulating an advance directive.

5. Re-discuss the patient's preferences for life-sustaining treatments every 6 months.
6. Initiate early referral to hospice or home care teams well in advance of the terminal phase of ALS to facilitate the work of the hospice team.
7. Be aware of the importance of spiritual issues for the quality of life and treatment choices. Establish a liaison with local pastoral care workers to be able to address the needs of the patient and relatives.
8. For symptomatic treatment of dyspnea and pain of intractable cause use opioids alone or in combination with benzodiazepines if anxiety is present. Titrating the dosages against the clinical symptoms will almost never result in a life-threatening respiratory depression (Sykes and Thorns, 2003; Class I A recommendation).
9. For treating terminal restlessness and confusion due to hypercapnia neuroleptics may be used, (e.g. chlorpromazine 12.5 mg every 4–12 h p.o., i.v. or p.r.).
10. Use oxygen only if symptomatic hypoxia is present.

Future developments

Being a syndrome with low incidence and short survival, most recommendations are Good Practice Points based on consensus of experts in the ALS field. More preferably randomized and double-blinded clinical trials are urgently needed to improve the management of ALS.

GOOD PRACTICE POINTS

Research Recommendations

1. Further studies of more specific diagnostic tools are needed, in particular in relation to cervical spondylotic myelopathy, inclusion body myositis and motor neuropathies.
2. There are no data on the effects of MD clinics on quality of life or care burden – the generation of such data would be beneficial.
3. Further studies are required to confirm the benefits of MD clinics, and to identify the factors that affect outcome.

4. Further studies are required to optimize the symptomatic treatment of ALS patients, in particular therapies for treating muscle cramps, drooling and bronchial secretions.
5. Better criteria for defining the use of PEG and PRG, and NIV and TV are urgently needed.
6. Further studies to evaluate the effects of PEG/PRG, cough-assisting devices and ventilation support on quality of life and survival are advocated.
7. Further studies are required to evaluate the language dysfunction and its treatment in ALS.
8. Studies of the medico-economical impact of more expensive procedures (NIV, TV, cough-assisting devices, advanced communication equipment) are needed.

Conflicts of interest

The present guidelines were prepared without external financial support. None of the authors report conflicting interests.

References

Abrahams S, Goldstein LH, Kew JJ et al. (1996). Frontal lobe dysfunction in amyotrophic lateral sclerosis. A PET study. Brain **119**:2105–2120.

Ackerman GM, Oliver D (1997). Psychosocial support in an outpatient clinic. Palliat Med **11**:167–168.

Aggarwal A, Nicholson G (2002). Detection of preclinical motor neurone loss in SOD1 mutation carriers using motor unit number estimation. J Neurol Neurosurg Psychiatry **73**:199–201.

Andersen G, Vestergaard K, Riis JO (1993). Citalopram for post-stroke pathological crying. Lancet **342:** 837–839.

Andersen PM, Forsgren L, Binzer M et al. (1996). Autosomal recessive adult-onset ALS associated with homozygosity for Asp90Ala CuZn-superoxide dismutase mutation. A clinical and genealogical study of 36 patients. Brain **119**:1153–1172.

Andersen PM, Nilsson P, Keränen M-L et al. (1997). Phenotypic heterogeneity in MND-patients with CuZn-superoxide dismutase mutations in Scandinavia. Brain **10:** 1723–1737.

Andersen PM, Gronberg H, Frankzen L, Funegard U (2001).External radiation of the parotid glands significantly reduces drooling in patients with motor neurone disease with bulbar paresis. J Neurol Sci **191**:111–114.

Andersen PM, Sims KB, Xin WW *et al.* (2003). Sixteen novel mutations in the gene encoding CuZn-superoxide dismutase in ALS. *Amyotroph Lateral Scler Other Motor Neuron Disord* **2:**62–73.

Andersen PM, Borasio GD, Dengler R *et al.* (2005) EFNS task force on management of amyotrophic lateral sclerosis: guidelines for diagnosing and clinical care of patients and relatives. An evidence-based review with good practice points. *Eur J Neurology* **12:**921–938.

Annane D, Chevrolet JC, Chevret S, Raphael JC (2000). Nocturnal mechanical ventilation for chronic hypoventilation in patients with neuromuscular and chest wall disorders. *Cochrane Database Syst Rev* CD001941.

Bak TH, Hodges JR (2004).The effects of motor neurone disease on language: further evidence. *Brain Lang* **89:**354–61.

Battistini S, Giannini F, Greco G *et al.* (2005). SOD1 mutations in amyotrophic lateral sclerosis Results from a multicenter Italian study. *J Neurol* **252:**782–788.

Belsh JM, Schiffman PL (1990). Misdiagnosis in patients with amyotrophic lateral sclerosis. *Arch Intern Med* **150:**2301–2305.

Bensimon G, Lacomblez L, Meininger V *et al.* (1994). A controlled trial of riluzole in amyotrophic lateral sclerosis. ALS/Riluzole Study Group. *N Engl J Med* **330:**585–591.

Bobowick AR, Brody JA (1973). Epidemiology of motor-neuron diseases. *N Engl J Med* **288:**1047–1055.

Borasio GD, Sloan R, Pongratz DE (1998). Breaking the news in amyotrophic lateral sclerosis. *J Neurol Sci* **160(Suppl 1):**S127–S133.

Borasio GD, Shaw PJ, Hardiman O, Ludolph AC, Sales Luis ML, Silani V, for the European ALS Study Group (2001a). Standards of palliative care for patients with amyotrophic lateral sclerosis: results of a European survey. *Amyotroph Lateral Scler Other Motor Neuron Disord* **2:**159–164.

Borasio GD, Voltz R, Miller RG (2001b). Palliative Care in Amyotrophic Lateral Sclerosis. In: *Palliative Care,* A. Carver and K. Foley, eds., Neurol Clin **19:**829–847.

Boukaftane Y, Khoris J, Moulard B *et al.* (1998). Identification of six novel SOD1 gene mutations in familial amyotrophic lateral sclerosis. *Can J Neurol Sci* **25:**192–196.

Bourke SC, Gibson GJ (2004). Non-invasive ventilation in ALS: current practice and future role. *Amyotroph Lateral Scler Other Motor Neuron Disord* **5:**67–71.

Bourke SC, Bullock RE, Williams TL, Shaw PJ, Gibson GJ (2003). Noninvasive ventilation in ALS: indications and effect on the quality of life. *Neurology* **61:**171–177.

Brainin M, Barnes M, Baron J.-C. *et al.* (2004). Guidance for the preparation of neurological management guidelines by EFNS scientific task forces – revised recommendations 2004. *Eur J Neurol* **11:**577–581.

Bromberg M (1999). Accelerating the diagnosis of amyotrophic lateral sclerosis. *The Neurologist* **5:**63–74.

Brooks BR, Miller RG, Swash M *et al.* (2000). El Escorial revisited: Revised criteria for the diagnosis of amyotrophic lateral sclerosis. *ALS and other motor neuron disorders* **1:**293–299.

Brooks BR, Thisted RA, Appel SH *et al.* (2004). Treatment of pseudobulbar affect in ALS with dextromethorphan/quinidine: A randomized trial. The AVP-923 ALS Study Group *Neurology* **63 :**1364–1370.

Bruera E, Sweeney C, Willey J *et al.* (2003). A randomized controlled trial of supplemental oxygen versus air in cancer patients with dyspnea. *Palliat Med* **17:**659–663.

Brugman F, Wokke JH, Vianney de Jong JM, Franssen H, Faber CG, Van den Berg LH (2005). Primary lateral sclerosis as a phenotypic manifestation of familial ALS. *Neurology* **64:**1778–1779.

Burton MJ (1991). The surgical management of drooling. *Dev Med Child Neurol* **33:** 1110–1116.

Camp-Bruno JA, Winsberg BF, Green-Parsons AR, Abrams JP (1989). Efficacy of benztropine therapy for drooling. *Dev Med Child Neurol* **31:**309–319.

Cazzolli PA, Oppenheimer EA (1996). Home mechanical ventilation for amyotrophic lateral sclerosis: nasal compared to tracheostomy-intermittent positive pressure ventilation. *J Neurol Sci* **139(Suppl):** 123–128.

Chio A (1999). Survey: an international study on the diagnostic process and its implications in amyotrophic lateral sclerosis. *J Neurol* **246(Suppl 3):**III1–5.

Chio A, Silani V, Italian ALS Stud Group (2001). ALS care in Italy: A nationwide study in neurological centres. *J Neurol Sci* **191:**145–150.

Chio A, Moral G, Balzarino C, Mutani R (2004). Interdisciplinary ALS Centres: Effect of survival and use of health services in a population-based survey. *Neurology* **2(Suppl):**S23.003 (Abstract).

Chio A, Galletti R, Finocchiaro C *et al.* (2004). Percutaneous radiological gastrostomy: a safe and effective method of nutritional tube placement in advanced ALS. *J Neurol Neurosurg Psychiatry* **75:**645–647.

Cobble M (1998). Language impairment in motor neurone disease. *J Neurol Sci* **160(Suppl 1):**S47–52.

Connolly PS, Shirley EA, Wasson JH, Nierenberg DW. (1992). Treatment of nocturnal leg cramps. A crossover trial of quinine vs vitamin E. *Arch Intern Med* **152:**1877–1880.

Cudkowicz ME, McKenna-Yasek D, Sapp PE *et al.* (1997). Epidemiology of mutations in superoxide dismutase in amyotrophic lateral sclerosis. *Ann Neurol* **41:**210–221.

Damian D, Tattersall MHN (1991). Letters to patients: Improving communication in cancer care. *Lancet* **338:**923–925.

Davenport RJ, Swingler RJ, Chancellor AM, Warlow CP (1996). Avoiding false positive diagnoses of motor neuron disease: lessons from the Scottish Motor Neuron Disease Register. *J Neurol Neurosurg Psychiatry* **60:**147–151.

Davies E, Hopkins A (1997). Good practice in the management of adults with malignant cerebral glioma: Clinical guidelines. Working Group. *Br J Neurosurg* **11:**318–330.

Dengler R (1999). Current treatment pathways in ALS: A European perspective. *Neurology* **53:** S4–10.

Desport JC, Preux PM, Truong CT, Courat L, Vallat JM, Couratier P (2000). Nutritional assessment and survival in ALS patients. *Amyotroph Lateral Scler Other Motor Neuron Disord* **1:**91–96.

Diener HC, Dethlefsen U, Dethlefsen-Gruber S, Verbeek P (2002). Effectiveness of quinine in treating muscle cramps: a double-blind, placebo-controlled, parallel-group, multicentre trial. *Int J Clin Pract* **56:**243–246.

Dogu O, Apaydin D, Sevim S et al. (2004). Ultrasound-guided versus 'blind' intraparotid injections of botulinum toxin-A for the treatment of sialorrhoea in patients with Parkinson's disease. *Clin Neurol Neurosurg* **106:**93–96.

Doyle D (1996). Breaking bad news. *J Royal Soc Med* **89:**590–591.

Drory VW, Goltsman E, Renik JG et al. (2001). The value of muscle exercise in patients with amyotrophic lateral sclerosis. *J Neurol Sci* **191:**133–137.

Evangelista T, Carvalho M, Conceicao I, Pinto A, de Lurdes M, Luis ML (1996). Motor neuropathies mimicking amyotrophic lateral sclerosis/motor neuron disease. *J Neurol Sci* **139(Suppl):**95–98.

Fong KY, Yu YL, Chan YW et al. (1996). Motor neuron disease in Hong Kong Chinese: Epidemiology and clinical picture. *Neuroepidemiology* **15:**239–245.

Forsgren L, Almay BG, Holmgren G, Wall S (1983). Epidemiology of motor neuron disease in northern Sweden. *Acta Neurol Scand* **68:**20–29.

Forshew, DA, Bromberg MB (2003). A survey of clinicians' practice in the symptomatic treatment of ALS. *Amyotrophic Lateral Scler Other Motor Neuron Disord* **4:**258–263.

Gallagher JP (1989). Pathologic laughter and crying in ALS: a search for their origin. *Acta Neurol Scand* **80:**114–117.

Garcia-Redondo A, Bustos F, Juan Y Seva B et al. (2002). Molecular analysis of the superoxide dismutase 1 gene in Spanish patients with sporadic or familial amyotrophic lateral sclerosis. *Muscle Nerve* **26:**274–278.

Gellera C (2001). Genetics of ALS in Italian families. *Amyotroph Lateral Scler Other Motor Neuron Disord.* **2(Suppl 1):**S43–46.

Giagheddu M, Puggioni G, Masala C et al. (1983). Epidemiologic study of amyotrophic lateral sclerosis in Sardinia, Italy. *Acta Neurol Scand* **68:**394–404.

Giess R, Naumann M, Werner E et al. (2000). Injections of botulinum toxin A into the salivary glands improve sialorrhoea in amyotrophic lateral sclerosis. *J Neurol Neurosurg Psychiatry* **69:**121–123.

Gunnarsson L-G, Palm R (1984). Motor neuron disease and heavy labour: an epidemiological survey of Värmland county, Sweden. *Neuroepidemiology* **3:**195–206.

Højer-Pedersen E, Christensen PB, Jensen NB (1989). Incidence and prevalence of motor neuron disease in two Danish counties. *Neuroepidemiology* **8:**151–159.

Haberlandt WF (1959). Genetic aspects of amyotrphic lateral sclerosis and progressive bulbar paralysis. *Acta Genet Med Gemell* **8:**369–373.

Hanayama K, Ishikawa Y, Bach JR (1997). Amyotrophic lateral sclerosis: successful treatment of of mucous plugging by mechanical insufflation-exsufflation. *Am J Phys Med Rehabil* **76:**338–339.

Harriman M, Morrison M, Hay J et al. (2001). Use of radiotherapy for control of sialorrhea in patients with amyotrophic lateral sclerosis. *J Otolaryngol* **30:**242–245.

Haverkamp LJ, Appel V, Appel SH (1995). Natural history of amyotrophic lateral sclerosis in a database population. Validation of a scoring system and a model for survival prediction. *Brain* **118:**707–719.

Heffernan C, Jenkinson C, Holmes T et al. (2004). Nutritional management in MND/ALS patients: an evidence based review. *Amyotroph Lateral Scler Other Motor Neuron Disord* **5:**72–83.

Hockstein NG, Samadi DS, Gendron K, Handler SD (2004). Sialorrhea: a management challenge. *Am Fam Physician* **69:**2628–2634.

Hyson HC, Johnson AM, Jog MS (2002). Sublingual atropine for sialorrhea secondary to parkinsonism: a pilot study. *Mov Disord* **17:**1318–1320.

Iannaccone S, Ferini-Strambi L (1996). Pharmacologic treatment of emotional lability. *Clin Neuropharmacol* **19:**532–535.

Ince PG, Lowe J, Shaw PJ (1998). Amyotrophic lateral sclerosis: current issues in classification, pathogenesis and molecular pathology. *Neuropathol Appl Neurobiol* **24:**104–117.

Jackson M, Al-Chalabi A, Enayat ZE, Chioza B, Leigh PN, Morrison KE (1997). Copper/zinc superoxide dismutase 1 and sporadic amyotrophic lateral sclerosis: analysis of 155 cases and identification of a novel insertion mutation. *Ann Neurol* **42:**803–807.

Jokelainen M (1977). Amyotrophic lateral sclerosis in Finland. II: Clinical characteristics. *Acta Neurol Scand* **56**:194–204.

Jones CT, Swingler RJ, Simpson SA, Brock DJ (1995). Superoxide dismutase mutations in an unselected cohort of Scottish amyotrophic lateral sclerosis patients. *J Med Genet* **32**:290–292.

Kesiktas N, Paker N, Erdogan N, Gulsen G, Bicki D, Yilmaz H (2004). The use of hydrotherapy for the management of spasticity. *Neurorehabil Neural Repair* **18**:268–273.

Lacomblez L, Bensimon G, Leigh PN *et al.* (1996). Dose-ranging study of riluzole in amyotrophic lateral sclerosis. Amyotrophic Lateral Sclerosis/Riluzole Study Group II. *Lancet* **347**:1425–1431.

Lee JRJ, Annegers JF, Appel S (1995). Prognosis of ALS and the effects of referral selection *J Neurol Sci* **132(2)**:207–215.

Li TM, Day SJ, Alberman E, Swash M (1986). Differential diagnosis of motoneurone disease from other neurological conditions. *The Lancet* **2**:731–733.

Li T-M, Alberman E, Swash M (1988). Comparison of sporadic and familial disease amongst 580 cases of motor neuron disease. *J Neurol Neurosurg Psychiatry* **51**:778–784.

Lima, A; Evangelista T, de Carvalho M (2003). Increased Creatine Kinase and Spontaneous Activity on Electromyography, in Amyotrophic Lateral Sclerosis. *Electromyogr Clin Neurophysiol* **43**:189–192.

Lind SE, Good MD. Seidel S, Csordas T, Good BJ (1989). Telling the diagnosis in cancer. *J Clin Oncol* **7**:583–589.

Lyall RA, Donaldson N, Polkey MI, Leigh PN, Moxham J (2001). Respiratory muscle strength and ventilatory failure in amyotrophic lateral sclerosis. *Brain* **124**:2000–2013.

Marquardt G, Seifert V (2002). Use of intrathecal baclofen for treatment of spasticity in amyotrophic lateral sclerosis. *J Neurol Neurosurg Psychiatry* **72**:275–276.

Mathus-Vliegen LM, Louwerse LS, Merkus MP, Tytgat GN, Vianney de Jong JM (1994). Percutaneous endoscopic gastrostomy in patients with amyotrophic lateral sclerosis and impaired pulmonary function. *Gastrointest Endosc* **40**:463–469.

McCluskey L, Casarett D, Siderowf A (2004). Breaking the news: a survey of ALS patients and their caregivers. *Amyotroph Lateral Scler Other Motor Neuron Disord* **5**:131–135.

Meininger V (1999). Getting the diagnosis right: beyond El Escorial. *J Neurol* **246** (suppl 3)**:**III10–III15.

Mier RJ, Bachrach SJ, Lakin RC, Barker T, Childs J, Moran M (2000). Treatment of sialorrhea with glycopyrrolate: A double-blind, dose-ranging study. *Arch Pediatr Adolesc Med* **154**:1214–1218.

Miller RG (2001). Examining the evidence about treatment in ALS/MND. *Amyotroph Lateral Scler Other Motor Neuron Disord* **2**:3–7.

Miller RG, Mitchell JD, Lyon M, Moore DH (2002). Riluzole for amyotrophic lateral sclerosis (ALS/motor neuron disease (MND). Cochrane Database Syst Rev **(2)**:CD001447.

Murphy J (2004). Communication strategies of people with ALS and their partners. *Amyotroph Lateral Scler Other Motor Neuron Disord* **5**:121–126.

Murray TJ, Pride S, Haley G (1974). Motor neuron disease in Nova Scotia. *CMA J* **110**:814–817.

Murros K, Fogelholm R (1983). Amyotrophic lateral sclerosis in middle-Finland: an epidemiological study. *Acta Neurol Scand* **67**:41–47.

Newall AR, Orser R, Hunt M (1996). The control of oral secretions in bulbar ALS/MND. *J Neurol Sci* **139(Suppl)**:43–44.

Niemann S, Joos H, Meyer T *et al.* (2004). Familial ALS in Germany: origin of the R115G SOD1 mutation by a founder effect. *J Neurol Neurosurg Psychiatry* **75**:1186–1188.

Norris FH Jr, U KS, Sachais B, Carey M. (1979). Trial of baclofen in amyotrophic lateral sclerosis. *Arch Neurol* **36**:715–716.

Oliver D, Borasio GD, Walsh D, eds. (2000). *Palliative Care in Amyotrophic Lateral Sclerosis*. Oxford University Press, Oxford.

Orrell RW, Habgood JJ, Gardiner I *et al.* (1997). Clinical and functional investigation of 10 missense mutations and a novel frameshift insertion mutation of the gene for copper-zinc superoxide dismutase in UK families with amyotrophic lateral sclerosis. *Neurology* **48**:746–751.

Poeck K (1996). Pathologisches lachen und weinen bei bulber amyotrophischer lateralsklerose. *Deutsche Med Wochenschr* **94**:310–314.

Porta M, Gamba M, Bertacchi G, Vaj P (2001). Treatment of sialorrhoea with ultrasound guided botulinum toxin A injection in patients with neurological disorders. *J Neurol Neurosurg Psychiatry* **70**:538–540.

Rosen AD (1978). Amyotrophic lateral sclerosis. Clinical features and prognosis. *Arch Neurol* **35**: 638–642.

Ross MA, Miller RG, Berchert L *et al.* (1998). Towards earlier diagnosis of ALS. Revised criteria. *Neurology* **50**:768–772.

Sancho J, Servera E, Diaz J, Marin J (2004). Efficacy of mechanical insufflation-exsufflation in medically stable patients with amyotrophic lateral sclerosis. *Chest* **125**:1400–1405.

dos Santos MT, de Oliveira LM (2004). Use of cryotherapy to enhance mouth opening in patients with cerebral palsy. *Spec Care Dentist* **24:**232–234.

Schiffer RB, Herndon RM, Rudick RA (1985). Treatment of pathological laughing and weeping with amitriptyline. *N Engl J Med* **312:**1480–1482.

Scott AG, Austin HE (1994). Nasogastric feeding in the management of severe dysphagia in motor neurone disease. *Palliat Med* **8:**45–49.

Shaw CE, Enayat ZE, Chioza BA *et al.* (1998). Mutations in all five exons of SOD-1 may cause ALS. *Ann Neurol* **43:**390–394.

Shaw AS, Ampong MA, Rio A, McClure J, Leigh PN, Sidhu PS (2004). Entristar skin-level gastrostomy tube: primary placement with radiologic guidance in patients with amyotrophic lateral sclerosis. *Radiology* **233:**392–399.

Stalpers LJ, Moser EC (2002). Results of radiotherapy for drooling in amyotrophic lateral sclerosis. *Neurology* **58:**1308.

Sykes N, Thorns A (2003). The use of opioids and sedatives at the end of life. *Lancet Oncology* **4:**312–318.

Talmi YP, Finkelstein Y, Zohar Y (1989). Reduction of salivary flow in amyotrophic lateral sclerosis with Scopoderm TTS. *Head Neck* **11:**565.

Talmi YP, Finkelstein Y, Zohar Y. (1990). Reduction of salivary flow with transdermal scopolamine: a four-year experience. *Otolaryngol Head Neck Surg* **103:**615–618.

Tan EK, Lo YL, Seah A, Auchus AP (2001). Recurrent jaw dislocation after botulinum toxin treatment for sialorrhoea in amyotrophic lateral sclerosis. *J Neurol Sci* **190:**95–97.

Thijs V, Peeters E, Theys P, Matthijs G, Robberecht W (2000). Demographic characteristics and prognosis in a Flemish amyotrophic lateral sclerosis population. *Acta Neurol Belg* **100:**84–90.

Thornton FJ, Fotheringham T, Alexander M, Hardiman O, McGrath FP, Lee MJ (2002). Amyotrophic lateral sclerosis: enteral nutrition provision–endoscopic or radiologic gastrostomy? *Radiology* **224:**713–717.

Traynor BJ, Codd MB, Corr B, Forde C, Frost E, Hardiman O (2000). Amyotrophic Lateral sclerosis mimic syndromes. *Arch Neurol* **57:**109–113.

Traynor BJ, Alexander M, Corr B *et al.* (2003). Effects of a multidisciplinary ALS clinic on survival. *J Neurol Neurosurg Psychiatry* **74:**1258–1261.

Wilbourn AJ (1998). Clinical neurophysiology in the diagnosis of amyotrophic lateral sclerosis: the Lambert and the El Escorial criteria. *J Neurol Sci* **160(Suppl 1):**S25–29.

Winterholler MG, Erbguth FJ, Wolf S, Kat S (2001). Botulinum toxin for the treatment of sialorrhoea in ALS: serious side effects of a transductal approach. *J Neurol Neurosurg Psychiatry* **70:**417–418.

Winterholler MG, Heckmann JG, Hecht M, Erbguth FJ (2002). Recurrent trismus and stridor in an ALS patient: successful treatment with botulinum toxin. *Neurology* **58:**502–503.

Previous guidelines or recommendations:

Gasser T, Dichgans M, Finsterer J *et al.* (2001). EFNS task force on molecular diagnosis of neurologic disorders. Part 1. *Eur J Neurol* **8:**299–314.

Howard RS, Orrell RW (2002). Management of motor neurone disease. *Postgrad Med J* **78:**736–741.

Jennings AL, Davies AN, Higgins JP, Gibbs JS, Broadley KE (2002). A systematic review of the use of opioids in the management of dyspnoea. *Thorax* **57:**939–944.

Leigh PN, Abrahams S, Al-Chalabi A *et al.* (2003). The management of motor neurone disease. *J Neurol Neurosurg Psychiatry* **70(Suppl IV):**iv32–iv47.

Miller RG, Rosenberg JA, Gelinas DF *et al.* (1999). Practice parameter: the care of the patient with amyotrophic lateral sclerosis (an evidence-based review): report of the Quality Standards Subcommittee of the American Academy of Neurology: ALS Practice Parameters Task Force. *Neurology* **52:**1311–1323.

CHAPTER 21

Post-polio syndrome

E. Farbu,*[a] N.E. Gilhus,[a] M.P. Barnes,[b] K. Borg,[c]
M. de Visser,[d] A. Driessen,[e] R. Howard,[f] F. Nollet,[g]
J. Opara,[h] E. Stalberg[i]

Abstract

Background Post-polio syndrome (PPS) is characterised by new or increased muscular weakness, atrophy, muscle pain and fatigue several years after acute polio.

Objectives To prepare diagnostic criteria for PPS, and to evaluate the existing evidence for therapeutic interventions.

Methods The Medline, EMBASE and ISI databases were searched. Consensus in the group was reached after discussion by e-mail.

We recommend Halstead's definition of PPS from 1991 as diagnostic criteria. Supervised, aerobic muscular training, both isokinetic and isometric is a safe and effective way to prevent further decline for patients with moderate weakness (Level B). Muscular training can also improve muscular fatigue, muscle weakness and pain. Training in a warm climate and non-swimming water exercises are particularly useful (Level B). Respiratory muscle training can improve pulmonary function. Recognition of respiratory impairment and early introduction of non-invasive ventilatory aids prevent or delay further respiratory decline and the need for invasive respiratory aid (Level C). Group training, regular follow-up and patient education are useful for the patients' mental status and well being. Weight loss, adjustment and introduction of properly fitted assistive devices should be considered (Good Practice Points). A small number of controlled studies of potential specific treatments for PPS have been completed, but no definitive therapeutic effect has been reported for the agents evaluated (pyridostigmine, corticosteroids, amantadine). Future randomised trials should particularly address the treatment of pain, which is commonly reported by PPS patients. There is also

*Present address: Neurocenter, Stavanger University Hospital, N-4068 Stavanger, Norway.

[a]Department of Neurology, Haukeland University Hospital, and University of Bergen, Bergen, Norway; [b]Academic Unit of Neurological Rehabilitation, Hunters Moor Hospital, Newcastle upon Tyne, UK; [c]Division of Rehabilitation Medicine, Department of Public Health Sciences and Danderyds University Hospital, Karolinska Intitutet, Karolinska Hospital, Stockholm, Sweden;

[d]Department of Neurology, Academic Medical Center, University of Amsterdam, the Netherlands; [e]Lt. Gen. Van Heutzlaan 6, 3743 JN Baarn, The Netherlands; [f]Department of Neurology, St. Thomas' Hospital, London, UK; [g]Department of Rehabilitation Medicine, Academic Medical Center, University of Amsterdam, the Netherlands; [h]Repty Rehab Centre. ul. Sniadeckio 1, PL 42-604 Tarnowskie Góry, Poland; [i]Department of Clinical Neurophysiology, University Hospital, Uppsala, Sweden.

a need for studies evaluating the long-term effects of muscular training.

Objectives

The aim was to develop a common definition of PPS and evaluate the existing evidence for the clinical effectiveness of therapeutic interventions and on this basis provide clinical guidelines for the management of PPS.

Background

Many patients with a history of previous polio experience new muscle weakness, new atrophy, fatigue, muscular and joint pain, and cold intolerance several years after acute paralytic poliomyelitis. A case of new atrophy and weakness many years after acute paralytic polio was first described in 1875 by Raymond (Raymond, 1875).

The term post-polio syndrome (PPS) was introduced by Halstead in 1985 to cover medical, orthopaedic, and psychological problems possibly or indirectly related to the long-term disability occurring many years after the acute episode. The criteria for PPS were:

1. Confirmed history of polio.
2. Partial or fairly complete neurological and functional recovery after the acute episode.
3. Period of at least 15 years with neurological and functional stability.
4. Two or more of the following health problems occurring after the stable period: extensive fatigue, muscle and/or joint pain, new weakness in muscles previously affected or unaffected, new muscle atrophy, functional loss, cold intolerance.
5. No other medical explanation found (Halstead and Rossi, 1985).

Halstead revised these criteria in 1991 and added 'gradual or abrupt onset of new neurogenic weakness' as a necessary criterion for PPS, with or without other co-existing symptoms (Halstead, 1991).

Dalakas redefined and narrowed the use of PPS in 1995. He combined the criteria for post-polio muscular atrophy (PPMA), that is, new muscular atrophy at least 15 years after the acute infection, and the following symptoms: fatigue and decreased endurance, increase in skeletal deformities and pain in joints (Dalakas, 1995). A third term, post-polio muscular dysfunction (PPMD), was introduced in 1996 with the following criteria:

1. History of paralytic polio; confirmed or not confirmed; partial or fairly complete functional recovery.
2. After a period of functional stability of at least 15 years development of new muscle dysfunction: muscle weakness, muscle atrophy, muscle pain, fatigue.
3. Neurological examination compatible with prior polio: lower motor neurone lesion; decreased or absent tendon reflexes; no sensory loss; compatible findings on EMG and/or MRI (Borg, 1996).

The symptoms reported for PPS are the same from all parts of the world. Muscle weakness, atrophy, generalised fatigue, post-exercise fatigue, muscle pain, fasciculations, cramps, cold intolerance, and joint pain dominate (Halstead and Rossi, 1985; Ivanyi et al., 1999; Jubelt and Agre, 2000; Chang and Huang, 2001; Farbu and Gilhus, 2001, 2002; Farbu et al., 2003; Rekand et al., 2003; Takemura et al., 2004). A history of previous paralytic polio seems to increase long-term mortality (Nielsen et al., 2003).

The prevalence of PPS has been reported from 15 to 80% of all patients with previous polio depending on the criteria applied and population studied (Halstead and Rossi, 1987; Ramlow et al., 1992; Dalakas, 1995; Halstead, 1998; Ivanyi et al., 1999; Burger and Marincek, 2000; Farbu et al., 2003). In many population-based studies, terms like 'late onset polio symptoms' have been used instead of PPS. Hospital-based studies use the term PPS, but in these studies it is always debatable whether the patient material is representative. Exact prevalence of PPS is therefore difficult to establish. For European populations, one Dutch study reported a prevalence of late onset polio symptoms of 46%, one study from Edinburgh reported a prevalence of more than 60%, in Estonia a prevalence of 52% has been reported, Norway 60%, and Denmark 63% (Lonnberg, 1993; Ivanyi *et al.*, 1999; Pentland *et al.*, 2000; Rekand *et al.*, 2003).

For symptomatic treatment and clinical purposes the difference between stable muscle weakness after polio and PPS often remains insignificant. Still, it would be of great benefit to have a consensus on the term PPS, both for clinical use, and for research. All three definitions are based on the principle of exclusion of other causes for new deterioration and new symptoms. Halstead claimed that two different symptoms, like joint pain and cold intolerance, were sufficient for a diagnosis of PPS, but later redefined and included new neurogenic muscle weakness as an obligatory criterion for the diagnosis. Dalakas proposed an even more focused neuromuscular approach where new atrophy was the cornerstone. Many patients report a sense of weakening in the muscles before it is detectable by clinical examination as new atrophy. These findings can be confirmed by isometric muscle strength evaluation and computer tomography imaging (Ivanyi *et al.*, 1998; Lygren *et al.*, 2005, unpublished observation). Atrophy is the end stage of new neuromuscular deterioration and by using this as a necessary criterion, patients in an earlier stage of neuromuscular deterioration will be excluded.

We suggest that the criteria for PPS used within the European Federation of Neurological Societies (EFNS) and Europe should be based on Halstead's definition from 1991 with emphasis on the new muscle weakness. The diagnosis of PPS is an exclusion diagnosis with no test or analysis specific for PPS, and the role of the investigation is to rule out every other possible cause for the new symptoms and clinical deterioration (Cashman *et al.*, 1987; Dalakas, 1995).

Role of clinical neurophysiology

Clinical neurophysiology is used for four main reasons. First, to establish typical lower motor neuron involvement (neurogenic electromyography (EMG) findings, normal sensory findings, and normal motor findings except for parameters reflecting muscle atrophy). Second, to exclude other causes. This is part of the PPS definition, and it is not uncommon to find patients in whom the initial diagnosis of polio must be revised. Third, to find concomitant nerve or muscle disorders, such as entrapments and radiculopathies. Fourth, to assess the degree of motor neuron loss. This cannot be quantified clinically, as loss of neurons may be completely masked by compensatory nerve sprouting and muscle fibre hypertrophy. Macro EMG studies have shown that loss of up to 50% of neurons may be compatible with a normal clinical picture (Stalberg and Grimby, 1995).

In longitudinal studies with macro EMG a continuous loss of neurons is demonstrated with exaggerated speed compared to normal age dependent degeneration (Grimby *et al.*, 1998). New weakness appears when the compensatory mechanisms are no longer sufficient, and occurs when macro motor unit potential (MUP) exceeds 20 times the normal size (Grimby *et al.*, 1998).

Search strategy

Medline via Pubmed, EMBASE, ISI and the Cochrane Library were searched from 1966 until 2004. Search terms were post-polio syndrome/post poliomyelitis/PPMA/PPMD/poliomyelitis in combination with management, therapy, treatment, medicaments, physiotherapy and intervention.

No meta-analyses of interventions for PPS were found when searching the databases.

Data were classified according to their scientific level of evidence as class I–IV (Brainin *et al.*, 2004). Recommendations are given as Level A to C according to the scheme for EFNS guidelines. When only class IV evidence was available but consensus could be reached the Task Force gives our recommendations as Good Practice Points (Brainin *et al.*, 2004). Consensus was reached mainly through e-mail correspondence.

A questionnaire about diagnosis, management, and care of post-polio patients was answered by the group members from The Netherlands, Norway, Poland, Sweden, and the United Kingdom.

Results

National surveys

None of the countries represented in this task force had formal national guidelines for PPS, for diagnosis or treatment. Diagnostic criteria applied were those of Halstead (Sweden), Borg (the Netherlands) and Dalakas (Norway). There were no national competence centres in any of the countries. Medical specialities involved were mainly physical medicine and rehabilitation, neurology, clinical neurophysiology, respiratory medicine and orthopaedics. Neurologists were involved in diagnosis whereas rehabilitation physicians were involved in long-term management and care. In the United Kingdom, PPS patients were mainly taken care of by their general practitioners with less contact with the secondary level of the health service.

Therapeutic interventions

Acetylcholinesterase inhibitors, steroids and amantadine

The effect of pyridostigmine in PPS has been investigated in four studies with particular emphasis on fatigue, muscular strength and quality of life. Two open pilot studies indicated a positive effect on fatigue (Trojan et al., 1993; Trojan and Cashman, 1995), but this was not confirmed in two double-blinded randomised controlled trials using a daily dose of 180 mg pyridostigmine (Trojan et al., 1999; Horemans et al., 2003). Horemans et al. reported a significant improvement in walking performance, but the difference in quadriceps strength was not significant as reported by Trojan et al. Hence, there is evidence at Class I that pyridostigmine is not effective in the management of fatigue and muscular strength in PPS. There are two randomised placebo controlled studies investigating the effect of high dose prednisolone (80 mg daily) and amantandine (200 mg daily) on muscular weakness and fatigue (prednisone) and fatigue (amantadine) (Dinsmore et al., 1995; Stein et al., 1995). They included a small number of patients, 17 and 23 respectively, and only Stein et al. included statistical power calculations. There was no significant effect on muscular strength or fatigue in any of these Class I studies.

Muscular training

It has been claimed that muscular overuse and training may worsen the symptoms in PPS and even provoke a further loss of muscular strength (Bennett and Knowlton, 1958). Many post-polio patients have been advised to avoid muscular overuse and intensive training (Halstead and Gawne, 1996; March of Dimes, 2000). Studies of muscle morphology and oxidative capacity in the tibialis anterior muscle indicate a high muscular activity due to gait and weight bearing (Borg and Henriksson, 1991; Grimby et al., 1996). When followed prospectively, the macro EMG MUP amplitude in the tibialis anterior muscle was found to be increased after 5 years, whereas there was no change in the macro MUP amplitude in the biceps brachii muscle (Sandberg and Stalberg, 2004). This indicates a more pronounced denervation–reinnervation process in the tibialis muscle, which may be due to daily use and higher muscle activities in the leg muscles. However, there are no prospective studies that show that increased muscle activity or training lead to loss of muscular strength compared to absence of training or less muscular activity. On the contrary, patients who reported regular physical activity had less symptoms and a higher functional level than physically inactive patients (Veicsteinas et al., 1998; Rekand et al., 2004). One randomised controlled trial reported significant improvement in muscular strength after a 12-week training programme with isometric contraction of hand muscles (Chan et al., 2003). Non-randomised trials with training programmes lasting from 6 weeks to 6 months involving both isokinetic, isometric and endurance muscular training have shown a significant increase in both isokinetic and isometric muscle strength (Einarsson, 1991; Ernstoff et al., 1996; Spector et al., 1996; Agre et al., 1997). No complications or side effects were reported. Hence, there is evidence at class II and III that supervised training programmes increase muscle strength in patients with post-polio syndrome. It should be added that the long-term effects (years) of training are not documented, and deserve prospective studies. For patients without cardiovascular disease, one randomised controlled study reported improved cardiovascular fitness after supervised exercise programmes using ergometer cycles (Jones *et al.*, 1989) (Class I). Aerobic training in upper extremities had beneficial effects on oxygen consumption, minute ventilation, power, and exercise time (Kriz *et al.*, 1992) (Class II). Aerobic walking exercises can help to economise movements and increase endurance without improvement in cardiovascular fitness (Dean and Ross, 1991). Ernstoff *et al.* reported an increase in work performance by reduction of heart rate during exercises; hence endurance training seems to improve cardiovascular conditioning (Class IV). It is important to emphasize that most exercise studies have been executed with supervision, submaximal work load, intermittent breaks, and rest periods between exercise sessions to prevent the likelihood of overuse effects. This is an important aspect for any PPS patient. With supervision we mean that particularly skilled therapists should advise the training participants with respect to work load, exercise technique, time consumption and rest periods during performances. Most of the participating patients in these studies were below 60 years of age. The effect of exercise programmes for subjects older than 60 years is therefore less documented.

One randomised controlled study of post-polio patients with pain, weakness, and fatigue in their shoulder muscles compared the effect of exercise only, exercise in combination with lifestyle modification, and lifestyle modification only (Klein *et al.*, 2002). All three groups improved after intervention, but a significant difference was found only for the two groups with exercise (Class II). The endpoints in this study were combinations of several symptoms. Further studies are needed to identify improvement on particular symptoms before conclusions are drawn regarding lifestyle modifications.

Treatment in a warm climate and training in water

Anecdotal reports from post-polio patients indicate a positive effect of a warm climate and of training in warm water with respect to pain and fatigue. One randomised controlled study reported a significant reduction in pain, health-related problems and depression for both groups after completing identical training programmes in either Norway or Tenerife (Strumse *et al.*, 2003). No significant difference in walking tests was seen. Both groups improved their walking skills, reduced their level of fatigue, depression, and health-related problems. However, the effect remained significantly longer in the Tenerife group (Class I).

Dynamic non-swimming water exercises for post-polio patients have been reported to reduce pain, improve cardiovascular conditioning, and increase subjective well-being in a controlled but not randomised study (Class III) (Willen *et al.*, 2001). A qualitative interview study (Class IV) indicated a positive effect on the self-confidence when performing group training in water (Willen and Scherman, 2002).

Respiratory aid

Reduced pulmonary function due to weak respiratory muscles and/or chest deformities may occur in patients with previous polio (Howard *et al.*, 1988; Kidd *et al.*, 1997). Patients with chest deformities have an increased risk of nocturnal hypoventilation and sleep-disordered breathing (Bergholtz, 1988; Howard *et al.*, 1988, Howard, 2003). The prevalence of respiratory impairment is highest among patients who were treated with artificial ventilation in the acute phase (Howard *et al.*, 1988). Shortness of breath is a common complaint in many post-polio patients, but is not necessarily related to respiratory impairment. Two hospital-based studies showed that respiratory function was normal in the majority of patients reporting shortness of breath, and cardiovascular deconditioning and being overweight were the most common causes for this symptom (Stanghelle *et al.*, 1993; Farbu *et al.*, 2003). Respiratory impairment can occur without shortness of breath and can present with daytime somnolence, morning headache, and fatigue (Dean *et al.*, 1991). There are no randomised trials evaluating the effect of respiratory aids. Reports indicate that early introduction of non-invasive respiratory aids like intermittent positive pressure ventilation (IPPV) or biphasic positive pressure (BIPAP) ventilators via mouthpiece or nasal application can stabilise the situation and prevent complications like chest infections, further respiratory decline and invasive ventilatory aid (tracheostomy) (Bergholtz *et al.*, 1988; Bach, 1995), and also improve exercise capacity (Vaz Fragoso *et al.*, 1992) (Class IV). If invasive ventilatory aid is needed, PPS patients with a tracheostomy and mechanical home ventilation are reported to have good perceived health despite severe physical disability (Markstrom *et al.*, 2002) (Class III). For patients already using intermittent respiratory aids, respiratory muscle training is useful (Klefbeck *et al.*, 2000) (Class IV). General precautions like stopping smoking, mobilisation of secretions, and cough assistance are beneficial (Bergholtz *et al.*, 1988).

Bulbar symptoms

Weakening of the bulbar muscles causing dysphagia, weakness of voice and vocal changes have been reported among patients with PPS (Sonies and Dalakas, 1991; Ivanyi *et al.*, 1994; Driscoll *et al.*, 1995; Abaza *et al.*, 2001). Case reports indicate that speech therapy and laryngeal muscle training are useful for these patients (Class IV) (Abaza *et al.*, 2001).

Weight control, assistive devices and lifestyle modifications

The importance of reducing weight, adaptation to assistive devices and modification of activities of daily living has been emphasised (Halstead *et al.*, 1995; Thorsteinsson, 1997; Jubelt and Agre, 2000; March of Dimes, 2000). The scientific evidence for these recommendations is limited, but there was consensus in our group that an individual with weak muscles benefits from losing excess weight, and that proper orthoses, walking sticks, and wheelchairs facilitate daily life activities (Good Practice Points). Participating in muscle training programmes and endurance training will, in many cases, also lead to weight loss, but there is no evidence that weight reduction alone can ameliorate symptoms. Patients with BMI (body mass index) >25 which is defined as overweight, did not report more symptoms than those of normal weight (Farbu *et al.*, 2003). On the other hand, a recent weight gain was found to be a predictive factor for PPS (Trojan *et al.*, 1994). Sleep disorders are

common among PPS patients (Farbu *et al.*, 2003), and can be a mix of obstructive sleep apnoea, frequency of tiredness on waking up and during the day, headache on waking up, daytime sleepiness, restless legs, and hypoventilation (Steljes *et al.*, 1990; Van Kralingen *et al.*, 1996; Hsu and Staats, 1998). It is widely accepted that obesity is related to obstructive sleep apnoea, and weight control is crucial for this disorder (Gami *et al.*, 2003). The number of patients receiving mechanical home ventilation because of obesity-induced hypoventilation has increased (Janssens *et al.*, 2003). From this perspective, there is a rationale for reducing excess weight in PPS patients (Class IV).

One pilot study reported that a change from metal braces to light weight carbon orthoses can be useful and increase walking ability in polio patients with new pareses (Heim *et al.*, 1997). Biomechanical analysis of the walking pattern can lead to optimal design of orthoses and improve function in the lower limbs (Class IV) (Perry and Clark, 1997).

Frequent periods of rest, energy conservation, and work simplification skills are thought to be useful for patients with fatigue (Packer *et al.*, 1991).

Coming to terms with new disabilities, educational interventions

New loss of function, increase in disability and handicap are common in post-polio patients (Ivanyi *et al.*, 1999; Nollet *et al.*, 1999; Farbu *et al.*, 2003). This can lead to reduced well-being and emotional stress. Group training with other post-polio patients, participation and regular follow-up at post-polio clinics can prevent a decline in mental status and give a more positive experience of the 'self' (Stanghelle and Festvag, 1997; Willen and Scherman, 2002)(Class III). Acceptance of assistive devices, environmental support and spending more time on daily tasks can facilitate coping with home and occupational life (Class III) (Thoren-Jonsson, 2001).

RECOMMENDATIONS

Level A: A small number of controlled studies of potential specific treatments for PPS have been completed, but no definitive therapeutic effect has been reported for the agents evaluated (pyridostigmine, steroids, and amantadine)

Level B: Supervised muscular training, both isokinetic and isometric, is a safe and effective way to prevent further decline of muscle strength in slightly or moderately weak muscle groups and can even reduce symptoms of muscular fatigue, muscle weakness and pain in selected post-polio patients. There are no studies evaluating the effect of muscular training in patients with severe weakness and the long-term effects of such training is not yet explored. Precautions to avoid muscular overuse should be taken with intermittent breaks, periods of rest between series of exercises and submaximal work load.

Training in a warm climate and non-swimming water exercises are particularly useful.

Level C: Recognition of respiratory impairment and early introduction of non-invasive ventilatory aids prevent or delay further respiratory decline and the need of invasive respiratory aids.

Respiratory muscle training can improve pulmonary function.

Group training, regular follow-ups and patient education are useful for the patients' mental status and well-being.

Good Practice Points: Weight loss, and adjustment and introduction of properly fitted assistive devices; but lack significant scientific evidence.

Conflicts of interests
The authors have reported no conflicts of interests.

References
Abaza MM, Sataloff RT, Hawkshaw MJ, Mandel S (2001). Laryngeal manifestations of postpoliomyelitis syndrome. *J Voice* **15**:291–294.

Agre JC, Rodriquez AA, Franke TM (1997). Strength, endurance, and work capacity after muscle strengthening exercise in postpolio subjects. *Arch Phys Med Rehabil* **78**:681–686.

Bach JR (1995). Management of post-polio respiratory sequelae. *Ann New York Acad Sci* **753**:96–102.

Bennett RL, Knowlton GC (1958). Overwork weakness in partially denervated skeletal muscle. *Clin Orthoped* **15**:22–29.

Bergholtz B, Mollestad SO, Refsum H (1988). [Post-polio respiratory failure. New manifestations of a forgotten disease]. *Tidsskrift for den Norske Laegeforening* **108**:2474–2475.

Borg K (1996). Post-polio muscle dysfunction 29th ENMC workshop 14–16 October 1994, Naarden, the Netherlands. *Neuromusc Disord* **6**:75–80.

Borg K, Henriksson J (1991). Prior poliomyelitis-reduced capillary supply and metabolic enzyme content in hypertrophic slow-twitch (type I) muscle fibres. *J Neurol Neurosurg Psychiatry* **54**:236–240.

Brainin M, Barnes M, Baron J-C, Gilhus NE, Hughes R, Selmaj K, Waldemar G (2004). Guidance for the preparation of neurological management guidelines by EFNS scientific task forces - revised recommendations 2004. *Euro J Neurol* **11**:1–6.

Burger H, Marincek C (2000). The influence of post-polio syndrome on independence and life satisfaction. *Disabil Rehabil* **22**:318–322.

Cashman NR, R. Maselli *et al.* (1987). Late denervation in patients with antecedent paralytic poliomyelitis. *New Engl J Med* **317**:7–12.

Chan KM, Amirjani N, Sumrain M, Clarke A, Strohschein FJ (2003). Randomized controlled trial of strength training in post-polio patients. *Muscle & Nerve* **27**:332–338.

Chang C-W, Huang S-F (2001). Varied clinical patterns, physical activities, muscle enzymes, electromyographic and histologic findings in patients with post-polio syndrome in Taiwan. *Spinal Cord* **39**:526–531.

Dalakas MC (1995). The post-polio syndrome as an evolved clinical entity. Definition and clinical description. *Ann New York Acad Sci* **753**:68–80.

Dean E, Ross J (1991). Effect of modified aerobic training on movement energetics in polio survivors. *Orthopedics* **14**:1243–1246.

Dean E, Ross J, Road DJ, Courtenay L, Madill KJ (1991). Pulmonary function in individuals with a history of poliomyelitis. *Chest* **100**:118–123.

Dinsmore S, Dambrosia J, Dalakas MC (1995). A double-blind, placebo-controlled trial of high-dose prednisone for the treatment of post-poliomyelitis syndrome. *Ann New York Acad Sci* **753**:303–313.

Driscoll BP, Gracco C, Coelho C, Goldstein J, Oshima K, Tierney E, Sasaki CT (1995). Laryngeal function in postpolio patients. *Laryngoscope* **105**:35–41.

Einarsson G (1991). Muscle conditioning in late poliomyelitis. *Arch Phys Med Rehabil* **72:**11–14.

Ernstoff B, Wetterqvist H, Kvist H, Grimby G (1996). Endurance training effect on individuals with postpoliomyelitis. *Arch Phys Med Rehabil* **77:**843–848.

Farbu E, Gilhus NE (2001). Polio as a socioeconomic and health factor. A paired sibling study. *J Neurol* **249:**404–409.

Farbu E, Gilhus NE (2002). Education, occupation, and perception of health amongst previous polio patients compared to their siblings. *Euro J Neurol* **9:**233–241.

Farbu E, Rekand T, Gilhus NE (2003). Post polio syndrome and total health status in a prospective hospital study. *Euro J Neurol* **10:**407–413.

Gami AS, Caples SM, Somers VK (2003). Obesity and obstructive sleep apnea. *Endocrinol Metabol Clin North Amer* **32:**869–894.

Gonzalez H, Khademi M, Andersson M, Piehl F, Wallstrom E, Borg K, Olsson T (2004). Prior poliomyelitis-IvIg treatment reduces proinflammatory cytokine production. *J Neuroimmunol* **150:**139–144.

Grimby L, Tollback A, Muller U, Larsson L (1996). Fatigue of chronically overused motor units in prior polio patients. *Muscle & Nerve* **19:**728–737.

Grimby G, Stalberg E, Sandberg A, Sunnerhagen KS (1998). An 8-year longitudinal study of muscle strength, muscle fiber size, and dynamic electromyogram in individuals with late polio. *Muscle & Nerve* **21:**1428–1437.

Halstead LS (1991). Assessment and differential diagnosis for post-polio syndrome. *Orthopedics* **14:**1209–1217.

Halstead LS (1998). Post-polio syndrome. *Sci Amer* **278:**42–47.

Halstead LS, Gawne AC (1996). NRH proposal for limb classification and exercise prescription. *Disabil Rehabil* **18:**311–316.

Halstead LS, Gawne AC, Pham BT (1995). National rehabilitation hospital limb classification for exercise, research, and clinical trials in post-polio patients. *Ann New York Acad Sci* **753:**343–353.

Halstead LS, Rossi CD (1985). New problems in old polio patients: results of a survey of 539 polio survivors. *Orthopedics* **8:**845–850.

Halstead LS, Rossi CD (1987). Post-polio syndrome: clinical experience with 132 consecutive outpatients. *Birth Defects Original Article Series* **23:**13–26.

Heim M, Yaacobi E, Azaria M (1997). A pilot study to determine the efficiency of lightweight carbon fibre orthoses in the management of patients suffering from post-poliomyelitis syndrome. *Clin Rehabil* **11:**302–305.

Horemans HLD, Nollet F, Beelen A, Drost G, Stegeman DF, Zwarts MJ, Bussmann JBJ, De Visser M, Lankhorst GJ (2003). Pyridostigmine in postpolio syndrome: No decline in fatigue and limited functional improvement. *J Neurol Neurosurg Psychiatry* **74:**1655–1661.

Howard RS, Wiles CM, Spencer GT (1988). The late sequelae of poliomyelitis. *Quart J Med* **66:**219–232.

Howard R (2003). Late post-polio functional deterioration. *Pract Neurol* **3:**66–77.

Hsu AA, Staats BA (1998). 'Postpolio' sequelae and sleep-related disordered breathing. *Mayo Clinic Proceedings* **73:**216–224.

Ivanyi B, Phoa SS, De Visser M (1994). Dysphagia in postpolio patients: a videofluorographic follow-up study. *Dysphagia* **9:**96–98.

Ivanyi B, Redekop W, De Jongh R, De Visser M (1998). Computed tomographic study of the skeletal musculature of the lower body in 45 postpolio patients. *Muscle & Nerve* **21:**540–542.

Ivanyi B, Nollet F, Redekop WK, De Haan R, Wohlgemuht M, Van Wijngaarden JK, De Visser M (1999). Late onset polio sequelae: disabilities and handicaps in a population-based cohort of the 1956 poliomyelitis outbreak in the Netherlands. *Arch Phys Med Rehabil* **80:**687–690.

Janssens J-P, Derivaz S, Breitenstein E, De Muralt B, Fitting J-W, Chevrolet J-C, Rochat T (2003). Changing patterns in long-term noninvasive ventilation: A 7-year prospective study in the Geneva Lake Area. *Chest* **123:**67–79.

Jones DR, Speier J, Canine K, Owen R, Stull A (1989). Cardiorespiratory responses to aerobic training by patients with postpoliomyelitis sequelae. *JAMA* **261:**3255–3258.

Jubelt B, Agre JC (2000). Characteristics and management of postpolio syndrome. *JAMA* **284:**412–414.

Kidd D, Howard RS, Williams AJ, Heatley FW, Panayiotopoulos CP, Spencer GT (1997). Late functional deterioration following paralytic poliomyelitis. *QJM: Monthly J Assoc Phys* **90:**189–196.

Klefbeck B, Lagerstrand L, Mattsson E (2000). Inspiratory muscle training in patients with prior polio who use part-time assisted ventilation. *Arch Phys Med Rehabil* **81:**1065–1071.

Klein MG, Whyte J, Esquenazi A, Keenan MA, Costello R (2002). A comparison of the effects of exercise and lifestyle modification on the resolution of overuse symptoms of the shoulder in polio survivors: a preliminary study. *Arch Phys Med Rehabil* **83:**708–713.

Kriz JL, Jones DR, Speier JL, Canine JK, Owen RR, Serfass RC (1992). Cardiorespiratory responses to upper extremity aerobic training by postpolio subjects. *Arch Phys Med Rehabil* **73:**49–54.

Lonnberg F (1993). Late onset polio sequelae in Denmark – presentation and results of a nation-wide survey of 3 607 polio survivors. *Scand J Rehabil Med Suppl* **28:**7–15.

Lygren H, Jones KO, Grenstad T, Dreyer V, Farbu E, Rekand T. Perceived disability, fatigue, pain, and measured isometric muscle strength in polio survivors. Physiotherpy Research International 2006, Submitted.

March of Dimes (2000). March of Dimes International Conference on Post Polio Syndrome. Identifying Best Practices in Diagnosis and Care. March of Dimes, White Plains, NY, USA.

Markstrom A, Sundell K, Lysdahl M, Andersson G, Schedin U, Klang B (2002). Quality-of-life evaluation of patients with neuromuscular and skeletal diseases treated with noninvasive and invasive home mechanical ventilation. *Chest* **122:** 1695–1700.

Nielsen NM, Rostgaard K, Juel K, Askgaard D, Aaby P (2003). Long-term mortality after poliomyelitis. *Epidemiology* **14:**355–360.

Nollet F, Beelen A, Prins MH, De Visser M, Sargeant AJ, Lankhorst GJ, De Jong BA (1999). Disability and functional assessment in former polio patients with and without postpolio syndrome. *Arch Physl Med Rehabil* **80:**136–143.

Packer TL, Martins I, Krefting L, Brouwer B (1991). Activity and post-polio fatigue. *Orthopedics* **14:**1223–1226.

Pentland B, Hellawel D, Benjamin J, Prasad R, Ainslie A (2000). *Health Bulletin* **58:**267–275.

Perry J, Clark D (1997). Biomechanical abnormalities of post-polio patients and the implications for orthotic management. *Neurorehabilitation* **8:**119–138.

Ramlow J, Alexander M, LaPorte R, Kaufmann C, Kuller L (1992). Epidemiology of the post-polio syndrome. *Amer J Epidemiol* **136:**769–786.

Raymond M (1875). Paralysie essentielle de l'enfance, atrophie musculaire consécutive. *Comptes Rendus de la Societé de la Biologie et de ses Filiales* **27:** 158.

Rekand T, Kôrv J, Farbu E, Roose M, Gilhus NE, Langeland N, Aarli JA (2003). Long term outcome after poliomyelitis in different health and social conditions. *Journal of Epidemiology and Community Health* **57:**368–372.

Rekand T, Kôrv J, Farbu E, Roose M *et al.* (2004). Lifestyle and late effects after poliomyelitis. A risk factor study on two populations. *Acta Neurol Scand* **109:**120–125

Sandberg A, Stalberg E (2004). Changes in macro electromyography over time in patients with a history of polio: a comparison of 2 muscles. *Arch Phys Med Rehabil* **85:**1174–1182.

Sonies BC, Dalakas MC (1991). Dysphagia in patients with the post-polio syndrome. *New Eng J Med* **324:**1162–1167.

Spector SA, Gordon PL, Feuerstein IM, Sivakumar K, Hurley BF, Dalakas MC (1996). Strength gains without muscle injury after strength training in patients with postpolio muscular atrophy. *Muscle & Nerve* **19:**1282–1290.

Stalberg E, Grimby G (1995). Dynamic electromyography and muscle biopsy changes in a 4-year follow-up: study of patients with a history of polio. *Muscle & Nerve* **18:**699–707.

Stanghelle JK, Festvag L, Aksnes AK (1993). Pulmonary function and symptom-limited exercise stress testing in subjects with late sequelae of poliomyelitis. *Scand J Rehabil Med* **25:**125–129.

Stanghelle JK, Festvag LV (1997). Postpolio syndrome: a 5 year follow-up. *Spinal Cord* **35:**503–508.

Stein DP, Dambrosia JM, Dalakas MC (1995). A double-blind, placebo-controlled trial of amantadine for the treatment of fatigue in patients with the post-polio syndrome. *Ann New York Acad Sci* **753:**296–302.

Steljes DG, Kryger MH, Kirk BW, Millar TW (1990). Sleep in postpolio syndrome. *Chest* **98:**133–140.

Strumse YAS, Stanghelle JK, Utne L, Ahlvin P, Svendsby EK (2003). Treatment of patients with postpolio syndrome in a warm climate. *Disabil Rehabil* **25:**77–84.

Takemura J, Saeki S, Hachisuka K, Aritome K (2004). Prevalence of post-polio syndrome based on a cross-sectional survey in Kitakyushu, Japan. *J Rehabil Med* **36:**1–3.

Thoren-Jonsson A-L (2001). Coming to terms with the shift in one's capabilities: a study of the adaptive process in persons with poliomyelitis sequelae. *Disabil Rehabil* **23:**341–351.

Thorsteinsson G (1997). Management of postpolio syndrome. *Mayo Clinic Proceedings* **72:**627–638.

Trojan DA, Gendron D, Cashman NR (1993). Anticholinesterase-responsive neuromuscular junction transmission defects in post-poliomyelitis fatigue. *J Neurol Sci* **114:**170–177.

Trojan DA, Cashman NR, Shapiro S, Tansey CM, Esdaile JM (1994). Predictive factors for postpoliomyelitis syndrome. *Arch Phys Med Rehabil* **75:**770–777.

Trojan DA, Cashman NR (1995). An open trial of pyridostigmine in post-poliomyelitis syndrome. *Canad J Neurol Sci* **22:**223–227.

Trojan DA, Collet J-P, Shapiro S, Jubelt B, Miller RG, Agre JC, Munsat TL, Hollander D, Tandan R, Granger C, Robinson A, Finch L, Ducruet T, Cashman NR (1999).

A multicenter, randomized, double-blinded trial of pyridostigmine in postpolio syndrome. *Neurology* **53:**1225–1233.

Van Kralingen KW, Ivanyi B, Van Keimpema ARJ, Venmans BJW, De Visser M, Postmus PE (1996). Sleep complaints in postpolio syndrome. *Arch Phys Med Rehabil* **77:**609–611.

Vaz Fragoso CA, Kacmarek RM, Systrom DM (1992). Improvement in exercise capacity after nocturnal positive pressure ventilation and tracheostomy in a post-poliomyelitis patient. *Chest* **101:**254–257.

Veicsteinas A, Sarchi P, Mattiotti S, Bignotto M, Belleri M (1998). Cardiorespiratory and metabolic adjustments during submaximal and maximal exercise in polio athletes. *Medicina Dello Sport* **51:**361–373.

Willen C, Scherman MH (2002). Group training in a pool causes ripples on the water: Experiences by persons with late effects of polio. *J Rehabil Med* **34:**191–197.

Willen C, Sunnerhagen KS, Grimby G (2001). Dynamic water exercise in individuals with late poliomyelitis. *Arch Phys Med Rehabil* **82:**66–72.

CHAPTER 22

Autoimmune neuromuscular conduction disorders

G.O. Skeie,[a] S. Apostolski,[b] A. Evoli,[c] N.E. Gilhus,[a]
I.K. Hart,[d] L. Harms,[e] D. Hilton-Jones,[f]
A. Melms,[g] J. Verschuuren,[h] H.W. Horge[i]

Abstract

Background Important progress has been made in our understanding of the cellular and molecular processes underlying the autoimmune neuromuscular transmission (NMT) disorders; myasthenia gravis (MG), Lambert–Eaton myasthenic syndrome (LEMS) and neuromyotonia (peripheral nerve hyperexcitability; Isaacs syndrome).

Objectives To prepare consensus guidelines for the treatment of the autoimmune NMT disorders.

Methods References retrieved from MEDLINE, EMBASE and the Cochrane Library were considered and statements prepared and agreed on by disease experts and a patient representative.

The proposed practical treatment guidelines are agreed upon by the Task Force

1. Anticholinesterase drugs should be the first drugs to be given in the management of MG (Good Practice Point).

2. Plasma exchange is recommended as a short-term treatment in MG, especially in severe cases to induce remission and in preparation for surgery (Recommendation Level B).

3. IvIg and plasma exchange are equally effective for the treatment of MG exacerbations (Recommendation Level A).

4. For patients with nonthymomatous autoimmune MG, thymectomy(TE) is recommended as an option to increase the probability of remission or improvement (Recommendation Level B).

5. Once thymoma is diagnosed TE is indicated irrespective of the severity of MG (Recommendation Level A).

6. Oral corticosteroids are first choice drugs when immunosuppressive drugs are necessary in MG (Good Practice Point).

7. In patients where long-term immunosuppression is necessary, azathioprine is recommended together with steroids to allow tapering the steroids to the lowest possible dose while maintaining azathioprine (Recommendation Level A).

8. 3,4-diaminopyridine is recommended as symptomatic treatment and IvIG has a positive

[a]Department of Neurology, University of Bergen, Norway; [b]Institute of Neurology, School of Medicine, University of Belgrade, Serbia and Montenegro; [c]Neuroscience Department, Catholic University, Rome, Italy; [d]University Department of Neurological Science, Walton Centre for Neurology and Neurosurgery, Liverpool, United Kingdom; [e]Universitätsmedizin Berlin Charité, Neurologische Klinik Berlin, Germany; [f]Radcliffe Infirmary, Oxford, United Kingdom; [g]Neurologische Klinik, Universität Tübingen, Germany; [h]Department of Neurology, LUMC, Leiden, The Netherlands; [i]Patient advocate, The Norwegian Muscular Disorders Association, Norway.

short-term effect in LEMS (Good Practice Point).

9. All neuromyotonia patients should be treated symptomatically with an antiepileptic drug that reduces peripheral nerve hyperexcitability (Good Practice Point).

10. Definitive management of paraneoplastic neuromyotonia and LEMS in treatment of the underlying tumour (Good Practice Point).

11. For immunosuppressive treatment of LEMS and NMT it is reasonable to adopt treatment procedures by analogy with MG (Good Practice Point).

Background and objectives

Autoimmune neuromuscular transmission (NMT) disorders are relatively rare, but often debilitating diseases. Myasthenia gravis (MG) is caused by auto antibodies against the acetylcholine receptor (AChR) at the neuromuscular junction. The autoimmune attack at the muscle endplate leads to NMT failure and muscle weakness. Lambert–Eaton myasthenic syndrome (LEMS) is caused by antibodies against the voltage-gated calcium channels (VGCC) at the presynaptic side of the muscle endplate. The antibodies inhibit acetylcholine(Ach) release and cause NMT failure and muscle weakness. Neuromyotonia (peripheral nerve hyperexcitability; Isaacs syndrome) is caused by antibodies to nerve voltage-gated potassium channels (VGKC) that produce nerve hyperexcitability and spontaneous and continuous skeletal muscle overactivity presenting as twitching and painful cramps and stiffness.

Our increased understanding of the basic mechanisms of neuromuscular transmission and autoimmunity has led to the development of novel treatment strategies. NMT disorders are now amenable to treatment and their prognoses are good. Treatment developed for other and more common antibody-mediated autoimmune disorders with similar pathogenetic processes have been applied also for NMT disorders. However, although present treatment strategies are increasingly underpinned by scientific evidence, they are still based partly on clinical experience. In this paper, we have reviewed the available literature on treatment for

the autoimmune NMT disorders and give evidence-based guidelines.

Materials and methods

Search strategy

MEDLINE 1966–2004 and EMBASE 1966–2004 were examined with appropriate MESH and free subject terms: 1. Myasthenia, 2. Myasthenia gravis, 3. Lambert Eaton , 4. Lambert Eaton myasthenic syndrome/LEMS, 5. Neuromyotonia, 6. Isaacs syndrome.

1–6 was combined with the terms: 7. Treatment, 8. Medication, 9. Therapy, 10. Controlled clinical trial, 11. Randomized controlled trial, 12. Clinical trial, 13. Multicenter study, 14. Meta analysis, 15. Cross-over studies, 16. Thymectomy, 17. Immunosuppression.

The Cochrane Central Register of Controlled Trials (CENTRAL) was also sought.

Articles in English that contained data that could be rated according to the guidance statement for neurological management guidelines of the European Federation of Neurological Societies (EFNS) were included (Brainin et al., 2004).

Information from patient and other voluntary organizations and existing guidelines including those from the American Academy of Neurology was reviewed and validated according to the above criteria. Finished and ongoing Cochrane data-based projects on LEMS treatment, immunosuppressive MG treatment, IvIg for MG, plasmapheresis for MG and corticosteroids for MG in addition to TE for MG were reviewed.

Methods for reaching consensus

Four members of the task force prepared parts of the manuscript and draft statements about the treatment of MG, LEMS and neuromyotonia. Evidence was classified as Class I to IV and recommendations as Level A to C according to the scheme agreed for EFNS guidelines (Brainin et al., 2004). When only class IV evidence was available but consensus could be reached the Task Force has offered advice as Good Practice Points (Brainin et al., 2004). The statements were revised and collated into a single document that was then revised iteratively until consensus was reached.

Myasthenia gravis

Myasthenia gravis (MG) is characterized by a fluctuating weakness of skeletal muscle with remissions and exacerbations (Vincent, 2002). In 85% of MG patients, the disease is caused by antibodies against the AChR at the postsynaptic side of the neuromuscular junction that cause transmission failure and produce destruction of the endplate. Of the 15% of generalized MG patients without AChR antibodies, 20–50% have antibodies against another synaptic antigen, muscle-specific tyrosine kinase [MuSK] (Hoch *et al.*, 2001). The remaining patients probably have antibodies against unknown antigens at the neuromuscular junction. MG is closely associated with thymic pathology. Fifteen per cent of MG patients have a thymoma and often have antibodies against additional striated muscle antigens such as titin (Aarli *et al.*, 1990) and ryanodine receptors (Mygland *et al.*, 1992). These antibodies are more common in thymoma and severe MG and are considered as useful markers for these conditions (Skeie *et al.*, 1995; Somnier *et al.*, 1999). A hypertrophic thymus is found in 60% of MG patients, typically young females, while most patients with debut after 50 years of age, have a normal or atrophic thymus.

MG often used to cause chronic, severe disability and had a high mortality. However, improved treatment allied with advances in critical care have transformed the long-term prognosis and life expectancy is now near normal (Gerber and Steinberg, 1976; Goulon *et al.*, 1989; Evoli *et al.*, 1996, 2002).

Symptomatic treatment

Acetylcholine esterase inhibitors (of which pyridostigmine is the most widely used) inhibit the breakdown of ACh at the neuromuscular junction. This increases the availability of ACh to stimulate AChR and facilitates muscle activation and contraction. These drugs are symptomatic treatments and most helpful when used as initial therapy in newly diagnosed MG patients, and as sole long-term treatment of milder, especially ocular, disease.

These drugs are usually well tolerated at standard doses of up to 60 mg five times per day. Adverse effects are caused by the increased concentration of ACh at both nicotinic and muscarinic synapses. The common muscarinic effects are gut hypermotility (stomach cramps, diarrhoea), increased sweating, excessive respiratory and gastrointestinal secretions (Shale *et al.*, 1983; Szathmary *et al.*, 1984), and bradycardia. The main nicotinic adverse effects are muscle fasciculations, and sometimes, cramps.

There are no placebo controlled randomized studies of these drugs, but case reports, case series and daily clinical experience demonstrate an objective and marked clinical effect (Class IV evidence). Although there is inadequate evidence for a formal recommendation, the Task Force agreed that an anticholinesterase drug should be the first-line treatment for all forms of MG (Class IV evidence, Good Practice Point).

The optimal dose is determined by the balance between clinical improvement and adverse effects, and can vary over time and with concomitant treatment. There is one report of additional effect of intranasally administered pyridostigmine, although this is not commercially available (Sghirlanzoni *et al.*, 1992) (Class III evidence).

Another symptomatic agent, ephedrine, increases ACh release. It has probably both less effect and more severe side effects than pyridostigmine (Sieb and Engel, 1993) (Class III evidence). Pyridostigmine should be preferred to ephedrine in the symptomatic treatment of MG (Recommendation Level C).

3,4-diaminopyridine releases ACh from nerve terminals and is used as a treatment for LEMS. In a double-blind, placebo-controlled trial the drug seemed effective in congenital (hereditary and non-immune) myasthenia patients. Juvenile MG patients did not respond (Anlar *et al.*, 1996) (Class III evidence). The drug is not recommended in autoimmune MG although it may prove useful in some forms of congenital myasthenia (Recommendation Level C).

Immune-directed treatment

Definitive MG treatments target the autoimmune response by suppressing the production of pathogenic antibodies or the damage induced by the antibodies. The aim of immunotherapy is to induce and then maintain remission. MG patients with a thymoma and other patients with anti-titin and anti-RyR antibodies usually have a severe disease (Skeie *et al.,* 1995; Romi *et al.,* 2000) (Class III evidence), thus, suggesting that more aggressive treatment strategies should be considered in these patients (Recommendation Level C).

Most MG treatment studies are insufficient. There is no consideration of whether patients have had thymectomy and it is not possible to extract from the data how many patients of a treatment arm have had thymectomy and how many have not. In non-operated patients, it is unknown how many of them had thymoma. In studies conducted before 1980, the percentage of patients with and without AChR antibodies is not known, and the MuSK antibodies were detected very recently. There are no controlled or prospective trials of immunosuppressive treatment in children and adolescents. Evidence suggests that each immunological subtype of MG may be associated with a different spectrum of clinical phenotypes and thymus pathologies that should be considered when designing optimum treatment strategies.

Plasma exchange

Antibodies are removed from patient sera by membrane filtration or centrifugation. The onset of improvement is within the first week and the effect lasts for 1–3 months. Short-term benefits of plasma exchange have been reviewed by Gajdos *et al.* (Cochrane review) (Gajdos *et al.* 2002) who conclude: 'There are no adequate randomized controlled trials, but many case series report short-term benefit from plasma exchange in myasthenia gravis, especially in myasthenic crisis'. Numerous reports have shown this (Dau, 1980; Olarte *et al.,* 1981; Perlo *et al.*1981) (all Class IV). The NIH consensus of 1986 states: 'the panel is persuaded that plasma exchange can be useful in strengthening patients with myasthenia gravis before thymectomy and during the postoperative period. It can also be valuable in lessening symptoms during initiation of immunosuppressive drug therapy and during an acute crisis' (Class IV evidence).

Therefore, sham controlled trials would be unethical. Plasma exchange is recommended as a short-term treatment in MG, especially in severe cases to induce remission and in preparation for surgery (Recommendation Level B).

There is one report on the use of repeated plasma exchange over a long period in refractory MG. It failed to show any cumulative long-term benefit of plasma exchange in combination with immunosuppressive drugs over immunosuppressive treatment alone (Gajdos *et al.,* 1983) (Class II evidence). A Cochrane review concludes that: 'There are no adequate randomized controlled trials to determine whether plasma exchange improves the long-term outcome from myasthenia gravis' (Gajdos *et al.,* 2002) (Class I evidence). Repeated plasma exchange is, thus, not recommended as a treatment to obtain a continuous and lasting immunosuppression in MG (Recommendation Level B).

Intravenous immunoglobulin

Intravenous immunoglobulin (IvIg) had a positive effect in several open studies especially in the acute phase of MG (Fateh-Moghadam *et al.,* 1984) (Class IV evidence). It has been used for the same indications as plasma exchange; rapidly progressive disease, preparation of weak patients for surgery including thymectomy, and as an adjuvant to minimize long-term side effects of oral immunosuppressive therapy (Dalakas, 1999). A recent Cochrane review compared the efficacy of IvIg compared to plasma exchange, other treatments, or placebo. It concluded: 'the only randomized controlled trial examining early treatment effects did not show a significant difference between IvIg and plasma exchange for the treatment of myasthenia gravis exacerbations'. Non-randomised evidence consistently favours the interpretation that they are equally effective in this situation (Gajdos *et al.,* 2003) (Class I evidence) (Recommendation Level A). Two multicentre randomized controlled studies suggest that, although efficacy is equal, side effects of IvIg may be fewer and less severe. Thus, IvIg may be the preferred option (Gajdos *et al.,* 1997) (Class I evidence). However, the controlled study by Gajdos *et al.,* (1997) used a lower volume of plasma exchange than usual for the treatment of

MG crisis, and the end point was improvement at a time-point set too late to allow proper assessment of whether one therapy worked quicker than the other. There are published abstracts but no papers suggesting that plasma exchange works faster in MG crisis.

In mild or moderate MG, no significant difference in efficacy of IvIg and placebo was found after 6 weeks. In moderate exacerbations of MG no statistically significant difference in efficacy was found between IvIg and methylprednisolone. Randomised controlled trials have not shown evidence of improved functional outcome or steroid-sparing effect with the repeated use of IvIg in moderate or severe stable MG (Gajdos *et al.*, 2003) (Class I evidence).

Clinical experience does, however, suggest that IvIg can be helpful in patients with severe MG who fail to respond to maximal tolerated doses of corticosteroids and/or immunosuppressive agents.

Thymectomy

There are several surgical approaches to Thymectomy (TE): full or partial sternotomy, transcervical and thoracoscopic. There are no randomised controlled studies for TE in MG.

It is difficult to compare the outcomes of the different operative techniques (confounding factors influenced both the controlled and the uncontrolled studies).

Despite the absence of randomised, well-controlled studies, TE in MG patients with and without thymoma is widely practised. Postoperative improvement can take months or years to appear, making it difficult to distinguish TE effects from those of immunosuppressive drugs, which are often used concomitantly. In a controlled study, a 34% remission and a 32% improvement rate were achieved after TE compared with 8% and 16% for matched patients without the operation (Buckingham *et al.*, 1976) (Class III evidence). As TE is an elective intervention, the patient should be in a clinically stable condition. The perioperative morbidity is very low and consists in wound healing disorders, bronchopneumonia, phrenic nerve damage and sternum instability with transsternal procedures.

The Quality Standard Subcommittee of the American Academy of Neurology (Gronseth and Barohn, 2000; 2002) analysed 28 articles written during 1953–1998 describing outcomes in 21 MG cohorts with or without TE (Class II evidence). Most series used the transsternal approach and the follow-up ranged from 3 to 28 years. There are a number of methodological problems in the studies including the definition of remission, the selection criteria, the medical therapy applied in both groups, and data on antibody status. However, 18 of the 21 cohorts showed improvement in MG patients who underwent TE compared with those who did not. The authors used median relative outcome rates and found that MG patients undergoing TE were twice as likely to attain medication-free remission, 1.6 times as likely to become asymptomatic, and 1.7 times as likely to improve. No study found a significant negative influence of TE on the outcome. A sub-group analysis after controlling for different single confounding variables yielded additional results. Patients with purely ocular manifestations did not benefit from TE. The outcome for younger TE patients was not significantly different from the total MG group. Mild MG (Ossermann grade 1–2) did not profit from surgery, while more severe cases (Ossermann grade 2b–4) were 3.7 times as likely to achieve remission after TE than those without surgery ($p < 0.0077$).

The widespread opinion that an early TE in the course of MG improves the chance of a quick remission is based on observations that lack detailed information and cannot be verified by meta-analysis. However, from pathogenic considerations it is tempting to assume that early TE should be preferred to TE after many years.

Gronseth *et al.* asserted unequivocally that 'for patients with nonthymomatous autoimmune MG, thymectomy is recommended as an option to increase the probability of remission or improvement'. Their recommendation is supported by this Task Force with the specification that patients with generalised MG and AChR antibodies are the group most likely to benefit (Recommendation Level B).

A future randomised trial to assess the efficacy of TE in the different clinical and immunological subgroups of MG patients is needed.

The indication for TE in AChR antibody negative MG patients is controversial. A retrospective cohort study displayed a similar post-operative course in AChR antibody negative and AChR antibody positive patients with a follow-up of at least 3 years (Guillermo *et al.*, 2004). Remission or improvement after TE occurred in 57% of AChR antibody negative patients and in 51% of AChR antibody positive patients. Another study (Evoli *et al.*, 2003) could not prove any effect of TE in 15 MuSK antibody positive patients, but the data do not permit any recommendations at present regarding TE in MG without AChR antibodies.

In MG patients with a thymoma the main aim of TE is to treat the tumour rather than for any effect on the MG. Once thymoma is diagnosed, TE is indicated irrespective of the severity of MG (Good Practice Point). Thymoma is a slow-growing tumour and TE should be performed only after stabilisation of the MG. After TE, the AChR-antibody titre usually falls less in patients with thymoma than in those with thymic hyperplasia (Reinhardt and Melms, 2000). The prognosis depends on early and complete tumour resection (Chen *et al.*, 2002).

Corticosteroids

In observational studies, remission or marked improvement is seen in 70–80% of MG patients treated with oral corticosteroids, usually prednisolone (Pascuzzi *et al.*, 1984) (Class IV evidence), but the efficacy has not been studied in double-blind, placebo-controlled trials. Steroids have side effects including weight gain, fluid retention, hypertension, diabetes, anxiety/depression/insomnia/psychosis, glaucoma, cataract, gastrointestinal haemorrhage and perforations, myopathy, increased susceptibility to infections and avascular joint necrosis. The risk of osteoporosis is reduced by giving bisphosphonate (Saag, 2004) (Class IV evidence), and antacids may prevent gastrointestinal complications. The Task Force agreed that oral prednisolone should be the first choice drug when immunosuppressive drugs are necessary in MG (Good Practice Point). Some patients have a temporary worsening of MG if prednisolone is started at a high dose. This steroid dip occurs after 4–10 days and sometimes can precipitate a MG crisis. Thus,

we recommend starting treatment at a low dose, 10–25 mg on alternate days, and increasing the dose gradually (10 mg per dose) to 60–80 mg on alternate days. If the patient is critically ill one should start on a high dose every day and use additional short-time treatments to overcome the temporary worsening. When remission occurs, usually after 4–16 weeks, the dose should be slowly reduced to the minimum effective dose given on alternate days (Good Practice Point).

Azathioprine

Azathioprine is in extensive use as an immunosuppressant. It is metabolized to 6-mercaptopurine, which inhibits DNA and RNA synthesis and interferes with T-cell function. The onset of therapeutic response may be delayed for 4–12 months, and maximal effect is obtained after 6–24 months. Azathioprine is usually well tolerated but idiosyncratic flu-like symptoms or gastrointestinal disturbances including pancreatitis occur in 10%, usually within the first few days of treatment. Some patients develop hepatitis with elevations of liver enzymes. Leucopenia, anaemia, thrombocytopenia or pancytopenia usually respond to drug withdrawal. Blood cell effects and hepatitis often do not recur after cautious reintroduction of the drug. Careful monitoring of full blood cell count and liver enzymes is mandatory and the dosage should be adjusted according to the results. About 11% of the population are heterozygous and 0.3% homozygous for mutations of the thiopurine methyltransferase gene and have an increased risk of azathioprine-induced myelosuppression.

One large double-blind randomised study has demonstrated the efficacy of azathioprine as a steroid sparing agent with a better outcome in patients on a combination of azathioprine and steroids than in patients treated with steroids alone (Palace *et al.*, 1998) (Class I evidence). It has an immunosupressive effect when used alone without steroids (Witte *et al.*, 1984) (Class III evidence). In a small randomized study, prednisone was associated with better and more predictable early improvement in muscle strength than azathioprine (Bromberg *et al.*, 1997) (Class III evidence). In patients where long-term immunosuppression is necessary, we recommend starting azathioprine together with steroids to allow tapering the steroids to the lowest dose possible, while maintaining azathioprine (Recommendation Level A).

Methotrexate

Methotrexate should be used in selected MG patients who do not respond to first choice immunosuppressive drugs (Good Practice Point). It is well studied in other autoimmune disorders, but there is no evidence of sufficient quality published for MG.

Cyclophosphamide

Cyclophosphamide is an alkylating agent with immunosuppressive properties. It is a strong suppressor of B-lymphocyte activity and antibody synthesis and at high doses it also affects T-cells. In a randomized, double-blind, placebo-controlled study including 23 MG patients, those on treatment had significantly improved muscle strength and a lower steroid dose compared with the placebo group. Intravenous pulses of cyclophosphamide allowed reduction of systemic steroids without deterioration of muscle strength or serious side effects (De Feo *et al.*, 2002). (Class II evidence). However, the relative high risk of toxicity including bone marrow suppression, opportunistic infections, bladder toxicity, sterility and neoplasms, limits the use of this medication to MG patients intolerant or unresponsive to steroids plus azathioprine, methotrexate, ciclosporin or mycophenolate mofetil (Recommendation Level B).

Ciclosporin

Ciclosporin has an immunosuppressive effect in both organ transplantation and autoimmune disorders. It is an inhibitor of T-cell function through inhibition of calcineurin signalling (Matsuda and Koyasu, 2000). Tindall *et al.* conducted a placebo-controlled double blind randomized study in 20 patients for 6 months with an open extension (Tindall *et al.*, 1987) (Class II evidence) (Tindall, 1992; Tindall *et al.*, 1993) (Class III evidence). The ciclosporin group had significantly improved strength and reduction in AChR antibody titre compared with the placebo group. Two open trials of 1 and 2 years treatment and one retrospective study all support the beneficial effect of ciclosporin (Goulon *et al.*, 1988, 1989; Bonifati and Angelini, 1997; Ciafaloni *et al.*, 2000) (Class III evidence). Ciclosporin is effective in MG, has significant side effects of nephrotoxicity and hypertension and should be considered only in patients intolerant or unresponsive to azathioprine (Recommendation Level B).

Mycophenolate mofetil

Mycophenolate mofetil's active metabolite, mycophenolic acid, is an inhibitor of purine nucleotide synthesis and impairs lymphocyte proliferation selectively. A few studies including a small double-blind placebo-controlled study of 14 patients have shown that mycophenolate mofetil is effective in patients with poorly controlled MG and as a steroid sparing medication (Hauser *et al.*, 1998; Meriggioli and Rowin, 2000, 2003; Chaudhry *et al.*, 2001; Ciafaloni *et al.*, 2001; Schneider *et al.*, 2001; Meriggioli *et al.*, 2003) (Class III, Class IV evidence). Mycophenolate mofetil should be tried in patients intolerant or unresponsive to azathioprine (Recommendation Level B).

FK506 (tacrolimus)

Tacrolimus (FK506) is a macrolide molecule of the same immunosuppressant class as ciclosporin. It inhibits the proliferation of activated T cells via the calcium–calcineurin pathway. FK506 also acts on ryanodine receptor-mediated calcium release from sarcoplasmic reticulum to potentiate excitation–contraction coupling in skeletal muscle (Timerman *et al.*, 1993). Case reports and a small open trial all showed a useful improvement of MG with minor side effects (Evoli *et al.*, 2002; Yoshikawa *et al.*, 2002; Konishi *et al.*, 2003; Takamori *et al.*, 2004) (Class III evidence). Interestingly, patients with anti-RyR antibodies (and potential excitation–contraction coupling dysfunction) had a rapid response to treatment indicating a symptomatic effect on muscle strength in addition to the immunosuppression (Takamori *et al.*, 2004). FK506 should be tried in MG patients with poorly controlled disease, especially in RyR antibody positive patients (Recommendation Level C).

Antibodies against leucocyte antigens

There are case reports of improvement of refractory MG with monoclonal antibodies against different lymphocyte subsets such as anti-CD20 (rituximab) (B-cell inhibitor) (Wylam *et al.*, 2003) (Class IV evidence), and anti-CD4 (T-cell inhibitor) (Ahlberg *et al.*, 1994) (Class IV evidence), both reporting good clinical outcome. These treatment strategies are promising, but more evidence is needed before any recommendations can be given.

Training, weight control and lifestyle modifications

The importance of reducing weight and modification of activities of daily living has been suggested, but there is no hard scientific evidence to this. There are reports that show some benefit of respiratory muscle training in MG (Weiner *et al.*, 1998) (Class III evidence) and strength training in mild MG (Lohi *et al.*, 1993) (Class III evidence). Physical training can be carried out safely in mild MG and produces some improvement of muscle force (Recommendation Level C).

MG is associated with a slightly increased rate of complications during birth and more frequent need of operative interventions (Hoff *et al.*, 2003) (Class II evidence). Transient neonatal MG occurs in 10–20% of children born to MG mothers. Maternal MG is also a rare cause of arthrogryphosis congenita and of recurrent miscarriages (Vincent *et al.*, 1995). Acetylcholine esterase inhibitors and immunosuppressive drugs should be continued during pregnancy when necessary for the MG, except for methotrexate, and also mycophenolate mofetil and other new drugs where no safety data are available (Ferrero *et al.*, 2005) (Good Practice Point). Effective immunosuppression can improve severe fetal MG-related conditions (Class III evidence). Women with MG should not be discouraged from conceiving, and pregnancy does not worsen the long-term outcome of MG (Batocchi *et al.*, 1999) (Class II evidence).

Recommendations for MG

After the diagnosis of MG is established an acetylcholine esterase inhibitor should be introduced. Thymoma patients should have thymectomy. AChR-antibody positive early-onset patients with generalized MG and insufficient response to pyridostigmine therapy should be considered for thymectomy, ideally within one year of disease onset. Immunosuppressive medication should be considered in all patients with progressive MG symptoms. We recommend starting with prednisolone covered by bisphosphonate and antacid. If long-term treatment with steroids is expected, a steroid-sparing agent, usually azathioprine, should be introduced. Non-responders or patients intolerant to this regime should be considered for treatment with one of the other recommended immunosuppressive drugs. Recommendation levels are generally B, C or Good Practice Points.

Lambert–Eaton myasthenic syndrome

Antibodies to peripheral nerve P/Q-type VGCC antibodies are present in the serum of at least 85% of Lambert–Eaton myasthenic syndrome (LEMS) patients (Motomura *et al.*, 1995). The disease is characterized by ascending muscle weakness that usually starts in the proximal lower limb muscles and is associated with sensory symptoms and autonomic dysfunction. Ptosis and ophthalmoplegia tend to be milder than in MG (Wirtz *et al.*, 2002). LEMS rarely causes respiratory failure (Wirtz *et al.*, 2002). In half of the patients LEMS is a paraneoplastic disease and a small cell lung carcinoma (SCLC) will be found (Wirtz *et al.*, 2005).

Symptomatic and immune-directed treatment

Evidence from small, randomised, controlled trials showed that both 3,4-diaminopyridine and IvIg improved muscle strength scores and compound muscle action potential amplitudes in LEMS patients (Maddison and Newsom-Davis, 2003) (Cochrane Review) (Class I evidence).

First-line treatment is 3,4-diaminopyridine (McEvoy *et al.*, 1989). An additional therapeutic effect may be obtained if combined with pyridostigmine. If symptomatic treatment is insufficient immunosuppressive therapy should be started, usually with a combination of prednisone and azathioprine. By analogy to MG, other drugs like ciclosporin or mycophenolate can be used, although evidence of benefit is limited to case series reports (Class IV evidence) (Recommendation Level C).

For patients with a paraneoplastic LEMS it is essential to treat the tumour. Chemotherapy is the first choice in SCLC and this will have an additional immunosuppressive effect. The presence of LEMS in a patient with SCLC improves tumour survival (Maddison et al., 1999). For a more detailed description of LEMS consult the Guidelines for the management of paraneoplastic disorders (EFNS guidelines).

Neuromyotonia (peripheral nerve hyperexcitability)/Isaacs syndrome

This commonest acquired form of generalised peripheral nerve hyperexcitability is autoimmune and caused by antibodies to nerve voltage-gated potassium channels (VGKC), although the only generally available assay detects these antibodies in only 30–50% of all patients (Hart et al., 2002). Neuromyotonia is paraneoplastic in up to 25% of patients and can predate the detection of neoplasia, usually thymus or lung, by up to 4 years (Hart et al., 1997). The clinical hallmark is spontaneous and continuous skeletal muscle overactivity presenting as twitching and painful cramps and often accompanied by stiffness, pseudomyotonia, pseudotetany and weakness (Newsom-Davis and Mills, 1993). One third of patients also have sensory features and up to 50% have hyperhidrosis suggesting autonomic involvement. Central nervous system features can occur (Morvan's syndrome) (Hart et al., 1997; Liguori et al., 2001).

Symptomatic and immune-directed treatment

Neuromyotonia usually improves with symptomatic treatment (Newsom-Davis and Mills, 1993), although evidence is case reports and case series (Class IV evidence). Carbamazepine,

phenytoin, lamotrigine and sodium valproate can be used, if necessary in combination.

Neuromyotonia often improves and can remit after treatment of an underlying cancer (Newsom-Davis and Mills, 1993). In patients whose symptoms are debilitating or refractory to symptomatic therapy, immunomodulatory therapies should be tried (Newsom-Davis and Mills, 1993; Hayat et al., 2000). Plasma exchange often produces useful clinical improvement lasting about 6 weeks accompanied by a reduction in EMG activity (Newsom-Davis and Mills, 1993) and a fall in VGKC antibody titres (Shillito et al., 1995). Single case studies suggest that IvIg can also help (Alessi et al., 2000). There are no good trials of long-term oral immunosuppression. However, prednisolone, with or without azathioprine or methotrexate, has been useful in selected patients (Newsom-Davis and Mills, 1993; Nakatsuji et al., 2000) (Class IV evidence) (Good Practice Point).

Conflicts of interest

None of the Task Force members reported any conflicts of interest.

References

Aarli JA, Stefansson K, Marton LS, Wollmann RL (1990). Patients with myasthenia gravis and thymoma have in their sera IgG autoantibodies against titin. *Clin Exp Immunol* **82**:284–288.

Ahlberg R, Yi Q, Pirskanen R, Matell G, Swerup C, Rieber EP, Riethmuller G, Holm G, Lefvert AK (1994). Treatment of myasthenia gravis with anti-CD4 antibody: improvement correlates to decreased T-cell autoreactivity. *Neurology* **44**:1732–1737.

Alessi G, De Reuck J, De Bleecker J, Vancayzeele S (2000). Successful immunoglobulin treatment in a patient with neuromyotonia. *Clin Neurol Neurosurg* **102**:173–175.

Anlar B, Varli K, Ozdirim E, Ertan M (1996). 3,4-diaminopyridine in childhood myasthenia: double-blind, placebo-controlled trial. *J Child Neurol* **11**:458–461.

Batocchi AP, Majolini L, Evoli A, Lino MM, Minisci C, Tonali P (1999). Course and treatment of myasthenia gravis during pregnancy. *Neurology* **52**:447–452.

Bonifati DM, Angelini C (1997). Long-term cyclosporine treatment in a group of severe myasthenia gravis patients. *J Neurol* **244**:542–547.

Brainin M, Barnes M, Baron JC, Gilhus NE, Hughes R, Selmaj K, Waldemar G (2004). Guidance for the preparation of neurological management guidelines by EFNS scientific task forces–revised recommendations 2004. *Eur J Neurol* **11**:577–581.

Bromberg MB, Wald JJ, Forshew DA, Feldman EL, Albers JW (1997). Randomized trial of azathioprine or prednisone for initial immunosuppressive treatment of myasthenia gravis. *J Neurol Sci* **150**:59–62.

Buckingham JM, Howard FM, Jr, Bernatz PE, Payne WS, Harrison EG, Jr, O'Brien PC, Weiland LH (1976). The value of thymectomy in myasthenia gravis: a computer-assisted matched study. *Ann Surg* **184**:453–458.

Chaudhry V, Cornblath DR, Griffin JW, O'Brien R, Drachman DB (2001). Mycophenolate mofetil: a safe and promising immunosuppressant in neuromuscular diseases. *Neurology* **56**:94–96.

Chen G, Marx A, Wen-Hu C, Yong J, Puppe B, Stroebel P, Mueller-Hermelink HK (2002). New WHO histologic classification predicts prognosis of thymic epithelial tumors: a clinicopathologic study of 200 thymoma cases from China. *Cancer* **95**:420–429.

Ciafaloni E, Nikhar NK, Massey JM, Sanders DB (2000). Retrospective analysis of the use of cyclosporine in myasthenia gravis. *Neurology* **55**:448–450.

Ciafaloni E, Massey JM, Tucker-Lipscomb B, Sanders DB (2001). Mycophenolate mofetil for myasthenia gravis: an open-label pilot study. *Neurology* **56**:97–99.

Dalakas MC (1999). Intravenous immunoglobulin in the treatment of autoimmune neuromuscular diseases: present status and practical therapeutic guidelines. *Muscle Nerve* **22**:1479–1497.

Dau PC (1980). Plasmapheresis therapy in myasthenia gravis. *Muscle Nerve* **3**:468–482.

De Feo LG, Schottlender J, Martelli NA, Molfino NA (2002). Use of intravenous pulsed cyclophosphamide in severe, generalized myasthenia gravis. *Muscle Nerve* **26**:31–36.

Evoli A, Batocchi AP, Tonali P (1996). A practical guide to the recognition and management of myasthenia gravis. *Drugs* **52**:662–670.

Evoli A, Di Schino C, Marsili F, Punzi C (2002). Successful treatment of myasthenia gravis with tacrolimus. *Muscle Nerve* **25**:111–114.

Evoli A, Tonali PA, Padua L, Monaco ML, Scuderi F, Batocchi AP, Marino M, Bartoccioni E (2003). Clinical correlates with anti-MuSK antibodies in generalized seronegative myasthenia gravis. *Brain* **126**:2304–2311.

Fateh-Moghadam A, Wick M, Besinger U, Geursen RG (1984). High-dose intravenous gammaglobulin for myasthenia gravis. *Lancet*, **1**:848–849.

Ferrero S, Pretta S, Nicoletti A, Petrera P, Ragni N (2005). Myasthenia gravis: management issues during pregnancy. *Eur J Obstet Gynecol Reprod Biol* **121**:129–138.

Gajdos P, Chevret S, Clair B, Tranchant C, Chastang C (1997). Clinical trial of plasma exchange and high-dose intravenous immunoglobulin in myasthenia gravis. Myasthenia Gravis Clinical Study Group. *Ann Neurol* **41**:789–796.

Gajdos P, Chevret S, Toyka K (2002). Plasma exchange for myasthenia gravis. *Cochrane Database Syst Rev* CD002275.

Gajdos P, Chevret S, Toyka K (2003). Intravenous immunoglobulin for myasthenia gravis. *Cochrane Database Syst Rev* CD002277.

Gajdos P, Simon N, de Rohan-Chabot P, Raphael JC, Goulon M (1983). [Long-term effects of plasma exchange in myasthenia. Results of a randomized study]. *Presse Med* **12**: 939–942.

Gerber NL, Steinberg AD (1976). Clinical use of immuno-suppressive drugs: part II. *Drugs* **11**:90–112.

Goulon M, Elkharrat D, Lokiec F, Gajdos P (1988). Results of a one-year open trial of cyclosporine in ten patients with severe myasthenia gravis. *Transplant Proc* **20**:211–217.

Goulon M, Elkharrat D, Gajdos P (1989). [Treatment of severe myasthenia gravis with cyclosporin. A 12-month open trial]. *Presse Med* **18**:341–346.

Gronseth GS, Barohn RJ (2000). Practice parameter: thymectomy for autoimmune myasthenia gravis (an evidence-based review): report of the Quality Standards Subcommittee of the American Academy of Neurology. *Neurology* **55**:7–15.

Gronseth GS, Barohn RJ (2002). Thymectomy for Myasthenia Gravis. *Curr Treat Options Neurol* **4**:203–209.

Guillermo GR, Tellez-Zenteno JF, Weder-Cisneros N, Mimenza A, Estanol B, Remes-Troche JM, Cantu-Brito C (2004). Response of thymectomy: clinical and pathological characteristics among seronegative and seropositive myasthenia gravis patients. *Acta Neurol Scand* **109**:217–221.

Hart IK, Maddison P, Newsom-Davis J, Vincent A, Mills KR (2002). Phenotypic variants of autoimmune peripheral nerve hyperexcitability. *Brain* **125**:1887–1895.

Hart IK, Waters C, Vincent A, Newland C, Beeson D, Pongs O, Morris C, Newsom-Davis J (1997). Autoantibodies detected to expressed K+ channels are implicated in neuromyotonia. *Ann Neurol* **41**:238–246.

Hauser RA, Malek AR, Rosen R (1998). Successful treatment of a patient with severe refractory myasthenia gravis using mycophenolate mofetil. *Neurology* **51**:912–913.

Hayat GR, Kulkantrakorn K, Campbell WW, Giuliani MJ (2000). Neuromyotonia: autoimmune pathogenesis and response to immune modulating therapy. *J Neurol Sci* **181:**38–43.

Hoch W, McConville J, Helms S, Newsom-Davis J, Melms A, Vincent A (2001). Auto-antibodies to the receptor tyrosine kinase MuSK in patients with myasthenia gravis without acetylcholine receptor antibodies. *Nat Med* **7:**365–368.

Hoff JM, Daltveit AK, Gilhus NE (2003). Myasthenia gravis: consequences for pregnancy, delivery, and the newborn. *Neurology* **61:**1362–1366.

Konishi T, Yoshiyama Y, Takamori M, Yagi K, Mukai E, Saida T (2003). Clinical study of FK506 in patients with myasthenia gravis. *Muscle Nerve* **28:**570–574.

Liguori R, Vincent A, Clover L, Avoni P, Plazzi G, Cortelli P, Baruzzi A, Carey T, Gambetti P, Lugaresi E, Montagna P (2001). Morvan's syndrome: peripheral and central nervous system and cardiac involvement with antibodies to voltage-gated potassium channels. *Brain* **124:**2417–2426.

Lohi EL, Lindberg C, Andersen O (1993). Physical training effects in myasthenia gravis. *Arch Phys Med Rehabil* **74:**1178–1180.

Maddison P, Newsom-Davis J (2003). Treatment for Lambert-Eaton myasthenic syndrome. *Cochrane Database Syst Rev* CD003279.

Maddison P, Newsom-Davis J, Mills KR, Souhami RL (1999). Favourable prognosis in Lambert-Eaton myasthenic syndrome and small-cell lung carcinoma. *Lancet* **353:**117–118.

Matsuda S, Koyasu S (2000). Mechanisms of action of cyclosporine. *Immunopharmacology* **47:**119–125.

McEvoy KM, Windebank AJ, Daube JR, Low PA (1989). 3,4-Diaminopyridine in the treatment of Lambert-Eaton myasthenic syndrome. *N Engl J Med* **321:**1567–1571.

Meriggioli MN, Ciafaloni E, Al-Hayk KA, Rowin J, Tucker-Lipscomb B, Massey JM, Sanders DB (2003). Mycophenolate mofetil for myasthenia gravis: an analysis of efficacy, safety, and tolerability. *Neurology* **61:**1438–1440.

Meriggioli MN, Rowin J (2000). Treatment of myasthenia gravis with mycophenolate mofetil: a case report. *Muscle Nerve* **23:**1287–1289.

Meriggioli MN, Rowin J (2003). Single fiber EMG as an outcome measure in myasthenia gravis: results from a double-blind, placebo-controlled trial. *J Clin Neurophysiol* **20:**382–385.

Motomura M, Johnston I, Lang B, Vincent A, Newsom-Davis J (1995). An improved diagnostic assay for Lambert-Eaton myasthenic syndrome. *J Neurol Neurosurg Psychiatry* **58:**85–87.

Mygland A, Tysnes OB, Matre R, Volpe P, Aarli JA, Gilhus NE (1992). Ryanodine receptor autoantibodies in myasthenia gravis patients with a thymoma. *Ann Neurol* **32:**589–591.

Nakatsuji Y, Kaido M, Sugai F, Nakamori M, Abe K, Watanabe O, Arimura K, Sakoda S (2000). Isaacs' syndrome successfully treated by immunoadsorption plasmapheresis. *Acta Neurol Scand* **102:**271–273.

Newsom-Davis J, Mills KR (1993). Immunological associations of acquired neuromyotonia (Isaacs' syndrome). Report of five cases and literature review. *Brain*, **116 (Pt 2):**453–469.

Olarte MR, Schoenfeldt RS, Penn AS, Lovelace RE, Rowland LP (1981). Effect of plasmapheresis in myasthenia gravis 1978–1980. *Ann N Y Acad Sci*, **377:**725–728.

Palace J, Newsom-Davis J, Lecky B (1998). A randomized double-blind trial of prednisolone alone or with azathioprine in myasthenia gravis. Myasthenia Gravis Study Group. *Neurology* **50:**1778–1783.

Pascuzzi RM, Coslett HB, Johns TR (1984). Long-term corticosteroid treatment of myasthenia gravis: report of 116 patients. *Ann Neurol* **15:**291–298.

Perlo VP, Shahani BT, Huggins CE, Hunt J, Kosinski K, Potts F (1981). Effect of plasmapheresis in myasthenia gravis. *Ann N Y Acad Sci* **377:**709–724.

Reinhardt C, Melms A (2000). Normalization of elevated CD4-/CD8- (double-negative) T cells after thymectomy parallels clinical remission in myasthenia gravis associated with thymic hyperplasia but not thymoma. *Ann Neurol* **48:**603–608.

Romi F, Skeie GO, Aarli JA, Gilhus NE (2000). The severity of myasthenia gravis correlates with the serum concentration of titin and ryanodine receptor antibodies. *Arch Neurol* **57:**1596–1600.

Saag KG (2004). Prevention of glucocorticoid-induced osteoporosis. *South Med J* **97:**555–558.

Schneider C, Gold R, Reiners K, Toyka KV (2001). Mycophenolate mofetil in the therapy of severe myasthenia gravis. *Eur Neurol* **46:**79–82.

Sghirlanzoni A, Pareyson D, Benvenuti C, Cei G, Cosi V, Lombardi M, Nicora M, Ricciardi R, Cornelio F (1992). Efficacy of intranasal administration of neostigmine in myasthenic patients. *J Neurol* **239:**165–169.

Shale DJ, Lane DJ, Davis CJ (1983). Air-flow limitation in myasthenia gravis. The effect of acetylcholinesterase inhibitor therapy on air-flow limitation. *Am Rev Respir Dis* **128:** 618–621.

Shillito P, Molenaar PC, Vincent A, Leys K, Zheng W, van den Berg RJ, Plomp JJ, van Kempen GT, Chauplannaz G, Wintzen AR *et al.* (1995). Acquired neuromyotonia: evidence for autoantibodies directed against K+ channels of peripheral nerves. *Ann Neurol* **38:**714–722.

Sieb JP, Engel AG (1993). Ephedrine: effects on neuromuscular transmission. *Brain Res* **623:** 167–171.

Skeie GO, Mygland A, Aarli JA, Gilhus NE (1995). Titin antibodies in patients with late onset myasthenia gravis: clinical correlations. *Autoimmunity* **20:**99–104.

Somnier FE, Skeie GO, Aarli JA, Trojaborg W (1999). EMG evidence of myopathy and the occurrence of titin autoantibodies in patients with myasthenia gravis. *Eur J Neurol* **6:** 555–563.

Szathmary I, Magyar P, Szobor A (1984). Air-flow limitation in myasthenia gravis. The effect of acetylcholinesterase inhibitor therapy on air-flow limitation. *Am Rev Respir Dis* **130:**145.

Takamori M, Motomura M, Kawaguchi N, Nemoto Y, Hattori T, Yoshikawa H, Otsuka K (2004). Anti-ryanodine receptor antibodies and FK506 in myasthenia gravis. *Neurology* **62:**1894–1896.

Timerman AP, Ogunbumni E, Freund E, Wiederrecht G, Marks AR, Fleischer S (1993). The calcium release channel of sarcoplasmic reticulum is modulated by FK-506-binding protein. Dissociation and reconstitution of FKBP-12 to the calcium release channel of skeletal muscle sarcoplasmic reticulum. *J Biol Chem* **268:**22992–22999.

Tindall RS (1992). Immunointervention with cyclosporin A in autoimmune neurological disorders. *J Autoimmun* **5(Suppl A):**301–313.

Tindall RS, Rollins JA, Phillips JT, Greenlee RG, Wells L, Belendiuk G (1987). Preliminary results of a double-blind, randomized, placebo-controlled trial of cyclosporine in myasthenia gravis. *N Engl J Med* **316:**719–724.

Tindall RS, Phillips JT, Rollins JA, Wells L, Hall K (1993). A clinical therapeutic trial of cyclosporine in myasthenia gravis. *Ann N Y Acad Sci* **681:** 539–551.

Vincent A (2002). Unravelling the pathogenesis of myasthenia gravis. *Nat Rev Immunol* **2:** 797–804.

Vincent A, Newland C, Brueton L, Beeson D, Riemersma S, Huson SM, Newsom-Davis J (1995). Arthrogryposis multiplex congenita with maternal autoantibodies specific for a fetal antigen. *Lancet* **346:**24–25.

Weiner P, Gross D, Meiner Z, Ganem R, Weiner M, Zamir D, Rabner M (1998). Respiratory muscle training in patients with moderate to severe myasthenia gravis. *Can J Neurol Sci* **25:**236–241.

Wirtz PW, Sotodeh M, Nijnuis M, Van Doorn PA, Van Engelen BG, Hintzen RQ, De Kort PL, Kuks JB, Twijnstra A, De Visser M, Visser LH, Wokke JH, Wintzen AR, Verschuuren JJ (2002). Difference in distribution of muscle weakness between myasthenia gravis and the Lambert-Eaton myasthenic syndrome. *J Neurol Neurosurg Psychiatry* **73:**766–768.

Wirtz PW, Willcox N, van der Slik AR, Lang B, Maddison P, Koeleman BP, Giphart MJ, Wintzen AR, Roep BO, Verschuuren JJ (2005). HLA and smoking in prediction and prognosis of small cell lung cancer in autoimmune Lambert-Eaton myasthenic syndrome. *J Neuroimmunol* **159:**230–237.

Witte AS, Cornblath DR, Parry GJ, Lisak RP, Schatz NJ (1984). Azathioprine in the treatment of myasthenia gravis. *Ann Neurol* **15:**602–605.

Wylam ME, Anderson PM, Kuntz NL, Rodriguez V (2003). Successful treatment of refractory myasthenia gravis using rituximab: a pediatric case report. *J Pediatr* **143:** 674–677.

Yoshikawa H, Mabuchi K, Yasukawa Y, Takamori M, Yamada M (2002). Low-dose tacrolimus for intractable myasthenia gravis. *J Clin Neurosci* **9:**627–628.

CHAPTER 23

Chronic inflammatory demyelinating polyradiculoneuropathy*

R.A.C Hughes,[a] P. Bouche[b], D.R. Cornblath,[c]
E. Evers,[d] R.D.M. Hadden,[e] A. Hahn,[f] I. Illa,[g]
C.L. Koski,[h] J.M. Léger,[i] E. Nobile-Orazio,[j]
J. Pollard,[k] C. Sommer,[l] P. Van den Bergh,[m]
P.A. van Doorn,[n] I.N. van Schaik[o]

Abstract

Background Numerous sets of diagnostic criteria have sought to define chronic inflammatory
demyelinating polyradiculoneuropathy (CIDP) and
randomized trials and systematic reviews of treatment have been published.

Objectives To prepare consensus guidelines on the
definition, investigation and treatment of CIDP.

Methods Disease experts and a patient representative considered references retrieved from MEDLINE
and Cochrane Systematic Reviews in May 2004
and prepared statements that were agreed to in an
iterative fashion.

The Task Force agreed on Good Practice Points
to define clinical and electrophysiological diagnostic criteria for CIDP with or without concomitant
diseases and investigations to be considered. The
principal treatment recommendations were:

1. Intravenous immunoglobulin (IVIg) or corticosteroids should be considered in sensory and
   motor CIDP (Recommendation Level B).
2. IVIg should be considered as the initial treatment in pure motor CIDP (Good Practice Point).
3. If IVIg and corticosteroids are ineffective plasma
   exchange (PE) should be considered (Recommendation Level A).
4. If the response is inadequate or the maintenance doses of the initial treatment are high,
   combination treatments or adding an immunosuppressant or immunomodulatory drug should
   be considered (Good Practice Point).
5. Symptomatic treatment and multidisciplinary
   management should be considered (Good Practice Point).

*Report of a joint task force of the European Federation
of Neurological Societies and the Peripheral Nerve
Society.

[a]King's College London School of Medicine, London,
UK; [b]Consultation de Pathologie Neuromusculaire
Groupe Salpétriére, France;
[c]Department of Neurology, John Hopkins University,
USA; [d]LCC Offices, Lincolnshire, UK; [e]King's College
London School of Medicine, UK; [f]Division of
Neurology, London Health Sciences Centre, Canada;
[g]Servei Neurologica, Hospital Universitari de la Sta Creu
i Sant Pau, Barcelona, Spain; [h]Department of Neurology,
Baltimore, USA; [i]Consultation de Pathologic
Neuromusculaire Groupe Hospitalier, Pitié Saltpétriére,
France; [j]Neurology, Milan University, Italy; [k]Neurology
Department, University of Sydney, Australia;
[l]Julius-Maximillians Universitat, Würzburg, Germany;
[m]Service de Neurologie, Laboratoire de Biologie
Neuromusculaire, Belgium; [n]Academic Medical Center,
University of Amsterdam, Netherlands; [o]Academic
Medical Center, University of Amsterdam, Netherlands.

European Journal of Neurology 2006, 13:326–332
Journal of the Peripheral Nervous System 2005, 10:220–228

Objectives

To construct guidelines for the definition, diagnosis and treatment of chronic inflammatory demyelinating polyradiculoneuropathy (CIDP) based on the available evidence and, where adequate evidence was not available, consensus.

Background

The first proposal for diagnostic clinical criteria for CIDP was published by Dyck *et al.* (1975, 1982) and included progressive course at 6 months, usually slowed nerve conduction velocities (and occurrence of conduction block), spinal fluid albumino-cytological dissociation, and nerve biopsy demonstrating segmental de- and remyelination, subperineurial or endoneurial oedema, and perivascular inflammation. Exclusion criteria were associated diseases, monoclonal gammopathy and evidence of hereditary neuropathy. This descriptive proposal was the basis for a formalized set of criteria (Barohn *et al.*, 1989). Mandatory inclusion and exclusion criteria reduced the required disease progression time to 2 months. Major laboratory criteria consisted of nerve biopsy abnormalities, motor conduction slowing to < 70% in two nerves, and spinal fluid protein > 450 mg/l. Fulfilment of all criteria was necessary for a definite diagnosis. Fulfilment of only two and one laboratory criteria led to the diagnostic categories of probable and possible, respectively. Research criteria were proposed by an American Academy of Neurology in 1991 (Ad Hoc Subcommittee of the American Academy of Neurology AIDS Task Force, 1991). Fulfilment of clinical, physiological, pathological and spinal fluid criteria led to three diagnostic categories (definite, probable and possible). Fulfilment of pathological criteria was necessary for a definite diagnosis. Physiological criteria for primary demyelination were very detailed, but restrictive when applied clinically as three of four nerve conduction parameters were required to be abnormal, even for the diagnosis of possible CIDP. On the other hand, the criteria for partial motor conduction block and abnormal temporal dispersion were probably not restrictive enough,

as suggested by the American Association of Electrodiagnostic Medicine (AAEM) consensus criteria for the diagnosis of partial conduction block (Olney, 1999). Patients who meet the American Academy of Neurology (AAN) research criteria certainly have CIDP, but many patients who clinicians diagnose as having CIDP do not meet these criteria. In research studies of therapy of CIDP, several different sets of diagnostic criteria for CIDP have been created. These have been reviewed in an addendum to this article, which is available on the Peripheral Nerve Society (PNS) website (http://pns.ucsd.edu/CIDP_GuideLines_Supplement.pdf). We offer the present diagnostic criteria to balance more evenly specificity (which needs to be higher in research than clinical practice) and sensitivity (which might miss treatable disease if set too high).

Since the first treatment trial of prednisone of Dyck and colleagues published in 1982 (Dyck *et al.*, 1982) a small body of evidence from randomised trials has accumulated to allow some evidence-based statements about treatments. These trials have been the subject of Cochrane reviews on which we have based some of our recommendations.

Search strategy

We searched MEDLINE from 1980 onwards on 24 July 2004 for articles on 'chronic inflammatory demyelinating polyradiculoneuropathy' and 'diagnosis' or 'treatment' or 'guideline' but found that the personal databases of Task Force members were more useful. We also searched the Cochrane Library in September 2004.

Methods for reaching consensus

Pairs of task force members prepared draft statements about definition, diagnosis and treatment that were considered at a meeting at the EFNS congress in September 2004. Evidence was classified as Class I to IV and recommendations as Level A to C according to the scheme agreed for EFNS guidelines (Brainin *et al.*, 2004). When only Class IV evidence was available but consensus could be reached the Task Force has offered advice as Good Practice Points (Brainin *et al.*, 2004). The statements were revised and collated into a single document that was then revised iteratively until consensus was reached.

Results

Diagnostic criteria for CIDP

New criteria are currently being developed for defining CIDP from first principles by a group led by CL Koski but in the meantime the Task Force was obliged to develop their own criteria based on consensus. Criteria for CIDP are closely linked to criteria for detection of peripheral nerve demyelination. At least 12 sets of electrodiagnostic criteria for primary demyelination have been published, not only to identify CIDP (for review, see van den Bergh and Piéret, 2004). Nerve biopsy, usually the sural sensory nerve, is considered useful for confirming the diagnosis, but is a mandatory criterion for a definite diagnosis of CIDP only in the American Academy of Neurology criteria. (Ad Hoc Subcommittee of the American Academy of Neurology AIDS Task Force, 1991). The available evidence indicates that sural nerve biopsy can provide supportive evidence for the diagnosis of CIDP, but positive findings are not specific and negative findings do not exclude the diagnosis. Increased spinal fluid protein occurs in at least 90% of patients. Therefore, increased protein levels can be used as a supportive but not mandatory criterion for the diagnosis. Integration of MRI abnormalities of nerve roots, plexuses, and peripheral nerves in diagnostic criteria for CIDP may enhance both sensitivity and specificity and may therefore be useful as a supportive criterion for the diagnosis. As most patients with CIDP respond to steroids, plasma exchange, or IVIg, a positive response to treatment may support the diagnosis and has been suggested as another diagnostic criterion (Latov, 2002). There is only class IV evidence concerning all these matters. Nevertheless the Task Force agreed on Good Practice Points to define clinical and electrophysiological diagnostic criteria for CIDP with or without concomitant diseases (tables 23.1–23.6).

Investigation of CIDP

Based on consensus expert opinion, CIDP should be considered in any patient with a progressive symmetrical or asymmetrical polyradiculoneuropathy in whom the clinical course is relapsing and remitting or progresses for more than two months, especially if there are positive sensory symptoms, proximal weakness, areflexia without wasting, or preferential loss of vibration or joint position sense. Electrodiagnostic tests are mandatory and the major features suggesting a diagnosis of CIDP are listed in table 23.2. Minor electrodiagnostic features are greater abnormality of median than sural nerve sensory action potentials, reduced sensory nerve conduction velocities and F-wave chronodispersion. If electrodiagnostic criteria for definite CIDP are not met initially, repeat electrodiagnostic testing in more nerves or at a later date, CSF examination, magnetic resonance imaging (MRI) of the spinal roots, brachial or lumbar plexus and nerve biopsy should be considered (table 23.6). The nerve for biopsy should be clinically and electrophysiologically affected and is usually the sural, but occasionally the superficial peroneal, superficial radial, or gracilis motor nerve. Sometimes the choice of nerve may be assisted by MRI. The minimal examination should include paraffin sections, immunohistochemistry and semi-thin resin sections. Electron microscopy and teased fibre preparations are highly desirable. There are no specific appearances. Supportive features are endoneurial oedema, macrophage-associated demyelination, demyelinated and to a lesser extent remyelinated nerve fibres, onion bulb formation, endoneurial mononuclear cell infiltration, and variation between fascicles. During the diagnostic work-up investigations to discover possible concomitant diseases should be considered (Good Practice Points, table 23.6).

Treatment of CIDP
Corticosteroids

In one unblinded RCT with 28 participants prednisone was superior to no treatment (Dyck *et al.*, 1982; Mehndiratta and Hughes, 2001) (Class II evidence). Six weeks of oral prednisolone starting at 60 mg daily produced benefit that was not

Table 23.1 Clinical diagnostic criteria.

I Inclusion criteria

A Typical CIDP

- Chronically progressive, stepwise, or recurrent symmetric proximal and distal weakness and sensory dysfunction of all extremities, developing over at least 2 months; cranial nerves may be affected, and
- Absent or reduced tendon reflexes in all extremities

B Atypical CIDP

One of the following, but otherwise as in A (tendon reflexes may be normal in unaffected limbs)

- Predominantly distal weakness (distal acquired demyelinating symmetric, DADS)
- Pure motor or sensory presentations, including chronic sensory immune polyradiculoneuropathy affecting the central process of the primary sensory neuron (Sinnreich *et al.* 2004)
- Asymmetric presentations (multifocal acquired demyelinating sensory and motor, MADSAM, Lewis–Sumner syndrome)
- Focal presentations (e.g. involvement of the brachial plexus or of one or more peripheral nerves in one upper limb)
- Central nervous system involvement (may occur with otherwise typical or other forms of atypical CIDP)

II Exclusion criteria

- Diphtheria, drug or toxin exposure likely to have caused the neuropathy
- Hereditary demyelinating neuropathy, known or likely because of family history, foot deformity, mutilation of hands or feet, retinitis pigmentosa, ichthyosis, liability to pressure palsy
- Presence of sphincter disturbance
- Multifocal motor neuropathy
- Antibodies to myelin associated glycoprotein

significantly different from that produced by a single course of IVIg 2.0 g/kg (Hughes *et al.*, 2001; van Schaik *et al.*, 2004) (Class II evidence). However, there are many observational studies reporting a beneficial effect from corticosteroids except in pure motor CIDP in which they have sometimes appeared to have a harmful effect (Donaghy *et al.*, 1994). Consequently, a trial of corticosteroids should be considered in all patients with significant disability (Recommendation Level B). There is no evidence and no consensus about whether to use daily or alternate day prednisolone or prednisone or intermittent high dose monthly intravenous or oral regimens (Bromberg and Carter, 2004).

Plasma exchange

Two small double-blind randomised controlled trials (RCTs) with altogether 47 participants showed that PE provides significant short-term benefit in

about two-thirds of patients but rapid deterioration may occur afterwards (Dyck *et al.*, 1986; Hahn *et al.*, 1996a; Mehndiratta *et al.*, 2004) (Class I evidence). Plasma exchange might be considered as an initial treatment (Recommendation Level A). However, because adverse events related to difficulty with venous access, use of citrate and haemodynamic changes are not uncommon, either corticosteroids or IVIg should be considered first (Good Practice Point).

Intravenous immunoglobulin

Meta-analysis of four double blind RCTs with altogether 113 participants showed that IVIg 2.0 g/kg produces significant improvement in disability lasting 2–6 weeks (van Doorn *et al.*, 1990; Vermeulen *et al.*, 1993; Hahn *et al.*, 1996b; Mendell *et al.*, 2001; van Schaik *et al.*, 2004) (Class I evidence). As the benefit from IVIg is short lived, treatment, which is expensive, needs to be repeated at

Table 23.2 Electrodiagnostic criteria.

I Definite: at least one of the following

A. At least 50% prolongation of motor distal latency above the upper limit of normal values in two nerves, or
B. At least 30% reduction of motor conduction velocity below the lower limit of normal values in two nerves, or
C. At least 20% prolongation of F-wave latency above the upper limit of normal values in two nerves (>50% if amplitude of distal negative peak CMAP < 80% of lower limit of normal values), or
D. Absence of F-waves in two nerves if these nerves have amplitudes of distal negative peak CMAPs at least 20% of lower limit of normal values + at least one other demyelinating parameter[a] in at least one other nerve, or
E. Partial motor conduction block: at least 50% amplitude reduction of the proximal negative peak CMAP relative to distal, if distal negative peak CMAP at least 20% of lower limit of normal values, in two nerves, or in one nerve + at least one other demyelinating parameter[a] in at least one other nerve, or
F. Abnormal temporal dispersion (>30% duration increase between the proximal and distal negative peak CMAP) in at least two nerves, or
G. Distal CMAP duration (interval between onset of the first negative peak and return to baseline of the last negative peak) of at least 9 ms in at least one nerve + at least one other demyelinating parameter[a] in at least one other nerve

II Probable

At least 30% amplitude reduction of the proximal negative peak CMAP relative to distal, excluding the posterior tibial nerve, if distal negative peak CMAP at least 20% of lower limit of normal values, in two nerves, or in one nerve + at least one other demyelinating parameter[a] in at least one other nerve

III Possible

As in I but in only one nerve

Note: To apply these criteria the median, ulnar (stimulated below the elbow), peroneal (stimulated below the fibular head) and tibial nerves on one side are tested. Temperatures should be maintained to at least 33°C at the palm and 30° C at the external malleolus. (Good Practice Points). Further technical details are given in the accompanying web document (www.blackwell-synergy.com/toc/ene/13/4) and see van den Bergh and Pieret, 2004).

[a] Any nerve meeting any of the criteria A–G

Table 23.3 Supportive criteria.

A. Elevated cerebrospinal fluid protein with leukocyte count < 10/mm^3 (Recommendation Level A)
B. Magnetic Resonance Imaging showing gadolinium enhancement and/or hypertrophy of the cauda equina, lumbosacral or cervical nerve roots, or the brachial or lumbosacral plexuses (Recommendation Level C)
C. Nerve biopsy showing unequivocal evidence of demyelination and/or remyelination in >= 5 or more fibres by electron microscopy or in >6 of 50 teased fibres
D. Clinical improvement following immunomodulatory treatment (Recommendation Level A)

intervals that need to be judged on an individual basis. Crossover trials have shown no significant short-term difference between IVIg and plasma exchange (Dyck *et al.*, 1994) or between IVIg and prednisolone (Hughes *et al.*, 2001), but the samples were too small to establish equivalence (both Class II evidence).

Immunosuppressive agents

No RCTs have been reported for any immunosuppressive agent except for azathioprine that showed no benefit when added to prednisone in 14 patients (Dyck *et al.*, 1985; Hughes *et al.*, 2004). Immunosuppressive agents (table 23.7) are often used together with corticosteroids to reduce the

Table 23.4 CIDP in association with concomitant diseases.

One of the following is present:

a. Conditions in which, in some cases, the pathogenesis and pathology are thought to be the same as in CIDP

- Diabetes mellitus
- HIV infection
- Chronic active hepatitis
- IgG or IgA monoclonal gammopathy of undetermined significance
- IgM monoclonal gammopathy without antibodies to myelin associated glycoprotein
- Systemic lupus erythematosus or other connective tissue disease
- Sarcoidosis
- Thyroid disease

b. Conditions in which the pathogenesis and pathology may be different from CIDP

- *Borrelia burgdorferi* infection (Lyme disease)
- IgM monoclonal gammopathy of undetermined significance with antibodies to myelin associated glycoprotein[a]
- POEMS syndrome
- Osteosclerotic myeloma
- Others (vasculitis, haematological and non-haematological malignancies, including Waldenström's macroglobulinaemia and Castleman's disease)

[a]Patients with antibodies to myelin associated glycoprotein are considered to have a disease with a different mechanism and are excluded. See table 23.1.

Table 23.5 Diagnostic categories.

Definite CIDP
Clinical criteria I A or B and II with electrodiagnostic criteria I; or
Probable CIDP + at least one supportive criterion; or
Possible CIDP + at least two supportive criteria

Probable CIDP
Clinical criteria I A or B and II with electrodiagnostic criteria II; or
Possible CIDP + at least one supportive criterion

Possible CIDP
Clinical criteria I A or B and II with electrodiagnostic criteria III
CIDP (definite, probable, possible) associated with concomitant diseases

need for IVIg or PE or to treat patients who have not responded to any of these treatments but there is only class IV evidence on which to base this practice (Hughes *et al.*, 2004). More research is needed before any recommendation can be made. In the meantime immunosuppressant treatment may be considered when the response to corticosteroids, IVIg or PE is inadequate (Good Practice Point).

Interferons

One crossover trial of interferon beta 1a for 12 weeks did not detect significant benefit (Hadden *et al.*, 1999), but the trial only included 10 patients. In a more recent non-randomised open study of intramuscular beta interferon 1a 30 mcg weekly 7 of 20 patients treated showed clinical improvement, 10 remained stable and 3 worsened (Vallat *et al.*, 2003). An open study of interferon alpha

Table 23.6 Investigations to be considered.

To identify CIDP
Nerve conduction studies
CSF cells and protein
MRI spinal roots, brachial plexus and lumbosacral plexus
Nerve biopsy

To detect concomitant diseases
Serum and urine paraprotein detection by immunofixation
  (repeating this should be considered in patients who are
  or become unresponsive to treatment)
Oral glucose tolerance test
Complete blood count
Renal function
Liver function
HIV antibody
Hepatitis B and C serology
Borrelia burgdorferi serology
C reactive protein
Anti-nuclear factor
Extractable nuclear antigen antibodies
Thyroid function
Angiotensin converting enzyme
Chest radiograph
Skeletal survey (repeating this should be considered in
  patients who are or become unresponsive to treatment)

To detect hereditary neuropathy
Examination of parents and siblings
PMP22 gene duplication or deletion (especially if slowing of
  conduction is uniform and no evidence of partial motor
  conduction block or abnormal temporal dispersion)
Gene mutations known to cause CMT1 or hereditary
  neuropathy with liability to pressure palsies

Table 23.7 Immunosuppressant and immunomodulatory drugs which have been reported to be beneficial in CIDP (Class IV evidence, see Hughes *et al.*, (2004) for review).

Anti-CD20 (rituximab)	Etanercept
Azathioprine	Interferon alpha
Cyclophosphamide	Interferon beta1a
Ciclosporin	Mycophenolate mofetil

showed benefit in 9 of 14 treatment-resistant patients (Gorson *et al.*, 1998) and there have been other favourable smaller reports. In the absence of evidence interferon treatment may be considered when the response to corticosteroids, IVIg or PE is inadequate (Good Practice Point).

Initial management (Good Practice Points)

Patients with very mild symptoms that do not or only slightly interfere with activities of daily living may be monitored without treatment. Urgent treatment with corticosteroids or IVIg should be considered for patients with moderate or severe disability, for example, when hospitalization is required or ambulation is severely impaired. Common initial doses of corticosteroids are prednisolone or prednisone 1 mg/kg or 60 mg daily but there is a wide variation in practice (Bromberg and Carter, 2004). The usual first dose of IVIg is 2.0 g/kg given as 0.4 g/kg on five consecutive days. Contraindications to corticosteroids will influence the choice towards IVIg and vice versa. For pure motor CIDP, IVIg treatment should be the first choice and if corticosteroids are used, patients should be monitored closely for deterioration.

Long-term management (Good Practice Points)

No evidence-based guideline can be given as none of the trials systematically assessed long-term management. Each patient requires assessment on an individual basis. For patients starting on corticosteroids a course of up to 12 weeks on their starting dose should be considered before deciding whether there is no treatment response. If there is a response, tapering the dose to a low maintenance level over one or two years and eventual withdrawal should be considered. For patients starting on IVIg, observation to discover the occurrence and duration of any response to the first course should be considered before embarking on further treatment. Between 15 and 30% of patients do not need further treatment. If patients respond to IVIg and then worsen, further and ultimately repeated doses should be considered. Repeated doses may be given over one or two days. The amount per course needs to be titrated according to the individual response. Repeat courses may be needed every 2–6 weeks. If a patient becomes stable on a regime of intermittent IVIg, the dose per course should be reduced before the frequency of administration is lowered. If frequent high dose IVIg is needed, the addition of corticosteroids or an immunosuppressive agent should be considered. Approximately 15% of patients fail to respond to any of these treatments. Some probably do not appear to respond because of severe secondary axonal degeneration that takes years to improve.

General treatment

There is a dearth of evidence concerning general aspects of treatment for symptoms of CIDP such as pain and fatigue. There is also a lack of research into the value of exercise and physiotherapy and the advice that should be offered concerning immunisations. International and national support groups offer information and support and physicians may consider putting patients in touch with these organisations at www.guillain-barre.com/ or www.gbs.org.uk (Good Practice Point).

RECOMMENDATIONS

Good Practice Points for defining diagnostic criteria for CIDP:

1. Clinical: typical and atypical CIDP (table 23.1)
2. Electrodiagnostic: definite, probable and possible CIDP (table 23.2)
3. Supportive: including CSF, MRI, nerve biopsy and treatment response (table 23.3)
4. CIDP in association with concomitant diseases (table 23.4)
5. Categories: definite, probable, and possible CIDP with or without concomitant diseases (table 23.5)

Good Practice Points for diagnostic tests

1. Electrodiagnostic tests are recommended in all patients (Good Practice Point)
2. CSF, MRI and nerve biopsy should be considered in selected patients (Good Practice Point)

3. Concomitant diseases should be considered in all patients but the choice of tests will depend on the clinical circumstances (table 23.6).

Recommendations for treatment
For induction of treatment

1. IVIg or corticosteroids should be considered in sensory and motor CIDP in the presence of troublesome symptoms (Level B). The presence of relative contraindications to either treatment should influence the choice (Good Practice Point).
2. The advantages and disadvantages should be explained to the patient who should be involved in the decision making (Good Practice Point).
3. In pure motor CIDP IVIg should be considered as the initial treatment (Good Practice Point).
4. If IVIg and corticosteroids are ineffective PE should be considered (Level A).

For maintenance treatment

1. If the first line treatment is effective continuation should be considered until the maximum benefit has been achieved and then the dose reduced to find the lowest effective maintenance dose (Good Practice Point).
2. If the response is inadequate or the maintenance doses of the initial treatment are high, combination treatments or adding an immunosuppressant or immunomodulatory drug may be considered (table 23.7) (Good Practice Point).
3. Advice about foot care, exercise, diet, driving and life style management should be considered. Neuropathic pain should be treated with drugs according to the EFNS guideline on treatment of neuropathic pain (Attal N, 2005 in preparation). Depending on the needs of the patient, orthoses, physiotherapy, occupational therapy, psychological support and referral to a rehabilitation specialist should be considered (Good Practice Points).
4. Information about patient support groups should be offered to those who would like it (Good Practice Point).

Conflicts of interest

The following authors have reported conflicts of interest as follows: R Hughes: personal none, departmental research grants or honoraria from Bayer, Biogen-Idec, Schering-LFB and Kedrion; D Cornblath: personal honoraria from Aventis Behring and Baxter; A Hahn: personal honoraria from Baxter, Bayer, Biogen-Idec; C Koski: personal honoraria from American Red Cross, Baxter, Bayer, ZLB-Behring; JM Léger: personal none, departmental research grants or honoraria from Biogen-Idec, Baxter, Laboratoire Français du Biofractionnement (LFB), Octapharma; E Nobile-Orazio: personal from Kedrion, Grifols, Baxter, LFB (and he has been commissioned by Kedrion and Baxter to give expert opinions to the Italian Ministry of Health on the use of IVIg in dysimmune neuropathies); J Pollard: departmental research grants from Biogen-Idec, Schering; P van Doorn: personal none, departmental research grants or honoraria from Baxter and Bayer. The other authors have nothing to declare.

References

Ad Hoc Subcommittee of the American Academy of Neurology AIDS Task Force. (1991). Research criteria for the diagnosis of chronic inflammatory demyelinating polyradiculoneuropathy (CIDP). *Neurology* **41**:617–618.

Barohn RJ, Kissel JT, Warmolts JR, Mendell JR (1989). Chronic inflammatory demyelinating polyradiculoneuropathy. Clinical characteristics, course, and recommendations for diagnostic criteria. *Arch Neurology* **46**:878–884.

Brainin M, Barnes M, Baron J-C, Gilhus NE, Hughes R, Selmaj K, Waldemar G (2004). Guidance for the preparation of neurological management guidelines by EFNS scientific task forces - revised recommendations 2004. *Euro J Neurol* **11**:577–581.

Bromberg MB, Carter O (2004). Corticosteroid use in the treatment of neuromuscular disorders: empirical and evidence-based data. *Muscle & Nerve* **30**:20–37.

Donaghy M, Mills KR, Boniface SJ, Simmons J, Wright I, Gregson N, Jacobs J (1994). Pure motor demyelinating neuropathy: Deterioration after steroid treatment and improvement with intravenous immunoglobulin. *J Neurol Neurosurg Psychiatry* **57**:778–783.

Dyck PJ, Daube J, O'Brien P, Pineda A, Low PA, Windebank AJ, Swanson C (1986). Plasma exchange in chronic inflammatory demyelinating polyradiculoneuropathy. *New Engl J Med* **314**:461–465.

Dyck PJ, Lais AC, Ohta M, Bastron JA, Okazaki H, Groover RV (1975). Chronic inflammatory polyradiculoneuropathy. *Proceedings of the Mayo Clinic* **50**:621–651.

Dyck PJ, Litchy WJ, Kratz KM, Suarez GA, Low PA, Pineda AA, Windebank AJ, Karnes JL, O'Brien PC (1994). A plasma exchange versus immune globulin infusion trial in chronic inflammatory demyelinating polyradiculoneuropathy. *Ann Neurol* **36**: 838–845.

Dyck PJ, O'Brien P, Swanson C, Low P, Daube J (1985). Combined azathioprine and prednisone in chronic inflammatory-demyelinating polyneuropathy. *Neurology* **35**:1173–1176.

Dyck PJ, O'Brien PC, Oviatt KF, Dinapoli RP, Daube JR, Bartleson JD, Mokri B, Swift T, Low PA, Windebank AJ (1982). Prednisone improves chronic inflammatory demyelinating polyradiculoneuropathy more than no treatment. *Ann Neurol* **11**:136–141.

Gorson KC, Ropper AH, Clark BD, Dew RB, III, Simovic D, Allam G (1998). Treatment of chronic inflammatory demyelinating polyneuropathy with interferon-alpha 2a. *Neurology* **50**:84–87.

Hadden RD, Sharrack B, Bensa S, Soudain SE, Hughes RAC (1999). Randomized trial of interferon beta-1a in chronic inflammatory demyelinating polyradiculoneuropathy. *Neurology* **53**:57–61.

Hahn AF, Bolton CF, Pillay N, Chalk C, Benstead T, Bril V, Shumak K, Vandervoort MK, Feasby TE (1996a). Plasma-exchange therapy in chronic inflammatory demyelinating polyneuropathy (CIDP): a double-blind, sham-controlled, cross-over study. *Brain* **119**:1055–1066.

Hahn AF, Bolton CF, Zochodne D, Feasby TE (1996b). Intravenous immunoglobulin treatment (IVIg) in chronic inflammatory demyelinating polyneuropathy (CIDP): a double-blind placebo-controlled cross-over study. *Brain* **119**:1067–1078.

Hughes RAC, Bensa S, Willison HJ, van den Bergh P, Comi G, Illa I, Nobile-Orazio E, van Doorn PA, Dalakas M, Bojar M, Swan AV, and the Inflammatory Neuropathy Cause and Treatment Group (2001). Randomized controlled trial of intravenous immunoglobulin versus oral prednisolone in chronic inflammatory demyelinating polyradiculoneuropathy. *Ann Neurol* **50**:195–201.

Hughes RAC, Swan AV, van Doorn PA (2004). Cytotoxic drugs and interferons for chronic inflammatory demyelinating polyradiculoneuropathy (Update). The Cochrane Database of Systematic Reviews Issue

4(CD003280). 2004. Chichester, UK: John Wiley & Sons, Ltd.

Latov N (2002). Diagnosis of CIDP. *Neurology* **59:**S2–S6.

Mehndiratta MM, Hughes RAC (2001). Corticosteroids for chronic inflammatory demyelinating polyradiculoneuropathy. The Cochrane Database of Systematic Reviews 3(CD 002062).

Mehndiratta MM, Hughes RAC, Agarwal P (2004). Plasma exchange for chronic inflammatory demyelinating polyradiculoneuropathy (Cochrane Review). The Cochrane Database of Systematic Reviews Issue 3(CD003906).

Mendell JR, Barohn RJ, Freimer ML, Kissel JT, King W, Nagaraja HN, Rice R, Campbell WW, Donofrio PD, Jackson CE, Lewis RA, Shy M, Simpson DM, Parry GJ, Rivner MH, Thornton CA, Bromberg MB, Tandan R, Harati Y, Giuliani MJ (2001). Randomized controlled trial of IVIg in untreated chronic inflammatory demyelinating polyradiculoneuropathy. *Neurology* **56:**445–449.

Olney RK (1999). Guidelines in Electrodiagnostic Medicine: Consensus criteria for the diagnosis of partial conduction block. *Muscle & Nerve* **22:** S225–S229.

Sinnreich M, Klein CJ, Daube JR, Engelstad J, Spinner RJ, Dyck PJB (2004). Chronic immune sensory polyradiculoneuropathy: A possibly treatable sensory ataxia. *Neurology* **63:**1662–1669.

Vallat JM, Hahn AF, Leger JM, Cros DP, Magy L, Tabaraud F, Bouche P, Preux PM (2003). Interferon beta-1a as an investigational treatment for CIDP. *Neurology* **60:**S23–S28.

van den Bergh PYK, Piéret F (2004). Electrodiagnostic criteria for acute and chronic inflammatory demyelinating polyradiculoneuropathy. *Muscle & Nerve* **29:**565–574.

van Doorn PA, Brand A, Strengers PF, Meulstee J, Vermeulen M (1990). High-dose intravenous immunoglobulin treatment in chronic inflammatory demyelinating polyneuropathy: a double-blind, placebo-controlled, crossover study [see comments]. *Neurology* **40:**209–212.

van Schaik IN, Winer JB, de Haan R, Vermeulen M (2004). Intravenous immunoglobulin for chronic inflammatory demyelinating polyneuropathy. Cochrane Database Syst.Rev. 2(CD001797).

Vermeulen M, van Doorn PA, Brand A, Strengers PFW, Jennekens FGI, Busch HFM (1993). Intravenous immunoglobulin treatment in patients with chronic inflammatory demyelinating polyneuropathy: A double blind, placebo controlled study. *J Neurol Neurosurg Psychiatry* **56:**36–39.

CHAPTER 24

Multifocal motor neuropathy*

I.N. van Schaik,[a] P. Bouche,[b] I. Illa,[c] J.M. Léger,[b]
P. Van den Bergh,[d] D.R. Cornblath,[e] E. Evers,[f]
R.D.M. Hadden,[g] R.A.C. Hughes,[h] C.L. Koski,[i]
E. Nobile-Orazio,[j] J. Pollard,[k] C. Sommer,[l]
P.A. van Doorn[m]

Abstract

Background Several diagnostic criteria for multifocal motor neuropathy (MMN) have been proposed in recent years and a beneficial effect of intravenous immunoglobulin (IVIg) and various other immunomodulatory drugs has been suggested in several trials and uncontrolled studies.

Objectives To prepare consensus guidelines on the definition, investigation and treatment of MMN.

Methods Disease experts and a patient representative considered references retrieved from MEDLINE

and the Cochrane Library in July 2004 and prepared statements that were agreed to in an iterative fashion.

The Task Force agreed on Good Practice Points to define clinical and electrophysiological diagnostic criteria for MMN and investigations to be considered. The principal recommendations and Good Practice Points were:

1. IVIg (2 g/kg given over 2–5 days) should be considered as the first line treatment (Recommendation Level A) when disability is sufficiently severe to warrant treatment.
2. Corticosteroids are not recommended (Good Practice Point).
3. If initial treatment with IVIg is effective, repeated IVIg treatment should be considered (Recommendation Level C). The frequency of IVIg maintenance therapy should be guided by the individual response (Good Practice Point).

---

*Report of a joint task force of the European Federation of Neurological Societies and the Peripheral Nerve Society

[a]Academic Medical Center, University of Amsterdam, Dept of Neurology, Amsterdam, the Netherlands; [b]Hospital de la Salpetriere, Dept of Neurology, Paris, France; [c]Hospital Sta Creu i Sant Pau, Universitat Autonoma de Barcelona, Dept of Neurology, Barcelona, Spain; [d]Cliniques Universitaires St-Luc, Universite Catholique de Louvain, Dept of Neurology, Brussels, Belgium; [e]Johns Hopkins University School of Medicine,

Journal of the Peripheral Nervous System 2006, 11:1–8

Dept of Neurology, Baltimore, USA; [f]Guillain-Barré Syndrome Support Group, Leicester, UK; [g]King's College Hospital, Dept of Neurology, London, UK; [h]King's College London School of Medicine, Dept of Neurology, London, UK; [i]University of Maryland, School of Medicine, Dept of Neurology, Baltimore, Maryland, USA; [j]University of Milan IRCCS Humanitas Clinical Institute, Dept of Neurological Sciences Dino Ferrari Center, Milan, Italy; [k]University of Sydney, Department of Medicine, Sydney, Australia; [l]University of Würzburg, Dept of Neurology, Wurzburg, Germany; [m]Erasmus Medical Center, Dept of Neurology, Rotterdam, the Netherlands.

Typical treatment regimens are 1 g/kg every 2–4 weeks or 2 g/kg every 4–8 weeks (Good Practice Point).

4. If IVIg is not or not sufficiently effective then immunosuppressive treatment may be considered. Cyclophosphamide, ciclosporin, azathioprine, interferon beta1a, or rituximab are possible agents (Good Practice Point).

5. Toxicity makes cyclophosphamide a less desirable option (Good Practice Point).

Objectives

To construct guidelines for the definition, diagnosis and treatment of multifocal motor neuropathy (MMN) based on the available evidence and, where adequate evidence was not available, consensus.

Background

Patients with a pure motor, asymmetric neuropathy with multifocal conduction blocks (CB) have been reported from 1986 onwards (Chad et al., 1986; Roth et al., 1986; Parry and Clarke, 1988). Pestronk and colleagues first introduced the term multifocal motor neuropathy and highlighted the association with IgM anti-ganglioside GM1 antibodies and the response to immune-modulating therapies (Pestronk et al., 1988). The diagnosis of MMN is based on clinical, laboratory and electrophysiological characteristics (Parry and Sumner, 1992; Van den Berg-Vos et al., 2000a; Nobile-Orazio, 2001; Nobile-Orazio et al., 2005). Several diagnostic criteria for this neuropathy have been proposed (Van den Berg-Vos et al., 2000c; Hughes, 2001; Olney et al., 2003). These criteria share the following clinical features: slowly progressive, asymmetric, predominantly distal weakness without objective loss of sensation in the distribution of two or more individual peripheral nerves, and absence of upper motor neuron signs. The hallmark of the disease is the presence of multifocal conduction block on electrophysiological testing outside the usual sites of nerve compression (Cornblath et al., 1991; Kaji and Kimura, 1991; Parry and Sumner, 1992; Parry, 1993; Van Asseldonk et al., 2003). Conduction block is a reduction in the amplitude or area (or both) of the compound muscle action potential (CMAP) obtained by proximal versus distal stimulation of motor nerves in the absence of or with only focal abnormal temporal dispersion (Cornblath et al., 1991; Nobile-Orazio, 2001; Kaji, 2003). The extent of reduction of the CMAP amplitude and/or area necessary for conduction block are still matters of debate. For this guideline, we present clinical and electrophysiological diagnostic criteria based on published criteria and consensus agreed upon by the task force.

MMN is a treatable disorder. A beneficial effect of various immunomodulatory drugs has been suggested in several uncontrolled studies (Pestronk et al., 1988; Krarup et al., 1990; Feldman et al., 1991; Hausmanowa-Petrusewicz et al., 1991; Chaudhry et al., 1993; Meucci et al., 1997; Van Es et al., 1997; Martina et al., 1999; Van den Berg-Vos et al., 2000b; Léger et al., 2005), and reviewed in a Cochrane systematic review (Umapathi et al., 2005). Four trials have shown high dose intravenous immunoglobulin (IVIg) therapy to be effective in MMN and this treatment currently is considered the standard treatment for MMN (Azulay et al., 1994; Van den Berg et al., 1995; Federico et al., 2000; Léger et al., 2001). These trials have also been reviewed in a Cochrane systematic review (van Schaik et al., 2005). This small body of evidence allowed some evidence-based statements about treatment.

Search strategy

We searched MEDLINE from 1980 onwards on 24 July 2004 for articles on ('multifocal motor neuropathy' and 'diagnosis' or 'treatment' or 'guideline') but found that the personal databases of Task Force members were more useful. We also searched the Cochrane Library in September 2004.

Methods for reaching consensus

Pairs of task force members prepared draft statements about definition, diagnosis and treatment that were considered at a meeting in September 2004. Evidence was classified as Class I to IV and recommendations as Level A to C according to the scheme agreed for EFNS guidelines (Brainin et al., 2004). When only Class IV evidence was available but consensus could be reached the Task Force has offered advice as Good Practice Points. The statements were revised and collated into a single document that was then revised iteratively until consensus was reached.

Results

Diagnostic criteria for MMN

The Task Force developed their own diagnostic criteria based on the published criteria (Parry and Sumner, 1992; Van den Berg-Vos et al., 2000a, 2000c; Nobile-Orazio, 2001; Hughes, 2001; Olney et al., 2003; Nobile-Orazio et al., 2005). The clinical criteria are listed in table 24.1. The main clinical features are weakness without objective sensory loss, slowly progressive or stepwise progressive

Table 24.1 Clinical criteria for MMN.

Core criteria (both must be present)

1. Slowly progressive or stepwise progressive, asymmetric limb weakness, or motor involvement having a motor nerve distribution in at least two nerves, for more than one month[a]
2. No objective sensory abnormalities except for minor vibration sense abnormalities in the lower limbs

Supportive clinical criteria

3. Predominant upper limb involvement[b]
4. Decreased or absent tendon reflexes in the affected limb[c]
5. Absence of cranial nerve involvement[d]
6. Cramps and fasciculations in the affected limb

Exclusion criteria

7. Upper motor neuron signs
8. Marked bulbar involvement
9. Sensory impairment more marked than minor vibration loss in the lower limbs
10. Diffuse symmetric weakness during the initial weeks
11. Laboratory: CSF protein >1 g/l

---

[a] Usually more than six months;
[b] At onset, predominant lower limb involvement account for nearly 10% of the cases;
[c] Slightly increased tendon reflexes, in particular in the affected arm have been reported and do not exclude the diagnosis of MMN provided criterion 7 is met;
[d] 12th nerve palsy reported.

course, asymmetric involvement of two or more nerves, and absence of upper motor neuron signs. Additional clinical criteria have also been proposed: no more than 7 of 8 affected limb regions, predominance of weakness in the upper limbs, decreased or absent tendon reflexes, and age of onset between 20 and 65 (Van den Berg-Vos et al., 2000a). These additional features were associated with a more frequent response to immunoglobulin therapy but it was unclear how they influenced diagnostic accuracy, and the absence of some of these features is not uncommon in patients with otherwise typical MMN (Nobile-Orazio et al., 2005). The Task Force decided not to include an age limit in the criteria.

The presence of conduction block (CB) in motor nerve fibres is the hallmark of the disease. The first papers defined CB as a 20–30% amplitude or area reduction if the distal CMAP duration did not exceed 15% greater than normal. In one of the main papers concerning the diagnostic criteria of MMN grading of CB was defined as definite or probable and in the other as definite, probable and possible (Van den Berg-Vos et al., 2000c; Hughes, 2001; Olney et al., 2003). There is only Class IV evidence concerning all these matters. Nevertheless, the Task Force agreed on Good Practice Points to define clinical and electrophysiological diagnostic criteria for MMN (tables 24.1 and 24.2).

Investigation of MMN

Based on consensus expert opinion, consideration of MMN should enter the differential diagnosis of any patient with a slowly or stepwise progressive asymmetrical limb weakness without objective sensory abnormalities, upper motor neuron or bulbar signs or symptoms. MMN should be differentiated from motor neuron disease, entrapment neuropathies, hereditary neuropathy with liability to pressure palsy, Lewis–Sumner syndrome, and chronic inflammatory demyelinating polyneuropathy, in particular its purely motor variant (Chad et al., 1986; Parry and Clarke, 1988; Pestronk et al., 1990; Veugelers et al., 1996; Beydoun, 1998; Saperstein et al., 1999; Parry, 1999; Ellis et al., 1999; Lewis, 1999; Molinuevo et al., 1999; Mezaki et al., 1999; Van den Berg-Vos et al., 2000c; Visser et al., 2002; Oh et al., 2005).

Table 24.2 Electrophysiological criteria for conduction block.[a]

1. Definite motor CB[a]

Negative CMAP area reduction on proximal versus distal stimulation of at least 50% whatever the nerve segment length (median, ulnar and peroneal). Negative CMAP amplitude on stimulation of the distal part of the segment with motor CB must be >20% of the lower limit of normal and >1 mV (baseline negative peak) and an increase of proximal negative peak CMAP duration must be ≤30%.

2. Probable motor CB[a]

Negative CMAP area reduction of at least 30% over a long segment of an upper limb nerve with an increase of proximal negative peak CMAP duration ≤30%;

OR

Negative CMAP area reduction of at least 50% (same as definite) with an increase of proximal negative peak CMAP duration >30%.

3. Normal sensory nerve conduction in upper limb segments with CB and normal SNAP amplitudes (see exclusion criteria).

[a] Evidence for conduction block must be found at sites distinct from common entrapment or compression syndromes.

Clinical examination and electrodiagnostic tests are mandatory and the features suggesting a diagnosis of MMN are listed under diagnostic criteria. A family history should be obtained. Other tests that can support the diagnosis MMN are CSF protein <1 g/l, anti-ganglioside GM1 antibodies (van Schaik et al., 1995; Taylor et al., 1996; Willison and Yuki, 2002) and increased signal intensity on T2-weighted MRI scans of the brachial plexus (Van Es et al., 1997; Van den Berg-Vos et al. 2000a, 2000c;. CSF, anti-ganglioside GM1 antibodies and MRI scans of the brachial plexus are not normally needed for patients fulfilling the clinical and electrodiagnostic criteria of MMN. Nerve biopsies are not routinely performed in MMN but can be useful in detecting an alternative cause (Bouche et al., 1995; Corse et al., 1996). Needle EMG, serum and urine paraprotein detection by immunofixation (Noguchi et al., 2003), thyroid function (Toscano et al., 2002), creatine kinase (Chaudhry et al., 1993; Van den Berg-Vos et al., 2000a), CSF cells and protein (Taylor et al., 2000; Van den Berg-Vos et al., 2000a) are investigations that can be helpful to discover concomitant disease or exclude other possible causes. This list is not complete and additional investigations should be guided by the clinical findings.

Treatment of MMN

The treatment options for people with MMN are sparse. In contrast to the response in CIDP, MMN does usually not respond to steroids or plasma exchange, and patients may worsen when they receive these treatments (Van den Berg et al., 1997; Carpo et al., 1998; Claus et al., 2000; Nobile-Orazio, 2001).

The efficacy of IVIg has been suggested by many open, uncontrolled studies. Four randomised controlled double-blind trials of IVIg for treating MMN have been done (Azulay et al., 1994; Van den Berg et al., 1995; Federico et al., 2000; Léger et al., 2001). These four RCTs included a total of 45 patients with MMN and have been summarized in a Cochrane systematic review (van Schaik et al., 2005). IVIg treatment is superior to placebo in inducing an improvement in muscle strength in patients with MMN (NNT 1.4, 95% CI 1.1–1.8)). As weakness is the only determinant of disability in patients with MMN, it is to be expected that in patients whose muscle strength improves after IVIg treatment, disability will improve as well. In a large retrospective study elevated anti-ganglioside GM1 antibodies and definite CB were significantly correlated with a favourable response to IVIg (Van den Berg-Vos et al., 2000a). In approximately a third of patients prolonged remission (>12 months) was established with IVIg alone; approximately half of patients need repeated IVIg infusions and, of them, half need additional immunosuppressive treatment.(Léger et al., 2005). Effectiveness declines during prolonged treatment, even when dosage is increased, probably due to ongoing axonal degeneration (Van den Berg *et al.*, 1998; Terenghi *et al.*, 2004). However, in one retrospective study, treatment with higher than normal maintenance doses of IVIg (1.6–2.0 g/kg given over 4–5 days) promoted reinnervation, decreased the number of conduction blocks and prevented axonal degeneration in ten MMN patients for up to 12 years (Vucic *et al.*, 2004).

Uncontrolled studies suggest a beneficial effect of cyclophosphamide (Pestronk *et al.*, 1988; Krarup *et al.*, 1990; Feldman *et al.*, 1991; Chaudhry *et al.*, 1993; Meucci *et al.*, 1997; Van Es *et al.*, 1997), interferon beta1a (Martina *et al.*, 1999; Van den Berg-Vos *et al.*, 2000b), and azathioprine (Hausmanowa-Petrusewicz *et al.*, 1991; Léger *et al.*, 2005). There is conflicting evidence for rituximab (Rojas-Garcia *et al.*, 2003; Rüegg *et al.*, 2004). Cyclophosphamide was not recommended by one group of experts because concern exists about its toxicity and lack of evidence of efficacy in MMN (Hughes, 2001).

Recommendations and Good Practice Points

Diagnostic criteria (Good Practice Points)

1. Clinical: the two core criteria and all exclusion criteria should be met (table 24.1).
2. Electrodiagnostic: definite or probable conduction block in at least two nerves (table 24.2).
3. Supportive: anti-GM1 antibodies, MRI, CSF and treatment response (table 24.3).
4. Categories: definite and probable MMN (table 24.4).

Diagnostic tests (Good Practice Points)

1. Clinical examination and electrodiagnostic tests should be considered in all patients.
2. Anti-ganglioside GM1 antibody testing, MRI of the brachial plexus, and CSF examination should be considered in selected patients.
3. Investigations to discover concomitant disease or exclude other possible causes should be considered but the choice of tests will depend on the individual circumstances.

Table 24.3 Supportive criteria.

1. Elevated IgM anti-ganglioside GM1 antibodies (Recommendation Level A).
2. Magnetic Resonance Imaging showing gadolinium enhancement and/or hypertrophy of the brachial plexuses (Good Practice Point).
3. Clinical improvement following IVIg treatment (Good Practice Point).

Table 24.4 Diagnostic categories.

Definite MMN
Clinical criteria 1, 2 and 7–11 (table 24.1) AND electrophysiological criteria 1 and 3 in one nerve (table 24.2).

Probable MMN
Clinical criteria 1, 2 and 7–11 AND electrophysiological criteria 2 and 3 in two nerves
Clinical criteria 1, 2 and 7–11 AND electrophysiological criteria 2 and 3 in one nerve AND at least one supportive criteria 1–3 (table 24.3).

Treatment

1. IVIg (2 g/kg given over 2–5 days) should be considered as the first line treatment (Level A) when disability is sufficiently severe to warrant treatment.
2. Corticosteroids are not recommended (Good Practice Point).
3. If an initial treatment with IVIg is effective, repeated IVIg treatment should be considered in selected patients (Level C). The frequency of IVIg maintenance therapy should be guided by the response (Good Practice Point). Typical treatment regimens are 1 g/kg every 2–4 weeks, or 2 g/kg every 1–2 months (Good Practice Point).
4. If IVIg is not or not sufficiently effective then immunosuppressive treatment may be considered. Cyclophosphamide, ciclosporin, azathioprine, interferon beta1a, or rituximab are possible agents (Good Practice Point).
5. Toxicity makes cyclophosphamide a less desirable option (Good Practice Point).

Conflicts of interest

The following authors have reported conflicts of interest: R Hughes: personal none, departmental research grants or honoraria from Bayer, Biogen-Idec, Schering-LFB and Kedrion; D Cornblath: personal honoraria from Aventis Behring and Baxter; C Koski: personal honoraria from American Red Cross, Baxter, Bayer, ZLB-Behring; JM Léger: personal none, departmental research grants or honoraria from Biogen-Idec, Baxter, Laboratoire Français du Biofractionnement (LFB), Octapharma; E Nobile-Orazio: personal from Kedrion, Grifols, Baxter, LFB (and he has been commissioned by Kedrion and Baxter to give expert opinions to the Italian Ministry of Health on the use of IVIg in dysimmune neuropathies); J Pollard: departmental research grants from Biogen-Idec, Schering; P van Doorn: personal none, departmental research grants or honoraria from Baxter and Bayer. The other authors have nothing to declare.

References

Azulay J-P, Blin O, Pouget J, Boucraut J, Billé-Turc F, Carles G, Serratrice G (1994). Intravenous immunoglobulin treatment in patients with motor neuron syndromes associated with anti-GM1 antibodies: a double-blind, placebo-controlled study. *Neurology* **44:**429–432.

Beydoun SR (1998). Multifocal motor neuropathy with conduction block misdiagnosed as multiple entrapment neuropathies. *Muscle Nerve* **21:**813–815.

Bouche P, Moulonguet A, Younes-Chennoufi AB, Adams D, Baumann N, Meininger V, Léger JM, Said G (1995). Multifocal motor neuropathy with conduction block: a study of 24 patients. *J Neurol Neurosurg Psychiatry* **59:**38–44.

Brainin M, Barnes M, Baron J-C, Gilhus NE, Hughes RAC, Selmaj K, Waldemar G (2004). Guidance for the preparation of neurological management guidelines by EFNS scientific task forces - revised recommendations 2004. *Eur J Neurol* **11:**577–581.

Carpo M, Cappellari A, Mora G, Pedotti R, Barbieri S, Scarlato G, Nobile-Orazio E (1998). Deterioration of multifocal motor neuropathy after plasma exchange. *Neurology* **50:**1480–1482.

Chad DA, Hammer K, Sargent J (1986). Slow resolution of multifocal weakness and fasciculation: a reversible motor neuron syndrome. *Neurology* **36:**1260–1263.

Chaudhry V, Corse AM, Cornblath DR, Kuncl RW, Drachman DB, Freimer ML, Miller RG, Griffin JW (1993). Multifocal motor neuropathy: response to human immune globulin. *Ann Neurol* **33:**237–242.

Claus D, Specht S, Zieschang M (2000). Plasmapheresis in multifocal motor neuropathy: a case report. *J Neurol Neurosurg Psychiatry* **68:**533–535.

Cornblath DR, Sumner AJ, Daube J, Gilliat RW, Brown WF, Parry GJ, Albers JW, Miller RG, Petajan J (1991). Conduction block in clinical practice. *Muscle Nerve* **14:** 869–871.

Corse AM, Chaudhry V, Crawford TO, Cornblath DR, Kuncl RW, Griffin JW (1996). Sural nerve pathology in multifocal motor neuropathy. *Ann Neurol* **39:**319–325.

Ellis CM, Leary S, Payan J, Shaw C, Hu M, O'Brien M, Leigh PN (1999). Use of human intravenous immunoglobulin in lower motor neuron syndromes. *J Neurol Neurosurg Psychiatry* **67:**15–19.

Federico P, Zochodne DW, Hahn AF, Brown WF, Feasby TE (2000). Multifocal motor neuropathy improved by IVIg: randomized, double-blind, placebo-controlled study. *Neurology* **55:**1256–1262.

Feldman EL, Bromberg MB, Albers JW, Pestronk A (1991). Immunosuppressive treatment in multifocal motor neuropathy. *Ann Neurol* **30:**397–401.

Hausmanowa-Petrusewicz I, Rowinska-Marcinska K, Kopec A (1991). Chronic acquired demyelinating motor neuropathy. *Acta Neurol Scand* **84:**40–45.

Hughes RAC (2001). 79th ENMC International Workshop: Multifocal motor neuropathy: 14–15 April 2000, Hilversum, The Netherlands. *Neuromusc Dis* **11:**309–314.

Kaji R (2003). Physiology of conduction block in multifocal motor neuropathy and other demyelinating neuropathies. *Muscle Nerve* **27:**285–296.

Kaji R, Kimura J (1991). Nerve conduction block. *Curr Opin Neurol Neurosurg* **4:**744–748.

Krarup C, Stewart JD, Sumner AJ, Pestronk A, Lipton SA (1990). A syndrome of asymmetric limb weakness with motor conduction block. *Neurology* **40:**118–127.

Léger JM, Chassande B, Musset L, Meininger V, Bouche P, Baumann N (2001). Intravenous immunoglobulin therapy in multifocal motor neuropathy: A double-blind, placebo-controlled study. *Brain* **124:**145–153.

Léger JM, Viala K, Cancalon F, Maisonobe T, Gruwez B, Waegemans T, Bouche P (2005). Are intravenous immunoglobulins a long-term therapy of multifocal motor neuropathy? A retrospective study of response to IVIg and its predictive criteria in 40 patients. *Neurology* **64(suppl 1):**A412.

Lewis RA (1999). Multifocal motor neuropathy and Lewis Sumner syndrome: two distinct entities. *Muscle Nerve* **22:**1738–1739.

Martina ISJ, Van Doorn PA, Schmitz PIM, Meulstee J, Van der Meché FGA (1999). Chronic motor neuropathies: response to interferon-β1a after failure of conventional therapies. *J Neurol Neurosurg Psychiatry* **66:**197–201.

Meucci N, Cappellari A, Barbieri S, Scarlato G, Nobile-Orazio E (1997). Long term effect of intravenous immunoglobulins and oral cyclophosphamide in multifocal motor neuropathy. *J Neurol Neurosurg Psychiatry* **63:**765–769.

Mezaki T, Kaji R, Kimura J (1999). Multifocal motor neuropathy and Lewis Sumner syndrome: a clinical spectrum. *Muscle Nerve* **22:**1739–1740.

Molinuevo JL, Cruz-Martinez A, Graus F, Serra J, Ribalta T, Valls-Sole J (1999). Central motor conduction time in patients with multifocal motor conduction block. *Muscle Nerve* **22:**926–932.

Nobile-Orazio E (2001). Multifocal motor neuropathy. *J Neuroimmunol* **115:**4–18.

Nobile-Orazio E, Cappellari A, Priori A (2005). Multifocal motor neuropathy: current concepts and controversies. *Muscle Nerve* **31:**663–680.

Noguchi M, Mori K, Yamazaki S, Suda K, Sato N, Oshimi K (2003). Multifocal motor neuropathy caused by a B-cell lymphoma producing a monoclonal IgM autoantibody against peripheral nerve myelin glycolipids GM1 and GD1b. *Br J Haematol* **123:**600–605.

Oh SJ, Claussen GC, Kim DS (2005). Motor and sensory demyelinating mononeuropathy multiplex (multifocal motor and sensory demyelinating neuropathy): a separate entity or a variant of chronic inflammatory demyelinating polyneuropathy? *J Periph Nerv Syst* **2:**362–369.

Olney RK, Lewis RA, Putnam TD, Campellone JVJ (2003). Consensus criteria for the diagnosis of multifocal motor neuropathy. *Muscle Nerve* **27:**117–121.

Parry GJ (1993). Motor neuropathy with multifocal conduction block. *Sem Neurol* **13:**269–275.

Parry GJ (1999). Are multifocal motor neuropathy and Lewis-Sumner syndrome distinct nosologic entities? *Muscle Nerve* **22:**557–559.

Parry GJ, Clarke S (1988). Multifocal acquired demyelinating neuropathy masquerading as motor neuron disease. *Muscle Nerve* **11:**103–107.

Parry GJ, Sumner AJ (1992). Multifocal motor neuropathy. In Dyck PJ, Thomas PK, Griffin JW (eds) *Peripheral Neuropathy*. WB Saunders Company, Philadelphia, pp. 671–684.

Pestronk A, Chaudhry V, Feldman EL, Griffin JW, Cornblath DR, Denys EH, Glasberg M, Kuncl RW, Olney RK, Yee WC (1990). Lower motor neuron syndromes defined by patterns of weakness, nerve conduction abnormalities, and high titer of antiglycolipid antibodies. *Ann Neurol* **27:**316–326.

Pestronk A, Cornblath DR, Ilyas AA, Baba H, Quarles RH, Griffin JW, Alderson K, Adams RN (1988). A treatable multifocal motor neuropathy with antibodies to GM1 ganglioside. *Ann Neurol* **24:**73–78.

Rojas-Garcia R, Gallardo E, de Andres I, Juarez C, Sanchez P, Illa I (2003). Chronic neuropathy with IgM anti-ganglioside antibodies: Lack of long term response to rituximab. *Neurology* **61:**1814–1816.

Roth G, Rohr J, Magistris MR, Ochsner F (1986). Motor neuropathy with proximal multifocal persistent conduction block, fasciculations and myokymia. Evolution to tetraplegia. *Eur Neurol* **25:**416–423.

Rüegg SJ, Fuhr P, Steck AJ (2004). Rituximab stabilizes multifocal motor neuropathy increasingly less responsive to IVIg. *Neurology* **63:**2178–2179.

Saperstein DS, Amato AA, Wolfe GI, Katz JS, Nations SP, Jackson CE, Bryan WW, Burns DK, Barohn RJ (1999). Multifocal acquired demyelinating sensory and motor neuropathy: the Lewis-Sumner syndrome. *Muscle Nerve* **22:**560–566.

Taylor BV, Gross L, Windebank AJ (1996). The sensitivity and specificity of anti-GM1 antibody testing. *Neurology* **47:**951–955.

Taylor BV, Wright RA, Harper CM, Dyck PJ (2000). Natural history of 46 patients with multifocal motor neuropathy with conduction block. *Muscle Nerve* **23:**900–908.

Terenghi F, Cappellari A, Bersano A, Carpo M, Barbieri S, Nobile-Orazio E (2004). How long is IVIg effective in multifocal motor neuropathy? *Neurology* **62:**666–668.

Toscano A, Rodolico C, Benvenga S, Girlanda P, Laura M, Mazzeo A, Nobile-Orazio E, Trimarchi F, Vita G, Messina C (2002). Multifocal motor neuropathy and asymptomatic Hashimoto's thyroiditis: first report of an association. *Neuromusc Dis* **12:**566–568.

Umapathi T, Hughes RAC, Nobile-Orazio E, Léger JM (2005). Immunosuppressant and immunomodulatory treatments for multifocal motor neuropathy (review). Cochrane Database Systematic Reviews 2005; Issue 3: art. No.: CD003217.pub2. DOI: 10.1002/14651858.CD003217.pub2.

Van Asseldonk JTH, Van den Berg LH, Van den Berg-Vos RM, Wieneke GH, Wokke JHJ, Franssen H (2003). Demyelination and axonal loss in multifocal motor neuropathy: distribution and relation to weakness. *Brain* **126:**186–198.

Van den Berg LH, Franssen H, Wokke JHJ (1998). The long-term effect of intravenous immunoglobulin treatment in multifocal motor neuropathy. *Brain* **121:**421–428.

Van den Berg LH, Kerkhoff H, Oey PL, Franssen H, Mollee I, Vermeulen M, Jennekens FG, Wokke JHJ (1995). Treatment of multifocal motor neuropathy with high dose intravenous immunoglobulins: a double blind, placebo controlled study. *J Neurol Neurosurg Psychiatry* **59**:248–252.

Van den Berg LH, Lokhorst H, Wokke JH (1997). Pulsed high-dose dexamethasone is not effective in patients with multifocal motor neuropathy. *Neurology* **48**:1135.

Van den Berg-Vos RM, Franssen H, Wokke JHJ, Van Es HW, Van den Berg LH (2000a). Multifocal motor neuropathy: diagnostic criteria that predict the response to immunoglobulin treatment. *Ann Neurol* **48**:919–926.

Van den Berg-Vos RM, Van den Berg LH, Franssen H, Van Doorn PA, Merkies ISJ, Wokke JHJ (2000b) Treatment of multifocal motor neuropathy with interferon-β1A. *Neurology* **54**:1518–1521.

Van den Berg-Vos RM, Van den Berg LH, Franssen H, Vermeulen M, Witkamp TD, Jansen GH, Van Es HW, Kerkhoff H, Wokke JHJ (2000c). Multifocal inflammatory demyelinating neuropathy: A distinct clinical entity? *Neurology* **54**:26–32.

Van Es HW, Van den Berg LH, Franssen H, Witkamp TD, Ramos LM, Notermans NC, Feldberg MA, Wokke JHJ (1997). Magnetic resonance imaging of the brachial plexus in patients with multifocal motor neuropathy. *Neurology* **48**:1218–1224.

van Schaik IN, Bossuyt PMM, Brand A, Vermeulen M (1995). The diagnostic value of GM1 antibodies in motor neuron disorders and neuropathies: a meta-analysis. *Neurology* **45**:1570–1577.

van Schaik IN, Van den Berg LH, de Haan R, Vermeulen M (2005). Intravenous immunoglobuline for multifocal motor neuropathy. Cochrane Database Systematic Reviews 2005; Issue 2: art. No.: CD004429.pub2. DOI: 10.1002/ 14651858.CD004429.pub2.

Veugelers B, Theys P, Lammens M, Van Hees J, Robberecht W (1996). Pathological findings in a patient with amyotrophic lateral sclerosis and multifocal motor neuropathy with conduction block. *J Neurol Sci* **136**:64–70.

Visser J, Van den Berg-Vos RM, Franssen H, Van den Berg LH, Vogels OJ, Wokke JH, de Jong JM, De Visser M (2002). Mimic syndromes in sporadic cases of progressive spinal muscular atrophy. *Neurology* **58**:1593–1596.

Vucic S, Black KR, Chong PST, Cros D (2004). Multifocal motor neuropathy. Decrease in conduction blocks and reinnervation with long-term IVIg. *Neurology* **63**:1264–1269.

Willison HJ, Yuki N (2002). Peripheral neuropathies and anti-glycolipid antibodies. *Brain* **125**:2591–2625.

CHAPTER 25

Paraproteinaemic demyelinating neuropathy*

R.D.M. Hadden,[a] E. Nobile-Orazio,[b] C. Sommer,[c]
A. Hahn,[d] I. Illa,[e] E. Morra,[f] J. Pollard,[g]
R. Hughes,[h] P. Bouche,[i] D. Cornblath,[j] E. Evers,[k]
C.L. Koski,[l] J.M. Léger,[m] P. Van den Bergh,[n]
P. van Doorn,[o] I.N. van Schaik[p]

Abstract

Background Paraprotein-associated neuropathies have heterogeneous clinical, neurophysiological, neuropathological and haematological features.

Objectives To prepare evidence-based and consensus guidelines on the clinical management of patients with both a demyelinating neuropathy and a paraprotein (paraproteinaemic demyelinating neuropathy, PDN).

Methods Search of MEDLINE and the Cochrane library, review of evidence and consensus agreement of an expert panel.

In the absence of adequate data, evidence-based recommendations were not possible but the panel agreed on the following Good Practice Points:

1. Patients with PDN should be investigated for a malignant plasma cell dyscrasia.
2. The paraprotein is more likely to be causing the neuropathy if the paraprotein is immunoglobulin M, antibodies are present in serum or on biopsy, or the clinical phenotype is chronic distal sensory neuropathy.
3. Patients with IgM PDN usually have predominantly distal and sensory impairment, with prolonged distal motor latencies, and often anti-myelin associated glycoprotein antibodies.
4. IgM PDN sometimes responds to immune therapies. Their potential benefit should be balanced against their possible side-effects and the usually slow disease progression.

*Report of a joint task force of the European Federation of Neurological Societies and the Peripheral Nerve Society

[a]Department of Neurology, King's College Hospital, London, UK; [b]Department of Neurological Science, University of Milan, Milan, Italy; [c]Department of Neurology, University of Würzburg, Würzburg, Germany; [d]Department of Clinical Neurological Sciences, University of Western Ontario, London, Canada; [e]Department of Neurology, Hospital Sta. Creu i Sant Pau, Barcelona, Spain; [f]Department of Haematology, Niguarda Hospital, Milan, Italy; [g]Department of Medicine, University of Sydney, Sydney, Australia; [h]Department of Neuroimmunology, King's College, London, UK; [i]Department of Neurophysiology, CHU Pitié-Salpêtrière, Paris, France; [j]Department of Neurology, Johns Hopkins University, Baltimore, MD, USA; [k]Lay member, Guillan-Barré Syndrome Support Group of the UK, UK; [l]Department of Neurology, University of Maryland, Baltimore, MD, USA; [m]Department of Neurology, Faculté de Médecine Pitié-Salpêtrière, Paris, France; [n]Department of Neurology, Clinique Universitaire St-Luc, Brussels, Belgium; [o]Department of Neurology, Erasmus Medical Centre, Rotterdam, The Netherlands; [p]Department of Neurology, Academic Medical Centre, Amsterdam, The Netherlands.

5. IgG and IgA PDN may be indistinguishable from chronic inflammatory demyelinating polyradiculoneuropathy, clinically, electrophysiologically, and in response to treatment.

6. For POEMS syndrome, local irradiation or resection of an isolated plasmacytoma, or melphalan with or without corticosteroids, should be considered, with haemato-oncology advice.

Objectives

To construct clinically useful guidelines for the diagnosis, investigation and treatment of patients with both a demyelinating neuropathy and a paraprotein (paraproteinaemic demyelinating neuropathy, PDN), based on the available evidence and, where evidence was not available, consensus.

Background

The neuropathies associated with paraproteins are difficult to classify, because of heterogeneity in the clinical and electrophysiological features of the neuropathy, the class, immunoreactivity, and pathogenicity of the paraprotein, and the malignancy of the underlying plasma cell dyscrasia (Yeung *et al.*, 1991; Latov, 1995; Ropper and Gorson, 1998). In the absence of an agreed diagnostic classification, it is not yet possible to provide specific diagnostic criteria, and treatment trials are more difficult to interpret.

Many patients with PDN have a neuropathy that is indistinguishable from chronic inflammatory demyelinating polyradiculoneuropathy (CIDP), and there is no consensus as to whether these should be considered the same or different diseases. We aim to be as inclusive as possible, but have chosen to concentrate on this guideline on demyelinating neuropathies. Axonal neuropathies with a paraprotein are not part of the scope of these guidelines but are mentioned briefly in the section 'Other neuropathy syndromes associated with paraproteinaemia'. As both paraproteins and neuropathies are common, it may be uncertain whether the paraprotein is causing the neuropathy or coincidental.

Search strategy

We searched MEDLINE from 1980 onwards on 24 July 2004 for articles on 'paraprotein(a)emic demyelinating neuropathy' and 'diagnosis' or 'treatment' or 'guideline' and used the personal databases of Task Force members. We searched the Cochrane Library in September 2004.

Methods for reaching consensus

Pairs of task force members prepared draft statements about classification, investigation and treatment that were considered at a meeting in September 2004. Evidence was classified as Class I to IV and recommendations as Level A to C (Brainin *et al.*, 2004). When only Class IV evidence was available but consensus could be reached the Task Force has offered advice as Good Practice Points. The statements were collated into a single document that was revised iteratively until unanimous consensus was reached.

Results

Any diagnostic classification of PDN must take account of the dimensions of clinical phenotype, immunoglobulin (Ig) class, presence of malignancy, antibodies to myelin associated glycoprotein (MAG), electrophysiological phenotype, and causal relationship of the paraprotein to the neuropathy (table 25.1). There is no consensus in the literature as to which should take precedence in classification. Here, we distinguish IgM from IgG and IgA PDN, because IgM PDN tends to have a typical clinical phenotype, pathogenic antibodies, a causal relationship between paraprotein and neuropathy, and the evidence about treatment is different. Nevertheless, there is significant overlap between the clinical and electrophysiological features of the neuropathy with different types of paraprotein.

Supplementary material, summarising some of the published evidence on investigation of PDN, is available online at *European Journal of Neurology*, www.blackwellpublishing.com (see Haddon *et al.*, 2006).

Table 25.1 Dimensions in classification of paraproteinaemic neuropathy.

1. Clinical phenotype
2. Immunoglobulin class
3. Monoclonal gammopathy of undetermined significance or malignant plasma cell dyscrasia
4. Presence of antibodies to myelin associated glycoprotein
5. Electrophysiology
6. Is paraprotein likely to be causing the neuropathy?

Table 25.2 Classification of haematological conditions with a paraprotein.

1) Malignant monoclonal gammopathies
   a) Multiple myeloma (*overt, asymptomatic (smouldering), non-secretory, or osteosclerotic*)
   b) Plasmacytoma (*solitary, extramedullary, multiple solitary*)
   c) Malignant lymphoproliferative disease:
      (1) Waldenström's macroglobulinaemia
      (2) Malignant lymphoma
      (3) Chronic lymphocytic leukaemia
   d) Heavy chain disease
   e) Primary amyloidosis (AL) (*with or without myeloma*)
2) Monoclonal gammopathy of undetermined significance

Investigation and classification of the paraprotein

Background

While some paraproteins (monoclonal gammopathy, monoclonal immunoglobulin) are detected by standard serum protein electrophoresis (SPEP), both serum immunoelectrophoresis (SIEP) and serum immunofixation electrophoresis (SIFE) are more sensitive techniques that detect lower paraprotein concentrations (Vrethem *et al.*, 1993; Keren, 1999). Heavy (IgM, IgG or IgA) and light chain (κ or λ) classes should be identified. A paraprotein indicates an underlying disease of plasma cells in bone marrow, which may be malignant (and may itself require treatment) or a monoclonal gammopathy of uncertain significance (MGUS, table 25.2, (International Myeloma Working Group, 2003). For detection of myeloma bone lesions, X-ray skeletal survey has similar sensitivity to Tc99m sesta-MIBI (2-methoxy-isobutyl-isonitrile), and both are superior to conventional radionuclide scintigraphy (Ludwig *et al.*, 1982; Balleari *et al.*, 2001; Alper *et al.*, 2003), although these studies did not distinguish osteolytic from osteosclerotic myeloma.

Recommended investigations

Table 25.3 suggests investigations to be considered in all patients with a paraprotein. SIFE should be performed in all cases of known paraprotein to define the heavy and light chain type, in all acquired demyelinating neuropathies, and if a paraprotein is suspected but not detected by standard SPEP.

Definition of MGUS

The definition of MGUS is different for IgM from IgG and IgA (table 25.4). Patients with IgM MGUS have alternatively been classified to have 'IgM-related disorders' if they have clinical features attributable to the paraprotein (such as neuropathy), or to have 'asymptomatic IgM monoclonal gammopathy' (Owen, 2003).

Good prognostic features suggesting a low risk of malignant transformation are:

a. IgM MGUS: normal full blood count (in particular, haemoglobin > 12.5 g/dL, lymphocytes < 4×10^9/L), absent (or only a small amount of) Bence-Jones protein in the urine, erythrocyte sedimentation rate (ESR) < 40 mm/h, monoclonal protein < 30 g/L (Morra *et al.*, 2004).

b. IgG/IgA MGUS: absent (or only a small amount of) Bence-Jones protein in the urine, no reduction of polyclonal serum immunoglobulin concentrations, ESR < 40 mm/h, <5% bone marrow plasma cell infiltration, monoclonal protein <20 g/L (Gregersen *et al.*, 2001; Cesana *et al.*, 2002).

Typical syndromes of paraproteinaemic demyelinating neuropathy

The most common types of PDN are those with demyelinating neuropathy and MGUS without non-neurological symptoms. The neuropathy is defined as demyelinating if it satisfies electrophysiological criteria for CIDP (Hughes *et al.*, 2005).

Table 25.3 Investigation of a paraprotein.

The following should be considered in all patients with a paraprotein

a) Serum immunofixation electrophoresis

b) Physical examination for peripheral lymphadenopathy, hepatosplenomegaly, macroglossia and signs of POEMS syndrome (see page 366)

c) Full blood count, renal and liver function, calcium, phosphate, erythrocyte sedimentation rate, C-reactive protein, uric acid, beta 2-microglobulin, lactate dehydrogenase, rheumatoid factor, serum cryoglobulins

d) Total immunoglobulin (Ig)G, IgA, IgM concentrations

e) Random urine collection for the detection of Bence–Jones protein (free light chains), and, if positive, 24-h urine collection for protein quantification

f) Radiographic X-ray skeletal survey (including skull, pelvis, spine, ribs, long bones (shoulder to wrist, and hip to ankle) to look for lytic or sclerotic lesions. If this is negative, then a Tc99m sestaMIBI (2-methoxy-isobutyl-isonitrile) scan if high degree of suspicion of myeloma (IgA lambda and IgG lambda paraproteins are more frequently associated with osteosclerotic myeloma)

g) Ultrasound or computed tomography of abdomen and chest (to detect lymphadenopathy, hepatosplenomegaly)

h) Consultation with a haematologist and bone marrow examination (morphology, immunophenotype and biopsy)

Table 25.4 Definition of monoclonal gammopathy of undetermined significance.

A) IgM-MGUS is defined by the presence of all of the following:

a) No lymphoplasmacytic infiltration on bone marrow biopsy, or equivocal infiltration with negative phenotypic studies

b) No signs or symptoms suggesting tumour infiltration (e.g. constitutional symptoms, hyperviscosity syndrome, organomegaly)

c) No evolution to malignant lymphoproliferative disease requiring treatment within 12 months from first detection of paraprotein

B) IgG or IgA-MGUS is defined by the presence of all of the following:

1. Monoclonal component ≤30 g/L

2. Bence–Jones proteinuria ≤1 g/24 h

3. No lytic lesions in bone

4. No anaemia, hypercalcaemia, or chronic renal insufficiency

5. Bone marrow plasma cell infiltration < 10%

6. No evolution to myeloma or other lymphoproliferative disease within 12 months after first detection of paraprotein

If there are subtle features of demyelination not meeting these criteria, further investigations should be considered to confirm evidence of immune-mediated demyelination (see section 'Cerebrospinal fluid and nerve biopsy').

IgM PDN
Clinical phenotype
Most patients with IgM PDN have the 'distal acquired demyelinating symmetrical' (DADS) clinical phenotype of predominantly distal, chronic (duration over 6 months), slowly progressive, symmetric, predominantly sensory impairment, with ataxia and relatively mild or no weakness, and often tremor (Class IV evidence) (Yeung et al., 1991; Maisonobe et al., 1996; Chassande et al., 1998; Simovic et al., 1998; Capasso et al., 2002; Magy et al., 2003). The DADS phenotype is most strongly associated with IgM anti-MAG antibodies, and some patients have more prominent ataxia with impairment predominantly of vibration and joint position sense. However, the clinical features do not correlate exactly with the paraprotein type: a minority of patients with IgM PDN have

proximal weakness with the phenotype more typical of IgG/IgA PDN, and some DADS patients do not have a paraprotein so that they are classified as having a variant of CIDP (Katz *et al.*, 2000).

Electrophysiology

Patients with the DADS clinical phenotype usually meet the definite electrophysiological criteria proposed for CIDP. They may also have additional specific electrophysiological features indicating uniform symmetrical and predominantly distal reduced conduction velocity, usually without conduction block (table 25.5, adapted from Kaku *et al.*, 1994; Notermans *et al.*, 2000; Capasso *et al.*, 2002).

Antibodies to myelin-associated glycoprotein and other neural antigens

Almost 50% of patients with IgM PDN have high titres of anti-MAG IgM antibodies (Nobile-Orazio *et al.*, 1994), more commonly associated with κ than λ light chains, and this is the best defined syndrome of PDN (Van den Berg *et al.*, 1996). Testing of antibodies to neural antigens should be considered in patients with IgM PDN (table 25.6).

IgG or IgA PDN

Patients with IgG or IgA PDN usually have both proximal and distal weakness, with motor and sensory impairment, indistinguishable clinically and electrophysiologically from typical CIDP. They usually have more rapid progression than DADS (Simovic *et al.*, 1998; Di Troia *et al.*, 1999; Magy *et al.*, 2003). However a minority of patients with

IgG or IgA PDN have the DADS clinical phenotype and associated electrophysiological features.

In patients with IgG or IgA paraprotein, no specific antibody has been consistently associated with demyelinating neuropathy, and therefore there is no need for antibody testing.

Other neuropathy syndromes associated with paraproteinaemia

This section briefly mentions other types of neuropathy associated with a paraprotein, including those with haematological malignancy, systemic symptoms or axonal electrophysiology, although these are not part of the main guidelines and not discussed in detail.

POEMS

POEMS (polyneuropathy, organomegaly, endocrinopathy, M-band and skin changes) syndrome usually has an underlying osteosclerotic myeloma, with IgA or IgG lambda paraprotein, but is sometimes associated with Castleman's disease. POEMS neuropathy has clinical features similar to CIDP. Many patients are initially thought to have CIDP or ordinary PDN, until POEMS is suggested by the presence of systemic features such as sclerotic bone lesions, hepatosplenomegaly, lymphadenopathy, endocrinopathy, papilloedema, skin changes (hypertrichosis, hyperpigmentation, diffuse skin thickening, finger clubbing, dermal haemangiomas, white nail beds) and oedema (Dispenzieri *et al.*, 2003).

Electrophysiology often shows a mixed demyelinating and axonal picture (Kelly, 1983). Features

Table 25.5 Electrophysiological features associated with the Distal Acquired Demyelinating Symmetric (DADS) clinical phenotype.

a) Uniform symmetrical reduction of conduction velocities; more severe sensory than motor involvement

b) Disproportionately prolonged distal motor latency (DML). This may be quantified by low terminal latency index (TLI). TLI is defined as distal velocity/intermediate velocity = distal distance/(motor conduction velocity × DML). TLI <= 0.25 is suggestive of the DADS phenotype

c) Severe involvement of peroneal nerves

d) Absent sural potential (i.e. less likely to have the 'abnormal median, normal sural' sensory action potential pattern)

e) Partial motor conduction block (i.e. proximal/distal compound muscle action potential amplitude ratio <0.5) is very rare

Table 25.6 Antibodies against neural antigens in patients with IgM PDN.

A. In patients with IgM PDN, testing for antibodies to myelin associated glycoprotein (MAG) should be considered. These antibodies may be considered to be:
   a. *definite* if Western Blot against human MAG is positive at a titre of 1/6400 or more
   b. *probable* if enzyme-linked immunosorbent assay (ELISA) against sulphated glucuronyl paragloboside (SGPG) or human MAG positive at high titre (usually 1/6400 or more, but depends on the laboratory and system used)
   c. *possible* if presence of complement fixing antibodies to peripheral nerve homogenate, or IgM binding to myelin detected by indirect immunohistochemistry or immunofluorescence of nerve sections (these methods are not specific and may also be positive in patients with high-titre anti-sulphatide IgM), or lower titres by (a) or (b)
B. In patients with IgM PDN without anti-MAG antibodies, testing for IgM antibodies against other neural antigens, including gangliosides GQ1b, GM1, GD1a and GD1b, SGPG and sulphatide, may be considered. The presence of these antibodies increases the probability of, but does not prove, a pathogenetic link between the paraprotein and the neuropathy. Their diagnostic relevance is not defined
C. In suspected CANOMAD, testing for anti-ganglioside antibodies should be considered (preferably by thin layer chromatography, but anti-GQ1b ELISA may be adequate)

that help to distinguish POEMS from CIDP include: reduced motor nerve conduction velocities more marked in intermediate than distal nerve segments (terminal latency index 0.35–0.5, the opposite of the DADS phenotype); rarity of conduction block; and compound muscle action potential amplitudes smaller in lower than upper limbs (Sung *et al.*, 2002).

There is no specific diagnostic test for POEMS, but if it is suspected then the following investigations should be considered: endocrine blood tests (thyroid, follicle stimulating hormone, luteinising hormone, glucose, prolactin, morning cortisol); ultrasound or computed tomography of abdomen and chest (organomegaly, lymphadenopathy); skin biopsy (may show distinctive glomeruloid haemangiomas in the dermis (Chan *et al.*, 1990)); serum vascular endothelial growth factor (Watanabe *et al.*, 1998); and nerve biopsy (may show uncompacted myelin lamellae (Vital *et al.*, 2003)).

Waldenström's macroglobulinaemia
Waldenström's macroglobulinaemia is defined by the presence of an IgM (usually κ) paraprotein (irrespective of concentration) and a bone marrow biopsy showing infiltration by lymphoplasmacytic lymphoma with a predominantly intertrabecular pattern, supported by appropriate immunophenotypic studies (Owen, 2003). The associated neuropathy is clinically heterogeneous, but sometimes associated with anti-MAG reactivity and clinical features of IgM anti-MAG neuropathy (Baldini *et al.*, 1994).

CANOMAD
The syndrome of chronic ataxic neuropathy with ophthalmoplegia, IgM monoclonal gammopathy, cold agglutinins and disialoganglioside (IgM anti-GD1b/GQ1b) antibodies (CANOMAD) is a rare neuropathy similar to the chronic Fisher syndrome, with mixed demyelinating and axonal electrophysiology (Willison *et al.*, 2001).

Other neuropathies with a paraprotein
Axonal neuropathy is often present in patients with MGUS, but the pathogenesis and causal relationship vary and it will not be considered further in these guidelines.

A few patients with cryoglobulinaemia (Vital *et al.*, 2000) or primary (AL) amyloidosis (Vital *et al.*, 2004) have demyelinating neuropathy, although far more have axonal neuropathy. AL-amyloidosis should be suspected in the presence of prominent neuropathic pain or dysautonomia, and may be demonstrated by biopsy of rectum, bone marrow, kidney or nerve, or fat aspirate.

In patients with lytic multiple myeloma (usually associated with IgA or IgG κ or λ paraprotein) neuropathy may be caused by heterogeneous mechanisms, including amyloidosis, metabolic and toxic insults, and cord or root compression due to vertebral collapse from lytic lesions (Kelly et al., 1981). Subacute weakness similar to Guillain-Barré syndrome may be caused by extensive infiltration of nerves or roots by lymphoma or leukaemia (Diaz-Arrastia et al., 1992).

Is the paraprotein causing the neuropathy?

A causal relationship is more likely with an IgM than an IgG or IgA paraprotein. Our Task Force has classified CIDP with a paraprotein separately from CIDP without a paraprotein, but there is still no consensus among experts as to whether IgG or IgA PDN may merely be CIDP with a co-incidental paraprotein. Malignant paraproteins may also cause a neuropathy, but the mechanism is incompletely understood. The only published criteria of causality were in a study in which all patients had the DADS phenotype, demyelinating physiology and MGUS (IgM or IgG) (Notermans et al., 2000). We modified these criteria extensively, and propose factors that suggest whether or not the paraprotein is likely to be causing the neuropathy (table 25.7).

Cerebrospinal fluid and nerve biopsy

Cerebrospinal fluid (CSF) examination and nerve biopsy may be helpful in selected circumstances (table 25.8, Good Practice Points), but are not usually necessary if there is clearly demyelinating physiology with MGUS. The CSF protein is elevated in 75–86% of patients with PDN (Notermans et al., 2000; Capasso et al., 2002). The presence of widely spaced myelin outer lamellae on electron microscopy is highly sensitive and specific for anti-MAG neuropathy. Immunoglobulin deposits may be identified on nerve structures (Vallat et al., 2000; Mehndiratta et al., 2004).

Treatment of paraproteinaemic demyelinating neuropathies

Monitoring of haematological disease

Patients with MGUS or asymptomatic Waldenström's macroglobulinaemia do not need treatment, unless required specifically because of neuropathy or other IgM-related conditions, according to a consensus panel guideline (Kyle et al., 2003). Whether they have a neuropathy or not, they should have regular haematological evaluation for early detection of malignant transformation, which occurs at approximately 1.3% per year. The following should be measured: paraprotein concentration, Bence Jones protein in the urine, serum immunoglobulin concentrations, ESR, creatinine, calcium, beta 2-microglobulin and full blood count, at a frequency of once a year for MGUS, every 6 months for asymptomatic Waldenström's macroglobulinaemia, or every 3 months if there is a higher risk of malignant transformation (Gregersen et al., 2001; Cesana et al., 2002; Morra et al., 2004) (Good Practice Point).

IgM PDN

A recent Cochrane review of anti-MAG paraproteinaemic neuropathy concluded that there is so far inadequate reliable evidence to recommend any particular immunotherapy (Lunn and Nobile-Orazio, 2003). The same conclusion may be extended to IgM paraprotein-associated neuropathy without anti-MAG antibodies. Based on evidence regarding the pathogenicity of anti MAG antibodies, therapy has been directed at reducing circulating IgM or anti-MAG antibodies by removal (plasma exchange, PE), inhibition (intravenous immunoglobulin, IVIg) or reduction of synthesis (corticosteroids, immunosuppressive, cytotoxic agents or interferon alpha). Only 5 controlled studies out of a total of 97 patients have been performed (Lunn and Nobile-Orazio, 2003).

Plasma exchange

In a review of uncontrolled studies or case reports (Nobile-Orazio et al., 2000), PE was temporarily effective in approximately half of the patients both alone and in combination with other therapies

Table 25.7 Causal relationship between paraprotein and demyelinating neuropathy.

1. *Highly probable* if IgM paraprotein (monoclonal gammopathy of uncertain significance (MGUS) or Waldenström's) and:

   a. high titres of anti-MAG or anti-GQ1b antibodies, or
   b. nerve biopsy shows IgM or complement deposits on myelin, or widely spaced myelin on electron microscopy

2. *Probable* if either:

   2a. IgM paraprotein (MGUS or Waldenström's) with high titres of IgM antibodies to other neural antigens (GM1, GD1a, GD1b, GM2, sulphatide, etc), and slowly progressive predominantly distal symmetrical sensory neuropathy, or
   2b. IgG or IgA paraprotein and nerve biopsy evidence (as in 1b but with IgG or IgA deposits)

3. *Less likely* when any of the following are present in a patient with MGUS and without anti-MAG antibodies (diagnosis may be described as "CIDP with coincidental paraprotein"):

   a) Time to peak of neuropathy <6 months
   b) Relapsing/remitting or monophasic course
   c) Cranial nerves involved (except CANOMAD)
   d) Asymmetry
   e) History of preceding infection
   f) Abnormal median with normal sural sensory action potential
   g) IgG or IgA paraprotein without biopsy features in 2b

Table 25.8 Cerebrospinal fluid (CSF) examination and nerve biopsy.

1. CSF examination is most likely to be helpful in the following situations:

   a) In patients with borderline demyelinating or axonal electrophysiology or atypical phenotype, where the presence of raised CSF protein would help to suggest that the neuropathy is immune-mediated
   b) The presence of malignant cells would confirm lymphoproliferative infiltration

2. Nerve biopsy (usually sural nerve) is most likely to be helpful when the following conditions are being considered:

   a) amyloidosis
   b) vasculitis (e.g. due to cryoglobulinaemia)
   c) malignant lymphoproliferative infiltration of nerves, or
   d) IgM PDN with negative anti-MAG antibodies, or IgG or IgA PDN with a chronic progressive course, where the discovery of widely-spaced myelin on electron microscopy or deposits of immunoglobulin and/or complement bound to myelin would support a causal relationship between paraprotein and neuropathy

However, clinical decisions on treatment are often made without a biopsy

(Class IV evidence). However, this was not confirmed in two controlled studies. In one, a randomised comparative open trial on 44 patients with neuropathy associated with IgM monoclonal gammopathy, 33 of whom had anti-MAG IgM, the combination of PE with chlorambucil was no more effective than chlorambucil alone (Oksenhendler *et al.*, 1995) (Class III). In a double-blind sham-controlled trial on 39 patients with neuropathy (axonal and demyelinating) associated with all classes of MGUS, PE was significantly effective overall, and in subgroups with IgG and IgA but not in the 21 patients with IgM MGUS (Dyck *et al.*, 1991) (Class II). In this study anti-MAG reactivity was not examined.

Corticosteroids

In a review of uncontrolled studies or case reports (Nobile-Orazio *et al.*, 2000), approximately half of the patients responded to corticosteroids given in association with other therapies, but corticosteroids were seldom effective alone (Class IV).

High-dose intravenous immunoglobulin

Intravenous immunoglobulin (IVIg) was effective in 2 of 11 patients in a randomised double-blind placebo-controlled trial (Dalakas *et al.*, 1996) (Class II). A multicentre double-blind cross-over trial of 22 patients with PDN with IgM MGUS, half of whom had anti-MAG IgM, showed significant improvement at 4 weeks with IVIg compared with placebo (Comi *et al.*, 2002) (Class II). The short duration of follow up leaves it unclear whether this was clinically useful. In an open study, 20 participants were randomised to IVIg or interferon alpha and only 1 of 10 treated with IVIg improved (Mariette *et al.*, 1997) (Class II).

Interferon-alpha

In the open comparative trial against IVIg, 8 of 10 patients with PDN and anti-MAG IgM improved with interferon-alpha (Mariette *et al.*, 1997) but the improvement was restricted to sensory symptoms (Class II). These results were not confirmed by the same authors in a randomized placebo-controlled study on 24 patients with PDN and anti-MAG IgM (Mariette *et al.*, 2000) (Class II).

Immunosuppressive therapies

In a review of uncontrolled studies or case reports (Nobile-Orazio *et al.*, 2000; Lunn and Nobile-Orazio, 2003), *chlorambucil* was effective in one third of patients when used alone and in a slightly higher proportion in combination with other therapies (Class IV).

Cyclophosphamide was rarely effective when used alone, but was effective in 40–100% of patients in two open trials using cyclic high-dose oral or intravenous cyclophosphamide together with corticosteroids (Notermans *et al.*, 1996) or PE (Blume *et al.*, 1995) (Class IV).

There are recent anecdotal reports on the efficacy of fludarabine (Sherman *et al.*, 1994; Wilson *et al.*, 1999), cladribine (Ghosh *et al.*, 2002), and high-dose chemotherapy followed by autologous bone marrow transplantation (Rudnicki *et al.*, 1998) in IgM PDN. These studies were limited to very small numbers and need to be confirmed in larger series.

Rituximab

The humanised monoclonal antibody (Rituximab) against the CD20 antigen was tested in several recent open pilot trials. In an open prospective study, over 80% of 21 patients with neuropathy with IgM antibodies to neural antigens (including 7 with PDN and anti-MAG IgM) improved in strength after 1 and 2 years, compared with none of 13 untreated patients (Pestronk *et al.*, 2003) (Class III). The average improvement in strength was 13% at 1 year and 23% at 2 years. However, it was not reported how many patients with anti-MAG antibodies improved, or whether Rituximab improved the sensory ataxia, the most frequently disabling feature. No response to Rituximab was observed in two patients, including one with an IgM monoclonal gammopathy-associated chronic motor neuropathy with anti-ganglioside IgM antibodies (Rojas-Garcia *et al.*, 2003). Six of nine patients with chronic polyneuropathy with IgM monoclonal gammopathy and anti-MAG IgM treated with Rituximab in an open phase II study had detectable improvement (defined as ≥ 2 points improvement in the Neuropathy Impairment Score), two remained stable and one worsened (Renaud *et al.*, 2003). However, only two patients had clinically useful improvement (≥ 10 points), and four had marginal improvement (5 or less) (Class IV).

GOOD PRACTICE POINTS

Treatment of IgM PDN

1. In patients without significant disability, consideration should be given to withholding immunosuppressive or immunomodulatory treatment, providing symptomatic treatment for tremor and paraesthesiae, and giving reassurance that symptoms are unlikely to worsen significantly for several years.

2. In patients with significant disability or rapid worsening, IVIg or PE should be considered as initial treatment, although their efficacy is unproven.
3. In patients with moderate or severe disability, immunosuppressive treatment should be considered, although its long-term efficacy remains unproven. Preliminary reports suggest that Rituximab may be a promising therapy.
4. More research is needed.

IgG and IgA PDN

In a review of uncontrolled studies on small series of patients (Nobile-Orazio *et al.*, 2002), 80% of those with CIDP-like neuropathy responded to the same immunotherapies used for CIDP (corticosteroids, PE and IVIg) as compared with 20% of those with axonal neuropathy (Nobile-Orazio *et al.*, 2002) (Class IV). The only randomized controlled trials, on 39 patients with neuropathy associated with MGUS including 18 with IgG or IgA MGUS and 21 with IgM (Dyck *et al.*, 1991), showed PE was efficacious compared with sham exchange in patients with IgG or IgA MGUS only (Class II). No distinction between demyelinating and axonal forms of neuropathy was made in terms of response to therapy.

GOOD PRACTICE POINTS

Treatment of IgG and IgA PDN
In patients with a CIDP-like neuropathy, the detection of IgG or IgA MGUS does not justify a different therapeutic approach from CIDP without a paraprotein.

POEMS

There are no controlled trials on the treatment of neuropathy in POEMS. Patients with a solitary plasmacytoma may benefit from local radiation or surgical excision. In a recent retrospective study on 99 patients with POEMS (including a review of previous studies) (Dispenzieri *et al.*, 2003), 74% of patients had some response to therapy (Class IV). Local radiation, performed only in patients with a localized or dominant plasmacytoma, was effective in 58% of 70 patients (54% improved, 4% stabilized) (Class IV). A combination of melphalan and corticosteroids was effective in 56% of 48 patients (44% improved, 12% stabilized) while corticosteroids alone were effective in 22% of 41 patients (Class IV). PE, azathioprine and ciclosporin were only effective when used in combination with corticosteroids. There is no evidence that PE, IVIg, or other immunosuppressive agents are effective when used alone. Tamoxifen, interferon alpha, alkylating agents and trans-retinoic acid have been used but the evidence is insufficient. Autologous peripheral blood stem cell transplantation induced neurological improvement or stabilization in 14 of 16 patients but has significant morbidity (Dispenzieri *et al.*, 2004).

GOOD PRACTICE POINTS

Treatment of POEMS
1. Patients should be managed in consultation with a haemato-oncologist.
2. Local radiation or surgery should be considered as the initial treatment for isolated plasmacytoma.
3. Melphalan (with or without corticosteroids) should be considered for patients with multiple or no detectable bone lesions.

Other syndromes

In the neuropathy associated with multiple myeloma, there are no controlled trials and little evidence of response to any treatment in anecdotal reports. There are no controlled treatment trials in the neuropathy associated with Waldenström's macroglobulinaemia.

Conflicts of interest

The following authors have reported conflicts of interest as follows: D Cornblath: personal honoraria from Aventis Behring and Baxter; R Hughes: personal none, departmental research grants or honoraria from Bayer, Biogen-Idec, Schering-LFB and Kedrion; C Koski: personal honoraria from American Red Cross, Baxter, Bayer, ZLB-Behring;

JM Léger: personal none, departmental research grants or honoraria from Biogen-Idec, Baxter, Laboratoire Français du Biofractionnement (LFB), Octapharma; E Nobile-Orazio: personal from Kedrion, Grifols, Baxter, LFB (and he has been commissioned by Kedrion and Baxter to give expert opinions to the Italian Ministry of Health on the use of IVIg in dysimmune neuropathies); J Pollard: departmental research grants from Biogen-Idec, Schering; P van Doorn: personal none, departmental research grants or honoraria from Baxter and Bayer. The other authors have nothing to declare.

Acknowledgement

We thank Dr Michael Lunn for his comments on the text.

References

Alper E, Gurel M, Evrensel T, Ozkocaman V, Akbunar T, Demiray M (2003). 99mTc-MIBI scintigraphy in untreated stage III multiple myeloma: comparison with X-ray skeletal survey and bone scintigraphy. *Nucl Med Commun* **24**:537–542.

Baldini L, Nobile-Orazio E, Guffanti A, Barbieri S, Carpo M, Cro L, Cesana B, Damilano I, Maiolo AT (1994). Peripheral neuropathy in IgM monoclonal gammopathy and Waldenstrom's macroglobulinemia: a frequent complication in elderly males with low MAG-reactive serum monoclonal component. *Am J Hematol* **45**:25–31.

Balleari E, Villa G, Garre S, Ghirlanda P, Agnese G, Carletto M, Clavio M, Ferrando F, Gobbi M, Mariani G, Ghio R (2001). Technetium-99m-sestamibi scintigraphy in multiple myeloma and related gammopathies: a useful tool for the identification and follow-up of myeloma bone disease. *Haematologica* **86**: 78–84.

Blume G, Pestronk A, Goodnough LT (1995). Anti-MAG antibody-associated polyneuropathies: improvement following immunotherapy with monthly plasma exchange and IV cyclophosphamide. *Neurology* **45**:1577–1580.

Brainin M, Barnes M, Baron JC, Gilhus NE, Hughes R, Selmaj K, Waldemar G (2004). Guidance for the preparation of neurological management guidelines by EFNS scientific task forces–revised recommendations 2004. *Eur J Neurol* **11**:577–581.

Capasso M, Torrieri F, Di Muzio A, De Angelis MV, Lugaresi A, Uncini A (2002). Can electrophysiology differentiate polyneuropathy with anti-MAG/SGPG antibodies from chronic inflammatory demyelinating polyneuropathy? *Clin Neurophysiol* **113**:346–353.

Cesana C, Klersy C, Barbarano L, Nosari AM, Crugnola M, Pungolino E, Gargantini L, Granata S, Valentini M, Morra E (2002). Prognostic factors for malignant transformation in monoclonal gammopathy of undetermined significance and smoldering multiple myeloma. *J Clin Oncol* **20**:1625–1634.

Chan JK, Fletcher CD, Hicklin GA, Rosai J (1990). Glomeruloid hemangioma. A distinctive cutaneous lesion of multicentric Castleman's disease associated with POEMS syndrome. *Am J Surg Pathol* **14**:1036–1046.

Chassande B, Leger JM, Younes-Chennoufi AB, Bengoufa D, Maisonobe T, Bouche P, Baumann N (1998). Peripheral neuropathy associated with IgM monoclonal gammopathy: correlations between M-protein antibody activity and clinical/electrophysiological features in 40 cases. *Muscle Nerve* **21**:55–62.

Comi G, Roveri L, Swan A, Willison H, Bojar M, Illa I, Karageorgiou C, Nobile-Orazio E, van den Bergh P, Swan T, Hughes R, Aubry J, Baumann N, Hadden R, Lunn M, Knapp M, Leger JM, Bouche P, Mazanec R, Meucci N, van der Meche F, Toyka K (2002). A randomised controlled trial of intravenous immunoglobulin in IgM paraprotein associated demyelinating neuropathy. *J Neurol* **249**:1370–1377.

Dalakas MC, Quarles RH, Farrer RG, Dambrosia J, Soueidan S, Stein DP, Cupler E, Sekul EA, Otero C (1996). A controlled study of intravenous immunoglobulin in demyelinating neuropathy with IgM gammopathy. *Ann Neurol* **40**:792–795.

Di Troia A, Carpo M, Meucci N, Pellegrino C, Allaria S, Gemignani F, Marbini A, Mantegazza R, Sciolla R, Manfredini E, Scarlato G, Nobile-Orazio E (1999). Clinical features and anti-neural reactivity in neuropathy associated with IgG monoclonal gammopathy of undetermined significance. *J Neurol Sci* **164**:64–71.

Diaz-Arrastia R, Younger DS, Hair L, Inghirami G, Hays AP, Knowles DM, Odel J G, Fetell MR, Lovelace RE, Rowland LP (1992). Neurolymphomatosis: a clinicopathologic syndrome re-emerges. *Neurology* **42**:1136–1141.

Dispenzieri A, Kyle RA, Lacy MQ, Rajkumar SV, Therneau TM, Larson DR, Greipp PR, Witzig TE, Basu R, Suarez GA, Fonseca R, Lust JA, Gertz MA (2003). POEMS syndrome: definitions and long-term outcome. *Blood* **101**:2496–2506.

Dispenzieri A, Moreno-Aspitia A, Suarez GA, Lacy MQ, Colon-Otero G, Tefferi A, Litzow MR, Roy V, Hogan WJ, Kyle RA, Gertz MA (2004). Peripheral blood stem cell transplantation in 16 patients with POEMS syndrome, and a review of the literature. *Blood* **104:** 3400–3407.

Dyck PJ, Low PA, Windebank AJ, Jaradeh SS, Gosselin S, Bourque P, Smith BE, Kratz KM, Karnes JL, Evans BA, *et al.* (1991). Plasma exchange in polyneuropathy associated with monoclonal gammopathy of undetermined significance. *N Engl J Med* **325:**1482–1486.

Ghosh A, Littlewood T, Donaghy M (2002). Cladribine in the treatment of IgM paraproteinemic polyneuropathy. *Neurology* **59:**1290–1291.

Gregersen H, Mellemkjaer L, Ibsen JS, Dahlerup JF, Thomassen L, Sorensen HT (2001). The impact of M-component type and immunoglobulin concentration on the risk of malignant transformation in patients with monoclonal gammopathy of undetermined significance. *Haematologica* **86:**1172–1179.

Hadden RDM, Nobile-Orazio E, Sommer C, Hahn A, Illa I, Morra E, Pollard J, Hughes RAC, Bouche P, Cornblath D, Evers E, Koski CL, Léger JM, Van den Bergh P, van Doorn P, van Schaik IN (2006). European Federation of Neurological Societies/Peripheral Nerve Society guideline on management of paraproteinaemic demyelinating neuropathies: report of a joint task force of the European Federation of Neurological Societies and the Peripheral Nerve Society. *Eur J Neurology* **13:** in press.

Hughes RAC, Bouche P, Cornblath DR, Evers E, Hadden RDM, Hahn A, Illa I, Koski CL, Léger JM, Nobile-Orazio E, Pollard J, Sommer C, Van den Bergh P, van Doorn PA, van Schaik IN (2005). European Federation of Neurological Societies/Peripheral Nerve Society guideline on management of chronic inflammatory demyelinating polyradiculoneuropathy. In press, *Eur J Neurol*, *J Periph Nerv System* and European Handbook of Neurolological Management.

International Myeloma Working Group (2003). Criteria for the classification of monoclonal gammopathies, multiple myeloma and related disorders: a report of the International Myeloma Working Group. *Br J Haematol* **121:**749–757.

Kaku DA, England JD, Sumner AJ (1994). Distal accentuation of conduction slowing in polyneuropathy associated with antibodies to myelin-associated glycoprotein and sulphated glucuronyl paragloboside. *Brain* **117 (Pt 5):**941–947.

Katz JS, Saperstein DS, Gronseth G, Amato AA, Barohn RJ (2000). Distal acquired demyelinating symmetric neuropathy. *Neurology* **54:**615–20.

Kelly JJ, Jr (1983). The electrodiagnostic findings in peripheral neuropathy associated with monoclonal gammopathy. *Muscle Nerve* **6:**504–509.

Kelly JJ, Jr, Kyle RA, Miles JM, O'Brien PC, Dyck PJ (1981). The spectrum of peripheral neuropathy in myeloma. *Neurology* **31:**24–31.

Keren DF (1999). Procedures for the evaluation of monoclonal immunoglobulins. *Arch Pathol Lab Med* **123:**126–132.

Kyle RA, Treon SP, Alexanian R, Barlogie B, Bjorkholm M, Dhodapkar M, Lister TA, Merlini G, Morel P, Stone M, Branagan AR, Leblond V (2003). Prognostic markers and criteria to initiate therapy in Waldenstrom's macroglobulinemia: consensus panel recommendations from the Second International Workshop on Waldenstrom's Macroglobulinemia. *Semin Oncol* **30:**116–120.

Latov N (1995). Pathogenesis and therapy of neuropathies associated with monoclonal gammopathies. *Ann Neurol* **37(Suppl 1):**S32–42.

Ludwig H, Kumpan W, Sinzinger H (1982). Radiography and bone scintigraphy in multiple myeloma: a comparative analysis. *Br J Radiol* **55:**173–181.

Lunn MP, Nobile-Orazio E (2003). Immunotherapy for IgM anti-Myelin-Associated Glycoprotein paraprotein-associated peripheral neuropathies. *Cochrane Database Syst Rev*: CD002827.

Magy L, Chassande B, Maisonobe T, Bouche P, Vallat JM, Leger JM (2003). Polyneuropathy associated with IgG/IgA monoclonal gammopathy: a clinical and electrophysiological study of 15 cases. *Eur J Neurol* **10:**677–685.

Maisonobe T, Chassande B, Verin M, Jouni M, Leger JM, Bouche P (1996). Chronic dysimmune demyelinating polyneuropathy: a clinical and electrophysiological study of 93 patients. *J Neurol Neurosurg Psychiatry* **61:** 36–42.

Mariette X, Chastang C, Clavelou P, Louboutin JP, Leger JM, Brouet JC (1997). A randomised clinical trial comparing interferon-alpha and intravenous immunoglobulin in polyneuropathy associated with monoclonal IgM. The IgM-associated Polyneuropathy Study Group. *J Neurol Neurosurg Psychiatry* **63:**28–34.

Mariette X, Brouet JC, Chevret S, Leger JM, Clavelou P, Pouget J, Vallat JM, Vial C (2000). A randomised double blind trial versus placebo does not confirm the benefit of alpha-interferon in polyneuropathy associated with monoclonal IgM. *J Neurol Neurosurg Psychiatry* **69:**279–280.

Mehndiratta MM, Sen K, Tatke M, Bajaj BK (2004). IgA monoclonal gammopathy of undetermined significance with peripheral neuropathy. *J Neurol Sci* **221:**99–104.

Morra E, Cesana C, Klersy C, Barbarano L, Varettoni M, Cavanna L, Canesi B, Tresoldi E, Miqueleiz S, Bernuzzi P, Nosari AM, Lazzarino M (2004). Clinical characteristics and factors predicting evolution of asymptomatic IgM monoclonal gammopathies and IgM-related disorders. *Leukemia* **18:**1512–1517.

Nobile-Orazio E, Casellato C, Di Troia A (2002). Neuropathies associated with IgG and IgA monoclonal gammopathy. *Rev Neurol (Paris)* **158:**979–987.

Nobile-Orazio E, Manfredini E, Carpo M, Meucci N, Monaco S, Ferrari S, Bonetti B, Cavaletti G, Gemignani F, Durelli L, *et al.* (1994). Frequency and clinical correlates of anti-neural IgM antibodies in neuropathy associated with IgM monoclonal gammopathy. *Ann Neurol* **36:**416–424.

Nobile-Orazio E, Meucci N, Baldini L, Di Troia A, Scarlato G (2000). Long-term prognosis of neuropathy associated with anti-MAG IgM M-proteins and its relationship to immune therapies. *Brain* **123(Pt 4):**710–717.

Notermans NC, Lokhorst HM, Franssen H, Van der Graaf Y, Teunissen LL, Jennekens FG, Van den Berg LH, Wokke JH (1996). Intermittent cyclophosphamide and prednisone treatment of polyneuropathy associated with monoclonal gammopathy of undetermined significance. *Neurology* **47:**1227–1233.

Notermans NC, Franssen H, Eurelings M, Van der Graaf Y, Wokke JH (2000). Diagnostic criteria for demyelinating polyneuropathy associated with monoclonal gammopathy. *Muscle Nerve* **23:**73–79.

Oksenhendler E, Chevret S, Leger JM, Louboutin JP, Bussel A, Brouet JC (1995). Plasma exchange and chlorambucil in polyneuropathy associated with monoclonal IgM gammopathy. IgM-associated Polyneuropathy Study Group. *J Neurol Neurosurg Psychiatry* **59:**243–247.

Owen RG (2003). Developing diagnostic criteria in Waldenstrom's macroglobulinemia. *Semin Oncol* **30:**196–200.

Pestronk A, Florence J, Miller T, Choksi R, Al-Lozi MT, Levine TD (2003). Treatment of IgM antibody associated polyneuropathies using rituximab. *J Neurol Neurosurg Psychiatry* **74:**485–489.

Renaud S, Gregor M, Fuhr P, Lorenz D, Deuschl G, Gratwohl A, Steck AJ (2003). Rituximab in the treatment of polyneuropathy associated with anti-MAG antibodies. *Muscle Nerve* **27:**611–615.

Rojas-Garcia R, Gallardo E, de Andres I, de Luna N, Juarez C, Sanchez P, Illa I (2003). Chronic neuropathy with IgM anti-ganglioside antibodies: lack of long term response to rituximab. *Neurology* **61:**1814–1816.

Ropper AH, Gorson KC (1998). Neuropathies associated with paraproteinemia. *N Engl J Med* **338:**1601–1607.

Rudnicki SA, Harik SI, Dhodapkar M, Barlogie B, Eidelberg D (1998). Nervous system dysfunction in Waldenstrom's macroglobulinemia: response to treatment. *Neurology* **51:**1210–1213.

Sherman WH, Latov N, Lange DE, Hays R, Younger DS (1994). Fludarabine for IgM antibody-mediated neuropathies (abstract). *Ann Neurol* **36:**326–327.

Simovic D, Gorson KC, Ropper AH (1998). Comparison of IgM-MGUS and IgG-MGUS polyneuropathy. *Acta Neurol Scand* **97:**194–200.

Sung JY, Kuwabara S, Ogawara K, Kanai K, Hattori T (2002). Patterns of nerve conduction abnormalities in POEMS syndrome. *Muscle Nerve* **26:**189–193.

Vallat JM, Tabaraud F, Sindou P, Preux PM, Vandenberghe A, Steck A (2000). Myelin widenings and MGUS-IgA: an immunoelectron microscopic study. *Ann Neurol* **47:**808–811.

Van den Berg L, Hays AP, Nobile-Orazio E, Kinsella LJ, Manfredini E, Corbo M, Rosoklija G, Younger DS, Lovelace RE, Trojaborg W, Lange DE, Goldstein S, Delfiner JS, Sadiq SA, Sherman WH, Latov N (1996). Anti-MAG and anti-SGPG antibodies in neuropathy. *Muscle Nerve* **19:**637–643.

Vital A, Lagueny A, Julien J, Ferrer X, Barat M, Hermosilla E, Rouanet-Larriviere M, Henry P, Bredin A, Louiset P, Herbelleau T, Boisseau C, Guiraud-Chaumeil B, Steck A, Vital C (2000). Chronic inflammatory demyelinating polyneuropathy associated with dysglobulinemia: a peripheral nerve biopsy study in 18 cases. *Acta Neuropathol (Berl)* **100:**63–68.

Vital C, Vital A, Bouillot S, Favereaux A, Lagueny A, Ferrer X, Brechenmacher C, Petry KG (2003). Uncompacted myelin lamellae in peripheral nerve biopsy. *Ultrastruct Pathol* **27:**1–5.

Vital C, Vital A, Bouillot-Eimer S, Brechenmacher C, Ferrer X, Lagueny A (2004). Amyloid neuropathy: a retrospective study of 35 peripheral nerve biopsies. *J Peripher Nerv Syst* **9:**232–241.

Vrethem M, Larsson B, von Schenck H, Ernerudh J (1993). Immunofixation superior to plasma agarose electrophoresis in detecting small M-components in patients with polyneuropathy. *J Neurol Sci* **120:**93–98.

Watanabe O, Maruyama I, Arimura K, Kitajima I, Arimura H, Hanatani M, Matsuo K, Arisato T, Osame M (1998). Overproduction of vascular endothelial growth factor/vascular permeability factor is causative in Crow-Fukase (POEMS) syndrome. *Muscle Nerve* **21:**1390–1397.

Willison HJ, O'Leary CP, Veitch J, Blumhardt LD, Busby M, Donaghy M, Fuhr P, Ford H, Hahn A,

Renaud S, Katifi HA, Ponsford S, Reuber M, Steck A, Sutton I, Schady W, Thomas PK, Thompson AJ, Vallat JM, Winer J (2001). The clinical and laboratory features of chronic sensory ataxic neuropathy with anti-disialosyl IgM antibodies. *Brain* **124:**1968–1977.

Wilson HC, Lunn MP, Schey S, Hughes RA (1999). Successful treatment of IgM paraproteinaemic neuropathy with fludarabine. *J Neurol Neurosurg Psychiatry* **66:**575–580.

Yeung KB, Thomas PK, King RH, Waddy H, Will RG, Hughes RA, Gregson NA, Leibowitz S (1991). The clinical spectrum of peripheral neuropathies associated with benign monoclonal IgM, IgG and IgA paraproteinaemia. Comparative clinical, immunological and nerve biopsy findings. *J Neurol* **238:**383–391.

CHAPTER 26

Limb girdle muscular dystrophies

F. Norwood,[a,b] M. de Visser,[c] B. Eymard,[d]
H. Lochmüller,[e] K. Bushby[a]

Abstract

Limb girdle muscular dystrophies (LGMDs) are termed as such as they share the characteristic feature of muscle weakness predominantly affecting the shoulder and pelvic girdles; their classification has been completely revised in recent years due to the elucidation of many of the underlying genetic and protein alterations in the various subtypes. An array of diagnostic measures is available but with varying ease of use and availability.

Several aspects of muscle cell function appear to be involved in the causation of muscle pathology. These cellular variations may confer some specific clinical features, thus permitting recognition of the LGMD subtype and hence directing appropriate levels of monitoring and intervention.

Despite an extensive literature on the individual limb girdle dystrophies, these publications may be impenetrable for the general neurologist in this increasingly complex field. The proposed guidelines suggest an approach to the diagnosis and monitoring of limb girdle dystrophies in a manner accessible to general neurologists.

Objectives

To provide guidelines for the best practice management of LGMDs based on the current state of clinical and scientific knowledge in the published literature.

Background

LGMD was first described as a clinical entity in 1954 by Walton and Natrass (Walton and Natrass, 1954). However it was not until the 1990s that linkage studies and the identification of the group of proteins associated with dystrophin at the sarcolemma began to demonstrate the heterogeneity of LGMDs. Classification of LGMDs was established through workshops held at the European Neuromuscular Centre (ENMC). The most recent classification is shown in table 26.1 (modified from Bushby and Beckmann, 2003). LGMDs are grouped into two sections, autosomal dominant (1) or recessive (2), and further subdivided into subtypes, each of which is known by a designated suffix allocated in chronological order of gene identification. As the genes and proteins involved in these disorders are identified, this locus-based approach is being superseded by a classification based on the underlying genetic defect.

[a]Institute of Human Genetics, Central Parkway, Newcastle upon Tyne, NE1 3BZ, United Kingdom; [b]King's Neuroscience Centre, King's College Hospital, London, United Kingdom; [c]Academic Medical Centre, University of Amsterdam, Department of Neurology, Amsterdam, Holland; [d]Hôpital de la Pitié, Salpétriere, Paris, France; [e]Genzentrum, Ludwig-Maximilians-Universität, Munich, Germany.

Table 26.1 105th ENMC workshop classification (from Bushby and Beckmann, 2003).

Disease	Mode of inheritance	Gene location	Gene symbol (gene product)
Limb-girdle MD, dominant	AD	5q22-q34	LGMD1A (=MYOT) (myotilin)
	AD (AR)	1q11-21	LGMD1B (=LMNA) (lamin A/C)
	AD (AR)	3p25	LGMD1C (=CAV3) (caveolin-3)
	AD	6q23	LGMD1D (CMD1F)
	AD	7q	LGMD1E
Limb-girdle, recessive	AR	15q15.1–q21.1	LGMD2A (=CAPN3) (calpain 3)
	AR	2p13	LGMD2B (=DYSF) (dysferlin)
	AR	13q12	LGMD2C (=SGCG) (γ-sarcoglycan)
	AR	17q12–q21.33	LGMD2D (=SGCA) (α-sarcoglycan)
	AR	4q12	LGMD2E (=SGCB) (β-sarcoglycan)
	AR	5q33-q34	LGMD2F (=SGCD) (δ-sarcoglycan)
	AR	17q11-q12	LGMD2G (=TCAP) (telethonin)
	AR	9q31-q34.1	LGMD2H (=TRIM32)
	AR	19q13.3	LGMD2I (=FKRP) (Fukutin related protein)
	AR	2q	LGMD2J (=TTN) (Titin)
	AR	9q34	LGMD2K (=POMT1)

With molecular clarification has come the increasing realisation that it is possible in some instances to recognise characteristic patterns of disease through thorough clinical assessment. Areas of particular importance are the involvement of the cardiac and respiratory systems but other features such as the presence of muscle hypertrophy, contractures and scapular winging may also be of diagnostic help. Prognosis for LGMDs is not uniform and thus timely intervention through early identification of potential complications may improve survival.

An array of diagnostic measures is available but with varying ease of use and availability; mutation analysis for some genes is a huge undertaking and analysis of expressed proteins may be complex. Nevertheless many causative mutations have been identified and it has been possible to work towards genotype–phenotype correlations. Genetic analysis has also extended the phenotypic range in several of the subtypes, with some genes producing hugely variable clinical features in affected individuals.

Search strategy

The following search protocols were employed with relevant keywords: MEDLINE for original papers and review articles (1985 to 2005); Cochrane database (www.cochrane.org/index0.htm); American Academy of Neurology (AAN) and European Federation of Neurological Sciences (EFNS) practice parameters or management guidelines (www.aan.com/professionals/practice/guideline/index.cfm; www.efns.org/); EMBASE, patient organisations (www.muscular-dystrophy.org; www.mdausa.org; www.mda.org.au); previous guidelines (www.inahta.org/inahta_web/index.asp; www.york.ac.uk/inst/crd/darehp.htm; www.g-i-n.net/index.cfm? fuseaction = membersarea).

Method for reaching consensus

The results of the literature review were evaluated by members of the task force; only those studies specific to LGMDs or the subtypes have been included. Older studies pre-1985 include cases of 'limb girdle dystrophy' but without accurate molecular diagnosis it is not possible to extract reliable data from these and so they have been excluded. All the evidence was categorised as class IV (Brainin *et al.*, 2004).

Results

LGMDs are relatively recent in their identification and clarification and efforts are ongoing with further genes and proteins expected to be discovered. In addition, the conditions are individually rare, some with only a few families identified. To date, no substantial randomised controlled trials of management of genetically defined LGMD have been published. However, as each condition becomes better understood, the phenotypic features of each become apparent through case reports and cohort studies and it is possible to recommend both general and specific Good Practice Points (Brainin *et al.*, 2004) for the management of LGMDs based on this knowledge.

Good Practice Points for management of LGMD

Aspects of care-Diagnosis

Clinical assessment

General principles

Thorough clinical assessment provides the basis for directing further investigation. Neonatal course, timing of developmental motor milestones and ability to rise from the floor/presence of Gowers' manoeuvre may all be of relevance. The ability to run, hop and jump and sporting ability may be significantly affected in childhood or may be normal until even middle age. The age of onset may vary both between and within subtypes and even between patients with the same mutation.

By definition, LGMDs have in common a predilection for involvement of the proximal musculature in the shoulder and pelvic girdles but these may be differentially affected, particularly in the early stages, and involvement of distal muscles may also occur. Rate of progression of the muscle weakness may not be linear.

Features such as spinal rigidity, scoliosis and limb contractures should be sought. Hypertrophy, usually of calf muscles but also of other limb muscles and even the tongue, may be present. Family history may suggest an autosomal dominant inheritance or consanguinity.

Although it is not possible to provide an absolute prediction of the clinical pattern, table 26.2 outlines the presence or absence of typical features in each LGMD to give a guide to the underlying diagnosis (Bushby, 1999; Beckmann *et al.*, 1999;

Laval and Bushby, 2004). Exceptions to the commonly recognised patterns can occur and the table should be seen as a guide only. It is also important to point out that for mutations in some of these genes, there is clinical heterogeneity. Specific examples of this include myotilin mutations (responsible for the rare LGMD1A and myofibrillar myopathy), cavcolin 3 mutations (reported with a range of presentations including hyper-CKaemia, LGMD1C and rippling muscle disease) and lamin A/C mutations, which are probably the most clinically variable of all, and have been reported in at least seven distinct diseases, in some of which muscle involvement may be minimal or absent. The variability in presentation for all of these conditions means that different family members, or indeed the same individual, may present with one or more manifestations of mutation in a particular gene.

Specific clinical pointers/indicators

In contrast to the congenital muscular dystrophies and myopathies, the only LGMD that may result in neonatal hypotonia is LGMD1B (lamin A/C). None of the LGMDs has been described in association with neonatal contractures. Those conditions that are most likely to present in early childhood are LGMD1B, 1C (caveolin-3 deficiency), the sarcoglycanopathies, LGMD2A (calpain deficiency) and some cases of LGMD2I. All of the LGMDs may result in a lifelong decreased sporting ability. This is less likely in LGMD2B (dysferlin deficiency) which in many patients is associated with a normal sporting ability until an abrupt onset of difficulty, occasionally preceded by a transient painful swelling of calf muscles.

Age of onset is relatively well-defined for some conditions: the mean age of onset for LGMD2A is in the early teens and in LGMD2B is $20 +/- 5$ years (Bushby *et al.*, 1999); however for others a much wider age range is found, such as in LGMD1C where age of onset may be from early childhood to the eighth decade depending on the phenotype (Woodman *et al.*, 2004). LGMD2C-F are also variable in their onset and progression; some patients (typically especially β and δ sarcoglycanopathies) may be as severely affected as patients with Duchenne muscular dystrophy

Table 26.2 Predominant clinical features for the most frequently occurring LGMDs.

Disease	Age of onset [1]	Weakness [2]	CK level [3]	Muscle hypertrophy [4]	Contractures [5]	Special features [6]	Respiratory [7]	Cardiac [8]
LGMD1A	c, d	Proximal/distal	A	No	No	Dysarthria	?	Yes?
LGMD1B	a, b	Proximal/distal	A	No	Yes		?	Yes A, CM
LGMD1C	a-d	Proximal/distal	B/C	Some cases	No	PIRCs, RMD	No	?
LGMD2A	a-c	Proximal	B/C	Some cases	Yes		No	No
LGMD2B	b, c	Proximal/distal	C	No	No		No	No
LGMB2C-F	a, b	Proximal	B/C	Yes	Secondary		Yes	Yes CM
LGMD2G	a, b	Proximal/distal	A-C	Some cases	No	Brazil	?	No
LGMD2H	b, c	Proximal	B	No	No	Hutterites	?	No
LGMD2I	a-d	Proximal	B/C	Yes	No		Yes	Yes CM
LGMD2J	a, b	Proximal/distal	B	No	No	Finnish	?	No?

[1] Range of age of onset in majority of patients: a = below age 10 years; b = 10–20 years; c = 20–40 years; d = over 40 years.

[2] Pattern of distribution of weakness in limb muscles.

[3] Range of creatine kinase (CK) level at diagnosis: A = normal or mildly elevated at less than 5x upper limit of normal; B = 5–10x upper limit of normal; C = over 10x upper limit of normal.

[4] Presence of muscle hypertrophy in limb muscles may occur.

[5] Presence of early fixed limb contractures may occur.

[6] Percussion-induced rapid muscle contractions (PIRCs); Rippling muscle disease (RMD).

[7] Presence of frequent respiratory complications.

[8] Presence of frequent cardiac complications: A = arrhythmia, CM = cardiomyopathy.

(DMD) whereas others are still ambulant into their 40s. Alpha-sarcoglycanopathy (LGMD2D) tends to be the mildest of the sarcoglycanopathies (Eymard et al., 1997).

Most LGMDs by definition involve predominantly proximal musculature, certainly once the full phenotype has evolved, but potential diagnostic difficulty could arise in, for example, the presence of only distal muscle involvement in the early stages of the Miyoshi type of dysferlin deficiency (although the characteristic gastrocnemius weakness is helpful) or in some patients with LGMD1B or 1C. An example of another useful discriminator is the relative preservation of hip abductor muscles in LGMD 2A (Pollit et al., 2001; Saenz et al., 2005) and the striking involvement of the posterior thigh muscles as shown on muscle magnetic resonance imaging (MRI) (Mercurio et al., 2005). Scapular winging is most characteristically seen in LGMD2A and 2C-F.

Associated features such as muscle hypertrophy may be observed quite frequently in LGMD1C, 2C-F and 2I (Fukutin related protein, FKRP). Calf hypertrophy is most common but other limb muscles may also be involved as may the tongue. The calf hypertrophy present in LGMD2I (in addition to the cardiac and respiratory involvement) resembles the Becker phenotype and has led to misdiagnosis of patients in the past. Macroglossia is seen in LGMD2C-F and 2I on occasion. Focal muscle atrophy is most typical of LGMD2A and LGMD2B.

Contractures are most common in LGMD1B where they may occur in childhood or develop over the course of the condition, representing an overlap with the autosomal dominant Emery–Dreifuss muscular dystrophy (EDMD) phenotype also caused by mutations in lamin A/C. Contractures may also be seen in LGMD2A but tend to be milder. Spinal rigidity is often a feature in LGMD1B and occasionally in LGMD2A (Pollitt *et al.*, 2001). Scoliosis is most often seen in LGMD2C-F, particularly once wheelchair dependence occurs.

Specific indicators include the reported dysarthria in the rare LGMD1A (myotilin) patients (Hauser *et al.* 2000). On the other hand, phenotypic variation within the same family as well as overlapping phenotypes are well-recognised; a mutation in a single LGMD gene such as caveolin-3 may produce one or more of a number of manifestations such as rippling muscles and percussion-induced repetitive contractions. This also occurs in the laminopathies where some members of the family may have partial lipodystrophy or peripheral neuropathy in addition to their muscle weakness, for example, whereas other members do not and indeed may have pure cardiac disease.

Intellectual impairment and facial weakness are not characteristically seen. A malignant hyperthermia reaction to general anaesthesia has been reported only in two patients from the Hutterite population who have mutations in FKRP (rather than TRIM32).

Geographical location of cases may also be helpful. LGMD2G (telethonin) has so far only been described in Brazilian patients (Moreira *et al.* 2000). LGMD 2H (TRIM32) is a relatively mild form seen in some areas of Canada with onset in the second or third decade and slow progression; most patients were still ambulant into their 50s (Frosk *et al.*, 2002). Sarcotubular myopathy is described in patients with the same TRIM 32 mutations (Schoser *et al.* 2005). LGMD2J (titin) was described in Finnish patients initially.

Cardiac involvement is very common in LGMD 1B, 2C-F and 2I whereas significant disease is infrequent in LGMD 1C, 2A and 2B. Cardiac complications may take the form of dysrhythmias or hypertrophic or dilated cardiomyopathy. Isolated familial hypertrophic cardiomyopathy has been described with CAV-3 mutations (Hayashi *et al.* 2004). Patients may be affected by both a dysrhythmia and cardiomyopathy, especially in LGMD1B. Respiratory muscle weakness does not necessarily accompany cardiac impairment; it is seen most often in LGMD 2C-F and in 2I where diaphragmatic involvement may be seen when patients are still ambulant but tends to be insignificant in 2A and 2B. Symptoms of nocturnal hypoventilation may herald the development of significant respiratory muscle weakness and need for intervention.

Investigation

Serum *creatine kinase* (CK) is a simple and useful investigation provided that non-muscle conditions are excluded first. The degree of elevation may be helpful in differentiating broadly between diagnoses; typically, it may be normal or only mildly raised in conditions such as LGMD1A and 1B, moderately raised (5–10x upper limit of normal) in LGMD1C, 2A, 2C-F and 2I and grossly raised (over 10X) in LGMD2B.

Neurophysiology studies are of little value in refining a diagnosis of LGMD. Nerve conduction studies can exclude a neuropathy if this causes diagnostic doubt in the early stages of presentation. Electromyography (EMG) usually shows myopathic features in patients with any type of LGMD with no ability to further specify the diagnosis. Laminopathy patients may additionally or exclusively have a peripheral neuropathy.

Muscle imaging with computed tomography (CT) or magnetic resonance imaging (MRI) is used increasingly to determine patterns of muscle involvement. No large studies of the LGMDs have been published but case reports and small series suggest characteristic patterns in some conditions. The most consistent examples are LGMD2A which selectively involves hip extensors and adductors (Mercurio *et al.*, 2005), involvement of the glutei in α-sarcoglycanopathy (Eymard *et al.*, 1997) and LGMD2J where loss of the thigh muscles and involvement of tibialis anterior is present (Udd *et al.*, 2005).

Muscle biopsy site(s) may be guided by imaging results. They are likely to yield the most useful information if they are undertaken on a

Table 26.3 Characteristic muscle biopsy findings in the LGMDs.

Disease	Protein	Histological features	Immunoanalysis: Primary changes	Secondary changes	Comments
LGMD1A	Myotilin	Dystrophic, inflammatory infiltrate, rimmed vacuoles	Myotilin normal, DGC intact	↓ laminin $\gamma1$	EM Z-line streaming
LGMD1B	Lamin A/C	Dystrophic	Lamin A/C usually normal	↓ laminin $\beta1$	
LGMD1C	Caveolin-3	Myopathic or dystrophic	↓ caveolin-3 labelling	↓ dysferlin	
LGMD2A	Calpain-3	Dystrophic	Absent, partial deficiency or normal	Calpain-3 degradation	
LGMD2B	Dysferlin	Dystrophic, inflammatory	↓ dysferlin	↓ calpain-3 in half	
LGMD2C	γ-sarcoglycan	Dystrophic	↓ γ-sarcoglycan	↓ other SG, dystrophin	
LGMD2D	α-sarcoglycan	Dystrophic	↓ α-sarcoglycan	↓ other SG, dystrophin	
LGMD2E	β-sarcoglycan	Dystrophic	↓ β-sarcoglycan	Severe ↓ other SG, dystrophin	
LGMD2F	δ-sarcoglycan	Dystrophic	↓ δ-sarcoglycan	Severe ↓ other SG, dystrophin	
LGMD2G	Telethonin	Dystrophic, rimmed vacuoles	Loss of telethonin labelling		
LGMD2H	TRIM32	Myopathic, sarcotubular			
LGMD2I	FKRP	Dystrophic	Often normal	↓ laminin $\alpha2$ and αDG	
LGMD2J	Titin	Myopathic, dystrophic, rimmed vacuoles	↓ titin	↓ calpain-3	

DGC:dystrophin–glycoprotein complex; αDG: alpha-dystroglycan; SG: sarcoglycans; EM: electron microscopy; ↓ = reduced level

clinically affected muscle but preferably not one that is 'end-stage'. Multiple biopsies may be performed. No studies compare open versus needle biopsies, although with the increasing number of immunohistochemical and immunoblotting procedures possible, it is important to obtain sufficient tissue to allow meaningful interpretation.

Muscle tissue should be analysed firstly with standard histological techniques. All LGMDs show dystrophic features with variation in fibre size, increased numbers of central nuclei and endomysial fibrosis. Inflammatory infiltrates are seen most commonly in dysferlin deficiency. Thus, there is the potential for diagnostic confusion and patients may have received a previous diagnosis of polymyositis. Rimmed vacuoles and Z line streaming may be seen in myotilin mutations as well as with mutations in the other genes causing myofibrillar myopathy. Table 26.3 summarises typical findings in each condition.

Immunohistochemistry and immunoblotting should be undertaken in a laboratory with sufficient expertise in both the performance and interpretation of these techniques. Immunohistochemical staining with a panel of antibodies ideally including all four anti-sarcoglycan antibodies may show one or more abnormalities. Demonstration of normal dystrophin staining is important (although there may be a mild secondary reduction in sarcoglycan deficiency). Quantitative analysis of proteins by Western blotting may be an additional useful technique for elucidating primary and secondary protein abnormalities (Anderson and Davison, 1999; Cooper *et al.*, 2003).

Primary changes on immunoanalysis may be clear and direct analysis specifically towards the underlying genetic defect, such as caveolin 3 reduction in LGMD1C. In other diseases, because of the interdependence of the sarcolemmal and associated proteins, disruption of one member of the complex or pathway may result in the concomitant loss of interacting proteins. This is particularly prominent in disorders of the dystrophin associated complex, where there may be reduction in all or many of the complex members, and secondary calpain3 reduction is seen in half of dysferlin deficiency patients and in patients with LGMD2J. These *secondary* changes may lead to diagnostic difficulty, particularly when direct assay for the primary defect is difficult.

In other situations, secondary changes may be the only clue to the underlying disorder. For example, in LGMD1B lamin A/C labelling is usually normal but there is frequently a secondary reduction in laminin-$\beta 1$ in adult patients. In LGMD2I, secondary reduction of laminin-$\alpha 2$ on immunolabelling was detected in most cases (Poppe *et al.*, 2003) and reduction in α-dystroglycan may also be seen and may correlate with the phenotype (Brown *et al.*, 2004). A deficiency of α ystroglycan is not specific for LGMD21 and may indicate the presence of a mutation in another glycosylation protein such as POMT1, the causative gene in LGMD2K (Balci *et al.* 2005). A summary of commonly observed primary and secondary changes is shown in table 26.3.

Immunoblotting has been the accepted test required for the diagnosis of LGMD2A (Fanin *et al.*, 2001). However there is variability in the quantity and function of calpain-3 protein detected on immunoblots, even for those patients in whom a calpain mutation is proven (Fanin *et al.*, 2004) and thus emphasis may shift to earlier analysis of the calpain-3 gene (Piluso *et al.*, 2005).

One group has developed a blood-based assay for dysferlin expression in monocytes, showing that this correlates with skeletal muscle expression. This potentially avoids the need for muscle biopsy although it is not in mainstream use at present (Ho *et al.*, 2002).

DNA analysis directed to provide confirmation of mutation in the affected gene(s) is the gold standard of diagnosis, and necessary to be able to offer carrier or presymptomatic testing to other family members. This is more straightforward in some forms of LGMD than others, depending to a large extent on whether or not there are commonly detected mutations or if mutations in different families tend to be unique. For example, the FKRP 'common mutation' C826A in LGMD2I can be detected readily in a diagnostic laboratory whereas some of the other causative genes are large, for example, dysferlin (55 exons), and screening for mutations is a formidable task. Thus mutation analysis in the lamin A/C, calpain-3, dysferlin and sarcoglycan genes may be restricted to those exons where most mutations have been detected previously; at present this is available only in selected laboratories. Mutation detection for the rarer types of LGMD may only be available on a research basis.

GOOD PRACTICE POINTS

Careful clinical assessment of factors such as the pattern of muscle involvement, associated features and family history should suggest likely diagnosi(e)s in a patient with LGMD. Confirmation of this should be achieved through the selective use of predominantly laboratory-based investigations, some of which are highly specialised and should only be undertaken in a laboratory with appropriate expertise. In some conditions this may be relatively straightforward but in others verification of the underlying mutation presently remains in the realm of the research laboratory. In the United Kingdom, patients may be referred for assessment to the centre for limb girdle muscular dystrophy (n.scag@ncl.ac.uk) funded by the National Specialist Commissioning Advisory Group (NSCAG).

Assessment and monitoring of adjunctive aspects

Respiratory management

Respiratory muscle weakness resulting in symptomatic hypoventilation and respiratory failure is found in a few of the LGMDs, most frequently in LGMD2I (Poppe *et al.*, 2003) and the sarcoglycanopathies. In LGMD2I and occasionally in the sarcoglycanopathies, respiratory failure may arise while the patient is still ambulant (Bushby and Beckmann, 2003; Poppe *et al.*, 2003).

There are no recommendations specific to the LGMDs but extrapolation from the monitoring and investigation of respiratory involvement in other neuromuscular conditions is helpful. Awareness of symptoms of respiratory insufficiency such as frequent chest infections, morning headache and daytime somnolence is important. Measurements of sitting (and supine if <80%) forced vital capacity (FVC) may be made in the outpatient clinic. Overnight pulse oximetry is recommended if the FVC is <60%. Annual influenza vaccination and prompt treatment of respiratory infections are suggested. Liaison with a respiratory physician with experience in the management of neuromuscular disorders is essential to ensure optimal timing of intervention with nocturnal home ventilation.

Cardiac management
The important issue of cardiac complications in LGMD as well as in other muscle conditions was considered at the 107th ENMC workshop (Bushby *et al.*, 2003). Cardiac involvement may manifest as a conduction defect and/or cardiomyopathy. In laminopathies, arrhythmias such as atrioventricular block, atrial paralysis and atrial fibrillation/flutter occur in the majority of patients by age 30 years and permanent pacing is required. However, even with permanent pacing, a recent paper cites a sudden death rate of 46% in lamin A/C mutation carriers and therefore recommends an implantable defibrillator (van Berlo *et al.*, 2005). Dilated cardiomyopathy arises in a third of laminopathy patients and is usually severe. Arrhythmias and hypertrophic or dilated cardiomyopathy are present in approximately 20% of sarcoglycanopathy patients. A third of LGMD 2I patients have a cardiomyopathy that is symptomatic. The remaining LGMDs do not characteristically show significant cardiac compromise.

Thus the ability to define precisely the underlying genetic defect allows a tailored approach to monitoring through better anticipation of the onset and progression of cardiac aspects. Monitoring and treatment of LGMD1B, 2C-F and 2I patients require close cardiological supervision. Electrocardiography and echocardiography are suggested as the standard initial investigations. In the absence of dedicated studies, treatment of heart failure is undertaken on general principles

with early use of angiotensin converting enzyme inhibitors. Anticoagulation may need consideration in patients with atrial fibrillation or standstill. For patients with particularly severe cardiac failure but relatively well-preserved respiratory function consideration of cardiac transplantation may be appropriate.

GOOD PRACTICE POINTS

Although serial monitoring of basic measurements of respiratory and cardiac function is attainable in the neurology outpatient setting, patients with a LGMD subtype known to place them at additional risk of cardiorespiratory complications ideally should be managed in conjunction with a respiratory physician and/or cardiologist. Intervention in the form of nocturnal ventilatory assistance for respiratory failure and with permanent pacing and/or management of developing cardiomyopathy may be life saving. The need to monitor for and treat complications as appropriate also applies to those patients in whom the underlying diagnosis is unknown as it follows that the attendant risk of cardiorespiratory complications is also unknown, but that general principles of management will apply.

Physical management
There are no papers relating specifically to LGMD and physiotherapy, exercise or orthotic use. The application of general principles is probably appropriate, as reviewed in Eagle (Eagle, 2002). Prevention of contracture development through stretching and splinting orthoses is important in maximising functional ability. Release of functionally limiting contractures (especially of the Achilles tendons) may be necessary especially in LGMD1B, LGMD2A or in childhood onset sarcoglycanopathy or LGMD2I. Scoliosis in LGMD occurs mainly after wheelchair dependence and attention should be paid to seating. The role of exercise is controversial but basic guidelines as for other types of muscular dystrophy would encourage gentle exercise within comfortable limits and the avoidance of prolonged immobility.

continued

Genetic counselling

Many patients seek medical advice due to concern for themselves, relatives or descendants. Delineation of the LGMD subtype allows knowledge of its autosomal dominant or recessive inheritance pattern to inform genetic counselling appropriately. Confirmation of the diagnosis in LGMD2I patients in particular has led to altered advice in some as previously they had been thought to be affected by Becker muscular dystrophy, an X-linked condition.

Drug treatment

There are no established drug treatments for LGMDs. Six patients with sarcoglycan-deficient muscular dystrophy took part in a double-blind, placebo-controlled crossover trial of creatine monohydrate. Thirty patients with other conditions were included. The mean improvement of 3% in muscle strength over the 8-week trial period was found to be significant but modest (Walter *et al.*, 2000). There are no relevant studies on the use of Co-enzyme Q10 (ubiquinone).

Corticosteroids have an established role in DMD boys (Moxley *et al.*, 2005); on this basis they have been used empirically in some patients with LGMD2C-F with reported improvement (Angelini *et al.*, 1998; Connolly *et al.*, 1998). As these conditions are so much rarer than DMD, it will not be possible to perform adequate treatment trials without collaboration among multiple neuromuscular centres.

Anti-inflammatory drugs have been suggested to suppress the inflammation seen in LGMD2B muscles. Trials in the animal model of LGMD2B are proposed and there is a randomised clinical trial underway in Germany.

Conflict of interests

None declared.

References

Anderson LVB, Davison K (1999). Multiplex Western blotting system for the analysis of muscular dystrophy proteins. *Am J Path* **154**(4):1017–1022.

Angelini C, Fanin M, Menegazzo E *et al.* (1998). Homozygous α-sarcoglycan mutation in two siblings: one asymptomatic and one steroid-responsive mild limb-girdle muscular dystrophy patient. *Muscle Nerve* **21**:769–775.

Balci B, Uyanik G, Dincer P, Gross C, Willer T, Talim B, *et al.* (2005). An autosomal recessive limb girdle muscular dystrophy (LGMD2) with mild mental retardation is allelic to Walker-Warburg syndrome (WWS) caused by a mutation in the POMT1 gene. 2005, *Neuromuscul Disord* **15**:271–275.

Beckmann JS, Brown RH, Muntoni F *et al.* (1999). 66th/67th ENMC sponsored international workshop: the limb-girdle muscular dystrophies. *Neuromusc Disorders* **9**:436–445.

Brainin M, Barnes M, Baron J-C *et al.* (2004). Guidance for the preparation of neurological management guidelines by EFNS scientific task forces – revised recommendations 2004. *Eur J Neurol* **11**:577–581.

Brown SC, Torelli S, Brockington M *et al.* (2004). Abnormalities in α-dystroglycan expression in MDC1C and LGMD2I muscular dystrophies. *Am J Path* **164**:727–737.

Bushby KMD (1999). Making sense of the limb-girdle muscular dystrophies. *Brain* **122**:1403–1420.

Bushby KMD, Beckmann JS (2003). The 105th ENMC sponsored workshop: pathogenesis in the non-sarcoglycan limb-girdle muscular dystrophies, Naarden, April 12–14, 2002. *Neuromusc Disorders* **13**:80–90.

Bushby K, Muntoni F, Bourke JP (2003). 107th ENMC international workshop: the management of cardiac involvement in muscular dystrophy and myotonic dystrophy. *Neuromusc Disorders* **13**:166–172.

Connolly AM, Pestronk A, Mehta S *et al.* (1998). Primary α-sarcoglycan deficiency responsive to immunosuppression over three years. *Muscle Nerve* **21**:1549–1553.

Cooper ST, Lo HP, North KN (2003). Single section Western blot. Improving the molecular diagnosis of the muscular dystrophies. *Neurology* **61**:93–97.

Eagle M (2002). Report on the Muscular Dystrophy Campaign workshop: Exercise in neuromuscular diseases. *Neuromusc Disorders* **12**:975–983.

Eymard B, Romero NB, Leturcq F *et al.* (1997). Primary adhalinopathy (alpha-sarcoglycanopathy): clinical, pathologic and genetic correlation in 20 patients with autosomal recessive muscular dystrophy. *Neurology* **48**(5):1227–1234.

Fanin M, Pegoraro E, Matsuda-Asada C *et al.* (2001). Calpain-3 and dysferlin protein screening in patients with limb-girdle dystrophy and myopathy. *Neurology* **56** (5):660–665.

Fanin M, Fulizio L, Nascimbeni AC *et al.* (2004). Molecular diagnosis in LGMD2A: mutation analysis or protein testing? *Hum Mutation* **24**:52–62.

Frosk P, Weiler T, Nylen E *et al.* (2002). Limb-girdle muscular dystrophy type 2H associated with mutation in TRIM32, a putative E3-ubiquitin-ligase gene. *Am J Hum Genet* **70:**663–672.

Hauser MA, Horrigan SK, Salmikangas P *et al.* (2000). Myotilin is mutated in limb girdle muscular dystrophy 1A. *Hum Mol Genet* **9**(14)**:**2141–2147.

Hayashi T, Arimura T, Ueda K *et al.* (2004). Identification and functional analysis of a caveolin-3 mutation associated with familial hypertrophic cardiomyopathy. *Biochem Biophys Res Commun* **313(1):** 178–184.

Ho M, Gallardo E, McKenna-Yasek D *et al.* (2002). A novel, blood-based diagnostic assay for limb girdle muscular dystrophy 2B and Miyoshi myopathy. *Ann Neurol* **51:**129–133.

Laval SH, Bushby KMD (2004). Limb-girdle muscular dystrophies – from genetics to molecular pathology. *Neuropathol Appl Neurobiol* **30:**91–105.

Mercurio E, Bushby K, Ricci E *et al.* (2005). Muscle MRI findings in patients with limb girdle muscular dystrophy with calpain 3 deficiency (LGMD2A) and early contractures. *Neuromusc Disorders* **15:**164–171.

Moreira ES, Wiltshire TJ, Faulkner G *et al.* (2000). Limb-girdle muscular dystrophy type 2G is caused by mutations in the gene encoding the sarcomeric protein telethonin. *Nat Genet* **24:**163–166.

Moxley RT, Ashwal S, Pandya S *et al.* (2005). Practice parameter: corticosteroid treatment of Duchenne dystrophy. *Neurology* **64:**13–20.

Piluso G, Politano L, Aurino S *et al.* (2005). Extensive scanning of the calpain-3 gene broadens the spectrum of LGMD2A phenotypes. *J Med Genet* **42:** 686-693.

Pollitt C, Anderson LVB, Pogue R *et al.* (2001). The phenotype of calpainopathy: diagnosis based on a multidisciplinary approach. *Neuromusc Disorders* **11:**287–296.

Poppe M, Cree L, Bourke J *et al.* (2003). The phenotype of limb-girdle muscular dystrophy type 2I. *Neurology* **60:**1246–1251.

Saenz A, Leturcq F, Cobo AM *et al.* (2005). LGMD2A: epidemiology and genotype-phenotype correlations based on a large mutational survey on the calpain 3 gene. *Brain* **128:**732–742.

Schoser BG, Frosk P, Engel AG *et al.* (2005) Commonality of TRIM32 mutation in causing sarcotubular myopathy and LGMD2H. *Ann Neurol* **57**(4)**:**591–595.

Udd B, Vihola A, Sarparanta J *et al.* (2005). Titinopathies and extension of the M-line mutation phenotype beyond distal myopathy and LGMD2J. *Neurology* **64:**636–642.

van Berlo JH, de Voogt WG, van der Kooi AJ *et al.* (2005). Meta-analysis of clinical characteristics of 299 carriers of LMNA gene mutations: do lamin A/C mutations portend a high risk of sudden death? *J Mol Med* **83**(1)**:**79–83.

Walter MC, Lochmuller H, Reilich P *et al.* (2000). Creatine monohydrate in muscular dystrophies: a double-blind, placebo-controlled clinical study. *Neurology* **54**(9)**:**1848–1850.

Walton J and Natrass F (1954). On the classification, natural history and treatment of the myopathies. *Brain* **77**(2)**:**169–231.

Woodman SE, Sotgia F, Galbiati F *et al.* (2004). Caveolinopathies. Mutations in caveolin-3 cause four distinct autosomal dominant muscle diseases. *Neurology* **62:**538–543.

CHAPTER 27

Neurological complications of HIV infection

P. Portegies,[a] L. Solod,[b] P. Cinque,[c]
A. Chaudhuri,[d] J. Begovac,[e] I. Everall,[f] T. Weber,[g]
M. Bojar,[h] P. Martinez-Martin,[i] P.G.E. Kennedy[d]

Abstract

The spectrum of neurological complications of HIV-infection has remained unchanged through the years, but its epidemiology has changed remarkably as a result of the introduction of highly active antiretroviral therapy (HAART). Guidelines for the diagnosis and treatment of cerebral toxoplasmosis, cryptococcal meningitis, progressive multifocal leukoencephalopathy, CMV encephalitis, CMV polyradiculomyelitis, tuberculous meningitis, primary CNS lymphoma, HIV dementia, HIV myelopathy and HIV polyneuropathy are given with a grading of evidence and recommendations.

Background and objectives

The introduction and widespread use of highly active antiretroviral therapy (HAART) for the treatment of HIV infection has resulted in dramatic reductions in morbidity, mortality and healthcare utilization (Kovacs et al., 1996; Hogg et al., 1998; Palella et al., 1998). Decreasing rates for opportunistic infections, including the neurological infections, have been reported. Diagnostic tools for these neurological complications have been greatly improved in the past 5–10 years. The therapeutic approach to the neurologic diseases has been influenced by the success of HAART. Together, these developments form the main reason for producing these new guidelines.

The objective of the study was to provide neurologists and others with evidence-based guidelines for the diagnosis and treatment of neurological complications of HIV infection.

Neurological complications

These guidelines deal with the most common neurological complications of HIV-infection. Although the epidemiology of neurological complications has changed considerably in recent years in the West, the spectrum has remained relatively unchanged. The most frequent opportunistic infections are cerebral toxoplasmosis, cryptococcal meningitis, progressive multifocal leukoencephalopathy (PML), tuberculous meningitis, cytomegalovirus (CMV) encephalitis and

[a]Department of Neurology, OLVG Hospital Amsterdam, the Netherlands; Department of Neurology, Academic Medical Centre, Amsterdam, the Netherlands; [c]Department of Infectious Diseases, San Raffaele Hospital, Milano, Italy; [d]Department of Neurology, University of Glasgow, Glasgow, Scotland, United Kingdom; [e]Department of Infectious Diseases, University of Zagreb, Croatia; [f]Institute of Psychiatry, London, United Kingdom; [g]Department of Neurology, Marienkrankenhaus, Hamburg, Germany; [h]Motol Hospital, Prague, Czech Republic; [i]Hospital de Getafe, Madrid, Spain.

CMV polyradiculomyelitis. Primary central nervous system (CNS) lymphoma has become less frequent, but is still an important cause of focal brain disease. The neurological diseases that are more directly related to HIV itself are HIV dementia, vacuolar myelopathy and peripheral neuropathy. HIV dementia is rare in patients who take HAART, but with resistance and compliance problems patients may become at risk. Peripheral neuropathy is still a frequent complication, not only in severely immunosuppressed patients. The role of antiretroviral drugs in the pathogenesis remains uncertain.

HAART

An increasing number of potent antiretroviral drugs are available (Richman, 2001). When used in combinations of three or four drugs, this treatment is called HAART. In most HIV-infected patients, especially treatment-naive patients, HAART is effective in rapidly reducing plasma levels of HIV-RNA, accompanied by a gradual increase in CD4 cell counts, sometimes to normal levels (Richman, 2001; Yeni et al., 2002). For many antiretroviral-naive patients, CD4 cell counts increase to levels at which the patients are no longer generally susceptible to serious opportunistic infections. As currently available antiretroviral regimens will not eradicate HIV, the goal of therapy is to durably inhibit viral replication so that the patient can attain and maintain an effective immune response to most potential microbial pathogens (De Luca et al., 2001; Yeni et al., 2002). The recently updated recommendations of the International AIDS Society-USA Panel advise the start of treatment in patients with symptomatic HIV disease and in patients with CD4 cell counts below 350 cells/ul or viral loads above 50 000–100 000 copies/ml (Yeni et al., 2002). The most commonly used regimens to start with contain two nucleoside reverse transcriptase (RT) inhibitors with either a non-nucleoside RT inhibitor or a single (or boosted) protease inhibitor. Antiretroviral activity is evaluated by assessing changes in CD4 cell count and viral load in the plasma. The availability of new drugs has widened the options for patients who fail to respond to their antiretroviral regimen. A patient with

one of the neurological complications described below has symptomatic HIV disease and HAART is indicated but the strength of the evidence for this recommendation varies from complication to complication.

The immune restoration itself, that is, the result of HAART, may have a beneficial effect on the neurological complication. For some of the neurological diseases (PML, HIV dementia), this has been documented in small uncontrolled studies. Besides HAART, disease-specific therapy for neurological complications is indicated, as discussed below. The duration of these specific treatments is determined by the level of immunosuppression. Before HAART became available, the treatment for acute infection had to be followed by lifelong secondary prophylaxis to prevent relapses (e.g. for toxoplasmosis, cryptococcosis). The recommendation in general now with HAART is that secondary prophylaxis can be discontinued if CD4 cell counts show a significant and sustained increase in both absolute and percentage terms, for example, if they have increased to above 200 cells/ul and have remained at that level for at least 3 months. Primary prophylaxis for neurological complications is not recommended.

Search strategy

A MEDLINE (National Library of Medicine) search of the relevant literature from 1966 to August 2002 was undertaken using various combinations of the following MeSH headings: HIV-1, acquired immunodeficiency syndrome, HIV-infections, toxoplasmosis cerebral, meningitis cryptococcal, leukoencephalopathy progressive multifocal, polyneuropathies, polyradiculopathy, encephalitis, myelitis transverse, lymphoma, central nervous system, cytomegalovirus infection, tuberculosis central nervous system, diagnosis, therapeutics, drug therapy. The following free text words were used: highly active antiretroviral therapy, cerebral toxoplasmosis, PML, CMV encephalitis, CMV polyradiculomyelitis, primary CNS lymphoma, HIV dementia, AIDS dementia, vacuolar myelopathy, HIV myelopathy and sensory neuropathy. Limitations included meta-analysis, randomized controlled trial, sensitivity and specificity, cohort studies, casecontrol studies.

Grading of recommendations

All members of the task force prepared one or more of the ten selected neurological complications. The material available from the literature review was integrated and summarized in graded recommendations. The recommendations were approved by all members.

Cerebral toxoplasmosis

Cerebral toxoplasmosis is a frequent cause of focal brain disease in HIV infection. *Toxoplasma gondii* is an obligate intracellular protozoan parasite in human beings. Toxoplasmic encephalitis is almost always caused by reactivation of *Toxoplasma gondii* cysts in brain parenchyma.

Diagnosis

A presumptive diagnosis of cerebral toxoplasmosis in HIV-infected patients is based on: (1) progressive neurological deficits, (2) contrast-enhancing mass lesion(s) on imaging studies [computed tomography/magnetic resonance imaging (CT/MRI)], (3) successful response within 2 weeks to specific treatment (see below) [Class IV]. Absence of one or more of these characteristics makes cerebral toxoplasmosis less likely. Those patients are possible candidates for brain biopsy. In clinical practice, most patients with mass lesion(s) are given 2 weeks of treatment anyway (including patients with negative serology or a single lesion). Cerebrospinal fluid (CSF) studies, including antibody studies and polymerase chain reaction (PCR) studies, have not produced conclusive results (Franzen *et al.*, 1997).

Treatment

Primary therapy for cerebral toxoplasmosis (Leport *et al.*, 1988; Danneman *et al.*, 1992; Katlama *et al.*, 1996a,b): pyrimethamine 200 mg load, then 50 mg/day (oral) with sulfadiazine 1 g four times daily (oral) (or clindamycin intravenous (i.v.) or oral 600 mg four times daily) with folinic acid 10 mg/day (oral) (Class IIa, Recommendation Level B).

Other possible combinations:

1 Trimethroprim/sulfamethoxazol oral or i.v. 2.5–5 mg/kg (TMP) q.i.d. [Class IIa] (Torre *et al.*, 1998).
2 Pyrimethamine (as above) plus clarithromycin 1 g twice daily [Class III].
3 Pyrimethamine (as above) plus azithromycin 600–1800 mg/day [Class III] (Jacobsen *et al.*, 2001).
4 Pyrimethamine (as above) plus dapsone 100 mg/day [Class III].
5 Atovaquone 750 mg four times daily (oral) [Class IIa] (Torres *et al.*, 1997).

For secondary prophylaxis (Leport *et al.*, 1988; Katlama *et al.*, 1996a): pyrimethamine 50 mg/day with sulfadiazine 500 mg four times daily (Class IIa, Recommendation Level B). Alternatives are: atovaquone 750 mg four times daily (oral) [Class IIa] [(Katlama *et al.*, 1996b) 13] or pyrimethamine 50 mg/day + sulfadiazine 500 mg four times daily, twice a week [Class IIa] (Podzamczer *et al.*, 1995).

The primary therapy is usually continued for 6 weeks, followed by secondary prophylaxis. Secondary prophylaxis can be stopped according to the recommendations described above.

Cryptococcal meningitis

Infection with the yeast *Cryptococcus neoformans* in HIV-infected individuals most often leads to a subacute meningitis. The initial infection is a pulmonary infection. In the immunosuppressed host dissemination occurs afterwards to many organ systems, including the CNS.

Diagnosis

A definitive diagnosis of cryptococcal meningitis is made by using any of the following methods:

1 Visualizing the fungus in the CSF using India ink (sensitivity 75–85%) [Class I].
2 Detecting cryptococcal antigen by latex agglutination assay in the CSF (sensitivity 95%) [Class I].
3 Positive CSF culture for *C. neoformans* [Class I].

Treatment

It is important to be alert (especially in the first week after the diagnosis has been made) for high

CSF pressures that may lead to blindness, coma, seizures etc. Removing 20–30 ml CSF by (repeated) spinal tap or (in severe cases) a lumbar drain for a few days may be necessary. Based on several randomized clinical trials (Larsen *et al.*, 1990; De Gans *et al.*, 1992; Saag *et al.*, 1992; Van der Horst *et al.*, 1997) the recommendation for treatment is: amphotericin B 0.7 mg/kg/day i.v. (with or without flucytosine 5-FC; 100 mg/kg/day orally) for 2 weeks [Class Ia]. This treatment is followed by: fluconazole 400 mg/day (or itraconazole 400 mg/day) (orally) to complete a course of 10 weeks (Class Ia, Recommendation Level A). The addition of flucytosine to amphotericin B did not significantly improve the mortality and clinical course in a randomized clinical trial (RCT); however, flucytosine was well tolerated and there was a trend to a better CSF sterilization with its use in this study (Van der Horst *et al.*, 1997). CSF examination should be repeated to confirm a therapeutic response (negative CSF culture).

For secondary prophylaxis fluconazole 200 mg/day (oral) (Class Ia, Recommendation Level A; Bozzette *et al.*, 1991; Powderly *et al.*, 1992; Saag *et al.*, 1999). Secondary prophylaxis can be stopped according to the recommendations described above.

Progressive multifocal leukoencephalopathy

Progressive multifocal leukoencephalopathy (PML) is a viral opportunistic infection of oligodendrocytes and astrocytes leading to demyelination in the CNS. The causative agent is a polyomavirus named JC virus. JC virus is ubiquitous in human beings and is usually acquired during adolescence (two-thirds have antibodies at age of 14 years).

Diagnosis

Slowly progressive focal neurological deficits with asymmetrical white matter abnormalities on MRI suggest PML. The lesions are non-enhancing, hyperintense on T2-weighted MRI, without mass effect. The subcortical 'U' fibres are characteristically involved. This diagnosis is strongly supported by positive CSF-PCR for JC virus DNA (sensitivity 72–100%; specificity 92–100%) [Class I] (Cinque

et al., 1997). If the CSF-PCR is negative, it is recommended to repeat CSF-PCR once or twice. Brain biopsy remains the final confirmatory test, but a positive CSF-PCR offers acceptable evidence.

Treatment

In patients who are being treated with HAART PML arrests or remits in approximately 50%, and survival is prolonged in these patients (Miralles *et al.*, 1998; Clifford *et al.*, 1999; De Luca *et al.*, 2000a, 2001). The course is progressive in the other 50%.

It has been suggested by several reports that cidofovir (5 mg/kg i.v. once weekly) offers an additional benefit [Class III] (De Luca *et al.*, 2000b; Marra *et al.*, 2002). Controlled clinical trials are lacking. Cidofovir should be considered as an experimental treatment.

CMV encephalitis

Cytomegalovirus belongs to the family of herpes viruses. CMV infection is endemic; the majority of HIV-infected adults have serologic evidence of prior CMV infection. Clinical syndromes in immunosuppressed patients include retinitis, gastrointestinal ulcers, encephalitis and polyradiculomyelitis.

Diagnosis

CMV encephalitis is suspected in an HIV-infected patient with (usually) a history of CMV disease (e.g. CMV retinitis), a clinically progressive encephalopathy and periventricular enhancement (ventriculitis) on imaging (CT/MRI) studies. The diagnosis is strongly supported by: (i) positive CSF-PCR for CMV-DNA (sensitivity 62–100%; specificity 89–100%) [Class I] (Cinque *et al.*, 1998) or (ii) positive CSF culture [Class I] (Cinque *et al.*, 1998), but in general CSF viral cultures are highly insensitive.

Brain biopsy is not a realistic option given the brainstem and periventricular localization of the encephalitis. CSF-PCR is the diagnostic test of choice.

Treatment

Induction treatment (for 3 weeks) (Anduze-Faris *et al.*, 2000): ganciclovir 5 mg/kg i.v. twice daily

[Class IV] or foscarnet 90 mg/kg i.v. twice daily [Class IV] or cidofovir 5 mg/kg i.v. every week; after two courses every 2 weeks [Class IV] or ganciclovir and foscarnet (dosages as above) (Class IV, Recommendation Level C).

Maintenance treatment (Anduze-Faris *et al.*, 2000): ganciclovir 5 mg/kg/day i.v. [Class IV].

CMV polyradiculomyelitis

This is the most common polyradiculomyelitis in AIDS. The most frequent manifestations are pain (low-back, sciatic), paresthesia, sphincter dysfunction, distal sensory loss, and progressive ascending weakness.

Diagnosis

CMV polyradiculomyelitis is suspected in an HIV-infected patient with (usually) a history of CMV disease (e.g. CMV retinitis), clinically a rapidly ascending polyradiculomyelitis and a highly characteristic CSF polymorphonuclear pleocytosis. The diagnosis is strongly supported by: (i) positive CSF-PCR for CMV-DNA (sensitivity 62–100%; specificity 89–100%) [Class I] (Cinque *et al.*, 1998) or (ii) positive CSF culture [Class I] (Cinque *et al.*, 1998), but in general CSF viral cultures are highly insensitive.

Treatment

Induction treatment (for 3 weeks) (Anduze-Faris *et al.*, 2000): ganciclovir 5 mg/kg i.v. b.i.d. [Class IV] or foscarnet 90 mg/kg i.v. b.i.d. [Class IV] or cidofovir 5 mg/kg i.v. every week; after two courses every 2 weeks [Class IV] or ganciclovir and foscarnet (dosages as above) (Class IV, Recommendation Level C).

Maintenance treatment (Anduze-Faris *et al.*, 2000): ganciclovir 5 mg/kg/day i.v. [Class IV].

Tuberculous meningitis

Infection with *Mycobacterium tuberculosis* is the leading cause of death worldwide among persons infected with HIV. Tuberculous meningitis and CNS tuberculomas are common complications. CNS tuberculosis in HIV disease is more frequent in developing countries.

Diagnosis

CNS tuberculosis has been described in 10–20% of patients with HIV-related tuberculosis. Lymphocytic pleocytosis, low glucose and raised protein are the typical features of tuberculous meningitis. Post-contrast brain scans show enhancement of the meninges and the periphery of the tuberculoma and on occasion, may reveal miliary lesions. Hydrocephalus may appear early. The diagnosis is based on demonstration of *Mycobacterium tuberculosis* in the CSF (Zuger and Lowy, 1997; Gordin, 1999): (i) culture (sensitivity 25–86%) [Class I] or (ii) CSF smear (ZN) (sensitivity 8–86%) [Class IV] or (iii) CSF-PCR (sensitivity 83–100%; specificity 88–100%) [Class II].

Treatment

Isoniazid 5 mg/kg/day, up to 300 mg/day and rifampicin 10 mg/kg/day up to 600 mg/day and pyrazinamide 15–30 mg/kg/day (max 2.5 g/day) and ethambutol 15–25 mg/kg/day up to 1600 mg/day (Class III, Recommendation Level A; Zuger and Lowy, 1997; Gordin, 1999).

Ethambutol can be substituted with streptomycin (15 mg/kg/day, up to 1 g/day i.m. or i.v.; max 2 months) or amikacin (15 mg/kg/day i.m. or i.v.). The role of steroids in HIV-positive tuberculous meningitis is unclear. The minimum duration of treatment is 6 months. Isoniazid may lead to pyridoxine deficiency and a sensorimotor distal polyneuropathy. Therefore pyridoxine 20 mg/day should be added to the regimen.

Primary CNS lymphoma

Primary CNS lymphoma is a non-Hodgkin's lymphoma that arises within and is confined to the nervous system. It is the second most frequent CNS mass lesion in adults with AIDS in western countries. Primary CNS lymphoma is associated with Epstein–Barr virus (EBV) infection. The transforming potential of the virus plays a role in the pathogenesis of this tumour.

Epstein–Barr virus has the potential to transform B lymphocytes after infection. This transforming potential of EBV is involved in the development of primary CNS lymphoma and other tumours. Cytological examination of the

CSF rarely reveals pathological cells and its value, although not well studied, seems limited. Data on other potential CSF markers of primary CNS lymphoma are inconclusive. Data on CD23 are promising and need further validation. These markers cannot be recommended as diagnostic tests in primary CNS lymphoma. Three small studies suggest that thallium-201 single photon emission computerized tomography (SPECT) is specific for primary CNS lymphoma. Two positron emission tomography (PET) studies show comparable results (O'Malley *et al.*, 1994; Ruiz *et al.*, 1994; Berry *et al.*, 1995; Cingolani *et al.*, 1998; Lorberboym *et al.*, 1998; Antinori *et al.*, 1999; Licho *et al.*, 2002). In conclusion, SPECT/PET study results are inconclusive, and these investigations cannot be recommended.

Diagnosis
A definitive diagnosis is made by histological examination of brain tissue (obtained by brain biopsy or at autopsy). In an HIV-infected individual with a single or multiple contrast-enhancing brain lesion(s) on CT or MRI not responding to anti-toxoplasmic therapy, a presumptive diagnosis can be supported by: positive CSF EBV-PCR (sensitivity 83–100%, specificity 93–100%) [Class II] (Cinque *et al.*, 1993, 1996; Arribas *et al.*, 1995; De Luca *et al.*, 1995).

Treatment
HAART improves neurological status and prolongs survival in patients with primary CNS lymphoma (Hoffman *et al.*, 2001). Besides HAART three other treatment options exist: (i) whole-brain irradiation and corticosteroids [Class III] (Baumgartner *et al.*, 1990; Goldstein *et al.*, 1991; Donahue *et al.*, 1995), (ii) intravenous methotrexate followed by whole brain radiation [Class III] (Jacomet *et al.*, 1997) or (iii) methotrexate, thiotepa, and procarbazine intravenously in combination with methotrexate intrathecally (Class III, Recommendation Level B; Forsyth *et al.*, 1994).

HIV dementia
HIV dementia is a syndrome of cognitive and motor dysfunction that has also been termed: AIDS dementia complex, HIV-associated cognitive-motor complex and AIDS dementia. Its paediatric counterpart is called progressive encephalopathy. The cognitive impairment is compatible with a subcortical dementia. Most patients with HIV dementia are severely immunosuppressed.

Diagnosis
The diagnosis is based on: (i) progressive cognitive impairment (with or without motor dysfunction), (ii) exclusion of CNS opportunistic infections and tumors (by CSF and CT/MRI) (Price, 1996; McArthur and Selnes, 1997) and is supported by: (1) high levels of HIV RNA in the CSF (above three log copies/ml) [Class III] (Brew *et al.*, 1997; Ellis *et al.*, 1997; McArthur *et al.*, 1997) and (2) diffuse, bilateral (often symmetrical) non-enhancing white-matter hyperintensities on MRI [Class III] (Levy *et al.*, 1986).

Treatment
Class III evidence for HAART (Foudraine *et al.*, 1998; Sacktor *et al.*, 2002) leads to a Level B recommendation. Most nucleosides and non-nucleosides (e.g. nevirapine) penetrate relatively well into the CSF; most protease inhibitors do not (with the exception of indinavir). It seems reasonable to include at least two drugs in the regimen that penetrate well (Enting *et al.*, 1998). The data are limited. Most combinations have not been well studied in HIV dementia.

HIV myelopathy
Spinal cord disease is observed in various stages of HIV infection. The most common type is HIV myelopathy (also named HIV-related vacuolar myelopathy). HIV myelopathy is a progressive non-segmental spinal cord disease. The diagnosis is one of exclusion.

Diagnosis
The diagnosis is based on: (i) progressive myelopathy without sensory level, (ii) absence of focal lesion or mass lesion in spinal cord or compression of spinal cord on MRI and (iii) negative human T-cell lymphotropic virus (HTLV-I) serology, (iv) normal serum vitamin B12, (v) negative CSF PCR

for herpesviruses, (vi) negative CSF syphilis tests (Di Rocco 1999; Thurnher *et al.*, 2000). All diagnostic tests have only class IV evidence.

Treatment

HAART [Class III] (Di Rocco *et al.*, 2000; Staudinger and Henry, 2000).

HIV polyneuropathy

Polyneuropathies do occur frequently in the course of HIV infection. The pathogenesis is poorly understood and treatment is largely restricted to symptomatic pain therapy.

Diagnosis

The most important neuropathy in HIV infection is the distal sensory polyneuropathy. Its pathogenesis is unclear. This neuropathy is indistinguishable from the toxic neuropathy caused by the nucleosides zalcitabine, didanosine, and stavudine. Symptoms of paraesthesiae and pain predominate; disability caused by loss of sensory or motor function is less prominent. Electrodiagnostic studies may be helpful in confirming the diagnosis but may not be necessary in all cases.

Treatment

Symptomatic treatment: (i) amitriptyline 25–100 mg/day [Class I], (ii) tramadol 50 mg three times daily to 100 mg four times daily [Class I] and (iii) carbamazepine 200 mg three or four times daily [Class I] (Sindrup and Jensen, 1999). Gabapentin is a promising drug (2400–3600 mg/day), but has not been studied in RCT.

Summary and conclusions

Despite the success of HAART, HIV-infected individuals are at risk for a variety of neurological complications. The risk for those complications increases with an increasing level of immunodeficiency. Those patients with CD4 cell counts below 200×10^6/ml are particularly at risk for opportunistic infections, lymphoma and HIV

dementia. Nucleic acid amplification in the CSF by PCR has greatly improved the diagnostic accuracy in PML, CMV infections, primary CNS lymphoma and HIV dementia. Besides HAART, specific treatment options are available for the majority of these complications. In general, the task force recommends rapidity in evaluating these patients to limit damage to the nervous system.

References

Anduze-Faris BM, Fillet AM, Gozlan J *et al.* (2000). Induction and maintenance therapy of cytomegalovirus central nervous system infection in HIV-infected patients. *AIDS* **14**:517524.

Antinori A, De Rossi G, Ammassari A *et al.* (1999). Value of combined approach with thallium-201 single-photon emission computed tomography and Epstein-Barr virus DNA polymerase chain reaction in CSF for the diagnosis of AIDS-related primary CNS lymphoma. *J Clin Oncol* **17**:554–560.

Arribas JR, Clifford DB, Fichtenbaum CJ, Roberts RL, Powderly WG, Storch GA (1995). Detection of Epstein-Barr virus DNA in cerebrospinal fluid for diagnosis of AIDS-related central nervous system lymphoma. *J Clin Microbiol* **33**:1580–1583.

Baumgartner JE, Rachlin JR, Beckstead JH *et al.* (1990). Primary central nervous system lymphomas: natural history and response to radiation therapy in 55 patients with acquired immunodeficiency syndrome. *J Neurosurg* **73**:206–211.

Berry I, Gaillard JF, Guo Z *et al.* (1995). Cerebral lesions in AIDS. What can be expected from scintigraphy? Cerebral tomographic scintigraphy using thallium-201: a contribution to the differential diagnosis of lymphomas and infectious lesions. *J Neuroradiol* **22**:218–228.

Bozzette SA, Larsen R, Chiu J *et al.* (1991). A controlled trial of maintenance therapy with fluconazole after treatment of cryptococcal meningitis in the acquired immunodeficiency syndrome. *N Engl J Med* **324**:580–584.

Brew B, Pemberton L, Cunningham P *et al.* (1997). Levels of human immunodeficiency virus type 1 RNA in cerebrospinal fluid correlate with AIDS dementia stage. *J Infect Dis* **175**:963–966.

Cingolani A, De Luca A, Larocca LM *et al.* (1998). Minimally invasive diagnosis of acquired immunodeficiency syndrome-related primary central nervous system lymphoma. *J Natl Cancer Inst* **90**:364–369.

Cinque P, Brytting M, Vago L *et al.* (1993). Epstein-Barr virus DNA in cerebrospinal fluid from patients with AIDS-related primary lymphoma of the central nervous system. *Lancet* **342:**398–401.

Cinque P, Vago L, Dahl H *et al.* (1996). Polymerase chain reaction on cerebrospinal fluid for diagnosis of virus-associated opportunistic diseases of the central nervous system in HIV-infected patients. *AIDS* **10:**951–958.

Cinque P, Scarpellini P, Vago L, Linde A, Lazzarin A (1997). Diagnosis of central nervous system complications in HIV-infected patients: cerebrospinal fluid analysis by the polymerase chain reaction. *AIDS* **11:**117.

Cinque P, Cleator GM, Weber T *et al.* for the European Union Concerted Action on Virus Meningitis and Encephalitis (1998). Diagnosis and clinical management of neurological disorders caused by cytomegalovirus in AIDS patients. *J Neurovirol* **4:**120–132.

Clifford DB, Yiannoutsos C, Glicksman M *et al.* (1999). HAART improves prognosis in HIV-associated progressive multifocal leukoencephalopathy. *Neurology* **52:**623–625.

Danneman B, McCutchan JA, Israelski D *et al.* (1992). Treatment of toxoplasmic encephalitis in patients with AIDS. A randomized trial comparing pyrimethamine plus clindamycin to pyrimethamine plus sulfadiazine. The California Collaborative Treatment Group. *Ann Intern Med* **116:**33–43.

De Gans J, Portegies P, Tiessens G *et al.* (1992). Itraconazole compared with amphotericin B plus flucytosine in AIDS patients with cryptococcal meningitis. *AIDS* **6:**185–190.

De Luca A, Antinori A, Cingolani A *et al.* (1995). Evaluation of cerebrospinal fluid EBV-DNA and IL-10 as markers for in vivo diagnosis of AIDS-related primary central nervous system lymphoma. *Br J Haematol* **90:**844–849.

De Luca A, Giancola ML, Ammassari A *et al.* (2000a). The effect of potent antiretroviral therapy and JC Virus load in cerebrospinal fluid on clinical outcome of patients with AIDS-associated Progressive Multifocal Leukoencephalopathy. *J Inf Dis* **182:**1077–1083.

De Luca A, Giancola ML, Ammassari A *et al.* (2000b). Cidofovir added to HAART improves virological and clinical outcome in AIDS-associated progressive multifocal leukoencephalopathy. *AIDS* **14:**117–121.

De Luca A, Giancola ML, Ammassari A *et al.* (2001). Potent anti-retroviral therapy with or without cidofovir for AIDS-associated progressive multifocal leukoencephalopathy: extended follow-up of an observational study. *J Neurovirol* **7:** 364–368.

Di Rocco A. (1999). Diseases of the spinal cord in human immunodeficiency virus infection. *Semin Neurol* **19:**151–155.

Di Rocco A, Geraci A, Tagliati M, Staudinger R, Henry K (2000). Remission of HIV myelopathy after highly active antiretroviral therapy. *Neurology* **55:**456.

Donahue BR, Sullivan JW, Cooper JS (1995). Additional experience with empiric radiotherapy for presumed human immunodeficiency virus-associated primary central nervous system lymphoma. *Cancer* **76:**328–332.

Ellis RJ, Hsia K, Spector Sa *et al.* (1997). Cerebrospinal fluid human immunodeficiency virus type 1 RNA levels are elevated in neurocognitive impaired individuals with acquired immunodeficiency syndrome: HIV Neurobehavioral Research Center Group. *Ann Neurol* **42:**679.

Enting RH, Hoetelmans RMW, Lange JMA, Burger DM, Beijnen JH, Portegies P (1998). Antiretroviral drugs and the central nervous system. *AIDS* **12:**1941–1955.

Forsyth PA, Yahalom J, DeAngelis LM (1994). Combined-modality therapy in the treatment of primary central nervous system lymphoma in AIDS. *Neurology* **44:**1473–1479.

Foudraine NA, Hoetelmans RMW, Lange JMA *et al.* (1998). Cerebrospinal fluid HIV-1 RNA and drug concentrations after treatment with lamivudine plus zidovudine or stavudine. *Lancet* **351:**1547–1551.

Franzen C, Altfeld M, Hegener P *et al.* (1997). Limited value of PCR for detection of *Toxoplasma gondii* in blood from human immunodeficiency virus-infected patients. *J Clin Microbiol* **35:**2639–2641.

Goldstein JD, Dickson DW, Moser FG *et al.* (1991). Primary central nervous system lymphomas in acquired immunodeficiency syndrome: a clinical and pathological study with results of treatment with radiation. *Cancer* **67:**2756–2765.

Gordin F (1999). *Mycobacterium tuberculosis*. In: Dolin R, Masur H, Saag MS, eds. AIDS Therapy. Churchill Livingstone, New York, pp. 359–374.

Hoffman C, Tabrizian S, Wolf E *et al.* (2001). Survival of AIDS patients with primary central nervous system lymphoma is dramatically improved by HAART-induced immune recovery. *AIDS* **15:**2119–2127.

Hogg RS, Heath KV, Yip B *et al.* (1998). Improved survival among HIV-infected individuals following initiation of antiretroviral therapy. *JAMA* **279:**450–454.

Jacobsen JM, Hafner R, Remington J *et al.* (2001). Dose-escalation, phase I/II study of zathromycin and pyrimethamine for the treatment of toxoplasmic encephalitis in AIDS. *AIDS* **15:**583–589.

Jacomet Ch, Girard P-M, Lebrette M-G, Leca Farese V, Montfort L, Rozenbaum W (1997). Intravenous methotrexate for primary central nervous system non-Hodgkin's lymphoma in AIDS. *AIDS* **11:**1725–1730.

Katlama C, De Wit S, O'Doherty E *et al.* (1996a). Pyrimethamine-clindamycin vs. pyrimethamine-sulfadiazine in acute and long-term therapy for toxoplasmic encephalitis in patients with AIDS. *Clin Infect Dis* **22:**268–275.

Katlama C, Mouthon B, Gourdon D, Lapierre D, Rousseau F (1996b). Atovaquone as long-term suppressive therapy for toxoplasmic encephalitis in patients with AIDS and multiple drug intolerance. Atovaquone Expanded Access Group. *AIDS* **10:**1107–1112.

Kovacs JA, Vogel S, Albert JM *et al.* (1996). Controlled trial of interleukin-2 infusions in patients infected with the human immunodeficiency virus. *N Engl J Med* **335:**1350–1356.

Larsen RA, Leal M, Chan L (1990). Fluconazole compared with amphotericin B plus flucytosine fpr cryptococcal meningitis in AIDS. *Ann Intern Med* **113:**183–187.

Leport C, Raffi F, Matheron S *et al.* (1988). Treatment of central nervous system toxoplasmosis with pyrimethamine/sulfadiazine combination in 35 patients with the acquired immunodeficiency syndrome. *Am J Med* **84:**94–100.

Levy RM, Rosenbloom S, Perrett LV (1986). Neuroradiologic findings in AIDS: a review of 200 cases. *Am J Roengenol* **147:**977–983.

Licho R, Litofsky NS, Senitko M, George M (2002). Inaccuracy of TI-201 brain SPECT in distinguishing cerebral infections from lymphoma in patients with AIDS. *Clin Nucl Med* **27:**81–86.

Lorberboym M, Wallach F, Estok L *et al.* (1998). Thallium-201 retention in focal intracranial lesions for differential diagnosis of primary lymphoma and nonmalignant lesions in AIDS patients. *J Nucl Med* **39:**1366–1369.

Marra Ch M, Rajijic N, Barker DE *et al.* (2002). A pilot study of cidofovir for progressive multifocal leukoencephalopathy in AIDS. *AIDS* **16:**1791–1797.

McArthur JC, Selnes OA (1997). Human immunodeficiency virus-associated dementia. In: Berger JR, Levy RM, eds. AIDS and the Nervous System, 2nd edn. Lippincott-Raven, Philadelphia, PA, pp. 527–567.

McArthur JC, McClernon DR, Cronin MF *et al.* (1997). Relationship between human immunodeficiency virus-associated dementia and viral load in cerebrospinal fluid and brain. *Ann Neurol* **42:**689.

Miralles P, Berenguer J, Garcia de Viedma D *et al.* (1998). Treatment of AIDS-associated progressive multifocal leukoencephalopathy with highly active antiretroviral therapy. *AIDS* **12:**2467–2472.

O'Malley JP, Ziessman HA, Kumar PN, Harkness BA, Tall JG, Pierce PF (1994). Diagnosis of intracranial lymphoma in patients with AIDS value of 201TI single-photon emission computed tomography. *Am J Roentgenol* **163:**417–421.

Palella FJ Jr, Delaney KM, Moorman AC *et al.* (1998). Declining morbidity and mortality among patients with advanced human immunodeficiency virus infection. *N Engl J Med* **338:**853–860.

Podzamczer D, Miro JM, Bolao F *et al.* (1995). Twice-weekly maintenance therapy with sulfadiazine-pyrimethamine to prevent recurrent toxoplasmic encephalitis in patients with AIDS. Spanish Toxoplasmosis Study Group. *Ann Intern Med* **123:**175–180.

Powderly WG, Saag MS, Cloud GA *et al.* (1992). A controlled trial of fluconazole or amphotericin B to prevent relapse of cryptococcal meningitis in patients with the acquired immunodeficiency syndrome. *N Engl J Med* **326:**793–798.

Price R (1996). Neurological complications of HIV infection. *Lancet* **348:**445–452.

Richman DD (2001). HIV chemotherapy. *Nature* **410:**995–1001.

Ruiz A, Ganz WI, Post MJD, Camp A, Landy H, Malin W (1994). Use of thallium[201] brain SPECT to differentiate cerebral lymphoma from Toxoplasma encephalitis in AIDS patients. *Am J Neuroradiol* **15:**1885–1894.

Saag MS, Powderly WG, Cloud GA *et al.* (1992). Comparison of amphotericin B with fluconazole in the treatment of acute AIDS-associated cryptococcal meningitis. *N Engl J Med* **326:**83–89.

Saag MS, Cloud GA, Graybill JR *et al.* (1999). A comparison of itraconazole versus fluconazole as maintenance therapy for AIDS-associated cryptococcal meningitis. National Institute of Allergy and Infectious Diseases Mycoses Study Group. *Clin Infect Dis* **28:**291–296.

Sacktor N, McDermott MP, Marder K *et al.* (2002). HIV-associated cognitive impairment before and after the advent of combination therapy. *J Neurovirol* **8:**136–142.

Sindrup SH, Jensen TS (1999). Efficacy of pharmacological treatments of neuropathic pain: an update and effect related to mechanism of drug action. *Pain* **83:**389–400.

Staudinger R, Henry K (2000). Remission of HIV myelopathy after highly active antiretroviral therapy. *Neurology* **54:**267–268.

Thurnher MM, Post MJ, Jinkins JR (2000). MRI of infections and neoplasms of the spine and spinal cord in 55 patients with AIDS. *Neuroradiology* **42:**551–563.

Torre D, Casari S, Speranza F *et al.* (1998). Randomized trial of trimethoprim-sulfamethoxazole versus pyrimethamine-sulfadiazine for therapy of toxoplasmic encephalitis in patients with AIDS. Italian Collaborative Study Group. *Antimicrob Agents Chemother* **42:**1346–1349.

Torres RA, Weinberg W, Stansell J *et al.* (1997). Atovaquone for salvage treatment and suppression of
toxoplasmic encephalitis in patients with AIDS. Ato-
vaquone/Toxoplasmic Encephalitis Study Group. *Clin
Infect Dis* **24:**422–429.

Van der Horst CM, Saag MS, Cloud GA *et al.* (1997). Treatment of cryptococcal meningitis associated with the
acquired immunodeficiency syndrome. *N Engl J Med*
337:15–21.

Yeni PG, Hammer SM, Carpenter ChCJ *et al.* (2002).
Antiretroviral Treatment for Adult HIV Infection in 2002.   Updated recommendations of
the International AIDS Society-USA Panel. *JAMA*
288:222–235.

Zuger A, Lowy FD (1997). Tuberculosis. In: Scheld WM,
Whitley RJ, Durack DT eds. Infections of the Central
Nervous System. Lippincott-Raven, Philadelphia, PA,
pp. 417–443.

CHAPTER 28

Encephalitis

I. Steiner,[a] H. Budka,[b] A. Chaudhuri,[c]
M. Koskiniemi, [d]K. Sainio,[e] O. Salonen,[f]
P.G.E. Kennedy[c,a]

Abstract

Background Viral encephalitis is a medical emergency. The spectrum of brain involvement and the prognosis are dependent mainly on the specific pathogen and the immunological state of the host. Although specific therapy is limited to only several viral agents, correct immediate diagnosis and introduction of symptomatic and specific therapy have a dramatic influence upon survival and reduce the extent of permanent brain injury in survivors.

Methods We searched MEDLINE (National Library of Medicine) for relevant literature from 1966 to May 2004. Review articles and book chapters were also included. Recommendations are based on this literature based on our judgment of the relevance of the references to the subject. Recommendations were reached by consensus. Where there was lack of evidence but consensus was clear we have stated our opinion as Good Practice Points.

Diagnosis should be based on medical history, examination followed by analysis of cerebrospinal fluid for protein and glucose contents, cellular analysis and identification of the pathogen by polymerase chain reaction (PCR) amplification and serology. Neuroimaging, preferably by MRI, is an essential aspect of evaluation. Lumbar puncture can follow neuroimaging when immediately available, but if this cannot be obtained at the shortest span of time it should be delayed only in the presence of strict contraindications. Brain biopsy should be reserved only for unusual and diagnostically difficult cases. All encephalitis cases must be hospitalized with access to intensive care units. Supportive therapy is an important basis of management. Specific, evidence-based, antiviral therapy is available for herpes encephalitis. Acyclovir might also be effective for varicella-zoster virus encephalitis, gancyclovir and foscarnet for cytomegalovirus encephalitis and pleconaril for enterovirus encephalitis. Corticosteroids as an adjunct treatment for acute viral encephalitis are not generally considered to be effective and their use is controversial. Surgical decompression is indicated for impending uncal herniation or increased intracranial pressure refractory to medical management.

[a]Laboratory of Neurovirology, Department of Neurology, Hadassah University Hospital, Jerusalem, Israel; [b]Institute of Neurology, Medical University of Vienna, Austria; [c]Department of Neurology, Institute of Neurological Sciences, Southern General Hospital, Glasgow, UK; [d]Department of Virology, Haartman institute, University of Helsinki, Finland; [e]Department of Clinical Neurophysiology, University of Helsinki, Finland; [f]Helsinki Medical Imaging Center, University of Helsinki, Finland.

Introduction

Clinical involvement of the central nervous system (CNS) is an unusual manifestation of human viral infection. The spectrum of brain involvement and the outcome of the disease are dependent on the specific pathogen, the immunological state of the host and a range of environmental factors. Although specific therapy is limited to only several viral agents, correct diagnosis and supportive and symptomatic treatment (when no specific therapy is available) are mandatory to ensure the best prognosis (for reviews see Koskiniemi *et al.* 2001; Chaudhuri and Kennedy, 2002; Redington and Tyler, 2002; Whitley and Gnann, 2002). This document addresses the optimal clinical approach to CNS infections caused by viruses.

Classification of evidence levels used in these guidelines for therapeutic interventions and diagnostic measures was according to Brainin *et al.* (2004) and detailed in tables 28.1 and 28.2a,b.

Methods

We searched MEDLINE (National Library of Medicine) for relevant literature from 1966 to May 2004. The search included reports of research in human beings only and in English. The search terms selected were: 'viral encephalitis', 'encephalitis', 'meningoencephalitis' and 'encephalopathy'. We then limited the search using the terms 'diagnosis', 'MR', 'PET', 'SPECT', 'EEG', 'cerebrospinal fluid', 'pathology', 'treatment' and 'antiviral therapy'. Review articles and book chapters were also included if they were considered to provide comprehensive reviews of the topic. The final choice of literature and the references included were based on our judgment of their relevance to this subject. Recommendations were reached by consensus of all Task Force participants (tables 28.1 and 28.2) and were also based on our own awareness and clinical experience. Where there was lack of evidence but consensus was clear we have stated our opinion as Good Practice Points (GPP).

Definitions and scope

Encephalitis is the presence of an inflammatory process in the brain parenchyma associated with clinical evidence of brain dysfunction. It can be

Table 28.1 Evidence classification scheme for the rating of recommendations for a therapeutic intervention.

Level A rating (established as effective, ineffective, or harmful) requires at least one convincing Class I study or at least two consistent, convincing Class II studies.

Level B rating (probably effective, ineffective, or harmful) requires at least one convincing Class II study or overwhelming Class III evidence.

Level C (possibly effective, ineffective, or harmful) rating requires at least two convincing Class III studies.

Table 28.2a Evidence classification scheme for a diagnostic measure.

Class I: A prospective study in a broad spectrum of persons with the suspected condition, using a 'gold standard' for case definition, where the test is applied in a blinded evaluation, and enabling the assessment of appropriate tests of diagnostic accuracy.

Class II: A prospective study of a narrow spectrum of persons with the suspected condition, or a well-designed retrospective study of a broad spectrum of persons with an established condition (by 'gold standard') compared to a broad spectrum of controls, where test is applied in a blinded evaluation, and enabling the assessment of appropriate tests of diagnostic accuracy.

Class III: Evidence provided by a retrospective study where either persons with the established condition or controls are of a narrow spectrum, and where test is applied in a blinded evaluation.

Class IV: Any design where test is not applied in blinded evaluation OR evidence provided by expert opinion alone or in descriptive case series (without controls).

Table 28.2b Evidence classification scheme for the rating of recommendations for a diagnostic measure.

Level A (established as useful/ predictive or not useful/ predictive) requires at least one convincing class I study or at least two consistent, convincing class II studies.

Level B (established as probably useful/ predictive or not useful/ predictive) requires at least one convincing class II study or overwhelming class III evidence.

Level C (established as possibly useful/ predictive or not useful/ predictive) requires at least two convincing class III studies.

due to a non-infective condition such as in acute disseminated encephalomyelitis (ADEM) or to an infective process, which is diffuse and usually viral. Herpes simplex virus type 1 (HSV-1), varicella zoster virus (VZV), Epstein–Barr virus (EBV), mumps, measles and enteroviruses are responsible for most cases of viral encephalitis in immunocompetent individuals (Koskiniemi *et al.*, 2001). Other non-viral infective causes of encephalitis may include such diseases as tuberculosis, rickettsial disease and trypanosomiasis, and will be discussed in the differential diagnosis section.

Encephalitis should be differentiated from encephalopathy which is defined as a disruption of brain function that is not due to a direct structural or inflammatory process. It is mediated via metabolic processes and can be caused by intoxications, drugs, systemic organ dysfunction (e.g. liver, pancreas) or systemic infection that spares the brain.

The structure of the nervous system determines a degree of associated inflammatory meningeal involvement in encephalitis, and therefore symptoms that reflect meningitis are invariable concomitants of encephalitis. Moreover, in textbooks and review articles the term viral meningo-encephalitis is often used to denote a viral infectious process of both the brain/spinal cord and the meninges.

Clinical manifestations and relevant environmental and personal information

The diagnosis of viral encephalitis is suspected in the context of a febrile disease accompanied by headache, altered level of consciousness and symptoms and signs of cerebral dysfunction. These may consist of abnormalities that can be categorized into four types: cognitive dysfunction (acute memory disturbances), behavioural changes (disorientation, hallucinations, psychosis, personality changes, agitation), focal neurological abnormalities (such as anomia, dysphasia, hemiparesis, hemianopia, etc.) and seizures. After the diagnosis is suspected, the approach should consist of obtaining a meticulous history and a careful general and neurological examination.

(1) *The history* is mandatory in the assessment of the patient with suspected viral encephalitis. It might be important to obtain the relevant information from an accompanying person (relative, friend, etc.) if the patient is in a confused, agitated and disoriented state. The geographical location as well as the recent travel history could be of relevance to identify causative pathogens that are endemic or prevalent in certain geographic regions (the recent example being severe acute respiratory syndrome, SARS). Likewise, seasonal occurrence can be important for other pathogens such as polio virus. Occupation may well be important (as in a case of a forestry worker with Lyme disease). Contact with animals such as farm animals would sometimes point to the cause, as animals serve as reservoirs for certain viruses (e.g. West Nile fever and the 1999 outbreak of the disease in New York). A history of insect or other animal bites can be relevant for arbovirus infection as well as rabies. Past contact with an individual afflicted by an infective condition is important. The medical status of the individual is of the utmost relevance. Thus, certain viral and non-viral pathogens cause encephalitis only or much more frequently in immune-suppressed individuals such as patients with AIDS or those who receive medications that

affect the immune system (e.g. cancer and organ transplant patients).

The mode of disease course up to the appearance of the neurological signs may provide clues to the aetiology. For example, enterovirus infection has a typical biphasic course. An associated abnormality outside the nervous system (bleeding tendency in haemorrhagic fever, the hydrophobia in rabies patients) may also point to a specific pathogen.

(2) General examination. Viral infection of the nervous system is almost always part of a generalised systemic infectious disease. Thus, other organs may be involved prior or in association with the CNS manifestations. Evidence for such an involvement should be obtained either from the history or during the examination. Skin rashes are not infrequent concomitants of viral infections, parotitis may be associated with mumps, gastrointestinal signs with enteroviral disease and upper respiratory findings may accompany influenza virus infection and HSV-1 encephalitis.

(3) Neurological examination. The findings relate to those of meningitis and disruption of brain parenchyma function. Thus, signs of meningeal irritation and somnolence reflect meningitis, while behavioural, cognitive and focal neurological signs and seizures reflect the disruption of brain function. Additional signs may include autonomic and hypothalamic disturbances, diabetes insipidus and the syndrome of inappropriate antidiuretic hormone secretion. The symptoms and signs are not a reliable diagnostic instrument to identify the causative virus. Likewise, the evolution of the clinical signs and their severity depend on host and other factors such as immune state and age and cannot serve as guidelines to identify the pathogen. In general, the very young and the very old have the most extensive and serious signs of encephalitis.

Diagnostic investigations

General
Peripheral blood count and cellular morphology are helpful in separating viral from non-viral infections. Lymphocytosis in the peripheral blood is common in viral encephalitis. Erythrocyte sedimentation rate is another non-specific test that is usually within normal range in viral infections. Other, general examinations such as chest x-ray, blood cultures, belong to the general work-up of febrile disease.

The auxiliary studies that examine viral infections of the nervous system include studies that characterise the extent and nature of CNS involvement (electroencephalography (EEG), and neuroimaging), microbiological attempts to identify the pathogen and histopathology and will be discussed here.

EEG is generally regarded as a non-specific investigation, although it is still sometimes a useful tool in certain situations. Thus, leukoencephalitides show more diffuse slow activity in the EEG and polioencephalitides more rhythmic slow activity (Vas and Cracco, 1990; Westmoreland, 1999). However, in practice this hardly helps in the differential diagnosis. Likewise, the EEG findings in postinfectious encephalitides differ from infectious encephalitis only in the time schedule of the abnormalities. The main benefit of EEG is to demonstrate cerebral involvement during the early state of the disease. Only in rare instances does the EEG show specific features that may give clues as to the diagnosis.

Acute viral encephalitis
The EEG is an early and sensitive indicator of cerebral involvement and usually shows a background abnormality prior to the initial evidence of parenchyma involvement on neuroimaging. This may in some instances be helpful in the differential diagnosis of aseptic meningitis. Often, focal abnormalities may be observed. During the acute phase, the severity of EEG abnormalities does not usually correlate with the extent of the disease. However, a fast improving EEG indicates a good prognosis and lack of improvement the opposite (Vas and Cracco, 1990; class IV). Although there may be seizures in the acute phase, interictal epileptiform EEG activity is a rarity. The EEG abnormalities usually subside more slowly than the clinical symptoms (Westmoreland, 1999).

Herpes simplex encephalitis (HSE)
In 80 per cent of the patients there is a typical finding in the EEG. In addition to the background

slowing there is a temporal focus showing periodic lateralized epileptiform discharges (PLEDs). This finding is temporary; it can be found during days 2–14 from the beginning of the disease, most often during days 5–10 (Lai and Gragasin, 1988). To detect this EEG finding often requires serial recordings. The repetition interval of these pseudoperiodic complexes is from 1 to 4 s; in newborns it can be faster with a frequency of 2 Hz. Also the localization in newborns may be other than temporal (Sainio *et al.*, 1983).

In brain-stem encephalitis the EEG mainly reflects the lowered consciousness and the abnormalities can be mild compared to the clinical state of the patient. Intermittent rhythmic delta activity (IRDA) has also been described in these patients.

In cerebellitis the EEG is mostly normal (Schmahmann and Sherman, 1998).

The EEG pattern in HIV infection of the brain is very variable, with background, paroxysmal and focal abnormalities (Westmoreland, 1999). Likewise the findings in ADEM are unspecific encephalitic abnormalities (Tenembaum *et al.*, 2002).

The EEG in subacute sclerosing panencephalitis (SSPE) shows a typical generalized periodic EEG pattern repeating with intervals between 4 and 15 s and synchronized with myoclonus of the patient (Westmoreland, 1999).

Neuroimaging of encephalitis

Magnetic resonance imaging (MRI). MRI is more sensitive and specific than CT for the evaluation of viral encephalitis. (Dun *et al.*, 1986; Schroth *et al.*, 1987; Marchbank *et al.*, 2000; Dale *et al.*, 2000; class IIIC). The advantages of MRI include the use of non-ionizing radiation, multiplanar imaging capability, improved contrast of soft tissue and high anatomical resolution. On the basis of previous data it should be the imaging technique of choice in determination of encephalitis. It allows earlier detection and treatment of inflammatory processes. MRI also provides valuable information for patient follow-up. In practical terms, however, many patients with suspicion of encephalitis often undergo CT scanning before neurological consultation.

A typical MRI protocol consists of routine T1 and T2 spin-echo sequences and a FLAIR (fluid-attenuation inversion recovery) sequence, which is considered extremely sensitive in detecting subtle changes in the early stages of an acute condition. Gradient-echo imaging, with its superior magnetic susceptibility, is also useful in detecting small areas of haemorrhage.

New MR imaging techniques are being applied to the study of various brain diseases. These technologies include procedures that can increase sensitivity to small, yet clinically relevant lesions, these techniques may be useful for imaging protocols of patients with suspicion of encephalitis:

1. *Diffusion- weighted MRI* (DWI) enables separation of cytotoxic from vasogenic oedema and distinguishes recent from old insult, which can often be difficult on routine T2 and FLAIR imaging.
2. *Low magnetization transfer Ratio* (MTR) reflects myelin damage, cell destruction or changes in water content.
3. *Magnetic resonance spectroscopy* (MRS) identifies and quantities concentration of various brain metabolites. Spectroscopy is capable of differentiating normal from pathologic brain and provides tissue specificity greater than that of imaging instances.
4. *Functional magnetic resonance imaging* (FMRI) uses very rapid scanning techniques that in theory can demonstrate alterations in blood oxygenation.

CT is recommended only as a screening examination with subtle clinical suspicion of encephalitis or when magnetic resonance imaging is unavailable (Dun *et al.*, 1986; Schroth *et al.*, 1987; Marchbank *et al.*, 2000; class IV).

Single photon emission tomography (SPECT) is more readily available than positron emission tomography (PET) and has been utilized in the study and diagnosis of encephalitis (Launes *et al.*, 1988). It can provide information about brain chemistry, cerebral neurotransmitters and brain function. It can also demonstrate hypoperfused tissue that seems normal on structural imaging.

Positron emission tomography (PET) though the gold standard in acquiring functional imaging data, remains a complex, costly and not readily available technique.

In summary, structural information is provided by CT scan and MRI while functional and metabolic data are provided by MRS, FMRI, SPECT and PET.

Imaging of specific disorders

(1) *Herpes simplex encephalitis (HSE)*. CT obtained early is often normal or subtly abnormal. Low attenuation, mild mass effect in temporal lobes and insula, haemorrhage and enhancement are late features. Follow-up scans 1–2 weeks after disease onset demonstrate progressively more widespread abnormalities with the involvement of contra lateral temporal lobe, insula and cingulate gyri. Contrast enhancement and changes of subacute haemorrhage may become readily apparent. MRI is much more sensitive in detecting early changes (Schroth *et al.*, 1987; Marchbank *et al.*, 2000; Chaudhuri and Kennedy, 2002; class IIIC). Involvement of cingulate gyrus and contra lateral temporal lobe is highly suggestive of herpes encephalitis. Typical early findings include gyral edema on T1–weighted (T1WI) imaging and high signal intensity in the temporal lobe or cingulate gyrus on T2WI, FLAIR and DWI and later haemorrhage. Hypointense on T1, hyperintense on T2WI, FLAIR, high signal on DWI are additional findings (Tsuchiya *et al.*, 1999; Ito *et al.*, 1999). In acute lesions, MRS reveals metabolic changes in relation to neuronal death such as a decrease of N-acetyl aspartate (NAA) signal. Resultant gliosis is reflected as an increase in inositol and creatine resonances. The reinstitution of a normal spectrum over time could then potentially be used as a marker of treatment efficacy (Menon *et al.*, 1990; Salvan *et al.*, 1999).

Neonatal HSV-2 infection often causes more widespread signal abnormalities than HSV-1 encephalitis, with periventricular white matter involvement and sparing of the medial temporal and inferior frontal lobes (Hinson and Tyor, 2001).

(2) *HIV-1*. CT demonstrates normal/mild atrophy with white matter hypodensity. MRI usually shows atrophy and non-specific white matter changes. MRS detects early decreases in levels of NAA and increases in choline-containing phospholipids (Cho) levels, even before abnormalities are detected by MRI and prior to clinical symptoms. Later, with cognitive dysfunction, further reductions in NAA and increases in Cho levels may be seen (Rudkin and Arnold, 1999). In the later stages of AIDS, the most common diseases affecting the brain parenchyma are secondary to opportunistic infection or malignancy and are predominantly focal. Neuroimaging is an important diagnostic tool for opportunistic infections. Toxoplasmosis (ring-enhancing mass(es) in basal ganglia), cryptococcosis (gelatinous 'pseudocysts'), meningoencephalitis, vasculitis, infarction, CMV-encephalitis (diffuse white matter hyperintensities), ventriculitis (ependymal enhancement), progressive multifocal leukoencephalopathy (PML, white matter hyperintensities that usually do not enhance), lymphoma (solitary or multifocal solid or ring-enhancing lesions either in deep grey and white matter or less frequent in subcortical areas) (Thurnher *et al.*, 2001; Yin *et al.*, 2001). MRS may be able to distinguish between these different space-occupying lesions based on their chemical profiles. 1H-magnetic resonance spectroscopy can serve to monitor the efficacy of antiretroviral therapy and may even be used to predict the responsiveness to drug therapy (Wilkinson *et al.*, 1997).

(3) CNS complications of *Varicella-zoster virus* infection (usually due to reactivation) include myelitis, encephalitis, large- and small-vessel arteritis, ventriculitis, and meningitis (Gilden *et al.*, 2000). Large vessel arteritis presents with ischaemic/haemorrhagic infarctions and MRI supported by angiography usually reveals these complications (Gilden *et al.*, 2000; Redington and Tyler, 2002).

(4) Miscellaneous viral infections. In *polio* and *coxsackie* virus infections, T2-weighted MRI may show hyperintensities in the midbrain and anterior horn of spinal cord (Shen *et al.*, 2000). In *Epstein–Barr virus (EBV)* infection hyperintensities in the basal ganglia and thalami may be observed on T2-weighted MRI (Shian and Chi, 1996). *West Nile virus* (WNV) can be associated with enhancement of leptomeninges, the periventricular areas, or both, on MRI (Sejvar *et al.*, 2003). T2-weighted MRI

of *Japanese encephalitis* can show hyperintensities in bilateral thalami, brainstem and cerebellum.

(5) *Acute disseminated encephalomyelitis (ADEM).* Initial CT may show low density, flocculent, asymmetric lesions with mild mass effect and contrast enhancement multifocal punctate or ring-enhancing lesions. However, CT is normal in 40% of cases. MRI is more sensitive and an essential diagnostic tool. T2WI and FLAIR scans present multifocal, usually bilateral, but asymmetric and large hyperintense lesions, involving peripheral white and grey matter. They do not usually involve the callososeptal interface. Contrast-enhanced T1-weighted images may show ring-enhancing lesions. Cranial nerves may enhance. DWI is variable. On MRS, NAA is transiently low and choline is normal (Dun *et al.*, 1986; Dale *et al.*, 2000; Bizzi *et al.*, 2001).

(6) MRI is also the most sensitive imaging tool for PML (Berger and Major, 1999). T2-weighted sequences initially show multiple, bilateral, non-enhancing, oval or round subcortical white matter hyperintensities in the parietooccipital area. Confluent white matter disease with cavitary change is a late manifestation of PML. Less common imaging manifestations of PML are unilateral white matter and thalamic or basal ganglia lesions.

(7) Rasmussen's encephalitis (RE) typically involves only one cerebral hemisphere, which becomes atrophic. The earliest CT and MRI abnormalities include high signal on T2-weighted MR images in cortex and white matter, cortical atrophy that usually involves the fronto insular region, with mild or severe enlargement of the lateral ventricle and moderate atrophy of the head of the caudate nucleus. Fluorodeoxyglucose PET has been reported to present hypometabolism; Tc-99m hexamethylpropyleamine oxime SPECT decreased perfusion and proton MRS reduction of NAA in the affected hemisphere. However, PET and SPECT findings are non-specific. MRI may become a valuable early diagnostic tool by demonstrating focal disease progression (Chiapparini *et al.* 2003).

(8) In paraneoplastic limbic encephalitis MRI FLAIR and DWI depicted bilateral involvement of the medial temporal lobes and multifocal involvement of the brain. T2-weighted turbo spin-echo images fail to show the changes (Thuerl, 2003).

Virological tests in encephalitis
General

The gold standard of diagnosis in encephalitis is virus isolation in cell culture, now to be replaced by the detection of specific nucleic acid from CSF or brain (Rowley *et al.*, 1990; Echevarria *et al.*, 1994; Lakeman and Whitley, 1995; Tebas *et al.*, 1998; class Ia). Intrathecal antibody production to a specific virus is similarly a strong evidence for aetiology (Levine *et al.*, 1978; Koskiniemi *et al.*, 2002; class Ib). Virus detection from throat, stool, urine or blood as well as systemic serological response like seroconversion or a specific IgM provides less strong evidence (Burke *et al.*, 1985; Koskiniemi *et al.*, 2001; class III). The CSF is a convenient specimen and is recommended for neurological viral diagnosis in general (Cinque and Linde, 2003). Brain biopsy is invasive and not used in routine clinical practice. At autopsy brain material will be obtained for virus isolation, nucleic acid and antigen detection as well as for immunohistochemistry and in situ hybridization.

Viral culture

Viral cultures from CSF and brain tissue as well as from throat and stool specimens are performed in four different cell lines: African green monkey cells, Vero cells, human amniotic epithelial cells and human embryonic skin fibroblasts. Cells are evaluated daily for cytopathic effect and the findings are confirmed by a neutralizing or an immunofluoresence antibody test. Viral cultures from CSF are positive in young children with enteroviral infection but only seldom, in less than 5%, in other cases (Muir and vanLoon, 1997; Storch, 2000; Class III). As brain biopsy is reserved only for unusual and diagnostically difficult cases, viral cultures are only rarely available from brain tissues.

Nucleic acid detection

For nucleic acid detection, polymerase chain reaction (PCR) technology provides the most convenient test. Assays for HSV-1, HSV-2, VZV, human herpesvirus 6 and 7, cytomegalovirus (CMV), Epstein–Barr virus (EBV), enteroviruses and respiratory viruses as well as for human immunodeficiency virus (HIV) can be performed from CSF samples or brain tissue. The primers are selected from a conserved region of the viral genome and the PCR product is identified by hybridisation with specific probes or by gel electrophoresis. Respiratory viruses' nucleic acid as well as *Chlamydia pneumoniae* and *Mycoplasma pneumoniae* can also be detected from throat samples and enterovirus nucleic acid from stool samples. These, however, cannot confirm the aetiology of encephalitis. PCR for *Chlamydia pneumoniae* can also be performed from a CSF sample. Detection of specific nucleic acid from the CSF depends on the timing of the CSF sample. The highest yield is obtained during the transient appearance of the virus in the CSF compartment during the first week after symptom onset, much less in the second week and only occasionally after that (Lakeman and Whitley, 1995; Koskiniemi *et al.*, 2002; Class I). In herpes simplex encephalitis the sensitivity is 96% and the specificity 99% when CSF is studied between 48 h and 10 days from the onset of symptoms (Lakeman and Whitley, 1995; Tebas *et al.*, 1998).

Instead of the single PCR tests, the multiplex PCRs are gaining ground in diagnostics (Tenorio *et al.*, 1993; Pozo and Tenorio, 1999). The sensitivity has been improved and it approaches that of the single PCRs and the specificities are equal. Real time PCR makes it possible to get the result in a shorter time while observing the yield cycle by cycle (Kessler *et al.*, 2000). The usage of microarrays for detection of viral nucleic acid is still expensive, but has the potential to become a regular diagnostic technique. Several microbes can be studied at the same time and identification of the genotype will be easier than using the current conventional methods.

Serological tests

Antibodies to HSV-1, HSV-2, VZV, CMV, HHV-6, HHV-7, CMV, EBV, respiratory syncytial virus (RSV), HIV, adeno, influenza A and B, rota, coxsackie B5, non-typed entero and parainfluenza 1 viruses as well as *Mycoplasma pneumoniae* are measured from serum and CSF by using enzyme immunoassay (EIA) tests and antibodies

for *Chlamydia pneumoniae* by microimmunofluorescence test (MIF) (MacCallum *et al.*, 1974; Levine 1978; Julkunen *et al.*, 1984; Socan *et al.*, 1994; Koskiniemi *et al.*, 1996, 2001; Gilden *et al.*, 1998; Class II). These tests are sensitive enough to detect even low amounts of antibodies from the CSF. The antibody levels in serum and CSF are compared with each other in the same dilution of 1:200. If the ratio of antibody levels is ≤ 20, it indicates intrathecal antibody production within the brain provided that no other antibodies are present in the CSF, that is, the blood brain barrier (BBB) is not damaged. The presence of several antibodies in the CSF suggests BBB breakdown, while the presence of specific IgM in the CSF indicates central nervous system disease (Burke *et al.*, 1985). The tests for measles, mumps and rubella are only occasionally needed in countries with effective vaccination programs. Tests for arboviruses and zoonooses will be useful in endemic areas (Burke *et al.*, 1985; Wahlberg *et al.*, 1989).

Antigen detection

Antigens of HSV, VZV and RSV, influenza A and B, parainfluenza 1 and 3, and adenoviruses can be studied from throat specimens with a conventional immunofluorescence (IF) test or with an EIA test and may provide a possible aetiology for encephalitis. In spite of promising initial results these tests are not helpful in diagnosis using CSF samples.

In conclusion: In a patient with suspected encephalitis obtaining serum and CSF for virological tests is the core of diagnostic procedure. Tests should include: PCR (single, multiplex or microarray) test for nucleic acid detection (from CSF) and serological tests for antibodies (from CSF and serum samples). In undiagnosed severe cases, PCR should be repeated after 3–7 days, and serological tests repeated after 2–4 weeks to show possible seroconversion or diagnostic increase in antibody levels. In children, viral culture from throat and stool samples as well as antigen detection for herpes and respiratory viruses are recommended during the first week. Viral culture from CSF is useful in children with suspected enteroviral or VZV disease if PCR tests are not available.

Histopathology

Encephalitis features a variety of histopathological changes in the brain, mainly depending upon the type of the infectious agent, the immunologic response by the host, and the stage of the infection. The aetiologic spectrum is strongly influenced by geography. It should also be noted that primary encephalitic processes may secondarily involve the meninges as well, with inflammatory infiltration resulting in usually mild CSF pleocytosis (lymphocytes with variable degree of activation, eventually plasmocytes). In encephalitis with a prominent necrotizing component, mixed CSF cellularity may also include granulocytes; this is frequently seen in HSV encephalitis, and CMV (peri)ventriculitis/myeloradiculitis of HIV patients.

The histopathological basis of encephalitis is the triad of damage to the parenchyma (usually nerve cell damage or loss, eventually demyelination), reactive gliosis, and inflammatory cellular infiltration (by haematogenous elements in the immunocompetent host) (Budka, 1997). This classical substrate is exemplified by (multi)nodular encephalitis, as in the majority of viral encephalitides consisting of nerve cell damage, followed by nerve cell death and neuronophagia; focal/nodular proliferation of astro- and microglia, and focal/nodular infiltration by lymphocytes, eventually macrophages. Thus, the classical encephalitic nodules are composed of the mixture of microglia, astrocytes and lymphocytes usually around affected neuron(s) (Budka, 1997).

Distribution and spread of these inflammatory changes are important for aetiologic considerations: six types of encephalitis may be distinguished, either focal or diffuse affecting either the gray matter, the white matter, or both (Love and Wiley, 2002). The encephalitic patterns include continuous polioencephalitis (e.g. in luetic general paresis) and patchy-nodular polioencephalitis (e.g. in poliomyelitis, rabies, acute encephalitis by flavi-, toga- and enteroviruses, HSV brainstem encephalitis), leukoencephalitis (e.g. in PML or HIV leukoencephalopathy), and panencephalitis (e.g. in bacterial septicemia with microabscesses, in Whipple's disease, SSPE, HIV encephalitis, and herpesviruses such as HSV, CMV and VZV

infection). Abscesses and granulomas may be randomly distributed in the brain. In addition to the inflammatory quality and characteristic distribution of tissue lesions, cytological features such as inclusion bodies (intranuclear in HSV, VZV encephalitis, PML and SSPE, cytoplasmic Negri bodies in rabies) or cytomegalic cell change in CMV disease give important diagnostic clues, especially when the involved cell type is considered: every viral infection of the nervous system usually features a fingerprint signature of selective vulnerability in the nervous system (Budka, 1997). However, immunosuppression and the effects of potent therapies have become notorious for being able to modify, blur or even wipe out the classical features of specific viral lesions.

The role of special techniques: Immunocytochemistry, in situ hybridization, PCR

Arguably, it is in the field of infections where the techniques of immunocytochemistry (ICC), *in situ* hybridization (ISH), and PCR have the most profound impact on neuropathological diagnosis. When done appropriately with adequate controls and adequate tissue selection, they provide an aetiologic diagnosis with high sensitivity and specificity (Budka, 1997; Johnson, 1998). Nevertheless, there are *caveats* for situations in which they may not be diagnostic:

- Production of the infectious agent may have burnt out, or its products may have become masked, resulting in negative ICC or ISH.
- Tissue preservation might be unsuitable for these techniques, e.g. ICC or ISH may be falsely negative on overfixed tissue, or nucleic acid amplification from paraffin embedded tissue by PCR may be blocked by yet unidentified factors.
- Since PCR and ISH are very sensitive techniques, positive results may just reflect the presence of genomic information resulting from dormant or latent, and not necessarily productive and pathogenic infection.

Therefore, prerequisites for the use of ICC, ISH, or PCR for neuropathological diagnosis of infections include simultaneous use of known positive and negative control tissues that were identically processed as the material to be examined; availability of reagents (antibodies, probes, primers) with defined specificities; adequate testing of reagents on control tissues for highest sensitivity and sensitivity (optimal signal to noise ratio) in the respective laboratory and experience with immunocytochemical antigen retrieval techniques such as enzyme digestion, microwave treatment or autoclaving (Budka, 1997).

Viruses may exert damage to the nervous system not only by productive virus infection of the nervous system, but by indirect means as well. The best example is the immune-mediated ADEM or postinfectious / perivenous encephalitis as a sequel of exanthematous viral disease of childhood (e.g. measles, varicella, rubella, mumps, influenza). This is very important for differential diagnosis from productive viral encephalomyelitis: multiple small demyelinated foci are arranged around small veins of the white matter, featuring cellular infiltration composed by lymphocytes, macrophages and microglia (Budka, 1997).

Other infective causes of meningoencephalitis and differential diagnosis

Clinical distinction between viral encephalitis and non-viral infective meningoencephalitis is difficult, often impossible. Epidemiological and demographic features, such as prevalent or emergent infections in the community, occupation, a history of travel and animal contacts may provide helpful clues. In acute bacterial meningitis, meningeal symptoms of intense headache, photophobia and vomiting appear early and are usually more severe than the encephalopathic features. Presence of multiple cranial neuropathies is also suggestive of a primary meningeal process. History of continued fever and a subacute onset of symptoms with progressive obtundation and/or features of raised intracranial pressure are more typical of suppurative intracranial infections such as brain abscess. Tuberculous meningitis (TBM) also presents similarly, and in children, symptoms of TBM are often subacute in onset. In a non-epidemic setting, the most common cause of focal encephalopathic findings is HSE; however among cases with biopsy

proven herpes encephalitis, there were no distinguishing clinical characteristics between patients positive for HSV and those who were negative (Whitley and Gnann, 2002).

ADEM, an autoimmune disease, with evidence of cell-mediated immunity to the myelin basic protein as its pathogenic basis (Behan *et al.*, 1968), is characterized by focal neurological signs and a rapidly progressive course in a usually apyrexial patient, usually with a history of febrile illness or immunisation preceding the neurological syndrome by days or weeks (post-infectious or post-vaccinal encephalomyelitis). It may be distinguished from infective encephalitis by the younger age of the patient, prodromal history of vaccination or infection, absence of fever at the onset of symptoms and the presence of multifocal neurological signs affecting optic nerves, brain, spinal cord and peripheral nerve roots. ADEM classically presents as a monophasic illness developing after certain viral infections or immunisations (post-infective and post-vaccinal ADEM). In the prodromal phase, patients experience migrainous-type headache with meningism. The disturbances of consciousness range from stupor and confusion to coma. There is usually preservation of the abdominal reflexes and patients have a mild fever often with peripheral blood pleocytosis. CSF shows lymphocytic pleocytosis, with mildly raised protein and may appear similar to the CSF in viral encephalitis. The clinical course of patients with Hashimoto's encephalopathy would fit a less aggressive form of recurrent ADEM (Chaudhuri and Behan, 2003).

CNS vasculitis can be part of a systemic disease or be confined to the nervous system. Systemic symptoms, aseptic meningitis and focal neurological deficit may occasionally simulate viral encephalitis. This is seen in both systemic vasculitis and primary CNS angiitis. In systemic vasculitis affecting the CNS it is usually possible to make a diagnosis based on a combination of systemic and CSF serologic and immunological tests and angiographic appearances of CNS vasculitis. In isolated angiitis diagnosis may be more challenging and even require brain and meningeal biopsy to secure the diagnosis where diagnostic uncertainties persist.

Pseudomigraine with pleocytosis. Acute confusion, psychosis and focal neurological deficit (hemiplegia, hemianaesthesia and aphasia) in association with migraine headache occur in the familial hemiplegic migraine (Feely *et al.*, 1982). Sterile CSF pleocytosis ('pseudomigraine') has been reported in migraine patients who may present similarly (Schraeder and Burns, 1980). It has been proposed that the CSF pleocytosis in some of these cases are due to recurrent predisposition to viral meningitis (Casteels-van Daele *et al.*, 1981). Pseudomigraine with pleocytosis and migraine coma are likely to represent reversible forms of ADEM (Chaudhuri and Behan, 2003).

Therapy

Anti-viral therapy

In two randomized controlled trials, acyclovir (10 mg/kg every 8 h given intravenously for 10 days) was found to be more effective than vidarabine (15 mg/kg/day) in improving survival rates of adult patients with biopsy proven HSE (Skoldenberg *et al.*, 1984; Whitley *et al.*, 1986). Acyclovir is a safe treatment and given the higher risk associated with diagnostic brain biopsy, it has become an established practice that treatment for viral encephalitis is commenced on suspicion before a specific aetiological diagnosis is possible (Chaudhuri and Kennedy, 2002). When given early in the clinical course of HSE before the patient becomes comatose, acyclovir reduces both mortality and morbidity in treated patients. Acyclovir is also the treatment of choice for neonatal HSE; however, there is no definitive evidence from trials that it is more effective than vidarabine. Acyclovir has a relatively short half-life in plasma and is usually given intravenously 10 mg/kg every 8 h in adults (total daily dose 30 mg/kg). The daily dose of acyclovir for neonatal HSE is 60 mg/kg (double the adult dose). As more than 80% of acyclovir in circulation is excreted unchanged in urine, renal impairment can rapidly precipitate acyclovir toxicity and therapeutic doses should be adjusted according to the renal clearance. Rare relapses of HSE have been reported after weeks to 3 months later when the duration of acyclovir treatment was

10 days or less (Davis, 2000). With conventional therapy, relapses of HSE may be higher than expected (5%) but do not occur if higher doses were administered for 21 days (Ito *et al.*, 2000). Although there have been no randomized trials, an accepted policy in clinical practice is to give acyclovir treatment for CSF PCR-positive HSE for 14 days in immunocompetent adult patients and 21 days for immunosuppressed patients. Use of vidarabine for HSE is limited to the unlikely and rare patients who cannot receive acyclovir because of side effects.

Besides HSV, acyclovir is also effective against VZV and the doses and duration of therapy for VZV encephalitis are similar to HSE (Good Practice Point, GPP). In CMV encephalitis, combination therapy with ganciclovir (5 mg/kg intravenously twice daily) with foscarnet (60 mg/kg every 8 h or 90 mg/kg every 12 h) is currently advised (GPP). Acyclovir is ineffective in CMV encephalitis. Antiretroviral therapy must be added or continued in HIV infected patients (Portegies, 2004).

No antiviral therapy is particularly effective in epizootic or enzootic viral encephalitis; however, because of the high mortality rate associated with B virus (cercopithecine herpesvirus) encephalitis in humans, it is currently proposed (Whitley and Gnann, 2002) that patients should be treated with intravenous acyclovir or ganciclovir.

Newer antivirals like valciclovir appear promising in HSV and VZV encephalitis but remain to be evaluated by formal trials (Biran and Steiner, 2002). Pleconaril is a new 'broad spectrum' antiviral with potential for use in enteroviral encephalitis and is undergoing clinical evaluation (Pevear *et al.*, 1999).

Corticosteroids

Large doses of corticosteroids (dexamethasone) as an adjunct treatment for acute viral encephalitis are not generally considered to be effective and their use is controversial. Probably the best evidence for steroid therapy is in VZV encephalitis. Primary VZV infection may cause severe encephalitis in immunocompetent children due to cerebral vasculitis (Hausler *et al.*, 2002). Vasculitis following primary and secondary VZV infection is recognized to lead to a chronic course in immunocompetent children and adults (granulomatous angiitis). HSE is occasionally complicated by severe, vasogenic cerebral oedema with CT or MRI evidence of midline shift where high dose steroids may have a role. Steroid pulse therapy with methylprednisolone has been observed to be beneficial in a small number of patients with acute viral encephalitis who had progressive disturbances of consciousness, an important prognostic factor for outcome (Nakano *et al.*, 2003).

Based on available data, combined acyclovir/ steroid treatment may be advised in immunocompetent individuals with severe VZV encephalitis and probably in other cases of acute viral encephalitis where progressive cerebral oedema documented by CT/MRI complicates the course of illness in the early phase (GPP). High dose dexamethasone or pulse methylprednisolone are both suitable agents. The duration of steroid treatment should be short (between 3 and 5 days) to minimize adverse effects (e.g. gastrointestinal haemorrhage, secondary fever and infections).

Although no randomized controlled trials have been performed, treatment with high dose steroids (intravenous pulses of methylprednisolone) and/or plasma exchange is usually the recommended treatment in ADEM (Cohen *et al.*, 2001; Class IV and GPP).

Surgical intervention

Surgical decompression for acute viral encephalitis is indicated for impending uncal herniation or increased intracranial pressure refractory to medical management (steroids and mannitol, GPP). Such intervention has been shown to improve outcome in HSE in individual cases (Yan, 2002).

General measures

All cases of acute encephalitis must be hospitalised. Like other critically ill patients, cases with acute viral encephalitis should have access to intensive care unit equipped with mechanical ventilators. Irrespective of the aetiology, supportive therapy for acute viral encephalitis is an important cornerstone of management (Chaudhuri and Kennedy, 2002). Seizures are controlled with intravenous phenytoin. Careful attention must be paid to the maintenance of respiration, cardiac rhythm, fluid balance, prevention of deep vein thrombosis, aspiration pneumonia, medical management of raised intracranial pressure and secondary bacterial infections. Secondary neurological complications in the course of viral encephalitis are common and include cerebral infarction, cerebral venous thrombosis, syndrome of inappropriate ADH secretion, aspiration pneumonia, upper gastrointestinal bleeding, urinary tract infections and disseminated intravascular coagulopathy.

Isolation for patients with community acquired acute infective encephalitis is not required. Consideration of isolation should be given for severely immunosuppressed patients, rabies encephalitis, patients with an exanthematous encephalitis and those with a contagious viral haemorrhagic fever.

Rehabilitation

Survivors of viral encephalitis and myelitis are a heterogenous group. Nature of the infective pathogen, variability in anatomic lesions and time to treatment contribute to outcome. Longitudinally designed case studies, reporting cognitive and psychosocial outcome of patients following herpes simplex virus encephalitis were conducted prior to current era of early diagnosis and effective therapy. While there are anecdotal case reports (Wilson *et al.*, 2001; Miotto, 2002 and others) there are very few studies on the outcome of rehabilitation following encephalitis (Moorthi *et al.*, 1999) to enable to draw any conclusions.

Preventive measures

Currently vaccines are available against a limited number of viruses with a potential to cause encephalitis. Universal immunization is recommended against mumps, measles, rubella and poliovirus. European travelers to specific geographic destinations (e.g. South East Asia) should receive advice regarding vaccination against rabies and Japanese encephalitis. Preventive measures against exotic forms of emerging paramyxovirus encephalitis (Nipah and Hendra viruses) are entirely environmental (sanitation, vector control and avoidance).

RECOMMENDATIONS

Diagnostic tests

Viral encephalitis is still an evolving discipline in medicine. The emergence of new, and re-emergence of old pathogens and the constant search for specific therapeutic measures, unavailable in most viral encephalitis cases, suggests that the following years will bring new developments in diagnosis and therapy. At present, adherence to a strict protocol of diagnostic investigations is recommended and includes:

Study	Findings	Level[a]	Class[b]
LP	Cells – 5–500 white blood cells, mainly lymphocytes; May be xanthochromic with red blood cells. Glucose – Normal (rarely reduced). Protein – >50 mg/dL	A	II
Serology	CSF and Serum	B	II
PCR	Major aid in diagnosis (CSF). May be false negative in the first 2 days of disease	A	I
EEG	Early and sensitive. Non-specific. May identify focal abnormalities	C	III
Imaging	MRI is usually more sensitive than CT, demonstrating high signal intensity lesion on T2-weighted and FLAIR images	B	II
Viral culture	Only rarely useful		
Brain biopsy	Highly sensitive. Not used routinely.	C	III and GPP

[a]Level of recommendation.
[a]Class of evidence.

RECOMMENDATIONS

Therapeutic interventions

The following are the specific and symptomatic therapeutic measures available for viral encephalitis

Interventions	Level[a]	Class[b]
Acyclovir for HSE	A	II
Acyclovir for suspected viral encephalitis	-	IV
Acyclovir for VZV encephalitis	-	IV
Gancylovir and/Foscarnet for CMV encephalitis	-	IV
Acyclovir or ganciclovir for B virus encephalitis	-	IV
Pleconaril for enterovirus encephalitis	-	NA
Corticosteroids for viral encephalitis		IV
Surgical decompression		IV

[a]Level of recommendation.
[a]Class of evidence.
NA, not available.

References

Behan PO, Geshwind N, Lamarche JB, et al. (1968). Delayed hypersensitivity to encephalitogenic protein in disseminated encephalitis. *Lancet* **ii**:1009–1012.

Berger JR, Major EO (1999). Progressive multifocal leukoencephalopathy. *Semin Neurol* **19**:193–200.

Biran I, Steiner I (2002). Herpes Encephalitis. *Current Treat Opt Infect Dis* **4**:271–276.

Bizzi A, Ulug AM, Crawford TO, Passe T, Bugiani M, Bryan RN, Barker PB (2001). Quantitative proton MR spectroscopic imaging in acute disseminated encephalomyelitis. *AJNR Am J Neuroradiol* **22**:1125–1130.

Brainin M, Barnes M, Baron JC, Gilhus NE, Hughes R, Selmaj K, Waldemar G (2004). Guidance for the preparation of neurological management guidelines by EFNS scientific task forces – revised recommendations 2004. *Eur J Neurol* **11**:577–581.

Budka H (1997). Viral infections. In: *Neuropathology – The Diagnostic Approach* (eds. Garcia JH, Budka H, McKeever PE, Sarnat HB, Sima AAF) St Louis: Mosby, pp. 353–391.

Burke DS, Nisalak A, Ussery MA, Laorakpongse T, Chantavibul S (1985). Kinetics of IgM and IgG responses to Japanese encephalitis virus in human serum and cerebrospinal fluid. *J Infect Dis* **151:**1093–1099.

Casteels-van Daele M, Standaert L, Boel M, Smeets E, Colaert J, Desmyter J (1981). Basilar migraine and viral meningitis. *Lancet* **i:**1366.

Chaudhuri A, Kennedy PG (2002). Diagnosis and treatment of viral encephalitis. *Postgrad Med J* **78:**575–583.

Chaudhuri A, Behan PO (2003). The clinical spectrum, diagnosis, pathpgenesis and treatment of Hashimoto's encephalopathy (recurrent acute disseminated encephalomyelitis). *Curr Med Chem* **10:**1645–1653.

Chiapparini L, Granata T, Farina L, Ciceri E, Erbetta A, Ragona F, Freri E, Fusco L, Gobbi G, Capovilla G, Tassi L, Giordano L, Viri M, Dalla Bernardina B, Spreafico R, Savoiardo M (2003). Diagnostic imaging in 13 cases of Rasmussen's encephalitis: can early MRI suggest the diagnosis? *Neuroradiology* **45:**171–183.

Cinque P, Linde A (2003). CSF Analysis in the diagnosis of viral meningitis and encephalitis. In *Clinical Neurovirology* (eds. Nath A, Berger JR), Marcel Dekker, Inc. New York, Basel, pp. 43–107.

Cohen O, Steiner-Birmanns B, Biran I., Abramsky O, Honigman S, Steiner I (2001). Recurrent acute disseminated encephalomyelitis tends to relapse at the previously affected brain site. *Arc Neurol* **58:**797–801.

Dale RC, de Sousa C, Chong WK, Cox TC, Harding B, Neville BG (2000). Acute disseminated encephalomyelitis, multiphasic disseminated encephalomyelitis and multiple sclerosis in children. *Brain* **123:**2407–2422.

Davis LE (2000). Diagnosis and treatment of acute encephalitis. *The Neurologist* **6:**145–159.

Dun V, Bale JF Jr, Zimmerman RA, Perdue Z, Bell WE (1986). MRI in children with postinfectious disseminated encephalomyelitis. *Magn Reson Imaging* **4:**25–32.

Echevarria JM, Casas I, Tenorio A, de Ory F, Martinez-Martin P (1994).Detection of varicella-zoster virus-specific DNA sequences in cerebrospinal fluid from patients with acute aseptic meningitis and no cutaneous lesions. *J Med Virol* **43:**331–335.

Feely MP, O'Hare J, Veale D, Callaghan N (1982). Episodes of acute confusion or psychosis in familial hemiplegic migraine. *Acta Neurol Scandinav* **65:**369–375.

Gilden DH, Bennett JL, Kleinschmidt-DeMasters BK, Song DD, Yee AS, Steiner I (1998). The value of cerebrospinal fluid antiviral antibody in the diagnosis of neurologic disease produced by varicella zoster virus. *J Neurol Sci* **159:**140–144.

Gilden DH, Kleinschmidt-DeMasters BK, LaGuardia JJ, Mahalingam R, Cohrs RJ (2000). Neurologic complications of the reactivation of varicella-zoster virus. *N Engl J Med* **342:**635–645.

Hausler M, Schaade L, Kemeny S, *et al.* (2002). Encephalitis related to primary varicella-zoster virus infection in immunocompetent children. *J Neurol Sci* **195:**111–116.

Hinson VK, Tyor WR (2001). Update on viral encephalitis. *Curr Opin Neurol* **14:**369–374.

Ito S, Hirose Y, Mokuno K (1999). The clinical usefulness of MRI diffusion weighted images in herpes simplex encephalitis-like cases. *Rinsho Shinkeigaku* **39:**1067–1070.

Ito Y, Kimura H, Yabuta Y, *et al.* (2000). Exacerbation of herpes simplex encephalitis after successful treatment with acyclovir. *Clin Infect Dis* **30:**185–187.

Johnson RT (1998). *Viral Diseases of the Nervous System.* 2nd ed. Lippincott Williams & Wilkins, Philadelphia.

Julkunen I, Kleemola M, Hovi T (1984). Serological diagnosis of influenza A and B infections by enzyme immuno assay: Comparison with the complement fixation test. *J Virol Methods* **1:**7–14.

Kessler HH, Muhlbauer G, Rinner B, Stelzl E, Berger A, Dorr HW, Santner B, Marth E, Rabenau H (2000). Detection of herpes simplex virus DNA by real-time PCR. *J Clin Microbiol* **38:**2638–2642.

Koskiniemi M, Gencay M, Salonen O, Puolakkainen M, Färkkilä M, Saikku P, Vaheri A and the Study Group (1996). *Chlamydia pneumoniae* associated with central nervous system infections. *Eur Neurol* **36:**160–163.

Koskiniemi M, Rantalaiho T, Piiparinen H, *et al.* (2001). Infections of the central nervous system of suspected viral origin: a collaborative study from Finland. *J Neurovirol* **7:**400–408.

Koskiniemi M, Piiparinen H, Rantalaiho T, Eranko P, Farkkila M, Raiha K, Salonen EM, Ukkonen P, Vaheri A (2002). Acute central nervous system complications in varicella zoster virus infections. *J Clin Virol* **25:**293–301.

Lai CW, Gragasin ME (1988). Electroencephalography in herpes simplex encephalitis. *J Clin Neurophysiol* **5:**87–103.

Lakeman FD, Whitley RJ (1995). Diagnosis of herpes simplex encephalitis: application of polymerase chain reaction to cerebrospinal fluid from brain-biopsied patients and correlation with disease. National Institute of Allergy and Infectious Diseases Collaborative Antiviral Study Group. *J Infect Dis* **171:**857–863.

Launes J, Nikkinen P, Lindroth L, Brownell AL, Liewendahl K, Iivanainen M (1988). Diagnosis of acute herpes simplex encephalitis by brain perfusion single photon emission computed tomography. *Lancet* **1:**1188–1191.

Levine D, Lauter CB, Lerner M (1978). Simultaneous serum and CSF antibodies in herpes simplex virus encephalitis. *JAMA* **240:**356–360.

Love S, Wiley CA (2002). Viral diseases. In: *Greenfield's Neuropathology* (eds. Graham DI, Lantos PL) 7th ed. London - New York - New Delhi: Arnold, vol. 2, pp. 1–105.

MacCallum FO, Chinn IJ, Gostling JVT (1974). Antibodies to herpes-simplex virus in the cerebrospinal fluid of patients with herpetic encephalitis. *J Med Microbiol* **7:**325–331.

Marchbank ND, Howlett DC, Sallomi DF, Hughes DV (2000). Magnetic resonance imaging is preferred in diagnosing suspected cerebral infections. *BMJ* **320:**187–188.

Menon DK, Sargentoni J, Peden CJ, Bell JD, Cox IJ, Coutts GA, Baudouin C, Newman CG (1990). Proton MR spectroscopy in herpes simplex encephalitis: assessment of neuronal loss. *J Comput Assist Tomogr* **14:**449–452.

Miotto EC (2002).Cognitive rehabilitation of naming deficits following viral meningo-encephalitis. *Arq Neuropsiquiatr* **60:**21–27.

Moorthi S, Schneider WN, Dombovy ML (1999).Rehabilitation outcomes in encephalitis–a retrospective study 1990–1997. *Brain Inj* **13:**139–146.

Muir P, vanLoon AM (1997). Enterovirus infections of the central nervous system. *Intervirology* **40:**153–166.

Nakano A, Yamasaki R, Miyazaki S, *et al.* (2003). Beneficial effect of steroid pulse therapy on acute viral encephalitis. *Eur Neurol* **50:**225–229.

Pevear DC, Tull TM, Seipel ME, Groarke JM (1999). Activity of pleoconaril against enteroviruses. *Antimicrob Agents Chemother* **43:**2109–2115.

Portegies P, Solod L, Cinque P, *et al.* (2004). Guidelines for the diagnosis and management of neurologic complications of HIV infection. *Eur J Neurol* **11:**297–304.

Pozo F, Tenorio A (1999). Detection and typing of lymphotropic herpesviruses by multiplex polymerase chain reaction. *J Virol Methods* **79:**9–19.

Redington JJ, Tyler KL (2002). Viral infections of the nervous system, 2002: update on diagnosis and treatment. *Arch Neurol* **59:**712–718.

Rowley AH, Whitley RJ, Lakeman FD, Wolinsky SM (1990). Rapid detection of herpes-simplex-virus DNA in cerebrospinal fluid of patients with herpes simplex encephalitis. *Lancet* **335:**440–441.

Rudkin TM, Arnold DL (1999). Proton magnetic resonance spectroscopy for the diagnosis and management of cerebral disorders. *Arch Neurol* **56:**919–926.

Sainio K, Granström ML, Pettay O, *et al.* (1983). EEG in neonatal herpes simplex encephalitis. *Electroenceph Clin Neurophysiol* **56:**556–561.

Salvan AM, Confort-Gouny S, Cozzone PJ, Vion-Dury J (1999). Atlas of brain proton magnetic resonance spectra. Part III: Viral infections. *J Neuroradiol* **26:**154–161.

Schmahmann JD, Sherman JC (1998). The cerebellar cognitive affective syndrome. *Brain* **121:**561–579.

Schraeder PL, Burns RA (1980). Hemiplegic migraine associated with an aseptic meningeal reaction. *Arch Neurol* **37:**377–379.

Schroth G, Kretzschmar K, Gawehn J, Voigt K (1987). Advantage of magnetic resonance imaging in the diagnosis of cerebral infections. *Neuroradiology* **29:** 120–126.

Sejvar JJ, Haddad MB, Tierney BC, Campbell GL, Marfin AA, Van Gerpen JA, Fleischauer A, Leis AA, Stokic DS, Petersen LR (2003). Neurologic manifestations and outcome of West Nile virus infection. *JAMA* **290:**511–515.

Shen WC, Tsai C, Chiu H, Chow K (2000). MRI of Enterovirus 71 myelitis with monoplegia. *Neuroradiology* **42:**124–127.

Shian WJ, Chi CS (1996). Epstein-Barr virus encephalitis and encephalomyelitis: MR findings. *Pediatr Radiol* **26:**690–693.

Skoldenberg B, Forsgren M, Alestig K, *et al.* (1984). Acyclovir versus vidarabine in herpes simplex encephalitis: randomized multicente study in consecutive Swedish patients. *Lancet* **2:**707–712.

Socan M, Beovic B, Kese D (1994). *Chlamydia pneumoniae* and meningoencephalitis. *N Engl J Med* **331:**406.

Storch AG (2000). Methodological overview. In *Essentials of Diagnostic Virology* (ed. Storch AG), Churchill Livinstone, New York, 1–23.

Tebas P, Nease RF, Storch GA (1998). Use of the polymerase chain reaction in the diagnosis of herpes simplex encephalitis: a decision analysis model. *Am J Med* **105:**287–295.

Tenembaum S, Chamoles N, Fejerman N (2002). Acute disseminated encephalomyelitis: a long-term follow-up study of 84 pediatric patients. *Neurology* **59:**1224–1231.

Tenorio A, Echevarria JE, Casas I, Echevarria JM, Tabares E (1993). Detection and typing of human herpesviruses by multiplex polymerase chain reaction. *J Virol Methods* **44:**261–269.

Thuerl C, Muller K, Laubenberger J, Volk B, Langer M (2003). MR imaging of autopsy-proved paraneoplastic limbic encephalitis in non-Hodgkin lymphoma. *AJNR Am J Neuroradiol* **24:**507–511.

Thurnher MM, Rieger A, Kleibl-Popov C, Settinek U, Henk C, Haberler C, Schindler E (2001). Primary central nervous system lymphoma in AIDS: a wider spectrum of CT and MRI findings. *Neuroradiology* **43:**29–35.

Tsuchiya K, Katase S, Yoshino A, Hachiya J (1999). Diffusion-weighted MR imaging of encephalitis. *AJR Am J Roentgenol* **173:**1097–1099.

Vas GA, Cracco JB (1990). Inflammatory encephalopathies. In D.D. Daly and T.A. Pedley (eds),*Current Practice of Clinical Electroencephalography*, 2nd ed. Raven Press, New York 1990; pp 386–389.

Westmoreland BF (1999). The EEG in cerebral inflammatory processes. In E. Niedermeyer and F. Lopes Da Silva (eds), *Electroencephalography*, 4th ed. Williams & Wilkins, Baltimore 1999; pp 302–316.

Wahlberg P, Saikku P, Brummer-Korvenkontio M (1989). Tick-borne viral encephalitis in Finland. The clinical features of Kumlinge disease during 1959–1987. *J Intern Med* **225:**173–177.

Whitley RJ, Alford CA, Hirsch MS, *et al.* (1986). Vidarabine versus acyclovir therapy in herpes simplex encephalitis. *N Eng J Med* **314:**144–149.

Whitley RJ, Gnann JW (2002). Viral encephalitis: familiar infections and emerging pathogens. *Lancet* **359:**507–514.

Wilkinson ID, Lunn S, Miszkiel KA, Miller RF, Paley MN, Williams I, Chinn RJ, Hall-Craggs MA, Newman SP, Kendall BE, Harrison MJ (1997). Proton MRS and quantitative MRI assessment of the short term neurological response to antiretroviral therapy in AIDS. *J Neurol Neurosurg Psychiatry* **63:**477–482.

Wilson BA, Gracey F, Bainbridge K (2001). Cognitive recovery from "persistent vegetative state": psychological and personal perspectives. *Brain Inj* **15:**1083–1092.

Yan HJ (2002). Herpes simplex encephalitis: the role of surgical decompression. *Surg Neurol* **57:**20–24.

Yin EZ, Frush DP, Donnelly LF, Buckley RH (2001). Primary immunodeficiency disorders in pediatric patients: clinical features and imaging findings. *AJR Am J Roentgenol* **176:**1541–1552.

CHAPTER 29

Treatment of neuropathic pain

N. Attal,[a,b] G. Cruccu,[a,c] M. Haanpää,[a,d]
P. Hansson,[a,e] T.S. Jensen,[a,f] T. Nurmikko,[g]
C. Sampaio,[h] S. Sindrup,[i] P. Wiffen[j]

Abstract

Background and objectives Neuropathic pain treatment remains unsatisfactory despite a substantial increase in the number of trials. This EFNS Task Force aimed at evaluating the existing evidence about the pharmacological treatment of neuropathic pain.

Methods Studies were identified using first the Cochrane Database then Medline. Trials were classified according to the aetiological condition. All Class I and II controlled trials (according to EFNS classification of evidence) were assessed, but lower class studies were considered in conditions that had no top level studies. Only treatments feasible in an outpatient setting were evaluated. Effects on pain symptoms/signs, quality of life and comorbidities were particularly searched for.

Results Most of the RCTs included patients with postherpetic neuralgia (PHN) and painful polyneuropathies (PPN) mainly due to diabetes. These trials provide Level A evidence for the efficacy of tricyclic antidepressants, gabapentin, pregabalin and opioids, with a large number of Class I trials, followed by topical lidocaine (in PHN) and the newer antidepressants venlafaxine and duloxetine (in PPN). A small number of controlled trials were performed in central pain, trigeminal neuralgia, other peripheral neuropathic pain states and multiple-aetiology neuropathic pains.

Conclusions The main peripheral pain conditions respond similarly well to tricyclic antidepressants, gabapentin and pregabalin, but some conditions, such as HIV-associated polyneuropathy, are more refractory. There are too few studies on central pain, combination therapy, and head-to-head comparison. For future trials, we recommend to assess quality of life and pain symptoms or signs with standardized tools.

[a]EFNS Panel Neuropathic Pain; [b]INSERM U-792, Centre d'Evaluation et de Traitement de la Douleur, Hôpital Ambroise Paré, AP-HP and Université Versailles-Saint-Quentin, France; [c]Department of Neurological Sciences, La Sapienza University, Rome, Italy; [d]Departments of Anaesthesiology and Neurosurgery, Pain Clinic, Helsinki University Hospital, Helsinki, Finland; [e]Department of Molecular Medicine and Surgery, Section of Clinical Pain Research and Pain Center, Department of Neurosurgery, Karolinska Institute, University Hospital, Stockholm, Sweden;

[f]Department of Neurology and Danish Pain Research Center, Aarhus University Hospital, Aarhus, Denmark; [g]Pain Research Institute, Division of Neurological Science, School of Clinical Sciences, University of Liverpool, United Kingdom; [h]Instituto de Farmacologia e Terapeutica Geral, Lisbon School of Medicine, University of Lisbon, Lisbon, Portugal; [i]Department of Neurology, Odense University Hospital, Odense, Denmark; [j]Cochrane Pain & Palliative Care Review Group, Oxford, UK.

Background and objectives

Despite the considerable increase in the number of randomized placebo-controlled trials in neuropathic pain over the last few years, the medical treatment of neuropathic pain is still far from being satisfactory, with less than half of the patients achieving significant benefit with any pharmacological drug (Dworkin *et al.*, 2003a; Finnerup *et al.*, 2005). Randomized controlled trials (RCT) have generally been performed in patients categorized according to their aetiologies. Most RCTs have been conducted in postherpetic neuralgia and painful polyneuropathy, whereas there are very few trials in other peripheral neuropathic pains–including trigeminal neuralgia–and central pain, and no RCTs in painful radiculopathies. Recently, therapeutic strategies aiming at selecting treatments by targeting the putative mechanisms of pain (mechanism-based strategies) have been proposed (Baron, 2000; Woolf and Max, 2001); yet, this approach remains difficult to apply in clinical practice (Attal, 2000; Hansson, 2003; Jensen and Baron, 2003).

Although well-conducted meta-analyses or systematic reviews on medical treatment of neuropathic pain have been recently published (Dworkin *et al.*, 2003a; Dubinsky *et al.*, 2004; Hempenstall *et al.*, 2005; Adriaensen *et al.*, 2005; Saarto and Wiffen, 2005; Finnerup *et al.*, 2005), there is still a lack of expert consensus on guidelines regarding the medical treatment of neuropathic pain. This may be mainly due to the heterogeneity of such pain in terms of aetiologies, symptoms, signs and underlying mechanisms.

The objectives of our Task Force were: (1) to examine all the RCTs performed in the various neuropathic pain conditions; (2) to evaluate the drug effects on pain symptoms, quality of life, and sleep, and adverse events; (3) to propose recommendations based on the results of these trials aiming at helping clinicians in their treatment choice for most neuropathic pain conditions; (4) to propose new studies that may help clarify unsolved issues.

Methods

We conducted an initial search through the central database in the Cochrane Library. Whenever the Cochrane search failed to find top level studies for a given neuropathic pain condition or a drug that was supposedly active on neuropathic pain, we expanded the search using Medline and other electronic databases (1966–to date), and checking reference lists published in meta-analyses, review articles, and other clinical reports. Furthermore, to get the most updated information, we also asked all the pharmaceutical companies producing drugs in this field to provide us with studies not yet published (Appendix A). Any reports retrieved from these contacts were pooled with the others for selection.

To provide the neurologist with clear indications regarding drug treatment for the most studied neuropathic pains, the Task Force decided to produce individual chapters for painful polyneuropathies, postherpetic neuralgia, trigeminal neuralgia, and central pain (spinal cord injury, post-stroke pain and multiple sclerosis), but to search and report also for the other less studied neuropathic conditions (post-traumatic/post-surgical nerve lesions, phantom limb pain, Guillain–Barré syndrome) and for neuropathic pains with multiple aetiology. Each chapter was assigned to two Task Force participants.

Classification of evidence Classification of evidence and recommendation grading adhered to the EFNS standards (Brainin *et al.*, 2004). In particular, Class I refers not only to adequate prospective randomized controlled trials, but also to adequately powered systematic reviews (SR).

Inclusion and exclusion criteria Included studies complied with the following criteria: (1) randomized or non-randomized but controlled Class I or II trials (lower class studies were evaluated in conditions in which no higher level studies were available); (2) pain relief considered as a primary outcome and measured with validated scales; (3) minimum sample of 10 patients; (4) treatment duration and follow-up clearly specified; (5) treatment assessed in repeated dose settings for at least 1 week; (6) treatment feasible in an outpatient setting (intravenous, subcutaneous, or intrathecal therapy or nerve blocks were not considered); (7) evaluating currently used drugs or drugs under clinical phase-III development: (8) including patients with pain secondary to a definite nervous system lesion/disease (definite neuropathic pain) (Rasmussen *et al.*, 2004) or classical trigeminal neuralgia; (9) full paper citations in English, Danish, French, Finnish, German, Italian, Portuguese, or Spanish.

Exclusion criteria were duplicated patient series, uncontrolled studies, pain without evidence of a nerve lesion, such as atypical facial pain, CRPS type I or low back pain, non-validated or unconventional outcome measures, non pharmacological intervention, treatments acting directly on the disease or pre-emptive treatments.

Information selected from the trials From articles meeting our search criteria, we extracted information regarding the efficacy on overall pain and main side effects, but also effects on pain symptoms or signs, quality of life and mood, whenever available. We also referred to recent well-conducted meta-analyses when analysis of these studies did not provide with additional information regarding these endpoints. We used the NNT (the number of patients needed to treat to obtain one responder to the active drug) with 95% confidence intervals (CI) for Class I/II studies to gain information regarding the overall efficacy of a drug. Unless otherwise specified, we used the NNT for 50% pain relief. These values were calculated for newer trials or extracted from recent meta-analyses performed by members of this Task Force (Sindrup *et al.*, 2005; Hempenstall *et al.*, 2005; Finnerup *et al.*, 2005) or the Cochrane database (Saarto and Wiffen, 2005; Wiffen *et al.*, 2005a–c). We did not use the Number Needed to Harm because of lack of uniform criteria for assessing harmful events (Finnerup *et al.*, 2005).

Results

Painful polyneuropathy

Painful polyneuropathy (PPN) is a common neuropathic pain condition. Diabetic polyneuropathy is the most classical example. Patients usually present with spontaneous and stimulus-evoked pains with a distal and symmetrical distribution (Otto *et al.*, 2003). Although one or more of the pain symptoms characteristics of neuropathic conditions are seen in the majority of the patients, the most frequent single pain symptom is deep aching pain (Otto *et al.*, 2003). Diabetic and non-diabetic PPN are similar in symptomatology and with respect to treatment response (Class I SR: *Sindrup and Jensen*, 2000). The only exceptions seem to concern HIV- and chemotherapy-induced neuropathy that are described separately.

Antidepressants Antidepressants have recently been reviewed in two Class I meta-analyses in neuropathic pain including PPN (Saarto and Wiffen, 2005; Sindrup *et al.*, 2005). Evidence for the efficacy of tricyclic antidepressants (TCAs: amitriptyline, clomipramine, desipramine, imipramine, table 29.1) has been compiled since they were first introduced in PPN about 30 years ago. Most data stem from relatively small crossover Class I or II trials, which may overestimate efficacy. The NNT for TCAs in painful polyneuropathy is 2.1 (CI 1.8–2.6) for drugs with balanced serotonin and noradrenalin reuptake inhibition and 2.5 (CI 1.9–3.6) for drugs that mainly inhibit noradrenaline reuptake (Sindrup *et al.*, 2005). In one trial, amitriptyline was slightly but significantly more effective than maprotiline (Class I: Vrethem *et al.*, 1997) whereas another trial failed to observe significant differences between clomipramine and desipramine (Class I: Sindrup *et al.*, 1990).

Selective serotonin reuptake inhibitors (SSRIs) or mianserin cause minor and clinically insufficient pain relief in four Class I trials (Class I SR: Sindrup *et al.*, 2005; Saarto and Wiffen, 2005), whereas serotonin-noradrenaline reuptake inhibitors (SNRIs) such as venlafaxine (150–225 mg/day) (Class I: Sindrup *et al.*, 2003; Rowbotham *et al.*, 2004; and duloxetine (60–120 mg/day) (Class I: Goldstein *et al.*, 2005; Raskin *et al.* 2005) are effective and have a better safety profile on the primary endpoint but much less effective on the proportion of responders than TCAs (see section 'Adverse events and indications for use'). In a head-to-head comparison, venlafaxine was as efficacious as the TCA imipramine (Class I: Sindrup *et al.*, 2003). With adequate dosing, the NNT is 4.6 (CI 2.9–10.6) for venlafaxine and 5.2 (CI 3.7–8.5) for duloxetine.

Table 29.1 Predominant mechanism of action of main drugs.

Drug	Predominant mechanism
Amitriptyline	TCA, balanced monoamine reuptake inhibition
Capsaicin (topical)	depolarizes the nervous membrane via vanilloid receptor type 1, initially stimulates then blocks skin nerve fibres
Carbamazepine	voltage-gated sodium-channel block
Clomipramine	TCA, balanced monoamine reuptake inhibition
Desipramine	TCA, predominantly noradrenaline reuptake inhibition
Dextromethorphan	NMDA-receptor antagonist
Duloxetine	SNRI, serotonin-noradrenaline reuptake inhibition
Gabapentin	binding to the $\alpha_{2\delta}$ subunit of presynaptic voltage-dependent calcium channels with reduced release of presynaptic transmitters
Imipramine	TCA, balanced monoamine reuptake inhibition
Lidocaine (topical)	block of peripheral sodium channels and thus of ectopic discharges.
Lamotrigine	presynaptic voltage-gated sodium-channel inhibition and thus reduced release of presynaptic transmitters
Memantine	NMDA-receptor antagonist
Nortriptyline	predominantly noradrenalin reuptake inhibition
Oxcarbazepine	voltage-gated sodium- and calcium-channel block
Oxycodone	$\mu-$opioid-receptor agonist
Pregabalin	binding to the $\alpha_{2\delta}$ subunit of presynaptic voltage-dependent calcium channels with reduced release of presynaptic transmitters
Topiramate	voltage-gated sodium-channel block and inhibition of glutamate release by an action on AMPA/kainate receptors
Tramadol	$\mu-$opioid-receptor agonist and monoamine reuptake inhibitor
Valproate	increase of GABA levels in brain and potentiation of GABA-mediated responses
Venlafaxine	SNRI, serotonin-noradrenaline reuptake inhibition

Antiepileptics Two small crossover double blind trials, published some 30 years ago, reported significant effects of carbamazepine (CBZ) in diabetic PPN, but their methods and reporting do not live up to current standards (Class III: Rull *et al.*, 1969; Wilton, 1974). One small double blind study (n = 16) reported similar efficacy of CBZ and nortriptyline-fluphenazine, but the small sample size might prevent showing a difference (Class II: Gomez-Perez *et al.*, 1996).

Oxcarbazepine (OXC) data were equivocal in PPN as judged by abstracts from the EFNS congress in 2004, with several still unpublished negative trials. However, in a recent double-blind parallel-group placebo trial of 16-week duration, OXC (300–1800 mg/day) was efficacious in diabetic PPN, with NNT = 5.9 (CI 3.2–42.2) (Class II: Dogra *et al.*, 2005).

Lamotrigine (LTG) has shown acceptable efficacy with NNT = 4 (CI 2.1–42) in diabetic PPN (Class I: Eisenberg *et al.*, 2001).

Topiramate failed to relieve diabetic PPN in three large controlled trials (Class I: Thienel *et al.*, 2004) and one later study found a marginal effect (Class I: Raskin *et al.*, 2004).

Data about valproate are controversial (Class I/II: Kochar *et al.*, 2002, 2004; Otto *et al.*, 2004) and its potential in PPN needs further scrutiny.

The antiepileptics with best evidence for efficacy in PPN are gabapentin (GBP) 1200–3600 mg/day and pregabalin 150–600 mg/day (Class I: Backonja *et al.*, 1998; Simpson, 2001; Lesser *et al.*, 2004; Rosenstock *et al.*, 2004). These drugs relieve diabetic PPN consistently across trials (overall NNT = 3.9, CI 3.2–5.1). Most of the initial pregabalin trials were flawed by exclusion of GBP non-responders, resulting in an enriched enrolment, but two recent Class I RCTs without this criterion still reported a similar efficacy (Richter *et al.*, 2005; Freynhagen *et al.*, 2005). Only one head-to-head controlled study compared GBP (1800 mg/day) to amitriptyline (75 mg/day). Because of an insufficient sample size, the order of efficacy and tolerability between these drugs could not be settled (Class II: Morello *et al.*, 1999). In one unpublished parallel group trial comparing pregabalin and amitriptyline to placebo, amitriptyline, but not pregabalin, was significantly better than placebo on the primary endpoint, but this may possibly be due to significant differences in baseline characteristics between the two active treatment groups (Class II: Pfizer, data on file).

Opioids Oxycodone (average doses 37–60 mg/day, range 10–99 mg/day), the only pure opioid assessed in PPN, is effective with a combined NNT = 2.6 (CI 1.9–4.1) (Class I: Watson *et al.*, 2003; Gimbel *et al.*, 2003). In these trials, patients previously receiving opioids were allowed to participate, which may enhance the proportion of opioid responders and reduce the incidence of side effects (see section 'Adverse events and indications for use'). Tramadol 200–400 mg/day, with opioid and monoaminergic effects, also relieves PPN effectively with an NNT = 3.4 (CI 2.3–6.4) (Class I: Harati *et al.*, 1998; Sindrup *et al.*, 1999a).

Others The antiarrhythmic drug mexiletine did not yield significant pain relief in four Class I–II trials in PPN (Class I SR: Finnerup *et al.*, 2005). Topical capsaicin gave discrepant results across five Class I–II studies that do not provide evidence for a clinically noticeable pain relief in PPN (Class I SR: Finnerup *et al.*, 2005). Furthermore, the intense burning sensation caused by this agent decreases compliance and may cause unblinding. The NMDA-antagonist memantine has not shown convincing efficacy in PPN (Class I: Sang *et al.*, 2002), while pain relief was found for the weak NMDA-antagonist dextromethorphan in two small trials (Nelson *et al.*, 1997; Sang *et al.*, 2002). Efficacy of levodopa has been reported in one small RCT (Class II: Ertas *et al.*, 1998). Other drugs assessed in PPN (aspirin, NSAIDs, topical clonidine) have

either limited or lack of efficacy on the basis of Class I– II trials or are not available for use (Class I SR: Sindrup and Jensen, 2000).

HIV-associated neuropathy and chemotherapy-induced neuropathy In HIV-associated neuropathy, two parallel-group RCTs did not show benefit from lamotrigine (300–600 mg/day) except in subgroups of patients depending on their use of concomitant antiretroviral therapy (ART) (Class I/II: Simpson *et al.*, 2000, 2003): the study with the largest sample (227 patients), which used stratified randomization, showed efficacy in the group receiving ART and had a high placebo response in the group not receiving ART (Simpson *et al.*, 2003), whereas the smaller study showed better effects in the group not receiving ART (Simpson *et al.*, 2000).

In one crossover RCT gabapentin (titrated to 2400 mg/day) improved pain and sleep with no significant difference from placebo (Class II: Hahn *et al.*, 2004).

There is evidence, from Class I/II studies that amitriptyline (Shlay *et al.*, 1998; Kieburtz *et al.*, 1998), topical lidocaine patches (Estanislao *et al.*, 2004), mexiletine (Kemper *et al.*, 1998; Kieburtz *et al.*, 1998) and capsaicin (Paice *et al.*, 2000) lack efficacy.

One Class II RCT performed in cisplatinum-induced neuropathy reported little benefit from nortriptyline (100 mg/day) on pain or paresthesias (except during the second period of treatment probably due to carryover effect), but the major limitation of this study is the lack of distinction between pain and paresthesia (Hammack *et al.*, 2002).

Combination therapy The usefulness of combination therapy has been assessed in two RCTs. The largest one, which also included patients with PHN, demonstrated synergistic effects of gabapentin–morphine combination, with better analgesia at lower doses of each drug than either as a single agent, but the additional effect of the combination was low (Class I: Gilron *et al.*, 2005). Another parallel-group study showed the superiority of gabapentin–venlafaxine combination on pain, mood and quality of life when compared with gabapentin plus placebo, but the study sample was very small (11 patients) (Class II: Simpson, 2001).

RECOMMENDATIONS

Treatments with established efficacy on the basis of Class I trials in PPN (with the exception of HIV-associated polyneuropathy) are TCAs, duloxetine, venlafaxine, gabapentin, pregabalin, strong opioids and tramadol (Level A). The SNRIs duloxetine and venlafaxine are recommended as second choice due to comparatively lower efficacy (based on NNT and one trial versus TCA), but are safer to use and have less contraindications than TCAs and may be preferred in patients with cardiac conditions. We recommend TCAs or gabapentin/pregabalin as first choice (see section "adverse effects and indications for use"). Second/third line therapy includes opioids (potential safety concerns in non cancer pain (see section 'Adverse events and indications for use') and lamotrigine (Level B). Treatments with weak efficacy or lack of efficacy include SSRIs, capsaicin, mexiletine, oxcarbazepine and topiramate (Level A). There is low strength of evidence and safety concerns for carbamazepine and insufficient support for the use of valproate.

HIV-associated polyneuropathy has been found refractory to most currently assessed drugs. This may be due to particular mechanisms of pain in this often progressive condition and to a high placebo response, observed in many trials. Only lamotrigine has been reported efficacious in a subgroup of patients receiving ART in one Class I trial, but a smaller Class II trial reported totally opposite results (Level B).

Postherpetic neuralgia

Postherpetic neuralgia (PHN) is a painful aftermath of herpes zoster. The most important risk factors for PHN are old age and severe acute pain. Patients with PHN commonly describe a constant generally burning pain, an intermittent pain with lancinating or shooting quality, and brush-induced allodynia is observed in nearly 90% of cases. In an individual patient, any component can be the most distressing feature of the pain (Nurmikko and Bowsher, 1990).

Antidepressants The TCAs amitriptyline (average dosages 65–100 mg/day), nortriptyline (average 89 mg), desipramine (average 65–73 mg) are effective in PHN on the basis of three Class I–II placebo-controlled trials with a combined NNT = 2.6 (CI 2.1–3.5) (Class I SR: Dubinsky *et al.*, 2004; Hempenstall *et al.*, 2005). In two small head-to-head comparative trials, the antidepressant maprotiline has been found slightly less effective than amiptryptline (Class II: Watson *et al.*, 1992) and nortriptyline as effective as amitriptyline, but better tolerated (Class II: Watson *et al.*, 1998). There are no RCTs of the efficacy of SSRIs or SNRIs in PHN.

Antiepileptics Gabapentin 1800–3600 mg/day (Class I: Rowbotham *et al.*, 1998; Rice *et al.*, 2001) and pregabalin 150–600 mg/day (Class I: Dworkin *et al.*, 2003b; Sabatowski *et al.*, 2004) have consistently shown efficacy in PHN, with an NNT of 4.4 (CI 3.3–6.1) for GBP and 4.9 (3.7–7.6) for pregabalin (Class I SR: Hempenstall *et al.*, 2005). Very good results have recently been obtained with valproate (Class II : Kochar *et al.* 2005).

Topical treatments Repeated application of lidocaine patches (5%) has shown efficacy in PHN patients in three placebo-controlled studies, all with short duration (up to 3 weeks) (Class II: Galer *et al.*, 1999, 2002; Wasner *et al.*, 2005). One crossover study (in 32 patients) did not report baseline levels of pain and used an enriched enrollment (i.e. only patients with clinical open label improvement with topical lidocaine were recruited) (Galer *et al.*, 1999). Two studies (Galer *et al.*, 2002; Wasner *et al.*, 2005; were post-hoc analyses from larger trials performed in multiple-aetiology neuropathic pain group (Class II: Meier *et al.*, 2003) or in PHN patients (unpublished).

Topical capsaicin 0.075% has been found effective, though to a small degree, in two parallel group RCTs with a combined NNT = 3.2 (CI 2.3–5.8) (Class I: Bernstein *et al.*, 1989; Watson *et al.*, 1993).

Opioids Oxycodone, morphine and methadone have shown efficacy on PHN in two crossover placebo-controlled RCTs (Class I: Watson and Babul, 1998; Raja et al., 2002). One non-placebo controlled parallel group study reported better efficacy of high versus low dosages of levorphanol in PHN patients (extracted from a larger group of patients with multiple-aetiology neuropathic pains) (Class I: Rowbotham et al., 2003). The combined NNT for strong opioids in PHN is estimated 2.7 (CI 2.1–3.7) (Class I SR: Hempenstell et al., 2005). In one trial comparing slow-release morphine (91 mg/day, range 15–225) and methadone (15 mg/day) with TCAs and placebo, pain relief was significantly greater with morphine than with nortriptyline, whereas the analgesic efficacy of methadone was comparable to that of TCAs (Raja et al., 2002). There were significantly more withdrawals during the opioid treatment than during the TCA treatment, but cognitive deterioration was seen only with TCAs.

Tramadol (mean dosage 275 mg/day, up to 400 mg/day) was shown to be moderately effective only on some measures of spontaneous pain intensity in PHN, with an NNT = 4.8 (CI 2.6–26.9) (Class I: Boureau et al., 2003); in this study, only patients with pain lasting for less than one year were included, thus several patients tended to recover spontaneously during the trial, which accounts for the high rate of placebo response.

Other treatments The NMDA-antagonists dextrometorphan and memantine, as well as the benzodiazepine lorazepam, are inefficacious in PHN (Class I/II: Max et al., 1988; Nelson et al., 1997; Eisenberg et al., 1998; Sang et al., 2002).

RECOMMENDATIONS

In PHN, drugs with established efficacy on the basis of several Class I or II trials include TCAs, gabapentin, pregabalin, strong opioids and topical lidocaine (Level A). We recommend TCAs and gabapentin/pregabalin as first line. Topical lidocaine has been found effective only in short-term Class II studies that used an enrichment phase or were post-hoc analyses from larger trials; thus the strength of evidence is lower for this drug. However, due to excellent tolerability, topical lidocaine may be proposed first line to elderly patients with allodynia and unable to tolerate systemic treatments. Despite established efficacy, strong opioids should be recommended as second choice because of potential safety concerns in non-cancer pain (see section 'Adverse events and indications for use'). Second/third line treatments include tramadol, valproate and capsaicin because of lower efficacy or limited strength of evidence (Level B). Drugs with weak efficacy or inefficacy include mexiletine and NMDA antagonists (Level A).

Trigeminal neuralgia

Trigeminal neuralgia (TN) typically presents with paroxysmal pain, with sudden, very brief attacks of pain (electric shocks). Pain may be spontaneous or evoked by innocuous stimuli in specific facial or intraoral areas (trigger zones). TN is divided into 'classical' (idiopathic) when secondary to vascular compression of the trigeminal nerve in the cerebellopontine angle or when no cause can be found, or 'symptomatic', when secondary in particular to cerebellopontine-angle benign masses or multiple sclerosis. Patients with symptomatic TN are considered to be less responsive to treatment (Cruccu and Truini, 2005).

Antiepileptics Phenytoin was the first drug used for TN, with positive effects, but there are only Class IV studies for this condition (Class I SR: Sindrup and Jensen, 2002).

Carbamazepine (CBZ) (200–1200 mg/day), the treatment of choice for TN, was studied 40 years ago in three placebo-controlled trials including a total of 150 patients, with an NNT = 1.8 (1.3–2.2) from one Class II and one Class III trial (Class I SR: Sindrup and Jensen, 2002; Wiffen et al., 2005b) and an effect on both the frequency and intensity of paroxysms in the largest study (Class II: Campbell et al., 1966). The use of CBZ is complicated by pharmacokinetic factors and sometimes severe adverse events, particularly in elderly patients (see section 'Adverse events and indications for use').

Oxcarbazepine (OXC) is commonly used as initial treatment for TN (Jensen, 2002). Its preference over CBZ is mainly related to its documented efficacy in epilepsy and accepted greater tolerability (Class I: Kutluay et al., 2003). Three double-blind RCTs compared OXC (average dose 1038 mg/day) versus CBZ (average dose 734 mg/day; Novartis, data on file). Only one of them was published in extenso (Class II: Liebel et al., 2001). In meta-analyses of these trials, including a total of 130 patients, the reduction in number of attacks and global assessment were equally good for both CBZ and OXC (88% of patients achieving a reduction of attacks by >50%), with no significant difference (SR Class II: Beydoun, 2000; Novartis, data on file). These studies are not placebo controlled, which impedes NNT calculations, and only the one published in extenso can be rated according to EFNS criteria.

The efficacy of both CBZ and OXC decreases over time (SR Class I: Sindrup and Jensen, 2002).

Lamotrigine (400 mg/day) has been found effective as add-on therapy on a composite index of efficacy in 14 patients (Class II: Zakrzewska et al., 1997). However, no statistical results are available on the intensity and frequency of paroxysms.

Several other antiepileptics (clonazepam, gabapentin, valproate) have been reported effective in small Class IV uncontrolled studies.

Other drugs Small Class II trials (10–15 patients) have shown that baclofen alone reduces the number of attacks (Fromm et al., 1984; Fromm and Terrence, 1987). Both tocainide and pimozide, reported to be as effective as or more effective than CBZ (Class II: Lindstrom and Lindblom, 1987; Lechin et al., 1989) are no longer used.

Ineffective therapy RCT-documented inefficacy in TN includes topical ophthalmic anaesthesia (Class I: Kondziolka et al., 1994) and topical capsaicin (Class III: Epstein and Marcoe, 1994). Tizanidine is less effective than CBZ (Class II/III: Vilming et al., 1986; Fromm et al., 1993).

Combination therapy Considering the relatively narrow mechanism of action of the available drugs, combination treatments might be useful, but there are no published studies comparing polytherapy with monotherapy (Nurmikko and Eldridge, 2001).

Symptomatic TN Only Class IV studies have reported beneficial effects of lamotrigine, gabapentin or topiramate on TN associated with multiple sclerosis (Class I SR: Sindrup and Jensen, 2002). All studies in TN secondary to cerebellopontine-angle tumours or other posterior fossa masses only deal with surgical treatment.

RECOMMENDATIONS

The two most widely used drugs in idiopathic TN are CBZ (200–1200 mg/day) (Level A) and OXC (600–1800 mg/day) (Level B). OXC poses less safety concerns. We recommend CBZ or OXC as first line and baclofen or lamotrigine as second/third line. Because TN typically lasts forever with periods of partial or complete remission and recurrence, the patients should be taught to adapt the dosage to the frequency of attacks. There is no evidence that combination therapies are advantageous. In patients non-responsive to medical treatment, surgical interventions have given excellent results. In fact, many patients cannot withstand several weeks of pharmacological testing and need prompt neurosurgical attention.

We encourage controlled studies in symptomatic TN.

Central pain

Central pain (CP) or central neuropathic pain is pain due to a lesion in the central nervous system. CP can be a consequence of stroke, spinal cord injury (SCI), multiple sclerosis (MS), but also other aetiologies (Boivie, 2005). Pain may be burning, shooting, aching, or pricking and is often accompanied by dysesthesia, hyperalgesia or allodynia, particularly to brush or cold (Attal and Bouhassira, 2005).

Tricyclic antidepressants Amitriptyline has been assessed in post-stroke and SCI pain. In 15 patients with post-stroke pain, amitriptyline 75 mg daily was superior to placebo (NNT = 1.7; CI 1.2–3.1) and to carbamazepine (800 mg), the latter being similar to placebo (Class I: Leijon and Boivie, 1989). In a large Class I study of patients with spinal cord injury pain ($n = 84$), amitriptyline (average dose 55 mg/day) was found to be ineffective, but the lack of effect might be due to inadequate assessment of neuropathic pain (Class I: Cardenas et al., 2002): the primary outcome was overall pain, and only regression analyses were used to determine if the effect of amitriptyline was influenced by the presence of neuropathic pain.

Antiepileptics In a Class I study of 30 patients with post-stroke pain, LTG (200 mg/day) significantly reduced pain intensity compared to placebo (Vestergaard et al., 2001). In patients with traumatic SCI, LTG up to 400 mg/day failed to induce a significant effect on spontaneous and evoked pain, but an effect was observed in a post-hoc analysis in patients with incomplete SCI (Class I: Finnerup et al., 2002).

In a small crossover trial of 20 patients with SCI pain, GBP up to 3600 mg was significantly effective (Class II: Levendoglu et al., 2004). Pregabalin (average dose 460 mg/day) was significantly efficacious in a large ($n = 137$) Class I parallel-group RCT in SCI (Pfizer, data on file).

In an RCT in SCI, there was no difference between valproate (up to 2400 mg/day for 3 weeks) and placebo (Class II: Drewes et al., 1994).

Opioids There is only one RCT on opioids, in multiple-aetiology peripheral or central pain: levorphanol at high dose (8.9 mg/day) was more effective than levorphanol at low dose (2.7 mg/day) in patients with central pain, but there was no placebo group (Class I: Rowbotham et al., 2003). There was no difference in response between patients with SCI, MS, PHN, or PPN, but patients with brain lesions had more early dropouts due to side effects compared with the others.

Others In a small crossover trial involving 11 SCI patients, mexiletine 450 mg/d was no better than placebo (Class II: Chiou-Tan et al., 1996). Low doses and small number of patients might play a role for lack of efficacy.

Cannabinoid treatment has recently been assessed in two RCTs on pain associated to MS. In one trial in 24 patients, the oral cannabinoid dronabinol (tetrahydrocannabinol, THC) 5–10 mg/day for 3 weeks, was superior to placebo with an NNT = 3.4 (CI 1.8–23.4) (Class I: Svendsen et al., 2004); dronabinol was effective on ongoing and paroxysmal pain, but not on mechanical allodynia. Cannabinoids delivered via an oromucosal spray (2.7 mg of THC, 2.5 mg of cannabidiol) are under clinical phase III development for pain due to MS. One parallel group placebo-controlled trial including 66 patients showed beneficial effects on pain and sleep (mean number of sprays 9.6, range 2–25), with an NNT = 3.7 (CI 2.2–13) (Class I: Rog et al., 2005). The patients included either had neuropathic or spasm-related pain and post-hoc analyses indicated a trend towards better effects in patients with painful muscle spasms.

RECOMMENDATIONS

Considering the small number of randomized controlled trials in CP and the generally small sample sizes, the treatment should be based on general principles for peripheral neuropathic pain treatment and for side effect profile. Currently, we may recommend gabapentin, pregabalin or tricyclic antidepressants as first choice for post-stroke or SCI pain (Level B, no level rating for pregabalin in the lack of published studies) and lamotrigine as second choice (Level B, but safety concerns, see section "advrse events and indications for use"). The level of evidence is lower for opioids in the lack of placebo-controlled studies. In central pain associated to MS, cannabinoids have shown significant efficacy (Level A), but may raise safety concerns (see section 'Adverse events and indications for use'). Therefore, we recommend initially a trial with other drugs found effective on other central pain conditions.

Less studied neuropathic pain conditions

RCTs in less studied neuropathic conditions encompassed pain due to cancer infiltration, phantom limb, post-surgical/post-traumatic nerve lesions, Guillain–Barré syndrome, or multiple-aetiology neuropathic pains.

Although many RCTs were performed in low back pain, no trial considered radiculopathy pain as a primary outcome. Regarding CRPS, most trials included patients with CRPS I or used sympathetic nerve blocks (Class I SR: Kingery, 1997). Trials in multiple-aetiology neuropathic pain included a large proportion of patients with CRPS or radiculopathy.

Neuropathic pain due to cancer infiltration Gabapentin (up to 1800 mg/day) in addition to opioids induced modest benefit on pain and dysesthesia in one large ($n = 121$) Class I RCT (Caraceni *et al.*, 2004); GBP was generally well tolerated, with no difference in dropouts compared to placebo. One RCT on low-dose amitriptyline (30–50 mg/day) for 10 days only, reported a modest effect on maximal but not average pain (Class II: Mercadante *et al.*, 2002).

Post-traumatic/post-surgical neuropathic pain Three studies were performed in post-mastectomy pain and one in mixed post-surgical pain related to cancer. One small ($n = 15$) Class II study showed efficacy of amitriptyline (25–100 mg) on pain, sleep and daily activities (Kalso *et al.*, 1996); side effects caused four early dropouts and most patients discontinued treatment after the study.

In one small ($n = 13$) Class II RCT, characterized by a remarkably high response to placebo, low-dose venlafaxine (37.5–75 mg/day) was effective on maximal pain and pain relief, but not on average pain (Tasmuth *et al.*, 2002). Topical capsaicin (0.075 %) was reported generally efficacious in a large Class I trial in post-surgical pain (Ellison *et al.*, 1997), whereas in a small Class II study in post-mastectomy pain it gave negative effects on steady pain and positive effects on jabbing pain, category pain intensity and pain relief (Watson and Evans, 1992). Both studies used a neutral placebo, which may induce a bias due to the burning sensation engendered by capsaicin.

There is evidence regarding the inefficacy of propranolol in post-traumatic nerve lesions (Class II: Scadding *et al.*, 1982) or cannnabinoid spray on pain after brachial plexus avulsion (Class I: Berman *et al.*, 2004).

Phantom limb pain In a small ($n = 19$) Class II RCT, GBP titrated to 2400 mg/day was effective on pain but had no effect on mood, sleep, or activities of daily living (Bone *et al.*, 2002). Morphine sulphate (70–300 mg/day) was effective in one small ($n = 12$) Class II RCT, but most patients and therapists recognized the active treatment, which might unmask the blinding; there was a significant reduction of attention in morphine-treated patients (Huse *et al.*, 2001).

There is evidence regarding the inefficacy of memantine 30 mg/day (Class I: Maier *et al.*, 2003) or amitriptyline 125 mg/day (Class II: Robinson *et al.*, 2004).

Guillain–Barré syndrome Two short-duration (7 days) Class II RCTs used gabapentin combined with opioids on demand. Gapapentin was superior to placebo in one study ($n = 18$; Pandey *et al.*, 2002) and superior to CBZ in another ($n = 36$; Pandey *et al.*, 2005), with rapid (day 2–3) reduction of both pain and opioid consumption. A systematic search by a consensus group on Guillain–Barré syndrome supports the use of GBP or CBZ in the intensive care unit in the acute phase, while appropriate opioids may be used but require careful monitoring of adverse effects in the setting of autonomic denervation (SR: Hughes *et al.*, 2005).

Multiple-aetiology neuropathic pains There is evidence for the efficacy of the antidepressants bupropion 150 mg (Class I: Semenchuck *et al.*, 2001), clomipramine (Class II: Panerai *et al.*, 1990), nortriptyline (Class II: Langohr *et al.*, 1982) and for topical lidocaine (Meier *et al.*, 2003, discussed in the section 'Effects on pain symptoms and signs'). Discrepant results were reported for mexiletine (Class I: Chabal *et al.*, 1992; Wallace *et al.*, 2000) with positive effects only on mechanical allodynia in one study (Wallace *et al.*, 2000). Results with the NMDA-antagonist riluzole were negative (Class II: Galer *et al.*, 2000).

Three RCTs examined the effects of opioids (Rowbotham *et al.*, 2003, see section 'Central pain'), dextromethorphan (negative results,

McQuay *et al.*, 1994, Class II) or GBP (Class II: Serpell, 2002) in patients with mixed peripheral or central pain. The GBP study was positive only at some time points on burning pain and hyperalgesia, but not on shooting pain; these poor results are possibly due to the inclusion of a large group of patients without evidence of nerve lesion (CRPS type I), who may be more refractory to the drug.

In two Class III trials, the aetiology was not mentioned at all, which makes any interpretation of the results impossible: one with lamotrigine 200 mg/day was negative and the other with capsaicin alone or combined with topical doxepine was positive on several pain symptoms (McCleane, 1999, 2000).

RECOMMENDATIONS

Several less studied neuropathic conditions, such as phantom limb pain, post-surgical neuropathic pain and Guillain–Barré syndrome, appear to be similarly responsive to most current drugs used in other neuropathic conditions (e.g. TCAs, GBP, opioids), but results are based on a limited number of generally Class II RCTs with small sample sizes (Level B). Neuropathic pain due to cancer infiltration seems to be more refractory to drug treatment, probably because it is a progressive condition.

Effects on pain symptoms and signs

Although most initial trials have considered neuropathic pain as a uniform entity, some newer trials have assessed various pain symptoms and signs of evoked pain. TCAs and SNRIs have been found similarly active on ongoing and paroxysmal pain in PPN or PHN (Class I/II: Watson *et al.*, 1992, 1998; Sindrup *et al.*, 2003; Goldstein *et al.*, 2005). The effect of antidepressants on symptoms or signs of evoked pain are controversial, with weak effects on brush-evoked allodynia compared to spontaneous pain (Class I/II: Kishore-Kumar *et al.*, 1990; Max *et al.*, 1991; Sindrup *et al.*, 2003) but positive effects on the subjective report of pains elicited by brush (Class II: Watson *et al.*, 1992, 1998) or pressure (Class I: Sindrup *et al.*, 2003).

The opioids oxycodone and tramadol have been found to relieve continuous pain, paroxysmal pain and symptoms of evoked pain (to touch) in three placebo controlled trials in PPN and PHN (Class I: Watson and Babul, 1998; Sindrup *et al.*, 1999; Watson *et al.*, 2003).

Lamotrigine has been reported effective on cold-evoked allodynia, though not on mechanical allodynia, in central post-stroke pain (Class I: Vestergaard *et al.*, 2001). GBP effects on distinct pain symptoms were investigated in a large group of patients with multiple-aetiology neuropathic pain, but this study had several limitations (see section 'Less studied neuropathic pain conditions'). In trigeminal neuralgia, CBZ was efficacious both on spontaneous and evoked attacks (Class II: Campbell *et al.*, 1966), and CBZ and OXC were found equally effective in reducing pain triggered by eating or drinking (Class I SR: Beydoun, 2002). A systematic review of RCTs reports that, although OXC reduced the number of spontaneous paroxysms in most patients, it did not succeed in suppressing the trigger-evoked pain in 42% of patients (Class I SR: Carazzana and Mikoshiba, 2003).

Efficacy of topical lidocaine has been reported on various symptoms (i.e. burning pain, dull pain, pain evoked by touch) (Galer *et al.*, 2002; Meier *et al.*, 2003, Class II), with a less prominent effect on touch-evoked pain than ongoing pain (Class II: Meier *et al.*, 2003). Surprisingly, this drug has recently been found more effective in allodynic PHN patients with major impairment of nociceptor function compared with those with no sensory loss (Wasner *et al.*, 2005, Class II).

Hence, many drugs appear to have different efficacy on the various symptoms and signs of neuropathic pain; however, because these trials had generally small sample sizes and used methods of assessment that often were not tested for reliability, these data need confirmation from large trials using standardized and validated measures (Cruccu *et al.*, 2004).

Effects on quality of life and comorbidities

Quality of life is usually impaired in patients with neuropathic pain, and this contributes to

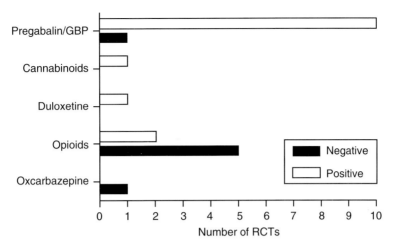

Figure 29.1. Quality of life/comorbidities
Number of Class I or II randomized controlled trials reporting positive (white) or negative (black) effects on most measures of quality of life and mood. Two studies with pregabalin (Richter *et al.*, 2005) or oxcarbazepine (Dogra *et al.*, 2005) had negative results on most measures of quality of life and mood, but found positive effects on sleep. Three additional studies with topical lidocaine (Meier *et al.*, 2003), pregabalin (Freynhagen *et al.*, 2005) or cannabinoids (Rog *et al.*, 2005) assessed sleep only (not shown here).

enhance the burden of pain. Notwithstanding previous EFNS guidelines that stressed its importance and detailed apt tools for assessment (Cruccu *et al.*, 2004), only some of the recent trials have adequately examined the effects of drug treatment on quality of life, sleep and comorbidities (figure 29.1). Significant effects on several measures of quality of life or sleep have been reported for pregabalin and gabapentin in several large Class I trials in PPN, PHN or SCI pain (Rowbotham *et al.*, 1998; Backonja *et al.*, 1998; Simpson, 2001; Serpell, 2002; Sabatowski *et al.*, 2004; Dworkin *et al.*, 2003b; Lesser *et al.*, 2004; Rosenstock *et al.*,2004; Freynhagen *et al.*, 2005, Gilron *et al.*, 2005; Pfizer, data on file), for duloxetine in PPN (Goldstein *et al.*, 2005, Class I) and for cannabinoids in multiple sclerosis (Svendsen *et al.*, 2004; Rog *et al.*, 2005, Class I) (Level A). One study found no significant effects of pregabalin on quality of life, but positive effects on sleep (Richter *et al.*, 2005, Class I). Pregabalin and gabapentin have also been found to improve some measures of mood (Class I: Backonja *et al.*, 1998; Rowbotham *et al.*, 1998; Rosenstock *et al.*, 2004; Sabatowski *et al.*, 2004 (Level A).

In contrast, strong opioids or tramadol have not shown significant effects on most measures of quality of life, mood or sleep in RCTs (Class I: Harati *et al.*, 1998; Watson and Babul, 1998; Boureau *et al.*, 2003; Gimbel *et al.*, 2003; Rowbotham *et al.*, 2003) with the exception of two studies (Class I: Watson *et al.*, 2003; Gilron *et al.*, 2005) (Level B). No effect on quality of life or mood has been reported for oxcarbazepine in one trial in PPN, but the drug had positive effects on sleep (Dogra *et al.*, 2005, Class II). Finally, one trial with topical lidocaine (Meier *et al.*, 2003, Class II) found no effects on quality of sleep in multiple-aetiology peripheral neuropathic pain (Level B).

Adverse events and indications for use

In this section, we present the main side effects observed with drugs with established efficacy in several trials of neuropathic pain and propose practical indications for use.

TCAs The most common side effects of TCAs are dry mouth, constipation, sweating, dizziness, disturbed vision, drowsiness, palpitation, ortho-static hypotension, sedation and urinary hesita-tion. More selective TCAs such as nortriptyline are better tolerated than the non-selective ones, with less anticholinergic effects and sedation (Class II: Watson *et al.*, 1998). A suspected association between TCA treatment and sudden cardiac death has raised concern; a recent epidemiological study found a slight increase in sudden cardiac death with TCA doses superior to 100 mg/day (Ray *et al.*, 2004). Therefore, caution is recommended for older patients, particularly those with cardiovascular risk factors (Dworkin *et al.*, 2003; Sindrup *et al.*, 2005). TCAs should be initiated at low dosages (10–25 mg in a single dose taken at bedtime) and then slowly titrated, as tolerated. Effective dosages are highly variable from one subject to another, the average dosage for amitriptyline being 75 mg/day. Whether TCA blood concentrations should be measured is still controversial (Class I SR: Sindrup *et al.*, 2005; Class II: Watson *et al.*, 1982; Kishore-Kumar *et al.*, 1990).

SNRIs Serotonin-noradrenaline reuptake inhibitors (duloxetine, venlafaxine) are safer to use than TCAs and are a better option in patients with car-diac disease. The relative risk for withdrawal is not significant and there is no need for drug level monitoring. The most frequently observed adverse events with duloxetine are nausea, somnolence, dry mouth, increased sweating, loss of appetite and weakness (Goldstein *et al.*, 2005, Class I). Although immediate release *venlafaxine* is associ-ated with adverse CNS and somatic symptoms such as agitation, diarrhoea, increased liver enzymes, hypertension, and hyponatremia (Class I SR: Deg-ner *et al.*, 2004), the extended release formulation seems to be far more tolerable, the main side effects being gastrointestinal disturbances (Class I: Rowbotham *et al.*, 2004; Sindrup *et al.*, 2003).

Adequate dosages of duloxetine range between 60 and 120 mg/day while doses of 20 mg/day are ineffective (Class I: Goldstein *et al.*, 2005). High doses of venlafaxine (150–225 mg/day) have been reported to be effective while lower doses (75 mg/day) are weakly or not effective (Class I/II: Tasmuth *et al.*, 2002; Rowbotham *et al.*, 2003).

Carbamazepine/Oxcarbazepine CBZ entails frequent adverse events, which include sedation, dizziness, gait abnormalities. Liver enzymes, blood cells, platelets and sodium levels must be monitored for at least 1 year, because of possible risk for hepati-tis, anaplastic effects or hyponatraemia. Induction of microsomal enzyme systems may influence the metabolism of several drugs.

In contrast to CBZ, OXC does not entail enzy-matic induction and there is little risk for crossed cutaneous allergy. In the first months of treatment, sodium levels must be monitored because OXC induces hyponatremia, particularly in the elderly (6% in a cohort of 54 patients) (Class I SR: Kutluay *et al.*, 2003). As regards other side effects, although a better tolerance has been claimed with OXC com-pared with CBZ (Carrazana and Mikoshiba, 2003; Beydoun, 2000, 2002), this notion lacks consis-tent evidence from Class I trials. In a recent trial in diabetic PPN, 27.5% of the OXC group discon-tinued treatment due to central or gastrointestinal side effects versus 8% with the placebo (Class II: Dogra *et al.*, 2005).

Both drugs should be initiated with low dosages and slowly increased up to efficacy or intoler-able side effects. Effective dosages range 200–1200 mg/day for CBZ and 600–1800 mg/day for OXC.

Gabapentin/Pregabalin The most common side effects of gabapentin and pregabalin include dizzi-ness, somnolence, peripheral oedema, and dry mouth, with a similar frequency for both drugs. While gabapentin is widely accepted as highly tol-erable even at high dosages (>2400 mg) (Class I SR: Wiffen *et al.*, 2005a,c), the reports on pre-gabalin change remarkably with the daily dose: with 150–300 mg there is almost no difference with placebo (Class I: Lesser *et al.*, 2004; Richter *et al.*, 2005), while the withdrawal rate reaches 20% with 600 mg (Class I: Dworkin *et al.*, 2003; Freynhagen *et al.*, 2005). Effective dosages range 1200–3600 mg/day for GBP and 150–600 mg/day for pregabalin. Gabapentin needs slow individ-ual titration with initial dosages of 300 mg/day (or less in elderly patients) while pregabalin can be titrated more rapidly and has a short onset of action (less than one week). Whereas GBP should be administered three times a day (t.i.d.), pregabalin can be administered twice a day (b.i.d.) because of concerns about tolerance or dependence issues.

Lamotrigine is generally well tolerated. Side effects include dizziness, nausea, headache and fatigue (Class I: Vestegaard *et al.*, 2001; Simpson, 2001; Eisenberg *et al.*, 2001, Finnerup *et al.*, 2002). However, it may induce potentially severe allergic skin reactions. In a meta-analysis collecting data from 572 patients, 9% of patients were withdrawn because of major adverse events, most commonly rash (Class I: Betts *et al.*, 1991). To minimize the occurrence of cutaneous rashes, a very slow dose titration is recommended: treatment should be initiated with 25 mg daily and increased by 25 mg every other week. The analgesic dosages of lamotrigine range 200–400 mg/day.

Opioids/tramadol The most common side effects of opioids are constipation, sedation and nausea. The risk of cognitive impairment has been reported to be negligible (Class I: Raja *et al.*, 2002; Rowbotham *et al.*, 2003), although morphine may impair attention at very high dosages (up to 300 mg/day) (Class II: Huse *et al.*, 2001). In RCTs on neuropathic pain, the side effect profile of opioids has been reported to be good, particularly for oxycodone (Class I: Babul, 1998; Raja *et al.*, 2002; Watson *et al.*, 2003; Gimbel *et al.*, 2003; Watson and Rowbotham *et al.*, 2003), sometimes with–surprisingly–a similar degree of side effects and number of dropouts in the active and placebo groups (Watson *et al.*, 2003; see also section 'Painful polyneuropathy'). However, less than 20% of patients continue with opioids after one year, because of an unfavourable balance between side effects and efficacy (Class I SR: Attal, 2000). According to recent European recommendations, opioids should be considered for chronic non-cancer pain as second line, if other reasonable therapies fail to provide adequate analgesia (Kalso *et al.*, 2003). Dosages of opioids should be titrated individually up to efficacy and side effects. Effective doses range 10–120 mg/day for oxycodone and 15–300 mg/day for morphine.

Tramadol has been reported to induce dizziness, dry mouth, nausea, constipation and somnolence with significantly more dropouts compared to placebo (Class I: Sindrup *et al.*, 1999; Boureau *et al.*, 2003; Rowbotham *et al.*, 2003). There is an increased risk of seizures in patients with a history of epilepsy or receiving drugs that may reduce the seizure threshold. Serotonergic syndrome (various combinations of myoclonus, rigidity, hyperreflexia, shivering, confusion, agitation, restlessness, coma, autonomic instability, fever, nausea, diarrhoea, flushing, and rarely, rhabdomyolysis and death) may occur if tramadol is used as an add-on treatment to other serotonergic medications (particularly SSRIs). Tramadol should be initiated at low dosages, particularly in the elderly patient (25 mg once daily) and then titrated as tolerated. The effective dosages range 200–400 mg/day.

The use of *lidocaine patches* is very safe with a very low systemic absorbtion and only local adverse effects (mild skin reactions) have been reported in RCTs (Class II: Galer *et al.*, 1999, 2002). Up to four patches per day for a maximum of 12 h may be used to cover the painful area (Class II: Meier *et al.*, 2003). Titration is not necessary.

Cannabinoids have been found generally well tolerated with low dosages (10 mg/day for dronabinol) and slow titration. Adverse events are mainly dizziness, dry mouth and sedation (Class I: Svendsen *et al.*, 2004; Rog *et al.*, 2005). However, the potential risk of physical dependence and tolerance warrants consideration with long-term use; one study found significant memory impairment with cannabinoids in spray (Rog *et al.*, 2005).

Final recommendations and issues for future trials

Selecting a first line medication in neuropathic pain should take into account not only the relative efficacy based at best on direct drug comparisons, but also the ratio efficacy/safety. The effect on different pain symptoms, comorbidities and quality of life should also be documented. So far, such assessment has been performed in a small number of studies for a few drugs only, and the evaluation of symptoms and signs used sometimes inadequate or non-validated methods (Cruccu *et al.*, 2004).

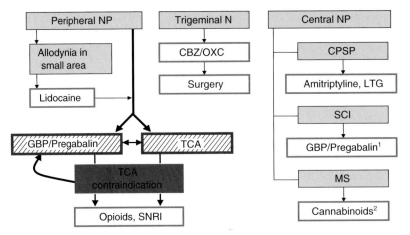

Figure 29.2. Simplified scheme
Top-level evidence (cross hatched boxes) is only available for peripheral pain (PPN and PHN). Both tricyclic antidepressants (TCA) and pregabalin/gabapentin (GBP) are first line, unless TCA are contraindicated. Topical lidocaine is indicated as add-on in patients with PHN having a small allodynic area. SNRI (duloxetine and venlafaxine) and opioids are second choice (SNRI have high-level evidence but a comparatively lower efficacy, opioids have high-level evidence but raise tolerability and safety concerns in long-term treatment for non-cancer chronic pain, lamotrigine has a lower level of evidence). Lower-level evidence is available for trigeminal neuralgia: we recommend the sodium-channel blockers carbamazepine (CBZ) and oxcarbazepine (OXC), then surgery. If the patient cannot or does not want to undergo surgery, then try add-on therapy with lamotrigine (LTG) or baclofen. Very few trials have been dealing with central pains; the best results have so far been achieved with amytriptyline and LTG in central post-stroke pain (CPSP), GBP and pregabalin in spinal cord injury (SCI), and cannabinoids in multiple sclerosis (MS). Mind, however that: (1) pregabalin data are still unpublished and, (2) cannabinoids, due to potential safety concerns, should be used after a negative trial with other drugs found beneficial in other central pain conditions. Combination therapies, which may well prove to be useful, are not indicated here because of insufficient available trials.

The effects of drugs on distinct peripheral neuropathic conditions share many similarities, with the exceptions of HIV-polyneuropathy and trigeminal neuralgia. Central pain has been much less studied. For this reason, the following recommendations concern mainly peripheral neuropathic pain and trigeminal neuralgia (figure 29.2). Recommendations pertaining to other conditions can be found in the above sections.

Drugs with best established efficacy and recommended as first line include TCAs, gabapentin, and pregabalin (Level A, Class I trials). TCAs seem to be more efficacious on the basis of NNT, but these values may have been overestimated and their superiority has not been confirmed by substantive head-to-head comparative trials. Contrary to common notion about their poor efficacy in neuropathic pain (McQuay, 2002), opioids have been found efficacious (Level A) but should only be proposed as second line based on recommendations for chronic non-cancer pain (Kalso *et al.*, 2003). Drugs with less established efficacy in various neuropathic conditions and recommended as second line include the SNRIs venlafaxine and duloxetine, lamotrigine, tramadol, and topical lidocaine. However, due to excellent tolerability, topical lidocaine may be preferred in PHN patients unable to tolerate systemic treatments. There is insufficient support for the use of carbamazepine and oxcarbazepine (with the noteworthy exception of trigeminal neuralgia), topiramate, the SSRIs, capsaicin with the exception of PHN and mexiletine, because of weak efficacy, discrepant results or safety concerns.

Regarding comorbidities and quality of life, only gabapentin, pregabalin and duloxetine have been adequately studied with positive effects, and may therefore be preferred in patients with severe impact of pain on quality of life or significant comorbidities (Level A), while lack of effects of opioids on these outcomes have been reported in most trials. Regarding pain symptoms or signs, only antidepressants and opioids/tramadol have so far been shown effective on ongoing and paroxysmal pain, while effects on touch-evoked pain have been reported for topical lidocaine and opioids/tramadol (Level B). The use of topical lidocaine should be preferred in patients with mechanical allodynia when the painful area is small.

Combination therapy may be proposed in cases of insufficient efficacy with monotherapy and should preferably use drugs with complementary mechanisms of action. It has been shown useful so far for gabapentin/morphine (Level A).

We propose the following strategy for new trials: (1) efficacy should be based on standardised and preferably internationally accepted endpoints and use standardised sets of tests for assessing efficacy (Cruccu *et al.*, 2004); in establishing such efficacy, not only overall pain, but also multiple pain symptoms or signs should be assessed; (2) universal and identical criteria for assessing harmful events should be obtained; (3) comparative trials of different drugs for specific pain conditions/mechanisms permit a solid way for presenting an algorithm for pain therapy; (4) the rationale for a combination therapy needs to be established.

Conflicts of interest

The following authors (initials) did trials or have been consultants for the following pharmaceutical companies:

NA: GlaxoSmithKline, Grunenthal, Novartis, Pfizer, Pierre Fabre, Sanofi-Aventis; GC: GlaxoSmithKline, Lundbeck, Janssen, Novartis, Pfizer; MH: Janssen-Cilag, Merck, Mundipharma, Organon, Orion, Pfizer, Sanofi; PH: Bioschwartz, GlaxoSmithKline, Lundbeck, Pfizer; TSJ: Eli Lilly, GlaxoSmithKline, Grunenthal, Lundbeck, Neurosearch, Pfizer; TN: Allergan, AstraZeneca, GlaxoSmithKline, GWPharma, Napp, Novartis, Pfizer, Renovis, SchwarzPharma; SS: Eli Lilly, GlaxoSmithKline, Grünenthal, Lundbeck, Novartis, Pierre Fabre, UCB Pharma.

The authors have no other conflicts to declare.

Acknowledgements

We wish to thank Cephalon, Endo, Forest Pharmaceuticals, Janssen & Johnson, Lundbeck, Novartis, Pfizer, Schwarz Pharma, UCB Pharma, and Wyeth, for providing us with documentation about their drug trials.

Appendix A:

Survey of pharmaceutical companies (see Methods)

Companies that were contacted:

Cephalon, Elan, Endo, Forest Pharmaceuticals, GSK, GW Pharma, Janssen & Johnson, Lilly, Lundbeck, Newron, Novartis, Pfizer, Schwarz Pharma, SigmaTau, UCB Pharma, Wallace Laboratories, Wyeth.

Companies that had relevant material and sent it to us:

Cephalon, Endo, Forest Pharmaceuticals, Janssen & Johnson, Lundbeck, Novartis, Pfizer, Schwarz Pharma, UCB Pharma, Wyeth.

References

Adriaensen H, Plaghki L, Mathieu C *et al.* (2005). Critical review of oral drug treatments for diabetic neuropathic pain-clinical outcomes based on efficacy and safety data from placebo-controlled and direct comparative studies. *Diabetes Metab Res Rev* **21**:231–240.

Attal N (2000). Chronic neuropathic pain: mechanisms and treatment. *Clin J Pain* **16(Suppl 3)**:S118–130.

Attal N, Bouhassira D (2005). Central Neuropathic pain. In *The Neurological Basis of Pain*. McGraw Hill, New York, pp 301–319.

Backonja M, Beydoun A, Edwards KR *et al.* (1998). Gabapentin for the symptomatic treatment of painful neuropathy in patients with diabetes mellitus: a randomized controlled trial. *JAMA* **280**:1831–1836 (Class I).

Baron R (2000). Neuropathic pain. The long path from mechanisms to mechanism-based treatment. *Anaesthesist* **49**:373–386.

Berman JS, Symonds C, Birch R (2004). Efficacy of two cannabis based medicinal extracts for relief of central neuropathic pain from brachial plexus avulsion: results of a randomised controlled trial. *Pain* **112**:299–306.

Bernstein JE, Korman NJ, Bickers DR *et al.* (1989). Topical capsaicin treatment of chronic postherpetic neuralgia. *J Am Acad Dermatol* **21**:265–270 (Class II).

Betts T, Goodwin G, Withers RM *et al.* (1991). Human safety of lamotrigine. *Epilepsia* **32(Suppl 2):**S17–21.

Beydoun A (2000). Safety and efficacy of oxcarbazepine: results of randomized, double-blind trials. *Pharmacotherapy* **20:**152S–158S.

Beydoun A (2002). Clinical use of tricyclic anticonvulsants in painful neuropathies and bipolar disorders. *Epilepsy Behav* **3:**S18–S22.

Boivie J (2005). Central Pain. In: *Wall and Melzack's Textbook of Pain*, SB MacMahon, M Koltzenburg (eds), Churchill Livingstone, Elsevier, pp 1057–1075.

Bone M, Critchley P, Buggy DJ (2002). Gabapentin in postamputation phantom limb pain: A randomized, double-blind, placebo-controlled, crossover study. *Reg Anesth Pain Med* **27:**481–486.

Boureau F, Legallicier P, Kabir-Ahmadi M (2003). Tramadol in post-herpetic neuralgia: a randomized, double-blind, placebo-controlled trial. *Pain* **104:**323–331 (Class I).

Brainin M, Barnes M, Baron JC *et al.* (2004). Guideline Standards Subcommittee of the EFNS Scientific Committee. Guidance for the preparation of neurological management guidelines by EFNS scientific task forces–revised recommendations. *Eur J Neurol* **11:**577–581.

Campbell FG, Graham JG, Zilkha KJ (1966). Clinical trial of carbamazepine (tegretol) in trigeminal neuralgia. *J Neurol Neurosurg Psychiatry* **29:**265–267.

Caraceni A, Zecca E, Bonezzi C *et al.* (2004). Gabapentin for neuropathic cancer pain: a randomized controlled trial from the Gabapentin Cancer Pain Study Group. *J Clin Oncol* **22:**2909–2917.

Cardenas DD, Warms CA, Turner JA *et al.* (2002). Efficacy of amitriptyline for relief of pain in spinal cord injury: results of a randomized controlled trial. *Pain* **96:**365–373 (Class I).

Carrazana E, Mikoshiba E (2003). Rationale and evidence for the use of oxcarbazepine in neuropathic pain. *J Pain Symptom Manag* **25:**S31–35.

Chabal C, Jacobson L, Mariano A *et al.* (1992). The use of oral mexiletine for the treatment of pain after peripheral nerve injury. *Anesthesiology* **76:**513–517 (Class I).

Chiou-Tan FY, Tuel SM, Johnson JC *et al.* (1996). Effect of mexiletine on spinal cord injury dysesthetic pain. *Am J Phys Med Rehabil* **75:**84–87 (Class I).

Cruccu G, Anand P, Attal N *et al.* (2004). EFNS guidelines on neuropathic pain assessment. *Eur J Neurol* **11:**153–162.

Cruccu G, Truini A (2005). Trigeminal neuralgia and orofacial pains. In: *The Neurological Basis of Pain*. McGraw Hill, New York, pp 401–414.

Degner D, Grohmann R, Kropp S, Ruther E, Bender S, Engel RR, Schmidt LG (2004). Severe adverse drug reactions of antidepressants: results of the German multicenter drug surveillance program AMSP. *Pharmacopsychiatry* **37(Suppl 1):**S39–S45.

Dogra S, Beydoun S, Mazzola J *et al.* (2005). Oxcarbazepine in painful diabetic neuropathy: a randomized, placebo-controlled study. *Eur J Pain* **9:**543–554 (Class II).

Drewes AM, Andreasen A, Poulsen LH (1994). Valproate for treatment of chronic central pain after spinal cord injury. A double-blind crossover study. *Paraplegia* **32:**565–569 (Class II).

Dubinsky RM, Kabbani H, El-Chami Z *et al.* (2004). Quality Standards Subcommittee of the American Academy of Neurology. Practice parameter: treatment of postherpetic neuralgia: an evidence-based report of the Quality Standards Subcommittee of the American Academy of Neurology. *Neurology* **63:**959–965.

Dworkin RH, Backonja M, Rowbotham MC *et al.* (2003a). Advances in neuropathic pain: diagnosis, mechanisms, and treatment recommendations. *Arch Neurol* **60:**1524–1534.

Dworkin RH, Corbin AE, Young JP Jr *et al.* (2003b). Pregabalin for the treatment of postherpetic neuralgia: a randomized, placebo-controlled trial. *Neurology* **60:**1274–1283 (Class I).

Eisenberg E, Kleiser A, Dortort A *et al.* (1998). The NMDA (N-methyl-D-aspartate) receptor antagonist memantine in the treatment of postherpetic neuralgia: a double-blind, placebo-controlled study. *Eur J Pain* **2:**321–327 (Class II).

Eisenberg E, Lurie Y, Braker C *et al.* (2001). Lamotrigine reduces painful diabetic neuropathy: a randomized, controlled study. *Neurology* **57:**505–509 (Class I).

Ertas M, Sagduyu A, Arac N *et al.* (1998). Use of levodopa to relieve pain from painful symmetrical diabetic polyneuropathy. *Pain* **75:**257–259 (Class II).

Ellison N, Loprinzi CL, Kugler J *et al.* (1997) Phase III placebo-controlled trial of capsaicin cream in the management of surgical neuropathic pain in cancer patients. *J Clin Oncol* **15:**2974–2980 (Class I).

Epstein JB, Marcoe JH. (1994). Topical application of capsaicin for treatment of oral neuropathic pain and trigeminal neuralgia. *Oral Surg Oral Med Oral Pathol* **77:**135–140 (Class III).

Estanislao L, Carter K, McArthur J *et al.* (2004). The Lidoderm-HIV Neuropathy Group. A Randomized Controlled Trial of 5% Lidocaine Gel for HIV-Associated Distal Symmetric Polyneuropathy. *J Acquir Immune Defic Syndr* **37:**1584–1586 (Class II).

Finnerup NB, Sindrup SH, Bach FW *et al.* (2002). Lamotrigine in spinal cord injury pain: a randomized controlled trial. *Pain* **96:**375–383 (Class I).

Finnerup NB, Otto M, McQuay HJ *et al.* (2005). Algorithm for neuropathic pain treatment: an evidence based proposal. *Pain* in press

Freynhagen R, Strojek K, Griesing T *et al.* (2005). Efficacy of pregabalin in neuropathic pain evaluated in a 12-week, randomised, double-blind, multicentre, placebo-controlled trial of flexible- and fixed-dose regimens. *Pain* **115**:254–263 (Class I).

Fromm GH, Terrence CF (1987). Comparison of L-baclofen and racemic baclofen in trigeminal neuralgia. *Neurology* **37**:1725–1728 (Class II).

Fromm GH, Terrence CF, Chattha AS (1984). Baclofen in the treatment of trigeminal neuralgia: double-blind study and long-term follow-up. *Ann Neurol* **15**:240–244 (Class II).

Fromm GH, Aumentado D, Terrence CF (1993). A clinical and experimental investigation of the effects of tizanidine in trigeminal neuralgia. *Pain* **53**:265–271 (Class II).

Galer BS, Rowbotham MC, Perander J *et al.* (1999). Topical lidocaine patch relieves postherpetic neuralgia more effectively than a vehicle topical patch: results of an enriched enrollment study. *Pain* **80**:533–538 (Class II).

Galer BS, Twilling LL, Harle J *et al.* (2000). Lack of efficacy of riluzole in the treatment of peripheral neuropathic pain conditions. *Neurology* **55**:971–975 (Class II).

Galer BS, Jensen MP, Ma T *et al.* (2002). The lidocaine patch 5% effectively treats all neuropathic pain qualities: results of a randomized, double-blind, vehicle-controlled, 3-week efficacy study with use of the neuropathic pain scale. *Clin J Pain* **18**:297–301 (Class II).

Gilron I, Bailey JM, Tu D *et al.* (2005). Morphine, gabapentin, or their combination for neuropathic pain. *N Engl J Med* **352**:1324–1334 (Class I).

Gimbel JS, Richrds P, Portenoy RK (2003). Controlled-release oxycodone for pain in diabetic neuropathy. A randomized controlled trial. *Neurology* **60**:927–934 (Class I).

Goldstein DJ, Lu Y, Detke MJ *et al.* (2005) Duloxetine versus placebo in patients with painful diabetic neuropathy. *Pain* **116**:109–118 (Class I).

Gomez-Perez FJ, Choza R, Rios JM *et al.* (1996). Nortriptyline-fluphenazine vs. carbamazepine in the symptomatic treatment of diabetic neuropathy. *Arch Med Res* **27**:525–529 (Class II).

Hahn K, Arendt G, Braun JS (2004). German Neuro-AIDS Working Group. A placebo-controlled trial of gabapentin for painful HIV-associated sensory neuropathies. *J Neurol* **251**:1260–1266 (Class II).

Hammack JE, Michalak JC, Loprinzi CL *et al.* (2002). Phase III evaluation of nortriptyline for alleviation of symptoms of cis-platinum-induced peripheral neuropathy. *Pain* **98**:195–203 (Class II).

Hansson P (2003). Difficulties in stratifying neuropathic pain by mechanisms. *Eur J Pain* **7**:353–357.

Harati Y, Gooch C, Swenson M *et al.* (1998). Edelman S, Greene D, Raskin P, Donofria P, Cornblath D, Sachdeo R, Siu CO, Kamin M. Double-blind randomized trial of tramadol for the treatment of diabetic neuropathy. *Neurology* **50**:1842–1846 (Class I).

Hardy JR, Rees EA, Gwilliam B, Ling J, Broadley K, A'Hern R (2001). A phase II study to establish the efficacy and toxicity of sodium valproate in patients with cancer-related neuropathic pain. *J Pain Symptom Manage* **1**:204–209 (Class II).

Hempenstall K, Nurmikko TJ, Johnson RW *et al.* (2005). Analgesic therapy in postherpetic neuralgia: a quantitative systematic review. *PLoS Med* **2**:628–644.

Hughes RA, Wijdicks EF, Benson E *et al.* (2005). Multidisciplinary Consensus Group. Supportive care for patients with Guillain–Barrè syndrome. *Arch Neurol* **62**:1194–1198.

Huse E, Larbig W, Flor H *et al.* (2001). Birbaumer N. The effect of opioids on phantom limb pain and cortical reorganization. *Pain* **90**:47–55. *J Clin Oncol* **22**:2909–2917 (Class II).

Jensen TS (2002). Anticonvulsants in neuropathic pain: rationale and clinical evidence. *Eur J Pain* **6(Suppl A)**:61–68.

Jensen TS, Baron R (2003). Translation of symptoms and signs into mechanisms in neuropathic pain. *Pain* **102**:1–8.

Kalso E, Tasmuth T, Neuvonen PJ (1996). Amitriptyline effectively relieves neuropathic pain following treatment of breast cancer. *Pain* **64**:293–302 (Class II).

Kalso E, Allan L, Dellemijn PL, Faura CC, Ilias WK, Jensen TS, Perrot S, Plaghki LH, Zenz M (2003). Recommendations for using opioids in chronic non-cancer pain. *Eur J Pain* **7**:381–386.

Kemper CA, Kent G, Burton S *et al.* (1998). Deresinski SC. Mexiletine for HIV-infected patients with painful peripheral neuropathy: a double-blind, placebo-controlled, crossover treatment trial. *J Acquir Immune Defic Syndr Hum Retrovirol* **19**:367–372 (Class I).

Kieburtz K, Simpson D, Yiannoutsos C *et al.* (1998). A randomized trial of amitriptyline and mexiletine for painful neuropathy in HIV infection. AIDS Clinical Trial Group 242 Protocol Team. *Neurology* **51**:1682–1688 (Class I).

Kingery WS (1997). A critical review of controlled clinical trials for peripheral neuropathic pain and complex regional pain syndromes. *Pain* **73**:123–139.

Kishore-Kumar R, Max MB, Schafer SC et al. (1990). Desipramine relieves postherpetic neuralgia. *Clin Pharmacol Ther* **47:**305–312 (Class II).

Kochar DK, Jain N, Agarwal RP et al. (2002). Sodium valproate in the management of painful polyneuropathy in type 2 diabetes–a randomized placebo controlled study. *Acta Neurol Scand* **106:**248–252 (Class II).

Kochar DK, Rawat N, Agrawal RP et al. (2004). Sodium valproate for painful diabetic neuropathy: a randomised double-blind placebo-controlled study. *QJM* **97:**33–38 (Class II).

Kochar DK, Garg P, Bumb RA et al. (2005). Divalproex sodium in the management of post-herpetic neuralgia: a randomized double-blind placebo-controlled study. *QJM* **98:**29–34.

Kondziolka D, Lemley T, Kestle JR et al. (1994). The effect of single-application topical ophthalmic anesthesia in patients with trigeminal neuralgia. A randomized double-blind placebo-controlled trial. *J Neurosurg* **80:**993–997 (Class I).

Kutluay E, McCague K, D'Souza J et al. (2003). Safety and tolerability of oxcarbazepine in elderly patients with epilepsy. *Epilepsy Behav* **4:**175–180.

Langohr HD, Stohr M, Petruch F (1982). An open and double-blind cross-over study on the efficacy of clomipramine (Anafranil) in patients with painful mono- and polyneuropathies. *Eur Neurol* **21:**309–317 (Class II).

Lechin F, van der Dijs B, Lechin ME et al. (1989). Pimozide therapy for trigeminal neuralgia. *Arch Neurol* **46:**960–963 (Class II).

Leijon G, Boivie J (1989). Central post-stroke pain–a controlled trial of amitriptyline and carbamazepine. *Pain* **36:**27–36 (Class I).

Lesser H, Sharma U, LaMoreaux L et al. (2004). Pregabalin relieves symptoms of painful diabetic neuropathy. *Neurology* **63:**2104–2110 (Class I).

Levendoglu F, Ogun CO, Ozerbil O et al. (2004). Gabapentin is a first line drug for the treatment of neuropathic pain in spinal cord injury. *Spine* **29:**743–751 (Class II).

Liebel JT, Menger N, Langohr H (2001). Oxcarbazepine in der Behandlung der Trigeminus neuralgie. *Nervenheilkunde* **20:**461–465 (Class II).

Lindstrom P, Lindblom U (1987). The analgesic effect of tocainide in trigeminal neuralgia. *Pain* **28:**45–50 (Class II).

Maier C, Dertwinkel R, Mansourian N et al. (2003). Efficacy of the NMDA-receptor antagonist memantine in patients with chronic phantom limb pain–results of a randomized double-blinded, placebo-controlled trial. *Pain* **103:**277–283 (Class I).

Max MB, Schafer SC, Culnane M et al. (1988). Amitriptyline, but not lorazepam, relieves postherpetic neuralgia. *Neurology* **38:**1427–1432 (Class II).

Max MB, Kishore-Kumar R, Schafer SC et al. (1991). Efficacy of desipramine in painful diabetic neuropathy: a placebo-controlled trial. *Pain* **45:**3–9 (Class I).

McCleane G (2000). Topical application of doxepin hydrochloride, capsaicin and a combination of both produces analgesia in chronic human neuropathic pain: a randomized, double-blind, placebo-controlled study. *Br J Clin Pharmacol* **49:**574–579 (Class III).

McCleane GJ (1999). 200 mg daily of lamotrigine has no analgesic effect in neuropathic pain: a randomised, double-blind, placebo controlled trial. *Pain* **83:**105–107 (Class III).

McQuay HJ (2002). Neuropathic pain: evidence matters. *Eur J Pain* **6(Suppl A):**11–18.

McQuay HJ, Carroll D, Jadad AR et al. (1994). Dextromethorphan for the treatment of neuropathic pain: a double-blind randomised controlled crossover trial with integral n-of-1 design. *Pain* **59:**127–133 (Class II).

Meier T, Wasner G, Faust M et al. (2003). Efficacy of lidocaine patch 5% in the treatment of focal peripheral neuropathic pain syndromes: a randomized, double-blind, placebo-controlled study. *Pain* **106:**151–158 (Class II).

Mercadante S, Arcuri E, Tirelli W et al. (2002). Amitriptyline in neuropathic cancer pain in patients on morphine therapy: a randomized placebo-controlled, double-blind crossover study. *Tumori* **88:**239–242 (Class II).

Morello CM, Leckband SG, Stoner CP et al. (1999). Randomized double-blind study comparing the efficacy of gabapentin with amitriptyline on diabetic peripheral neuropathy pain. *Arch Intern Med* **159:**1931–1937 (Class II).

Nelson KA, Park KM, Robinovitz E et al. (1997). High-dose oral dextromethorphan versus placebo in painful diabetic neuropathy and postherpetic neuralgia. *Neurology* **48:** 1212–1218 (Class I).

Nurmikko T, Bowsher D (1990). Somatosensory findings in postherpetic neuralgia. *J Neurol Neurosurg Psychiatry* **53:**135–141.

Nurmikko TJ, Eldridge PR (2001). Trigeminal neuralgia-pathophysiology, diagnosis and current treatment. *Br J Anaesth* **87:**117–132.

Otto M, Bach FW, Jensen TS et al. (2004). Valproic acid has no effect on pain in polyneuropathy: a randomized controlled trial. *Neurology* **62:**285–288 (Class I).

Otto M, Bak S, Bach FW et al. (2003). Pain phenomena and possible mechanisms in patients with painful polyneuropathy. *Pain* **101:**187–192.

Paice JA, Ferrans CE, Lashley FR *et al.* (2000). Topical capsaicin in the management of HIV-associated peripheral neuropathy. *J Pain Symptom Manage* **19**:45–52 (Class I).

Pandey CK, Bose N, Garg G *et al.* (2002). Gabapentin for the treatment of pain in Guillain–Barre syndrome: a double-blinded, placebo-controlled, crossover study. *Anesth Analg* **95**:1719–1723 (Class II).

Pandey CK, Raza M, Tripathi M *et al.* (2005). The comparative evaluation of gabapentin and carbamazepine for pain management in Guillain-Barre syndrome patients in the intensive care unit. *Anesth Analg* **101**:220–225 (Class II).

Panerai AE, Monza G, Movilia P *et al.* (1990). A randomized, within-patient, cross-over, placebo-controlled trial on the efficacy and tolerability of the tricyclic antidepressants chlorimipramine and nortriptyline in central pain. *Acta Neurol Scand* **82**:34–38 (Class II).

Raja SN, Haythornwaite JA, Pappagallo M *et al.* (2002). Opioids versus antidepressants in postherpetic neuralgia. *Neurology* **59**:1015–1021 (Class I).

Raskin P, Donofrio PD, Rosenthal NR *et al.* (2004). Topiramate vs placebo in painful diabetic polyneuropathy: analgesic and metabolic effects. *Neurology* **63**:865–873 (Class I).

Raskin J, Pritchett YL, Wang F *et al.* (2005). A double-blind, randomized multicenter trial comparing duloxetine with placebo in the management of diabetic peripheral neuropathic pain. *Pain Med* **6**:346–356.

Rasmussen PV, Sindrup SH, Jensen TS *et al.* (2004). Symptoms and signs in patients with suspected neuropathic pain. *Pain* **110**:461–469.

Ray WA, Meredith S, Thapa PB *et al.* (2004). Cyclic antidepressants and the risk of sudden cardiac death. *Clin Pharmacol Ther* **75**:234–241.

Rice ASC, Maton S (2001). Post Herpetic Neuralgia Study Group. Gabapentin in postherpetic neuralgia; a randomised, double-blind, controlled study. *Pain* **94**:215–224 (Class I).

Richter RW, Portenoy R, Sharma U *et al.* (2005). Relief of diabetic peripheral neuropathy with pregabalin: a randomised placebo-controlled trial. *J Pain* **6**:253–260 (Class I).

Robinson LR, Czerniecki JM, Ehde DM *et al.* (2004). Trial of amitriptyline for relief of pain in amputees: results of a randomized controlled study. *Arch Phys Med Rehabil* **85**:1–6 (Class II).

Rog DJ, Nurmikko TJ, Friede T *et al.* (2005). Randomized, controlled trial of cannabis-based medicine in central pain in multiple sclerosis. *Neurology* **65**:812–819 (Class I).

Rosenstock J, Tuchmann M, LaMoreaux L *et al.* (2004). Pregabalin for the treatment of painful diabetic peripheral neuropathy: a double-blind, placebo-controlled trial. *Pain* **110**:628–638 (Class I).

Rowbotham MC, Harden N, Stacey B *et al.* (1998). Gabapentin for treatment of postherpetic neuralgia. *JAMA* **280**:1837–1843 (Class I).

Rowbotham MC, Twilling L, Davies PS *et al.* (2003). Oral opioid therapy for chronic peripheral and central neuropathic pain. *N Eng J Med* **348**:1223–1232 (Class II).

Rowbotham MC, Goli V, Kunz NR *et al.* (2004). Venlafaxine extended release in the treatment of painful diabetic neuropathy: a double-blind, placebo-controlled study. *Pain* **110**:697–706 (Class I).

Rull JA, Quibrera R, Gonzalez-Millan H *et al.* (1969). Symptomatic treatment of peripheral diabetic neuropathy with carbamazepine (Tegretol): double blind crossover trial. *Diabetologia* **5**:215–218 (Class I).

Saarto T, Wiffen P (2005). Antidepressants for neuropathic pain. *Cochrane Database Syst Rev* **20**(3):CD005454.

Sabatowski R, Galvez R, Cherry DA *et al.* (2004). Pregabalin reduces pain and improves sleep and mood disturbances in patients with post-herpetic neuralgia: results of a randomised, placebo-controlled clinical trial. *Pain* **109**:26–35 (Class I).

Sang CN, Booher S, Gilron I *et al.* (2002). Dextromethorphan and memantine in painful diabetic neuropathy and postherpetic neuralgia. Efficacy and dose-response trials. *Anesthesiology* **96**:1053–1061 (Class I).

Scadding JW, Wall PD, Parry CB *et al.* (1982). Clinical trial of propranolol in post-traumatic neuralgia. *Pain* **14**:283–292 (Class II).

Semenchuk MR, Sherman S, Davis B (2001). Double-blind, randomized trial of bupropion SR for the treatment of neuropathic pain. *Neurology* **57**:1583–1588 (Class I).

Serpell MG (2002). Neuropathic pain study group. Gabapentin in neuropathic pain syndromes: a randomised, double-blind, placebo-controlled trial. *Pain* **99**:557–566 (Class II).

Shlay JC, Chaloner K, Max MB *et al.* (1998). Acupuncture and amitriptyline for pain due to HIV-related peripheral neuropathy: a randomized controlled trial. Terry Beirn Community Programs for Clinical Research on AIDS. *JAMA* **280**:1590–1595 (Class I).

Simpson DA (2001). Gabapentin and venlafaxine for the treatment of painful diabetic neuropathy. *J Clin Neuromusc Dis* **3**:53–62 (Class II).

Simpson DM, Olney R, McArthur JC *et al.* (2000). A placebo-controlled trial of lamotrigine for painful HIV-associated neuropathy. *Neurology* **54**:2115–2119 (Class II).

Simpson DM, McArthur JC, Olney R *et al.* (2003). Lamotrigine for HIV-associated painful sensory neuropathies: A placebo-controlled trial. *Neurology* **60:**1508–1514 (Class I).

Sindrup SH, Jensen TS (1999). Efficacy of pharmacological treatments of neuropathic pain: an update and effect related to mechanism of action. *Pain* **83:** 389–400.

Sindrup SH, Jensen TS (2000). Pharmacologic treatment of pain in polyneuropathy. *Neurology* **55:**915–920.

Sindrup SH, Jensen TS (2002). Pharmacotherapy of trigeminal neuralgia. *Clin J Pain* **18:**22–27.

Sindrup SH, Gram LF, Skjold T *et al.* (1990). Clomipramine vs desipramine vs placebo in the treatment of diabetic neuropathy symptoms. A double-blind cross-over study. *Br J Clin Pharmacol* **30:**683–691 (Class I).

Sindrup SH, Andersen G, Madsen C *et al.* (1999). Tramadol relieves pain and allodynia in polyneuropathy: a randomised, double-blind, controlled trial. *Pain* **83:**85–90 (Class I).

Sindrup SH, Bach FW, Madsen C *et al.* (2003). Venlafaxine versus imipramine in painful polyneuropathy. A randomized, controlled trial. *Neurology* **60:**1284–1289 (Class I).

Sindrup SH, Otto M, Finnerup NB *et al.* (2005). Antidepressants in the treatment of neuropathic pain. *Basic Clin Pharmacol Ther* **96:**399–409.

Svendsen KB, Jensen TS, Bach FW (2004). The cannabinoid dronabinol reduces central pain in Multiple Sclerosis. A randomised double-blind placebo controlled cross-over trial. *BMJ* **329:**253–261 (Class I).

Tasmuth T, Hartel B, Kalso E (2002). Venlafaxine in neuropathic pain following treatment of breast cancer. *Eur J Pain* **6:**17–24 (Class II).

Thienel U, Neto W, Schwabe SK *et al.* (2004). Topiramate Diabetic Neuropathic Pain Study Group. Topiramate in painful diabetic polyneuropathy: findings from three double-blind placebo-controlled trials. *Acta Neurol Scand* **110:**221–231.

Vestergaard K, Andersen G, Gottrup H *et al.* (2001). Lamotrigine for central poststroke pain: A randomized controlled trial. *Neurology* **56:**184–190 (Class I).

Vilming ST, Lyberg T, Lataste X (1986). Tizanidine in the management of trigeminal neuralgia. *Cephalalgia* **6:**181–182 (Class III).

Vrethem M, Boivie J, Arnqvist H *et al.* (1997). A comparison a amitriptyline and maprotiline in the treatment of painful polyneuropathy in diabetics and nondiabetics. *Clin J Pain* **13:**313–323 (Class I).

Wallace MS, Magnuson S, Ridgeway B (2000). Efficacy of oral mexiletine for neuropathic pain with allodynia: a double-blind, placebo-controlled, crossover study. *Reg Anesth Pain Med* **25:**459–467 (Class I).

Wasner G, Kleinert A, Binder A *et al.* (2005). Postherpetic neuralgia: topical lidocaine is effective in nociceptor-deprived skin. *J Neurol* **252:**677–686 (Class II).

Watson CP, Evans RJ (1992). The postmastectomy pain syndrome and topical capsaicin: a randomized trial. *Pain* **51:**375–379 (Class II).

Watson CP, Babul N (1998). Efficacy of oxycodone in neuropathic pain: a randomized trial in postherpetic neuralgia. *Neurology* **50:**1837–1841 (Class I).

Watson CP, Evans RJ, Reed K *et al.* (1982). Amitryptiline versus placebo in post-herpetic neuralgia. *Neurology* **32:**671–673 (Class II).

Watson CP, Chipman M, Reed K *et al.* (1992). Amitriptyline versus maprotiline in postherpetic neuralgia: a randomized, double-blind, crossover trial. *Pain* **48:**29–36 (Class II).

Watson CP, Tyler KL, Bickers DR *et al.* (1993). A randomized vehicle-controlled trial of topical capsaicin in the treatment of postherpetic neuralgia. *Clin Ther* **15:**510–526 (Class I).

Watson CP, Vernich L, Chipman M *et al.* (1998). Nortriptyline versus amitriptyline in postherpetic neuralgia: a randomized trial. *Neurology* **51:**1166–1171 (Class II).

Watson CP, Moulin D, Watt-Watson J *et al.* (2003). Controlled-release oxycodone relieves neuropathic pain: a randomized controlled trial in painful diabetic neuropathy. *Pain* **105:**71–78 (Class I).

Wiffen P, McQuay H, Edwards J *et al.* (2005a). Gabapentin for acute and chronic pain. *Cochrane Database Syst Rev* **20**(3):CD005452.

Wiffen P, McQuay H, Moore R (2005b). Carbamazepine for acute and chronic pain. *Cochrane Database Syst Rev* **20**(3):CD005451.

Wiffen P, Collins S, McQuay H *et al.* (2005c). Anticonvulsant drugs for acute and chronic pain. *Cochrane Database Syst Rev* **20**(3):CD001133.

Wilton TD (1974). Tegretol in the treatment of diabetic neuropathy. *S Afr Med J* **48:** 869–872 (Class III).

Woolf CJ, Max MB (2001). Mechanism-based pain diagnosis: issues for analgesic drug development. *Anesthesiology* **95:**241–249.

Zakrzewska JM, Chaudhry Z, Nurmikko TJ *et al.* (1997). Lamotrigine (lamictal) in refractory trigeminal neuralgia: results from a double-blind placebo controlled crossover trial. *Pain* **73:**223–230 (Class II).

CHAPTER 30

Acute relapses of multiple sclerosis

F. Sellebjerg,[a] D. Barnes,[b] G. Filippini,[c]
R. Midgard,[d] X. Montalban,[e] P. Rieckmann,[f]
K. Selmaj,[g] L.H. Visser,[h] P. Soelberg Sørensen[a]

Abstract

Background Relapses, exacerbations or attacks of multiple sclerosis (MS) are the dominating features of relapsing–remitting MS, but are also observed in patients with secondary progressive MS. High-dose methylprednisolone is the routine therapy for relapses at present, but other treatments are also in current use.

Objectives The objective of the task force was to review the literature on treatment of MS relapses to provide evidence-based treatment recommendations.

Methods Review of the literature with classification of evidence according to the European Federation of Neurological Societies (EFNS) guidelines for scientific task forces.

Recommendations Short-term, high-dose methylprednisolone treatment should be considered for the treatment of relapses of MS (Recommendation Level A). The optimal glucocorticoid treatment regimen, in terms of clinical efficacy and adverse events, remains to be established. A more intense, interdisciplinary rehabilitation programme should be considered as this probably further improves recovery after treatment with methylprednisolone (Recommendation Level B). Plasma exchange is probably efficacious in a subgroup of patients with severe relapses not responding to methylprednisolone therapy, and should be considered in this patient subgroup (Recommendation Level B). There is a need for further randomised, controlled trials to establish the optimal treatment regimen for relapses of MS.

Background

Relapses, exacerbations or attacks of multiple sclerosis (MS) are the dominating feature of relapsing–remitting MS, but are also observed in patients with secondary progressive MS with superimposed relapses. Even patients with primary progressive MS may experience relapses (Lublin and Rheingold, 1996; Confavreux *et al.*, 2000). In the McDonald criteria for the diagnosis of MS, a relapse

---

[a]Danish MS Centre, Copenhagen University Hospital, Denmark; [b]Department of Neurology, Atkinson Morley's Hospital, Wimbledon, United Kingdom; [c]Unit of Epidemiology and Clinical Trial Centre, Istituto Nazionale Neurologico C. Besta, Milan, Italy; [d]Department of Neurology, Molde Hospital, Norway;

[e]Clinical Neuroimmunology Unit, University Hospital Vall d'Hebron, Barcelona, Spain; [f]Department of Neurology, Julius-Maximilians University of Würzburg, Germany; [g]Department of Neurology, Medical University of Lodz, Poland; [h]Department of Neurology, St. Elisabeth Hospital, Tilburg, The Netherlands.

is defined as 'an episode of neurological disturbance of the kind seen in MS, when the clinicopathological studies have established that the causative lesions are inflammatory and demyelinating in nature' (McDonald *et al.*, 2001). An attack should last for at least 24 h and, according to the McDonald criteria, there should be expert opinion that the event is not a pseudoattack as might be caused by an increase in body temperature or infection. Multiple episodes of paroxysmal symptoms, for example, tonic spasms or trigeminal neuralgia occurring over not less than 24 h, may also constitute a relapse. Although the majority of relapses improve to some extent, incomplete recovery is an important determinant of irreversible neurological impairment in MS at least in the earlier stages of MS (Confavreux *et al.*, 2003; Lublin *et al.*, 2004).

Glucocorticoid treatment is recommended as the first-line treatment of MS relapses in North American guidelines and in the recommendations of a European consensus group on therapy in MS (Goodin *et al.*, 2002; Multiple Sclerosis Therapy Consensus Group, 2004). Other treatments for MS relapses have also been studied in clinical trials. The aim of the European Federation of Neurological Societies (EFNS) task force on treatment of MS relapses was to review the current literature on relapse treatment. Important issues to consider were whether treatment of MS relapses: (1) can improve the speed of recovery; (2) can influence long-term recovery; (3) can influence subsequent disease activity; (4) has significant side effects. Furthermore, the task force sought to provide guidelines on whether all relapses should be treated and how relapses during pregnancy should be managed.

Search strategy

We searched literature databases (Embase and PubMed), in English, for papers using the search terms 'multiple sclerosis', 'attack', 'relapse', 'exacerbation' and 'treatment' in November 2004. The Cochrane Library and the reference lists of individual papers were searched for studies not identified in the Embase and PubMed searches. Studies of various treatments for patients suffering from relapses of MS were considered for the guidelines and were

rated as class I to class IV studies according to the recommendations for EFNS scientific task forces (Brainin *et al.*, 2004).

Method for reaching consensus

The results of the literature searches were circulated by e-mail to the task force members for comments. The task force chairman prepared a first draft of the manuscript based on the results of the literature review and comments from the task force members. The draft and the recommendations were discussed during telephone conferences until consensus was reached within the task force. Recommendations were rated from A to C according to the EFNS guidelines for scientific task forces (Brainin *et al.*, 2004). Where there was insufficient evidence to support firm recommendations the term 'Good Practice Point' was used.

Results

Effect of glucocorticoid and adrenocorticotrophic hormone (ACTH) treatment on MS relapses

Glucocorticoid or ACTH treatment of MS relapses was analysed in a Cochrane review that included results from six randomised, placebo-controlled clinical trials of either ACTH (two trials), intravenous (i.v.) methylprednisolone treatment (three trials) or oral methylprednisolone treatment (one trial) (Miller *et al.*, 1961; Rose *et al.*, 1970; Durelli *et al.*, 1986; Milligan *et al.*, 1987; Filipovic *et al.*, 1997; Sellebjerg *et al.*, 1998). All trials reported a benefit in terms of rate of recovery compared to placebo (Filippini *et al.*, 2000). A similar conclusion was reached in another meta-analysis, which used less stringent criteria for study inclusion than the Cochrane review (Brusaferri and Candelise, 2000).

Three trials have compared the relative efficacy of i.v. methylprednisolone and ACTH treatment in MS relapses (Abbruzzese *et al.*, 1983; Barnes *et al.*, 1985; Thompson *et al.*, 1989). One study including 14 patients treated with i.v. methylprednisolone (1 g daily for 7 days) and 11 patients treated with intramuscular (IM) ACTH (80 units, 60 units, 40 units and 20 units daily, each for 1 week) reported more rapid improvement (after 3 and 28 days) after i.v. methylprednisolone treatment than after ACTH treatment, but there was no significant difference after 3 months (Barnes *et al.*, 1985). The patient blinding and the primary outcome were not clearly defined, however, for which reason this study should be considered a class III study. One class II study compared the administration of 1 g of methylprednisolone once daily for 3 days to ACTH treatment (80 units for 7 days, 40 units for 4 days and 20 units for 3 days) in 61 patients, and found no difference in terms of rate of recovery or final outcome after 12 weeks (Thompson *et al.*, 1989). A class III study including 60 patients, treated with either i.v. methylprednisolone (20 mg/kg day 1–3, 10 mg/kg day 4–7, 5 mg/kg day 8–10, and 1 mg/kg day 11–15) or ACTH (1 mg i.v. daily for 15 days), also did not provide evidence of any difference in the efficacy of ACTH and methylprednisolone treatment (Abbruzzese *et al.*, 1983). These three studies found no major differences in adverse events between methylprednisolone and ACTH treatment. Thus there is no evidence of any major difference in the efficacy of ACTH and methylprednisolone treatment from comparative studies, but the clinical trials were too small to rule out some difference in efficacy. Indeed, in the Cochrane review it was suggested that methylprednisolone treatment could still confer greater benefit than treatment with ACTH, and the administration of methylprednisolone is simpler than the more prolonged treatment with ACTH (Filippini *et al.*, 2000).

In a separate meta-analysis (Miller *et al.*, 2000) of three double-blind, randomised, controlled trials comparing methylprednisolone treatment (500 mg or more daily) to placebo, it was concluded that treatment with i.v. methylprednisolone (15 mg/kg day 1–3, 10 mg/kg day 4–6, 5 mg/kg day 7–9, 2.5 mg/kg day 10–12 , 1 mg/kg day 13–15 followed by oral prednisone tapered slowly over 120 days; Durelli *et al.*, 1986), i.v. methylprednisolone without a tapering dose (500 mg once daily for 5 days; Milligan *et al.*, 1987), or oral methylprednisolone (500 mg once daily for 5 days followed by 400, 300, 200, 100, 64, 48, 32, 16, 8, and 8 mg once daily the subsequent 10 days; Sellebjerg *et al.*, 1998) resulted in significantly faster recovery

than did treatment with placebo (table 30.1). The two first trials provided follow-up data in a placebo-controlled design for 15 days (Durelli *et al.*, 1986) and 28 days (Milligan *et al.*, 1987). The oral methylprednisolone study found significant differences between the methylprednisolone and the placebo group after 8 weeks, but there was no significant difference in the outcome after 1 year (Sellebjerg *et al.*, 1998). In the latter trial there was no evidence that the 1-year risk of subsequent relapses was influenced by oral high-dose methylprednisolone treatment.

Specific glucocorticoids, dose, and route of administration

The clinical trials of glucocorticoid treatment in relapses of MS have mainly assessed the effect of methylprednisolone treatment. Two trials have compared the effect of methylprednisolone treatment given i.v. or orally. One class III study compared the effect of methylprednisolone (500 mg once daily for 5 days) given orally or i.v. in 35 patients with an MS relapse, and found no significant difference in recovery between the two treatment arms after 5 and 28 days (Alam *et al.*, 1993). Another study (class I) compared the effect of oral methylprednisolone (48 mg daily for 7 days, 24 mg daily for 7 days, and 12 mg daily for 7 days) to treatment with i.v. methylprednisolone (1 g daily for 3 days) (Barnes *et al.*, 1997). In this study, recovery from the relapse was similar in the 38 patients in the i.v. treatment group and the 42 patients in the oral treatment group at all time points for up to 24 weeks of follow-up. The relapse rate the following 2 years was also similar in the oral and i.v. treatment group (Sharrack *et al.*, 2000).

Oral tapering doses of glucocorticoids have been used in many trials, but none have compared the outcome of a relapse in patients treated with tapering doses of glucocorticoids or placebo following short-term high-dose treatment.

Three studies have compared i.v. methylprednisolone treatment given in different doses. One class III study found that recovery was faster after treatment with i.v. methylprednisolone (1 g once daily for 5 days) than after a single 1 g dose of

Table 30.1 Summary of three randomised, placebo-controlled trials comparing methylprednisolone (MP) treatment to placebo in patients with relapses of MS (Durelli *et al.*, 1986; Milligan *et al.*, 1987; Sellebjerg *et al.*, 1998). Data are changes in Kurtzke EDSS scores from baseline (mean and standard deviation in brackets) or differences (mean and 95% confidence intervals in brackets) between MP and placebo reported in a meta-analysis (Miller *et al.*, 2000).

Study and treatment	Change from baseline	Difference (MP vs. placebo)
Day 5–7		
Durelli, placebo ($n = 8$)	0(0)	
i.v. methylprednisolone ($n = 12$)	−1.00(0.6)	−1.00 (−1.45 to −0.55)
Milligan, placebo ($n = 9$)	−0.28(0.51)	
i.v. methylprednisolone ($n = 13$)	−1.46(1.38)	−1.18(−2.19 to −0.17)
Sellebjerg, placebo ($n = 25$)	−0.06(0.44)	
Oral methylprednisolone ($n = 26$)	−0.58(0.82)	−0.52(−0.89 to −0.14)
Pooled difference:		−0.76 (standard error 0.14)
Day 21–28		
Durelli, placebo ($n = 8$)	−0.38(0.52)	
i.v. methylprednisolone ($n = 12$)	−2.04(1.48)	−1.67(−2.82 to −0.51)
Milligan, placebo ($n = 8$)	−0.25(1.22)	
i.v. methylprednisolone ($n = 13$)	−2.04(1.51)	−1.79(−3.11 to −0.46)
Sellebjerg, placebo ($n = 25$)	−0.38(0.81)	
Oral methylprednisolone ($n = 26$)	−0.94(0.90)	−0.56(−1.04 to −0.08)
Pooled difference:		−0.85 (standard error 0.21)

i.v. methylprednisolone (Bindoff *et al.*, 1988). Two other studies (both class III) have compared the effect of different doses of i.v. methylprednisolone in relapses of MS on a panel of different outcome measures. In the first study, treatment with i.v. methylprednisolone at a dose of 500 mg once daily for 5 days was compared to treatment with 2000 mg once daily for 5 days in thirty-one patients with a relapse of MS (Oliveri *et al.*, 1998). There was no difference in the efficacy of the low dose and the high dose of methylprednisolone in terms of clinical recovery or short-term suppression of magnetic resonance imaging (MRI) disease activity, but it was suggested that the high dose resulted in more pronounced suppression of MRI disease activity after 1 and 2 months. In the second study, i.v. methylprednisolone at a dose of 1 g or 2 g once daily for 5 days was compared in 24 patients who were followed up with clinical and neurophysiologic studies for 21 days after randomisation to one of the two treatment arms (Fierro *et al.*, 2002). This study showed no significant differences between the two methylprednisolone doses on the majority of diverse outcome measures, but a few favoured the higher dose over the lower dose. Two studies have compared the effect of treatment with different doses of methylprednisolone and dexamethasone in relapses of MS (Milanese *et al.*, 1989; La Mantia *et al.*, 1994). Due to the small sample sizes and the differences in the baseline characteristics of the patients randomised to the different treatment arms, the results of these two studies are difficult to interpret.

Glucocorticoid treatment of acute optic neuritis

In the North American Optic Neuritis Treatment Trial (ONTT) 457 patients were randomised to receive treatment with i.v. methylprednisolone (250 mg four times daily for 3 days followed by oral prednisone, 1 mg/kg for 11 days, 20 mg on day 15, and 10 mg on days 16 and 18), oral prednisone (1 mg/kg for 14 days, 20 mg on day 15, and 10 mg on days 16 and 18), or oral placebo

(Beck *et al.*, 1992). Treatment allocation was not blinded in patients randomised to treatment with i.v. methylprednisolone, while prednisone treatment and placebo was given in a double-blind design. Thus, the study was regarded as a class II study investigating the efficacy of methylprednisolone treatment, but as a class I study in the comparison of oral prednisone and placebo. The study found no significant effect of i.v. methylprednisolone or oral prednisone treatment on the recovery of visual acuity, but the recovery of contrast sensitivity and visual fields was significantly faster in patients treated with i.v. methylprednisolone. After 6 months, patients treated with i.v. methylprednisolone had still recovered slightly better than patients treated with placebo, but no significant treatment effect was seen at follow-up after 1 year (Beck *et al.*, 1993a). Oral prednisone treatment had no effect on the recovery from acute optic neuritis in neither the ONTT nor a Danish class I study of oral prednisolone versus placebo in 128 patients with acute optic neuritis (Beck *et al.*, 1992; J.L. Frederiksen, personal communication). Treatment with oral methylprednisolone (100 mg, 80 mg, 60 mg, 40 mg, 30 mg, 20 mg, 10 mg, and 5 mg daily for 3 days each) was not better than treatment with oral thiamine (100 mg daily for 24 days) on any of several outcome measures in a class II study including 38 patients with acute optic neuritis (Trauzettel-Klosinski *et al.*, 1993).

Two additional studies (class I) have compared the effect of treatment with high-dose methylprednisolone in acute optic neuritis. One study included 60 patients with acute optic neuritis who were treated with oral high-dose methylprednisolone (500 mg once daily for 5 days followed by 400, 300, 200, 100, 64, 48, 32, 16, 8, and 8 mg once daily the subsequent 10 days) or oral placebo (Sellebjerg *et al.*, 1999). Oral methylprednisolone treatment resulted in significantly better recovery of spatial visual function (visual acuity and contrast sensitivity), colour vision function, and visual symptoms after 1 week, but only borderline significant effects were observed after 3 weeks, and after 8 weeks there was no evidence of an effect of oral methylprednisolone treatment (Sellebjerg *et al.*, 1999). In a study of 66 patients with acute optic neuritis treatment with i.v. methylprednisolone

(1 g once daily for 3 days) did not improve the outcome from acute optic neuritis after 26 weeks on neither a panel of visual function and neurophysiologic variables nor on MRI outcome measures (Kapoor *et al.*, 1998).

A controversial finding in the ONTT was that patients treated with i.v. methylprednisolone appeared to have a lower risk of developing MS during 2 years of follow-up than patients treated with placebo. This was not statistically significant in the original trial report (Beck *et al.*, 1992), but reached a significance level of $p = 0.03$ (not corrected for multiple comparisons) in a *post hoc* analysis where the baseline status of many patients had been reclassified (Beck *et al.*, 1993b; Goodin 1999). It was also suggested that oral prednisone treatment was associated with an increased risk of recurrent optic neuritis, but not an increased risk of subsequently developing MS (Beck *et al.*, 1992 and 1993b). As there was no blinding to methylprednisolone treatment, and as the effect of treatment on MS risk was only observed after reanalysis and reclassification of the initial data, this part of the ONTT must be regarded as a class III study. Another class III study (a retrospective natural history study) has suggested that i.v. methylprednisolone treatment (1 g once daily for 3 days) could actually increase the risk of subsequently developing MS (Herishanu *et al.*, 1989). In the latter study, a surprisingly low risk of conversion to MS was, however, observed in the control group of untreated patients and patients treated with oral prednisone.

Glucocorticoid treatment in MS subgroups

Whether subgroups of patients with MS relapses may benefit more from glucocorticoid treatment has been addressed only in few studies. It has been suggested that patients with more severe relapses are more likely to respond to treatment with i.v. methylprednisolone (class IV evidence, Nos *et al.*, 2004). Another uncontrolled (class IV) study suggested that patients with high cerebrospinal fluid (CSF) concentrations of myelin basic protein (MBP) are more likely to improve after i.v. methylprednisolone treatment (Whitaker *et al.*, 1993). This finding was confirmed using 1-week follow-up data in a *post hoc* analysis of patients included in two randomised, placebo-controlled trials of oral high-dose methylprednisolone treatment (Sellebjerg *et al.*, 2003). However, the additional benefit of methylprednisolone treatment in patients with high CSF concentrations of MBP was not sustained at follow-up after 8 weeks, while patients who had an active gadolinium-enhanced MRI at baseline appeared to benefit from treatment even at follow-up after 8 weeks (class III evidence, Sellebjerg *et al.*, 2003).

Side effects of glucocorticoid treatment

In the placebo-controlled trials serious adverse events were not observed after high-dose methylprednisolone treatment. (Durelli *et al.*, 1986; Milligan *et al.*, 1987; Sellebjerg *et al.*, 1998). Milligan *et al.* (1987) did not report the precise frequency of adverse events, but noted that treatment was surprisingly free from serious adverse events. Those most frequently reported were a slight reddening of the face, transient ankle swelling, and a metallic taste in the mouth during infusion. In the Cochrane review it was concluded that the oral administration of methylprednisolone is associated with a higher frequency of side effects (mainly gastrointestinal and psychic disorders), and that oral administration should be avoided for this reason (Filippini *et al.*, 2000). In the study of Durelli *et al.* (1986), the incidence of elevated mood and insomnia increased during the study from 2 out of 11 patients (18%) treated with intravenous high-dose methylprednisolone at day 5 to 5 out of 11 patients (45%) at day 15. In the study of oral high-dose treatment with an oral tapering dose and a total treatment duration of 15 days, disturbed sleep was observed in 65% and slight mood changes in 23% (Sellebjerg *et al.*, 1998), which is not significantly different from the frequency observed by Durelli and coworkers. In the study by Durelli and coworkers (1986) gastrointestinal side effects were not reported, but all patients received prophylactic antacid treatment. In the study of oral high-dose methylprednisolone treatment gastrointestinal side effects (mainly heartburn not requiring symptomatic treatment) was observed in 38% of patients treated with oral methylprednisolone and 8% in the placebo group (Sellebjerg *et al.*, 1998). The only randomised comparison of i.v. and

oral treatment with methylprednisolone at equivalent doses did not report the exact frequency of side effects, but found that the side effects (including gastrointestinal side effects) of oral and i.v. methylprednisolone treatment were similar (Alam *et al.*, 1993). This is supported by the results of a smaller, non-randomised class III study comparing treatment with i.v. methylprednisolone and oral prednisone at equivalent doses, which also failed to detect any difference in the side effects of oral and i.v. treatment (Metz *et al.*, 1999).

In a review of 240 patients who had been treated with one or more courses of i.v. methylprednisolone (1 g daily for 5 days followed by 10 days of oral prednisone treatment), minor infections were observed in four patients; one patient had a single seizure within 12 h of treatment, eleven patients were noted to have glucosuria during treatment, five had gastrointestinal symptoms that required antacid or H2 antagonist treatment, three patients had an exacerbation of acne, ankle oedema was recorded in two patients, and one patient was hypertensive during treatment. A feeling of well being was common (frequency not given), and four patients had episodes of euphoria whereas two patients were depressive. Transient facial flushing, a transient disturbance of taste, distal paraesthesia, insomnia, and mild weight gain occurred in a significant proportion of patients, but the exact frequency was not stated (Lyons *et al.*, 1988).

Severe side effects of methylprednisolone treatment are rare, but psychosis, acute pancreatitis, and anaphylactoid reactions to i.v. treatment have been reported (Pryse-Phillips *et al.*, 1984; Chrousos *et al.*, 1993; van den Bergh *et al.*, 1997). Short-term methylprednisolone treatment in patients with MS appears to be safe in terms of long-term effects on bone mineralization, but pulsed methylprednisolone treatment has marked short-term effects on bone metabolism, and the available studies do not entirely rule out adverse effects on bone structure (Dovio *et al.*, 2004).

Other treatments

A single class I crossover study of 22 patients with severe relapses of inflammatory demyelination (including 12 with MS) who were refractory to treatment with high-dose methylprednisolone suggested a beneficial effect of treatment with plasma exchange (Weinshenker *et al.*, 1999). In this study there was 'moderate' or 'marked' improvement during plasma exchange treatment in 8 out of 19 patients (42%), whereas such improvement was observed only after 1 out of 17 courses (6%) of sham treatment (*p*=0.01). An effect of plasma exchange on 10 patients with acute optic neuritis who had not improved after high-dose i.v. methylprednisolone treatment has also been reported in an open (class IV) study (Ruprecht *et al.*, 2004).

A Cochrane review and studies of treatment with intravenous immunoglobulin (IVIG) have shown that prophylactic treatment may result in a decrease in the number of relapses in patients with relapsing–remitting MS (Sørensen *et al.*, 2002; Gray *et al.*, 2003). A single class IV study of IVIG treatment in relapses of MS suggested that as many as 68% of patients improved within 24 h of treatment (Soukop and Tschabitscher, 1986). Two recent studies have investigated if IVIG treatment as add-on to therapy with high-dose i.v. methylprednisolone is superior to add-on placebo treatment (Sørensen *et al.*, 2004: class I study; Visser *et al.*, 2004: class II study). Both studies were negative on primary and secondary end-points. In addition, a randomised class I trial of treatment with IVIG or placebo in 68 patients with acute optic neuritis failed to detect any treatment effect (Roed *et al.*, 2005). Similarly, whereas treatment with natalizumab appears to lower the frequency of relapses in MS, natalizumab was not efficacious in the treatment of relapses in a randomised, placebo-controlled class I study of 180 patients with an MS relapse (O'Connor *et al.*, 2004).

A single class II study compared the effect of multidisciplinary rehabilitation to the effect of 'standard therapy' in a randomised clinical trial design, where both treatment arms received i.v. methylprednisolone treatment. The study suggested that a multidisciplinary team rehabilitation programme results in better functional recovery after 3 months than does treatment with i.v. methylprednisolone in a 'standard' setting (Craig *et al.*, 2003).

Treatment of relapses during pregnancy

There are no specific studies on relapse treatment in pregnant patients with MS, but short-term treatment with glucocorticoids is generally considered safe in pregnant women, and treatment may be considered in patients with a relapse of sufficient severity to warrant treatment, although treatment during the first trimester should probably be avoided (class IV evidence: Ferrero *et al.*, 2004).

RECOMMENDATIONS

There is consistent evidence from several class I studies and meta-analyses for a beneficial effect of glucocorticoid treatment in relapses of MS. Hence, treatment with intravenous or oral methylprednisolone in a dose of at least 500 mg daily for 5 days should be considered for treatment of relapses (Level A). Treatment with i.v. methylprednisolone (1 g once daily for 3 days) should be considered as an alternative treatment (Good Practice Point; Multiple Sclerosis Therapy Consensus Group, 2004). Treatment with i.v. methylprednisolone (1 g once daily for 3 days with an oral tapering dose) may be considered for treatment of acute optic neuritis (Level B).

There is no evidence of major differences in the efficacy of methylprednisolone treatment given i.v. or orally in terms of clinical efficacy or side effects, but prolonged, oral treatment may possibly be associated with a higher prevalence of side effects. Furthermore, due to the low number of patients included in the available clinical trials, some efficacy differences between the i.v. and oral route of administration cannot be excluded. The optimal dosage, the specific glucocorticoid to be used, and whether to use a taper after initial pulse therapy, has not been adequately addressed in randomised, controlled trials. This implies a need for new, randomised studies assessing risk/benefit ratios and adverse effects of specific glucocorticoids, dose, and route of administration for treatment of MS relapses.

There is insufficient data to clearly define patient subgroups who are more likely to respond to methylprednisolone treatment, but treatment may be more efficacious in patients with clinical, MRI, or CSF evidence (increased MBP concentration in CSF) indicating higher disease activity (Recommendation Level C). Administration of treatment in an inpatient or outpatient setting has not been addressed in clinical trials, but consideration should be given to administering the first course of methylprednisolone as an inpatient (Good Practice Point).

In patients who fail to respond to therapy with methylprednisolone in the dose range used in the randomised, placebo-controlled trials (Durelli et al., 1986; Milligan et al., 1987; Filipovic et al., 1997; Sellebjerg et al., 1998), treatment with higher doses (up to 2 g daily for 5 days) should be considered (Recommendation Level C; Multiple Sclerosis Therapy Consensus Group, 2004).

Patients with inflammatory demyelination, including patients with MS, who have not responded to treatment with methylprednisolone may benefit from plasma exchange treatment, but only about one third of treated patients are likely to respond. This treatment regimen should probably be restricted to a subgroup of patients with severe relapses (Recommendation Level B). A randomised, controlled study specifically addressing the effect of plasma exchange in patients with severe relapses of MS not responding to methylprednisolone treatment would be desirable.

A more intense, interdisciplinary rehabilitation programme should be considered after treatment with i.v. methylprednisolone as evidence from a single trial suggests that this probably further improves recovery (Recommendation Level B).

There is insufficient data to support the use of IVIG therapy as monotherapy for relapses of MS. Treatment with IVIG as an add-on to treatment of MS relapses with methylprednisolone or as monotherapy for acute optic neuritis is not efficacious (Recommendation Level A). Neither is natalizumab as monotherapy efficacious in MS relapses.

Conflicts of interest

Finn Sellebjerg has received a travel grant and an unrestricted research grant from Pharmacia.

References

Abbruzzese G, Gandolfo C, Loeb C (1983). 'Bolus' methylprednisolone versus ACTH in the treatment of multiple sclerosis. *Ital J Neurol Sci* **2:**169–172.

Alam SM, Kyriakides T, Lawden M, Newman PK (1993). Methylprednisolone in multiple sclerosis: a comparison of oral with intravenous therapy at equivalent high dose. *J Neurol Neurosurg Psychiatry* **56:**1219–1220.

Barnes D, Hughes RAC, Morris RW et al. (1997). Randomised trial of oral and intravenous methylprednisolone in acute relapses of multiple sclerosis. *Lancet* **349:**902–906.

Barnes MP, Bateman DE, Cleland PG, et al. (1985). Intravenous methylprednisolone for multiple sclerosis in relapse. *J Neurol Neurosurg Psychiatry* **48:**157–159.

Beck RW, Cleary PA, Anderson MM et al. (1992). A randomized, controlled trial of corticosteroids in the treatment of acute optic neuritis. *N Engl J Med* **326:**581–588.

Beck RW, Cleary PA, the Optic Neuritis Study Group (1993a). Optic neuritis treatment trial. One-year follow-up results. *Arch Neurol* **111:**773–775.

Beck RW, Cleary PA, Trobe JD et al. (1993b). The effect of corticosteroids for acute optic neuritis on the subsequent development of multiple sclerosis. *N Engl J Med* **329:**1764–1749.

Bindoff L, Lyons PR, Newman PK, Saunders M (1988). Methylprednisolone in multiple sclerosis: a comparative dose study. *J Neurol Neurosurg Psychiatry* **51:**1108–1109.

Brainin M, Barnes M, Baron J-C, et al. (2004). Guidance for the preparation of neurological management guidelines by ENFS scientific task forces – revised recommendations 2004. *Eur J Neurol* **11:**577–581.

Brusaferri F, Candelise L (2000). Steroids for multiple sclerosis and optic neuritis: a meta-analysis of randomized controlled clinical trials. *J Neurol* **247:**435–442.

Chrousos GA, Kattah JC, Beck RW, Cleary PA, and the Optic Neuritis Study Group (1993). Side effects of glucocorticoid treatment. *JAMA* **269:**2110–2112.

Confavreux C, Vukusic S, Moreau T, Adeleine P (2000). Relapses and progression of disability in multiple sclerosis. *N Engl J Med* **343:**1430–1438.

Confavreux C, Vukusic S, Adeleine P (2003). Early clinical predictors and progression of irreversible disability in multiple sclerosis: an amnesic process. *Brain* **126:**770–782.

Craig J, Young CA, Ennis M, Baker G, Boggild M (2003). A randomised controlled trial comparing rehabilitation against standard therapy in multiple sclerosis patients receiving intravenous steroid treatment. *J Neurol Neurosurg Psychiatry* **74:**1225–1230.

Dovio A, Perazzolo L, Osella G et al. (2004). Immediate fall of bone formation and transient increase of bone resorption in the course of high-dose, short-term glucocorticoid therapy in young patients with multiple sclerosis. *J Clin Endocrin Metab* **89:**4923–4928.

Durelli L, Cocito D, Riccio A (1986). High-dose intravenous methylprednisolone in the treatment of multiple sclerosis. *Neurology* **36:**238–243.

Ferrero S, Pretta S, Ragni N (2004). Multiple sclerosis: management issues during pregnancy. *Eur J Obstet Gynecol Reprod Biol* **115:**3–9.

Fierro B, Salemi G, Brighina F et al. (2002). A transcranial magnetic stimulation study evaluating methylprednisolone treatment in multiple sclerosis. *Acta Neurol Scand* **105:**152–157.

Filippini G, Brusaferri F, Sibley WA, et al. (2000). Corticosteroids or ACTH for acute exacerbations in multiple sclerosis. *Cochrane Database Syst Rev* CD001331.

Filipovic SR, Drulovic J, Stojsavljevic N, Levic Z (1997). The effects of high-dose intravenous methylprednisolone on event-related potentials in patients with multiple sclerosis. *J Neurol Sci* **152:**147–153.

Goodin DS (1999). Perils and pitfalls in the interpretation of clinical trials: a reflection on the recent experience in multiple sclerosis. *Neuroepidemiology* **18:**53–63.

Goodin DS, Frohman EM, Garmany GP, et al. (2002). Disease modifying therapies in multiple sclerosis. Report of the therapeutics and technology assessment subcommittee of the American Academy of Neurology and the MS council for clinical practice guidelines. *Neurology* **58:**169–177.

Gray O, McDonnell GV, Forbes RB (2003). Intravenous immunoglobulins for multiple sclerosis. *Cochrane Database Syst Rev* CD002936.

Herishanu YO, Badarna S, Sarov B, Abarbanel JM, Segal S, Bearman JE (1989). A possible harmful late effect of methylprednisolone therapy on a time cluster of optic neuritis. *Acta Neurol Scand* **80:**569–574.

Kapoor R, Miller DH, Jones SJ, et al. (1998). Effects of intravenous methylprednisolone on outcome in MRI-based prognostic subgroups in acute optic neuritis. *Neurology* **50:**230–237.

Kiziltas S, Imeryüz N, Gürkan T, et al. (1998). Corticosteroid therapy augments gastroduodenal permeability to sucrose. *Am J Gastroenterol* **93:**2420–2425.

La Mantia L, Eoli M, Milanese C, et al. (1994). Double-blind trial of dexamethasone versus methylprednisolone in multiple sclerosis acute relapses. *Eur Neurol* **34:**199–203.

Levic Z, Micic D, Nikolic J et al. (1996). Short-term high-dose steroid therapy does not affect the hypothalamic-pituitary-adrenal axis in relapsing multiple sclerosis patients. Clinical assessment by the insulin tolerance test. *J Endocrinol Invest* **19:**30–34.

Lublin FD, Reingold SC (1996). Defining the clinical course of multiple sclerosis: results of an international survey. *Neurology* **46:**907–911.

Lublin FD, Baier M, Cutter G (2003). Effect of relapses on development of residual deficit in multiple sclerosis. *Neurology* **61:**1528–1532.

Lyons PR, Newman PK, Saunders M (1988). Methylprednisolone therapy in multiple sclerosis: a profile of adverse events. *J Neurol Neurosurg Psychiatry* **51:**285–287.

McDonald WI, Compston A, Edan G, et al. (2001). Recommended diagnostic criteria for multiple sclerosis: guidelines from the international panel on the diagnosis of multiple sclerosis. *Ann Neurol* **50:**121–127.

Metz LM, Sabuda D, Hilsden RJ, Enns R, Meddings JB (1999). Gastric tolerance of high-dose pulse oral prednisone in multiple sclerosis. *Neurology* **53:**2093–2096.

Milanese C, La Mantia L, Salmaggi A, et al. (1989). Double-blind randomised trial of ACTH versus dexamethasone versus methylprednisolone in multiple sclerosis bouts. *Eur Neurol* **29:**10–14.

Miller H, Newell DJ, Ridley A (1961). Multiple sclerosis: Treatment of acute exacerbations with corticotrophin (A.C.T.H.). *Lancet* **2:**1120–1122.

Miller DM, Weinstock-Guttman B, Béthoux F, et al. (2000). A meta-analysis of methylprednisolone in recovery from multiple sclerosis exacerbations. *Mult Scler* **6:**267–273.

Milligan NM, Newcombe R, Compston DAS (1987). A double-blind controlled trial of high dose methylprednisolone in patients with multiple sclerosis: 1. clinical effects. *J Neurol Neurosurg Psychiatry* **50:**511–516.

Miro J, Amada JA, Pesquera C, Lopez-Cordovilla JJ, Berciano J (1990). Assessment of the hypothalamic-pituitary-adrenal axis function after corticosteroid therapy for MS relapses. *Acta Neurol Scand* **81:**524–528.

Multiple Sclerosis Therapy Consensus Group (2004). Escalating immunotherapy of multiple sclerosis. *J Neurol* **251:**1329–1339.

Nos C, Sastre-Garriga J, Borras C, Rio J, Tintoré M, Montalban X (2004). Clinical impact of intravenous methylprednisolone in attacks of multiple sclerosis. *Mult Scler* **10:**413–416.

O'Connor PW, Goodman A, Willmer-Hulme, et al. (2004). Randomized multicenter trial of natalizumab in acute MS relapses. Clinical and MRI effects. *Neurology* **62:**2038–2043.

Oliveri RL, Valentino P, Russo C et al. (1998). Randomized trial comparing two different high doses of methylprednisolone in MS. *Neurology* **50:**1833–1836.

Pryse-Phillips WEM, Chandra RK, Rose B (1984). Anaphylactoid reaction to methylprednisolone pulsed therapy for multiple sclerosis. *Neurology* **34:**1119–1121.

Roed HG, Langkilde A, Sellebjerg F, et al. (2005). A double-blind, randomized, placebo-controlled trial of intravenous immunoglobulin treatment in acute optic neuritis. *Neurology.* In press.

Rose AS, Kuzma JW, Kurtzke JF, *et al.* (1970). Cooperative study in the evaluation of therapy in multiple sclerosis: ACTH vs. placebo. *Neurology* **20**:1–59. (Class I).

Ruprecht K, Klinker E, Dintelmann T, Rieckmann P, Gold R (2004). Plasma exchange for severe optic neuritis. Treatment of 10 patients. *Neurology* **63**: 1081–1083.

Sellebjerg F, Frederiksen JL, Nielsen PM, Olesen J (1998). Double blind, randomized, placebo-controlled study of oral, high-dose methylprednisolone in attacks of MS. *Neurology* **51**:529–534.

Sellebjerg F, Nielsen HS, Frederiksen JL, Olesen J (1999). A randomized, controlled trial of oral high-dose methylprednisolone in acute optic neuritis. *Neurology* **52**:1479–1484.

Sellebjerg F, Jensen CV, Larsson HBW, Frederiksen JL (2003). Gadolinium-enhanced MRI predicts response to methylprednisolone in MS. *Mult Scler* **9**:102–107.

Sharrack B, Hughes RAC, Morris RW *et al.* (2000). The effect of oral and intravenous methylprednisolone treatment on subsequent relapse rate in multiple sclerosis. *J Neurol Sci* **173**:73–77.

Soukop W, Tschabitscher H (1986). Gammaglobulintherapie bei Multipler Sklerose. *Wien Med Wochenschr* **136**:477–480.

Sørensen PS, Haas J, Sellebjerg F, *et al.* (2004). Intravenous immunoglobulins as add-on treatment to methylprednisolone for acute relapses in multiple sclerosis. *Neurology* **63**:2028–2033.

Thompson AJ, Kennard C, Swash M, *et al.* (1989). Relative efficacy of intravenous methylprednisolone and ACTH in the treatment of acute relapse in MS. *Neurology* **39**:969–971.

Trauzettel-Klosinski S, Axman D, Diener HC (1993). The Tübingen study on optic neuritis – a prospective, randomized and controlled trial. *Clin Vision Sci* **8**:385–394.

van den Berg JSP, van Eikema Hommes OR, Wuis EW, Stapel S, van der Valk PGM (1997). Anaphylactoid reaction to intravenous methylprednisolone in a patient with multiple sclerosis. *J Neurol Neurosurg Psychiatry* **63**:813–814.

Visser LH, Beekman R, Tijssen CC, *et al.* (2004). A randomized, double-blind, placebo-controlled pilot study of IV immune globulins in combination with i.v. methylprednisolone in the treatment of relapses in patients with MS. *Mult Scler* **10**:89–91.

Weinshenker BG, O'Brien PC, Petterson TM, *et al.* (1999). A randomized trial of plasma exchange in acute central nervous system inflammatory demyelinating disease. *Neurology* **46**:878–886.

Whitaker JN, Layton BA, Herman PK, Kachelhofer RD, Burgard S, Bartolucci AA (1993). Correlation of myelin basic protein-like material in cerebrospinal fluid of multiple sclerosis patients with their response to glucocorticoid treatment. *Ann Neurol* **33**:10–17.

CHAPTER 31

Status epilepticus

H. Meierkord,[a] P. Boon,[b] B. Engelsen,[c] K. Göcke,[d]
S. Shorvon,[e] P. Tinuper,[f] M. Holtkamp[a]

Abstract

The objective of the current paper was to review the literature and discuss the degree of evidence for various treatment strategies for status epilepticus in adults. We searched MEDLINE and EMBASE for relevant literature from 1966 to January 2005. Furthermore, the Cochrane Central Register of Controlled Trials (CENTRAL) was sought. Recommendations are based on this literature and on our judgement of the relevance of the references to the subject. Recommendations were reached by informative consensus approach. Where there was a lack of evidence but consensus was clear we have stated our opinion as Good Practice Points (GPP). The preferred treatment pathway for generalised convulsive status epilepticus (GCSE) is intravenous (i.v.) administration of 4 mg lorazepam or 10 mg diazepam directly followed by 15–18 mg/kg phenytoin or equivalent fosphenytoin. If seizures continue more than 10 min after first injection another 4 mg lorazepam or 10 mg diazepam is recommended. Refractory GCSE is treated by anaesthetic doses of midazolam, propofol or barbiturates; the anaesthetics are titrated against an EEG burst suppression pattern for at least 24 h. The initial therapy of NCSE depends on the type and the cause. In most cases of absence SE a small i.v. dose of lorazepam or diazepam will terminate the attack. Complex partial status epilepticus is initially treated as GCSE, however, when refractory further non-anaesthetising substances should be given instead of anaesthetics. In subtle status epilepticus i.v. anaesthesia is required.

Background

Incidence, mortality and morbidity

Generalised convulsive status epilepticus (GCSE) and non-convulsive status epilepticus (NCSE) are important neurological conditions potentially associated with significant mortality and morbidity rates. Annual incidence rates of GCSE range between 3.6 and 6.6 per 100 000 and of NCSE between 2.6 and 7.8 per 100 000 (Coeytaux et al., 2000; Knake et al., 2001; Vignatelli et al., 2003). Mortality and morbidity rates of SE are heavily influenced by the underlying aetiology and it is therefore difficult to give reliable figures for the condition itself (Coeytaux et al., 2000; Wu et al., 2002; Shneker and Fountain, 2003). In particular,

[a]Department of Neurology, Charité-Universitätsmedizin Berlin, Berlin, Germany; [b]Department of Neurology, Ghent University Hospital, Ghent, Belgium; [c]Department of Neurology, Haukeland University Hospital, Bergen, Norway; [d]Deutsche Epilepsievereinigung e.V., Berlin, Germany; [e]Institute of Neurology, University College London, London, United Kingdom; [f]Department of Neurological Sciences, University of Bologna, Bologna, Italy.

mortality of NCSE after profound brain damage is high and usually due to the injury itself (Shneker and Fountain, 2003). However, there is general agreement that immediate and effective treatment is required. First line anticonvulsants like benzodiazepines and phenytoin fail to terminate SE in 31–50% of cases (Treiman *et al.*, 1998; Mayer *et al.*, 2002; Holtkamp *et al.*, 2005b). Status epilepticus continuing after such failure is termed refractory status epilepticus and represents an even more difficult clinical problem.

Drug treatment approaches in this situation are based on retrospective series, case reports and expert opinions. The goal of this paper is to summarise published treatment options for generalised convulsive and non-convulsive status epilepticus. Post-anoxic myoclonus is not considered in this guideline as there is no agreement regarding its epileptic nature. The focus of this article is on critical care situations in adults and status epilepticus in children is not considered.

Mechanisms

The basic processes generating SE may be seen as a failure of the normal mechanisms that terminate seizures. Reduced inhibition and persistent excessive excitation create interactions that produce and sustain ongoing seizure activity. Pronounced excitation via glutamate analogues leads to prolongation of seizures (Najm *et al.*, 2000) and gamma-aminobutyric acid (GABA) antagonists such as picrotoxin and bicuculline may also provoke SE (Jones-Davis and Macdonald, 2003), both impairing the usual mechanism by which seizures terminate. During prolonged seizure activity dynamic changes in $GABA_A$ receptor function have been described resulting in progressive receptor insensitivity (Kapur and Macdonald, 1997). Absence SE with 3-Hz spike-wave discharges are induced by excessive inhibition (Snead, III, 1995). This form of SE does not lead to the neuronal injury seen with excessive excitation (Fountain, 2000).

Search strategy

One member of the Task Force Panel (HM) searched available published reports from 1966 to 2005 using the database MEDLINE and EMBASE (last search in January 2005). The search was limited to papers published in English. The subject term 'status epilepticus' was combined with the terms 'controlled clinical trial', 'randomised controlled trial', 'multicentre study', meta analysis' and 'cross over study'. Furthermore, the Cochrane Central Register of Controlled Trials (CENTRAL) was sought. Finally, the websites of the World Health Organisation (WHO), the International League against Epilepsy (ILAE) and the American Neurological Association (ANA) were explored to look for additional information.

Evaluation of published literature

The evidence for therapeutic interventions (class I–IV) and the rating of recommendations (Level A–C) were classified by using the definitions previously reported (Brainin *et al.*, 2004).

Methods for reaching consensus

The other members of the task force read the first draft of the recommendations and discussed changes (informative consensus approach). Where there was a lack of evidence but consensus was clear we have stated our opinion as Good Practice Points (GPP).

Definitions

The time that has to evolve to define ongoing epileptic activity as 'status epilepticus' is as yet not generally agreed upon. The Commission on Classification and Terminology of the International League Against Epilepsy defines status epilepticus as 'a seizure [that] persists for a sufficient length of time or is repeated frequently enough that recovery between attacks does not occur' (Commission on Classification and Terminology of the International League Against Epilepsy, 1981). Experimental studies have shown irreversible neuronal damage after about 30 min of continuing epileptic activity (Meldrum and Horton, 1973). Therefore, this time window has been adopted by the majority of authors (Shorvon, 1994; Coeytaux *et al.*, 2000; Knake *et al.*, 2001). On the other hand, some clinical data indicate that spontaneous cessation of generalised convulsive seizures is unlikely after 5 min (Theodore *et al.*, 1994; Shinnar *et al.*, 2001) and therefore acute treatment with anticonvulsants is required. Consequently, Lowenstein *et al.* have proposed an operational definition of SE that is based on a duration of 5 min (Lowenstein *et al.*, 1999). Currently, clinical studies are based on 5 min (Alldredge *et al.*, 2001), 10 min (Treiman *et al.*, 1998; Mayer *et al.*, 2002) or 30 min (America's Working Group on Status Epilepticus, 1993; Knake *et al.*, 2001) of ongoing epileptic activity to define status epilepticus. The diagnosis of non-convulsive status epilepticus is based on a change in behaviour and/or mental state from baseline and an associated electroencephalogram (EEG) with epileptiform discharges (Kaplan, 1996). There is currently no generally accepted duration of electro-clinical alterations incorporated in the diagnostic criteria of NCSE.

NCSE includes subtypes such as absence status, complex partial status epilepticus and subtle generalised status epilepticus. The latter evolves from overt generalised convulsive status epilepticus and is characterised by coma and ongoing electrographic seizure activity without any or with subtle convulsive movements (Treiman *et al.*, 1998). Absence status epilepticus with 3-Hz spike-wave discharges is a more benign type of status epilepticus and is not further considered in this paper.

An appropriate definition of refractory status epilepticus also is still missing. The failure of two (Prasad *et al.*, 2001; Mayer *et al.*, 2002) or three (Cascino, 1996; Lowenstein and Alldredge, 1998) anticonvulsants has been suggested in combination with a minimal duration of the condition of 1 h (Hanley and Kross, 1998; Mayer *et al.*, 2002) or 2 h (Stecker *et al.*, 1998; Prasad *et al.*, 2001) or regardless of the time that has elapsed since onset (America's Working Group on Status Epilepticus, 1993; Lowenstein and Alldredge, 1998).

Results

Literature and data on treatment
Initial treatment of generalised convulsive status epilepticus
High level evidence for the initial pharmacological treatment of generalised convulsive status

epilepticus (GCSE) has been given in three randomised controlled trials (RCT) that are indicated below. In 384 patients with GCSE, i.v. administration of 0.1 mg/kg lorazepam was successful in 64.9% of cases, 15 mg/kg phenobarbital in 58.2% of cases, and 0.15 mg/kg diazepam followed by 18 mg/kg phenytoin in 55.8% of cases; the efficacy of these anticonvulsants was not significantly different (Treiman *et al.*, 1998) (class I). The same trial has shown that in pairwise comparison initial monotherapy with 18 mg/kg phenytoin is significantly less effective than administration of lorazepam. Another RCT has focussed on the pre-hospital treatment of GCSE performed by paramedics (Alldredge *et al.*, 2001) (class I). Patients were administered 2 mg IV lorazepam, 5 mg IV diazepam, or placebo; the injection of identical doses of benzodiazepines was repeated when seizures continued for more than 4 min. Lorazepam terminated SE in 59.1% of cases and was as effective as diazepam (42.6%). Both drugs were significantly superior to the administration of placebo (21%). An earlier RCT on 81 episodes of all clinical forms of SE compared i.v. administration of 4 mg lorazepam vs. 10 mg diazepam that were repeated when seizures continued or recurred after 10 min (Leppik *et al.*, 1983) (class I). In episodes of GCSE with or without focal onset ($n = 39$) thirteen episodes responded to lorazepam after the first administration and three after the second while three episodes did not respond. With diazepam fourteen episodes responded to the first administration and two to the second while four episodes did not respond.

Initial treatment of non-convulsive status epilepticus
The pharmacological treatment of subtle SE has been addressed in a RCT with 134 patients (Treiman *et al.*, 1998) (class I). The i.v. administration of lorazepam (0.1 mg/kg), diazepam (0.15 mg/kg) followed by phenytoin (18 mg/kg), phenobarbital (18 mg/kg), and phenytoin (18 mg/kg) terminated SE in 8–24% of cases, only. Success rates were not significantly different between the drugs or drug combinations tested. However, key criterion for study entry was the evidence of subtle SE at the time of evaluation,

regardless of prior treatment. Though not further specified, it can be assumed that in some of the patients anticonvulsants have been administered before. Further RCT or other prospective data focussing on the treatment of subtle or other forms of NCSE are missing. Even retrospective studies usually do not address this frequent subgroup of SE.

Side effects of initial treatment of status epilepticus
Safety issues of the common initial anticonvulsants have been compared in patients with generalised convulsive SE as well as in patients with non-convulsive subtle SE (Treiman *et al.*, 1998) (class I). In GCSE hypoventilation was observed in 10–17% of cases, hypotension in 26–34% of cases, and cardiac arrhythmias in 2–7% of cases. These side effects were more frequent in subtle SE and ranged between 3 and 59% of cases. Distribution of side effects was not significantly different in patients treated with lorazepam, diazepam followed by phenytoin, phenobarbital, and phenytoin in overt and subtle SE. Out-of-hospital administration of benzodiazepines compared to placebo did not result in more complications such as arterial hypotension, cardiac dysrhythmia, or respiratory intervention (Alldredge *et al.*, 2001) (class I). These side effects occurred in 10.6% of patients treated with lorazepam, 10.3% of patients treated with diazepam, and 22.5% of patients given placebo.

Refractory status epilepticus
The rationale for treating refractory SE with anaesthesia is that prolonged electrographic seizure activity, in experimental animal models, results in brain damage (Walker *et al.*, 1999; Holtkamp *et al.*, 2005a). To what extent this occurs in human SE is not known, but it is for this reason that most authorities recommend general anaesthesia to obtain burst suppression on the EEG (i.e. the absence of electrographic seizure activity) if initial therapy has not controlled the SE within 1–2 h. However, there are no studies comparing anaesthetic therapy with continuing non-anaesthetising anticonvulsants. The therapeutic decision is based on the type of status epilepticus, comorbidity and prognostic issues. This is of

special relevance in patients with non-convulsive forms of status epilepticus as the risks of anaesthesia (e.g. arterial hypotension, gastroparesis, immunosuppression etc.) may be greater than the risks of ongoing non-convulsive epileptic activity (Kaplan, 2000). In view of the lack of controlled studies the decision on further treatment is based on a few retrospective studies and expert opinions. Retrospective studies have analysed the further treatment options after failure of initial anticonvulsants (Mayer *et al.*, 2002). It should be noted that treatment pathways were naturally influenced by multiple variables such as aetiology, age and comorbidity. In 26 episodes of RSE, after failure of first- and second-line drugs 23 episodes were treated with a third-line drug that was non-anaesthetising in all but one case. In 12 of these episodes seizures were controlled, but 11 patients needed further more aggressive treatment (Mayer *et al.*, 2002) (class IV). These data indicate that the majority of patients with status epilepticus refractory to initial anticonvulsants was treated with further non-anaesthetising anticonvulsants that were successful in approximately half of the patients. However, these data did not differentiate between GCSE and NCSE.

The lowest class of evidence available is based on experts' opinions. Two surveys have been performed, one on the treatment of GCSE among American neurologists (Claassen *et al.*, 2003) and another one on the management of refractory GCSE and CPSE among epileptologists and critical care neurologists in Austria, Germany and Switzerland (Holtkamp *et al.*, 2003). American neurologists did not agree on how to proceed in pharmacological treatment of SE after failure of benzodiazepines and phenytoin or fosphenytoin: more than 80% would not directly proceed to an anaesthetic (43% administer phenobarbital and 16% valproic acid), while 19% would directly administer an anaesthetic (Claassen *et al.*, 2003) (class IV). However, this survey did not include the management of refractory CPSE. The European survey revealed that after failure of benzodiazepines and phenytoin two thirds of the participants would administer in GCSE as well as in CPSE another non-anaesthetising anticonvulsant, the majority preferred phenobarbital. Immediate administration of an anaesthetic was preferred by 35% in GCSE and by 16% in CPSE (Holtkamp *et al.*, 2003) (class IV). Three fourths of the experts did not administer anaesthetics in refractory CPSE at all, while all did at some time point in GCSE. Administration of anaesthetics was withheld in CPSE: more than 60% of the participants administer anaesthetics not earlier than 60 min after onset of status compared to only 21% of participants waiting that long in GCSE.

Further non-anaesthetising anticonvulsants
Though phenobarbital has been assessed in the initial anticonvulsive treatment (Treiman *et al.*, 1998) of status epilepticus, sufficient data on the efficiency of the substance after failure of benzodiazepines and phenytoin/fosphenytoin are missing. Doses of 20 mg/kg infused at a rate of 30–50 mg/min are used.

The role of i.v. valproic acid in the treatment of SE is yet to be defined. Valproic acid is a non-sedating substance that has not caused hypotension or respiratory suppression and has been reported to be effective in generalised convulsive and non-convulsive status epilepticus (Sinha and Naritoku, 2000) (class IV). In a retrospective study that included 63 patients efficacy rates of 63% were reported and favourable tolerance of rapid administration raging from 200 to 500 mg/min (Limdi *et al.*, 2005) (class IV). Loading doses of 25–45 mg/kg have been suggested (Venkataraman and Wheless, 1999) (class IV) and infusion rates up to 6 mg/kg/min (Hodges and Mazur, 2001) (class IV). However, at present, there is inadequate data to justify its use before phenytoin.

Anaesthetising anticonvulsants
Most authorities recommend administering anaesthetic agents to a depth of anaesthesia that produces a burst suppression pattern in the EEG (Holtkamp *et al.*, 2003) (class IV) or an isoelectric EEG (Kaplan, 2003). Studies are needed in this area, as these issues give rise to ethically highly problematic decisions.

Barbiturates, midazolam and propofol are commonly used in refractory SE (Holtkamp *et al.*, 2003) (class IV). There have been no randomised controlled trials comparing these treatment options. A systematic review of drug therapy for refractory status epilepticus including barbiturates, midazolam, and propofol assessed data on 193 patients from 28 retrospective trials in an attempt to clarify this issue (Claassen *et al.*, 2002) (class IV). Pentobarbital was more effective than either propofol or midazolam in preventing breakthrough seizures (12 versus 42%). However, in most studies barbiturates were titrated against an EEG burst suppression pattern while midazolam and propofol was administered to obtain EEG seizure cessation. Accordingly, side effects such as arterial hypotension were significantly more frequently seen with pentobarbital compared to midazolam and propofol (77 versus 34%). Overall mortality was 48% but there was no association between drug selection and the risk of death.

RECOMMENDATIONS

General initial management
General management approaches in generalised convulsive, complex partial, and subtle status epilepticus should include: assessment and control of the airways and of ventilation, arterial blood gas monitoring to see if there is metabolic acidosis and hypoxia requiring immediate treatment through airway management and supplemental oxygen, ECG and blood pressure monitoring. Other measures include: Intravenous glucose and thiamine as required, emergency measurement of antiepileptic drug levels, electrolytes and magnesium, a full haematological screen, and measures of hepatic and renal function. The cause of the status should be identified urgently and may require treatment in its own right (Good Practice Point).

Initial pharmacological treatment of GCSE and NCSE
The initial therapy of NCSE depends on the type and the cause. Subtle status epilepticus evolving from GCSE is refractory by nature and its further treatment is described below. Complex partial status epilepticus should be treated initially as GCSE. The preferred treatment pathway is i.v. administration of 4 mg lorazepam, this dose is

repeated if seizures continue more than 10 min after first injection. If necessary, additional phenytoin (15–18 mg/kg) or equivalent fosphenytoin is recommended. Alternatively, 10 mg diazepam directly followed by 15–18 mg/kg phenytoin or equivalent fosphenytoin can be given, if seizures continue more than 10 min after injection another 10 mg diazepam is recommended. If necessary, additional lorazepam (4–8 mg) should be administered (Level A).

General management of refractory status epilepticus
GCSE that does not respond to initial anticonvulsant substances needs to be treated in an intensive care unit (GPP).

Pharmacological treatment for refractory GCSE and subtle status epilepticus
In GCSE and subtle status epilepticus we suggest to proceed immediately to the infusion of anaesthetic doses of midazolam, propofol, or barbiturates because of the increasing risk of brain and systemic damage. Due to poor evidence we can not recommend which of the anaesthetic substances should be administered first. We recommend the titration of the anaesthetic against an EEG burst suppression pattern. This goal should be maintained for at least 24 h. Simultaneously, initiation of the chronic medication that the patient will be treated with in future should be initiated (GPP).

Barbiturates Thiopental starting with a 100–200 mg bolus over 20 s, then further 50 mg boluses every 2–3 min until seizures are controlled, infusion rate of 3–5 mg/kg/h. Pentobarbital (the first metabolite of thiopental) is marketed in the United States as the alternative to thiopental and is given as a bolus dose of 10–20 mg/kg followed by an infusion of 0.5–1 mg/kg/h increasing to 1–3 mg/kg/h.

Midazolam Effective initial i.v. doses of midazolam are a 0.2 mg/kg bolus, followed by continuous infusion at rates of 0.1–0.4 mg/kg/h.

Propofol Intravenous bolus of 2 mg/kg followed by a continuous infusion of 5–10 mg/kg/h.

Exceptions Elderly patients in whom intubation and artificial ventilation would not be justified. In these cases non-anaesthetising anticonvulsants may be tried (see below) (GPP).

Pharmacological treatment for refractory NCSE
In complex partial status epilepticus, the time that has elapsed until termination of status is less critical compared to GCSE. Thus, general anaesthesia due to its possible severe complications should be postponed and non-anaesthetising anticonvulsants may be tried before (GPP).

Phenobarbital: 20 mg/kg i.v. administration of additional boluses requires intensive care conditions.

Valproic acid: i.v. bolus of 25–45 mg/kg followed by maximum rates up to 6 mg/kg/min.

If the treatment regimen includes the administration of anaesthetics then the same protocol applies as described for refractory generalised convulsive status epilepticus.

Conflicts of interest

Hartmut Meierkord, Paul Boon, Bernt Engelsen, Klaus Göcke, Simon Shorvon, Paolo Tinuper and Martin Holtkamp, all declare no conflict of interest.

References

Alldredge BK, Gelb AM, Isaacs SM *et al.* (2001). A comparison of lorazepam, diazepam, and placebo for the treatment of out-of-hospital status epilepticus. *N Engl J Med* **345**:631–637.

America's Working Group on Status Epilepticus (1993). Treatment of convulsive status epilepticus. Recommendations of the Epilepsy Foundation of America's Working Group on Status Epilepticus. *JAMA* **270**:854–859.

Brainin M, Barnes M, Baron JC *et al.* (2004). Guidance for the preparation of neurological management guidelines by EFNS scientific task forces–revised recommendations 2004. *Eur J Neurol* **11**:577–581.

Cascino GD (1996). Generalized convulsive status epilepticus. *Mayo Clin Proc* **71**:787–792.

Claassen J, Hirsch LJ, Emerson RG, Mayer SA (2002). Treatment of refractory status epilepticus with pentobarbital, propofol, or midazolam: a systematic review. *Epilepsia* **43**:146–153.

Claassen J, Hirsch LJ, Mayer SA (2003). Treatment of status epilepticus: a survey of neurologists. *J Neurol Sci* **211**:37–41.

Coeytaux A, Jallon P, Galobardes B, Morabia A (2000). Incidence of status epilepticus in French-speaking Switzerland: (EPISTAR). *Neurology* **55**:693–697.

Commission on Classification and Terminology of the International League Against Epilepsy (1981). Proposal for revised clinical and electroencephalographic classification of epileptic seizures. *Epilepsia* **22**:489–501.

Fountain NB (2000). Status epilepticus: risk factors and complications. *Epilepsia* **41(Suppl 2):**S23–S30.

Hanley DF, Kross JF (1998). Use of midazolam in the treatment of refractory status epilepticus. *Clin Ther* **20**:1093–1105.

Hodges BM, Mazur JE (2001). Intravenous valproate in status epilepticus. *Ann Pharmacother* **35**:1465–1470.

Holtkamp M, Masuhr F, Harms L, Einhaupl KM, Meierkord H, Buchheim K (2003). The management of refractory generalised convulsive and complex partial status epilepticus in three European countries: a survey among epileptologists and critical care neurologists. *J Neurol Neurosurg Psychiatry* **74**:1095–1099.

Holtkamp M, Matzen J, van Landeghem F, Buchheim K, Meierkord H (2005a). Transient loss of inhibition precedes spontaneous seizures after experimental status epilepticus. *Neurobiol Dis* **19**:162–170.

Holtkamp M, Othman J, Buchheim K, Meierkord H (2005b). Predictors and prognosis of refractory status epilepticus treated in a neurological intensive care unit. *J Neurol Neurosurg Psychiatry* **76**:534–539.

Jones-Davis DM, Macdonald RL (2003). GABA(A) receptor function and pharmacology in epilepsy and status epilepticus. *Curr Opin Pharmacol* **3**:12–18.

Kaplan PW (1996). Nonconvulsive status epilepticus. *Semin Neurol* **16**:33–40.

Kaplan PW (2000). No, some types of nonconvulsive status epilepticus cause little permanent neurologic sequelae (or: "the cure may be worse than the disease"). *Neurophysiol Clin* **30**:377–382.

Kaplan PW (2003). Nonconvulsive status epilepticus. *Neurology* **61**:1035–1036.

Kapur J, Macdonald RL (1997). Rapid seizure-induced reduction of benzodiazepine and Zn2+ sensitivity of hippocampal dentate granule cell GABAA receptors. *J Neurosci* **17**:7532–7540.

Knake S, Rosenow F, Vescovi M *et al.* (2001). Incidence of status epilepticus in adults in Germany: a prospective, population-based study. *Epilepsia* **42**:714–718.

Leppik IE, Derivan AT, Homan RW, Walker J, Ramsay RE, Patrick B (1983). Double-blind study of lorazepam and diazepam in status epilepticus. *JAMA* **249**:1452–1454.

Limdi NA, Shimpi AV, Faught E, Gomez CR, Burneo JG (2005). Efficacy of rapid IV administration of valproic acid for status epilepticus. *Neurology* **64**:353–355.

Lowenstein DH, Alldredge BK (1998). Status epilepticus. *N Engl J Med* **338**:970–976.

Lowenstein DH, Bleck T, Macdonald RL (1999). It's time to revise the definition of status epilepticus. *Epilepsia* **40**:120–122.

Mayer SA, Claassen J, Lokin J, Mendelsohn F, Dennis LJ, Fitzsimmons BF (2002). Refractory status epilepticus: frequency, risk factors, and impact on outcome. *Arch Neurol* **59**:205–210.

Meldrum BS, Horton RW (1973). Physiology of status epilepticus in primates. *Arch Neurol* **28**:1–9.

Najm IM, Ying Z, Babb T *et al.* (2000). Epileptogenicity correlated with increased N-methyl-D-aspartate receptor subunit NR2A/B in human focal cortical dysplasia. *Epilepsia* **41**:971–976.

Prasad A, Worrall BB, Bertram EH, Bleck TP (2001). Propofol and midazolam in the treatment of refractory status epilepticus. *Epilepsia* **42**:380–386.

Shinnar S, Berg AT, Moshe SL, Shinnar R (2001). How long do new-onset seizures in children last? *Ann Neurol* **49**:659–664.

Shneker BF, Fountain NB (2003). Assessment of acute morbidity and mortality in nonconvulsive status epilepticus. *Neurology* **61**:1066–1073.

Shorvon S (1994). Status epilepticus: its clinical features and treatment in children and adults. Cambridge: Cambridge University Press.

Sinha S, Naritoku DK (2000). Intravenous valproate is well tolerated in unstable patients with status epilepticus. *Neurology* **55**:722–724.

Snead OC, III (1995). Basic mechanisms of generalized absence seizures. *Ann Neurol* **37**:146–157.

Stecker MM, Kramer TH, Raps EC, O'Meeghan R, Dulaney E, Skaar DJ (1998). Treatment of refractory status epilepticus with propofol: clinical and pharmacokinetic findings. *Epilepsia* **39**:18–26.

Theodore WH, Porter RJ, Albert P *et al.* (1994). The secondarily generalized tonic-clonic seizure: a videotape analysis. *Neurology* **44**:1403–1407.

Treiman DM, Meyers PD, Walton NY *et al.* (1998). A comparison of four treatments for generalized convulsive status epilepticus. Veterans Affairs Status Epilepticus Cooperative Study Group. *N Engl J Med* **339**:792–798.

Venkataraman V, Wheless JW (1999). Safety of rapid intravenous infusion of valproate loading doses in epilepsy patients. *Epilepsy Res* **35**:147–153.

Vignatelli L, Tonon C, D'Alessandro R (2003). Incidence and short-term prognosis of status epilepticus in adults in Bologna, Italy. *Epilepsia* **44**:964–968.

Walker MC, Perry H, Scaravilli F, Patsalos PN, Shorvon SD, Jefferys JG (1999). Halothane as a neuroprotectant during constant stimulation of the perforant path. *Epilepsia* **40:**359–364.

Wu YW, Shek DW, Garcia PA, Zhao S, Johnston SC (2002). Incidence and mortality of generalized convulsive status epilepticus in California. *Neurology* **58:**1070–1076.

Previous guidelines or recommendations

America's Working Group on Status Epilepticus (1993). Treatment of convulsive status epilepticus. Recommendations of the Epilepsy Foundation of America's Working Group on Status Epilepticus. *JAMA* **270:**854–859.

CHAPTER 32

Alcohol-related seizures

G. Bråthen,[a] E. Ben-Menachem,[b] E. Brodtkorb,[a]
R. Galvin,[c] J.C. Garcia-Monco,[d] P. Halasz,[e]
M. Hillbom,[f] M.A. Leone,[g] A.B. Young[h]

Abstract

Despite being a considerable problem in neurological practice and responsible for one third of
seizure-related admissions, there is little consensus
as to the optimal investigation and management of
alcohol-related seizures. The final literature search
was undertaken in September 2004. Consensus recommendations are given graded according to the
EFNS guidance regulations. To support the history
taking, use of a structured questionnaire is recommended. When the drinking history is inconclusive, elevated values of carbohydrate-deficient
transferrin and/or gammaglutamyl transferase can
support a clinical suspicion. A first epileptic seizure
should prompt neuroimaging (CT or MRI). Before
starting any carbohydrate containing fluids or
food, patients presenting with suspected alcohol
overuse should be given prophylactic thiamine
parenterally. After an alcohol withdrawal seizure
(AWS), the patient should be observed in hospital for at least 24 h and the severity of withdrawal
symptoms needs to be followed. For patients with
no history of withdrawal seizures and mild to
moderate withdrawal symptoms, routine seizure
preventive treatment is not necessary. Generally,
benzodiazepines are efficacious and safe for primary and secondary seizure prevention; diazepam
or, if available, lorazepam, is recommended.
The efficacy of other drugs is insufficiently documented. Concerning long-term recommendations
for non-alcohol dependant patients with partial
epilepsy and controlled seizures, small amounts
of alcohol may be safe. Alcohol-related seizures
require particular attention both in the diagnostic
work-up and treatment. Benzodiazepines should
be chosen for the treatment and prevention of
recurrent AWS.

Background It has been known since Hippocratic
times that alcohol overuse causes epileptic seizures
(Lloyd, 1978). The nature of this relationship is
complex and poorly understood. Despite being a
considerable problem in neurological practice and
responsible for one third of seizure-related admissions (Earnest and Yarnell, 1976; Hillbom, 1980;
Bråthen *et al.*, 1999; Jallon *et al.*, 1999), there is little consensus as to the optimal investigation and
management of alcohol related seizures. Furthermore, different treatment traditions and policies

[a]Department of Neurology and Clinical
Neurophysiology, Trondheim University Hospital,
Norway; [b]Institute of Clinical; Neuroscience,
SU/Sahlgrenska Hospital, Gothenburg, Sweden;
[c]Department of Neurology, Cork University Hospital,
Ireland; [d]Servicio de Neurologia, Hospital de Galdacano,
Spain; [e]National Institute of Psychiatry and Neurology,
Epilepsy Center, Budapest, Hungary; [f]Department of
Neurology, Oulu University Hospital, Finland; [g]Clinica
Neurologica, Ospedale Maggiore; della Carità, Novara,
Italy; [h]Castle Craig Hospital, Blyth Bridge, West Linton,
Peebleshire, UK.

European Journal of Neurology 2005, 12:575–581

exist, and vary from country to country. These guidelines summarize the current evidence for the diagnosis and management of alcohol-related seizures.

Methods The task force systematically searched MEDLINE, EMBASE, the Cochrane databases, and several other sources for relevant trials related to a set of pre-defined key questions. The final search was done in September 2004. Recent papers of high relevance were reviewed. Consensus was reached by discussions during meetings of the Task Force at EFNS congresses and at a separate workshop. The evidence and recommendation levels are graded according to the current guidance (Brainin *et al.*, 2004). Some important aspects of patient management that lack the evidence required for recommendations have been included; these are marked Good Practice Point, for 'Good Practice Points'. Details of the literature search, method for reaching consensus and additional information on the development of this guideline is available on the Task Force homepage on the European Federation of Neurological Societies (EFNS) website (http://www.efns.org).

Results

Diagnosis of alcohol-related seizures
History taking
Unless alcohol withdrawal symptoms are unequivocally present, the clinical diagnosis of an alcohol-related seizure can only be made by obtaining a drinking history that indicates alcohol overuse prior to the seizure. As patients frequently underreport true levels of alcohol consumption, there is a need to control for this bias. Therefore, whenever possible, a relative or friend should be asked about the recent alcohol intake.

Several other legal or illegal pharmacological agents may influence the tendency to have seizures, either because of withdrawal (e.g. benzodiazepines) or because of a direct neurotoxic effect (e.g. antipsychotics, antidepressants, or stimulant drugs). These factors may complicate the clinical picture and should be considered in the diagnosis of alcohol-related seizures.

A good drinking history includes both the quantity and frequency of alcohol intake and changes in drinking pattern, at least during the previous 5 days, as well as the time of the last alcohol intake (Good Practice Point).

Questionnaires
Structured questionnaires have been developed to reveal and grade excessive alcohol consumption as well as alcohol overuse and dependence. To be clinically useful a questionnaire needs to be both brief and reliable. Probably the most commonly applied instrument is CAGE, which is the acronym for a simple four question item, (available on http://www.efns.org). It is brief, easily memorized and has reasonably fair accuracy (Mayfield *et al.*, 1974). However, it fails to detect binge drinking, which is probably best assessed by directly asking for the largest number of drinks in a single drinking occasion (Matano *et al.*, 2003). The Alcohol Use Disorders Identification Test (AUDIT) includes this item. It is a 10-item questionnaire which requires a 2–3 min interview and provides a fine-pitched grading (0–40) of alcohol use and overuse. For patient populations with lower drinking levels, it has higher accuracy than other questionnaires (MacKenzie *et al.*, 1996; Fiellin *et al.*, 2000) but is not easily memorized and may be perceived as too long for routine use in busy medical settings. A handful of brief versions, e.g. AUDIT-C, FAST, and AUDIT-PC, consisting of three to five AUDIT items, or Five-SHOT, a combination of AUDIT and CAGE items, have all shown good accuracy compared with AUDIT (Piccinelli *et al.*, 1997; Bush *et al.*, 1998; Seppä *et al.*, 1998; Hodgson *et al.*, 2003). Other questionnaires, such as the Brief Michigan Alcoholism Screening Test (Brief MAST; MacKenzie *et al.*, 1996), and the Munich Alcoholism Test (MALT; Feuerlein *et al.*, 1977) have widespread use, but do not offer better accuracy than AUDIT or its brief versions, and their use in a routine clinical setting is more demanding.

RECOMMENDATIONS

Questionnaires offer high diagnostic accuracy for alcohol overuse (Level A). To identify patients with alcohol-related seizures and binge drinking, brief versions of AUDIT are recommended as they are accurate and easy to use in busy clinical settings (Level A).

Biomarkers

For detection of alcohol overuse, questionnaire-based interviews are reported to be more sensitive than any biomarker (Bernadt *et al.*, 1982; Aertgeerts *et al.*, 2002). However, in cases where information on recent alcohol consumption is unavailable or considered unreliable, markers of alcohol consumption can increase the accuracy of the clinical diagnosis (Bråthen *et al.*, 2000; Martin *et al.*, 2002).

Carbohydrate-deficient transferrin (CDT) and gammaglutamyl transferase (GGT) are sensitive markers for alcohol overuse, although GGT is less specific than CDT. Systematic literature reviews have been inconclusive as to which marker is better (Salaspuro, 1999; Scouller *et al.*, 2000). Both CDT and GGT show poor accuracy as screening instruments for alcohol-related seizures in unselected seizure populations (Bråthen *et al.*, 2000). Attempts to combine the tests have lead to slightly increased sensitivity (Sillanaukee and Olsson, 2001; Anttila *et al.*, 2003). As the current intoxication level is important information with potential treatment consequences (Savola *et al.*, 2004), blood alcohol should be measured in patients with suspected alcohol-related seizures (Good Practice Point).

RECOMMENDATIONS

CDT and GT have a potential to support a clinical suspicion of alcohol overuse when the drinking history is inconclusive (Level A). Because of poor accuracy in unselected populations, biomarkers should not be applied as general screening instruments (Level C).

Patient examination and observation

The clinical examination should be focused on features distinctive of either epilepsy or withdrawal

Table 32.1 Early (<72 h) post-ictal signs and symptoms after seizures because of epilepsy and alcohol withdrawal seizures.

	Epilepsy	Early alcohol withdrawal
Consciousness level	Post-ictal sleep/drowsiness	Sleeplessness
Mood	Calm	Anxiety, unrest, nightmares
Tremor	No	Yes
Sweating	No	Yes
Blood pressure	Normal	Elevated
Pulse rate	Normal	Elevated (>90)
Temperature	Normal/light fever	Fever
Arterial blood	Normal	Respiratory alkalosis[a]
EEG	Pathology[b]	Normal, low amplitude
Questionnaires	Normal scores	Normal or elevated scores

[a]Respiratory alkalosis may be masked by seizure-induced metabolic acidosis, but it will reappear within 2 h after cessation of convulsions (Orringer *et al.*, 1977).
[b]Initial post-ictal slowing in most patients. Inter-ictal epileptiform discharges in approximately 50% (FIRST Group, 1993).

seizures (table 32.1). To predict the severity of alcohol withdrawal, the revised Clinical Institute Withdrawal Assessment Scale (CIWA-Ar) can be applied (Sullivan *et al.*, 1989). The CIWA-Ar takes 2–5 min to administer and grades withdrawal severity on a scale from 0 to 67 (available as appendix to this guideline on http://www.efns.org). More than 90% of alcohol withdrawal seizures (AWS) occur within 48 h of cessation of a prolonged drinking bout (Victor and Brausch, 1967; Bråthen *et al.*, 1999). Patients should be observed in hospital for at least 24 h, after which a clinical risk assessment should be made with respect to development of symptoms of alcohol withdrawal (Good Practice Point).

For the general treatment of the alcohol withdrawal syndrome readers should refer to recent guidelines on the topic [Mayo-Smith *et al.*, 1997; Claassen and Adinoff, 1999; Scottish

Intercollegiate Guidelines Network (SIGN), 2002; Mayo-Smith *et al.*, 2004].

RECOMMENDATIONS

The CIWA questionnaire can be applied to grade the severity of withdrawal symptoms and give support to the decision on whether to keep or discharge the patient (Level A).

Neuroimaging

The diagnostic yield of cerebral computed tomography (CT) after a first alcohol-related seizure is high, mainly because patients overusing alcohol have a high incidence of structural intracranial lesions (Earnest *et al.*, 1988; Schoenenberger and Heim, 1994). Seizures that occur later than 48 h after intake of the last drink may indicate other potential aetiologies than simple alcohol withdrawal, such as subdural haematoma, brain contusion, or mixed drug and alcohol overuse (Hillbom and Hjelm-Jäger, 1984). When patients present repeatedly with clinically typical alcohol-related seizures, reimaging is not necessary, but changes in seizure type and frequency, seizure occurrence more than 48 h after cessation of drinking, or other unusual features should prompt repeat neuroimaging (Good Practice Point).

RECOMMENDATIONS

Although it may seem obvious that a given seizure is alcohol-related, if it is a first known seizure, the patient should have brain imaging (CT or MRI) without and with contrast (Level C).

Electroencephalography

The incidence of electroencephalography (EEG) abnormalities (slow or epileptiform activity) is lower amongst patients with AWS than in those with seizures of other aetiology. Therefore, EEG pathology suggests that the seizure may not have been caused exclusively by alcohol withdrawal (Victor and Brausch, 1967; Sand *et al.*, 2002).

RECOMMENDATIONS

EEG should be recorded after a first seizure. Subsequent to repeated AWS, EEG is considered necessary only if an alternative aetiology is suspected (Level C).

Patient management

Subsequent to the acute treatment of alcohol-related seizures, attention should be given to other potential complications of alcohol overuse such as thiamine deficiency, electrolyte disturbances, acute intracranial lesions, infections, and development of the alcohol withdrawal syndrome, potentially leading to delirium tremens. Apart from acute intracranial lesions, which fall outside the scope of these guidelines, these factors are addressed below.

Thiamine therapy

Prolonged heavy drinking causes reduced absorption and increased excretion of thiamine. Only 5–14% of patients with Wernicke's encephalopathy are diagnosed in life (Torvik *et al.*, 1982; Blansjaar and van Dijk, 1992). The majority (approximately 80%) of those who show CNS lesions caused by thiamine deficiency are chronic alcohol overusers (Torvik *et al.*, 1982; Harper *et al.*, 1986).

Thiamine is a comparatively harmless vitamin, the diagnosis of thiamine deficiency is difficult, and the consequences of not treating may be severe. Therefore, the threshold for starting therapy should be low. Oral administration is insufficient as the intestinal thiamine absorption may be severely impaired (Holzbach, 1996). In a recent Cochrane review, only one sufficiently large randomized double-blind trial on the preventive effects of different doses of thiamine could be identified (Ambrose *et al.*, 2001), from which it could only be concluded that a daily dose of 200 mg thiamine was better than 5 mg (Day *et al.*, 2004). For the treatment of imminent or manifest Wernicke's encephalopathy, uncontrolled trials and empirical clinical practice suggest a daily dose of at least 200 mg thiamine parenterally for minimum 3–5 days. In our experience, patients with

Wernicke's encephalopathy may benefit from continued treatment for more than 2 weeks (Good Practice Point).

RECOMMENDATIONS

Before starting any carbohydrate containing fluids or food, patients presenting with known or suspected alcohol overuse should be given prophylactic thiamine in the emergency room (Level B).

Treatment of electrolyte disturbances

Because of large fluid intake (beer), hyponatremia may develop in alcohol overusers. The serious disorder of central pontine myelinolysis is thought to be triggered by osmotic gradients in the brain, a situation that may well result from attempts to correct this electrolyte disturbance rapidly (Lampl and Yazdi, 2002). Hyponatremia in alcohol overusers generally shows a benign clinical course (Mochizuki *et al.*, 2003), and usually repairs with cessation of alcohol intake and re-institution of a normal diet (Kelly *et al.*, 1998). If infusion is considered necessary, according to a retrospective study the rate of serum sodium correction should not exceed 10 mmol/day (Saeed *et al.*, 2002). The evidence is insufficient for treatment recommendations.

Hypomagnesemia and respiratory alkalosis seem to be associated with alcohol withdrawal, and correction of hypomagnesemia may raise the seizure threshold in the initial phase of alcohol withdrawal (Victor, 1973). Unresponsiveness to parenteral thiamine therapy is a possible consequence of hypomagnesemia (Traviesa, 1974). However, there is not sufficient evidence to recommend routine correction of hypomagnesemia.

Should all patients with symptoms of alcohol withdrawal be offered seizure prophylactic treatment?

Patients with mild-to-moderate alcohol withdrawal symptoms (CIWA < 10) can successfully be detoxified with supportive care only (Whitfield *et al.*, 1978). Supportive treatment includes a calm, reassuring atmosphere, dim light, coffee restriction, and hydration.

The mean incidence of seizures in patients receiving placebo during trials on drugs for prevention of AWS is approximately 8% (Hillbom *et al.*, 2003). These data originate from selected patients in need of treatment for alcoholism; the general seizure risk during uncomplicated alcohol withdrawal is probably lower. As seizures during previous detoxifications increase the risk for seizures during subsequent withdrawals (Lechtenberg and Worner, 1990; Mayo-Smith and Bernard, 1995), patients with these characteristics will probably benefit from prophylactic treatment regardless of the current withdrawal symptom severity.

RECOMMENDATIONS

For patients with no history of withdrawal seizures and mild to moderate withdrawal symptoms, routine seizure preventive treatment is not recommended (Level B). Patients with severe alcohol withdrawal symptoms, regardless of seizure occurrence, should be treated pharmacologically (Level C).

Drug options for primary prevention of alcohol withdrawal seizures

An ideal drug for symptom relief during detoxification from alcohol should display fast loading, long duration, minor side-effects, low toxicity, few interactions, minimal overuse potential, and high efficacy in preventing both withdrawal symptoms in general as well as seizures. Drugs should be available in more than one form, liquid being particularly useful for some patients. Apart from overuse potential, benzodiazepines (BZD) fulfil all the above listed criteria for an ideal drug. BZD are cheap, widely available, and have a well-documented safety profile.

In a meta-analysis of controlled trials for primary prevention of AWS, a highly significant risk reduction for seizures with BZD compared with placebo was demonstrated (Hillbom *et al.*, 2003). Drugs with rapid onset of action (diazepam, lorazepam, alprazolam) seem to have higher overuse potential than those with slower onset of action (chlordiazepoxide, oxazepam, halazepam). For the purpose of reducing the risk of seizures because of BZD withdrawal and reducing rebound withdrawal symptoms after discontinuation, long-acting drugs should be preferred to short-acting ones (Mayo-Smith, 1997; Hillbom *et al.*, 2003). However, short-acting BZDs may have advantages for patients with respiratory insufficiency. Symptom-triggered treatment has been reported to be as effective as fixed-dose or loading therapy, resulting in lower doses and shorter treatment time (Saitz *et al.*, 1994; Jaeger *et al.*, 2001).

Lorazepam has some advantages over diazepam. Despite a shorter half-life it has longer duration of action because it is less accumulated in lipid stores. However, its onset of action is slightly slower than that of diazepam. Many other drugs and drug combinations are being used, including carbamazepine, chlormethiazole, sodium valproate, gamma-hydroxybutyrate, and clonidine, all for which the documentation is generally poor (Robinson *et al.*, 1989; Saitz *et al.*, 1994; Holbrook *et al.*, 1999; Hillbom *et al.*, 2003).

RECOMMENDATIONS

When pharmacological treatment is necessary, benzodiazepines should be chosen for the primary prevention of seizures in a person with alcohol withdrawal, as well as for treatment of the alcohol withdrawal syndrome. The drugs of choice are lorazepam and diazepam. Although lorazepam has some pharmacological advantages to diazepam, the differences are minor and, as i.v. lorazepam is largely unavailable in Europe, diazepam is recommended. Other drugs for detoxification should only be considered as add-ons (Level A).

Secondary prevention of withdrawal seizures

Following a withdrawal seizure, the recurrence risk within the same withdrawal episode is 13–24% (Hillbom *et al.*, 2003). Consequently, there is a good rationale for treating these patients as soon as possible in order to prevent subsequent seizures. Lorazepam reduces recurrence risk significantly (D'Onofrio *et al.*, 1999). Phenytoin did not prevent relapses in patients who had one or

more seizures during the same withdrawal episode (Hillbom *et al.*, 2003).

RECOMMENDATIONS

Benzodiazepines should be used for the secondary prevention of AWS (Level A). Phenytoin is not recommended for prevention of AWS recurrence (Level A). The efficacy of other antiepileptics for secondary prevention of AWS is undocumented.

Alcohol-related status epilepticus

Alcohol withdrawal is one of the commonest causes of status epilepticus (SE), and SE may be the first manifestation of alcohol-related seizures. Although SE has probably a better prognosis when alcohol-related (Alldredge and Lowenstein, 1993), it increases the risk for subsequent epilepsy (Hesdorffer *et al.*, 1998). One recent study indicates that lorazepam may be superior to diazepam for the treatment of out-of-hospital SE (Alldredge *et al.*, 2001). In another study comparing four treatments, lorazepam was considered easier to use but not more efficacious than diazepam, phenobarbital or phenytoin (Treiman *et al.*, 1998).

RECOMMENDATIONS

For the initial treatment of alcohol-related status epilepticus, i.v. lorazepam is safe and efficacious. When unavailable, i.v. diazepam is a good alternative (Level A).

Management of epilepsy in patients with current alcohol overuse

The comprehensive management of these patients includes careful counselling and information about the seizure precipitating effect of alcohol, particularly the concurrent withdrawal of alcohol and AEDs. Prescription of AEDs to alcohol overusers is often a fruitless undertaking which may increase their seizure problems because of poor compliance, drug overuse and drug-alcohol interactions (Hillbom and Hjelm-Jäger, 1984). The ideal drug for such patients should be well tolerated in combination with alcohol and have a benign side-effect profile, including safety in overdose (Malcolm *et al.*, 2001), and have a suppressive effect on drinking behaviour. In a few small studies, carbamazepine, valproic acid and gabapentin have each been reported to reduce alcohol consumption (Mueller *et al.*, 1997; Brady *et al.*, 2002; Voris *et al.*, 2003), and topiramate has recently been shown to reduce craving for alcohol (Johnson *et al.*, 2003). Prophylactic AED treatment should only be considered after recurrent epileptic seizures clearly unrelated to alcohol intake, following the usual guidelines for AED treatment. The available data do not allow for recommendations on this topic.

How much alcohol can a patient with epilepsy safely consume?

In various European countries, different advice has been given as to whether patients with epilepsy should abstain totally from alcohol (Höppener, 1990). Only one randomized controlled clinical study (Höppener *et al.*, 1983) has addressed this particular issue; an intake of one to three drinks each containing 9.8 g ethanol (standard alcohol units; see Turner, 1990) up to three times a week did not increase seizure susceptibility in treated patients with partial epilepsy. Another study suggested a seizure risk proportional to the alcohol intake level (Mattson *et al.*, 1990).

Alcohol sensitivity may vary between epilepsy syndromes. Generalized epilepsies, in particular juvenile myoclonic epilepsy, seem to be more sensitive to alcohol, sleep deprivation and in particular the combination of these factors (Pedersen and Petersen, 1998).

RECOMMENDATIONS

For the majority of patients with partial epilepsy and controlled seizures, and in the absence of any history of alcohol overuse, an intake of one to three standard alcohol units, one to three times a week, is safe (Level B).

Conflicts of interest

The present guidelines were developed without external financial support. None of the authors report conflicting interests.

References

Aertgeerts B, Buntinx F, Ansoms S, Fevery J (2002). Questionnaires are better than laboratory tests to screen for current alcohol abuse or dependence in a male inpatient population. *Acta Clin Belg* **57:** 241–249.

Alldredge BK, Lowenstein DH (1993). Status epilepticus related to alcohol abuse. *Epilepsia* **34:**1033–1037.

Alldredge BK, Gelb AM, Isaacs SM *et al.* (2001). A comparison of lorazepam, diazepam, and placebo for the treatment of out-of-hospital status epilepticus. *N Engl J Med* **345:**631–637.

Ambrose ML, Bowden SC, Whelan G (2001). Thiamin treatment and working memory function of alcoholdependent people: preliminary findings. *Alcohol Clin Exp Res* **25:**112–116.

Anttila P, Järvi K, Latvala J, Blake JE, Niemelä O (2003). A new modified γ-%CDT method improves the detection of problem drinking: studies in alcoholics with or without liver disease. *Clin Chim Acta* **338:** 45–51.

Bernadt MW, Mumford J, Taylor C, Smith B, Murray RM (1982). Comparison of questionnaire and laboratory tests in the detection of excessive drinking and alcoholism. *Lancet* **i:**325–328.

Blansjaar BA, van Dijk JG (1992). Korsakoff-Wernicke syndrome. *Alcohol Alcohol* **27:**435–437.

Bråthen G, Brodtkorb E, Helde G, Sand T, Bovim G (1999). The diversity of seizures related to alcohol use. A study of consecutive patients. *Eur J Neurol* **6:** 697–703.

Bråthen G, Bjerve K, Brodtkorb B, Bovim G (2000). Validity of carbohydrate-deficient transferrin and other markers as diagnostic aids in the detection of alcohol-related seizures. *J Neurol Neurosurg Psychiatry* **68:**342–348.

Brady KT, Myrick H, Henderson S, Coffey SF (2002). Use of divalproex in alcohol relapse prevention: a pilot study. *Drug Alcohol Depend* **67:**323–330.

Brainin M, Barnes M, Baron J-C *et al.* (2004). Guidance for the preparation of neurological management guidelines by EFNS scientific task forces – revised recommendations. *Eur J Neurol* **11:**577–581.

Bush K, Kivlahan DR, McDonnel MB, Fihn SD, Bradley KA (1998). The AUDIT alcohol consumption questions (AUDIT-C): an effective brief screening test for problem drinking. *Arch Intern Med* **16:**1789–1795.

Claassen CA, Adinoff B (1999). Alcohol withdrawal syndrome. Guidelines for management. *CNS Drugs* **12:**279–291.

D'Onofrio G, Rathlev NK, Ulrich AS, Fish SS, Freedland ES (1999). Lorazepam for the prevention of recurrent seizures related to alcohol. *N Engl J Med* **340:** 915–919.

Day E, Bentham P, Callaghan R, Kuruvilla T, George S (2004). Thiamine for Wernicke-Korsakoff Syndrome in people at risk from alcohol abuse (Cochrane review). *Cochrane Database Syst Rev* **1:**CD004033.

Earnest MP, Yarnell P (1976). Seizure admissions to a city hospital: the role of alcohol. *Epilepsia* **17:**387–393.

Earnest MP, Feldman H, Marx JA, Harris BS, Biletch M, Sullivan LP (1988). Intracranial lesions shown by CT in 259 cases of first alcohol related seizure. *Neurology* **38:**1561.

Feuerlein W, Ringer C, Kufner H, Antons K (1977). Diagnose des Alkoholismus. Der Münchner Alkoholismustest (MALT). Munch Med Wochenschr **119:** 1275–1286.

Fiellin DA, Reid MC, O'Connor PG (2000). Screening for alcohol problems in primary care: a systematic review. *Arch Intern Med* **160:**1977–1989.

FIRST Group (1993). Randomized clinical trial on the efficacy of antiepileptic drugs in reducing the risk of relapse after a first unprovoked tonic-clonic seizure. *Neurology* **43:**478–483.

Harper CG, Giles M, Finlay-Jones R (1986). Clinical signs in the Wernicke-Korsakoff complex: a retrospective analysis of 131 cases diagnosed at necropsy. *J Neurol Neurosurg Psychiatry* **49:**341–345.

Hesdorffer DC, Logroscino G, Cascino G *et al.* (1998). Risk of unprovoked seizure after acute symptomatic seizure: effect of status epilepticus. *Ann Neurol* **44:**908–912.

Hillbom ME (1980). Occurrence of cerebral seizures provoked by alcohol abuse. *Epilepsia* **21:**459–466.

Hillbom ME, Hjelm-Jäger M (1984). Should alcohol withdrawal seizures be treated with anti-epileptic drugs? *Acta Neurol Scand* **69:**39–42.

Hillbom M, Pieninkeroinen I, Leone M (2003). Seizures in alcohol-dependent patients. Epidemiology, pathophysiology and management. *CNS Drugs* **17:** 1013–1030.

Hodgson RJ, John B, Abbasi T *et al.* (2003). Fast screening for alcohol misuse. *Addict Behav* **28:**1453–1463.

Holbrook AM, Crowther R, Lotter A, Cheng C, King D (1999). Meta-analysis of benzodiazepine use in the treatment of acute alcohol withdrawal. *CMAJ* **160:** 649–655.

Holzbach E (1996). Thiamine absorption in alcoholic delirium patients. *J Stud Alcohol* **57:**581–584.

Höppener RJ (1990). The effect of social alcohol use on seizures in patients with epilepsy. In: Porter RJ, Mattson RH, Cramer JA, Diamond I, eds. *Alcohol and Seizures. Basic Mechanisms and Clinical Concepts.* F.A. Davis Company, Philadelphia, pp. 222–232.

Höppener RJ, Kuyer A, van der Lugt PJM (1983). Epilepsy and alcohol: the influence of social alcohol intake on seizures and treatment in epilepsy. *Epilepsia* **24:** 459–471.

Jaeger TM, Lohr RH, Pankratz VS (2001). Symptomtriggered therapy for alcohol withdrawal syndrome in medical inpatients. *Mayo Clin Proc* **76:**695–701.

Jallon P, Smadja D, Cabre P, Le Mab G, Bazin M (1999). EPIMART: prospective incidence study of epileptic seizures in newly referred patients in a French Caribbean island (Martinique). *Epilepsia* **40:** 1103–1109.

Johnson BA, Ait-Daoud N, Bowden CL *et al.* (2003). Oral topiramate for treatment of alcohol dependence: a randomised controlled trial. *Lancet* **361:** 1677–1685.

Kelly J, Wassif W, Mitchard J, Gardner WN (1998). Severe hyponatremia secondary to beer potomania complicated by central pontine myelinolysis. *Int J Clin Pract* **52:**585–587.

Lampl C, Yazdi K (2002). Central pontine myelinolysis. *Eur Neurol* **47:**3–10.

Lechtenberg R, Worner T (1990). Seizure risk with recurrent alcohol detoxification. *Arch Neurol* **47:**535–538.

Lloyd G (1978). *Hippocratic Writings.* Penguin Books, Middlesex, UK, pp. 222.

MacKenzie D, Langa A, Brown T (1996). Identifying hazardous or harmful alcohol use in medical admissions: a comparison of Audit, CAGE and Brief MAST. *Alcohol Alcohol* **31:**591–599.

Malcolm R, Myrick H, Brady KT, Ballenger JC (2001). Update on anticonvulsants for the treatment of alcohol withdrawal. *Am J Addict* **10(Suppl):**16–23.

Martin MJ, Heyermann C, Neumann T *et al.* (2002). Pre-operative evaluation of chronic alcoholics assessed for surgery of the upper digestive tract. *Alcohol Clin Exp Res* **26:**836–840.

Matano RA, Koopman C, Wanat SF, Whitsell SD, Borgrefe A, Westrup D. (2003). Assessment of binge drinking of alcohol in highly educated employees. *Addict Behav* **28:**1299–1310.

Mattson RH, Fay ML, Sturman JK, Cramer JA, Wallace JD, Mattson EM (1990). The effect of various patterns of alcohol use on seizures in patients with epilepsy.

In: Porter RJ, Mattson RH, Cramer JA, Diamond I, eds. *Alcohol and Seizures. Basic Mechanisms and Clinical Concepts*. F.A. Davis Company, Philadelphia, pp. 233–240.

Mayfield D, Mcleod G, Hall P (1974). The CAGE questionnaire: validation of a new alcoholism screening instrument. *Am J Psychiatry* **131:**1121–1123.

Mayo-Smith MF for the American Society of Addiction Medicine Working Group on Pharmacological Management of Alcohol Withdrawal (1997). Pharmacological management of alcohol withdrawal. A meta-analysis and evidence-based practice guideline. *JAMA* **278:** 144–151.

Mayo-Smith MF, Bernard D (1995). Late onset seizures in alcohol withdrawal. *Alcohol Clin Exp Res* **19:**656–659.

Mayo-Smith MF, Beecher LH, Fischer TL *et al.* (2004). Management of alcohol withdrawal delirium. An evidencebased practice guideline. *Arch Intern Med* **164:**1405–1412.

Mochizuki H, Masaki T, Miyakawa T *et al.* (2003). Benign type of central pontine myelinolysis in alcoholism: clinical, neuroradiological and electrophysiological findings. *J Neurol* **250:**1077–1083.

Mueller TI, Stout RL, Rudden S *et al.* (1997). A double-blind, placebo-controlled pilot study of carbamazepine for the treatment of alcohol dependence. *Alcohol Clin Exp Res* **21:**86–92.

Orringer CE, Eustace JC, Wunsch CD, Gardner LB (1977). Natural history of lactic acidosis after grand-mal seizures. A model for the study of an anion-gap acidosis not associated with hyperkalemia. *N Engl J Med* **297:**796–799.

Pedersen SB, Petersen KA (1998). Juvenile myoclonic epilepsy: clinical and EEG features. *Acta Neurol Scand* **97:**160–163.

Piccinelli M, Tessari E, Bortolomasi M *et al.* (1997). Efficacy of the alcohol use disorders identification test as a screening tool for hazardous alcohol intake and related disorders in primary care: a validity study. *BMJ* **314:**420–427.

Robinson BJ, Robinson GM, Maling TJ, Johnson RH (1989). Is clonidine useful in the treatment of alcohol withdrawal? *Alcohol Clin Exp Res* **13:**95–98.

Saeed BO, Beaumont D, Handley GH, Weaver JU (2002). Severe hyponatremia: investigation and management in a district general hospital. *J Clin Pathol* **55:** 893–896.

Saitz R, Mayo-Smith MF, Roberts MS, Redmond HA, Bernard DR, Calkins DR (1994). Individualized treatment for alcohol withdrawal. A randomized double-blind controlled trial. *JAMA* **272:**519–523.

Salaspuro M (1999). Carbohydrate-deficient transferrin as compared to other markers of alcoholism: a systematic review. *Alcohol* **19:**261–271.

Sand T, Bråthen G, Michler R, Brodtkorb E, Helde G, Bovim G (2002). Clinical utility of EEG in alcohol-related seizures. *Acta Neurol Scand* **105:**18–24.

Savola O, Niemelä O, Hillbom M (2004). Blood alcohol is the best indicator of hazardous alcohol drinking in young adults and working aged patients with trauma. *Alcohol Alcohol* **39:**340–345.

Schoenenberger RA, Heim SM (1994). Indication for computed tomography of the brain in patients with first uncomplicated generalised seizure. *BMJ* **309:** 986–989.

Scottish Intercollegiate Guidelines Network (SIGN) (2002). The Management of Harmful Drinking and Alcohol Dependence in Primary Care. SIGN, Edinburgh, (SIGN publication No. 74).

Scouller K, Conigrave KM, Macaskill P, Irwig L, Whitfield JB (2000). Should we use carbohydrate-deficient transferrin instead of G-Glutamyltransferase for detecting problem drinkers? A systematic review and metaanalysis. *Clin Chem* **46:**1894–1902.

Seppä K, Lepisto J, Sillanaukee P (1998). Five-shot questionnaire on heavy drinking. *Alcohol Clin Exp Res* **22:**1788–1791.

Sillanaukee P, Olsson U (2001). Improved diagnostic classification of alcohol abusers by combining carbohydratedeficient transferrin and -glutamyltransferase. *Clin Chem* **47:**681–685.

Sullivan JT, Sykora K, Schneiderman J, Naranjo CA, Sellers EM (1989). Assessment of alcohol withdrawal: the revised Clinical Institute Withdrawal Assessment for Alcohol scale (CIWA-AR). *Br J Addict* **84:**1353–1357.

Torvik A, Lindboe CF, Rogde S (1982). Brain lesions in alcoholics: a neuropathological study with clinical correlations. *J Neurol Sci* **56:**233–248.

Traviesa DC (1974). Magnesium deficiency: a possible cause of thiamine refractoriness in Wernicke-Korsakoff encephalopathy. *J Neurol Neurosurg Psychiatry* **37:** 959–962.

Treiman DM, Meyers PD, Walton NY *et al.* (1998). A comparison of four treatments for generalized convulsive status epilepticus. Veterans Affairs Status Epilepticus Cooperative Study Group. *N Engl J Med* **339:**792–798.

Turner C (1990). How much alcohol is in a "standard drink?" An analysis of 125 studies. *Br J Addict* **85:** 1171–1175.

Victor M (1973). The role of hypomagnesemia and respiratory alkalosis in the genesis of alcohol withdrawal symptoms. *Ann N Y Acad Sci* **215:**235–248.

Victor M, Brausch C (1967). The role of abstinence in the genesis of alcoholic epilepsy. *Epilepsia* **8**:1–20.

Voris J, Smith NL, Rao SM, Thorne DL, Flowers QJ (2003). Gabapentin for the treatment of ethanol withdrawal. *Subst Abus* **24**:129–132.

Whitfield CL, Thompson G, Lamb A, Spencer V, Pfeifer M, Browning-Ferrando M ((1978). Detoxification of 1024 alcoholic patients without psychoactive drugs. *JAMA* **239**:1409–1410.

CHAPTER 33

Brain metastases

R. Soffietti,[a] P. Cornu,[b] J.Y. Delattre,[c] R. Grant,[d]
F. Graus,[e] W. Grisold,[f] J. Heimans,[g]
J. Hildebrand,[h] P. Hoskin,[i] M. Kalljo,[j]
P. Krauseneck,[k] C. Marosi,[l] T. Siegal,[m] C. Vecht[n]

Abstract

Background Brain metastases represent one of the most frequent neurological complications of systemic cancer, being increased in frequency over time as a result of advances in neuroimaging procedures and improvement of the overall survival.

Objectives The objectives have been to establish evidence-based guidelines and identify controversies regarding the management of patients with brain metastases.

Methods The collection of scientific data was obtained by consulting the Cochrane Library, bibliographic databases, overview papers and previous guidelines from Scientific Societies and Organisations. Moreover the views of the Members of the Task Force on several critical issues were investigated by means of an e-mail questionnaire.

A tissue diagnosis by stereotactic or open surgery should be obtained when the primary tumour is unknown or CT/MRI do not show the typical aspect of a brain metastasis (Level B). Dexamethasone is the corticosteroid of choice for patients with symptoms/signs attributable to cerebral oedema (Good Practice Point). Anticonvulsants should not be prescribed prophylactically (Level A). Low molecular weight heparin is indicated for venous thromboembolism (Level A). Surgery should be considered in patients with up to three brain metastases in an accessible location, large size and considerable mass effect (Good Practice Point). Surgery is effective in prolonging the survival of patients with single brain metastasis when the systemic disease is absent/controlled and the performance status is high (Level A). Stereotactic radiosurgery should be considered in patients with metastases of 3–3.5 cm of maximum

[a]Department of Neurology and Oncology, San Giovanni Battista Hospital and University, Torino, Italy; [b]Department of Neurosurgery, Pitié-Salpétrière and University, Paris, France; [c]Department of Neurology, Pitié-Salpétrière, Paris, France; [d]Department of Neurology, Western General Hospital and University, Edinburgh, United Kingdom; [e]Service of Neurology, Hospital Clinic, Villaroel, Barcelona Spain; [f]Department of Neurology, Kaiser-Franz-Josef Spital, Vienna Austria; [g]Department of Neurology, Academisch Ziekenhuis V.U., Amsterdam, The Netherlands; [h]Consultant Neurologist, Brussel, Belgium; [i]Department of Radiotherapy, Mount Vernon Hospital and University, Northwood, Middlesex, United Kingdom; [j]Department of Neurology, University Hospital, Helsinki, Finland; [k]Neurologische Clinic, Bamberg, Germany; [l]Division Oncology, Vienna General Hospital and University, Vienna, Austria; [m]Neuro-Oncology Clinic, Hadassah Hebrew University, Jerusalem, Israel; [n]Department of Neurology, Med Center Haaglanden, The Hague, The Netherlands.

diameter and/or located in critical areas and/or with comorbidities precluding surgery (Level B). The role of adjuvant whole brain radiotherapy (WBRT) after surgery or radiosurgery remains to be clarified. In case of absent/controlled systemic cancer and Karnofsky Performance score of 70 or more (table 33.1), one can either withhold initial WBRT if close follow-up with magnetic resonance imaging (MRI) is performed or deliver early WBRT with fractions of 1.8–2 Gy to a total dose of 40 55 Gy to avoid late neurotoxicity (Good Practice Point). WBRT alone is the treatment of choice for patients with single or multiple brain metastases not amenable to surgery or radiosurgery (Level B). Chemotherapy may be the initial treatment for patients with brain metastases from chemosensitive tumours, while radiation therapy, with or without chemotherapy, is still the treatment of choice for patients needing a palliation of neurological symptoms (Good Practice Point).

Objectives

The primary objective has been to establish evidence-based guidelines in regard to the management of patients with brain metastases. The secondary objective has been to identify areas where there are still controversies and clinical trials are needed.

Background

Brain metastases represent an important cause of morbidity and mortality for cancer patients. Brain metastases are more common than primary brain tumours. The incidence of brain metastases has increased over time as a consequence of the increase in overall survival for many types of cancer and the improved detection by MRI. Brain metastases may occur in 20–40% of patients with cancer, being symptomatic during life in 60–75%. In adults the primary tumours most likely to metastatize to the brain are located, in decreasing order, in the lung (minimum 50%), breast (15–25%), skin (melanoma) (5–20%), colon-rectum and kidney, but in general any malignant tumour is able to metastatize to the brain. The primary site is unknown in up to 15% of patients. Brain metastases are more often diagnosed in patients with known malignancy (metachronous presentation). Less frequently (up to 30%) brain metastases are diagnosed either at the time of primary tumour diagnosis (synchronous presentation) or before the discovery of the primary tumour (precocious presentation). High performance status, solitary brain metastasis, absence of systemic metastases, controlled primary tumour and younger age (<60–65 years) are the most important favourable prognostic factors (Gaspar et al.,1997; Lagerwaard et al., 1999). Based on these factors the Radiation Therapy Oncology Group (US) has identified subgroups of patients with different prognosis (recursive partitioning analysis (RPA) Class I, II, III) (Gaspar et al., 1997). Neurocognitive functions are prognostically important as well (Murray et al., 2000; Meyers et al., 2004). The prognosis is similar for patients with both known and unknown primary tumour (Rudà et al., 2001).

Search strategy

We searched: the Cochrane Library to date; Medline–Ovid (January 1966 to date); Medline–ProQuest; Medline-EIFL; Embase–Ovid (January 1990 to date); CancerNet; Science Citation Index (ISI). We used specific and sensitive keywords, as well as combinations of keywords, and publications in any language of countries represented in the Task Force. We also collected guidelines from National and European multidisciplinary neuro-oncological Societies and Groups (from Italy, France, Netherlands, Germany and the United Kingdom). Moreover we performed an investigation (by e-mail questionnaire) regarding the views of Members of the Task Force on several critical issues, reflecting the different national situations (10 countries) and specialisations (eleven neurologists, one neurosurgeon, one radiation oncologist, one medical oncologist).

Method for reaching consensus

The scientific evidence of papers collected from the literature was evaluated and graded according to

Table 33.1 Karnofsky Performance Status (KPS).

KPS 100	Normal; no complaints; no evidence of disease
KPS 90	Able to carry on normal activity; minor signs or symptoms of disease
KPS 80	Normal activity with effort; some signs or symptoms of disease
KPS 70	Cares for self; unable to carry on normal activity or to do active work
KPS 60	Requires occasional assistance, but is able to care for most personal needs
KPS 50	Requires considerable assistance and frequent medical care
KPS 40	Disabled; requires special care and assistance
KPS 30	Severely disabled; hospitalization is indicated, although death not imminent
KPS 20	Very sick; hospitalization necessary; active support treatment is necessary
KPS 10	Moribund; fatal processes progressing rapidly
KPS 0	Death

Brainin *et al.*, 2004, and recommendations were given according to the same paper. When sufficient evidence for recommendation A-C was not available, we considered a recommendation to be a "Good Practice Point" if agreed by all Members of the Task Force. When analysing results and drawing recommendations, at any stage the differences were resolved by discussions and, if persisting, were reported in the text.

Results

Diagnosis

Headache (40–50%), focal neurological deficits (30–40%) and seizures (15–20%) are the most common presenting symptoms. A minority of patients have an acute "strokelike" onset, more often related to an intratumoural haemorrhage (melanoma, choriocarcinoma and renal carcinoma). Altered mental status or impaired cognition are seen in patients with multiple metastases and/or increased intracranial pressure, sometimes resembling a metabolic encephalopathy. Contrast-enhanced MRI is more sensitive than enhanced CT (including double-dose delayed contrast) or unenhanced MRI in detecting brain metastases, particularly when located in the posterior fossa or very small (Schellinger *et al.*, 1999) (Class II evidence). Double or triple doses of gadolinium-based contrast agents are better than single doses, but increasing the dose may lead to an increased number of false-positive findings (Sze *et al.*, 1998) (Class III evidence).

There are no pathognomonic features on CT or MRI that distinguish brain metastases from primary brain tumours (more commonly malignant gliomas and lymphomas) or non-neoplastic conditions (abscesses, infections, demyelinating diseases, vascular lesions). A peripheral location, spherical shape, ring enhancement with prominent peritumoural oedema and multiple lesions all suggest metastatic disease: these characteristics are helpful but not diagnostic, even in patients with a positive history of cancer. Diffusion-weighted (DW) MR imaging may be useful for the differential diagnosis of ring-enhancing cerebral lesions (restricted diffusion in abscesses compared to unrestricted diffusion in cystic or necrotic glioblastomas or metastases), but the findings are not specific (Desprechins *et al.*, 1999; Hartmann *et al.*, 2001) (Class III evidence). In patients with either histologically confirmed or radiologically suspected brain metastases and a negative history of cancer chest CT is more sensitive than chest radiograph in detecting a synchronous lung tumour (more commonly a non-small cell cancer) (Class III evidence). CT of the abdomen occasionally shows an unsuspected cancer. Further investigations are almost never fruitful without positive features in the patient's history or localizing signs on the physical examination to suggest a primary site (Van de Pol *et al.*, 1996) (Class III evidence). Whole-body fluorodeoxyglucose positron emission tomography (FDG PET) is a sensitive tool for detecting a "probable" primary tumour by visualizing foci of abnormal uptake, more often in the lung (Klee *et al.*, 2002) (Class III evidence), but the specificity in differentiating malignant tumours from benign or inflammatory lesions is relatively low.

Supportive care

Most neurologists use dexamethasone to control cerebral oedema, largely because of its minimal mineralocorticoid effect and long half-life. Patients are generally managed with starting doses of 4–8 mg per day (Vecht et al., 1994) (Class II evidence). Up to 75% of patients with brain metastases show marked neurological improvement within 24–72 h after beginning dexamethasone. Any other corticosteroid is effective if given in equipotent doses. Side effects from chronic dexamethasone administration, including myopathy, are frequent and contribute to disability. When used as the sole form of treatment, dexamethasone produces about one month's remission of symptoms and slightly increases the 4–6-week median survival of patients who receive no treatment at all (Cairncross and Posner, 1983).

The need for anticonvulsant medication is clear in patients who have experienced a seizure by the time their brain tumour is diagnosed. Although many clinicians routinely place patients with brain metastases on prophylactic antiepileptic drugs (AEDs), the evidence (Class I) does not support this practice. The Quality Standards Subcommittee of the American Academy of Neurology (AAN) has reported on anticonvulsant prophylaxis in patients with newly diagnosed brain tumours, including brain metastases (Glantz et al., 2000). Twelve studies, either randomized controlled trials or cohort studies, investigating the ability of prophylactic AEDs (phenytoin, phenobarbital, valproic acid) to prevent first seizures, have been examined, and none have demonstrated efficacy. Subtherapeutic levels of anticonvulsants were extremely common and the severity of side effects appeared to be higher (20–40%) in brain tumour patients than in the general population receiving anticonvulsants, probably because of drug interactions (Class II evidence). Phenytoin, carbamazepine and phenobarbital stimulate the cytochrome P450 system and accelerate the metabolism of corticosteroids and chemotherapeutic agents such as nitrosoureas,

paclitaxel, cyclophosphamide, topotecan, irinotecan, thiotepa, adriamycin and methotrexate, and thus reduce their efficacy. The role of prophylactic anticonvulsants remains to be addressed specifically in some subgroups of patients who have a higher risk of developing seizures, such as those with metastatic melanoma, haemorrhagic lesions and multiple metastases. For patients who underwent a neurosurgical procedure the efficacy of prophylaxis has not been proven (Kuijlen et al., 1996) (Class II evidence), and the AAN recommends to withdraw AEDs at 1 week after surgery. The efficacy of novel AEDs (levetiracetam, topiramate, gabapentin, oxcarbazepine, lamotrigine) in controlling epileptic seizures has not been extensively investigated.

Anticoagulant therapy is the standard treatment for acute venous thromboembolism (VTE) in cancer patients. For initial therapy subcutaneous low-molecular weight heparin (LMWH) is as effective and safe as intravenous unfractionated heparin (UFH) (Gould et al., 1999) (Class I evidence). LMWH is more effective than oral anticoagulant therapy (warfarin) in preventing recurrent VTE in cancer patients (Lee et al., 2003) (Class I evidence). The duration of anticoagulant therapy has not been specifically addressed in cancer patients. A prophylaxis with either UFH or LMWH reduces the risk of VTE in patients undergoing major surgery for cancer (Class II evidence).

Treatment of single brain metastasis
Surgery

Three randomized trials have compared surgical resection followed by WBRT with WBRT alone (Patchell et al., 1990; Vecht et al., 1993; Mintz et al., 1996). The first two studies have shown a survival benefit for patients receiving the combined treatment (median survival 9–10 months versus 3–6 months). In the Patchell study, patients who received surgery displayed a lower rate of local relapses (20% versus 52%) and a longer time of functional independence. The third study, which included more patients with an active systemic disease and a low Karnofsky performance status, did not show any benefit with the addition of surgery. Therefore, there is Class I evidence that the survival benefit of surgical resection is limited to the sub-group of patients with controlled systemic disease and good performance status. Surgical resection allows in the majority of patients an immediate relief of symptoms of intracranial hypertension, a reduction of focal neurological deficits and seizures, and a rapid steroid taper. Gross total resection of a brain metastasis can be achieved with lower morbidity using contemporary image guided systems, such as preoperative functional MRI, intraoperative neuronavigation and cortical mapping (Black and Johnson, 2004) (Class IV evidence). The combined resection of a solitary brain metastasis and a synchronous non small-cell lung carcinoma (stage I and II) is increasingly performed, yielding a median survival of at least 12 months, with 10–30% of patients surviving at 5 years (Kelly and Bunn, 1998) (Class III evidence). In selected patients with local relapse of a single brain metastasis and good performance status, re-operation affords a neurological improvement and prolongation of survival (Black and Johnson, 2004) (Class III evidence).

Stereotactic radiosurgery

Stereotactic radiosurgery (SRS) permits the delivery of a single high dose of radiation to a target of 3–3.5 cm of maximum diameter by using gamma-knife (multiple cobalt sources) or linear accelerator (Linac) through a stereotactic device. The rapid dose fall-off of SRS minimizes the risk of damage to the surrounding normal nervous tissue. In patients with newly diagnosed brain metastases a decrease of symptoms, a local tumour control (defined as shrinkage or arrest of growth) at 1 year of 80–90% and a median survival of 6–12 months have been reported (Warnick et al., 2004; Soffietti et al., 2005) (Class II evidence). Metastases from radioresistant tumours, such as melanoma, renal cell carcinoma and colon cancer, respond to SRS as well as do metastases from radiosensitive tumours. Radiosurgery allows the treatment of brain metastases in almost any location. The type of radiosurgical procedure, gamma-knife or Linac-based, does not have an impact on the results (Sneed et al., 2002). A randomized trial has shown that SRS combined with WBRT (radiosurgical boost) is superior to WBRT alone in terms of survival (Andrews et al., 2004) (Class II evidence). Survival following radiosurgery is comparable to that achieved with surgery (Warnick et al., 2004; Soffietti et al., 2005) (Class II evidence). SRS is less invasive than surgery and can be accomplished in an outpatient setting, and thus offers cost effectiveness advantages over surgery; on the other hand, patients with large lesions may require chronic steroid administration. Radiosurgery is effective for patients with brain metastases that have recurred following conventional WBRT (Shaw et al., 2000) (Class II evidence).

Hypofractionated stereotactic radiotherapy can be an alternative to SRS.

Acute (early) and chronic (late) complications following radiosurgery for brain metastases are relatively modest (Gelblum et al., 1998). Acute reactions (due to oedema) occur in 7–10% of patients, more often within 2 weeks of treatment, and include headache, nausea and vomiting, worsening of pre-existent neurological deficits and seizures. These reactions are generally reversible with steroids. Chronic complications consist of haemorrhage and radionecrosis (1–17%), requiring re-operation in up to 4% of patients. Radiographically, a transient increase in the size of the irradiated lesion, with increasing oedema and mass effect, with or without radionecrosis, cannot be distinguished from a tumour progression: FdG-PET (Chao et al., 2001) and MR spectroscopy (Rock et al., 2004) can give additional information .

Whole-brain radiotherapy after surgery or radiosurgery (adjuvant WBRT)

It is still controversial whether adjuvant WBRT, whose rationale is that of destroying microscopic metastatic deposits at the original tumour site or at distant intracranial locations, is necessary after complete surgical resection or radiosurgery. Time-consuming fractionated treatment, possible long-term neurotoxicity and availability of effective salvage treatments at recurrence are the main arguments against WBRT. Adjuvant WBRT after complete surgical resection significantly reduces local and distant CNS relapses (18% versus 70%), without affecting overall survival or functionally independent survival (Patchell et al., 1998) (Class I evidence). A modest survival benefit for the addition of WBRT has been found in the subset of patients without evidence of extracranial disease (Patchell *et al.*, 1998). WBRT in conjunction with radiosurgery improves local control and reduces the risk of new distant brain metastases, but most studies (non-randomized) support the viewpoint that the combination of radiosurgery and WBRT does not improve the overall survival, except for patients without evidence of extracranial disease (Class II evidence). WBRT may cause early adverse effects (fatigue, alopecia, eustachian tube dysfunction) and late neurotoxicity. Long-term survivors after WBRT frequently develop radiographic changes on CT or MRI, including cortical atrophy, ventriculomegaly and hyperintensity of the periventricular white matter in T2 and FLAIR images. Up to 11% of patients have clinical symptoms such as memory loss progressing to dementia, frontal gait disorders and urinary incontinence. The risk of late neurotoxicity is higher with hypofractionated schedules of radiotherapy (size fraction >2 Gy) (De Angelis *et al.*, 1989).

Whole-brain radiotherapy alone

Median survival after WBRT alone is 3–6 months. Different fractionation schedules, ranging from 20 Gy in 1 week to 50 Gy in 4 weeks, yield comparable results (Borgelt *et al.*, 1980; Hoskin and Brada, 2001) (Class II evidence). Nausea, vomiting, headache, fever and transient worsening of neurological symptoms in the initial phase of therapy may be observed.

The treatment of multiple brain metastases

Median survival after WBRT alone is 2–6 months, with good palliation of symptoms including headache, motor deficits, confusional states and cranial nerve palsies. Hypofractionated treatments are generally employed, most commonly 30 Gy in ten fractions or 20 Gy in five fractions. In patients with poor prognostic factors supportive care only is frequently prescribed. Radiosurgery is an alternative to WBRT in patients with up to three brain metastases. WBRT with radiosurgery boost

improves functional independence but not survival in patients with two or three lesions (Andrews *et al.*, 2004) (Class I evidence). Among new radiosensitizers used in conjunction with standard WBRT, motexafin-gadolinium and RSR 13 have shown a benefit in prolonging time to neurologic/neurocognitive progression in patients with brain metastases from lung and in those of RPA Class II breast cancer respectively (Mehta *et al.*, 2003; Shaw *et al.*, 2003; Suh *et al.* 2006) (Class III evidence). When the number of brain metastases is limited (up to three), the lesions are accessible and the patients are relatively young, in good neurological condition and with a controlled systemic disease, complete surgical resection yields results that are comparable to those obtained in single lesions (Pollock *et al.*, 2003) (Class III evidence).

The role of chemotherapy

Chemosensitivity is the critical factor for the response of brain metastases to chemotherapeutic agents (Soffietti *et al.*, 2005): brain metastases are often as responsive as the primary tumour and extracranial metastases; higher response rates are observed when newly diagnosed, chemotherapy-naïve patients are treated; response rate of brain and systemic cancer declines with second and third-line therapy; response to chemotherapy of brain metastases from mostly chemosensitive tumours (small-cell lung carcinoma, germ cell tumours, lymphomas) is of the same order of that observed after radiotherapy. The blood–brain barrier penetration is a limiting factor in micrometastases and for molecular targeted agents. The combination of radiotherapy and chemotherapy may improve the response rate and/or the progression-free survival, but not the overall survival (Robinet *et al.*, 2001; Antonadou *et al.*, 2002; Verger *et al.*, 2005) (Class I evidence).

Emerging treatments

Emerging treatments of brain metastases, which are still confined to an investigational setting, include both local and systemic approaches.

An innovative modality of postoperative local irradiation is the Gliasite Radiation Therapy

System, consisting of an inflatable balloon placed in the resection cavity at the time of tumour debulking and filled with an acqueous solution of Iodine-125. The dose delivered is up to 60 Gy at 1 cm and the device is explanted after 3–6 days of treatment. A multicenter phase II study on single brain metastasis has been completed in the United States, and the preliminary analysis indicates that the procedure is relatively safe and the local recurrence rate could be significantly reduced (Rogers *et al.*, 2004). Local chemotherapy, utilizing BCNU-impregnated biodegradable polymers placed in the resection cavity, has recently entered a clinical trial in the United States.

Novel cytotoxic drugs, such as temozolomide, fotemustine, capecitabine, etc, are being investigated, alone or in combination, in brain metastases from different tumour types (Soffietti *et al.*, 2005). Among molecular targeted agents, preliminary encouraging results in brain metastases from non small-cell lung cancer have been reported with gefitinib (ZD 1839), an oral epidermal growth factor receptor (EGFR) tyrosine kinase inhibitor (Ceresoli *et al.*, 2004). Novel molecular agents, targeting angiogenesis and/or proliferation and/or invasion and/or apoptosis will be available for clinical trials in the near future.

RECOMMENDATIONS

1. Diagnosis

- When neurological symptoms and/or signs develop in a patient with known systemic cancer, brain metastases must always be suspected. Careful medical history and physical examination with special emphasis on the presence/activity of the systemic disease and the general physical condition (estimation of the performance status) are recommended. All these recommendations are Good Practice Points.
- CT (including double-dose delayed contrast) is inferior to MRI, but it is sufficient when it shows multiple brain metastases. Contrast-enhanced MRI is indicated when (a) surgery or radiosurgery are considered for one or two metastases on contrast-enhanced CT and a KPS $\geq$ 70 (b) contrast-enhanced CT is negative but the history is strongly suggestive for the presence of brain metastases in a patient with established malignant disease (c) CT is not conclusive to eliminate non-neoplastic lesions (abscesses, infections, demyelinating diseases, vascular lesions). All these recommendations are Level B.
- Diffusion MRI is useful for the differential diagnosis of ring-enhancing lesions (Level C).
- EEG is indicated in patients who suffer from seizures that cannot be classified as epileptic (Good Practice Point).
- Tissue diagnosis (by stereotactic or open surgery) should be obtained when (a) the primary tumour is unknown (b) the systemic cancer is well controlled and the patient is a long-term survivor (c) lesions on MRI do not show the typical aspect of brain metastases (d) there is clinical suspicion of an abscess (fever, meningism) (Level B). In patients with unknown primary tumour, CT of the chest/abdomen and mammography are recommended by most Members of the Task Force, but a further extensive evaluation is not appropriate in the absence of specific symptoms or indications from the brain biopsy (Good Practice Point). FDG PET can be useful for detecting the primary tumour (Good Practice Point). The histopathologic studies on the brain metastasis may provide valuable information in indicating a likely organ of origin and guiding further specialized diagnostic work-up: in this regard immunohistochemical staining to detect tissue-, organ-, or tumour-specific antigens is useful (Good Practice Point).
- CSF cytology is needed when the coexistence of a carcinomatous meningitis is suspected (Good Practice Point).

continued

2. Supportive care

- Dexamethasone is the corticosteroid of choice and twice-daily dosing is sufficient (Good Practice Point). In most cases, starting doses should not exceed 4–8 mg per day, but patients with severe symptoms, including impaired consciousness or other signs of increased intracranial pressure, may benefit from higher doses such as 16 mg/day or even more (Level B). An attempt to reduce the dose should be undertaken within 1 week of initiation of treatment; if possible, steroids should be weaned off within 2 weeks. If complete weaning off is not possible, the lowest possible dose should be looked for. Asymptomatic patients do not require steroids. Steroids may reduce the acute side-effects of radiation therapy. All these recommendations are Good Practice Points.

- Anticonvulsants should not be prescribed prophylactically (Level A). In patients who suffer from epileptic seizures and need a concomitant treatment with chemotherapeutics, enzyme-inducing antiepileptic drugs (EIAEDs) should be avoided (Level B).

- In patients with venous thromboembolism low-molecular weight heparin is effective and well tolerated for both initial therapy and secondary prophylaxis (Level A). A duration of the anticoagulant treatment ranging from 3 and 6 months is recommended (Good Practice Point). Prophylaxis in patients undergoing surgery is recommended (Level B).

3. Treatment of single brain metastasis

- Surgical resection should be considered in patients with single brain metastasis in an accessible location, especially when the size is large, the mass effect is considerable and an obstructive hydrocephalus is present (Good Practice Point). Surgery is recommended when the systemic disease is absent/controlled and the Karnofsky Performance score is 70 or more (Level A). When the combined resection of a solitary brain metastasis and a non small-cell lung carcinoma (stage I and II) is feasible, surgery for the brain lesion should come first, with a maximum delay between the two surgeries not exceeding 3 weeks (Good Practice Point). Patients with disseminated but controllable systemic disease (i.e. bone metastases from breast cancer) or with a radioresistant primary tumour (melanoma, renal cell carcinoma, colon cancer) may benefit from surgery (Good Practice Point). Surgery at recurrence is useful in selected patients (Level C).

- Stereotactic radiosurgery should be considered in patients with metastases of a diameter of ≤3–3.5 cm and/or located in eloquent cortical areas, basal ganglia, brain stem or with comorbidities precluding surgery (Level B). Gamma-knife or linear accelerator (Linac) is equally effective (Level B). Stereotactic radiosurgery may be effective at recurrence after prior radiation treatment (Level B).

- The role of adjuvant WBRT after surgery or radiosurgery remains to be clarified. In case of absent/controlled systemic disease and Karnofsky Performance score of 70 or more, one can either withhold initial WBRT if close follow up with MRI (every 3–4 months) is performed or deliver early WBRT with fractions of 1.8–2 Gy to a total dose of 40–55 Gy to avoid late neurotoxicity (Good Practice Point).

- WBRT alone is the therapy of choice for patients with active systemic disease and/or poor performance status and should employ hypofractionated regimens such as 30 Gy in ten fractions or 20 Gy in five fractions (Level B). For elderly patients with poor performance status WBRT can be withheld and supportive care only employed (Good Practice Point).

4. The treatment of multiple brain metastases: In patients with up to three brain metastases, good performance status (KPS of 70 or more) and controlled systemic disease, stereotactic radiosurgery is an alternative to WBRT (Level B), while surgical resection is an option when the lesions are in an accessible location (Level C). In patients with more than three brain metastases WBRT with hypofractionated regimens is the treatment of choice (Level B). In bedridden patients it should be considered to withhold active radiation treatment and restrict therapy to supportive care (Good Practice Point).

5. The role of chemotherapy: Chemotherapy may be the initial treatment for patients with brain metastases from chemosensitive tumours, like small-cell lung cancers, lymphomas, germ cell tumours and breast cancers, especially for chemo-naïve patients or if an effective chemotherapy schedule for the primary is still available (Good Practice Point). Radiation therapy, with or without chemotherapy, is still the treatment of choice for patients needing a palliation of neurological symptoms (Good Practice Point).

Conflicts of interest

None of the Members of the Task Force, including the chairperson, had any form of conflict of interest.

References

Andrews DW, Scott CB, Sperduto PW, Flanders AE, Gaspar LE, Schell MC, Wasik-Werner M, Demas W, Ryu J, Bahary JP, Souhami L, Rotman M, Mehta M, Curran J (2004). Whole brain radiation therapy with or without stereotactic radiosurgery boost for patients with one to three brain metastases: phase III results of the RTOG randomised trial. *The Lancet* **363:**1665–1672.

Antonadou D, Paraskevaidis M, Sarris G, Coliarakis N, Economou I, Karageorgis P, Throuvalas N (2002). Phase 2 randomized trial of temozolomide and concurrent radiotherapy in patients with brain metastases. *J Clin Oncol* **20:**3644–3650.

Black PM and Johnson MD (2004). Surgical resection for patients with solid brain metastases: current status. *J Neuro Oncol* **69:**119–124.

Borgelt BB, Gelber RD, Kramer S, Brady LW, Chang CH, Davis LW, Perez CA, Hendrickson FR (1980). The palliation of brain metastases: final results of the first two studies by the Radiation Therapy Oncology Group. *Int J Radiat Oncol Biol Phys* **6:**1–9.

Brainin M, Barnes M, Baron JC, Gilhus NE, Hughes R, Selmaj K, Walderman G (2004). Guidance for the preparation of neurological management guidelines by EFNS scientific task forces - revised recommendations 2004. *Eur J Neurol* **11:**577–581.

Cairncross JG, Posner JB (1983). The management of brain metastases. Walker MD (ed) *Oncology of the Nervous System*. Martinus Nijhoff, Boston, pp 342–377.

Ceresoli G, Cappuzzo F, Gregorc V, Bartolini S, Crinò L, Villa E (2004). Gefitinib in patients with brain metastases from non-small cell lung cancer: a prospective trial. *Ann Oncol* **15:**1042–1047.

Chao ST, Suh JH, Raja S, Lee SY, Barnett G (2001). The sensitivity and specificity of FDG PET in distinguishing recurrent brain tumor from radionecrosis in patients treated with stereotactic radiosurgery. *Int J Cancer* **96:**191–197.

De Angelis LM, Delattre JY, Posner JB (1989). Radiation-induced dementia in patients cured of brain metastases. *Neurology* **39:**789–796.

Desprechins B, Stadnik T, Koerts G, Shabana W, Breucq C, Osteux M (1999). Use of diffusion-weighted MR imaging in the differential diagnosis between intracerebral necrotic tumors and cerebral abscesses. *AJNR Am J Neuroradiol* **20:**1252–1257.

Gaspar L, Scott C, Rotman M, Asbell S, Phillips T, Wasserman T, McKenna WG, Byhardt R (1997). Recursive partitioning analysis (RPA) of prognostic factors in three Radiation Therapy Oncology Group (RTOG) brain metastases trials. *Int J Radiat Oncol Biol Phys* **37:**745–751.

Gelblum DY, Lee H, Bilsky M, Pinola C, Longford S, Wallner K (1998). Radiographic findings and morbidity in patients treated with stereotactic radiosurgery. *Int J Radiat Oncol Biol Phys* **42:**391–395.

Glantz MJ, Cole BF, Forsyth PA, Recht LD, Wen PA, Chamberlain MC, Grossman SA, Cairncross JG (2000). Practice parameter: anticonvulsant prophylaxis in patients with newly diagnosed brain tumors. Report of the Quality Standards Subcommittee of the American Academy of Neurology. *Neurology* **54:**1886–1893.

Gould MK, Dembitzer AD, Doyle RL, Hastie TJ, Garber AM (1999). Low-molecular-weight heparins compared with unfractionated heparin for treatment of acute deep venous thrombosis. A meta-analysis of randomized, controlled trials. *Ann Intern Med* **130**(10):800–809.

Hartmann M, Jansen O, Heiland S, Sommer C, Munkel K, Sartor K (2001). Restricted diffusion within ring enhancement is not pathognomonic for brain abscess. *AJNR Am J Neuroradiol* **22**:1738–1742.

Hoskin PJ and Brada M (2001). Radiotherapy for brain metastases. *Clin Oncol* **13**:91–94.

Kelly K, Bunn PA (1998). It is time to reevaluate our approach to the treatment of brain metastases in patients with non-small cell lung cancer? *Lung Cancer* **20**:85–91.

Klee B, Law I, Hoigaard L, Kosteljanetz M (2002). Detection of unknown primary tumours in patients with cerebral metastases using whole-body 18F-fluorodeoxyglucose positron emission tomography. *Eur J Neurol* **9**:657–662.

Kuijlen JM, Teernstra OP, Kessels AG, Herpers MJ, Beuls EA (1996). Effectiveness of antiepileptic prophylaxis used with supratentorial craniotomies: a meta-analysis. *Seizure* **5**:291–298.

Lagerwaard FJ, Levendag PC, Nowak PJ, Eijkenboom WM, Hanssens PE, Schmitz PI (1999). Identification of prognostic factors in patients with brain metastases: a review of 1292 patients. *Int J Radiat Oncol Biol Phys* **43**:795–803.

Lee AY, Levine MN, Baker RI, Bowden C, Kakkar AK, Prins M (2003). Low-molecular-weight heparin versus coumarin for the prevention of recurrent venous thromboembolism in cancer. *N Engl J Med* **349**:146–153.

Mehta M, Rodrigus P, Terhaard C, Rao A, Suh J, Roa W, Sohuami L, Beziak A, Leibenhaut M, Komaki R, Schultz C, Timmerman R, Curran W, Smith J, Phan SC, Miller R, Renschler M (2003). Survival and neurologic outcomes in a randomized trial of motexafin–gadolinium and whole-brain radiation therapy in brain metastases. *J Clin Oncol* **21**:2529–2536.

Meyers CA, Smith JA, Bezjak A (2004). Neurocognitive function and progression in patients with brain metastases treated with whole brain radiation and motexafin gadolinium: results of a randomized phase III trial. *J Clin Oncol* **22**:157–165.

Mintz AH, Kestle J, Rathbone MP, Gaspar L, Hugenholtz H, Fisher B, Duncan G, Skingley P, Foster G, Levine M (1996). A randomized trial to assess the efficacy of surgery in addition to radiotherapy in patients with a single cerebral metastasis. *Cancer* **78**:1470–1476.

Murray KJ, Scott C, Zachariah B, Michalski JM, Demas W, Vora NL, Whitton A, Movsas B (2000). Importance of the Mini-Mental Status Examination in the treatment of patients with brain metastases: a report from the Radiation Therapy Oncology Group protocol. *Int J Radiat Oncol Biol Phys* **48**:59–64.

Patchell RA, Tibbs PA, Walsh JW, Dempsey RJ, Maruyama Y, Kryscio RJ, Markesbery WR, Macdonald JS, Young B (1990). A randomized trial of surgery in the treatment of single metastases to the brain. *N Engl J Med* **322**:494–500.

Patchell RA, Tibbs PA, Regine WF, Dempsey RJ, Mohiuddin M, Kryscio RJ, Markesbery WR, Foon KA, Young B (1998). Postoperative radiotherapy in the treatment of single brain metastases to the brain. *JAMA* **280**:1485–1489.

Pirzkall A, Debus J, Lohr F, Fuss M, Rhein B, Engenhart-Cabillic R, Wannenmaker M (1998). Radiosurgery alone or in combination with whole-brain radiotherapy for brain metastases. *J Clin Oncol* **16**:3563–3569.

Pollock BE, Brown PD, Foote RL, Stafford SL, Schomberg PJ (2003). Properly selected patients with multiple brain metastases may benefit from aggressive treatment of their intracranial disease. *J Neuro Oncol* **61**:73–80.

Robinet G, Thomas P, Breton JL, Lena H, Gouva S, Dabouis G, Bennouna J, Souquet PJ, Balmes P, Thiberville L, Fournel P, Quoix E, Riou R, Rebattu P, Perol M, Paillotin D, Mornex F (2001). Results of a phase III study of early versus delayed whole brain radiotherapy with concurrent cisplatin and vinorelbine combination in inoperable brain metastases of non-small cell lung cancer: Groupe Francais de Pneumocancerologie (GFPC) protocol 95-1. *Ann Oncol* **12**:59–67.

Rock JP, Scarpace L, Hearshen D, Gutierrez J, Fisher JL, Rosenblum M, Mikkelsen T (2004). Associations among magnetic resonance spectroscopy, apparent diffusion coefficients, and image-guided histopathology with special attention to radiation necrosis. *Neurosurgery* **54**:1111–1117.

Rogers LR, Rock JR, Sills A, Vogelbaum M, Ewend M, Shaw E (2004). Final results of a phase II study of resection and gliasite brachytherapy for a single brain metastasis. *Neuro-Oncology* **6**(4): 363.

Rudà R, Borgognone M, Benech F, Vasario E, Soffietti R (2001). Brain metastases from unknown primary tumor. *J Neurol* **248**:394–398.

Schellinger PD, Meinck HM, Thron A (1999). Diagnostic accuracy of MRI compared to CT in patients with brain metastases. *J Neurooncol* **44**:275–281.

Shaw E, Scott C, Souhami L, Dinapoli R, Kline R, Loeffler J, Farnan N (2000). Single dose radiosurgical treatment of recurrent previously irradiated primary brain tumors and brain metastases: final report of RTOG protocol 90-05. *Int J Radiat Oncol Biol Phys* **47**:291–298.

Sneed PK, Suh JH, Goetsch SJ, Sanghavi SN, Chappell R, Buatti JM, Regine WF, Weltman E, King VJ, Breneman JC, Sperduto PW, Mehta MP (2002). A multi-institutional review of radiosurgery alone vs. radiosurgery with whole brain radiotherapy as the initial management of brain metastases. *Int J Radiat Oncol Biol Phys* **53:**519–526.

Soffietti R, Costanza A, Laguzzi E, Nobile M, Rudà R (2005). Radiotherapy and chemotherapy of brain metastases. *J Neuro-Oncol* **75 (1):**1–12.

Sze G, Johnson C, Kawamura Y, Goldberg SN, Lange R, Friedland RJ, Wolf RJ (1998). Comparison of single- and triple-dose contrast material in the MR screening of brain metastases. *AJNR* **19:**821–828.

Suh J, Stea B, Nabid A, Kresl J, Fortim A, Mercier J, Senzer N, Chang E, Boyd A, Cagnoni P and Shaw E (2006). Phase III study of efaproxiral as an adjunct to whole-brain radiation therapy for brain metastases. *J Clin Oncol* **24:**106–114.

Van de Pol M, van Aalst VC, Wilmink JT, Twijnstra A (1996). Brain metastases from an unknown primary tumor: which diagnostic procedures are indicated? *J Neurol Neurosurg Psychiatr* **61:**321–323.

Vecht CJ, Haaxma-Reiche H, Noordijk EM, Padberg GW, Voormolen JH, Hoekstra FH, Tans JT, Lambooij N, Metsaars JA, Wattendorff AR (1993). Treatment of single brain metastasis: radiotherapy alone or combined with neurosurgery? *Ann Neurol* **33:**583–590.

Vecht CJ, Hovestadt A, Verbiest HB, van Vliet JJ, van Putten WL (1994). Dose-effect relationship of dexamethasone on Karnofsky performance in metastatic brain tumors: a randomized study of doses of 4, 8, and 16 mg per day. *Neurology* **44:**675–680.

Verger E, Gil M, Yaya R, Vinolas L, Villa S, Pujol T, Quintò L, Graus F (2005). Temozolomide and concomitant whole brain radiotherapy in patients with brain metastases: a phase 2 trial. *Int J Radiation Oncology Biol. Phys* **61:**185–191.

Warnick RE, Darakchiev BJ, Breneman JC (2004). Stereotactic radiosurgery for patients with solid brain metastases: current status. *J Neuro Oncol* **69:**125–137.

CHAPTER 34

Paraneoplastic syndromes

C.A. Vedeler,[a] J.C. Antoine,[b] B. Giometto,[c] F. Graus,[d] W. Grisold,[e] I.K. Hart,[f] J. Honnorat,[g] P.A.E. Sillevis Smitt,[h] J.J.G.M. Verschuuren,[i] R Voltz[j] for the Paraneoplastic Neurological Syndrome Euronetwork

Abstract

Background Paraneoplastic neurological syndromes (PNS) are remote effects of cancer on the nervous system.

Objectives An overview of the management of classical PNS, that is, paraneoplastic limbic encephalitis, subacute sensory neuronopathy, paraneoplastic cerebellar degeneration, paraneoplastic opsoclonus-myoclonus, Lambert-Eaton myasthenic syndrome and paraneoplastic peripheral nerve hyperexitability is given. Myasthenia gravis and paraproteinemic neuropathies are not included in this report.

Methods No evidence-based recommendations were possible, but Good Practice Points were agreed by consensus.

Urgent investigation is indicated, especially in CNS syndromes, to allow tumour therapy to be started early and prevent progressive neuronal death and irreversible disability. Onconeural antibodies are of great importance in the investigation of PNS and can be used to focus the tumour search. PDG-PET is useful if the initial radiological tumour screen is negative. Early detection and treatment of the tumour is the approach that seems to offer the greatest chance for PNS stabilization. Immune therapy usually has no or modest effect on the CNS syndromes, whereas such therapy is beneficial for PNS affecting the neuromuscular junction. Symptomatic therapy should be offered to all patients with PNS.

Background

Paraneoplastic neurological syndromes (PNS) were initially defined as neurological syndromes of unknown cause that often antedate the diagnosis of an underlying, usually not clinically evident, cancer. In the last two decades, the discovery

[a]Department of Neurology, Haukeland University Hospital and Department of Clinical Medicine, University of Bergen, Norway; [b]Department of Neurology, Hopital Bellevue, Saint Etienne, France; [c]Department of Neurology and Psychiatry (2 Neurologic Clinic) University of Padua, Padua, Italy; [d]Service of Neurology, Institut d'Investigacio Biomedica August Pi i Sunyer (IDIBAPS), Hospital Clinic, University of Barcelona, Barcelona, Spain; [e]Ludwig Boltzmann Institut fur Neuroonkologie, Vienna, Linz, Austria; [f]Neuroimmunology Group, Department of Neurological Science, Liverpool, United Kingdom; [g]Ataxia Research Center, Neurology B, Hospital Neurologique, Lyon, France; [h]Department of Neurology, Erasmus University Medical Center, Rotterdam, The Netherlands; [i]Department of Neurology, Leiden University Medical Center, Leiden, The Netherlands; and [j]Department of Palliative Medicine, University of Cologne, Germany.

Table 34.1 Paraneoplastic neurological syndromes and their therapy.

Paraneoplastic syndrome	Common associated therapy	Onconeural antibodies	Response to symptomatic tumours	Response to immunotherapy	Response to tumour therapy
Limbic encephalitis	SCLC Testicular Breast Hodgkin's Thymoma	Hu Ma2 CV2/CRMP5 Amphiphysin VGKC, but not specific for paraneoplasia	Yes	Variable. Ma2 and onconeural antibody negative patients seem to respond best	Yes, patients often stabilize if treated early
Subacute sensory neuronopathy	SCLC Breast Ovarian Sarcoma Hodgkin's	Hu CV2/CRMP5	Yes	Rare	Yes, especially when treated early
Cerebellar degeneration	Ovary Breast SCLC Hodgkin's	Yo Hu Tr CV2/CRMP5 VGCC, but not specific for paraneoplasia	Yes	Rare	Yes, especially in Hodgkin's
Opsoclonus-myoclonus	Lung Breast Gynecological Melanoma Histocytoma Neuroblastoma in children	Ri Hu Ma2 Amphiphysin Often none, especially in children	Yes	Occasionally in adults. Often in children	Yes
Lambert-Eaton myasthenic Syndrome	SCLC	VGCC, but not specific for paraneoplasia	Yes	Yes	Yes
Peripheral nerve hyperexcitability	Thymoma SCLC NonSCLC Hodgkin's Plasmacytoma	VGKC, but not specific for paraneoplasia	Yes	Yes	Yes

that many PNS are associated with antibodies against neural antigens expressed by the tumour (onconeural antibodies) has suggested that some PNS are immune mediated. PNS are rare and occur in less than 1% of patients with cancer. However, the diagnosis and treatment is important because the disability caused by the PNS is often severe and the correct diagnosis usually leads to the discovery of a small tumour with a chance of being cured (table 34.1). Recently, recommended diagnostic criteria for PNS have been published by the PNS Euronetwork (Graus *et al.*, 2004). In this paper, the European Federation of Neurological Societies (EFNS) Task force, as part of the PNS Euronetwork, has outlined guidelines for the management of classical PNS.

Methods

The Task Force considered the different syndromes known as paraneoplastic and chose to focus on classical PNS (Graus *et al.*, 2004): paraneoplastic limbic encephalitis (PLE), subacute sensory neuronopathy (SSN), paraneoplastic cerebellar degeneration (PCD) and paraneoplastic opsoclonus-myoclonus (POM), as well as Lambert-Eaton myasthenic syndrome (LEMS) and paraneoplastic peripheral nerve hyperexitability (PPNH). Myasthenia gravis has not been included and will be reported together with a broader overview of LEMS and PNH in a separate Task Force report on treatment of neuromuscular disorders. Paraproteinemic neuropathies have previously been evaluated by a EFNS Task force (Willison *et al.*, 2000). Paraneoplastic retinopathy and dermatomyositis have not been included in this report. Search strategies have included English literature from the following databases: Cochrane Library, Med Line, Pub-Med (last search 15 December 2004). The key words used for the search included 'limbic encephalitis', 'sensory neuronopathy', 'cerebellar ataxia', 'opsoclonus-myoclonus', 'Lambert-Eaton myasthenic syndrome', 'neuromyotonia' in combination with 'investigation' and 'therapy'. All evidence available was evaluated as Class IV- case reports, case series, and expert opinion (Brainin *et al.*, 2004). Thus, no recommendations reach Level A, B or C (Brainin *et al.*, 2004). However, Good Practice Points were agreed by consensus.

Paraneoplastic limbic encephalitis

Clinical features

Paraneoplastic limbic encephalitis (PLE) is characterized by the acute, or subacute, onset of symptoms that suggest involvement of the limbic system. Patients may develop short-term memory loss or amnesia, become disoriented, or may show psychosis including visual or auditory hallucinations, or paranoid obsession. Confusion, depression and anxiety are also common. Generalized or partial complex seizures are seen in about 50% of patients. In the majority of patients, the symptoms antedate the diagnosis of a tumour by a mean of 3–5 months. PLE is preferentially associated with small cell lung cancer (SCLC) (40%), germ cell tumors of the testis (20%), breast cancer (8%), Hodgkin's lymphoma, thymoma and immature teratoma (Gultekin *et al.*, 2000).

Investigation

Magnetic resonance imaging (MRI) alterations in PLE are seen in about 60% of patients, but the figure is probably much higher if fluid attenuation inversion recovery (FLAIR) sequences are included in the study. The MRI features are most evident on coronal sections and typically consist of abnormal high-signal intensity on T2 sequences in one or both medial temporal lobe(s). On T1 sequences the temporal-limbic area may be hypointense and atrophic and rarely enhance with contrast injection (Dirr *et al.*, 1990). In the absence of MRI abnormalities, fluorodeoxyglucose-positron emission tomography (FDG-PET) studies should show an increased tracer activity in the medial temporal lobe, which may reflect an acute stage of the inflammatory process (Provenzale *et al.*, 1998). In 45% of patients, electroencephalogram (EEG) reveals epileptic abnormalities from the temporal lobe, but in the majority of patients it shows unilateral or bilateral temporal slow waves. Cerebrospinal fluid (CSF) examinations show inflammatory signs (e.g. pleocytosis, oligoclonal bands) in about 60% of patients.

Onconeuronal antibodies may be found in the serum and CSF of about 60% of patients with PLE. The most frequent onconeuronal antibodies are: anti-Hu, anti-Ma2 (with or without anti-Ma1), anti-CV2/CRMP5 and anti-amphiphysin. Seventy-eight per cent of patients with PLE and anti-Hu have symptoms that suggest a dysfunction in areas of the nervous system other than the limbic system. In fact, PLE may be the presenting or the predominant disorder of patients with paraneoplastic encephalomyelitis (PEM) or the 'anti-Hu syndrome'. These patients usually are older than 40 years, and the related tumour is a SCLC.

Patients with only Ma2 antibodies are usually male, younger than 40 years and clinically present with symptoms of diencephalic and upper brainstem dysfunction. The MRI evaluation is more likely to present abnormalities in medial temporal lobes, hypothalamus, basal ganglia, thalamus or upper brainstem collicular region (Dalmau *et al.*, 2004). CV2/CRMP5 antibodies are instead detected in patients with thymoma or SCLC (Yu *et al.*, 2001). Voltage-gated potassium channel (VGKC) antibodies can be associated with PLE and thymoma or with non-paraneoplastic LE (Buckley *et al.*, 2001; Pozo-Rosich *et al.*, 2003; Vincent *et al.*, 2004).

Patients older than 40 years, smokers and with Hu antibody have to be investigated for the presence of a SCLC. Anti-Hu positive patients could also have extrathoracic tumours, but these can be considered responsible for PLE only when they express Hu antigens (Graus *et al.*, 2001). The absence of Hu antibody does not rule out the presence of SCLC, however, in patients older than 40 years, and without onconeural antibodies, the more frequently associated tumours are: breast cancer, non-SCLC tumours and thymoma. Imaging studies to detect SCLC include high resolution CT of the chest and PDG-PET if the CT scan is negative (Linke *et al.*, 2004; Younes-Mhenni *et al.*, 2004). Special attention must be addressed to abnormal lymph nodes in the mediastinum. Bronchoscopy is usually negative. In male patients younger than 40 years, the detection of Ma2 antibodies suggests the presence of testicular cancer which should be evaluated with ultrasound.

Therapy

Early detection and treatment of the underlying tumour is the approach that offers the greatest chance for neurological improvement or symptom stabilization. In men with only Ma2 antibodies elective orchidectomy and serial examination of the testicle to rule out in situ carcinomas is indicated in patients at high risk of testicular cancer such as the presence of calcifications or undescended testicle. The increasing evidence that PLE is immune-mediated has prompted the use of immune therapies. There are no reports that indicate which kind of immune therapy should be used. Patients are usually treated with one or more of the following: intravenous immunoglobulin, plasma exchange or steroids (Gultekin *et al.*, 2000). PLE without onconeural antibodies and those with Ma2 antibodies (with or without anti-Ma1) seem to

respond better to immune therapy (Gultekin *et al.*, 2000). Symptomatic therapy of PLE is directed against epilepsy and psychiatric symptoms.

Subacute sensory neuronopathy

Clinical features

Several neuropathies have been reported as paraneoplastic, but only subacute sensory neuronopathy (SSN) is regarded as a classical PNS (Graus *et al.*, 2004). SSN is associated with SCLC in 70–80% of cases, but may also occur with breast cancer, ovarian cancer, sarcoma, or Hodgkin's disease (Horwich *et al.*, 1977). SSN precedes the overt clinical manifestations of the cancer with a median delay of 4.5 months (Graus *et al.*, 2001). The onset of SSN is usually subacute and rapidly progressive over weeks before a plateau phase is reached. The distribution is frequently multifocal or asymmetrical. Symptoms consist of pain and paraesthesiae (Graus *et al.*, 2001). Upper limbs are usually affected first or almost invariably involved with the evolution. Sensory loss, especially affecting deep sensation, often leads to severe sensory ataxia and tendon reflexes are absent. Sensory loss may also affect the face, chest, or abdomen. Many patients become bedridden, but an indolent course has been reported (Graus *et al.*, 1994). SSN occurs in 74% of patient with PEM and is predominant in 50–60% and clinically pure in 24% (Graus *et al.*, 2001). Autonomic neuropathy including digestive pseudo-obstruction is frequent.

Investigation

CSF analysis may show elevated protein concentration, pleocytosis and sometimes oligoclonal bands. Electrophysiologically, the hallmark is a severe and diffuse alteration of sensory nerve action potentials that are either absent or markedly reduced (Camdesssance *et al.*, 2002). Motor conduction velocities can be mildly altered. Nerve biopsy is usually not necessary, but may sometimes be helpful to distinguish SSN from multiple mononeuropathy due to vasculitis (Younger *et al.*, 1994).

Hu antibodies are most often associated with SSN. Their estimated specificity in the diagnosis of cancer in patients suspected to have SSN is 99%, but the sensitivity is 82% (Molinuevo *et al.*, 1998).

The absence of Hu antibodies does not exclude the presence of an underlying cancer. CV2/CRMP5 antibodies also occur with peripheral neuropathies (Antoine *et al.*, 2001). In this setting, the neuropathy is usually sensory or sensori-motor in which upper limbs are less frequently involved, but often associated with cerebellar ataxia (Honnorat *et al.*, 1996; Yu *et al.*, 2001). The electrophysiological pattern is axonal or mixed axonal and demyelinating. SCLC, neuroendocrine tumours, and thymoma are usually associated with CV2/CRMP5 antibodies. When high resolution CT of the chest is negative, FDG-PET is recommended (Linke *et al.*, 2004; Younes-Mhenni *et al.*, 2004).

Therapy

In a retrospective study of 200 patients with PEM/SSN, treatment of the tumour was an independent predictor of improvement and stabilization of the neurological disorder (Graus *et al.*, 2001) arguing that an early diagnosis of the cancer may give the patients the best chance of stabilizing the neurological disorder. Although occasional reports indicate that immunosuppressive treatment may improve patients with SSN and Hu antibodies, a larger series failed to demonstrate a clear benefice of intravenous immunoglobulin, steroids, plasma exchange, or cyclophosphamide, alone or in combination (Keime-Guibert *et al.*, 2000). Symptomatic treatment is directed against neuropathic pain, sensory ataxia and dysautonomic manifestation such as orthostatic hypotension.

Paraneoplastic cerebellar degeneration

Clinical features

Paraneoplastic cerebellar degeneration (PCD) is characterised by subacute development of a severe pancerebellar dysfunction. Cerebellar signs usually begin with gait ataxia and, over a few weeks or months, progress to severe, usually symmetrical truncal and limb ataxia, with dysarthria and often nystagmus (Peterson *et al.*, 1992). Occasionally, the onset is rapid, within a few hours or days. Vertigo is common, and many patients complain of diplopia. The cerebellar deficit usually stabilizes,

but, the patient is then often severely incapacitated and most become bed-bound in the first 3 months after diagnosis. PCD is preferentially associated with ovarian cancer, breast cancer, SCLC, or Hodgkin's disease.

Investigation

Brain MRI studies are initially normal, but can demonstrate cerebellar atrophy in the latter stages of the disease. CSF examination shows inflammatory signs without cancer cells (e.g. pleocytosis, oligoclonal bands) in about 60% of PCD patients.

Yo antibodies are most frequently associated with PCD. These patients are mainly female with an average age of 61 years. The associated cancer is ovary, breast, or other gynecological malignancies. Patients with Hu antibodies differ from those with anti-Yo in terms of a frequent association with SCLC, the same frequency in male and female, and often other neurological manifestations as part of PEM (Graus *et al.*, 2001). Between 13% and 20% of patients with Hu antibodies present with a subacute cerebellar syndrome that, in the initial stage, cannot be differentiated from PCD (Graus *et al.*, 2001). Neuropathy is observed in 60% of patients with PCD and CV2/CRMP5 antibodies (Honnorat *et al.*, 1996; Yu *et al.*, 2001) and such antibodies are observed in about 7% of patients with PCD (Mason *et al.*, 1997). Patients with CV2/CRMP5 antibodies are mainly male (70%) with an average age of 62 years. The most frequently associated tumour is SCLC (60%). Tr antibodies are markers of patients with PCD and Hodgkin's disease, which is the third most common associated cancer with PCD, after SCLC and ovarian cancer. Unlike other antibodies, anti-Tr usually disappears after treatment of the tumour or, in a few patients, are only found in the CSF (Bernal *et al.*, 2003). Ri antibodies are mainly observed in patients with cerebellar ataxia and paraneoplastic opsoclonus-myoclonus (POM). The associated cancers are breast or lung cancer. Some cases of PCD have been reported in association with antibodies against amphiphysin, Ma2, Zic4, mGluR1 or VGCC (Shams'ili *et al.*, 2003; Graus *et al.*, 2002, 2004;. When VGCC antibodies are present, LEMS can be associated with PCD (Mason *et al.*, 1997; Fukuda *et al.*, 2003). The absence of onconeural antibodies cannot rule out the diagnosis of PCD, as only 50% of patients with PCD harbor such antibodies (Mason *et al.*, 1997).

If a SCLC is suspected, the tumour is generally demonstrated by high resolution CT of the chest. Special attention must be addressed to abnormal lymph nodes in the mediastinum. Bronchoscopy is usually negative. The use of FDG-PET should be reserved to patients with onconeural antibodies when conventional imaging fails to identify a tumour (Linke *et al.*, 2004; Younes-Mhenni *et al.*, 2004). In the patients without onconeural antibodies the sensitivity and specificity of FDG-PET is poorer. If a gynecological tumour is suspected careful breast and pelvic examination, mammography and pelvic CT are recommended. If no malignancy is revealed with this initial work-up, surgical exploration and removal of ovaries may be warranted, particularly in postmenopausal women with Yo antibodies (Peterson *et al.*, 1992).

Therapy

The best chance to at least stabilize the syndrome is to treat the underlying tumour (Shams'ili *et al.*, 2003). Immune therapy is rarely effective, but few patients have been reported with improvement after intravenous immunoglobulin, steroids or plasmapheresis (Keime-Guibert *et al.*, 2000; Widdess-Walsh *et al.*, 2003; Vernino *et al.*, 2004). Patients with anti-Tr and Hodgkin's disease are more likely to improve than those with other antibodies (Bernal *et al.*, 2003). In patients with Yo antibodies, the prognosis is worse in patients with ovarian cancer and better in patients with breast cancer (Rojas *et al.*, 2000). The prognosis is also better in PCD patients without onconeural antibodies than in patients with Hu antibodies (Mason *et al.*, 1997). Symptomatic treatment of cerebellar ataxia includes neurorehabilitation with speech and swallowing therapy, and modest additional gains can be seen with propranolol or antiepileptic drugs.

Paraneoplastic opsoclonus-myoclonus

Clinical features

Opsoclonus means involuntary eye movements in any direction. It does not remit in darkness and

with eyes closed and may occur intermittently or, if more severe, constantly. In paraneoplastic opsoclonus-myoclonus (POM), opsoclonus is often accompanied by cerebellar signs such as gait ataxia and limb myoclonus, the so-called dancing eyes, dancing feet syndrome and encephalopathy (Anderson *et al.*, 1988; Buttner *et al.*, 1997; Straube *et al.*, 2004). In contrast to most paraneoplastic syndromes, the course of POM may be remitting and relapsing (Anderson *et al.*, 1988; Dropcho *et al.*, 1993).

In infants, the most common associated tumour is neuroblastoma (Mitchell *et al.*, 2002; Gambini *et al.*, 2003). In adults it is either lung cancer, breast cancer, or a gynecological cancer such as ovary or uterus (Bataller *et al.*, 2001; Voltz, 2002; Darnell and Posner, 2003). The association with other tumours on single case basis has been reported, such as melanoma (Berger and Mehari, 1999) or malignant fibrous histiocytoma (Zamecnik *et al.*, 2004).

Investigation

Brain MRI studies are normal while examination of the CSF may show mild pleocytosis and protein elevation. Most infant (Antunes *et al.*, 2000; Pranzatelli *et al.*, 2002) and adult patients do not harbour a clearly defined onconeural antibody (Bataller *et al.*, 2001; Bataller *et al.*, 2003). In those who do, anti-Hu, anti-amphiphysin, anti-Ri or anti-Ma2 may be found (Bataller *et al.*, 2001; Prestigiacomo *et al.*, 2001; Wong *et al.*, 2001; Wirtz *et al.*, 2002).

In children, the search for an occult neuroblastoma should include imaging of the chest and abdomen (CT-scan or MRI), urine catecholamine measurements (VMA and HVA) and metaiodobenzylguanidine (MIBG) scan (Swart *et al.*, 2002). When negative, the evaluation should be repeated after several months (Hayward *et al.*, 2001).

Initial investigation in adult patients suspected of POM should be directed at tumours associated with this condition, that is, high resolution CT of the chest and abdomen and gynecological examination and mammography in women (Bataller *et al.*, 2001). When this evaluation is negative, FDG-PET should be considered (Linke *et al.*, 2004; Younes-Mhenni *et al.*, 2004).

Therapy

Tumour therapy is the mainstay of management (Bataller *et al.*, 2001). In the pediatric population, POM may improve following treatment with adrenocorticotropic hormone (ACTH), steroids, or intravenous immunoglobulin, but residual CNS signs are frequent (Hayward *et al.*, 2001; Rudnick *et al.*, 2001; Mitchell *et al.*, 2002). In contrast to idiopathic OM, no clear advantage of immune therapy has been demonstrated in adult POM (Bataller *et al.*, 2001). Improvement following steroids, cyclophosphamide, azathioprine, intravenous immunoglobulin, plasma exchange or plasma filtration with a protein A column has been described in single cases (Dropcho *et al.*,1993; Nitschke *et al.*, 1995; Jongen *et al.*, 1988; Wirtz *et al.*, 2002). Symptomatic therapy of nystagmus and oscillopsia includes the use of various antiepileptic drugs, baclofen or propranolol (Straube *et al.*, 2004). Myoclonus can be treated with antiepileptic drugs.

Lambert-Eaton myasthenic syndrome

Clinical features

In more than 90% of the patients, muscle weakness starts proximal in the legs. Weakness can spread to other skeletal muscles in a caudo-cranial order, but only rarely leads to need for artificial respiration. Ptosis and ophthalmoplegia tend to be milder than in myasthenia gravis (Wirtz *et al.*, 2002). Autonomic dysfunction is characterized by the presence of a dry mouth, dryness of the eyes, blurred vision, impotence, constipation, impaired sweating, or orthostatic hypotension (O'Neill *et al.*, 1988). The autonomic dysfunction is mostly mild to moderate, in contrast to the severe disabling autonomic dysfunction sometimes found in SSN/PEM. In rare cases, patients with Lambert-Eaton myasthenic syndrome (LEMS) and SCLC develop PCD (Mason *et al.*, 1997; Fukuda *et al.*, 2003).

Investigation

Electrophysiological studies show a reduced amplitude of the compound muscle action potential after nerve stimulation with decrement at low frequency stimulation (3 Hz) of more than 10%, and an increment of more than 100% after maximum voluntary contraction of the muscle for 15 s. High frequency stimulation at > 20 Hz also produces an increased increment, but is painful and not usually necessary. Anti-P/Q-type VGCC antibodies are present in the serum of at least 85% of the patients (Motomura *et al.*, 1995). These antibodies are found in both forms of LEMS, with or without SCLC. Antibodies to N-type VGCC have also been found in the serum, but their contribution to the muscle weakness or autonomic dysfunction is probably small. They are not used for diagnostic purposes.

In half of the LEMS patients, SCLC will be found, mostly within 2 years. A retrospective study of 77 patients with LEMS, showed that patients who had been smoking and were HLA-B8-negative had a 69% chance of developing SCLC. On the other hand, none of 24 patients who never smoked and were HLA-B8-positive developed SCLC (Wirtz *et al.*, 2005). However, it is recommended that all patients are examined by high resolution chest CT, and possibly also by bronchoscopy and PDG-PET if the CT scan is negative. This is especially important for patients with high risk of SCLC (smoking and HLA-B8 negative). Follow-up should be continued with CT scans every 6 months for at least 4 years.

Therapy

For patients with a SCLC it is important to treat the tumour. Specific tumour therapy in a small retrospective series resulted in recovery from the neurological syndrome within 6–12 months (Chalk *et al.*, 1990). One patient remained tumour free after radiotherapy and local resection at 12 years. Chemotherapy which is the first choice of tumour treatment will also have an immunosuppressive effect on LEMS. It has been shown that the presence of LEMS in patients with SCLC improves survival (Maddison *et al.*, 1999). Symptomatic treatment consists of 3,4-diaminopyridine (McCoy *et al.*, 1989) and additional therapeutic effect may be obtained if combined with pyridostigmin. If this treatment is not sufficient, steroids, azathioprine, plasma exchange and intravenous immunoglobulin should be considered.

Paraneoplastic peripheral nerve hyperexcitability

Clinical features

The commonest form of PNH (neuromyotonia; Isaacs' syndrome) is autoimmune and often caused by antibodies to VGKC (Hart *et al.*, 1997). Paraneoplastic peripheral nerve hyperexcitability (PPNH) is present in up to 25% of the patients and can predate the detection of a tumour by up to 4 years (Hart *et al.*, 2002). In a study of sixty patients, seven (12%) had a thymoma with myasthenia gravis (MG), two (3%) had a thymoma without clinical MG, four (7%) had a SCLC, and one (2%) had a lung adenocarcinoma (Hart *et al.*, 2002). PPNH can also occur with Hodgkin's disease (Caress *et al.*, 1997; Lahrmann *et al.*, 2001) and plasmacytoma (Zifko *et al.*, 1994).

The clinical hallmark of PNH is spontaneous and continuous skeletal muscle overactivity usually presenting as twitching and painful cramps and often accompanied by various combinations of stiffness, pseudomyotonia, pseudotetany, and weakness (Newsom-Davis and Mills, 1993). About 33% of patients also have sensory features and up to 50% have hyperhidrosis suggesting autonomic involvement. CNS features can occur, ranging from personality change and insomnia to a psychosis with delusions, hallucinations, and autonomic disturbance (Morvan's syndrome).

Investigation

EMG helps to confirm PNH and excludes other causes of continuous muscle overactivity such as stiff limb syndromes (Newsom-Davis and Mills, 1993). Nerve conduction studies may characterize an underlying peripheral neuropathy (Newsom-Davis and Mills, 1993; Hart *et al.*, 2002).

There is no antibody that indicates whether PNH is paraneoplastic. VGKC antibodies are found in about 35% of all acquired PNH patients, although this rises to 80% in those with thymoma (Hart *et al.*, 1997). VGKC antibodies can also be associated with PLE and thymoma without PNH, or with non-paraneoplastic LE (Buckley *et al.*, 2001; Pozo-Rosich *et al.*, 2003; Vincent *et al.*, 2004). Hu antibodies can be helpful as one PPNH patient had SCLC (Toepfer *et al.*, 1999). Serum and urine screening for a paraprotein can help identify a plasmacytoma (Zifko *et al.*, 1994).

Most adults warrant a post contrast CT mediastinum scan as up to 15% of patients have a thymoma, sometimes in the absence of MG or AChR antibodies (Hart *et al.*, 2002). This is combined with a high resolution CT of the chest as about 10% of PNH patients will have a SCLC or adenocarcinoma (Hart *et al.*, 2002). Chest CT may also help detect Hodgkin's disease (Caress *et al.*, 1997; Lahrmann *et al.*, 2001). When the initial tumour screen is negative and malignancy is still suspected, PDG-PET is the investigation of choice. Monitoring for up to 4 years is indicated in those at risk of lung cancer (Hart *et al.*, 2002).

Treatment

PPNH often improves and can remit after treatment of cancer (Newsom-Davis and Mills, 1993; Zifko *et al.*, 1994; Caress *et al.*, 1997; Toepfer *et al.*, 1999). The demonstration that most cases of PNH are autoimmune has led to trials of immunomodulatory therapies in patients, including a few with thymoma (Newsom-Davis and Mills, 1993; Hayat *et al.*, 2000) whose symptoms are debilitating or refractory to symptomatic therapy. Plasma exchange often produces useful clinical improvement lasting about 6 weeks accompanied by a reduction in EMG activity (Newsom-Davis and Mills, 1993) and a fall in VGKC antibody titres (Shillito *et al.*, 1995). Experience suggests that intravenous immunoglobulin can also help (Alessi *et al.*, 2000) despite reports that it worsened PNH in one patient (Ishii *et al.*, 1994) and was less effective than plasma exchange in another (van den Berg *et al.*, 1999). By analogy with LEMS, selected patients with severe PPNS refractory to other treatments may benefit from serial immunomodulatory therapy every 6–8 weeks.

Prednisolone, with or without azathioprine or methotrexate, has been useful in selected autoimmune PNH patients (Newsom-Davis and Mills, 1993; Nakatsuji *et al.*, 2000) including a few patients with thymoma-associated PPNH who did not improve after thymectomy (Newsom-Davis and Mills, 1993). All forms of PNH, including paraneoplastic, usually improve with symptomatic treatment using various anti-epileptic drugs (Newsom-Davis and Mills, 1993).

GOOD PRACTICE POINTS

- Patients with PNS most often present with neurological symptoms before an underlying tumour is detected. Onconeural antibodies should be sought in sera from patients with suspected PNS. The antibodies are important for the diagnosis and tumour search.
- Radiological investigations for tumours, such as high resolution CT for the detection of SCLC, are important, but should be followed by PDG-PET if no tumour is found.
- Patients should also be followed at regular intervals, for example every 6 months for up to 4 years, to search for tumour in cases where the initial tumour screen was negative.
- Early detection and treatment of the tumour is the approach that seems to offer the greatest chance for PNS stabilization. This is done in cooperation with a oncologist, pulmologist, gynecologist, or pediatrician depending on the associated tumour.
- Immune therapy (steroids, plasma exchange or intravenous immunoglobulin) usually has no or modest effect on PLE, SSN, or PCD.
- Children with POM may respond to immune therapy, whereas no clear evidence of such therapy has been shown in adults with POM.
- Patients with LEMS or PPNH usually improve with immune therapy.
- Symptomatic therapy should be offered to all patients with PNS.

Acknowledgements

This study was supported by grant QLG1-CT-2002-01756 of the European Commission.

References

Alessi G, De Reuck J, De Bleecker J, Vancayzeele S (2000). Successful immunoglobulin treatment in a patient with neuromyotonia. *Clin Neurol Neurosurgery* **102**:173–175.

Anderson NE, Budde-Steffen C, Rosenblum MK et al. (1988). Opsoclonus, myoclonus, ataxia, and encephalopathy in adults with cancer: a distinct paraneoplastic syndrome. *Medicine* **67**:100–109.

Antoine JC, Honnorat J, Camdesssance JP et al. (2001). Paraneoplastic anti-CV2 antibodies react with peripheral nerve and are associated with a mixed axonal and demyelinating peripheral neuropathy. *Ann Neurol* **49**:214–221.

Antunes NL, Khakoo Y, Matthay KK et al. (2000). Antineuronal antibodies in patients with neuroblastoma and paraneoplastic opsoclonus-myoclonus. *J Pediatr Hematol Oncol* **22**:315–320.

Bataller L, Graus F, Saiz A, Vilchez JJ (2001). Clinical outcome in adult onset idiopathic or paraneoplastic opsoclonus-myoclonus. *Brain* **124**:437–443.

Bataller L, Rosenfeld MR, Graus F, Vilchez JJ et al. (2003). Autoantigen diversity in the opsoclonus-myoclonus syndrome. *Ann Neurol* **53**:347–353.

Berger JR, Mehari E (1999). Paraneoplastic opsoclonus-myoclonus secondary to malignant melanoma. *J Neurooncol* **41**:43–45.

Bernal F, Shams'ili S, Rojas I et al. (2003). Anti-Tr antibodies as markers of paraneoplastic cerebellar degeneration and Hodgkin's disease. *Neurology* **60**:230–234.

Brainin M, Barnes M, Baron J-C, Gilhus NE, Hughes R, Selmaj K, Waldemar G (2004). Guidance for the preparation of neurological management guidelines by EFNS scientific task forces – revised recommendations 2004. *Eur J Neurol* **11**:577–581.

Buckley C, Oger J, Clover L et al. (2001). Potassium channel antibodies in two patients with reversible limbic encephalitis. *Ann Neurol* **50**:74–79.

Buttner U, Straube A, Handke V (1997). [Opsoclonus and ocular flutter]. *Nervenarzt* **68**:633–637.

Camdesssance JP, Antoine JC, Honnorat J et al. (2002). Paraneoplastic peripheral neuropathy associated with anti-Hu antibodies. A clinical and electrophysiological study of 20 patients. *Brain* **125**:166–175.

Caress JB, Abend WK, Preston DC, Logigian EL (1997). A case of Hodgkin's lymphoma producing neuromyotonia. *Neurology* **49**:258–259.

Chalk CH, Murray NM, Newsom-Davis J, O'Neill JH, Spiro SG (1990). Response of the Lambert-Eaton myasthenic syndrome to treatment of associated small-cell lung carcinoma. *Neurology* **40**:1552–1556.

Dalmau J, Graus F, Villarejo A et al. (2004). Clinical analysis of anti-Ma2-associated encephalitis. *Brain* **127**:1831–1844.

Darnell JC, Posner JB (2003). Paraneoplastic syndromes involving the nervous system. *N Engl J Med* **349**:1543–1554.

Dirr LY, Elster AD, Donofrio PD, Smith M (1990). Evolution of brain abnormalities in limbic encephalitis. *Neurology* **40:**1304–1306.

Dropcho EJ, Kline LB, Riser J (1993). Antineuronal (anti-Ri) antibodies in a patient with steroid-responsive opsoclonus-myoclonus. *Neurology* **43:**207–211.

Fukuda T, Motomura M, Nakao Y, Shiraishi H, Yoshimura T, Iwanaga K, Tsujihata M, Eguchi K (2003). Reduction of P/Q-type calcium channels in the postmortem cerebellum of paraneoplastic cerebellar degeneration with Lambert-Eaton myasthenic syndrome. *Ann Neurol* **53:**21–28.

Gambini C, Conte M, Bernini G *et al.* (2003). Neuroblastic tumors associated with opsoclonus-myoclonus syndrome: histological, immunohistochemical and molecular features of 15 Italian cases. *Virchows Arch* **442:**555–562.

Graus F, Bonaventura I, Uchya M *et al.* (1994). Indolent anti-Hu-associated paraneoplastic sensory neuropathy. *Neurology* **44:**2258–2261.

Graus F, Keime-Guibert F, Reòe R *et al.* (2001). Anti-Hu-associtaed paraneoplastic encephalomyelitis: analysis of 200 patients. *Brain* **124:**1138–1148.

Graus F, Lang B, Pozo-Rosich P *et al.* (2002). P/Q type calcium channel antibodies in paraneoplastic cerebellar degeneration with lung cancer. *Neurology* **59:** 764–766.

Graus F, Delattre JY, Antoine JC *et al.* (2004). Recommended diagnostic criteria for paraneoplastic neurological syndromes. *J Neurol Neurosurg Psychiatry* **75:**1135–1140.

Gultekin SH, Rosenfeld MR, Voltz R *et al.* (2000). Paraneoplastic limbic encephalitis: neurological symptoms, immunological findings and tumor association in 50 patients. *Brain* **123:**1481–1494.

Hart IK, Waters C, Vincent A *et al.* (1997). Autoantibodies detected to expressed potassium channels are implicated in neuromyotonia. *Ann Neurol* **41:** 238–246.

Hart IK, Maddison P, Newsom-Davis J *et al.* (2002). Phenotypic variants of peripheral nerve hyperexcitability. *Brain* **125:**1887–1895.

Hayat GR, Kulkantrakorn K, Campbell WW, Giuliani MJ (2000). Neuromyotonia: autoimmune pathogenesis and response to immune modulating therapy. *J Neurol Sci* **181:**38–43.

Hayward K, Jeremy RJ, Jenkins S, Barkovich AJ *et al.* (2001). Long-term neurobehavioral outcomes in children with neuroblastoma and opsoclonus-myoclonus-ataxia syndrome: relationship to MRI findings and anti-neuronal antibodies. *J Pediatr* **139:**552–559.

Horwich MS, Cho L, Porro RS, Posner JB (1977). Subacute sensory neuropathy: a remote effect of carcinoma. *Ann Neurol* **2:**7–19.

Honnorat J, Antoine JC, Derrington E *et al.* (1996). Antibodies to a subpopulation of glial cells and a 66 kDa developmental protein in patients with paraneoplastic neurological syndromes. *J Neurol Neurosurg Psychiatry* **61:**270–278.

Ishii A, Hayashi A, Ohkoshi N *et al.* (1994). Clinical evaluation of plasma exchange and high dose intravenous immunoglobulin in a patient with Isaacs' syndrome. *J Neurol Neurosurg Psychiatry* **57:**840–842.

Jongen JL, Moll WJ, Sillevis Smitt PA *et al.* (1988). Anti-Ri positive opsoclonus-myoclonus-ataxia in ovarian duct cancer. *J Neurol* **245:**691–692.

Keime-Guibert F, Graus F, Fleury A *et al.* (2000). Treatment of paraneoplastic neurological syndromes with antineuronal antibodies (anti-Hu, anti-Yo) with a combination of immunoglobulins, cyclophosphamide, and methylprednisolone. *J Neurol Neurosurg Psychiatry* **68:**479–482.

Lahrmann H, Albrecht G, Drlicek M *et al.* (2001). Acquired neuromyotonia and peripheral neuropathy in a patient with Hodgkin's disease. *Muscle Nerve* **24:**834–838.

Linke R, Schroeder M, Helmberger T, Voltz R (2004). Antibody-positive paraneoplastic neurologic syndromes: value of CT and PET for tumor diagnosis. *Neurology* **63:**282–286.

Maddison P, Newsom-Davis J, Mills KR, Souhami RL (1999). Favourable prognosis in Lambert-Eaton myasthenic syndrome and small-cell lung carcinoma. *Lancet* **353:**117–118.

Mason WP, Graus F, Lang B *et al.* (1997). Small-cell lung cancer, paraneoplastic cerebellar degeneration and the Lambert-Eaton myasthenic syndrome. *Brain* **120:**1279–1300.

McEvoy KM, Windebank AJ, Daube JR, Low PA (1989). 3,4-Diaminopyridine in the treatment of Lambert-Eaton myasthenic syndrome. *N Engl J Med* **321:**1567–1571.

Mitchell WG, Davalos-Gonzalez Y, Brumm VL *et al.* (2002). Opsoclonus-ataxia caused by childhood neuroblastoma: developmental and neurologic sequelae. *Pediatrics* **109:**86–98.

Molinuevo JL, Graus F, Serrano C *et al.* (1998). Utility of anti-Hu antibodies in the diagnosis of paraneoplastic sensory neuropathy. *Ann Neurol* **4:**976–980.

Motomura M, Johnston I, Lang B *et al.* (1995). An improved diagnostic assay for Lambert-Eaton myasthenic syndrome. *J Neurol Neurosurg Psychiatry* **58:**85–87.

Nakatsuji Y, Kaido M, Sugai F et al. (2000). Isaacs' syndrome successfully treated by immunoadsorption plasmapheresis. *Acta Neurol Scand* **102:**271–273.

Newsom-Davis J, Mills KR (1993). Immunological associations of acquired neuromyotonia (Isaacs' syndrome). Report of five cases and literature review. *Brain* **116:**453–469.

Nitschke M, Hochberg F, Dropcho E (1995). Improvement of paraneoplastic opsoclonus-myoclonus after protein A column therapy. *N Engl J Med* **332:**192.

O'Neill JH, Murray NM, Newsom-Davis J (1988). The Lambert-Eaton myasthenic syndrome. A review of 50 cases. *Brain* **111:**577–596.

Peterson K, Rosenblum MK, Kotanides H, Posner JB (1992). Paraneoplastic cerebellar degeneration. I. A clinical analysis of 55 anti-Yo antibody-positive patients. *Neurology* **42:**1931–1937.

Pozo-Rosich P, Clover L, Saiz A et al. (2003). Voltage-gated potassium channel antibodies in limbic encephalitis. *Ann Neurol* **54:**530–533.

Pranzatelli MR, Tate ED, Wheeler A et al. (2002). Screening for autoantibodies in children with opsoclonus-myoclonus-ataxia. *Pediatr Neurol* **27:**384–387.

Prestigiacomo CJ, Balmaceda C, Dalmau J (2001). Anti-Ri-associated paraneoplastic opsoclonus-ataxia syndrome in a man with transitional cell carcinoma. *Cancer* **91:**1423–1428.

Provenzale JM, Barboriak DP, Coleman RE (1998). Limbic encephalitis: comparison of FDG PET and MRI findings. *Am J Roentgenol* **18:**1659–1660.

Rojas I, Graus F, Keime-Guibert F et al. (2000). Long-term clinical outcome of paraneoplastic cerebellar degeneration and anti-Yo antibodies. *Neurology* **55:**713–715.

Rudnick E, Khakoo Y, Antunes NL et al. (2001). Opsoclonus-myoclonus-ataxia syndrome in neuroblastoma: clinical outcome and antineuronal antibodies-a report from the Children's Cancer Group Study. *Med Pediatr Oncol* **36:**612–622.

Shams'ili S, Grefkens J, de Leeuw B et al. (2003). Paraneoplastic cerebellar degeneration associated with antineuronal antibodies: analysis of 50 patients. *Brain* **126:**1409–1418.

Shillito P, Molenaar PC, Vincent A et al. (1995). Acquired neuromyotonia: evidence for autoantibodies directed against K+ channels of peripheral nerves. *Ann Neurol* **38:**714–722.

Straube A, Leigh RJ, Bronstein A et al. (2004). EFNS task force-therapy of nystagmus and oscillopsia. *Eur J Neurol* **11:**83–89.

Swart JF, de Kraker J, van der Lely N (2002). Metaiodobenzylguanidine total-body scintigraphy required for revealing occult neuroblastoma in opsoclonus-myoclonus syndrome. *Eur J Pediatr* **161:**255–258.

Toepfer M, Schroeder M, Unger JM et al. (1999). Neuromyotonia, myoclonus, sensory neuropathy and cerebellar symptoms in a patient with antibodies to neuronal nucleoproteins (anti-Hu-antibodies). *Clin Neurol Neurosurg* **101:**207–209.

van den Berg JS, van Engelen BG, Boerman RH, de Baets MH (1999). Acquired neuromyotonia: superiority of plasma exchange over high-dose intravenous human immunoglobulin. *J Neurol* **246:**623–625.

Vernino S, O'Neill BP, Marks RS et al. (2004). Immunomodulatory treatment trial for paraneoplastic neurological disorders. *Neuro-oncol* **6:**55–62.

Vincent A, Buckley C, Schott JM et al. (2004). Potassium Channel antibody-associated encephalopathy: a potentially immunotherapy-responsive form of encephalitis. *Brain* **127:**701–712.

Voltz R (2002). Paraneoplastic neurological syndromes: an update on diagnosis, pathogenesis, and therapy. *Lancet Neurol* **1:**294–305.

Widdess-Walsh P, Tavee JO, Schuele S, Stevens GH (2003). Response to intravenous immunoglobulin in anti-Yo associated paraneoplastic cerebellar degeneration: case report and review of the literature. *J Neurooncol* **63:**187–190.

Willison HJ, Ang W, Gilhus NE et al. (2000). EFNS Task force report: a questionairre-based survey on the service provision and quality assurance for deterniniation of diagnostic autoantibody tests in European neuroimmunology centres. European Federation of Neurological Societies. *Eur J Neurol* **7:**625–628.

Wirtz PW, Sotodeh M, Nijnuis M et al. (2002). Difference in distribution of muscle weakness between myasthenia gravis and the Lambert-Eaton myasthenic syndrome. *J Neurol Neurosurg Psychiatry* **73:**766–768.

Wirtz PW, Sillevis Smitt PA, Hoff JI et al. (2002). Anti-Ri antibody positive opsoclonus-myoclonus in a male patient with breast carcinoma. *J Neurol* **249:**1710–1712.

Wirtz PW, Willcox N, van der Slik AR et al. (2005). HLA and smoking in prediction and prognosis of small cell lung cancer in autoimmune Lambert-Eaton myasthenic syndrome. *J Neuroimmunol* **159:**230–237.

Wong AM, Musallam S, Tomlinson RD et al. (2001). Opsoclonus in three dimensions: oculographic, neuropathologic and modelling correlates. *J Neurol Sci* **189:**71–81.

Younes-Mhenni S, Janier MF, Cinotti L et al. (2004). FDG-PET improves tumour detection in patients with paraneoplastic neurological syndromes. *Brain* **127:**2331–2338.

Younger DS, Dalmau J, Inghirami G *et al.* (1994). Anti-Hu-associated peripheral nerve and muscle microvasculitis. *Neurology* **44:**181–183.

Yu Z, Kryzer TJ, Grisemann GE *et al.* (2001). CRMP-5 neuronal autoantibody: marker of lung cancer and thymoma-related autoimmunity. *Ann Neurol* **49:**146–154.

Zamecnik J, Cerny R, Bartos A *et al.* (2004). Paraneoplastic opsoclonus-myoclonus syndrome associated with malignant fibrous histiocytoma: neuropathological findings. *Cesk Patol* **40:**63–67.

Zifko U, Drlicek M, Machacek E *et al.* (1994). Syndrome of continuous muscle fiber activity and plasmacytoma with IgM paraproteinemia. *Neurology* **44:**560–561.

CHAPTER 35

Nystagmus and oscillopsia

A. Straube,[a] R.J. Leigh,[b] A. Bronstein,[c] W. Heide,[d]
P. Riordan-Eva,[e] C.C. Tijssen,[f] I. Dehaene,[g]
D. Straumann[h]

Abstract

An overview of possible treatment options for oculomotor disorders that prevent clear vision is given. Downbeat nystagmus, upbeat nystagmus, seesaw nystagmus, periodic alternating nystagmus, acquired pendular nystagmus and saccadic oscillations such as opsoclonus/ocular flutter are discussed. In addition, superior oblique myokymia and vestibular paroxysmia are reviewed. All treatment recommendations available in the literature are classified as class C only. In general, only some of the patients benefit from the treatment.

Introduction

The ocular motor system serves to hold images steady on the retina (especially the central fovea). Abnormal eye movements may cause excessive motion of images on the retina, leading to blurred vision and to the illusion that the seen world is moving (oscillopsia). Abnormal eye movements may also interfere with spatial localization and the ability to make accurate limb movements. In clinical practice, the identification of specific abnormalities of eye movements is often useful in the topological diagnosis of a broad range of disorders that affect the brain. Although we now know quite a lot about the anatomy, physiology and pharmacology of the ocular motor system, our treatment options for abnormal eye movements remain fairly limited. Most drug treatments are based on case reports. Only a few controlled trials have been published in recent years, and they were all based on a small number of subjects, and not all patients respond positively to the treatment. Thus, all treatment recommendations have to be classified as Class C (Hilgers, 2001). The goal of the paper is to summarize all published treatment options for nystagmus and oscillopsia as well as to provide a short overview of the definition and pathophysiology of certain distinct ocular motor syndromes.

[a]Department of Neurology, University of Munich, Munich, Germany; [b]Department of Neurology, Case Western Reserve University, Cleveland, OH, United States; [c]Academic Department of Neuro-Otology, Imperial College of Science, Technology and Medicine, London, United Kingdom; [d]Department of Neurology, University at Lübeck, Lübeck, Germany; [e]Department of Ophthalmology, King's College Hospital, London, United Kingdom; [f]Department of Neurology, St Elisabeth Hospital, Tilburg, The Netherlands; [g]Department of Neurology, Algemeen Hospital, Brugge, Belgium; [h]Department of Neurology, University of Zurich, Zurich, Switzerland.

A large part of this review concerns nystagmus, which is defined as repetitive, to-and-fro involuntary eye movements that are initiated by slow drifts of the eye. Physiological nystagmus that occurs during rotation of the body in space acts to *preserve* clear vision. In contrast, pathological nystagmus causes the eyes to drift away from the target, thus degrading vision. One form, pendular nystagmus, consists of to-and-fro quasi-sinusoidal oscillations. More commonly, nystagmus consists of an alternation of unidirectional drifts away from the target and their correction by fast movements (saccades), which temporarily bring the visual target back to the fovea; this is jerk nystagmus. Nystagmus should be distinguished from inappropriate saccades that prevent steady fixation. Saccades are fast movements, and the smeared retinal signal due to these movements is largely ignored. However, patients in whom abnormal saccades repeatedly misdirect the fovea often complain of difficulty in reading.

Methods

One member of the Task Force Panel (AS) searched through all available published information using the database Med-Line (last search March 2003). The search was restricted to papers published in English, French, or German. The key words used for the search included the following sequences: 'nystagmus and therapy', 'treatment of ocular motor disorders' and 'treatment of double vision'. All published papers were included, as only a limited number of controlled studies are available. The other members of the task force read the first draft of the recommendation and discussed changes (informative consensus approach).

Supranuclear ocular motor disorders

Central vestibular disorders

The vestibulo-ocular reflex (VOR) normally generates eye rotations, after a short latency, in the same plane as the head rotation that elicits them. Disorders of the vestibular *periphery* cause nystagmus in a direction that is determined by the pattern of involved labyrinthine semicircular canals. The complete, unilateral loss of one labyrinth causes a mixed horizontal-torsional nystagmus that is suppressed by visual fixation. *Central* vestibular disorders may also cause an imbalance of these reflexes, leading to upbeat, downbeat, or torsional nystagmus (see below). Another consequence of vestibular disease is a change in the size (gain) of the overall dynamic VOR response. As a result of this change, patients complain of oscillopsia during rapid head movements. A VOR gain larger than 1 (eye speed exceeds head speed) results from a disinhibition of the brainstem circuits responsible for the VOR and is caused by vestibulo-cerebellar dysfunction. Loss of peripheral vestibular function causes impaired vision and oscillopsia during locomotion, due to the inability to compensate for the high-frequency head perturbations that occur with each footfall.

Downbeat nystagmus

Downbeat nystagmus is a central form of vestibular nystagmus that is often present when the eyes are close to the central position; it usually increases on downgaze and especially on lateral gaze. It also often becomes evident or is increased by placing the patient in a head-hanging position, or by tipping the head forward. In patients with cerebellar atrophy, some authors found that downbeat nystagmus is more prominent in prone than in supine body position (Marti *et al.*, 2002), but this could not be confirmed by others (Bronstein *et al.*, 1987). Visual fixation has little effect on its slow-phase speed; convergence may suppress or enhance it in some patients. In general, the nystagmus is accompanied by a vestibulocerebellar ataxia with a tendency to fall backward (Büchele *et al.*, 1983). Lesions that cause downbeat nystagmus occur in the vestibulocerebellum bilaterally and in the underlying medulla (Leigh and Zee, 1999). The pathophysiological mechanism of downbeat nystagmus appears to be due to a central imbalance of the vertical VOR (Baloh and Spooner, 1981) or due to an abnormality of the vertical-torsional gaze-holding mechanism - the 'neural integrator for eye movements' (Glasauer *et al.*, 2003).

Aetiology

The most common cause of downbeat nystagmus is cerebellar degeneration (hereditary, sporadic, or paraneoplastic). Other important causes are Chiari malformation and drug intoxication (especially the anticonvulsants and lithium). Multiple sclerosis (MS) is an uncommon cause, and a congenital form is rare (Halmagyi *et al.*, 1983). In practice cerebellar atrophy, ArnoldChiari malformation, various cerebellar lesions (MS, vascular, tumors), and idiopathic causes account for approximately one-fourth of the cases each (Bronstein *et al.*, 1987). Downbeat nystagmus occurs in the channelopathy episodic ataxia type 2, for which a new treatment option has recently been developed (Strupp and Schüler, 2002).

Upbeat nystagmus

Upbeat nystagmus is present with the eyes close to the central position and usually increases on upgaze. Vertical smooth pursuit is usually disrupted by the nystagmus. In some patients the upbeat nystagmus changes to downbeat nystagmus during convergence.

Aetiology

Probable causes of upbeat nystagmus are lesions in the ascending pathways from the anterior canals (and/or the otoliths) at the pontomesencephalic or pontomedullary junction, near the perihypoglossal nuclei (Fisher *et al.*, 1983). Upbeat nystagmus is most often seen after medullary lesions (Stahl *et al.*, 2000). The main causes are MS, tumours of the brainstem, Wernicke's encephalopathy, cerebellar degeneration and intoxication (e.g. nicotine).

RECOMMENDATIONS

Downbeat nystagmus. No studies on the natural course of downbeat nystagmus are available. In non-placebo-controlled studies with a limited number of patients, administration of the GABA-A agonist clonazepam (0.5 mg per os (p.o.) three times daily; Currie and Matsuo, 1986), the GABA-B agonist baclofen (10 mg p.o. three times daily)

(Dieterich *et al.*, 1991), and gabapentin (probably calcium channel blocker) (Averbuch-Heller *et al.*, 1997) had positive effects and reduced downbeat nystagmus. Intravenous injection of the cholinergic drug physostigmine (Ach-esterase inhibitor) worsened downbeat nystagmus in five patients. This effect was partially reversed in one patient by the anticholinergic drug biperiden, suggesting that anticholinergic drugs might be beneficial, as was shown in a double-blind study on intravenous scopolamine (Barton *et al.*, 1994). In isolated patients with a craniocervical anomaly, a surgical decompression by removal of part of the occipital bone in the region of the foramen magnum was beneficial (Pedersen *et al.*, 1980; Spooner and Baloh, 1981; personal observation). Recent placebo-controlled studies (Strupp *et al.*, 2003) have suggested that the potassium channel blocker 3,4-diaminopyridine may be effective in downbeat nystagmus. As downbeat nystagmus is generally less pronounced in upward gaze, base-down prisms sometimes help to reduce oscillopsia during reading.

Upbeat nystagmus. Treatment with baclofen (5–10 mg p.o. three times daily) resulted in an improvement in several patients (Dieterich *et al.*, 1991).

Seesaw nystagmus

Seesaw nystagmus is a rare pendular or jerk oscillation. One half cycle consists of elevation and intorsion of one eye with synchronous depression and extorsion of the other eye. During the next half cycle there is a reversal of the vertical and torsional movements. The frequency is lower in the pendular (2–4 Hz) than in the jerk variety.

Aetiology

Jerk hemi-seesaw nystagmus has been attributed to unilateral meso-diencephalic lesions (Halmagyi *et al.*, 1994), affecting the interstitial nucleus of Cajal and its vestibular afferents from the vertical semicircular canals (Endres *et al.*, 1996; Rambold *et al.*, 1999). The pendular form is associated with lesions affecting the optic chiasm. Loss of crossed visual input seems to be the crucial element in the pathophysiology of pendular seesaw nystagmus (Stahl *et al.*, 2000).

RECOMMENDATIONS

Alcohol had a beneficial effect (1.2 g/kg body weight) in two patients (Frisèn and Wikkelso, 1986; Lepore, 1987), as did clonazepam (Carlow, 1986). Recently, Averbruch-Heller *et al.* (1997) reported on three patients with a seesaw component to their pendular nystagmus, who improved on gabapentin.

Periodic alternating nystagmus

Periodic alternating nystagmus is a spontaneous horizontal beating nystagmus, the direction of which changes periodically. Periods of oscillation range from 1 s to 4 min, typically 1–2 min. When the nystagmus amplitude gradually decreases, the nystagmus reverses its direction, and then the amplitude increases again. During the nystagmus patients often complain of increasing/decreasing oscillopsia.

Aetiology

Patients with periodic alternating nystagmus commonly have vestibulocerebellar lesions. Their nystagmus also disrupts visual fixation, being present also during normal viewing. These observations and animal experiments support the idea that this type of nystagmus is caused by lesions of the inferior cerebellar vermis (nodulus and uvula), leading to a disinhibition of the GABA-ergic velocity-storage mechanism, which is mediated in the vestibular nuclei (Waespe *et al.*, 1985; Furman *et al.*, 1990). The underlying aetiologies are craniocervical anomalies, MS, cerebellar degenerations or tumours, brainstem infarction, anticonvulsant therapy and bilateral visual loss.

RECOMMENDATIONS

In general, periodic alternating nystagmus does not improve spontaneously. Several case reports describe a positive effect of baclofen, a GABA-B

---

agonist, in a dose of 5–10 mg p.o. three times daily (Halmagyi *et al.*, 1980; Larmande and Larmande, 1983; Isago *et al.*, 1985; Carlow, 1986; Nuti *et al.*, 1986). Furthermore, phenothiazine and barbiturates have been found to be effective in single cases (Nathanson *et al.*, 1953; Isago *et al.*, 1985). Periodic alternating nystagmus due to bilateral visual loss resolves if vision is restored (Cross *et al.*, 1982; Jay *et al.*, 1985).

Non-vestibular supranuclear oculomotor disorders

Acquired pendular nystagmus

Acquired pendular nystagmus (APN) is a quasi-sinusoidal oscillation that may have a predominantly horizontal, vertical, or mixed trajectory (i.e. circular, elliptical, or diagonal); it can predominantly be either monocular or binocular (Gresty *et al.*, 1982; Traccis *et al.*, 1990; Leigh *et al.*, 1992; Lopez *et al.*, 1996). The frequency of this type of nystagmus is 2–7 Hz (Zee, 1985), and often the nystagmus is associated with head titubation (not synchronized with the nystagmus), trunk and limb ataxia, or visual impairment.

Aetiology

Acquired pendular nystagmus occurs with several disorders of myelin (MS, toluene abuse, PelizaeusMerzbacher disease), as a component of the syndrome of oculopalatal tremor (myoclonus), in Whipple's disease (Leigh and Zee, 1999); the two more common aetiologies in the adult are MS and brainstem stroke (Lopez *et al.*, 1996). On the basis of observations that the nystagmus is often dissociated and that eye movements other than optokinetic nystagmus and voluntary saccades are also disturbed, a lesion in the brainstem near the oculomotor nuclei has been suggested (Gresty *et al.*, 1982). Alternatively, an inhibition of the inferior olive due to lesions of the 'Mollaret triangle' (Lopez *et al.*, 1996) or an instability of the gaze-holding network (neural integrator) has been proposed; this suggestion has received experimental modelling support (Das *et al.*, 2000) and has led to the proposal of potential therapies (Stahl *et al.*, 2000).

RECOMMENDATIONS

Most reports (case reports or case series) state that anticholinergic treatment with trihexyphenidyl (20–40 mg p.o. daily) is effective (Herishanu and Louzoun, 1986; Jabbari et al., 1987), but in a double-blind study by Leigh et al. (1991a) only one of six patients showed improvement from this oral treatment, whereas three patients showed a decrease in nystagmus and improvement of visual acuity during treatment with tridihexethyl chloride (a quaternary anticholinergic that does not cross the blood–brain barrier). In contrast, Barton et al. (1994) found in a double-blind trial that scopolamine (0.4 mg intravenous (i.v.)) decreased the nystagmus in all five tested patients with acquired pendular nystagmus. However, there are even observations that scopolamine may make the pendular nystagmus worse in some patients (Kim et al., 2001). In three other patients the combination with lidocaine (100 mg i.v.) decreased nystagmus (Ell et al., 1982; Gresty et al., 1982). Recently, Starck et al. (1997) reported an improvement in three of ten patients who received a scopolamine patch (containing 1.5 mg scopolamine, released at a rate of 0.5 mg per day). The same authors failed to observe further improvement when scopolamine and mexiletine (400–600 mg p.o. daily) were given in combination. The most effective substance in their study was memantine, a glutamate antagonist, which significantly improved the nystagmus in all nine tested patients (15–60 mg p.o. daily). Two patients responded to clonazepam (3×0.5–1.0 mg p.o. daily), a GABA-A agonist (Starck et al., 1997). Two other groups have reported benefit with GABA-ergic drugs. Traccis et al. (1990) showed improvement in one of three patients with APN and cerebellar ataxia due to MS when treated with isoniazid (800–1000 mg p.o. daily) and glasses with prisms that induced convergence. This observation was not confirmed by other investigators (Leigh et al., 1994). Gabapentin substantially improved the nystagmus (and visual acuity) in 10 of 15 patients (Averbruch-Heller et al., 1997). Gabapentin was superior to vigabatrin in a small series of patients (Bandini et al., 2001). Interestingly, Mossman et al. (1993) described two patients who benefited from intake of alcohol but not from other substances. The necessary blood levels were 20–35 mmol/l. Recently, a beneficial effect of cannabis was also reported (Schon et al., 1999; Dell'Osso, 2000).

Practically, treatment should start with memantine in a dosage of 15–60 mg p.o. or alternatively 300–400 mg gabapentin three times daily. If there is no or only a small effect, benzodiazepines like clonazepam (0.5–1.0 mg p.o. three times daily) can be tried. Further possibilities are scopolamine patches or trihexyphenidyl. However, side effects are a major limitation of anticholinergic therapy.

Opsoclonus and ocular flutter

Opsoclonus consists of repetitive bursts of conjugate saccadic oscillations, which have horizontal, vertical and torsional components. During each burst of these high-frequency oscillations, the movement is continuous, without any intersaccadic interval. These oscillations are often triggered by eye closure, convergence, pursuit and saccades; amplitudes range up to 2–15°; (overview in Leigh and Zee, 1999). In ocular flutter the same pattern is restricted to the horizontal plane. The ocular symptoms are often accompanied by cerebellar signs, such as gait and limb myoclonus (the 'dancing feet, dancing eyes syndrome').

Aetiology

A functional disturbance of active saccadic suppression by the pontine omnipause neurons is the most probable pathophysiological mechanism. As histological abnormalities of these neurons have not been shown (Ridley et al., 1987), a functional lesion of the glutaminergic cerebellar projections from the fastigial nuclei to the omnipause cells is a likely cause for their disinhibition. Opsoclonus can be observed in benign cerebellar encephalitis (post-viral, e.g. coxsackie B37; postvaccinal), or as a paraneoplastic symptom (infants, neuroblastoma; adults, carcinoma of the lung, breast, ovary, or uterus).

In addition to therapy for any underlying process such as tumour or encephalitis, treatment with immunoglobulins or prednisolone may be occasionally effective (Pless and Ronthal, 1996). Four of five patients with square-wave oscillations, probably a related fixation disturbance, showed an improvement on therapy with valproic acid (Traccis *et al.*, 1997). In single cases an improvement has been observed during treatment with propranolol (40–80 mg p.o. three times daily), nitrazepam (15–30 mg p.o. daily), and clonazepam (0.5–2.0 mg p.o. three times daily) (overview in Leopold, 1985; Carlow, 1986). Nausieda *et al.* (1981) reported a dramatic improvement in one patient after the administration of 200 mg thiamine i.v.; no further descriptions of the patient are given in the paper.

Spontaneous remissions, which can last for days up to years, are typical of superior oblique myokymia but there are several reports that anticonvulsants, especially carbamazepine, have a therapeutic effect. Carbamazepine (200–400 mg p.o. three or four times daily) or, less often, phenytoin (250–400 mg p.o. daily) are recommended (Susac *et al.*, 1973; Rosenberg and Glaser, 1983). Gabapentin has also been reported to be effective (Tomsak *et al.*, 2002). Long-term studies on the continued effectiveness of these drugs are not available. Rosenberg and Glaser (1983) described a decrease in the efficacy of the treatment after a month in some patients. Beta-blockers, even topically, have been reported to be effective (Tyler and Ruiz, 1990; Bibby *et al.*, 1994).

In chronic cases that did not improve with anticonvulsants, tenotomy of the superior oblique muscle was performed, but usually it necessitates inferior oblique surgery as well (Palmer and Shults, 1984; Brazis *et al.*, 1994). Surgical decompression of the IV nerve has also been reported to be beneficial but may result in superior oblique palsy (Samii *et al.*, 1998; Scharwey *et al.*, 2000).

Practically, treatment should be started with carbamazepine (200–400 mg p.o. three to four times daily) or phenytoin (250–400 mg p.o. daily). The side effects and the risk of such therapy are the same as when used to treat trigeminal neuralgia.

Nuclear and infranuclear ocular disorders
Superior oblique myokymia

Superior oblique myokymia consists of paroxysmal monocular high-frequency oscillations. In the primary gaze position and in abduction these oscillations are mainly torsional, but when the eyes are in adduction the oscillations have a vertical component. Voluntary eye movements, as when looking down, can provoke the oscillations. The patients usually complain of oscillopsia during these paroxysmal attacks.

Aetiology
The pathophysiology of this condition is not totally clear. Analogous to hemifacial spasm and trigeminal neuralgia, vascular compression of the IV nerve (Lee, 1984; Hashimoto *et al.*, 2001; Yousry *et al.*, 2002), or alternatively spontaneous discharges in the IV nerve nucleus (Hoyt and Keane, 1962) or of the superior oblique muscle may be responsible (Leigh *et al.*, 1991b).

Paroxysmal vestibular episodes

Clinically, the patients describe short, repeated, paroxysmal attacks of to-and-fro vertigo lasting for seconds to maximally minutes, which can sometimes be provoked by particular head positions. Other symptoms can be tinnitus, hyperacusis, or facial contractions during the attacks. Clinical examination between the attacks may reveal signs of permanent vestibular deficit, hypoacusis, or facial paresis on the affected side (Brandt and Dieterich, 1994; Straube *et al.*, 1994).

Aetiology
High-resolution magnetic resonance imaging may show the compression of the VII nerve by an artery

(most often AICA) or seldom a vein in the region of the root entry zone of the vestibular nerve in some patients, but this can also be seen in subjects without symptoms. The neuropathological mechanism may be peripheral ephaptic transmission that takes place in the part of the cranial nerve still containing central myelin (derived from oligodendroglia), if the nerve has direct contact with a blood vessel. This hypothesis is supported by the analysis of epidemiological data that show a correlation of the incidence of the syndrome with the anatomical length of the central myelin (De Ridder *et al.*, 2002). Another theory is that the pulsation of the blood vessel causes an afferent sensory inflow that then causes a false central response.

RECOMMENDATIONS

As initial therapy, an anticonvulsant [carbamazepine (slow release formulation) 2 × 200–800 mg p.o. daily; phenytoin 250–400 mg p.o. daily, lamotrigine 100–400 mg p.o. daily] should be given (Brandt, 1999). In general, a positive response to antiepileptic drugs can be achieved with low dosages. If the symptoms do not cease, a surgical approach may be considered (Jannetta *et al.*, 1984). There are no satisfactory follow-up studies, and the diagnostic criteria have not yet been fully established.

References

Averbuch-Heller L, Tusa RJ, Fuhry L *et al.* (1997). A double-blind controlled study of gabapentin and baclofen as treatment for acquired nystagmus. *Ann Neurol* **41**:818–825.

Baloh RW, Spooner JW (1981). Downbeat nystagmus. A type of central vestibular nystagmus. *Neurology* **31**:304–310.

Bandini F, Castello E, Mazzella L, Mancardi GL, Solaro C (2001). Gabapentin but not vigabatrin is effective in the treatment of acquired nystagmus in multiple sclerosis: How valid is the GABAergic hypothesis? *J Neurol Neurosurg Psychiatry* **71**:107–110.

Barton JJS, Huaman AG, Sharpe JA (1994). Muscarinic antagonists in the treatment of acquired pendular and downbeat nystagmus: a double-blind, randomized trial of three intravenous drugs. *Ann Neurol* **35**:319–325.

Bibby K, Deane JS, Farnworth D, Cappin J (1994). Superior oblique myokymia: a topical solution? *Br J Ophthalmol* **78**:882.

Brandt T (1999). *Vertigo. Its Multisensory Syndromes.* 2nd edn. Springer-Verlag, London.

Brandt T, Dieterich M (1994). Vestibular paroxysmia: vascular compression of the eighth nerve? *Lancet* **26**:798–799.

Brazis PW, Miller NR, Henderer JD, Lee AG (1994). The natural history and results of treatment of superior oblique myokymia. *Arch Ophthalmol* **112**:1063–1067.

Bronstein AM, Miller DH, Rudge P, Kendall BE (1987). Down beating nystagmus: magnetic resonance imaging and neuro-otological findings. *J Neurol Sci* **81**:173–184.

Büchele W, Brandt T, Degner D (1983). Ataxia and oscillopsia in downbeat-nystagmus vertigo syndrome. *Adv Oto-Rhino Laryngol* **30**:291–297.

Carlow TJ (1986). Medical treatment of nystagmus and ocular motor disorders. *Int Ophthalmol Clin* **26**:251–264.

Cross SA, Smith JL, Norton EW (1982). Periodic alternating nystagmus clearing after vitrectomy. *J Clin Neuroophthalmol* **2**:511.

Currie J, Matsuo V (1986). The use of clonazepam in the treatment of nystagmus induced oscillopsia. *Ophthalmology* **93**:924–932.

Das VE, Oruganti P, Kramer PD, Leigh RJ (2000). Experimental tests of a neural-network model for ocular oscillations caused by disease of central myelin. *Exp Brain Res* **133**:189–197.

De Ridder D, Moller A, Verlooy J, Cornelissen M, De Ridder L (2002). Is the root entry/exit zone important in microvascular compression syndromes? *Neurosurgery* **51**:427–433.

Dell'Osso LF (2000). Suppression of pendular nystagmus by smoking cannabis in a patient with multiple sclerosis. *Neurology* **13**:2190–2191.

Dieterich M, Straube A, Brandt T, Paulus W, Büttner U (1991). The effects of baclofen and cholinergic drugs on upbeat and downbeat nsytagmus. *J Neurol Neurosurg Psychiatry* **54**:627–632.

Ell J, Gresty M, Chambers BR, Frindley L (1982). Acquired pendular nystagmus: characteristics, pathophysiology and pharmacological modification. In: Roucoux A, Crommeilinck M, eds. *Physiological and Pathological Aspects of Eye Movements.* Dr W. Junk Publ., The Hague, Boston, and London, pp. 89–98.

Endres M, Heide W, Kompf D (1996). See-saw nystagmus. Clinical aspects, diagnosis, pathophysiology: observations in 2 patients. *Nervenarzt* **67**:484–489.

Fisher A, Gresty M, Chambers B, Rudge P (1983). Primary position upbeating nystagmus: a variety of central positional nystagmus. *Brain* **106:**949–964.

Frisèn L, Wikkelso C (1986). Posttraumatic seesaw nystagmus abolished by ethanol ingestion. *Neurology* **36:**841–844.

Furman JMR, Wall C, Pang D (1990). Vestibular function in periodic alternating nystagmus. *Brain* **113:**1425–1439.

Glasauer S, Hoshi M, Kempermann U, Eggert T, Büttner U (2003). Three-dimensional eye position and slow phase velocity in humans with downbeat nystagmus. *J Neurophysiol* **89:**338–354.

Gresty M, Ell JJ, Findley LJ (1982). Acquired pendular nystagmus: its characteristics, localising value and pathophysiology. *J Neurol Neurosurg Psychiatry* **45:**431–439.

Halmagyi MG, Rudge P, Gresty MA (1980). Treatment of periodic alternating nystagmus. *Ann Neurol* **8:**609–611.

Halmagyi MG, Rudge P, Gresty MA, Sanders MD (1983). Downbeating nystagmus. A review of 62 cases. *Arch Neurol* **40:**777–784.

Halmagyi GM, Aw ST, Dehaene I, Curthoys IS, Todd MJ (1994). Jerk-waveform see-saw nystagmus due to unilateral meso-diencephalic lesion. *Brain* **117:**775–788.

Hashimoto M, Ohtsuka K, Hoyt WF (2001). Vascular compression as a cause of superior oblique myokymia disclosed by thin-slice magnetic resonance imaging. *Am J Ophthalmol* **31:**676–677.

Herishanu Y, Louzoun Z (1986). Trihexyphenidyl treatment of vertical pendular nystagmus. *Neurology* **36:**82–84.

Hilgers R-D (2001) Qualitätsbeurteilung von Studien zur klinischen Effektivität. In: Lauterbach KW, Schrappe M, eds. *Gesundheitsökonomie, Qualitätsmanagement und Evidence-based Medicine.* Schattauer, Stuttgart, pp. 89–95.

Hoyt WF, Keane JR (1962). Superior oblique myokymia: report and discussion of five cases of benign intermittent uniocular microtremor. *Arch Ophthalmol* **84:**461–467.

Isago H, Tsuboya R, Kataura A (1985). A case of periodic alternating nystagmus: with special reference to the efficacy of baclofen treatment. *Auris Nasus Larynx* **12:**15–21.

Jabbari B, Rosenberg M, Scherokman B, Gunderson CH, McBurney JW, McClintock W (1987). Effectiveness of trihexyphenidyl against pendular nystagmus and palatal myoclonus: evidence of cholinergic dysfunction. *Mov Disord* **2:**93–98.

Jannetta PJ, Møller MD, Møller AR (1984). Disabling positional vertigo. *N Engl J Med* **310:**1700–1705.

Jay WM, Williams BB, De Chicchis A (1985). Periodic alternating nystagmus clearing after cataract surgery. *J Clin Neuroophthalmol* **5:**149–152.

Kim JI, Averbuch-Heller L, Leigh RJ (2001). Evaluation of transdermal scopolamine as treatment for acquired nystagmus. *J Neuro-ophthalmology* **21:**188–192.

Larmande P, Larmande A (1983). Action du baclofene sur le nystagmus alternant periodique. *Bull Mem Soc Fr Ophtalmol* **94:**390–393.

Lee JP (1984). Superior oblique myokymia: a possible etiologic factor. *Arch Ophthalmol* **102:**1178–1179.

Leigh RJ, Zee DS (1999). *The Neurology of Eye Movements*, 3rd edn. Oxford University Press, New York.

Leigh RJ, Burnstine TH, Ruff RL, Kasmer RJ (1991a). The effect of anticholinergic agents upon acquired nystagmus: a double-blind study of trihexyphenidyl and tridihexethyl chloride. *Neurology* **41:**1737–1741.

Leigh RJ, Tomsak RL, Seidman SH, Dell'Osso LF (1991b). Superior oblique myokymia. Quantitative characteristics of the eye movements in three patients. *Arch Ophthalmol* **109:**1710–1713.

Leigh RJ, Tomsak RL, Grant MP *et al.* (1992). Effectiveness of botulinum toxin administered to abolish acquired nystagmus. *Ann Neurol* **32:**633–642.

Leigh RJ, Averbuch-Heller L, Tomsak RL, Remler BF, Yaniglos SS, Dell'Osso LF (1994). Treatment of abnormal eye movements that impair vision: strategies based on current concepts of physiology and pharmacology. *Ann Neurol* **36:**129–141.

Leopold HC (1985). Opsoklonus- und Myoklonie-Syndrom. Klinische und elektronystagmographische Befunde mit Verlaufsstudien. *Fortschritte der Neurologie, Psychiatrie* **53:**42–54.

Lepore FE (1987). Ethanol-induced resolution of pathologic nystagmus. *Neurology* **37:**877.

Lopez LI, Bronstein AM, Gresty MA, Du Boulay EP, Rudge P (1996). Clinical and MRI correlates in 27 patients with acquired pendular nystagmus. *Brain* **119:**465–472.

Marti S, Palla A, Straumann D (2002). Gravity dependence of ocular drift in patients with cerebellar downbeat nystagmus. *Ann Neurol* **52:**712–721.

Mossman SS, Bronstein AM, Rudge P, Gresty MA (1993). Acquired pendular nystagmus suppressed by alcohol. *Neuro-ophthalmology* **13:**99–106.

Nathanson M, Bergman PS, Bender MB (1953). Visual disturbances as the result of nystagmus on direct forward gaze. Effect of amobarbital sodium. *Arch Neurol Psychiatry* **69:**427–435.

Nausieda PA, Tanner CM, Weiner WJ (1981). Opsoclonic cerebellopathy. A paraneoplastic syndrome responsive to thiamine. *Arch Neurol* **38:**780–782.

Nuti D, Ciacci G, Giannini F, Rossi A, Frederico A (1986). Aperiodic alternating nystagmus: report of two cases and treatment by baclofen. *Ital J Neurol Sci* **7**:453–459.

Palmer EA, Shults WT (1984). Superior oblique myokymia: preliminary results of surgical treatment. *J Pediatr Ophthalmol* (Strabismus) **21**:91–101.

Pedersen RA, Troost BT, Abel LA, Zorub D (1980). Intermittent down beat nystagmus and oscillopsia reversed by suboccipital craniectomy. *Neurology* **30**:1232–1242.

Pless M, Ronthal M (1996). Treatment of opsoclonus-myoclonus with high-dose intravenous immunoglobulin. *Neurology* **46**:583–584.

Rambold H, Helmchen C, Büttner U (1999). Unilateral muscimol inactivations of the interstitial nucleus of Cajal in the alert rhesus monkey do not elicit seesaw nystagmus. *Neurosci Lett* **272**:75–78.

Ridley A, Kennard C, Scholtz CL, Büttner-Ennever JA, Summers B, Turnbull A (1987). Omnipause neurons in two cases of opsoclonus associated with oat cell carcinoma of the lung. *Brain* **110**:1699–1709.

Rosenberg MI, Glaser JS (1983). Superior oblique myokymia. *Ann Neurol* **13**:667–669.

Samii M, Rosahl SK, Carvalho GA, Krzizok T (1998). Microvascular decompression for superior oblique myokymia: first experience. *J Neurosurg* **89**:1020–1024.

Scharwey K, Krzizok T, Samii M, Rosahl SK, Kaufmann H (2000). Remission of superior oblique myokymia after microvascular decompression. *Ophthalmologica* **214**:426–428.

Schon F, Hart PE, Hodgson TL *et al.* (1999). Suppression of pendular nystagmus by smoking cannabis in a patient with multiple sclerosis. *Neurology* **53**:2209–2210.

Spooner JW, Baloh RW (1981). ArnoldChiari malformation. Improvement in eye movements after surgical treatment. *Brain* **104**:51–60.

Stahl JS, Averbuch-Heller L, Leigh RJ (2000). Acquired nystagmus. *Arch Ophthalmol* **118**:544–549.

Starck M, Albrecht H, Pöllmann W, Straube A, Dieterich M (1997). Drug therapy of acquired nystagmus in multiple sclerosis. *J Neurol* **244**:916.

Straube A, Büttner U, Brandt T (1994). Recurrent attacks with skew deviation, torsional nystagmus and contraction of the left frontalis muscle. *Neurology* **44**:177–178.

Strupp M, Schüler O (2002). Improvement of downbeat nystagmus and postural imbalance by 3,4-diaminopyridine, a prospective, placebo-controlled study. *J Vestibular Res* **11**:226.

Strupp M, Schüler O, Krafczyk S *et al.* (2003). Treatment of downbeat nystagmus with 3,4-diaminopyridine a prospective, placebo-controlled, double-blind study. *Neurology* **61**:165–170.

Susac JO, Smith JL, Schatz NJ (1973). Superior oblique myokymia. *Arch Neurol* **29**:432–434.

Tomsak RL, Kosmorsky GA, Leigh RJ (2002). Gabapentin attenuates superior oblique myokymia. *Am J Ophthalmol* **133**:721–723.

Traccis S, Rosati G, Monaco MF, Aiello IN, Agnetti V (1990). Successful treatment of acquired pendular elliptical nystagmus in multiple sclerosis with isoniazid and base-out prisms. *Neurology* **40**:492–494.

Traccis S, Marras MA, Puliga MV *et al.* (1997). Square-wave jerks and square-wave oscillations: treatment with valproic acid. *Neuro-ophthalmology* **18**:51–58.

Tyler RD, Ruiz RS (1990). Propranolol in the treatment of superior oblique myokymia. *Arch Ophthalmol* **108**:175–176.

Waespe W, Cohen B, Raphan T (1985). Dynamic modification of the vestibuloocular reflex by the nodulus and uvula. *Science* **228**:199–202.

Yousry I, Dieterich M, Naidich TP, Schmid UD, Yousry TA (2002). Superior oblique myokymia: magnetic resonance imaging support for the neurovascular compression hypothesis. *Ann Neurol* **51**:361–368.

Zee DS (1985). Mechanisms of nystagmus. *Am J Otolaryngol* **(Suppl)**:30–34.

CHAPTER 36

Orthostatic hypotension

H. Lahrmann,[a] P. Cortelli,[b] M. Hilz,[c]
C.J. Mathias,[d] W. Struhal,[a] M. Tassinari[b]

Abstract

Orthostatic (postural) hypotension (OH) is a common, yet under diagnosed disorder. It may contribute to disability and even death. It can be the initial sign, and lead to incapacitating symptoms in primary and secondary autonomic disorders. These range from visual disturbances and dizziness to loss of consciousness (syncope) after postural change. Evidence-based guidelines for the diagnostic workup and the therapeutic management (non-pharmacological and pharmacological) are provided based on the EFNS guidance regulations. The final literature research was performed in March 2005.

For diagnosis of OH, a structured history taking and measurement of blood pressure (BP) and heart rate in supine and upright position are necessary. OH is defined as fall in systolic BP below 20 mmHg and diastolic BP below 10 mmHg of baseline within 3 min in the upright position. Passive head-up tilt testing is recommended if the active standing test is negative, especially if the history is suggestive of OH, or in patients with motor impairment. The management initially consists of education, advice and training on various factors that influence blood pressure. Increased water and salt ingestion effectively improves OH. Physical measures include leg crossing, squatting, elastic abdominal binders and stockings, and careful exercise. Fludrocortisone is a valuable starter drug. Second line drugs include sympathomimetics, such as midodrine, ephedrine, or dihydroxyphenylserine. Supine hypertension has to be considered.

Background

Orthostatic (postural) hypotension (OH) is a frequent cause of syncope and may contribute to morbidity, disability and even death, because of the potential risk of substantial injury (Mathias, 2003). It may be the initial sign of autonomic failure and cause major symptoms in many primary and secondary diseases of the autonomic nervous system (ANS) (e.g. pure autonomic failure (PAF), multiple system atrophy (MSA), Parkinson's disease and diabetic autonomic neuropathy). It occurs frequently in elderly patients because of therapy (vasoactive drugs, antidepressants), reduced fluid

[a]Department of Neurology, Kaiser Franz Josef Hospital; L. Boltzmann Institute for Neurooncology, Vienna, Austria; [b]Neurological Department, University of Bologna, Bologna, Italy; [c]Neurological Department, University Erlangen-Nuremberg, Erlangen, Germany; Department of Neurology, New York University, School of Medicine, NY, USA; [d]Neurovascular Medicine Unit, Imperial College London at St. Mary's Hospital; Autonomic Unit, National Hospital for Neurology and Neurosurgery, Queen Square; and Institute of Neurology, University College London, London, UK.

intake and decreased ANS function. In Parkinson's disease the prevalence of OH may be as high as 60% (Senard *et al.*, 2001). Characteristic symptoms of OH include light-headedness, visual blurring, dizziness, generalized weakness, fatigue, cognitive slowing, leg buckling, coat-hanger ache, and gradual or sudden loss of consciousness. Falls with injuries may result.

Orthostatic hypotension is defined by consensus as a fall in blood pressure (BP) of at least 20 mmHg systolic and 10 mm Hg diastolic within 3 min in the upright position (Schatz *et al.*, 1996). This reduces perfusion pressure of organs, especially above heart level, such as the brain. Neurogenic OH results from impaired cardiovascular adrenergic function. The lesion can be postganglionic as in PAF, or preganglionic as in MSA. Other causes of OH are low intravascular volume (blood or plasma loss, fluid or electrolyte loss), impaired cardiac function due to structural heart disease, and vasodilatation, due to drugs, alcohol, heat (Mathias *et al.*, 2003).

Objectives

Orthostatic hypotension is an under diagnosed disorder. Many new treatment options, pharmacological and non-pharmacological, have been published in recent years. Evidence-based guidelines for clinical and laboratory diagnostic workup, and therapeutic management of OH are provided for physicians involved in the care of such patients.

Methods

Electronic search strategies used the following databases: Cochrane library, Medline, Pub Med, and various internet search routines, for English publications. Key search terms included 'orthostatic hypotension', 'syncope', 'hypotension' and 'therapy', 'treatment' or 'diagnosis', and first year availability of each referenced literature database until March 2005. References classified by evidence levels were selected by one individual and checked by another investigator. Where there was a lack of evidence but consensus was clear, we have stated our opinion as Good Practice Points (GPP) (Brainin *et al.*, 2004).

Diagnostic strategies

Tests to investigate OH are considered here and not general investigations of the ANS. A limitation is a paucity of randomised and blind studies. The wide variation of test methods, protocols and equipment in autonomic laboratories make comparison of results difficult (Lahrmann *et al.*, 2005).

The history is of particular importance and has a high diagnostic value (pre-existing disease, detailed description of sequence of symptoms). The initial clinical evaluation should include a detailed physical and neurological examination, 12-lead ECG recording, routine laboratory testing and BP measurements while supine and upright. Non-neurogenic causes of OH must be considered, as they can exacerbate neurogenic OH.

The cardiovascular responses to standing may be investigated by recording BP and heart rate while supine and for up to 3 min while upright. Passive head-up tilt testing (HUT) is recommended if the active standing test is negative, especially if the history is suggestive of OH, and in patients with motor impairment, as in Parkinson's disease, MSA and spinal cord lesions. Tilt tables with foot board support, and if available, devices providing non-invasive, automatic and ideally continuous heart rate and BP measurements are recommended (Mathias and Bannister, 2002).

Protocol:

- Orthostatic testing should take place in a quiet room, at a temperature between 20 and 24 °C. The patient should rest while supine for ideally 5 min before HUT is started. Emptying the bladder before testing is recommended.
- Passive HUT to an angle between 60° and 80° for 3 min is recommended for the diagnosis of OH (Ravits, 1997; Chandler and Mathias, 2002).
- HUT is considered positive if systolic BP falls below 20 mmHg and diastolic BP below 10 mmHg of baseline. If symptoms occur, the patient should be tilted back to the supine position immediately.
- Measurement of plasma noradrenaline levels while supine and upright may be of value.

- In contrast with cardiologic guidelines pharmacological provocation with sublingual nitroglycerine or intravenous isoproterenol is not recommended to diagnose OH as it reduces sensitivity and will result in false positive outcomes (Ravits, 1997).
- Combination of HUT and physiological measures, such as lower body negative pressure application, as used in neurally-mediated syncope, is not recommended for diagnosis of OH.

HUT is a safe procedure for the diagnosis of OH (Brignole *et al.*, 2001). However, as syncope and arrhythmias have been described, the investigating staff should be adequately trained to recognise such problems. Resuscitation equipment and a team experienced in cardiac life support should be available at short notice (GPP).

RECOMMENDATIONS

All Level C
- Structured history taking
- Detailed physical examination
- 12-lead ECG recording
- Routine laboratory testing
- BP measurements while supine and upright
- Cardiologic referral, if heart disease or abnormal ECG is present or suspected
- Active standing or HUT, ideally with continuous assessment of BP and HR for 3 min
- Further ANS screening tests, with other appropriate investigations, depending on the possible aetiology of the underlying disorder (Mathias, 2003).

Management

Many new treatment options for OH have been studied in the last decade. Controlled trials have been performed for drugs and physical therapy. However, many of these studies included only small groups of patients with a variety of disorders that cause OH, and different diagnostic criteria have been used. If not noted otherwise, studies are classified as Class IV (Brainin *et al.*, 2004).

General principles

In addition to head up postural change, BP is influenced by many stimuli in everyday life. These include a hot environment, carbohydrate rich meals and exercise. The physiological mechanisms and individual strategies to avoid OH and syncope should be explained to the patients and caregivers. The following recommendations are mainly a result of panel consensus and qualified as GPP.

Elevated environmental temperatures, a hot bath or shower, and sauna should be avoided as they cause venous pooling. Prolonged recumbence during daytime and sudden head up postural change, particularly in the morning, when BP may be lowered by nocturnal polyuria, should be avoided (Mathias *et al.*, 1986). Postprandial hypotension may increase OH (vasodilatation in splanchnic vessels). Large meals, especially carbohydrate rich, and alcohol should be avoided. A carefully controlled and individualised exercise training (swimming, aerobics, and, if possible, cycling and walking) often improves OH.

Supine hypertension

Supine hypertension may be a problem, resulting from medication and/or being part of the disease. Therefore, 24-h measurement of BP is best before and if needed after starting a new therapy. Patients may self-monitor BP, daily at about the same time, and when they experience symptoms. Pressor medications should be avoided after 6 p.m. and the bed head elevated (20–30 cm). On occasion, short acting antihypertensive drugs may be considered (e.g. nitro-glycerine sublingual).

Non-pharmacological treatment

Avoidance of factors that may induce OH is recommended first line, particularly in mild forms. Educating the patients and carers on the mechanisms of OH is important. The next step includes a range of non-pharmacological strategies.

Patients should be advised to move to head-up position slowly, sit on the edge of the bed for some minutes after recumbence and activate calf muscles while supine. Physical counter manoeuvres can be applied immediately at the onset of presyncopal symptoms. They need to be explained and trained individually. In case of motor disabilities and compromised balance, as in the cerebellar forms of MSA, programmes with appropriate aids have to be developed. Leg crossing with tension of the thigh, buttock and calf muscles (party position), bending over forward to reduce the orthostatic difference between the heart and brain and compress the splanchnic vessels by increasing abdominal pressure, squatting to reduce blood pooling are effective in temporarily reducing OH (Wieling *et al.*, 1993; ten Harkel *et al.*, 1994; Bouvette *et al.*, 1996; Smit *et al.*, 1999; van Dijk *et al.*, 2005). Not all patients can perform these manoeuvres and sitting or lying down, and using a cane that can be folded into a tripod chair (Smit *et al.*, 1999), are useful. Elastic stockings and abdominal compression bands reduce venous pooling and have been shown effective in small studies (Denq *et al.*, 1997; Tanaka *et al.*, 1997). Sleeping with head-end of the bed elevated (20–30 cm), particularly in combination with low dose fludrocortisone, improves OH (van Lieshout *et al.*, 2000).

To compensate for renal salt loss a liberal intake of salt, at least 8 g (150 mmol) of sodium chloride daily, if needed as salt tablets (starting dose 500 mg three times a day (t.i.d.)), are recommended. Water repletion (2–2.5 l/day) is important, while 500 ml of water is effective in raising BP immediately (Mathias and Young, 2004).

Cardiac pacing is not recommended in neurogenic OH (Sahul *et al.*, 2004).

Pharmacological treatment
Plasma expansion
Fludrocortisone

Fludrocortisone acetate is a synthetic mineralocorticoid with minimal glucocorticoid effects. It increases renal sodium reabsorbtion and expands plasma volume. Sensitisation of alpha-adrenoceptors may augment the action of noradrenaline. After oral administration, fludrocortisone is readily absorbed and peak plasma levels are reached within 45 min. Elimination half-life is around 7 h.

Review of clinical studies No Class I and II studies were identified. One class III (Campbell *et al.*,1975) and one class IV (Hoehn, 1975) study have shown an increase in BP and improvement of symptoms.

RECOMMENDATIONS

Level C
- Fludrocortisone as first line drug-monotherapy of OH (0.1–0.2 mg per day).
- Full benefit requires a high dietary salt and adequate fluid intake.
- Combination of a high salt diet, head-up tilt sleeping (20–30 cm) and a low dose of fludrocortisone (0.1–0.2 mg) is an effective means of improving OH (van Lieshout *et al.*, 2000).

Mild dependent oedema can be expected and fludrocortisone should be used with caution in patients with a low serum albumin. Higher doses of fludrocortisone can result in fluid overload and congestive heart failure, severe supine hypertension and hypokalaemia (Schatz *et al.*, 1976). To prevent hypokalaemia food rich in potassium such as fruits, vegetables, poultry, fish and meat is advisable. Headache may occur, especially while supine.

Alpha receptor agonists

There are many sympathomimetic drugs that act on alpha-adrenoceptors. Midodrine has been investigated extensively. Adrenaline (epinephrine) and noradrenaline (norepinephrine) are inactive when administered orally, and rapidly inactivated in the body after infusion. Common adverse effects of sympathomimetics with a central action, such as ephedrine, are tachycardia, anxiety, restlessness, insomnia and tremor. Dry mouth, impaired blood circulation to the extremities, supine hypertension, and cardiac arrhythmias may occur.

Midodrine

Midodrine is a prodrug with an active metabolite, desglymidodrine, that is a peripherally acting alpha-1-adrenoceptor agonist. It increases BP via vasoconstriction. Midodrine does not cross the blood–brain barrier after oral administration and does not increase heart rate. The absolute bioavailability is 93% and the elimination half-life of desglymidodrine is 2–3 h. The duration of action of midodrine is approximately 4 h. It is excreted mainly in urine.

Review of clinical studies Class I: One dose-response study (Wright *et al.*, 1998) and two studies with a total number of 259 patients investigating the efficacy, safety and tolerability of long-term midodrine application (Jankovic *et al.*, 1993; Low *et al.*, 1997) were identified. An increase in orthostatic BP and decrease in OH-related symptoms were reported.

Class III: Efficacy and safety were higher with midodrine than with ephedrine (Fouad-Tarazi *et al.*, 1995).

Class IV: Midodrine reduced exercise-induced OH in PAF (Schrage *et al.*, 2004).

RECOMMENDATIONS

All Level A

- Midodrine is recommended for mono- or combined therapy (e.g. with fludrocortisone).
- Initial dosage is 2.5 mg orally 2–3 times daily increasing gradually up to 10 mg t.i.d.
- Supine hypertension is a common (25%) adverse effect and may be severe. The last dose should be administered at least 4 h before going to sleep and BP should be monitored.
- Adverse effects are piloerection (goose bumps, 13%), scalp or general pruritus (10 and 2%), scalp or general paraesthesia (9% each), urinary retention (6%) and chills (5%).

Some patients worsen on midodrine, maybe due to adrenoceptor desensitization (Kaufmann *et al.*, 1988). It should be administered with caution in patients with hepatic dysfunction and is contraindicated in severe heart disease, acute renal failure, urinary retention, phaeochromocytoma and thyrotoxicosis (McClellan *et al.*, 1998).

DOPS

Dihydroxyphenylserine (DOPS) is a prodrug that is converted by dopadecarboxylase to noradrenaline.

Review of clinical studies Class I: Administration of 200 mg and 400 mg L-DOPS daily improved OH symptoms in 146 chronic haemodialysis patients (Akizawa *et al.*, 2002). In short-term (4 weeks,

$n = 86$) and long-term studies (24–52 weeks, $n = 74$) the efficacy of L-DOPS (400 mg/day) for OH after dialysis was demonstrated (Iida *et al.*, 2002).

Class III: In 20 patients with familial amyloid neuropathy L-threo-DOPS effectively improves orthostatic tolerance (Carvalho *et al.*, 1997). DL-DOPS improved OH in 10 patients with central and peripheral ANS disorders (Freeman *et al.*, 1999). In 19 patients with severe OH L-DOPS improved BP and orthostatic tolerance (Kaufmann *et al.*, 2003). In 26 MSA and 6 PAF patients 300 mg of L-threo-DOPS given twice daily were effective in controlling symptomatic OH (Mathias *et al.*, 2001).

RECOMMENDATIONS

Level A

In a dosage between 200 mg and 400 mg per day L-DOPS reduces OH. It is the only effective treatment of dopamine beta-hydroxylase deficiency. In all studies reviewed, no major side effects were reported. Future studies will have to investigate which patient groups benefit most from this drug.

Octreotide

The somatostatin analogue octreotide inhibits release of gastrointestinal peptides, some of which have vasodilatatory properties. It is administered subcutaneously starting with 25–50 mg.

Review of clinical studies Four Class III studies were identified: In 18 PAF patients octreotide reduced postural, postprandial and exertion-induced hypotension, without causing or increasing nocturnal hypertension (Alam *et al.*, 1995). Octreotide improved OH in MSA patients after acute and chronic administration (Bordet *et al.*, 1994 and 1995). The combination of midodrine and octreotide was more effective in reducing OH than either drug alone (Hoeldtke *et al.*, 1998).

> ## RECOMMENDATIONS
>
> ### Level C
> Subcutaneous doses of 25–150 mg half an hour before a meal may be used to reduce postprandial OH. It does not increase supine hypertension. Nausea and abdominal cramps may occur.

Other treatment options

For the drugs listed below there is no clear evidence for use in OH. Many are recommended as GPP and warrant future studies.

Ephedrine, that acts on alpha- and beta-adrenergic receptors, is recommended by the authors, as it reduces OH in many patients, particularly with central lesions like MSA (15 mg t.i.d.). *Yohimbine*, an alpha-2-adrenoceptor antagonist with central and peripheral effects, has been used in refractory OH (6 mg daily) (Jordan *et al.*, 1998, Class III). *Dihydroergotamine* (DHE), a direct alpha-adrenoceptor agonist stimulating constriction of venous capacity vessels, has shown some benefit and may be used in severe OH (3–5 mg t.i.d. oral) (Level C: Conte *et al.*, 1976, Class III; Lubke *et al.*, 1976, Class III; Victor *et al.*, 2002, Class IV). *Desmopressin*, a vasopressin analogue, acts on renal tubular vasopressin-2 receptors, diminishing nocturnal polyuria, and may be applied as nasal spray (10–40 μg) or orally (100–400 μg) at night (Mathias *et al.*, 1986, Class IV). *Erythropoietin* is recommended in anaemic patients (Hoeldtke and Streeten, 1993; Biaggioni *et al.*, 1994; Perera *et al.*, 1995). *Indomethacin*, a prostaglandin synthetase inhibitor, has been used in severe OH (75–150 mg/day) (Kochar and Itskovitz, 1978, Class IV; Jordan *et al.*, 1998, Class III).

Summary

- OH is defined as fall in BP within 3 min of active standing or HUT.
- The key to managing OH is individually tailored therapy. The goal of treatment is to improve the patient's functional capacity and quality of life, preventing injury, rather than to achieve a target BP.

- Management of patients with OH consists of education, advice and training on various factors that influence blood pressure, and special aspects that have to be avoided (foods, habits, positions and drugs).
- Physical measures include leg crossing, squatting, elastic abdominal binders and stockings, and careful exercise (GPP).
- Increased water (2–2.5 l/day) and salt ingestion (> 8g or 150 mmol per day) effectively improve OH.
- Fludrocortisone is a valuable starter drug (0.1–0.2 mg per day, Level C). Second line drugs include sympathomimetics, such as midodrine (start with 2.5 mg b.i.d and increase to 10 mg t.i.d, Level A) or ephedrine (15 mg t.i.d., GPP). DOPS (200–400 mg daily, Level A) reduces OH with only minor side effects. It is an effective treatment in dopamine beta-hydroxylase deficiency.
- Supine hypertension has to be considered.
- Individual testing with a series of drugs, based on the risk of side effects, pharmacological interactions and probability of response in the individual patient, may be considered when the measures shown here are not satisfactory.

Conflicts of interest

The present guidelines were developed without external financial support. None of the authors reports conflicting interests.

References

Akizawa T, Koshikawa S, Iida N, Marumo F, Akiba T, Kawaguchi Y, Imada A, Yamazaki C, Suzuki M, Tubakihara Y (2002). Clinical effects of L-threo-3,4-dihydroxyphenylserine on orthostatic hypotension in hemodialysis patients. Nephron 90:384–390.

Alam M, Smith G, Bleasdale-Barr K, Pavitt DV, Mathias CJ (1995). Effects of the peptide release inhibitor, octreotide, on daytime hypotension and on nocturnal hypertension in primary autonomic failure. *J Hypertens* **13**:1664–1669.

Biaggioni I, Robertson D, Krantz S, Jones M, Haile V (1994). The anemia of primary autonomic failure and its reversal with recombinant erythropoietin. *Ann Intern Med* **121**:181–186.

Bordet R, Benhadjali J, Libersa C, Destee A (1994). Octreotide in the management of orthostatic hypotension in multiple system atrophy: pilot trial of chronic administration. *Clin Neuropharmacol* **17:**380–383.

Bordet R, Benhadjali J, Destee A, Belabbas A, Libersa C (1995). Octreotide effects on orthostatic hypotension in patients with multiple system atrophy: a controlled study of acute administration. *Clin Neuropharmacol* **18:**83–89.

Bouvette CM, McPhee BR, Opfer-Gehrking TL, Low PA (1996). Role of physical countermaneuvers in the management of orthostatic hypotension: efficacy and biofeedback augmentation. *Mayo Clin Proc* **71:**847–853.

Brainin M, Barnes M, Baron JC, Gilhus NE, Hughes R, Selmaj K, Waldemar G (2004). Guidance for the preparation of neurological management guidelines by EFNS scientific task forces–revised recommendations 2004. *Eur J Neurol* **11:**577–581.

Brignole M, Alboni P, Benditt D *et al.* (2001). Guidelines on management (diagnosis and treatment) of syncope. *Eur Heart J* **22:**1256–1306.

Campbell IW, Ewing DJ, Clarke BF (1975). 9-Alpha-fluorohydrocortisone in the treatment of postural hypotension in diabetic autonomic neuropathy. *Diabetes* **24:**381–384.

Carvalho MJ, van den Meiracker AH, Boomsma F, Man in 't Veld AJ, Freitas J, Costa O, de Freitas AF (1997). Improved orthostatic tolerance in familial amyloidotic polyneuropathy with unnatural noradrenaline precursor L-threo-3,4-dihydroxyphenylserine. *J Auton Nerv Syst* **62:**63–71.

Chandler MP, Mathias CJ (2002). Haemodynamic responses during head-up tilt and tilt reversal in two groups with chronic autonomic failure: pure autonomic failure and multiple system atrophy. *J Neurol* **249:**542–548.

Conte JJ, Fournie GJ, Maurette MH (1976). Dihydroergotamine: an effective treatment for postural hypotension due to antihypertensive drugs (ganglion-blocking agents excepted). *Cardiology* **61(Suppl 1):**342–349.

Denq JC, Opfer-Gehrking TL, Giuliani M, Felten J, Convertino VA, Low PA (1997). Efficacy of compression of different capacitance beds in the amelioration of orthostatic hypotension. *Clin Auton Res* **7:**321–326.

Fouad-Tarazi FM, Okabe M, Goren H (1995). Alpha sympathomimetic treatment of autonomic insufficiency with orthostatic hypotension. *Am J Med* **99:**604–610

Freeman R, Landsberg L, Young J (1999). The treatment of neurogenic orthostatic hypotension with 3,4-DL-threo-dihydroxyphenylserine: a randomized, placebo-controlled, crossover trial. *Neurology* **53:**2151–2157.

Hoeldtke RD, Streeten DH (1993). Treatment of orthostatic hypotension with erythropoietin. *N Engl J Med* **329:**611–615.

Hoeldtke RD, Horvath GG, Bryner KD, Hobbs GR (1998). Treatment of orthostatic hypotension with midodrine and octreotide. *J Clin Endocrinol Metab* **83:**339–343.

Hoehn MM (1975). Levodopa-induced postural hypotension. Treatment with fludrocortisone. *Arch Neurol* **32:**50–51.

Iida N, Koshikawa S, Akizawa T, Tsubakihara Y, Marumo F, Akiba T, Kawaguchi Y, Imada A, Yamazaki C, Suzuki M (2002). Effects of L-threo-3,4-dihydroxyphenylserine on orthostatic hypotension in hemodialysis patients. *Am J Nephrol* **22:**338–346.

Jankovic J, Gilden JL, Hiner BC, Kaufmann H, Brown DC, Coghlan CH, Rubin M, Fouad-Tarazi FM (1993). Neurogenic orthostatic hypotension: a double-blind, placebo-controlled study with midodrine. *Am J Med* **95:**38–48.

Jordan J, Shannon JR, Biaggioni I, Norman R, Black BK, Robertson D (1998). Contrasting actions of pressor agents in severe autonomic failure. *Am J Med* **105:**116–124.

Kaufmann H, Brannan T, Krakoff L, Yahr MD, Mandeli J (1988). Treatment of orthostatic hypotension due to autonomic failure with a peripheral alpha-adrenergic agonist (midodrine). *Neurology* **38:**951–956.

Kaufmann H, Saadia D, Voustianiouk A, Goldstein DS, Holmes C, Yahr MD, Nardin R, Freeman R (2003). Norepinephrine precursor therapy in neurogenic orthostatic hypotension. *Circulation* **108:**724–728.

Kochar MS, Itskovitz HD (1978). Treatment of idiopathic orthostatic hypotension (Shy-Drager syndrome) with indomethacin. *Lancet* **1:**1011–1014.

Lahrmann H, Magnifico F, Haensch CA, Cortelli (2005). Autonomic Nervous System Laboratories: A European Survey. *Eur J Neurol* **12:**375–379.

Low PA, Gilden JL, Freeman R, Sheng KN, McElligott MA (1997). Efficacy of midodrine vs placebo in neurogenic orthostatic hypotension: a randomized, double-blind multicenter study. *JAMA* **277:**1046–1051. Correction. ibid.; **278:**388.

Lubke KO (1976). A controlled study with Dihydergot on patients with orthostatic dysregulation. *Cardiology* **61(Suppl 1):**333–341.

Mathias CJ (2003). Autonomic diseases: clinical features and laboratory evaluation. *J Neurol Neurosurg Psychiatry* **74(Suppl 3):**iii31–41.

Mathias CJ, Young TM (2004). Water drinking in the management of orthostatic intolerance due to orthostatic hypotension, vasovagal syncope and postural tachycardia syndrome. *Euro J Neurol* **11:**613–619.

Mathias CJ, Fosbraey P, da Costa DF, Thornley A, Bannister R (1986). The effect of desmopressin on nocturnal polyuria, overnight weight loss, and morning postural hypotension in patients with autonomic failure. *Br Med J (Clin Res Ed)* **293:**353–354.

Mathias CJ, Senard JM, Braune S, Watson L, Aragishi A, Keeling JE, Taylor MD (2001). L-theo-dihydroxphenylserine (L-threo-DOPS, droxidopa) in the management of neurogenic orthostatic hypotension: a multi-national, multi-centre, dose-ranging study in multiple system atrophy and pure autonomic failure. *Clin Auton Res* **11:**235–242.

Mathias CJ, Bannister R (2002). Investigation of autonomic disorders. In Mathias CJ and Bannister R, eds., *Autonomic Failure. A Textbook of Clinical Disorders of the Autonomic Nervous System.* 4th edn. Oxford: Oxford University Press. pp 169–195.

McClellan KJ Wiseman LR, Wilde MI (1998). Midodrine: a review of its therapeutic use in the management of orthostatic hypotension. *Drugs Aging* **12:**76–86.

Perera R, Isola L, Kaufmann H (1995). Effect of recombinant erythropoietin on anemia and orthostatic hypotension in primary autonomic failure. *Clin Auton Res* **5:**211–213.

Ravits JM (1997). AAEM minimonograph #48: autonomic nervous system testing. *Muscle Nerve* **20:**919–937.

Sahul ZH, Trusty JM, Erickson M, Low PA, Shen WK (2004). Pacing does not improve hypotension in patients with severe orthostatic hypotension–a prospective randomized cross-over pilot study. *Clin Auton Res* **14:**255–258.

Schatz IJ, Miller MJ, Frame B (1976). Corticosteroids in the management of orthostatic hypotension. *Cardiology* **61(Suppl 1):**280–289.

Schatz IJ *et al.* (1996) Consensus statement on the definition of orthostatic hypotension, pure autonomic failure and multiple system atrophy. *Clin Auton Res* **6:**125–126.

Schrage WG, Eisenach JH, Dinenno FA, Roberts SK, Johnson CP, Sandroni P, Low PA, Joyner MJ (2004). Effects of midodrine on exercise-induced hypotension and blood pressure recovery in autonomic failure. *J Appl Physiol* **97:**1978–1984.

Senard JM, Brefel-Courbon C, Rascol O, Montastruc JL (2001). Orthostatic hypotension in patients with Parkinson's disease: pathophysiology and management. *Drugs Aging* **18:**495–505.

Smit AA, Wieling W, Opfer-Gehrking TL, Emmerik-Levelt HM, Low PA (1999). Patients' choice of portable folding chairs to reduce symptoms of orthostatic hypotension. *Clin Auton Res* **9:**341–344.

Tanaka H, Yamaguchi H, Tamai H (1997). Treatment of orthostatic intolerance with inflatable abdominal band. *Lancet* **349:**175.

ten Harkel AD, van Lieshout JJ, Wieling W (1994). Effects of leg muscle pumping and tensing on orthostatic arterial pressure: a study in normal subjects and patients with autonomic failure. *Clin Sci* (Lond) **87:**553–558.

van Dijk N, de Bruin IGJM, Gisolf J, Bruin-Bon HACM, Linzer M, van Lieshout JJ, Wieling W (2005). Hemodynamic effects of legcrossing and skeletal muscle tensing during free standing in patients with vasovagal syncope. *J Appl Physiol* **98(2):**584–590

van Lieshout JJ, ten Harkel AD, Wieling W (2000). Fludrocortisone and sleeping in the head-up position limit the postural decrease in cardiac output in autonomic failure. *Clin Auton Res* **10:**35–42.

Victor RG, Talman WT (2002). Comparative effects of clonidine and dihydroergotamine on venomotor tone and orthostatic tolerance in patients with severe hypoadrenergic orthostatic hypotension. *Am J Med* **112:**361–368.

Wieling W, van Lieshout JJ, van Leeuwen AM (1993). Physical manoeuvres that reduce postural hypotension in autonomic failure. *Clin Auton Res* **3:**57–65.

Wright RA, Kaufmann HC, Perera R, Opfer-Gehrking TL, McElligott MA, Sheng KN, Low PA (1998). A double-blind, dose response study of midodrine in neurogenic orthostatic hypotension. *Neurology* **51:**120–124.

CHAPTER 37

Cerebral venous and sinus thrombosis

K. Einhäupl,[a] M.-G. Bousser,[b] S.F.T.M. de Bruijn,[c]
J.M. Ferro,[d] I. Martinelli,[e] F. Masuhr,[a] J. Stam[f]

Abstract

Background Cerebral venous and sinus thrombosis (CVST) is a rare disease that accounts for less than 1% of all strokes. Diagnosis is still frequently overlooked or delayed due to the wide spectrum of clinical symptoms and the often subacute or lingering onset. Current therapeutic measures that are used in clinical practice include the use of anticoagulants such as dose-adjusted intravenous heparin or body weight-adjusted subcutaneous low-molecular-weight heparin, the use of thrombolysis, and symptomatic therapy including control of seizures and elevated intracranial pressure.

Methods We searched MEDLINE (National Library of Medicine), the Cochrane Central Register of Controlled Trials (CENTRAL) and the Cochrane Library to review the strength of evidence to support these interventions and the preparation of recommendations on the therapy of CVST based on the best available evidence. Review articles and book chapters were also included.

Recommendations were reached by consensus. Where there was a lack of evidence but consensus was clear we stated our opinion as Good Practice Points.

Patients with CVST without contraindications for anticoagulation should be treated either with body weight-adjusted subcutaneous low-molecular-weight heparin (LMWH) or dose-adjusted intravenous heparin (Good Practice Point). Concomitant intracranial haemorrhage related to CVST is not a contraindication for heparin therapy. The optimal duration of oral anticoagulation after the acute phase is unclear. Oral anticoagulation may be given for 3 months if CVST was secondary to a transient risk factor, for 6–12 months in patients with idiopathic CVST and in those with 'mild' hereditary thrombophilia. Indefinite AC should be considered in patients with two or more episodes of CVST and in those with one episode of CVST and 'severe' hereditary thrombophilia (Good Practice Point).

There is insufficient evidence to support the use of either systemic or local thrombolysis in patients with CVST. If patients deteriorate despite adequate anticoagulation and other causes of deterioration have been ruled out, thrombolysis may be a

---

[a]Department of Neurology, Charité, Humboldt-University Berlin, Germany; [b]Department of Neurology, Hôpital Lariboisière, France; [c]Department of Neurology, Haga Hospital, The Hague and LUMC, Leiden, The Netherlands; [d]Department of Neurology, Hospital Santa Maria, Lisboa, Portugal; [e]A. Bianchi Bonomi Hemophilia and Thrombosis Center, IRCCS Maggiore Hospital, University of Milan, Italy; [f]Department of Neurology, Academic Medical Centre Amsterdam, The Netherlands.

therapeutic option in selected cases, possibly in those without intracranial haemorrhage (Good Practice Point). There are no controlled data about the risks and benefits of certain therapeutic measures to reduce an elevated intracranial pressure (with brain displacement) in patients with severe CVST. Antioedema treatment (including hyperventilation, osmotic diuretics, craniectomy) should be used as life-saving interventions (Good Practice Point).

Background and objectives

Cerebral venous and sinus thrombosis (CVST) is a rare condition that accounts for less than 1% of all strokes. The exact incidence in adults is unknown as population-based studies are not available but one can expect 5–8 cases per year in a tertiary care centre (Bousser *et al.*, 1985; Einhäupl *et al.*, 1990). A Canadian study reported an incidence of 0.67 cases per 100.000 children below 18 years and 43% of the reported cases were seen in neonates (deVeber *et al.*, 2001). The peak incidence in adults is in their third decade with a male/female ratio of 1.5–5 per year (Einhäupl *et al.*, 1990; de Bruijn *et al.* 2001). Diagnosis is still frequently overlooked or delayed due to the wide spectrum of clinical symptoms and the often subacute or lingering onset. Headache is the most frequent symptom of CVST and occurs in almost 90% of all cases (Ferro *et al.*, 2004). The headache may be of acute onset (thunderclap headache) and may be clinically indistinguishable from headache in patients with subarachnoid haemorrhage (de Bruijn *et al.*, 1996). Focal or generalized seizures are far more frequently seen in CVST than in arterial stroke and occur in 40% of all patients with an even higher incidence (76%) in peripartum CVST (Cantu and Barrinagarrimenteria, 1993; Ferro *et al.*, 2004). Focal neurological signs (including focal seizures) are the most common finding in CVST. They include central motor and sensory deficits, aphasia or hemianopsia and occur in 40–60% of all cases. In patients with focal deficits together with headache, seizures or an altered consciousness CVST should always be considered. The syndrome of isolated intracranial hypertension (IIH) with headache, vomiting and blurred vision due to papilloedema is the most homogeneous pattern of clinical presentation accounting for 20–40% of CVST cases. Stupor or coma are found in 15–19% of patients at hospital admission (Mehraein *et al.*, 2003; Ferro *et al.*, 2004) and are usually seen in cases with extensive thrombosis or affection of the deep venous system with bilateral thalamic involvement. Of all clinical signs reported in CVST, coma at admission is the most consistent and strongest predictor of a poor outcome (de Bruijn *et al.*, 2001; Ferro *et al.*, 2004).

Intra-arterial four-vessel angiography has long been the gold standard for establishing the diagnosis of CVST but today magnetic resonance imaging (MRI) and magnetic resonance angiography (MRA) are regarded the best tools both for the diagnosis and follow up of CVST (for review see Masuhr *et al.*, 2004). Cranial computed tomography (CCT) alone is not sufficient but diagnosis can be established in combination with CT angiography although the use of iodinated contrast fluid and ionising radiation remains a disadvantage that makes it inappropriate for follow-up examinations.

Current therapeutic measures that are used in clinical practice include the use of anticoagulants such as dose-adjusted intravenous heparin or body weight-adjusted subcutaneous low-molecular-weight heparin, the use of thrombolysis, and symptomatic therapy including control of seizures and elevated intracranial pressure. Particularly the use of heparin has long been a matter of debate. Whereas anticoagulation is effective in the treatment and prevention of extracerebral venous thrombosis, the high rate of spontaneous intracranial haemorrhages seen in patients with CVST cause many physicians to hesitate to administer heparin because of safety concerns. More recently, the introduction of local thrombolysis has stirred the discussion about the optimal therapy of patients with CVST (Bousser, 1999).

The aim of the present Task Force was to review the strength of evidence to support these interventions and the preparation of recommendations on the therapy of CVST based on the best available evidence for the efficacy and safety of anticoagulant therapy, thrombolysis and symptomatic therapy.

Materials and methods

Search strategy

MEDLINE 1966–2004 and EMBASE 1966–2004 were examined with appropriate MESH and free subject terms: 1. cerebral venous and sinus thrombosis, 2. cerebral venous thrombosis, 3. cortical vein thrombosis, 4. intracranial thrombosis.

1–4 was combined with the terms: 5. treatment, 6. medication, 7. therapy, 8. controlled clinical trial, 9. randomised controlled trial, 10. multicenter study, 11. meta analysis, 12. anticoagulation, 13. thrombolysis, 14. local thrombolysis, 15. antiepileptic therapy, 16. intracranial pressure, 17. steroids, 18. hyperventilation, 19. osmotic diuretics, 20. craniectomy, 21. decompressive surgery.

The Cochrane Central Register of Controlled Trials (CENTRAL) and the Cochrane Library and references of selected articles were also searched. Review articles and book chapters were also included if they were considered to provide comprehensive reviews of the topic. The search included reports of research in human beings only and in the English language. The literature search was performed by K.E. and F.M. who also prepared a first draft of the manuscript. The manuscript was sent via e-mail and was reviewed by all members of the Task Force and suggestions and corrections were incorporated. Recommendations were reached by consensus of all Task Force members and were also based on our own awareness and clinical experience. Where there was a lack of evidence but consensus was clear we stated our opinion as Good Practice Points. The final draft of the manuscript was approved by all members of the Task Force.

The classification for evidence levels for therapeutic interventions were made according to the guidance for the preparation of neurological management guidelines by EFNS scientific task forces (Brainin *et al.*, 2004).

Treatment

Heparin therapy

The rationale of anticoagulant therapy in CVST is to avoid thrombus extension, to favour spontaneous thrombus resolution and to prevent pulmonary embolism particularly in patients with concomitant extracranial deep vein thrombosis. At the same time anticoagulation (AC) may promote or worsen intracranial haemorrhage (ICH) which occurs in 40–50% of patients with CVST (de Bruijn *et al.*, 1999; Ferro *et al.*, 2004) and which may be the main reason to withhold AC. In addition, AC is always associated with an increased risk for extracranial bleeding complications.

There are only two small controlled trials that compared the efficacy and safety of AC with placebo for the treatment of CVST. Both trials chose an unfavourable outcome as the main criterion to evaluate the efficacy of AC instead of a good outcome (e.g. Rankin Scale 0–1) which might have been a better choice in a condition with a much better prognosis than arterial stroke. In addition, the 3 months follow-up for the evaluation of the functional outcome may have been too short as major improvement of the patients with CVST can be observed far beyond.

The first study (Einhäupl *et al.*, 1991) compared dose-adjusted intravenous heparin with placebo in 20 patients (10 patients in each treatment group). Eight patients in the heparin group recovered completely and none died whereas only one patient in the placebo group recovered fully and three patients died. Treatment assessment was performed by using a specially developed CVST severity scale that contained the items headache, focal signs, seizures and level of consciousness. Using this scale, there was a significant difference between the two groups after 3 days in favour of the active treatment and the difference remained significant after 3 months. Three patients with previous ICH recovered completely and no new haemorrhages occurred in the heparin group whereas in the placebo group two patients with pre-treatment ICH died and two new haemorrhages were observed. There were no major extracranial haemorrhages in the heparin group and one probable case of fatal pulmonary embolism in the control group.

The outcome assessment was criticized (Stam *et al.*, 1991) because the CVST severity scale was not validated as a final outcome measure in neurological patients. Using death and dependency as clearly defined outcome parameters, the difference between the two groups would not be significant. Nevertheless, the study did show some benefit and even more important demonstrated the safety of AC in patients with CVST.

The second randomized trial compared body weight-adjusted subcutaneous low-molecular-weight heparin (LMWH) with placebo in 60 patients with CVST (de Bruijn *et al.*, 1999). A poor outcome – defined as death or Barthel index <15 – was observed after 3 weeks in 6 of the 30 patients treated with LMWH (20%) compared to 7 of the 29 controls (24%). After 3 months, three patients (10%) in the LMWH group and six patients (21%) in the placebo group had a poor outcome that corresponded to a non-significant absolute risk reduction of 11% in favour of the active treatment. No new ICH or secondary worsening of the 15 patients with pretreatment haemorrhage were observed in the LMWH group. There was one major extracerebral haemorrhage in the heparin group and one probable case of fatal pulmonary embolism in the control group.

A meta-analysis of these two trials showed that the use of AC led to an absolute risk reduction in death or dependency of 13% (confidence interval −30 to +3%) with a relative risk reduction of 54% (Stam *et al.*, 2001). Although this difference did not reach statistical significance both trials showed a consistent and clinically meaningful trend in favour of AC and demonstrated the safety of anticoagulant therapy. Thus, data from controlled trials favour the use of anticoagulation in patients with CVST because it may reduce the risk of a fatal outcome and severe disability and does not promote ICH at least in the small number of patients in the trials.In patients with isolated intracranial hypertension (and proven CVST) and threatened vision with the need for repeated lumbar punctures to remove cerebrospinal fluid (CSF) to obtain a normal closing pressure, AC should be withheld until 24 h after the last lumbar puncture.

It is unclear, whether treatment with full-dose intravenous heparin or subcutaneously applied LMWH is equally effective for CVST. A meta-analysis that compared the efficacy of fixed dose subcutaneous LMWH versus adjusted dose unfractionated heparin for extracerebral venous thromboembolism found LMWH to be superior and significantly less major bleeding complications

(van Dongen *et al.*, 2004). Further advantages include the route of administration that increases the mobility of patients and the lack of laboratory monitoring and subsequent dose adjustments. A possible advantage of dose-adjusted intravenous heparin therapy particularly in critically ill patients may be the fact that the activated partial thromboplastin time normalizes within 1–2 h after discontinuation of the infusion if complications occur or surgical intervention is necessary.

GOOD PRACTICE POINTS

Current evidence shows that patients with CVST without contraindications for anticoagulation should be treated either with body weight-adjusted subcutaneous LMWH (180 anti-factor Xa U/kg/24 h administered by two subcutaneous injections daily) or dose-adjusted intravenous heparin with an at least doubled activated partial thromboplastin time. Concomitant intracranial haemorrhage related to CVST is not a contraindication for heparin therapy. For the reasons mentioned above, LMWH should be preferred in uncomplicated CVST cases.

Thrombolysis

There is currently no evidence from randomized controlled trials about the efficacy and safety of either systemic or local thrombolytic therapy in patients with CVST. Thrombolytic therapy has the potential to provide faster restitution of venous outflow and positive effects of local thrombolytic treatment of CVST have increasingly been reported from uncontrolled series (Horowitz *et al.*, 1995; Kim and Suh, 1997; Frey *et al.*, 1999, Wasay *et al.*, 2001). Patients were either treated with heparin and urokinase or heparin and recombinant tissue plasminogen activator (rtPA) that may carry less bleeding complications due to its clot selectiveness and shorter half-life. Two uncontrolled studies that used rtPA in combination with dose-adjusted intravenous heparin included a total of 21 patients (Kim and Suh, 1997; Frey *et al.*, 1999). In the Korean study (Kim and Suh, 1997) that included nine patients, a mean total dose of 135 mg (range 50–300 mg) rtPA was used compared to 46 mg (range 23–128 mg) in the American study (Frey *et al.*, 1999) which included 12 patients. Both studies placed a microcatheter directly into the thrombus via the transfemoral vein and performed a bolus injection of rtPA followed by continuous infusion. In the two studies combined, rapid (mean time of 20 h in the Korean and 29 h in the American study) and complete recanalization was achieved in 15 of 21 patients and 14 of 21 patients showed a complete clinical recovery. However there were two extracerebral bleeding complications in the Korean study and two patients with pretreatment ICH in the American study worsened because of increased intracerebral bleeding that required surgery in one case. Thus, although recanalization was rapidly achieved, local thrombolysis may carry a higher risk of bleeding complications compared to AC particularly if pretreatment ICH is present (Bousser, 1999). Controlled trials that compare heparin therapy and local thrombolysis are lacking and there is no evidence that clinical outcome is better than with heparin alone. Currently, local thrombolysis may be a therapeutic option for patients at high risk for a poor outcome despite heparin therapy. The International Study on Cerebral Vein and Dural Sinus Thrombosis (ISCVT) recently identified coma on admission and thrombosis of the deep venous system apart from underlying causes as the most important predictors for a poor clinical outcome (Ferro *et al.*, 2004). More than 80% of the included 624 adult patients were treated with AC. Comatose patients may define a subgroup of patients with CVST who are at high risk of death despite AC (Mehraein *et al.*, 2003). Under this particular condition, the effect of AC may come too late to prevent irreversible brain damage and these patients may possibly benefit from thrombolytic therapy. A recently published systematic review on the use of thrombolytics in CVST suggested a possible benefit in such severe cases (Canhão *et al.*, 2003). Thirty-eight of the reported patients were comatose at the start of thrombolytic therapy, of whom six (13%) died. Intracranial haemorrhage occurred in 17% and was associated with clinical deterioration in 5% of cases. In comparison, a retrospective analysis found that 8 (53%) of the 15 patients with stupor or coma at the start of dose-adjusted intravenous heparin therapy died

(Mehraein *et al.*, 2003). In the ISCVT, 12 (38%) of the 31 comatose patients died (Ferro *et al.*, 2004). However, the results of the review were based on case reports and uncontrolled case series and there are yet no established clinical criteria for the use of thrombolytics in CVST. A controlled randomized trial is warranted to further study the efficacy and safety of thrombolysis in CVST. However, such a trial will be difficult to perform in single centres because of the small number of severe patients, particularly in countries and centres with early diagnosis of CVST. Only an international multicentre trial may be able to clarify the role of thrombolysis in the treatment of CVST.

GOOD PRACTICE POINTS

There is insufficient evidence to support the use of either systemic or local thrombolysis in patients with CVST. If patients deteriorate despite adequate anticoagulation and other causes of deterioration have been ruled out, thrombolysis may be a therapeutic option in selected cases, possibly in those without intracranial haemorrhage. The optimal substance (urokinase or rtPA), dosage, route (systemic or local), or method of administration repeated bolus or bolus plus infusion) are not known.

Oral anticoagulation

Controlled data about the benefit and optimal duration of oral AC in patients with CVST are not available but most authors recommend continued anticoagulation after the acute phase. In the ISCVT median time on oral AC after discharge was 7.7 months (Ferro *et al.*, 2004). A recently published MRI follow-up study of 33 patients suggested that recanalization occurs within the first 4 months after CVST irrespective of further AC. These data may provide some guidance on the duration of AC but whether incomplete or absent recanalization increases the risk of recurrence is not known. No relapses occurred in two follow-up studies that showed incomplete or no recanalization in more than 40% of the patients (Strupp *et al.*, 2002; Baumgartner *et al.*, 2003).

Analogous to patients with extracerebral venous thrombosis, oral AC with a target INR of 2.0–3.0

may be given for 3 months if CVST was secondary to a transient (reversible) risk factor and for 6–12 months if it was idiopathic (Büller et al., 2004). However, the risk of recurrence of CVST may be lower than that of extracerebral venous thrombosis. In the ISCVT, 2.2% of all patients had a recurrent sinus thrombosis with a median follow-up of 16 months (Ferro et al., 2004) and prolonged AC may expose some patients to an unnecessary bleeding risk although there was also a risk of 4.3% for other thrombotic events during follow-up including 2.5% of pelvic or limb venous thrombosis and 0.5% of pulmonary embolism.

Oral AC is also recommended for 6–12 months in patients with extracerebral venous thrombosis and a 'mild' hereditary thrombophilia such as protein C and S deficiency, heterozygous factor V Leiden or prothrombin G20210A mutations. Long-term treatment should be considered for patients with a 'severe' hereditary thrombophilia that carries a high risk of recurrence, such as antithrombin deficiency, homozygous factor V Leiden mutation, or two or more thrombophilic conditions. Indefinite AC is also recommended in patients with two or more episodes of idiopathic objectively documented extracerebral venous thrombosis (Büller et al., 2004). Thus, in the absence of controlled data the decision on the duration of anticoagulant therapy must be based on individual hereditary and precipitating factors as well as on the potential bleeding risks of long-term AC. Regular follow-up visits should be performed after termination of AC and patients should be informed about early signs (headache) indicating a possible relapse.

GOOD PRACTICE POINTS

There are insufficient data about the optimal duration of oral anticoagulation in patients with CVST. Analogous to patients with a first episode of extracerebral venous thrombosis, oral AC may be given for 3 months if CVST was secondary to a transient risk factor, for 6–12 months in patients with idiopathic CVST and in those with 'mild' hereditary thrombophilia. Indefinite AC should be considered in patients with two or more episodes of CVST and in those with one episode of CVST and 'severe' hereditary thrombophilia.

Symptomatic treatment

Symptomatic therapy includes the use of antiepileptic drugs, management of increased intracranial pressure, the control of psychomotor agitation and analgesic treatment.

Control of seizures

There are no data regarding the effectiveness of a prophylactic use of antiepileptic drugs (AED) in patients with CVST. Whereas some authors recommend prophylactic treatment (Einhäupl and Masuhr, 1994) because of the high incidence of seizures (and series of seizures or even status epilepticus) and their possible detrimental effects on the metabolic situation during the acute phase of the disease, others restrict the use of anticonvulsants to patients with seizures (Ameri and Bousser, 1992). A recently published study identified focal sensory deficits and the presence of focal oedema or ischaemic/haemorrhagic infarcts on admission CCT/MRI as significant predictors of early symptomatic seizures (Ferro et al., 2003). Although data are insufficient to give recommendations, these findings suggest that prophylactic treatment with AED may be a therapeutic option for those patients whereas it is not warranted when there are no focal neurological deficits and no focal parenchymal lesions on brain scan (e.g. patients with isolated intracranial hypertension). If no antiepileptic treatment has been performed before the first seizure occurs, effective concentrations of AEDs should be achieved rapidly because series of seizures frequently occur in patients with CVST.

The risk of residual epilepsy after CVST is low compared to the high rate of patients with early seizures. Reported incidences range from 5–10.6% (Preter et al., 1996; Ferro et al., 2003,2004). In the Portuguese series (Ferro et al., 2003), all late seizures occurred within the first year. A haemorrhagic lesion in the acute brain scan was the strongest predictor of post-acute seizures. In all series together, late seizures were more common in patients with early symptomatic seizures than in those patients with none. Thus, prolonged treatment with AED for one year may be reasonable for patients with early seizures and haemorrhagic lesions on admission brain scan whereas in patients without these risk factors AED therapy may be tapered off gradually after the acute stage.

GOOD PRACTICE POINTS

Prophylactic antiepileptic therapy may be a therapeutic option in patients with focal neurological deficits and focal parenchymal lesions on admission CT/MRI. The optimal duration of treatment for patients with seizures is unclear.

Treatment of elevated intracranial pressure

Although brain swelling is observed in about 50% of all patients with CVST on CCT, minor brain oedema needs no other treatment than AC which improves the venous outflow sufficiently to reduce intracranial pressure in most patients (Ameri and Bousser, 1992; Einhäupl and Masuhr, 1994). In patients with isolated intracranial hypertension and threatened vision, a lumbar puncture with sufficient cerebrospinal fluid (CSF) removal to obtain a normal closing pressure should be performed before starting AC 24 h after the puncture. There are no controlled data but acetazolamide may be considered in patients with persistent papilloedema. In a few patients vision continues to deteriorate despite repeated lumbar punctures and/or acetazolamide. In these cases shunting procedures (lumboperitoneal, ventriculoperitoneal shunts or optic nerve fenestration) should be considered.

Antioedema treatment is necessary in only 20% of patients and should be carried out according to general principles of therapy of raised intracranial pressure (head elevation at about 30 degrees, hyperventilation with a target $PaCO_2$ pressure of 30–35 mmHg, intravenous application of osmotic diuretics). However one should keep in mind, that osmotic substances might be harmful in venous outflow obstruction, as they are not as quickly eliminated from the intracerebral circulation as in other conditions. The use of tris-hydroxy-methly-aminomethane (THAM) which decreases

intracranial pressure after intravenous administration via an alkalotic vasoconstriction may be a therapy option in ventilated patients. Restricted volume intake for treatment of brain oedema must be avoided, as these measures can cause an additional deterioration of blood viscosity. Steroids can not be generally recommended for treatment of elevated intracranial pressure, as their efficacy is unproven and they may be harmful through their promotion of the thrombotic process. Most recently, no benefit of steroids was found in a case-control study of the ISCVT (Canhão et al., 2004).

In severe cases with threatening transtentorial brain herniation due to a unilateral large haemorrhagic infarct, decompressive surgery may be the only way to save the patient's life. Local thrombolysis seems no treatment option in such cases because of the incalculable risk of further ICH extension with an additional detrimental effect on intracranial pressure. Stefini and co-workers (Stefini et al., 1999) reported three patients with fixed dilated pupils due to transtentorial herniation who underwent decompressive surgery two of whom recovered with only minor neurological sequelae. The haemorrhagic infarct should not be removed because neuronal damage is often less pronounced in CVST-related haemorrhage explaining the possible reversibility of even severe clinical symptoms (Villringer et al., 1994).

GOOD PRACTICE POINTS

In patients with isolated intracranial hypertension and threatened vision possible therapeutic measures may include one or more lumbar punctures, acetazolamide and incidentally CSF-shunting procedures. There are no controlled data about the risks and benefits of certain therapeutic measures (e.g. steroids, decompressive surgery) to reduce an elevated intracranial pressure (with brain displacement) in patients with CVST. Antioedema treatment should be carried out according to general principles of therapy of raised intracranial pressure. In a very small subgroup of patients who deteriorate especially in the presence of large intracerebral haemorrhages, decompressive craniectomy might

continued

be an alternative treatment option in the future. At present this therapy needs further investigation and should be regarded as experimental.

Conflicts of interest

K. Einhäupl was the principal investigator of the treatment trial with unfractionated heparin (Einhäupl et al., 1991). J. Stam and S.T.F.M. de Bruijn were principal investigators of the CVST Study Group Trial (De Bruijn SFTM et al., 1999).

References

Ameri A, Bousser MG (1992). Cerebral venous thrombosis. *Neurol Clin* **10**:87–111.

Baumgartner RW, Studer A, Arnold M, Georgiadis D (2003). Recanalisation of cerebral venous thrombosis. *J Neurol Neurosurg Psychiatry* **74**:459–461.

Bousser MG, Chiras J, Bories J, Castaigne P (1985). Cerebral venous thrombosis - a review of 38 cases. *Stroke* **16**:199–213.

Bousser MG (1999). Cerebral venous thrombosis. Nothing, heparin, or local thrombolysis? *Stroke* **30**:481–483.

Brainin M, Barnes M, Baron J-C, Gilhus NE, Hughes R, Selmaj K, Waldemar G (2004). Guidance for the preparation of neurological management guidelines by EFNS scientific task forces – revised recommendations 2004. *Eur J Neurol* **11**:577–581.

Büller HR, Agnelli G, Hull RH, Hyers TM, Prins MH, Raskob GE (2004). Antithrombotic therapy for venous thromboembolic disease. The seventh ACCP conference on antithrombotic and thrombolytic therapy. *Chest* **126**:401S–428S.

Canhão P, Falcão F, Ferro JM (2003). Thrombolytics for cerebral sinus thrombosis. A systematic review. *Cerebrovasc Dis* **15**:159–166.

Canhão P, Cortesão A, Cabral M, Ferro J, Stam J, Bousser MG, Barinagarrementeria F, for the ISCVT Investigators (2004). Are steroids useful for the treatment of cerebral venous thrombosis ? ISCVT results. *Cerebrovasc Dis* **17(Suppl 5)**:16.

Cantu C, Barrinagarrimenteria F (1993) Cerebral Venous thrombosis associated with pregnancy and puerperium.Review of 67 cases. *Stroke* **24**:1880–1884.

De Bruijn SFTM, Stam J, Kapelle LJ for the Cerebral Venous Sinus Thrombosis Study Group (1996). Thunderclap headache as first symptom of cerebral venous sinus thrombosis. *Lancet* **348**:1623–1625.

De Bruijn SFTM, Stam J for the Cerebral Venous Sinus Thrombosis Study Group (1999). Randomized, placebo-controlled trial of anticoagulant treatment with low-molecular-weight heparin for cerebral sinus thrombosis. *Stroke* **30**:484–488.

De Bruijn SFTM, de Haan RJ, Stam J for the Cerebral Venous Sinus Thrombosis Study Group (2001). Clinical features and prognostic factors of cerebral venous and sinus thrombosis in a prospective series of 59 patients. *J Neurol Neurosurg Psychiatry* **70**:105–108.

deVeber G, Andrew M, Adams C, for the Canadian Pediatric Ischemic Stroke Study Group (2001). Cerebral sinovenous thrombosis in children. *N Engl J Med* **345**:417–423.

Einhäupl KM, Villringer A, Meister W, Mehraein S, Garner C, Pellkofer M, Haberl RL, Pfister HW, Schmiedek P (1991). Heparin treatment in sinus venous thrombosis. *Lancet* **338**:597–600.

Einhäupl KM, Villringer A, Haberl RL, Pfister W, Deckert M, Steinhoff H, Schmiedek P (1990) Clinical spectrum of sinus venous thrombosis. In: Einhäupl K, Kempski O, Baethmann A (eds) Cerebral sinus thrombosis. Experimental and clinical aspects. Plenum Press, New York, pp 149–155.

Einhäupl KM, Masuhr F (1994). Cerebral venous and sinus thrombosis - an update. *Eur J Neurol* **1**:109–126.

Ferro JM, Correia M, Rosas MJ, Pinto AN, Neves G for the Cerebral Venous Thrombosis Portuguese Collaborative Study Group (2003). Seizures in cerebral vein and dural sinus thrombosis. *Cerebrovasc Dis* **15**:78–83.

Ferro JM, Canhão P, Stam J, Bousser MG, Barinagarrementeria F, for the ISCVT Investigators (2004) Prognosis of cerebral vein and dural sinus thrombosis. Results of the International Study on Cerebral Vein and Dural Sinus Thrombosis (ISCVT). *Stroke* **35**:664–670.

Frey IL, Muro GJ, McDougall CG, Dean BL, Jahnke HK (1999). Cerebral venous thrombosis. Combined intrathrombus rtPA and intravenous heparin. *Stroke* **30**:489–494.

Horowitz M, Purdy P, Unwin H, Carstens G, Greenlee R, Hise J, Kopitnik T, Batjer H, Rollins N, Samson D (1995). Treatment of dural sinus thrombosis using selective catheterisation and urokinase. *Ann Neurol* **38**:58–67.

Kim SY, Suh JH (1997). Direct endovascular thrombolytic therapy for dural sinus thrombosis: infusion of alteplase. *Am J Neuroradiol* **18**:639–645.

Masuhr F, Mehraein S, Einhäupl K (2004). Cerebral venous and sinus thrombosis. *J Neurol* **251**:11–23.

Mehraein S, Schmidtke K, Villringer A, Valdueza JM, Masuhr F (2003). Heparin treatment in cerebral sinus and venous thrombosis: patients at risk of fatal outcome. *Cerebrovasc Dis* **15**:17–21.

Preter M, Tzourio C, Ameri A, Bousser MG (1996). Long-term prognosis in cerebral venous thrombosis – Follow-up of 77 patients. *Stroke* **27**:243–246.

Stam J, Lensing AWA, Vermeulen M, Tijssen JGP (1991). Heparin treatment for cerebral venous and sinus thrombosis. *Lancet* **338**:1154.

Stam J, de Bruijn SFTM, deVeber G (2001). Anticoagulation for cerebral sinus thrombosis. The Cochrane Database of Systematic Reviews Issue 4. Art. No.: CD002005.

Stefini R, Latronico N, Cornali C, Rasulo F, Bollati A (1999). Emergent decompressive craniectomy in patients with fixed dilated pupils due to cerebral venous and dural sinus thrombosis: report of three cases. *Neurosurgery* **45**:626–629.

Strupp M, Covi M, Seelos K, Dichgans M, Brandt T (2002). Cerebral venous thrombosis: correlation between recanalization and clinical outcome – a long-term follow-up of 40 patients. *J Neurol* **249**:1123–1124.

Van Dongen CJJ, van den Belt AGM, Prins MH, Lensing AWA (2004). Fixed dose subcutaneous low molecular weight heparins versus adjusted dose unfractionated heparin for venous thromboembolism. The Cochrane Database of Systematic Reviews Issue 4. Art. No.: CD001100.

Villringer A, Mehraein S, Einhäupl KM (1994). Pathophysiological aspects of cerebral sinus venous thrombosis. *J Neuroradiol* **21**:72–80.

Wasay M, Bakshi R, Kojan S, Bobustuc G, Dubey N, Unwin DH (2001). Nonrandomized comparison of local urokinase thrombolysis versus systemic heparin anticoagulation for superior sagittal sinus thrombosis. *Stroke* **32**:2310–2317.

CHAPTER 38

Cerebral vasculitis

N.J. Scolding,[a] H. Wilson,[b] R. Hohlfeld,[c]
C. Polman,[d] I. Leite,[e] N.E. Gilhus[f]

Abstract

Background Cerebral vasculitis is rare, difficult to diagnose and without firm evidence for best clinical practice.

Objectives To examine ongoing clinical practice in Europe and generate robust practical guidelines for diagnosis and treatment.

Methods Clinical information was collected from experts in 15 European countries, and a thorough Medline search was undertaken.

The Task Force agreed on Good Practice Points for diagnosis and therapy:

- A brain biopsy is recommended for diagnostic purposes when cerebral vasculitis is still suspected after a thorough examination.
- Cerebral angiography has limited sensitivity and specificity for cerebral vasculitis.
- Induction treatment should be given using high-dose corticosteroids and cyclophosphamide.
- Long-time maintenance treatment should be given using low-dose corticosteroids and azathioprine.

Multicentre prospective studies are needed both for diagnostic and treatment purposes.

Introduction

Cerebral vasculitis is an uncommon disorder that offers unusual problems for the neurologist. It is notoriously difficult to recognise, producing a wide range of possible neurological symptoms and signs and no typical or characteristic features (Moore and Fauci, 1981; Moore, 1998; Scolding, 1999). Potential clinical patterns that might facilitate recognition have been proposed (Scolding *et al.*, 1997), but are yet to be tested prospectively on large numbers of patients, and their value in consequence remains to be substantiated.

Suspicion of the disorder having been entertained, confirmation or exclusion of cerebral vasculitis presents a second serious – and in some

[a]Institute of Clinical Neurosciences, Department of Neurology, University of Bristol, Frenchay Hospital, Bristol, United Kingdom; [b]Dept of Neurology, Royal Free Hospital, Pond Street, London, UK; [c]Klinikum Grosshadern, Munich, Germany; [d]Free University Hospital, MB Amsterdam, Netherlands; [e]Department of Neurology, Hospital Geral Santo Antonio, Portugal; [f]Department of Neurology, Haukeland University Hospital, Bergen, Norway.

cases, quite insurmountable – set of problems. There are no serological or other blood or spinal fluid laboratory tests of any sensitivity or specificity; imaging by CT or MRI is likewise lacking in sensitivity; angiography is of questionable use (Calabrese and Mallek, 1988; Hankey, 1991; Greenan *et al.*, 1992; Vollmer *et al.*, 1993; Alhalabi and Moore, 1994; Stone *et al.*, 1994; Scolding *et al.*, 1997). Finally, whilst intuitively this is a disorder most neurologists would regard as eminently treatable, there are no therapeutic trials to provide an evidence base for this assumption.

This combination of difficulties in recognition and in diagnosis, in a disorder that is serious and indeed not uncommonly fatal, and yet (probably) highly treatable, emphasises the importance of attempting to address the clinical problem of cerebral vasculitis (Joseph and Scolding, 2002). It is, however, an uncommon disorder – there are no epidemiological data, but an estimate has been hazarded of an incidence of 1–2 million per year – creating additional difficulties; even two or three neurological centres collaborating are unlikely to accumulate sufficient numbers of patients within a workable time frame for useful studies.

Methods

The European Federation of Neurological Societies (EFNS) Scientist Panel on Neuroimmunology considered that a European collaborative cohort might offer a powerful means of beginning to address the problems outlined above. A Task Force on Cerebral Vasculitis was established to improve the recognition, diagnosis and management of cerebral vasculitis throughout Europe. This will be achieved by providing guidelines whose confirmation will ultimately depend on the establishment of a sound evidence base. A European-wide survey of current clinical practice was included.

A simple 10-point questionnaire covering various aspects of the diagnosis and management of cerebral vasculitis was sent to 51 expert neurologists in 26 European countries. Replies were received from 29 (57%) experts, from 15 countries.

Statements about diagnosis and treatment were discussed among the Task Force members. Evidence was classified according to the EFNS

guidelines (Brainin *et al.*, 2004). As very few relevant controlled studies exist on the topic, the recommendations given should be regarded as Good Practice Points (Brainin *et al.*, 2004), where advice is given on the basis of consensus in our group and available evidence.

Results of survey

The cumulative number of patients given the diagnosis of cerebral vasculitis by the 29 responding expert neurologists is approximately 140 per year, a mean of 4.8 cases per neurologist per year.

Dependence on cerebral angiography varied widely, but 11of 29 neurologists (38%) based this diagnosis on angiography in over 75% of cases; a mean of 50% of patients throughout Europe had been diagnosed as having cerebral vasculitis based on angiography. Only three neurologists depended on cerebral biopsy in 80% or more of cases; conversely 12 of 25 neurologists (48%) based diagnosis on biopsy in more than 20% of cases. Most neurologists committed between 0 and 5 patients to biopsy per year, a mean of 2.3 biopsies per year. Only 13 of 29 neurologists (45%) recommended biopsy if there was an identifiable lesion. Of the remainder, most used non-dominant frontal or temporal open biopsy, usually ensuring that parenchymal and meningeal tissue were included.

Eighty per cent of the patients with the diagnosis of cerebral vasculitis received steroids (orally or intravenously) alone as 'first line treatment', and cyclophosphamide only if steroids failed. Most of the remaining neurologists used cyclophosphamide as first line therapy. Fourteen used cyclophosphamide as second line treatment, others using azathioprine (3), intravenous immunoglobulin (2), methotrexate (1), and other 'potent immunosuppressive' agents (2). Only four respondents treated patients with potent immunosuppressive agents 'only if biopsy-proven', 84% administering such treatment without tissue confirmation of the diagnosis. All acknowledged the difficulties of assessing the therapeutic response - variably relying on clinical imaging, spinal fluid and blood tests, particularly erythrocyte sedimentation rate (ESR) and C-reactive protein levels.

All 29 neurologists were interested in participating in further collaborative European research.

Conclusions and Discussion

Even European neurologists with particular interest in cerebral vasculitis see only a handful of cases per year. Nevertheless, the cumulative experience of some 140 cases per year emphasises the potential power of the pooled response. A large prospective study would offer a number of valuable opportunities.

First, an analysis of the clinical features may provide means of improving the recognition of cerebral vasculitis. Three clinical patterns have been previously suggested (Scolding *et al.*, 1997). First, patients may present with acute, sub-acute or recurrent encephalopathy; the second is presentation with features of a focal, space-occupying lesion. Third, patients may exhibit a clinical picture that in many ways resembles multiple sclerosis – a relapsing, remitting course, often including brain stem episodes and optic neuropathy, and often with multifocal white matter lesions on MRI scanning and oligoclonal bands on cerebrospinal fluid (CSF) analysis (table 38.1). However, these patterns were suggested from an analysis of only 10–12 cases, and though reference to retrospective case series suggests the patterns might accommodate virtually all cases of cerebral vasculitis, their true value remains to be proven by large prospective studies. Whether these or indeed better patterns might usefully aid recognition of cerebral vasculitis cannot be determined on the basis of small studies on pooled retrospective series with the case-selection biases they carry.

The value of a number of laboratory or imaging investigative procedures similarly requires a prospective study. Specifically, the negative predictive power of tests such as a normal ESR, or normal C-reactive protein (Scolding *et al.*, 1997), or normal spinal fluid analysis (Calabrese and Mallek, 1988; Hankey, 1991; Scolding *et al.*, 1997), together with the positive predictive power of these tests – or combinations of various test results with particular clinical and/or imaging features – all these also require prospective studies including relatively large numbers of patients.

There was particular variation in relation to the diagnostic weight given to cerebral angiography. In many instances, there was radiological uncertainty concerning the distinction between 'vasculopathy' and 'vasculitis'. Angiography is a test limited in both sensitivity and specificity in the diagnosis of cerebral vasculitis: retrospective series suggest a sensitivity of only 24–33% (Hankey, 1991; Vollmer *et al.*, 1993; Calabrese and Mallek, 1988; Koo and Massey, 1988; Alrawi *et al.*, 1999), with a specificity of a similar order – a number of inflammatory, metabolic, malignant or other vasculopathies can accurately mimic angiitis.

There was a corresponding limited reliance on brain biopsy for diagnosis. In a few instances this was explained by local factors, such as difficulties in access to neurosurgical intervention. This test too is, of course, limited in sensitivity, and necessarily entails some iatrogenic risk (Barza and Pauker, 1980; Chu *et al.*, 1998). However, a recent retrospective study of some 61 patients biopsied for suspected cerebral vasculitis has usefully illuminated this topic (Alrawi *et al.*, 1999). No patient suffered any significant morbidity as a result of the procedure. Thirty-six per cent of the patients were confirmed as having cerebral vasculitis, but no less usefully and importantly, 39% biopsies showed an alternative, unsuspected diagnosis – lymphoma

Table 38.1 Cerebral vasculitis: suggested clinical patterns of presentation that might facilitate recognition (Scolding *et al.*, 1997).

- Acute or sub-acute encephalopathy, with headache with an acute confusional state, progressing to drowsiness and coma.
- Intracranial mass lesion - with headache, drowsiness, focal signs and (often) raised intracranial pressure.
- Superficially resembling atypical multiple sclerosis (*MS-plus*) in phenotype - with a relapsing-remitting course, and features such as optic neuropathy and brain stem episodes, but also accompanied by other features less common in multiple sclerosis: seizures, severe and persisting headaches, encephalopathic episodes, or stroke-like episodes.

(six cases), multiple sclerosis (two cases), or infection (seven cases, including toxoplasmosis, herpes, and also two cases of cerebral abscess. Biopsy failed to yield a clear diagnosis in 25% of patients in this study, though even here, biopsy might arguably not be described as 'non-contributory', at least decreasing the likelihood of the alternative diagnoses mentioned above.

This valuable retrospective study also provided some evidence first that biopsy of normal-appearing tissue was no less likely to yield diagnostic information than biopsy targeted upon discrete lesions (Alrawi *et al.*, 1999). The numbers (20 biopsies of normal appearing tissue, 40 of radiologically apparent lesions) were not very large and again a more substantial prospective study would be useful.

What lessons may be learnt, and does this preliminary and rather informal survey yield any provisional recommendations? First, the results confirm the relative uncommonness of the disorder, but emphasise the potential strength of a collaborative effort, in which, additionally, there emerged considerable enthusiasm. According to current practice, 140 patients are given this diagnosis annually by the 29 responding neurologists, with perhaps 20–40 of these having biopsy confirmation. Expanding the collaborating neurologist pool – and several regional specialists have, since this survey, expressed interest in joining – would yet further increase the power of any prospective study of both diagnostic approaches and of therapy.

Second, the wide variation in current clinical practice is of interest. The very limited sensitivity and specificity of cerebral angiography has arguably been underemphasised in the past; some series of cerebral vasculitis patients have

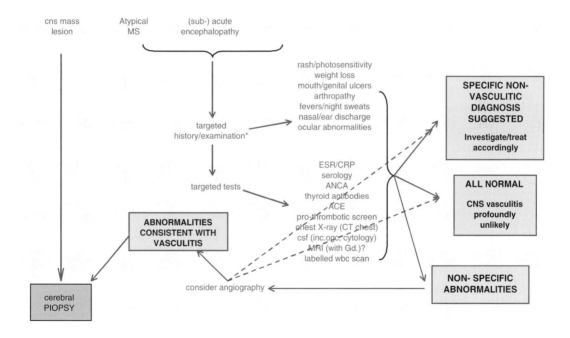

Figure 38.1. A diagnostic approach to suspected cerebral vasculitis

indeed rested wholly upon this investigation for diagnosis. There has also perhaps been historically an overemphasis on the value of steroids. While there have been no prospective placebo-controlled trials of immunosuppressive treatment in cerebral vasculitis (or indeed in the systemic vasculitides), large retrospective series of patients with systemic Wegener's granulomatosis, or with microscopic polyangiitis provide clear support for their use (Hoffman *et al.*, 1990, 1992; Adu *et al.*, 1997; Scolding, 2000). There is some merit in the argument that the absence of tissue confirmation properly directs neurologists away from prescribing cyclophosphamide, and towards steroids, but responding neurologists in this survey indicated that it was not this factor that inhibited their use of potent immunosuppressives; only 3 of 29 neurologists used cyclophosphamide as part of their first line therapeutic regimen.

Whether cyclophosphamide is best given by intravenous pulses or continuous oral therapy is not established (Cupps, 1990; Adu *et al.*, 1997), and this question could of course usefully be incorporated into a large prospective study. Most regimes recommend an induction course of between 10 and 16 g cumulative dose; (retrospective) studies of patients with systemic vasculitis and other inflammatory disorders suggest that bladder carcinoma, perhaps the most notorious and serious toxic effect of cyclophosphamide, may be restricted very largely to patients who have received cumulative dose in excess of 100 g (Talar *et al.*, 1996).

From a practical perspective, we now feel able to propose the diagnostic approach outlined below (figure 38.1), and a pragmatic approach to therapy (Savage *et al.*, 1997; Jayne *et al.*, 2003) when a tissue diagnosis of cerebral vasculitis has been confirmed (table 38.2). These represent, in our view, reasonable syntheses emerging from the currently available evidence, but this evidence is not adequate for formal recommendations (Joseph and Scolding, 2002; Brainin *et al.*, 2004). We suggest therefore that a further, prospective pan-European study of cerebral vasculitis is needed, and could carry sufficient power to confirm or improve this management approach: it is also likely to yield valuable insights into the recognition, diagnosis

Table 38.2 Cerebral vasculitis: a common treatment regime.

Induction Regime (3 months)	Maintenance Regime (continued for a further 10 months)
High dose steroids Intravenous methyl prednisolone, 1 g/day for 3 days	Alternate day steroids 10–20 mg prednisolone
Plus Oral* cyclophosphamide 2.0 mg/kg§ (max 200 mg/day)	Plus Azathioprine[a] (2 mg/kg/day) instead of cyclophos
Then Oral prednisolone 60 mg/day (after intravenous methyl prednisolone), decreasing at weekly intervals by 10 mg increments to 10 mg/day if possible	

[a]Methotrexate (10–25 mg once weekly) is an alternative to azathioprine.

and treatment of this difficult, unusual and often very serious neurological disorder.

References

Adu D, Pall A, Luqmani RA, Richards NT, Howie AJ, Emery P, Michael J, Savage CO Bacon PA (1997). Controlled trial of pulse versus continuous prednisolone and cyclophosphamide in the treatment of systemic vasculitis. *QJM* **90**:401–409.

Alhalabi M, Moore PM (1994). Serial angiography in isolated angiitis of the central nervous system. *Neurology* **44**:1221–1226.

Alrawi A, Trobe J, Blaivas M, Musch DC (1999). Brain biopsy in primary angiitis of the central nervous system. *Neurology* **53**:858–860.

Barza M, Pauker SG (1980). The decision to biopsy, treat, or wait in suspected herpes encephalitis. *Ann Intern Med* **92**:641–649.

Brainin M, Barnes M, Baron JC, Gilhus NE, Hughes R, Selmaj K, Waldemar G (2004). Guidance for the preparation of neurological management guidelines by EFNS scientific task forces–revised recommendations 2004. *Eur J Neurol* **11**:577–581.

Calabrese LH, Mallek JA (1988). Primary angiitis of the central nervous system. Report of 8 new cases, review of the literature, and proposal for diagnostic criteria. *Medicine* **67:**20–39.

Chu CT, Gray L, Goldstein LB, Hulette CM (1998). Diagnosis of intracranial vasculitis: a multi-disciplinary approach. *J Neuropathol Exp Neurol* **57:**30–38.

Cupps TR (1990). Cyclophosphamide: to pulse or not to pulse? [editorial; comment]. *Am J Med* **89:**399–402.

Greenan TJ, Grossman RI, Goldberg HI (1992). Cerebral vasculitis: MR imaging and angiographic correlation. *Radiology* **182:**65–72.

Hankey G (1991). Isolated angiitis/angiopathy of the CNS. Prospective diagnostic and therapeutic experience. *Cerebrovasc Dis* **1:**2–15.

Hoffman GS, Leavitt RY, Fleisher TA, Minor JR, Fauci AS (1990). Treatment of Wegener's granulomatosis with intermittent high-dose intravenous cyclophosphamide. *Am J Med* **89:**403–410.

Hoffman GS, Kerr GS, Leavitt RY, Hallahan CW, Lebovics RS, Travis WD, Rottem M, Fauci AS (1992). Wegener granulomatosis: an analysis of 158 patients. *Ann Intern Med* **116:**488–498.

Jayne D, Rasmussen N, Andrassy K, Bacon P, Tervaert JW, Dadoniene J, Ekstrand A, Gaskin G, Gregorini G, De GK, Gross W, Hagen EC, Mirapeix E, Pettersson E, Siegert C, Sinico A, Tesar V, Westman K, Pusey C (2003). A randomized trial of maintenance therapy for vasculitis associated with antineutrophil cytoplasmic autoantibodies. *N Engl J Med* **349:**36–44.

Joseph FG, Scolding NJ (2002). Cerebral vasculitis – a practical approach. *Pract Neurol* **2:**80–93.

Koo EH, Massey EW (1988). Granulomatous angiitis of the central nervous system: Protean manifestations and response to treatment. *J Neurol Neurosur Psych* **51:**1126–1133.

Moore PM (1998). Central nervous system vasculitis. *Curr Opin Neurol* **11:**241–246.

Moore PM, Fauci AS (1981). Neurologic manifestations of systemic vasculitis. A retrospective and prospective study of the clinicopathologic features and responses to therapy in 25 patients. *Am J Med* **71:**517–524.

Savage CO, Harper L, Adu D (1997). Primary systemic vasculitis. *Lancet* **349:**553–558.

Scolding NJ (1999). Cerebral vasculitis, in *Immunological and Inflammatory Diseases of the Central Nervous System* (Scolding NJ, ed), pp. 210–258. Butterworth-Heinemann, Oxford.

Scolding NJ (2000). Systemic inflammatory diseases and the nervous system, in *New Treatments in Neurology* (Scolding NJ, ed), pp. in. Butterworth Heinemann, Oxford.

Scolding NJ, Jayne DR, Zajicek JP, Meyer PAR, Wraight EP, Lockwood CM (1997). The syndrome of cerebral vasculitis: recognition, diagnosis and management. *Q J Med* **90:**61–73.

Stone JH, Pomper MG, Roubenoff R, Miller TJ, Hellmann DB (1994). Sensitivities of noninvasive tests for central nervous system vasculitis: a comparison of lumbar puncture, computed tomography, and magnetic resonance imaging. *J Rheumat* **21:**1277–1282.

Talar WC, Hijazi YM, Walther MM, Linehan WM, Hallahan CW, Lubensky I, Kerr GS, Hoffman GS, Fauci AS, Sneller MC (1996). Cyclophosphamide-induced cystitis and bladder cancer in patients with Wegener granulomatosis. *Ann Intern Med* **124:**477–484.

Vollmer TL, Guarnaccia J, Harrington W, Pacia SV, Petroff OAC (1993). Idiopathic granulomatous angiitis of the central nervous system: diagnostic challenges. *Arch Neurol* **50:**925–930.

Neurological problems in liver transplantation

M. Guarino,[a] J. Benito-Leon,[b] J. Decruyenaere,[c]
E. Schmutzhard,[d] K. Weissenborn,[e] A. Stracciari[a]

Abstract

Background Neurological impairment after orthotopic liver transplantation (OLT) is common and represents a major source of morbidity and mortality. The diagnosis and management of neurological problems occurring after OLT are difficult and evidence-based guidelines for this task are currently lacking.

Methods A Task Force was set up under the auspices of the European Federation of Neurological Societies to devise guidelines to prevent and manage neurological problems in OLT. We selected six major neurological problems and approached them combining an evidence-based scientific literature analysis with a search for consensus by means of a Delphi process.

Results Search results were translated into a series of recommendations constituting a basis for better care of patients with neurological complications after OLT.

Background and objectives

Neurological problems are reported in 13–47% of patients after orthotopic liver transplantation (OLT) (Stracciari and Guarino, 2001). Most neurological complications occur early after surgery and increase the risk of mortality (Pujol *et al.*, 1994; Guarino *et al.*, 1996). The spectrum of clinical presentations is wide and the aetiology heterogeneous. Management is empirical and currently based mainly on practical experience, lacking evidence derived from scientific literature. Our study aimed to devise a uniform management protocol across different centres involved in the neurological care of liver transplanted patients. We considered some topics highly relevant in clinical practice: immunosuppression neurotoxicity, seizures, central pontine myelinolysis, cerebrovascular disorders, neuromuscular disorders and cerebral infections. Our guidelines mainly address the prevention, diagnosis and management of problems emerging in the first 6 months after surgery.

Search strategy

Assessment of reliable scientific literature and search of consensus by means of a Delphi process (Jones and Hunter, 1995) were applied. Literature

[a]Neurology Unit, S. Orsola-Malpighi University Hospital, Bologna, Italy; [b]Department of Neurology, Móstoles General Hospital, Móstoles, Madrid, Spain;

European Journal of Neurology 2006, 13:2–9

[c]Department of Intensive Care Medicine, Ghent University Hospital, Ghent, Belgium; [d]Department of Neurology, Innsbruck Medical University, Innsbruck, Austria; [e]Department of Neurology, Hannover University Hospital, Hannover, Germany.

on selected topics was systematically reviewed by two of us (MG, AS) through the MEDLINE database of the National Library of Medicine from 1969, Cochrane Library, existing guidelines (National Clinical Clearinghouse, Scottish Intercollegiate Guidelines Network, National Institute of Clinical Excellence) and textbooks. On the basis of literature analysis and the suggestions of panel members, a large number of statements were identified and submitted to the participants, who had to rank their agreement using a scoring system of 0–9 points, where 0–3 was disagreement, 4–6 uncertain, 7–9 agreement. Agreement had to be obtained with a maximum of three rounds. An 80% agreement level among members was set as acceptable. The material obtained by the Delphi process was integrated and summarized in graded recommendations. The literature was surveyed continuously up to December 2004 to update the recommendations that were approved by all members.

Grading of recommendations

The literature analysis is presented giving the class of evidence (I–IV), according to European Federation of Neurological Societies (EFNS) guidelines (Brainin *et al.*, 2004).

The recommendation section includes statements classified in levels A–C derived from classes I–III of evidence according to EFNS guidelines when feasible. For those clinical areas exhibiting Class IV scientific evidence, recommendations were based on the agreement obtained by the Delphi process and indicated in the text as Good Practice Points (GPP).

Results

Immunosuppression neurotoxicity

The most commonly used immunosuppressants in OLT are the calcineurin inhibitors cyclosporine (CS) and tacrolimus (FK506). Mycophenolate mofetil and sirolimus have recently been introduced. Corticosteroids, OKT3 and antithymocyte globulin complete the immunosuppressive regimen. Neurotoxicity is mainly associated with CS and FK506, amounting to 10–30% for CS (Guarino *et al.*, 1999) and up to 32% for FK506

(Wijdicks *et al.*, 1994). Sirolimus and mycophenolate mofetil lack the neurotoxicity of calcineurin inhibitors (Kniepeiss *et al.* 2003; Moreno *et al.*, 2003; Maramottom and Wijdicks, 2004). Neurotoxicity often occurs early after surgery, not always related to high plasma levels. Manifestations are various, mainly affecting the central nervous system, and are usually distinguished in minor (tremor, headache, insomnia, paresthesiae) and major (encephalopathy, akinetic mutism, seizures, speech disorders, polyneuropathy, myopathy).

Literature analysis

Several predisposing factors have been advocated: hypocholesterolaemia (De Groen *et al.*, 1989), hypomagnesaemia (Thompson *et al.*, 1984), hypertension (Textor *et al.*, 1994) [Class IV], and hepatic encephalopathy (Pujol *et al.* 1994; Guarino *et al.*, 1999) [Class III]. New oral formulations of CS (Neoral) (Wijdicks *et al.*, 1999) as well as delayed starting and low-dosage regimens (Gomez *et al.*, 1996) seem to attenuate the severity of neurotoxicity, whereas it could be exacerbated by concomitant treatments (i.e. metoclopramide) (Trzepacz *et al.*, 2000; Prescott *et al.*, 2004) [Class III, IV]. Magnetic resonance imaging (MRI) may reveal nonenhancing high-resolution T2 images mainly involving posterior white matter. However, CS and FK506-related pontine abnormalities, similar to central pontine myelinolysis (CPM), have also been reported (Kaaber *et al.*, 1995; Fryer *et al.*, 1996; Rodriguez *et al.*, 1998; Ravaioli *et al.*, 2003), sometimes associated with an insidious speech disorder that may rapidly evolve into mutism and locked-in syndrome [Class IV]. Given its sensitivity in revealing cerebral white matter abnormalities, MRI supports the diagnosis of neurotoxicity (Appignani *et al.*, 1996; Bianco *et al.*, 2004) [Class II, IV].

To treat neurotoxicity, a reduction of doses and conversion from CS to FK506 and vice versa have been suggested (Pratschke *et al.*, 1997; Abouljoud *et al.*, 2002) [Class IV].

The recent use of novel combinations of drugs (calcineurin inhibitors plus mycophenolate mofetil or sirolimus) allows lower dosages of CS and FK506 (McAlister *et al.*, 2001) without weakening the immunosuppression efficacy [Class IV]. The same occurs with the implementation of so-called

CS and FK506 sparing regimens by switching to mycophenolate mofetil (Pfitzman *et al.*, 2003) or sirolimus (Kniepeiss *et al.*, 2003) [Class IV].

In most cases, these approaches lead to a resolution of symptoms and reversal of neuroimaging abnormalities (Appignani *et al.*, 1996; Bianco *et al.*, 2004; Ravaioli *et al.*, 2003) [Class IV]. However, some patients with irreversible deficits are occasionally seen, especially if the immunosuppressive regimen is not changed promptly (Casanova *et al.*, 1997) [Class IV].

Minor side effects are usually transient and self-limiting. Headache, tremor, paresthesiae, and insomnia are successfully managed with symptomatic conventional treatment (Stracciari and Guarino, 2001) [Class IV]. However, a change in the immunosuppressive regimen has occasionally been necessary in refractory headache (Rozen *et al.*, 1996) [Class IV].

OKT3 neurotoxicity usually presents with headache, rarely with a transient aseptic meningitis and exceptionally with a diffuse encephalopathy (Parizel *et al.*, 1997). The use of lower doses or pre-treatment with steroids, antihistaminic drugs or indomethacin may decrease the severity of symptoms (Rossi *et al.*, 1993) [Class IV]. Acute side effects of corticosteroids include behavioural and mood disorders, while chronic use may lead to myopathy, both reversible with adjustment of therapy (Rosener, 1996) [Class IV].

RECOMMENDATIONS

Cyclosporine and tacrolimus neurotoxicity: prevention requires minimum efficacious doses, oral administration as soon as possible, strict plasma levels monitoring (including metabolites), electrolytes imbalance (i.e. hypomagnesemia) and hypertension check and correction, and attention to pharmacological interactions (Level C). Brain MRI is the choice diagnostic tool (Level B) and should be performed as soon as severe neurotoxicity is suspected (Good Practice Point). In case of major side effects, prompt switching to a non calcineurin inhibitor (e.g. sirolimus) is indicated (Good Practice Point). Secondary options include conversion from cyclosporine to tacrolimus and

vice versa (Good Practice Point). Minor complications require switching only in case of intractable and invalidating symptoms. Generally, their treatment should follow the guidelines for these disorders, administering drugs lacking both hepatotoxicity and interference with immunosuppressants (e.g. gabapentin for paresthesiae, riboflavin for migraine prophylaxis) (Good Practice Point).

OKT3 neurotoxicity: prevention consists of administering minimal dosages and pre-medication with corticosteroids (Good Practice Point). Aseptic meningitis does not need treatment, because it is usually self-limiting. Encephalopathy requires antioedema agents and very rarely OKT3 withdrawal (Good Practice Point).

Corticosteroid neurotoxicity: severe acute behavioural disorders may be treated by a temporary reduction and/or withdrawal of intravenous steroid administration. Brief regimens of low-dose neuroleptics (e.g. haloperidol, olanzapin, quetiapin, risperidon) may be considered (Good Practice Point).

Seizures

Seizure incidence is about 5% (Wijdicks *et al.*, 1996a; Guarino *et al.*, 1999; Choi *et al.*, 2004). Most are generalized tonic-clonic, but a focal onset may have escaped observation. Convulsive or non-convulsive status epilepticus is rare. Seizures occur early after surgery. Causes are drugs, acute metabolic derangement, hypoxic-ischemic injury, cerebral lesions, sudden withdrawal of narcotic agents, inadvertent discontinuation or changes in anticonvulsant drugs in epileptics. Immunosuppressant toxicity is the main aetiology (Guarino *et al.*,1996; Wijdicks *et al.*, 1996a).

Literature analysis

Preventive measures mainly focus on the control of metabolic parameters and correct drug management. The diagnostic approach includes a wide spectrum of tests to cover all possible causes (Wijdicks *et al.*, 1996a; Wszolek and Steg, 1997) [Class IV]. Cerebral MRI is suggested as the investigation of choice to search for seizure aetiology in the general population (Scottish Intercollegiate Guidelines Network, 2004) [Class II]. This also seems applicable in liver transplanted patients, as MRI can help in detecting immunosuppressant-related brain damage. No randomized controlled trials are available on the use of antiepileptic drugs in liver transplanted patients. Treatment can be problematic both because of the interference between most antiepileptics and immunosuppressants and the usual need for intravenous therapy. Among intravenous anticonvulsants, phenytoin is preferred (Adams *et al.*, 1987; Wijdicks *et al.*, 1996a) [Class IV]. Among oral antiepileptics, gabapentin (Wszolek and Steg, 1997) and levetiracetam (Chabolla *et al.*, 2003) are of interest both for their efficacy and lack of hepatic induction [Class IV]. Prognostic studies report a favourable outcome both for survival and absence of seizure recurrence after a short period of therapy (3 months) in most cases (Wijdicks *et al.*, 1996a; Choi *et al.*, 2004) [Class III, IV].

RECOMMENDATIONS

Seizure prevention requires close monitoring of metabolic parameters (in particular electrolytes) and immunosuppressant levels, and caution in managing discontinuation or adjustment of epileptogenic drugs (Good Practice Point). The diagnostic approach should routinely include laboratory tests, EEG and neuroimaging. Cerebrospinal fluid (CSF) examination is indicated when central nervous system infection is suspected (Good Practice Point). Brain MRI is the current standard of reference (Level B). When MRI is not available or contraindicated, computerized tomography (CT) can be applied (Level C). The first-line intravenous antiepileptic drug is phenytoin whose administration in adults should not exceed 50 mg/min to obtain serum levels between 10 and 20 mcg/ml (Good Practice Point). When oral administration is possible, new antiepileptics could be considered, for example, gabapentin or levetiracetam (Good Practice Point). Status epilepticus must be managed according to guidelines for the general population (Treiman *et al.*, 1998) (Level A). In most cases, antiepileptic therapy can be suspended after three months (Level C).

Central pontine myelinolysis

CPM is a symmetrical demyelinating lesion at the centre of the pons seen usually in alcoholics and malnourished patients, attributed to a rapid correction of hyponatraemia (Martin, 2004). CPM has been reported in 1–8% of liver transplanted patients (Wijdicks *et al.*, 1996b; Guarino *et al.*, 1996; Bonham *et al.*, 1998; Bronster *et al.*, 2000). The high incidence in OLT is likely favoured by the usual hyponatraemic state of patients with cirrhosis and by the large replacement of fluids during the operation, leading to a sharp increase in plasma levels of sodium. CPM occurs early after surgery. Clinical manifestations do not differ from non liver transplanted patients, including insidious misleading presentations (Wijdicks *et al.*, 1996b) or paucisymptomatic pictures (Kato *et al.*, 2002). A high mortality has been reported (Abbasoglu *et al.*, 1998; Yu *et al.*, 2004).

Literature analysis

Hyponatraemia and an abrupt rise in serum sodium (> 18 mM/L/24–48 h) are significantly related to the occurrence of CPM in liver transplanted patients (Abbasoglu *et al.*, 1998; Yu *et al.*, 2004) [Class IV]. There is no definite therapy for CPM. Sporadic suggestions include the use of steroids and intravenous immunoglobulins with some benefit. Re-inducing hyponatraemia in the very early phase of CPM has been also proposed (Oya *et al.*, 2001) [Class IV]. Prevention is based on a slow correction of perioperative hyponatraemia (Abbasoglu, 1998; Yu *et al.*, 2004), not exceeding 8 mM/L/day (Martin, 2004). Transplantation at an early stage of the liver disease has also been suggested (Yu *et al.*, 2004) [Class IV]. MRI is currently the best investigation (Ruzek *et al.*, 2004) [Class IV]. Serial MRI could be needed because the appearance of the lesion may be delayed (Bronster *et al.*, 2000) [Class IV].

RECOMMENDATIONS

Given enough time before OLT, hyponatraemia should be corrected slowly. The variations in serum sodium concentration must be carefully monitored and controlled before and during surgery to avoid major fluctuations (Good Practice Point). If the patient is hyponatremic when undergoing OLT, a perioperative hourly correction rate at or below 0.5 mM/L/h should be maintained. The correction rate should not exceed 8 mM/L/day (Good Practice Point). MRI should be performed early and repeated if negative (Good Practice Point).

Neuromuscular disorders

Neuromuscular disorders present with focal or generalized weakness. Focal weakness includes mononeuropathies, with an incidence of 2–13% (Wijdicks *et al.*, 1996c; Campellone *et al.*, 1998a; Santilli *et al.*, 1999) and brachial plexopathy whose incidence is 1–5.8% (Katirij *et al.*, 1989; Guarino *et al.*, 1996; Santilli *et al.*, 1999). Axonal involvement is common. Invasive procedures, perioperative positioning and rarely compressive masses (e.g. haematoma) are the main causes. Generalized weakness occurs in 1.5–10% of patients (Guarino *et al.*, 1996; Wijdicks *et al.*, 1996c; Campellone *et al.*, 1998b; Mirò *et al.*, 1999; Santilli *et al.*, 1999; Reazaigua-Delclaux *et al.*, 2002) and consists of axonal or demyelinating polyneuropathy and necrotizing myopathy, mainly related to immunosuppression neurotoxicity (Goy *et al.*, 1989; Ayres *et al.*, 1994; Bronster *et al.*, 1995b) and critical illness (Mirò *et al.*, 1999; Campellone and Lacomis, 1999; Reazaigua-Delclaux *et al.*, 2002). Guillain-Barré syndrome (El-Sabrout *et al.*, 2001; Colle *et al.*, 2002) and chronic inflammatory demyelinating polyneuropathy (Taylor *et al.*, 1995; Echaniz-Laguna *et al.*, 2004) are also reported.

Literature analysis

No systematic studies have analysed the risk factors for neuromuscular complications in OLT. Diabetes and alcoholism do not seem to increase the risk of perioperative mononeuritis (Campellone *et al.*, 1998a) [Class III]. High doses of corticosteroids and use of non-depolarizing neuromuscular blocking agents are reported to favour quadriplegia after OLT (Campellone *et al.*, 1998b; Mirò *et al.*, 1998) [Class III]. Diagnosis is mainly based on conventional electrophysiological study, muscular enzymes assessment and CSF examination. Nerve

or muscle biopsy should also be considered. Prognosis is usually good (Wijdicks *et al.*, 1996c; Mirò *et al.*, 1998; Reazaigua-Delclaux 2002) [Class IV], but some patients need mechanical supports to walk (Campellone *et al.*, 1998b). Prevention of perioperative neuropathy is focused on careful perioperative nursing (Warner, 1998) [Class IV]. Minimizing the use of corticosteroids and neuromuscular blocking agents in a critical illness setting has proven of help in preventing neuromuscular disorders (Motomura, 2003) [Class IV]. Treatment includes a change of immunosuppression when neurotoxicity is the cause (Ayres *et al.*, 1994; Bronster *et al.*, 1995a) [Class IV], and conventional therapy in case of Guillain-Barré syndrome (El-Sabrout *et al.*, 2001) or chronic inflammatory demyelinating polyneuropathy (Taylor *et al.*, 1995) [Class II]. No specific treatment exists for critical illness neuromuscular disorders. Customary general measures for critical illness usually applied in intensive care units (e.g. insulin therapy) can reduce mortality and morbidity (Van den Berghe *et al.*, 2001) [Class II].

RECOMMENDATIONS

Perioperative Mononeuropathies: prevention implies caution during catheterisation, avoiding blinded cannulations and external compressions by blood pressure cuff or tourniquet (Good Practice Point).

To reduce perioperative malpositioning it is indicated to maintain the arms at less than 90° of abduction, to maintain the arms at less than 30° of extension when combined with abduction, padding of the exposed nerves (i.e. at the level of fibular head, popliteal space, calcaneus, under forearms, under hands), frequent repositioning during prolonged surgery. Patients should be instructed to avoid postures potentially compressing or stretching the nerves (Good Practice Point).

Generalized weakness: prevention requires avoiding when possible the prolonged use of non-depolarizing neuromuscular blocking agents and minimizing the use of high dose intravenous corticosteroids (Level C). In case of calcineurin inhibitors toxicity, prompt switching to a different agent (e.g. sirolimus) is recommended (Good Practice Point). Customary general measures for critical illness, including aggressive insulin-therapy, and conventional management of Guillain-Barré syndrome and chronic inflammatory demyelinating polyneuropathy are indicated (Level B).

Cerebrovascular disorders

Acute cerebrovascular disorders occur in 2–6.5% of OLT recipients, mostly with cerebral haemorrhage (Wijdicks *et al.*, 1995; Guarino *et al.*, 1996; Wang *et al.*, 2000), usually within 2 months after surgery (Singh *et al.*, 1994; Guarino *et al.*, 1996; Wang *et al.*, 2000). Focal deficits may be obscured by diffuse encephalopathy. Several risk factors are recognised, those directly associated with hepatic failure such as coagulation disturbances and those secondary to immunosuppressive therapy such as hypercholesterolaemia, diabetes, hypertension (Adair, 1999; Singh *et al.*, 1994; Wang *et al.*, 2000). Perioperative events, such as cerebral hypoperfusion and massive transfusion, may also favour cerebrovascular injury (Wang *et al.*, 2000; Plachky *et al.*, 2004). Causes of cerebral bleeding include aspergillus angiopathy and mycotic aneurysms (Singh *et al.*, 1994; Wang *et al.*, 2000).

Literature analysis

Adjustment of cerebrovascular risk factors before, during and post-OLT is the main preventive measure (Adair, 1999; Wang *et al.*, 2000) [Class IV].

Diagnosis and treatment are similar to that adopted in the general population; attention is paid to the search for infection as a cause of acute cerebrovascular disorders, to institute prompt antimicrobial therapy (Adair, 1999) [Class III–IV].

RECOMMENDATIONS

Prevention includes correction of coagulopathies before surgery (e.g. administration of platelets and blood products but with caution due to the risk of consumptive coagulopathy), avoiding perioperative cerebral hypoperfusion and control of cerebrovascular risk factors after OLT (especially hypertension) (Good Practice Point). According to general guidelines, CT scan is the preferred diagnostic test in early phases of acute cerebrovascular disorders, especially to detect haemorrhage (Level C). MRI, despite its greater sensitivity, is often not tolerated or is not applicable immediately after OLT, but it should be considered to characterize some vascular lesions or to rule out other aetiologies (Good Practice Point).

A search for bacteriemia or fungemia to detect infection should be routinely applied (Good Practice Point). General treatment of cerebrovascular disorders in OLT should not differ from that applied in the general population (Good Practice Point). Concomitant antifungal treatment should be given in the presence of angiopathy related to central nervous system infections (Level C).

Central nervous system infections

Central nervous system infections in liver transplanted patients are favoured by immuno suppression. The incidence is estimated in 5% (Tolkoff-Rubin *et al.*, 1999; Singh and Husain, 2000), with a high mortality (Bronster *et al.*, 2000). Lysteria monocytogenes, Aspergillus fumigatus and Criptococcus neoformans are the most commonly involved pathogens (Singh and Husain, 2000). Viral infections are very rare, related to herpesvirus-6 and cytomegalovirus (Singh and Husain, 2000). Progressive multifocal leukoencephalopathy has been occasionally reported (Bronster *et al.*, 1995). Most central nervous system infections are metastatic from other sites (mainly gastrointestinal tract and lung). Clinical patterns include meningitis, encephalitis, abscesses, or a combination.

Literature analysis

Neuroimaging, spinal tap after excluding increased intracranial pressure, and the search for signs of systemic infection are the core of diagnosis. Brain biopsy can be performed in individual cases (Bonham *et al.*, 1998; Tolkoff-Rubin *et al.*, 1999) [Class IV]. CSF-Polymerase Chain Reaction is crucial in detecting viral infections (Portegies *et al.*, 2004) [Class I]. Prevention focuses on eradicating infection in donor and recipients and avoiding nosocomial contamination (Stone and Schaffner, 1990; Tolkoff-Rubin *et al.*, 1999; Soave, 2001) [Class III]. No data are available suggesting the need for specific prophylactic antimicrobial strategies for central nervous system infection. Treatment is based on guidelines for immunocompromised patients (Saag *et al.*, 2000; Ascioglu *et al.*, 2002; Herbrecht *et al.*, 2002; Bohme *et al.*, 2003; Dewhurst, 2004; Portegies *et al.*, 2004; Schwartz and Thiel, 2004) and OLT centres' experience (Tolkoff-Rubin *et al.*, 1999; Wu *et al.*, 2002) [Class III, II]. Antimicrobial agents can interfere with drugs used in livertransplanted patients (e.g. voriconazole with tacrolimus and sirolimus, phenytoin and carbamazepine; amphotericin B with CS) (Venkataramanan *et al.*, 2002).

RECOMMENDATIONS

An early in-depth diagnostic approach is advocated, including brain CT/MRI, lumbar puncture and possibly brain biopsy, and the search for extracerebral sources of infection (Good Practice Point). CSF-Polymerase Chain Reaction is essential for viral infections (Level A). Prompt administration of therapy, upon suspicion of the diagnosis without definitive proof is needed to control infection (Good Practice Point). An exhaustive search for latent infection in donor and recipients is required, including close monitoring for intestinal strongyloidiasis in patients who have lived for long periods in tropical or subtropical countries (Level C). Exposure to hospital contamination must be avoided (Level C). Specific drug protocols to prevent brain infections are not required (Good Practice Point). Treatment of neurolisteriosis consists of prolonged administration of ampicillin plus gentamicin; second choice includes trimethoprim-sulfamethoxazole (Level C). For brain nocardiosis prolonged administration of trimethoprim-sulfamethoxazole is suggested (Level C). For brain aspergillosis, the first choice drug is voriconazole: initially, 6 mg/kg IV every 12 h in two doses, then 4 mg/kg IV every 12 h, switching to oral dosing (same dosage) as tolerated and clinically justified; maintenance regimen consists of 200–300 mg orally every 12 h. Duration of intravenous therapy should be between 6 and 27 days, followed by oral administration for 4–24 weeks (Level A). In case of intolerance, contraindications or therapy failure: liposomal amphotericin B (1–5 mg/Kg/day) or capsofungin 50 mg/day (loading dose: 70 mg day 1) or itraconazole (except after voriconazole) (Level B). Surgical resection may be considered. First line treatment for cryptococcal meningitis is a combination of liposomal amphotericin B plus 5-flucitosin. Schedule treatment includes: induction with amphotericin B (0.7 mg/kg/day) and flucytosine (150 mg/kg/day) for 2 weeks, followed by consolidation with fluconazole for 8–10 weeks (400–800 mg/day), followed by 6–12 months at lower doses of lower doses of fluconazole (200 mg/day) (Level A). Treatment for herpesvirus-6 and cytomegalovirus encephalitis is ganciclovir and foscarnet, either alone or in combination (Level C). For progressive multifocal leukoencephalopathy cidofovir is a possible option (Good Practice Point).

Conflicts of interest

We declare that we have no conflict of interest in connection with this paper.

Acknowledgement

We are indebted to Roberto D'Alessandro and Alessandro Liberati for their helpful methodological suggestions.

References

Abbasoglu O, Goldstein RM, Vodapally MS *et al.* (1998). Liver transplantation in hyponatremic patients with emphasis on central pontine myelinolysis. *Clin Transplant* **12:**263–269.

Aboulioud MS, Kumar MS, Brayman KL, Emre S, Bynon JS; OLN study group (2002). Neoral rescue therapy in transplant patients with intolerance to tacrolimus. *Clin Transplant* **16:**168–172.

Adair JC (1999). Cerebrovascular disorders. In (EFM Wijdicks, ed.), *Neurologic Complications in Organ Transplant Recipients*, Butterworth-Heineman, pp 193–216.

Adams DH, Gunson B, Honigsberger L *et al.* (1987). Neurological complications following liver transplantation. *Lancet* **1**:949–951.

Appignani BA, Bhadella RA, Blacklow SC, Wang AK, Roland SF, Freeman RB (1996). Neuroimaging findings in patients on immunosuppressive therapy: experience with tacrolimus toxicity. *Am J Roentgenol* **166**:683–688.

Ascioglu S, Rex JH, de Pauw B *et al.* (2002). Defining opportunistic invasive fungal infections in immunocompromised patients with cancer and hematopoietic stem cell transplants: an international consensus. *Clin Infect Dis* **34**:7–14.

Ayres RCS, Dousset B, Wixon S, Buckels JAC, McMaster P, Mayer AD (1994). Peripheral neuropathy with tacrolimus. *Lancet* **343**:862–863.

Bianco F, Fattaposta F, Locuratolo N *et al.* (2004). Reversible diffusion MRI abnormalities and transient mutism after liver transplantation. *Neurology* **62**:981–983.

Bohme A, Ruhnke M, Buchheidt DT *et al.* (2003). Treatment of fungal infections in hematology and oncology–guidelines of the Infectious Diseases Working Party (AGIHO) of the German Society of Hematology and Oncology (DGHO). *Ann Hematol* **82 (Suppl 2)**:S133–140.

Bonham CA, Dominguez EA, Fukui MB *et al.* (1998). Central nervous system lesions in liver transplant recipients: prospective assessment of indications for biopsy and implications for management. *Transplantation* **66**:1596–1604.

Brainin M, Barnes M, Baron J-C *et al.* (2004). Guidance for the preparation of neurological management guidelines by EFNS scientific task forces – revised recommendations 2004. *Eur J Neurol* **11**:577–581.

Bronster DJ, Yonover P, Stein J, Scelsa SN, Miller CM, Sheiner PA (1995a). Demyelinating sensorimotor polyneuropathy after administration of FK506. *Transplantation* **59**:1066–1068.

Bronster DJ, Lidov MW, Wolfe D, Schwartz ME, Miller CM (1995b). Progressive multifocal leukoencephalopathy after orthotopic liver transplantation. *Liver Transpl Surg* **1**:371–372.

Bronster DJ, Emre S, Boccagni P, Sheiner PA, Schwartz ME, Miller CM (2000). Central nervous system complications in liver transplant recipients–incidence, timing, and long-term follow-up. *Clin Transplant* **14**:1–7.

Campellone JV, Lacomis D, Giuliani MJ, Kramer DJ (1998a). Mononeuropathies associated with liver transplantation. *Muscle Nerve* **21**:896–901.

Campellone JV, Lacomis D, Kramer DJ, Van Cott AC, Giuliani MJ (1998b). Acute myopathy after liver transplantation. *Neurology* **50**:46–53.

Campellone JV, Lacomis D (1999). Neuromuscular disorders. In (EFM Wijdicks, ed.), *Neurologic Complications in Organ Transplant Recipients*, Butterworth-Heineman, pp 169–192.

Casanova B, Prieto M, Deya E *et al.* (1997). Persistent cortical blindness after cyclosporine leukoencephalopathy. *Liver Transpl Surg* **3**:638–640.

Chabolla DR, Harnois DM, Meschia JF (2003). Levetiracetam monotherapy for liver transplant patients with seizures. *Transplant Proc* **35**:1480–1481.

Choi EJ, Kang JK, Lee SA, Kim KH, Lee SG, Andermann F (2004). New-onset seizures after liver transplantation: clinical implications and prognosis in survivors. *Eur Neurol* **52**:230–236.

Colle I, Van Vlierberghe H, Troisi R *et al.* (2002). Campylobacter-associated Guillain-Barre syndrome after orthotopic liver transplantation for hepatitis C cirrhosis: a case report. *Hepatol Res* **24**:205.

De Groen PC (1989). Cyclosporine: a review and its specific use in liver transplantation. *Mayo Clin Proc* **64**:680–689.

Dewhurst S (2004). Human herpesvirus type 6 and human herpesvirus type 7 infections of the central nervous system. *Herpes* **11(Suppl 2)**:105A–111A.

Echaniz-Laguna A, Battaglia F, Ellero B, Mohr M, Jaeck D (2004). Chronic inflammatory demyelinating polyradiculoneuropathy in patients with liver transplantation. *Muscle Nerve* **30**:501–504.

El-Sabrout RA, Radovancevic B, Ankoma-Sey V, Van Buren C (2001). Guillain-Barrè syndrome after solid organ transplantation. *Transplantation* **71**:1311–1316.

Fryer JP, Fortier MV, Metrakos P *et al.* (1996). Central pontine myelinolysis and cyclosporine neurotoxicity following liver transplantation. *Transplantation* **61**:658–661.

Gomez R, Moreno E, Loinaz C *et al.* (1996). Liver transplantation with a twenty-four delay and an initial low dose of cyclosporine. *Hepato-Gastroenterology* **43**:435–439.

Goy JJ, Stauffer JC, Deruaz JP *et al.* (1989). Myopathy as possible side-effect of cyclosporin. *Lancet* **1**:1446–1447.

Guarino M, Stracciari A, Pazzaglia P *et al.* (1996). Neurological complications of liver transplantation. *J Neurol* **243**:137–142.

Guarino M, Stracciari A, D'Alessandro R *et al.* (1999). A prospective study on the neurological complications after liver transplantation. *Gastroenterol Int* **12**:140–145.

Herbrecht R, Denning DW, Patterson TF *et al.* (2002). Voriconazole versus amphotericin B for primary therapy of invasive aspergillosis. *N Engl J Med* **347**:408–415.

Jones J, Hunter D (1995). Consensus methods for medical and health services research. *BMJ* **311:**376–380.

Kabeer MH, Filo RS, Milgrom ML (1995). Central pontine myelinolysis following orthotopic liver transplant: association with cyclosporin toxicity. *Postgrad Med J* **71:**239–241.

Katirji MB (1989). Brachial plexus injury following liver transplantation. *Neurology* **39:**736–738.

Kato T, Hattori H, Nagato M *et al.* (2002). Subclinical central pontine myelinolysis following liver transplantation. *Brain Dev* **24:**179–182.

Kniepeiss D, Iberer F, Grasser B, Schaffellner S, Tscheliessnigg KH (2003). Sirolimus and mycophenolate mofetil after liver transplantation. *Transpl Int* **16:**504–509.

Maramottom BV, Wijdicks EF (2004). Sirolimus may not cause neurotoxicity in kidney and transplant recipients. *Neurology* **63:**1958–1959.

Martin RJ (2004). Central pontine and extrapontine myelinolysis: the osmotic demyelination syndromes. *J Neurol Neurosurg Psychiatry* **75(Suppl 3):**22–28.

McAlister VC, Peltekian KM, Malatjalian DA *et al.* (2001). Orthotopic liver transplantation using low-dose tacrolimus and sirolimus. *Liver Transpl* **7:**701–708.

Mirò O, Salmeron JM, Masanes F *et al.* (1999). Acute quadriplegic myopathy with myosin-deficient muscle fibres after liver transplantation. *Transplantation* **67:**1144–1151.

Moreno JM, Rubio E, Gomez A *et al.* (2003). Effectiveness and safety of mycophenolate mofetil as monotherapy in liver transplantation. *Transplant Proc* **35:**1874–1876.

Motomura M (2003). Critical illness polyneuropathy and myopathy. *Rinsho Shinkeigaku* **43:**802–804.

Oya S, Tsutsumi K, Ueki K, Kirino T (2001). Reinduction of hyponatremia to treat central pontine myelinolysis. *Neurology* **57:**1931–1932.

Parizel PM, Snoek H-W, van den Hauwe L *et al.* (1997). Cerebral complications of murine monoclonal CD3 antibody (OKT3): CT and MRI findings. *Am J Neuroradiol* **18:**1935–1938.

Pfitzman R, Klupp J, Langrehr *et al.* (2003). Mycophenolate mofetil for immunosuppression after liver transplantation: a follow-up study of 191 patients. *Transplantation* **76:**130–136.

Plachky J, Hofer S, Volkmann M, Martin E, Bardenheuer HJ, Weigand MA (2004). Regional cerebral oxygen saturation is a sensitive marker of cerebral hypoperfusion during orthotopic liver transplantation. *Anesth Analg* **99:**344–349.

Portegies P, Solod L, Cinque P *et al.* (2004). Guidelines for the diagnosis and management of neurological complications of HIV infection. *Eur J Neurol* **11:**297–304.

Pratschke J, Neuhaus R, Tullius SG *et al.* (1997). Treatment of cyclosporine-related adverse effects by conversion to tacrolimus after liver transplantation. *Transplantation* **64:**938–940.

Prescott WA Jr, Callahan BL, Park JM (2004). Tacrolimus toxicity associated with concomitant metoclopramide therapy. *Pharmacotherapy* **24:**532–537.

Pujol A, Graus F, Rimola A *et al.* (1994). Predictive factors of inhospital CNS complications following liver transplantation. *Neurology* **44:**1226–1230.

Ravaioli M, Guarino M, Stracciari A *et al.* (2003). Speech disorder related to tacrolimus-induced pontine myelinolysis after orthotopic liver transplantation. *Transpl Int* **16:**605–607.

Rezaiguia-Delclaux, Lefaucher JP, Zakkouri M, Duvoux C, Duvaldestin P, Stephan F (2002). Severe acute polyneuropathy complicating orthotopic liver allograft failure. *Transplantation* **74:**880–882.

Rodriguez J, Benito-Leon J, Molina JA, Ramos A, Bermejo F (1998). Central pontine myelinolisis associated with cyclosporin in liver transplantation. *Neurologia* **13:**437–440.

Rosener M, Martin E, Zipp F, Dichgans J, Martin R (1996). Neurological side-effects of pharmacologic corticoid therapy. *Nervenarzt* **67:**983–986.

Rossi SJ, Schroeder TJ, Hariharan S, First MR (1993). Prevention and management of the adverse effects associated with immunosuppressive therapy. *Drug Saf* **9:**104–131.

Rozen TD, Wijdicks EFM, Hay JH (1996). Treatment-refractory cyclosporine-associated headache. Relief with conversion to FK-506. *Neurology* **47:**1347.

Ruzek KA, Campeau NG, Miller GA (2004). Early diagnosis of central pontine myelinolysis with diffusion-weighted imaging. *AJNR* **25:**210–213.

Saag MS, Graybill RJ, Larsen RA *et al.* (2000). Practice guidelines for the management of cryptococcal disease. *Clin Infect Dis* **30:**710–718.

Santilli IM, Jann S, Sterzi R *et al.* (1999). Neuromuscular complications of orthotopic liver transplantation. *Gastroenterol Int* **12:**151–154.

Schwartz S, Thiel E (2004). Update on the treatment of cerebral aspergillosis. *Ann Hematol* **831:**S42–S44.

Scottish Intercollegiate Guidelines Network – SIGN (2004). Diagnosis and management of epilepsy in adults.

Singh N, Yu VL, Gayowski T (1994). Central nervous system lesions in adult liver transplant recipients: clinical review with implications for management. *Medicine* **73:**110–118.

Singh N, Husain S (2000). Infections of the central nervous system in transplant recipients. *Transpl Infect Dis* **2**:101–111.

Soave R (2001). Prophylaxis strategies for solid organ transplantation. *Clin Infect Dis* **33(Suppl 1)**:26–31.

Stone WJ, Schaffner W (1990). Strongyloides infections in transplant recipients. *Semin Respir Infect* **5**:58–64.

Stracciari A, Guarino M (2001). Neuropsychiatric complications of liver transplantation. *Met Brain Dis* **16**:3–11.

Taylor BV, Wijdicks EFM, Poterucha JJ, Weisner RH (1995). Chronic inflammatory demyelinating polyneuropathy complicating liver transplantation. *Ann Neurol* **38**:828–831.

Textor SC, Canzanello VJ, Taler SJ *et al.* (1994). Cyclosporine-induced hypertension after transplantation. *Mayo Clin Proc* **69**:1182–1193.

Thompson CB, June CH, Sullivan KM, Thomas ED (1984). Association between cyclosporin neurotoxicity and hypomagnesaemia. *Lancet* **17**:1116–1120.

Tolkoff-Rubin NE, Hovingh KG, Rubin RH (1999). Central nervous system infections. In: Wijdicks EFM, ed. *Neurologic Complications in Organ Transplant Recipients*. Boston: Butterworth Heinemann, pp 141–168.

Treiman DM, Meyers PD, Walton NY *et al.* (1998). A comparison of four treatments for generalized convulsive status epilepticus. Veterans Affairs Status Epilepticus Cooperative Study Group. *N Engl J Med* **339**:792–798.

Trzepacz PT, Gupta B, Di Martini A (2000). Pharmacologic issues in organ transplantation: psychopharmacology and neuropsychiatric medication side effects. In: Trzepacz PT, Di Martini A, eds, *The Transplant Patient*. Cambridge University Press, pp 187–213.

Van den Berghe G, Wouters P, Weekers F *et al.* (2001). Intensive insulin treatment reduced mortality and morbidity in critically ill patients. *N Engl J Med* **345**:1359–1367.

Venkataramanan R, Zang S, Gayowski T, Singh N (2002). Voriconazole inhibition of the metabolism of tacrolimus in a liver transplant recipient and in human liver microsomes. *Antimicrob Agents Chemother* **46**:3091–3093.

Wang WL, Yang ZF, Lo CM, Liu CL, Fan ST (2000). Intracerebral hemorrhage after liver transplantation. *Liver Transpl* **6**:345–348.

Warner MA (1998). Perioperative neuropathies. *Mayo Clin Proc* **73**:567–574.

Wijdicks EFM, Wiesner RH, Dahlke LJ, Kron RAF (1994). FK506-induced neurotoxicity in liver transplantation. *Ann Neurol* **35**:498–501.

Wijdicks EFM, De Groen PC, Wiesner RH, Kron RAF (1995). Intracerebral hemorrhage in liver transplant recipients. *Mayo Clin Proc* **70**:443–446.

Wijdicks EFM, Plevak DJ, Wiesner RH, Steers JL (1996a). Causes and outcome of seizures in liver transplant recipients. *Neurology* **47**:1523–1525.

Wijdicks EFM, Blue PR, Steers JL, Wiesner RH (1996b). Central pontine myelinolysis with stupor alone after orthotopic liver transplantation. *Liver Transpl Surg* **2**:14–16.

Wijdicks EFM, Litchy WJ, Wiesner RH, Krom RA (1996c). Neuromuscular complications associated with liver transplantation. *Muscle Nerve* **19**:696–700.

Wijdicks EFM, Dahlke LJ, Wiesner RH (1999). Oral cyclosporine decreases severity of neurotoxicity in liver transplant recipients. *Neurology* **52**:1708–1710.

Wszolek ZK, Steg RE (1997). Seizures after orthotopic liver transplantation. *Seizure* **6**:31–39.

Wu G, Vilchez RA, Eidelman B *et al.* (2002). Cryptococcal meningitis: an analysis among 5521 consecutive organ transplant recipients. *Transpl Infect Dis* **4**:183–188.

Yu J, Zheng SS, Liang TB, Shen Y, Wang WL, Ke QH (2004). Possible causes of central pontine myelinolysis after liver transplantation. *World J Gastroenterol* **10**:2540–2543.

CHAPTER 40

Fatty acid mitochondrial disorders

C. Angelini,[a] A. Federico,[b] H. Reichmann,[c]
A. Lombes,[d] P. Chinnery,[e] D. Turnbull[e]

Abstract

Guidelines in the diagnosis and current dietary treatment of long-chain fatty acid (LCFA) defects have been collected according to evidence-based medicine. Since the identification of carnitine and carnitine palmitoyltransferase deficiency more than 25 years ago nearly every enzymatic step required for β-oxidation has been associated with an inherited metabolic disorder. These disorders effectively preclude the use of body fat as energy source. Clinical consequence can range from no symptoms to severe manifestations including cardiomyopathy, hypoglycaemia, peripheral neuropathy and sudden death. A diet high in carbohydrates with medium-chain triglycerides (MCT) and reduced amount of LCFA has a beneficial effect (class IV evidence), and in appropriate deficiency states carnitine and riboflavin are used.

Background

Lipid storage myopathies (LSM) represent various disease entities whose biochemical defect falls into diverse aetiology (Vockley and Whiteman, 2002); these disorders might be due either to defects of the carnitine membrane carrier or to enzymatic defects in beta-oxidation energy supply. L-carnitine, CPT I, carnitine acyltranslocase and CPT II provide a mechanism whereby long-chain fatty acyl (LCFA)-CoAs are transferred from the cytosol inside the mitochondria where they undergo beta-oxidation. A series of enzymes bound to the mitochondrial inner membrane or soluble in cytosol transform fatty acyl-CoA into acetyl-CoA (figure 40.1). A mitochondrial trifunctional protein associated to the inner mitochondrial membrane has been found that performs three different enzymatic activities for LCFA oxidation. The presentation of disorders is done according to the pathway of LCFA transfer and oxidation.

Search strategy

The task force for metabolic disorders systematically searched the Medline database using key words and examined textbooks and existing guidelines. According to the guidance for the preparation of neurological management by the EFNS task force (Brainin et al., 2004), articles were included if they contained data that could be rated according to grades of recommendation for treatment classified in terms of evidence-based medicine. Most

[a]Department of Neurology, University of Padova, Italy; [b]Department of Neurological and Behavioural Sciences, University of Siena, Italy; [c]Neurologischen Universitaetsklinik Universitaetsklinikum Carl Gustav Carus der Technischen Universität Dresden; [d]Unite de recherche INSERM 153, Hopital de la Salpetriere, Paris; [e]Department of Neurology, The University of Newcastle upon Tyne, United Kingdom.

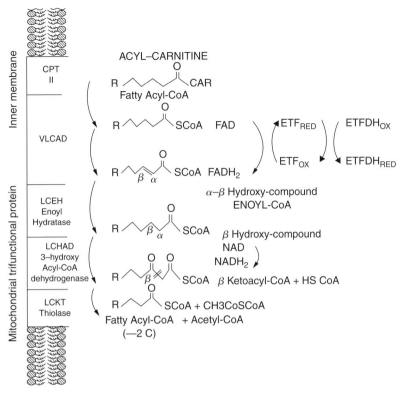

Figure 40.1. Pathway of LCFA oxidation by enzymes in the inner mitochondrial membrane. The other cofactor and enzymes are either in cytosol or mitochondrial matrix.

guideline recommendations in this document are derived from case reports (class IV evidence), as no large trials have been conducted in fatty acid disorders and therefore these guidelines reflect consensus in opinions of experts in the field (class IV). The consensus was reached analysing series of treated patients and in discussing pre-existing guidelines.

Results

Carnitine palmytoyl transferase deficiency (CPT 2)

In the most typical presentations CPT 2 deficiency is seen in young adults (Supplementary Table 1 available at the *European Journal of Neurology*, www.blackwellpublishing.com; see Angelini *et al.* 2006) experiencing episodes of muscle pain and rhabdomyolysis triggered by prolonged exercise or cold. The disease is autosomal recessive and is mostly seen in males, however intolerance to

exercise might be observed also in carriers of CPT 2 mutations suggesting a dominant negative effect of this tetrameric protein (Orngreen *et al.*, 2005).

The rhabdomyolitic attacks triggered by fasting or cold consist of pain, stiffness without cramps and highly elevated CK levels (up to 50.000 U) reflecting muscle necrosis. This may lead to acute renal failure.

GOOD PRACTICE POINTS

Preventing myoglobinuric episodes is important and this can be achieved by avoiding strenuous exercise during fasting or cold. During an attack 5% glucose solution is useful as an alternative metabolic fuel. Some guidelines for the treatment of rhabdomyolysis are according to published guidelines, that is, a standard treatment protocol for myoglobinuria (Better and Stein, 1990): intravenous infusion of hypotonic sodium chloride and sodium bicarbonate (sodium chloride 110 mmol/litre and bicarbonate 40 mmol/litre) in 5% glucose solution to which 10 g mannitol/litre is added in a 20% solution. The solution should be infused into a young adult of 75 kg weight at the rate of 12 litres per day to obtain a diuresis of 8 litres per day and to keep pH above 6.5. This therapeutic regimen will control both hyperkaleamia and acidosis and therefore might prevent acute renal failure.

Carnitine transport defects

Primary L-carnitine deficiency syndromes are rare biochemical disorders and can be classified on the basis of clinical and biochemical criteria in muscle carnitine deficiency and systemic carnitine deficiency. A carnitine deficiency syndrome should be suspected in a patient with lipid storage myopathy when the following symptoms are present: hypogliceamia, with or without ketoacidosis with a Reye-like syndrome, myalgias, weakness, abnormal fatiguability and cardiomyopathy with left axis deviation (Tein *et al.*, 1990; Nezu *et al.*, 1999).

Primary systemic carnitine deficiency is a well-recognised treatable entity of childhood (Supplementary table 2 available at the *European Journal of Neurology*, www.blackwellpublishing.com) characterised by progressive cardiomyopathy, lipid storage myopathy and attacks of hypoglycaemia, hepatomegaly with Reye-like syndrome that may lead to permanent brain damage (Chapoy *et al.*, 1980).

Diagnosis

In several cases, a defect of carnitine 'high affinity' transport (OCNT2 gene) has been demonstrated in cultured fibroblasts and genomic DNA can be screened for mutations (Tang *et al.*, 1999; Wang *et al.*, 2000).

Guidelines for therapy
Carnitine supplementation corrects cardiomyopathy and other clinical signs (Tein *et al.*, 1990). In some cases, this treatment might avoid cardiac transplant. The L-carnitine dose may vary from 100 to 600 mg/kg/day on the basis of the calculated carnitine depletion from muscle, liver,

heart and kidney. Individually adjusted dose may require plasma levels measurement. No side effects are noted for L-carnitine supplementation except occasional diarrhoea or fishy body odour, in some cases a medium-chain triglyceride diet may be added (class IV evidence).

Muscle carnitine deficiency
In primary muscle carnitine deficiency the clinical syndrome is confined to the skeletal muscle (Engel and Angelini, 1973; Vergani and Angelini, 1999); the clinical features are episodes of fluctuating muscle weakness, affecting mostly limb and neck muscles, causing severe myalgia.

Diagnostic guidelines and therapy

The patients show on fasting and on a high fat diet appropriate ketogenesis; biochemical features are low muscle carnitine in muscle (below 15%); absence of organic aciduria. Carnitine concentration in plasma and liver are normal; there is 'in vitro' stimulation by L-carnitine of labelled palmitate and oleate oxidation.

Although much is known about mechanisms of carnitine transport, data on muscle-specific transport (low affinity) in human muscle carnitine deficiency cases are still scanty. In one childhood case an abnormal low affinity carnitine transport (Vergani and Angelini, 1999) was found in cultured muscle; this could be due to either a delayed maturation or an abnormal carnitine carrier protein. The available evidence indicates that low muscle content is the result of a genetic defect of the sarcolemmal carnitine transporter. Therefore, muscle carnitine deficiency could be caused by an abnormal low affinity carrier or by a low number of sarcolemmal carnitine carriers. It is distinct by carnitine insufficiency and by the absence of acylcarnitines elevation in plasma or urine.

Treatment with L-carnitine replacement and MCT diet has been successful in a number of cases (class IV evidence).

Defects of beta-oxidation

Defects of fatty acids oxidation may affect muscle alone or in conjunction with signs in other tissues, that is, liver, heart (Supplementary Table 3 available at the *European Journal of Neurology*, www.blackwellpublishing.com). For many of the different enzyme deficiencies the clinical features are similar in some patients. This is reflected by exercise-induced muscle pain and rhabdomyolysis. The diagnosis is often suggested by characteristic patterns of organic acids excreted in the urine, which are specific for various enzymatic blocks.

Enzymatic and immunochemical analysis performed in fibroblasts and in muscle and liver mitochondria will confirm the diagnosis. In-born errors of beta-oxidation are:

1. Very Long-chain Acyl-CoA Dehydrogenase Deficiency (LCHAD or VLCAD)
2. Medium-Chain Acyl-CoA Dehydrogenase Deficiency (MCAD)
3. Short-Chain Acyl-CoA Dehydrogenase Deficiency (SCAD)
4. Riboflavin-responsive disorders of beta-oxidation (RR-HAD).

Guidelines for laboratory diagnosis of fatty acid oxidation defects

Dicarboxylic aciduria is a distinct finding associated with a metabolic block of beta-oxidation. The substrates are converted to dicarboxylic acids by the combined action of omega-oxidation in endoplasmic reticulum and by peroxisomal beta-oxidation.

The metabolic intermediates derived from the enzymatic block can be detected in the urine and blood; often they are formed only during a metabolic crisis. The qualitative and quantitative study of the organic acids produced in the patients is indicated with gas chromatography-mass spectrometry (GC-MS) analysis: acyl-carnitines can be revealed in patients with organic aciduria due to the activity of acyl-carnitine-transferase and their pattern of appearance in plasma and urine is a useful diagnostic test. They are especially important in diagnosis β-oxidation blocks such as VCLAD or MCAD deficiency. Other secondary metabolites, produced by enzymatic reactions that free CoA from acyl residues, can be detected in patients' urine: glycine derivatives like hexanoyl-glycine or phenylpropionyl-glycine are pathognomic of MCAD deficiency. The presence of glycine or acyl-carnitine derivatives in the urine indicates

an increased accumulation of acyl-CoAs in the mitochondria. Glutaric aciduria type 2 is pathognomic of riboflavin responsive LSM. Fat accumulation in muscle biopsy depends upon diet and activity level; therefore analysis of metabolites is a crucial part and can be associated to the study of labelled fatty acid oxidation and appropriate enzyme studies in fibroblasts.

Very long-chain acyl-CoA dehydrogenase deficiency
VLCAD deficiency has been mostly described in children (Hale *et al.*, 1985). The patients reported so far can be grouped according to their clinical course: a first group has onset in the first few months of life and shows a high mortality; a second group is characterised by recurrent episodes of coma after fasting, but presents no cardiomyopathy; a third group presents with late onset rhabdomyolysis and myalgia after muscle exercise.

Deficient patients cannot oxidise C18 to C16 fatty acids, whereas they can normally utilise shorter fatty acids (shorter than C14). The disease is inherited as an autosomal recessive trait. The common mutation for LCHAD deficiency is (1538 G > C). Onset of symptoms is in the first year of life, characterised by intermittent hypoglycaemia, lethargy and coma. The typical presentation is a progressive lethargy, evolving into coma during a fasting or during a febrile episode associated with vomiting and diarrhoea that induces a catabolic state. Hepatomegaly, cardiomyopathy, and muscle weakness are usually observed. Exercise-induced myoglobinuria is a possible presentation (Olgivie *et al.*, 1994; Orngreen *et al.*, 2004). Cardiologic involvement is frequent. Other distinctive laboratory findings include hypoglycaemia, hypoketonuria, high serum ammonia, and slight elevation of serum aminotransferases. Low ketones during severe hypoglycaemia strongly suggest a specific defect of fatty acid oxidation. Liver biopsy, when performed, reveals an increase in both macro- and microvesicular fat and mitochondrial abnormalities.

Trifunctional enzyme deficiency
Three adults patients from a family with recurrent rhabdomyolysis and peripheral neuropathy were reported (Schaefer *et al.*, 1996). A low-fat/high

carbohydrate diet was beneficial in one patient reducing the frequency of rhabdomyolytic episodes.

Medium-chain acyl-CoA-dehydrogenase deficiency
MCAD deficiency (OMIM number 22274) is the most common error of fatty oxidation found in the United States, United Kingdom and Northern Europe. It is manifested by a recurrent syndrome of somnolence, vomiting, coma, hypoglycaemia, fatty infiltration of the liver and dicarboxylic aciduria. The crises are often precipitated by intercurrent infections. Patients cannot oxidise the medium-chain fatty acids (C12 to C6). The disorder becomes life threatening during episodes of stress or fasting (Supplementary table 4 available at the *European Journal of Neurology*, www.blackwellpublishing.com), which result in decreased caloric intake or increased catabolism.

MCAD deficiency has been found in cases of Reye-like syndrome and in some cases of sudden infant death syndrome (SIDS). The first episodes of the disorder occur in the first 12–18 months of life. Incidence in the two sexes is similar. The mortality rate is 25% but can reach 60% in cases with later onset (second year of life). In half of the families there was a high incidence of death in infancy.

Hepatomegaly due to fatty liver has been described in some cases. Seizures have been reported, but it should be noted that the patients may have normal development and growth, and no clinical sign of cardiomyopathy or myopathy. During the crisis, all patients develop hypoketotic hypoglycemia, with increased ratio of FFA-to-ketone bodies, elevated serum aminotransferases and mild hyperammonaemia, probably due to increased proteolysis. Plasma and tissue carnitine is low (25% of control in liver and muscle), with increased acyl/free carnitine ratio. The secondary carnitine insufficiency observed in MCAD-deficient patients is due not only to increased excretion of acyl-carnitines, with depletion of tissue carnitine, but also to defective reabsorption in the kidney.

Molecular biology
Several laboratories have identified the molecular aetiology of MCAD deficiency as a common point

mutation in the locus lp31 (chromosome 1). The mutation, an A to G transition at nucleotide 985, leads to a substitution of lysine with glutamic acid of the mature protein dehydrogenase. It has been observed that patients with MCAD synthesise a normal-size MCAD precursor, which is usually targeted to the mitochondria. A small group (10%) of mutation carrier is completely asymptomatic.

GOOD PRACTICE POINTS

The treatment is similar in LCHAD and MCAD deficiency: fasting and long intervals between meals should be avoided; a high-carbohydrate, low-fat diet should be administered and L-carnitine supplementation can be useful in preventing secondary carnitine insufficiency (Type IV evidence). Prevention is important, considering the high incidence of the disease (1/8930 in a newborn screening program in Pennsylvania) and the good prognosis in patients under adequate dietary control. The best prevention is the identification of the patients during the asymptomatic period, possibly at birth. Screening of all newborns can be achieved by searching for the typical metabolites in the urine. In Pennsylvania (Ziadeh *et al.*, 1995) a dry blood spot test on Guthrie cards of newborn babies has been proposed analysing blood acyl carnitines using GC/MS. On peripheral blood DNA the identification of the A to G mutation, present in 90% of the patients, is obtained by restriction analysis (NcoI) of the relevant sequence amplified by the polymerase chain reaction. Data obtained after the initial screening indicate that there is a high prevalence of the mutated allele in babies of German and British heritage, whereas this mutation has been rarely found in newborns of the Mediterranean area. These data suggest that the mutation occurred in a single progenitor of a Germanic tribe. Prenatal diagnosis is possible using the same molecular analysis.

Short-chain acyl-CoA dehydrogenase deficiency
Few patients with SCAD deficiency have been described. In SCAD deficiency the dicarboxylic aciduria is not striking. Many shorter chain length fatty acid residues are seen, such as

ethylmalonic, butyric and methylsuccinic acids. In these patients, the oxidation of C4 to C6 fatty acids is compromised. As MCAD catalyses 50% of C4 dehydrogenation, the diagnosis may be difficult and may require inhibition of MCAD with specific antisera. SCAD deficiency is associated with different clinical phenotypes: a severe infantile form (Coates *et al.*, 1988) and a late onset myopathic picture.

Riboflavin-responsive multiple acyl-CoA-dehydrogenase defects (RR - MAD)

This is a relatively common LSM presenting in adult life with fluctuating episodes of profound weakness, associated with carnitine insufficiency and glutaric aciduria and usually underdiagnosed that responds dramatically to riboflavin (Antozzi *et al.*, 1994; Vergani *et al.*, 1996, 1999).

Both SCAD and MCAD activity are low in skeletal muscle and mitochondria of these patients that present with a LSM (Antozzi *et al.*, 1994; Vergani *et al.*, 1996), therefore this entity is called riboflavin responsive multiple acyl-CoA-dehydrogenase deficiency (Supplementary Table 5 available at the *European Journal of Neurology*, www.blackwellpublishing.com).

It is difficult to explain the improvement of patients and the enzyme changes observed during riboflavin treatment. Riboflavin-responsive multiple acyl-CoA dehydrogenase deficiency may be due to different mechanism(s). Riboflavin enters as a coenzyme not only in acyl-CoA dehydrogenase but also in Complex I and Complex II of the respiratory chain. Possible mechanisms of riboflavin deficiency include (a) decreased cellular riboflavin uptake and decreased FAD synthesis; (b) decreased FAD transport into mitochondria; (c) abnormal binding of FAD to apoenzymes; (d) increased catabolism of FAD for increased FADPase. The biochemical study in mitochondria and muscle of FAD and FMM levels reveals different mechanism(s) in patients with riboflavin deficiency (Vergani *et al.*, 1999).

GOOD PRACTICE POINTS

It is important to recognise these patients as they improve after riboflavin treatment (100–200 mg/day). Several cases of LSM-associated beta-oxidation defects have been reported due to multiple acyl CoA dehydrogenase deficiencies that were riboflavin responsive (class IV evidence).

Evidence that a biochemical defect involving the oxidation of short-chain fatty acids causes a deficiency of both SCAD, MCAD and FAD and FMN cofactor depletion in biopsied muscle mitochondria has to be found in most cases, especially in those who are riboflavin responsive (Vergani *et al.*, 1999).

GOOD PRACTICE POINTS

Treatment of Fatty Acid Disorders

The main caution in defects of mitochondrial β-oxidation is the avoidance of fasting (class IV evidence). By not allowing patients in such disorders to become dependent for energy needs on β-oxidation the accumulation of toxic intermediate metabolites is avoided and development of most critical symptoms is minimized. Fat consumption should be restricted to 25% of total calories and the intake should be a reduced amount of LCFA (class IV evidence). Increased caloric intake from carbohydrates may be necessary during intermittent illness due to increased metabolic demands on the body. A low fat/high carbohydrate diet is beneficial in reducing rhabdomyolitic episodes in several disorders of fatty acid metabolism including CPT2 deficiency (Orngreen *et al.*, 2003) and trifunctional enzyme deficiency (Schaefer *et al.*, 1996).

The current dietary treatment of LCFA defects (high carbohydrate with medium-even-chain triglycerides and reduced long-chain fats) represent evidence provided by expert opinion alone or by descriptive case series without controls. It is difficult to perform double blind studies to prevent cardiomyopathy, rhabdomyolysis and muscle weakness. A possible alternative diet has been proposed by replacing dietary medium-even-chain fatty acids by medium-odd-chain fatty acids (Roe *et al.*, 2002), or by precursors of acetyl-CoA such as by the anaplerotic effect of propionyl-CoA* to restore energy production and improve cardiac and skeletal muscle function.

*The anaplerotic capacity of propionyl CoA refers to the possibility of providing direct energy to the Krebs cycle, being a precursor of acetyl-CoA.

Conflicts of interest

The authors have no conflict of interest in this Chapter.

Acknowledgements

This paper was prepared as part of a European Biobank Network.

References

Angelini C, Vergani L, Martinuzzi A (1992). Clinical and Biochemical aspects of carnitine deficiency and insufficiency: transport defects and inborn errors of beta-oxidation. *Crit Rev Clin Lab Sci* **29:**217–242.

Angelini C, Federico A, Reichmann H, Lombes A, Chinnery P, Turnbull D (2006). Task force guidelines handbook: EFNS guidelines on diagnosis and management of fatty acid mitochondrial disorders. *Eur J Neurology* **13:**in press.

Antozzi C, Garavaglia B, Mora M *et al.* (1994). Late-onset riboflavin responsive myopathy with combined multiple acyl-CoA dehydrogenase and respiratory chain deficiency. *Neurology* 2153–2158.

Better OS, Stein GH (1990). Early management of shock and prophylaxis of acute renal failure in traumatic rhabdomyolisis. *New Engl J Med* **322:**825–829.

Brainin M, Barnes M, Baron JC, Gilhus NE, Hughes R, Selmaj K, Waldemar G (2004). Guidance for the preparation of neurological management guidelines by EFNS scientific task forces–revised recommendations 2004. *Eur J Neurol* **11:**577–581.

Chapoy PR, Angelini C, Brown WJ, Stiff J, Shug AL, Cederbaum SD (1980). Systemic carnitine deficiency: a treatable inherited lipid storage disease presenting as recurrent Reye's syndrome. *New Engl J Med* **303:**1389–1394.

Coates PM, Acili DE, Finocchiaro G, Tanaka K, Winter SC (1988). Genetic deficiency of short chain acylcoenzyme A dehydrogenase in cultured fibroblasts from a patient with muscle carnitine deficiency and severe skeletal muscle weakness. *J Clin Invest* **81:**171–175.

Engel AG, Angelini C (1973). Carnitine deficiency of human skeletal muscle with associated lipid storage myopathy: reports of a new syndrome. *Science* **179:**899–902.

Hale DE, Batshaw MC, Coates P *et al.* (1985). Long-chain Acylcoenzyme A dehydrogenase deficiency: an inherited cause of no ketotic hypoglicemia. *Paediatric Res* **19:**666–671.

Nezu J, Tamai I, Oku A, Ohashi R, Yabuuchi H, Hashimoto N, Nikaido H, Sai Y, Koizumi A, Shoji Y, Takada G, Matsuishi T, Yoshino M, Kato H, Ohura T, Tsujimoto G, Hayakawa J, Shimane M, Tsuji A (1999). Primary systemic carnitine deficiency is caused by mutations in a gene encoding sodium ion-dependent carnitine transporter. *Nat Genet* **21(1):**91–94.

Olgivie I, Pourfarzam M, Jackons S *et al.* (1994). Very long-chain acyl-Coenzyrne A dehydrogenase deficiency presenting with exercise induced myoglobinuria. *Neurology* **44:**463–473.

Orngreen MC, Ejstrup R, Vissing J (2003). Effect of diet on exercise tolerance in carnitine palmitoyltransferase II deficiency. *Neurology* **61:**559–561.

Orngreen MC, Norgaard MG, Sacchetti M, van Engelen BG, Vissing J (2004). Fuel utilization in patients with very long-chain acyl-coa dehydrogenase deficiency. *Ann Neurol* **56:**279–283.

Orngreen MC, Duno M, Ejstrup R, Christensen E, Schwartz M, Sacchetti M, Vissing J (2005). Fuel utilization in subjects with carnitine palmitoyltransferase 2 gene mutations. *Ann Neurol* **57:**60–66.

Roe CR, Sweetman L, Roe DS, David F, Brunengraber H (2002). Treatment of cardiomyopathy and rhabdomyolysis in long-chain fat oxidation disorders using an anaplerotic odd-chain triglyceride. *J Clin Invest* **110:**259–269.

Schaefer J, Jackson S, Dick DJ, Turnbull DM (1996). Trifunctional enzyme deficiency: adult presentation of a usually fatal beta-oxidation defect. *Ann Neurol* **40:**597–602.

Tang NL, Ganapathy V, Wu X, Hui J, Seth P, Yuen PM, Wanders RJ, Fok TF, Hjelm NM (1999). Mutations of OCTN2, an organic cation/carnitine transporter, lead to deficient cellular carnitine uptake in primary carnitine deficiency. *Hum Mol Genet* **8:**655–660.

Tein L, De Vivo C, Brieman F *et al.* (1990). Impaired skin fibroblast carnitine uptake in primary systemic carnitine deficiency manifested by childhood carnitine-responsive cardiomyopathy. *Paediatric Res* **28:**247–255.

Vergani L, Angelini C (1999). Infantile lipid storage myopathy with nocturnal hypoventilation shows abnormal low-affinity muscle carnitine uptake in vitro. *Neuromusc Disord* **9(5):**320–322.

Vergani L, Angelini C, Pegoraro E *et al.* (1996). Hereditary protein C deficiency associated with riboflavin responsive lipid storage myopathy. *Euro J Neurol* **3:** 61–65.

Vergani L, Barile M, Angelini C *et al.* (1999). Riboflavin therapy: biochemical heterogeneity in two adult lipid storage myopathies. *Brain* **122:**2401–2411.

Vockley J, Whiteman DA (2002). Defects of mitochondrial beta-oxidation: a growing group of disorders. *Neuromuscul Disord* **12(3):**235–246.

Wang Y, Taroni F, Garavaglia B, Longo N (2000). Functional analysis of mutations in the OCTN2 transporter causing primary carnitine deficiency: lack of genotype-phenotype correlation. *Hum Mutat* **16:** 401–407.

Ziadeh R, Hoffman EP, Finegold DN *et al.* (1995). Medium-chain acyl-CoA dehydrogenase deficiency in Pennsylvania: neonatal screening shows high incidence and unexpected mutation frequencies. *Paediatric Res* **37:**675–678.

CHAPTER 41

Narcolepsy

M. Billiard,[a] C. Bassetti,[b] Y. Dauvilliers,[c]
L. Dolenc-Grošelj,[d] G.J. Lammers,[e] G. Mayer,[f]
T. Pollmächer,[g] P. Reading,[h] K. Sonka[i]

Abstract

Background Management of narcolepsy with or
without cataplexy relies on several classes of drugs,
namely stimulants for excessive daytime sleepiness
and irresistible episodes of sleep, antidepressants
for cataplexy and hypnosedative drugs for disturbed nocturnal sleep. In addition behavioural
measures can be of notable value. Guidelines on
the management of narcolepsy have already been
published. However, contemporary guidelines are
necessary given the growing use of modafinil to
treat excessive daytime sleepiness in Europe within
the last 5–10 years, and the decreasing need for
amphetamines and amphetamine-like stimulants;
the extensive use of new antidepressants in the
treatment of cataplexy, apart from consistent randomized placebo-controlled clinical trials; and the
present re-emergence of gammahydroxybutyrate
(GHB) under the name sodium oxybate, as a treatment of all major symptoms of narcolepsy.

Methods A task force composed of the leading specialists of narcolepsy in Europe was appointed.
This task force conducted an extensive review of
pharmacological and behavioural trials available in
the literature. All trials were analysed according to
their class evidence.

Recommendations concerning the treatment of
each single symptom of narcolepsy as well as general recommendations were made. Modafinil is the
first-line pharmacological treatment of excessive
daytime sleepiness and irresistible episodes of sleep
in association with behavioural measures. However, based on several large randomized controlled
trials showing the activity of sodium oxybate not
only on cataplexy but also on excessive daytime
sleepiness and irresistible episodes of sleep, it is
likely that there is a growing tendency to use it
for the later indications if it is registered. Given
the availability of modafinil and the foreseen availability of sodium oxybate, the place of other
compounds will become fairly limited. Since its
recent registration for cataplexy sodium oxybate
has now become the first line treatment of cataplexy. Second line treatments are antidepressants,

[a]School of Medicine, University of Montpellier,
Montpellier, France; [b]Neurology Department, University
Hospital, Zurich, Switzerland; [c]Neurology Department,
Guide Chauliac Hospital, Montpellier, France; [d]Institute
of Clinical Neurophysiology, Division of Neurology,
University Medical Center, Ljubljana, Slovenia;
[e]Department of Neurology and Clinical
Neurophysiology, Leiden University, Medical Center,

Leiden, The Netherlands; [f]Hephata Klinik, Department
of Neurology, Schwalmstadt-Treysa, Germany; [g]Zentrum
für Psychiatrie und Psychotherapie, Klinikum
Ingolstadt, Ingolstadt, Germany; [h]The James Cook
University Hospital, Middlesbrough, United Kingdom;
[i]Department of Neurology, Charles University, Prague,
Czech Republic.

either tricyclics or newer antidepressants, the later being increasingly used these past years despite few or no randomized placebo-controlled clinical trials. As for disturbed nocturnal sleep the best option is still hypnotics until sodium oxybate is registered. Psychostimulants should be considered either if modafinil causes adverse effects or if there is insufficient or decreasing activity. The first-line treatment of cataplexy remains tricyclic antidepressants for a majority of sleep specialists. However, the alternative treatment sodium oxybate is based on several large search-randomized controlled trials and it might become the drug of choice when it is registered in Europe. A series of other compounds, such as norepinephrine/serotonine, norepinephrine and serotonine uptake blockers are increasingly used despite few or no randomized placebo-controlled clinical trials.

Objectives

The treatments used for narcolepsy, either pharmacological or behavioural, are diverse. However, the quality of the published clinical evidences supporting them varies widely and studies comparing the efficacy of different substances are lacking. Several treatments are used on an empirical basis, specially antidepressants for cataplexy, due to the fact that these medications are already used widely in depressed patients, leaving little motivation from the manufacturers to investigate efficacy in relatively rare indications. Others, in particular the more recently developed substances, such as modafinil or sodium oxybate, are evaluated in large randomized placebo-controlled trials. Our objective was to reinforce the use of those drugs evaluated in randomized placebo-controlled trials and to reach a consensus, as much as possible, on the use of other available medications.

Background

Narcolepsy is a disabling syndrome, first described by Westphal (1877) and Gelineau (1880). Excessive daytime sleepiness is the main symptom of narcolepsy. It includes a feeling of sleepiness waxing and waning throughout the day and episodes of irresistible sleep recurring daily or almost daily.

Cataplexy is the second commonest symptom of narcolepsy and the most specific one. It is defined as a sudden loss of voluntary muscle tone with preserved consciousness triggered by emotion. Its frequency is extremely variable from one or less per year to several per day. Other symptoms referred to as auxiliary symptoms are less specific and not essential for the diagnosis. They include hypnagogic and hypnopompic hallucinations, visual perceptual experiences occurring at sleep onset or on awakening, sleep paralysis, a transient generalized inability to move or to speak during the transition from wakefulness to sleep or vice-versa, and disturbed nocturnal sleep with frequent awakenings and parasomnias. Obesity, headache, memory/concentration difficulties, depressed mood, psychosocial problems and accidents are additional common features of narcolepsy.

The prevalence of narcolepsy is estimated around 25 per 100 000 in Caucasian populations. It is often extremely incapacitating, interfering with every aspect of life, in work and social settings.

Excessive daytime sleepiness is life long although it diminishes with age as assessed by the multiple sleep latency test, an objective test of sleepiness based on 20-min polygraphic recording sessions repeated every 2 h, four or five times a day. Cataplexy may vanish after a certain time spontaneously or with treatment. Hypnagogic hallucinations and sleep paralysis are most often temporary. Disturbed nocturnal sleep has no spontaneous tendency to improve with time.

In the revised International Classification of Sleep Disorders (2005), two forms of narcolepsy are distinguished: narcolepsy with cataplexy and narcolepsy without cataplexy.

The essential diagnostic criteria of narcolepsy with cataplexy are:

A. The patient has a complaint of excessive daytime sleepiness occurring almost daily for at least 3 months.
B. A definite history of cataplexy, defined as sudden and transient episodes of loss of muscle tone triggered by emotions, is present.
C. The diagnosis of narcolepsy with cataplexy should, whenever possible, be confirmed by

nocturnal polysomnography followed by a multiple sleep latency test (MSLT). The mean sleep latency on MSLT is less than or equal to 8 min and two or more sleep onset REM periods (SOREMPs) are observed following sufficient nocturnal sleep (minimum 6 h) during the night prior to the test. Alternatively, hypocretin-1 levels in the CSF are less than or equal to 110 pg/ml, or one third of mean normal control values.

D. The hypersomnia is not better explained by another sleep disorder, medical or neurological disorder, mental disorder, medication use, or substance use disorder.

The diagnostic criteria of narcolepsy without cataplexy include criteria A and D, while criteria B and C are as follows:

B. Typical cataplexy is not present, although doubtful or atypical cataplexy-like episodes may be reported.
C. The diagnosis of narcolepsy without cataplexy must be confirmed by nocturnal polysomnography followed by an MSLT. In narcolepsy without cataplexy, the mean sleep latency on MSLT is less than or equal to 8 min and two or more SOREMPs are observed following sufficient nocturnal sleep (minimum 6 h) during the night prior to the test.

Recent years have been characterized by several breakthroughs in the understanding of the pathophysiology of the condition. First, there have been the discoveries of a mutation of the hypocretin type 2 receptor in the autosomal recessive canine model of narcolepsy and of a narcoleptic phenotype in the orexin (hypocretin) knockout mice. Then came the observation of lowered or undetectable levels of hypocretin-1 in the CSF of most human narcoleptics and the finding that sporadic narcolepsy, in dogs and humans, may also be related to a deficiency in the production of hypocretin-1 ligands. The undetectable hypocretin-1 levels seem to be the consequence of a selective degeneration of hypocretin cells in the lateral hypothalamus. An autoimmune aetiology is hypothesized. However, direct evidence for such a mechanism is still lacking.

Compared to these advances there has been no revolutionary new treatments developed for excessive daytime sleepiness or cataplexy in the last few years, except for the recent trials with intravenous immunoglobulin (IVIg). However, there are several reasons for producing contemporary guidelines on the management of narcolepsy. First, modafinil has been used in Europe for over 10 years, decreasing the need to use amphetamine and amphetamine-like stimulants. Second, the newer antidepressants are now widely used in the treatment of cataplexy. Third, sodium oxybate, a drug previously referred to as gamma-hydroxybutyrate has been registered for use in cataplexy and is currently submitted for use in all symptoms of narcolepsy.

The first effort in standardizing the treatment of narcolepsy was the 'Practice parameters for the use of stimulants in the treatment of narcolepsy' (Standards of Practice Committee of the American Academy of Sleep Medicine, 1994). Seven years later an update of these practice parameters for the treatment of narcolepsy grading the evidence available and modifying the 1994 practice parameters was published, (Standards of Practice Committee of the American Academy of Sleep Medicine, 2001). Finally, Guidelines on the diagnosis and management of narcolepsy in adults and children were prepared for the United Kingdom (Briton *et al.* 2002).

Methods and search strategy

The best available evidence to address each question was sought, with the classification scheme by type of study design according to the EFNS Guidance document (Brainin *et al.*, 2004). If the highest level of evidence was not sufficient or required updating the literature search was extended to the lower adjacent level of evidence. Several databases were used including Cochrane library, MEDLINE, EMBASE and Clinical Trials until September 2004. Previous guidelines for treatment were sought. Each member of the Task force was assigned a special task, primarily based on symptoms of narcolepsy (excessive daytime sleepiness and irresistible episodes of sleep, cataplexy, hallucinations and sleep paralysis, disturbed nocturnal sleep, parasomnias) and also on associated features (obstructive sleep apnea hypopnea syndrome, periodic limb movements in sleep, neuropsychiatric symptoms) and special treatments (behavioural and experimental).

Methods for reaching consensus

Each member of the Task force was first invited to send his own contribution to the chairman. Then a meeting gathering seven of the nine members of the Task force was scheduled during the V International Symposium on Narcolepsy in Ascona, Switzerland, 10–15 October 2004. A draft of the Guidelines was then prepared by the chairman and circulated among all members of the task force for comments. On receipt of these comments the chairman prepared the final version that was circulated again among members for endorsement.

Results

Excessive daytime sleepiness and irresistible episodes of sleep

Modafinil and methylphenidate have the indication narcolepsy. Sodium oxybate is currently submitted for all symptoms of narcolepsy. All other drugs are 'off-label'.

(1) Modafinil (N06BA05)

Modafinil is a (2-[(diphenylmethyl) sulfinyl] acetamide) chemically unrelated to CNS stimulants such as amphetamine and methylphenidate. Involvement of adrenergic alpha1 stimulation (Lin *et al.*, 1992), indirect and direct interactions of dopamine systems (Mignot *et al.*, 1994; Ferraro *et al.*, 1996; Dauvilliers *et al.*, 2001; Wisor *et al.*, 2001) and involvement of serotonergic/GABAergic mechanisms (Ferraro *et al.*, 1996) have been suggested as possible mechanisms of action. Elimination half-life is 10–12 h.

Four major class I evidence studies (Billiard *et al.*, 1994, 50 patients; Broughton *et al.*, 1997, 70 patients; U.S. Modafinil in narcolepsy multicenter study groups 1998 and 2000, 285 and 273 patients) have shown the efficacy of modafinil on excessive daytime sleepiness at doses, 300, 200

and 400 mg/day. The key points of these studies were a reduction of daytime sleepiness, an overall benefit noted by physicians as well as by patients, and a significant improvement in maintaining wakefulness measured by the MWT, with the 300 mg/day dose (Billiard *et al.*, 1994); a significant decrease of the likelihood of falling asleep measured by the Epworth Sleepiness Scale (ESS), a reduction of irresistible episodes of sleep and of severe somnolence as assessed by the sleep log and a significant improvement in maintaining wakefulness measured with the MWT, with both 200 and 400 mg/day doses (Broughton *et al.*, 1997); consistent improvements in subjective measures of sleepiness (ESS) and in clinician assessed change in the patient's condition (Clinical Global Impression or CGI), significant improvement in maintaining wakefulness (MWT) and in decreasing sleepiness judged on the MSLT with both the 200 and the 400 mg/day doses (U.S. Modafinil in Narcolepsy multicenter study groups 1998 and 2000).

Three further studies have dealt with open label extension data. Beusterien *et al.* (1999) reported significantly high scores on 10 of 17 health related quality of life scales in 558 narcoleptic patients on modafinil 400 mg/day dose, with positive treatment effects sustained over the 40-week extension period. Moldofsky *et al.* (2000) reported on 69 patients who entered a 16-week open label extension, followed by a randomized placebo-controlled 2-week period of assessment. Mean sleep latencies on the MWT were 70% longer in the modafinil group compared to placebo. The latency to sleep decreased from 15.3 to 9.7 min in the group switched from modafinil to placebo, and the ESS score increased from 12.9 to 14.4. Mitler *et al.* (2000) reported on 478 patients who were enrolled in two 40-week open label extension studies. The majority of patients (75%) received modafinil 400 mg daily. Disease severity improved in >80% of patients throughout the 40-week study.

According to a class I evidence study (Schwartz *et al.*, 2003) in which the efficacy of modafinil 400 mg once daily, 400 mg given in a split dose, or 200 mg once daily was compared, the 400 mg split-dose regimen improved wakefulness significantly in the evening compared with the 200 mg and 400 mg once daily regimen (both $p < 0.05$).

Although co-administration of drugs is very common in the treatment of narcolepsy with cataplexy, there is little systematic evidence to support particular combinations. In volunteers there appears to be no pharmacokinetic interactions between modafinil and d-amphetamine or methylphenidate.

In the randomized trials adverse effects were minimal. In the Broughton *et al.* study (1997), the modafinil 400 mg group had more nauseas and nervousness than the modafinil 200 mg and placebo groups. In the U.S. Modafinil Multicenter Study Group 1998 trial, headache was reported in the treatment groups with a frequency of 52% in the modafinil 200 mg/day, 51% in the modafinil 400 mg/day and 36% in the placebo groups, respectively. However, it is our experience that headache usually disappears after several weeks. In the U.S. Modafinil multicenter study group 2000 trial, modafinil was associated with nausea and rhinitis in 11–13% of the subjects compared with 2–3% in the placebo group.

There is no reported evidence that tolerance develops to the effects of modafinil on excessive daytime sleepiness, although some clinicians have observed it. Similarly, it is generally accepted that modafinil has a low abuse potential. On rare occasions worsening of cataplexy with modafinil has been observed.

The possibility of induction of human hepatic cytochrome P450 enzymes by modafinil should be borne in mind. For example modafinil increases the metabolism of the oral contraceptives (Palovaara *et al.*, 2000) and a product containing 50 μg or higher ethinyloestradiol should be prescribed.

Teratology studies performed in animals did not provide any evidence of harm to the foetus (FDA B-category). However, modafinil is not recommended in narcoleptic pregnant women as clinical studies are still insufficient.

Behavioural treatments

Although non-pharmacological treatments of narcolepsy have more or less always been part of an integrative treatment concept, very little systematic studies have been performed investigating the impact of such approaches on the symptomatology of narcoleptic patients.

Five class II evidence studies and three class III evidence studies investigated the effects of various sleep-wake schedules on excessive daytime sleepiness and sleep in narcoleptic patients. However, most of these studies were extremely heterogeneous and only two studies (Rogers and Aldrich, 1993; Rogers *et al.*, 2001) looked at the effects of a behavioural regime in a clinically meaningful time range (2–4 weeks). All other studies considered only acute (1–2 days) manipulations. Among those, a study by Mullington and Broughton (1993) tested two napping strategies, a single long nap placed 180° out of phase with the nocturnal midsleep time (i.e. with the midnap point positioned 12 h after the nocturnal midsleep time) and five naps positioned equidistantly throughout the day, with the midnap time of the third nap set at 180° out of phase with the nocturnal midsleep and the others equidistant between the hours of morning awakening and evening sleep onset. The two protocols tested resulted in a reaction time improvement, but no difference between long and multiple naps was disclosed. Most experts agree that patients should live a regular life: go to bed at the same hour each night and rise at the same time each day.

RECOMMENDATIONS

First-line pharmacological treatment of excessive daytime sleepiness and irresistible episodes of sleep should rely on modafinil, 100–400 mg per day, given in two doses, one in the morning and one early in the afternoon (Level A). In a few cases dosage should be increased up to 300 mg twice a day. Increase of the daily dosage above 600 mg is in general not advisable. However there is a growing tendency in the USA to use sodium oxybate as first line treatment of excessive daytime sleepiness, and this could be the case in Europe as well if sodium oxybate is registered for "narcolepsy" (including cataplexy, excessive daytime sleepiness and disturbed nocturnal sleep). The starting dose is 4.5 g/night, divided into two equal doses of 2.25 g/night. The dose may be increased to a maximum of 9 g/night, divided into two equal doses of 4.5 g/night by increments of 1.5 g. Two weeks are recommended between dosage increments. Many patients will start to feel better within the first few days but they will not have their optimal response for a few weeks. Most patients will have about 75% of the improvement that they are going to see at any given dose after about four weeks, but to get maximal response at any given dose may take as long as 8 to 12 weeks. If modafinil or sodium oxybate is unsatisfactory the alternative drug can be added. Given these different possibilities the place left for other compounds becomes extremely limited.

Behavioural treatment measures are always advisable. Essentially, the studies available support on a B level the recommendation to take planned naps during the day, as naps decrease sleep tendency and shorten reaction time. Because of varying performance demands and limitations on work or home times for taking them, naps are best scheduled on a patient by patient basis.

Second-line treatment should be considered either in case of adverse effects such as disabling headache or nervousness or if there is insufficient efficacy, either from the outset of treatment or subsequently. Choice of second-line medication depends on personal preference and availability of the drug in the particular country. Methylphenidate, slow release, starting with 5–10 mg up to 60 mg/day, mazindol, starting with 1 mg up to 6 mg/day, are the main alternatives (Level B). In cases where these drugs are ineffective or unavailable, the use of d-amphetamine slow release or methamphetamine, under close control (Level B) is recommended. Although co-administration of drugs is common in the treatment of narcolepsy there is little systematic evidence to support particular combinations. In volunteers there appear to be no pharmacological interactions between modafinil and dexamphetamine or methylphenidate. Finally, the order of preference may have to be totally reconsidered if sodium oxybate becomes available, following agreement from European authorities (Level A), provided patients are warned of the risk of abuse if the drug is taken at high doses.

(2) Amphetamines and amphetamine-like CNS stimulants

Amphetamine (N06BA01*)

At low doses the main effect of amphetamine is to release dopamine and to a lesser extent norepinephrine and serotonine. At higher doses monoaminergic depletion and inhibition of reuptake occurs. The d-isomer of amphetamine is more specific for dopaminergic transmission and is a better stimulant compound. Methamphetamine is more lipophilic than d-amphetamine and therefore has more central and fewer peripheral effects than d-amphetamine. The elimination half-life of these drugs is between 10 and 30 h.

Five reports concerned the use of amphetamines. Three class II evidence studies (Shindler et al., 1985; Mitler et al., 1990, 1993) showed that d-amphetamine and methamphetamine are effective treatments of excessive daytime sleepiness in short-term use (up to 4 weeks) at starting doses of 15–20 mg increasing up to 60 mg/day. One class IV evidence study (Chen et al., 1995) showed that long-term drug treatment would result in only minor reduction in irresistible sleep episode propensity.

The main adverse effects are minor irritability, hyperactivity, mood changes, headache, palpitations, sweating, tremors, anorexia and insomnia (Mitler et al., 1994). Doses of amphetamine > 60–100 mg daily often cause serious toxic effects including 'very fast thinking', 'difficulty controlling burst of thoughts', 'bursts of verbal aggressiveness'. Psychotic reactions occur in less than 1% of subjects (Guilleminault, 1993). There are conflicting views on the risk of developing hypertension under chronic administration.

Tolerance to amphetamine effect may develop in up to one third of patients (Guilleminault, 1993). There is little or no evidence of abuse and addiction in narcoleptic patients (Parkes and Dahlitz, 1993).

The FDA classifies drugs as A (controlled studies in humans have shown no risk), B (controlled studies in animals have shown no risk), C (controlled studies in animals have shown risk),

---

*Anatomical Therapeutic Chemical (ATC) nomenclature.

D (controlled studies in humans have shown risk) according to their embryotoxic and teratogenic effects. Dextroamphetamine, with a FDA-D classification and methamphetamine, with a FDA-C classification, are contraindicated during conception and pregnancy.

Amphetamines are controlled drugs.

Methylphenidate (N06BA04)
Similar to the action of amphetamine methylphenidate induces dopamine release, but in contrast, it does not have any major effect on monoamine storage. The clinical effect of methylphenidate is supposed to be similar to that of amphetamines. However, clinical experience would argue for a slight superiority of amphetamines. In comparison with amphetamine, methylphenidate has a much shorter elimination half-life (2–7 h) and the daily dose may be divided into 2–3 parts. A sustained release form is available and can be useful for some patients.

There were five reports on the use of methylphenidate. There was only one class II evidence study showing significant improvement in all dosages (10, 30, 60 mg/day) compared to baseline (Mitler *et al.*, 1986). According to a class IV evidence study (Yoss and Daly, 1959) methylphenidate conveyed good to excellent response in 68% of cases and according to another one (Honda *et al.*, 1979) methylphenidate produced marked to moderate improvement in 90% of cases. On the Maintenance of Wakefulness Test (MWT) the sleep latencies were increased to 80% of controls with a 60 mg daily dose (Mitler *et al.*, 1990).

Adverse effects are the same as with amphetamines. However, methylphenidate probably has a better therapeutic index than d-amphetamine with less reduction of appetite or increase in blood pressure (Guilleminault *et al.*, 1974).

Tolerance may develop. Abuse potential is low in narcoleptic patients.

Methyphenidate has no FDA classification because no adequate animal or human studies have been performed. It is contraindicated in pregnant women.

(3) Gamma-hydroxybutyrate (GHB), Sodium oxybate (in its most recent designation) (N07XX04)

GHB is a natural neurotransmitter/neuromodulator that may act through its own receptors and via stimulation of GABA-B receptors. A major effect may be silencing of dopaminergic neurons. Its elimination half-life is 90–120 min.

Broughton and Mamelak (1979) were the first to suggest that GHB was useful to control cataplexy, enhance daytime alertness and improve night sleep in narcoleptic patients. In 1989 Scrima *et al.* published the first reports of a class II evidence study showing no effect of GHB at a dose of 25–50 mg/kg, twice a night, on subjective estimates of sleep latency at night and on the Stanford Sleepiness Scale (SSS). Later on an evidence class 1 study (Lammers *et al.*, 1993) found a substantial improvement of all parameters of subjective daytime sleepiness with two nocturnal doses of 30 mg/kg, although MSLT results were not significantly different from placebo. The main potential problem with GHB is abuse potential. GHB is misused in athletes due to its metabolic effects (growth hormone releasing effect) and it has been used as a 'date rape' drug because of its rapid sedating effects. However, the monitored prescription programme in the United States revealed that this is very low risk in narcoleptic patients. Cases of overdose or severe withdrawal symptoms are occasionally observed in emergency rooms. Adverse effects, in particular when using high doses, may be enuresis and somnambulism. Waking up while the drug is still centrally active may result in dizziness and gait problems.

Gamma-hydroxybutyrate has recently re-emerged as a major treatment for narcolepsy with cataplexy under the name sodium oxybate (the terms 'GHB', '4-hydroxybutyric acid, sodium salt', and 'sodium oxybate' are completely synonymous). Four class I evidence studies (U.S. Xyrem Multicenter Study Group, 2002 and 2003; Mamelak *et al.* 2004; The Xyrem International Study Group 2005) have shown reduced excessive daytime sleepiness, increased level of alertness and ability to concentrate and a recent class I evidence study has shown sodium oxybate and modafinil to be equally efficacious for the treatment of excessive daytime sleepiness (data on file at Orphan Medical). Starting dose is 3–4.5 g/night. Full therapeutic benefit generally occurs at the 6–9 g/night doses. This drug is only available in liquid form and must be taken twice a night.

Most commonly reported adverse effects are nausea, which usually goes away after a few days, nocturnal enuresis which may persist intermittently, confusional arousals and headache. Of concern is the above mentioned abuse potential of GHB. While there is no clear evidence of emergence of dependence in patients taking sodium oxybate at therapeutic doses, this possibility cannot be excluded.

Animal studies have shown no evidence of teratogenicity (FDA B-category). However, the potential risk for humans is unknown, and sodium oxybate is not recommended during pregnancy.

(4) Other compounds

Pemoline (N06BA05)

Pemoline, an oxazolidine derivative with long half-life (12 h) and mild action, selectively blocks dopamine reuptake and only weakly stimulates dopamine release.

There were two reports on the use of pemoline in narcoleptic patients. According to a class II evidence study (Mitler *et al.*, 1986) using three dosages (18.75; 56.25 and 112.50 mg/day) pemoline did not improve wakefulness but it did improve ability to perform Wilkinson Addition and Digit-Symbol Substitution tests on a 112.50 mg daily dose. According to a class IV evidence study (Honda and Hishikawa, 1980) there was a moderate to marked improvement in sleepiness in 65% of narcoleptic subjects.

Pemoline is usually better tolerated than d-amphetamine or methamphetamine in terms of adverse effects (minimal sympathomimetic effects) and tolerance (Honda and Hishikawa, 1980). Due to potential lethal hepatotoxicity, the medication has been withdrawn in several countries.

Pemoline is classified as FDA B-category (no risk in animal studies), but there have been no controlled studies in humans, so that the drug is not recommended during pregnancy.

Mazindol (A08AA06)

Mazindol is an imidazolidine derivative with pharmacological effects similar to the amphetamines. It is a weak releasing agent for dopamine, but it also blocks dopamine and norepinephrine reuptake with high affinity. Its elimination half-life is around 10 h.

There were five reports on the use of mazindol in treating excessive daytime sleepiness in narcoleptic patients. According to a class II evidence study (Shindler *et al.*, 1985) mazindol was effective in reducing sleepiness at a dose of 2 + 2 mg/day (during 4 weeks) in 53–60% of subjects. In addition several class IV evidence studies (Parkes and Schachter, 1979; Iijima *et al.*, 1980; Vespignani *et al.*, 1984; Alvarez *et al.*, 1991) have shown significant improvement of sleepiness in 50–75% of patients. Clinical experience suggests to start treatment at a low dosage of 1 mg/day which may be effective in individual patients.

Adverse effects include dry mouth, nervousness, constipation, and less frequently nausea, vomiting, headache, dizziness, tachycardia and excessive sweating. Rare cases of pulmonary hypotension and valvular abnormalities have been reported. For this reason it has been withdrawn from the market in several countries. The use in narcolepsy is still warranted according to most experts, but as second-line treatment and with close monitoring. Tolerance is uncommon and abuse potential may be low (Parkes and Schachter, 1979). Mazindol is also classified as FDA B-category, without controlled studies in humans. It is not recommended in pregnant women.

Phenelzine (N06AF03)

Phenelzine is a non-selective MAOI that can cause hypertensive crises if tyramine or dopamine-containing food or sympathomimetic agents are ingested concurrently.

Wyatt *et al.* (1971) administered phenelzine (60–90 mg/day) for 1 year to seven narcoleptic patients who previously had unsatisfactory responses to more conventional forms of therapy. All patients noted improvement in cataplexy and irresistible episodes of sleep, although three continued to experience some drowsiness.

However, there is the above mentioned risk of hypertensive crisis and the necessity to avoid some drugs and to adhere to certain dietary restriction that makes this medication unsuitable for long-term treatment.

Selegiline (N04BOD1)

Selegiline is a potent irreversible MAO-B selective inhibitor. It is metabolically converted to desmethyl selegiline, amphetamine and methamphetamine. The elimination half-life of the main metabolites is variable, 2.5 h for desmethyl selegiline, 18 h for amphetamine and 21 h for methamphetamine. According to one class I evidence study (Hublin *et al.*, 1994) selegiline, 10–40 mg daily, reduced irresistible episodes of sleep and sleepiness up to 45%, and according to another one (Mayer and Meier-Ewert, 1995) selegiline at a dose of at least 20 mg/day caused a significant improvement of daytime sleepiness and a reduction of irresistible episodes of sleep, as well as a dose-dependent REM suppression during nighttime sleep and naps. The results were similar in a class IV evidence study (Reinish *et al.*, 1995) showing improvement in 73% of patients. Use of selegiline is limited by potentially sympathomimetic adverse effects and interaction with other drugs. Co-administration of triptans and serotonin specific reuptake inhibitors is contraindicated. Abuse potential is low (Hublin *et al.*, 1994; Mayer and Meier-Ewert,
1995).

Selegiline is another FDA B-category drug without controlled studies in humans. It is not recommended in pregnant women.

Monoamine oxidase inhibitors

Monoamine oxidase inhibitors (MAOIs) inhibit the oxidative deamination of the three classes of biogenic amines: noradrenergic, dopaminergic and 5-HT.

Cataplexy

Only one of the medications listed below has the indication 'cataplexy'. All other medications are 'off-label'.

(1) Gammahydroxybutyrate (GHB), sodium oxyate (in its most recent designation) (N07XX04)

According to a class II evidence study (Scrima *et al.*, 1989) GHB at a dose of 25–50 mg/kg, twice at night, reduced cataplexy in 50% of 20 subjects. Later on a class I evidence study (Lammers, 1993) showed a significant reduction in the number of cataplectic attacks per day with GHB two daily doses of 30 mg/kg at night in 24 subjects. Adverse effects were rather limited with one patient reporting a single period of protracted sleep paralysis in combination with hypnagogic hallucination in the first week of treatment and another patient reporting loss of weight in the first two weeks of treatment with GHB.

U.S. Xyrem Multicenter Study Groups 2002 and 2003 (class I evidence) have shown a significant dose dependent reduction of the number of cataplectic attacks in large samples of patients (136 in the first one and 118 in the second) in doses of sodium oxybate, 3–9 g nightly in two doses, which were significant at 4 weeks and maximal after 8 weeks. In addition, the U.S. Xyrem Multicenter Study Group 2004 was conducted to demonstrate the long-term efficacy of sodium oxybate for the treatment of cataplexy. Fifty-five narcoleptic patients with cataplexy who had received continuous treatment with sodium oxybate for 7–44 months (mean: 21 months) were enrolled in a double-blind treatment withdrawal paradigm. During the 2-week double-blind phase, the abrupt cessation of sodium oxybate therapy in the placebo group resulted in a significant increase in the number of cataplexies compared to the patients who remained on sodium oxybate. Ultimately the Xyrem International Study Group (2005) conducted a study with 228 adult narcolepsy with cataplexy patients randomized to receive 4.5, 6 or 9 g sodium oxybate nightly or placebo for 8 weeks. Compared to placebo, doses of 4.5, 6 and 9 g sodium oxybate for 8 weeks resulted in statistically significant median decreases in weekly cataplexy attacks of 57.0, 65.0 and 84.7% respectively.

Adverse effects, nausea, vomiting, headache, dizziness, sleepiness, paresthesia, tremor, enuresis were generally mild, and only dizziness occurred at a significant level ($p < 0.5$). Patients showed no evidence of tolerance.

Behavioural therapy

The single non-pharmacological approach known to specifically reduce the frequency and severity of cataplexy, which however has not been empirically studied, is to avoid precipitating factors. Because cataplexy is tightly linked to strong, particularly positive, emotions, the most important precipitating factor is social contact. Indeed, social withdrawal is frequently seen in narcolepsy and helpful in reducing cataplexy, but it can hardly be considered as a recommendation or 'treatment'.

both excessive daytime sleepiness and cataplexy (Level A). However rare, serious adverse effects have been reported with mazindol and selegiline may have sympathomimetic adverse effects and interaction with other drugs. In general there are no clear dosage recommendations for anticataplectic medications, except for tricyclics and sodium oxybate, and the dose has to be titrated according to the effect on cataplexies and adverse effects. There is no accepted behavioural treatment of cataplexy. However, advice to some subjects should include the avoidance of known triggers, whenever possible.

RECOMMENDATIONS

Based on several class 1 evidence (Level A rating) studies, first line pharmacological treatment of cataplexy is sodium oxybate at a starting dose of 4.5 g/night divided into two equal doses of 2.25 g/night. The dose may be increased to a maximum of 9 g/night, divided into two equal doses of 4.5 g/night, by increments of 1.5 g. Two weeks are recommended between dosage increments. Delays of efficacy are as pointed out in treating excessive daytime sleepiness. Second line pharmacological treatments are antidepressants. Tricyclic antidepressants, particularly clomipramine (10–75 mg), are the most potent anticataplectic drugs. However, they have the drawback of anticholinergic adverse effects. Starting dosage should always be as low as possible. Selective serotonine reuptake inhibitors are slightly less active but have less adverse effects. The norepinephrine/serotonine reuptake inhibitor venlafaxine is widely used today but lacks any published clinical evidence of efficacy. Norepinephrine reuptake inhibitors, reboxetine and atomotexine, also lack published clinical evidence. As for viloxazine it is probably less potent but may have less adverse effects than the SSRIs. Sodium oxybate benefits from published class I evidence (Level A) studies, but has not yet received licensing approval. It could become first-line treatment of cataplexy pending its approval. Mazindol and selegiline have the advantage of being partially effective for

(2) Monoamine non-specific uptake inhibitors (N06AA)

The first use of tricyclics for treating cataplexy dates back to 1960 with imipramine(Akimoto *et al.*, 1960). It was followed by desmethylimipramine(Hishikawa *et al.*, 1965), clomipramine (Passouant and Baldy-Moulinier, 1970) and protryptiline (Schmidt *et al.*, 1977).

Clomipramine, a drug that is principally a serotoninergic reuptake inhibitor, but metabolizes rapidly into desmethyl clomipramine, an active metabolite with principally adrenergic reuptake inhibitory properties, has been the most widely evaluated for cataplexy, with one class III evidence study (Schachter and Parkes, 1980) and four class IV evidence studies (Passouant and Baldy-Moulinier, 1970; Shapiro, 1975; Guilleminault *et al.*, 1976; Chen *et al.*, 1995). All these studies have shown a complete abolition or decrease in severity and frequency of cataplexy at doses of 25–75 mg daily. However, low doses of 10–20 mg daily are often very effective and it is always advisable to start with them.

Reported adverse effects consist in anticholinergic effects including dry mouth, sweating, constipation, tachycardia, weight increase, hypotension, difficulty in urinating and impotence. One trial (Guilleminault *et al.*, 1976) mentioned the development of tolerance after 4.5 months. Patients may experience with tricyclics a worsening or 'de novo' onset of REM sleep behaviour disorder. Moreover, there is a risk, if the tricyclics are suddenly withdrawn, of a marked increase in number and severity of cataplectic attacks, a situation referred to as 'rebound cataplexy', or even 'status cataplecticus'. Tolerance to the effects of tricyclics may develop.

Animal studies have not shown teratogenic properties and epidemiological studies performed in a limited number of women have not shown any risk of malformation in the fœtus (FDA B-category). However, newborns of mothers submitted to long standing treatment with high doses of antidepressants may show symptoms of atropine intoxication. Thus, if cataplexy is mild, it is advisable to cease the anti-cataplectic drug before conception. When cataplexy is severe the risk of injury during pregnancy may be greater than the risks caused to the infant by the drug.

(3) Newer antidepressants
Serotonin specific uptake inhibitors (SSRIs) (N06AB)
These compounds are much more selective than tricyclic antidepressants towards the serotoninergic transporter, although most of them have affinities for other monoamine transporters at 10–100 times higher concentrations. In comparison with tricyclics higher doses are required and effects less pronounced (Nishino and Mignot, 1997).

According to a class I evidence study (Schrader *et al.*, 1986) femoxetine, 600 mg/day, reduced cataplexy. In addition two class III evidence studies (Langdon *et al.*, 1986; Frey and Narbonne 1994) have shown fluoxetine (20–60 mg/day) and one class III evidence study (Schachter and Parkes, 1980) has shown fluvoxamine (25-200 mg/day) to be mildly active on cataplexy.

Adverse effects are less pronounced than with tricyclics. They include CNS excitation, gastrointestinal upset, movement disorders and sexual difficulties. The risk of marked increase in number and severity of cataplectic attacks has been documented after discontinuation of SSRIs (Poryazova *et al.*, 2005). Tolerance to SSRIs does not develop.

Studies performed in animals did not provide any evidence of malformation (FDA B- category). However clinical studies are not sufficient to assess a possible risk for the human fœtus. Thus the use of SSRIs is not recommended in narcoleptic pregnant women.

Norepinephrine uptake inhibitors
In a class III evidence study (Guilleminault *et al.*, 1986), viloxazine (N06AX09) at a 100 mg dose daily significantly reduced cataplexy. The main advantage of this compound rests on its limited adverse effects (nausea and headache in one subject only out of 22).

In a class IV evidence study (Larrosa *et al.*, 2001), reboxetine (N06AX18) at a daily dose of 2–10 mg, significantly reduced cataplexy. Treatment was generally well tolerated, with only minor adverse effects being reported (dry mouth, hyperhydrosis, constipation, restlessness). Atomoxetine (N06BA09) (36–100 mg/day) has been used anecdotally with success on cataplexy. Of note however, atomoxetine has been shown to slightly but significantly increase heart rate and blood pressure in large samples. Thus caution is needed.

Norepinephrine/serotoninergic uptake inhibitor
Venlafaxine (N06AX16) (150–375 mg/day), was given to four subjects, for a period of 2–7 months (Smith *et al.*, 1996). Initial improvement in both excessive daytime sleepiness and cataplexy was reported by all subjects.

No subjective adverse effects were observed apart from slight insomnia in two subjects. Increased heart rate and blood pressure are potential adverse effects. Tolerance was reported in one subject.

Venlafaxine is not recommended in pregnant narcoleptic women.

Other compounds
Mazindol (A08AA06)
Mazindol has an anticataplectic property in addition to its alerting effect. According to a class II evidence study (Schindler *et al.*, 1985) mazindol at a dose of 2+2 mg/day (during 4 weeks) did not alter the frequency of cataplexy. On the other hand, in one class IV evidence study (Iijima *et al.*, 1986) the 'percentage of efficacy' was 50% and in another class IV evidence study (Vespignani *et al.*, 1984) 85% of subjects reported significant improvement on cataplexy.

Potential adverse effects have been reviewed above.

Phenelzine (N06AF03)

As already pointed out, Wyatt *et al.* (1971) administered phenelzine (60–90 mg/day) for 1 year, to seven narcoleptic patients who previously had unsatisfactory response to more conventional forms of therapy (class IV evidence study). All patients noted improvement in cataplexy.

Selegiline (N04B0D1)

Selegiline has a potent anticataplectic effect in addition to its relatively good alerting effect. According to one class 1 evidence study selegiline reduced cataplexy up to 89% at a dose of 10–40 mg (Hublin *et al.*, 1994) and, according to a second one, reduced cataplexy significantly at a dose of 10 mg × 2 (Mayer and Meier-Ewert, 1995). Adverse effects and interaction with other drugs have been referred to above.

Amphetamine (N06BA01)

As previously indicated, the main effect of amphetamines is to release dopamine and to a lesser extent norepinephrine and serotonine. The effect of amphetamine on norepinephrine neurons, in particular, may help to control cataplexy. This may be an important factor in patients who switch from amphetamine to modafinil and find that mild cataplexy is no longer controlled.

Hallucinations and sleep paralysis

Treatment of hallucinations and sleep paralysis is considered as a treatment of REM-associated phenomena. Most studies have focused much more on the treatment of cataplexy. Improvement of cataplexy is most often associated with reduction of hallucinations and sleep paralysis. One class I evidence study (Lammers *et al.*, 1993) focused on the effects of GHB on irresistible sleep episodes, awakenings at night, cataplexy, hallucinations and sleep paralysis. There was a reduction of the daily number of hallucinations, while the effect on sleep paralysis could not be assessed due to the low incidence of this item during the baseline period.

There are no reports on attempts to modify the occurrence of these symptoms by behavioural techniques.

RECOMMENDATIONS

Recommendations are as for cataplexy.

Poor sleep
Benzodiazepines (N05CD) and non-benzodiazepines (N05CF)

A single class III evidence study (Thorpy *et al.*, 1992) has shown an improvement of sleep efficiency and overall sleep quality with triazolam 0.25 mg given for two nights only. Adverse effects were not recorded. No effect of improved sleep on excessive daytime sleepiness was recorded. No study has been performed with either zopiclone or zolpidem or zaleplon.

Gamma-hydroxybutyrate (GHB), Sodium oxybate (in its most recent designation) (N07XX04)

Studies performed with GHB 25–30 mg/kg at night have shown either a decrease of subjective arousals (Scrima *et al.*, 1989), or a decrease of the number of awakenings (Lammers *et al.*, 1993), or a decrease of sleep fragmentation (Mamelak *et al.*, 1986).

The U.S. Xyrem studies have shown a significant decrease of the number of night-time awakenings, with sodium oxybate 9 g (U.S. Xyrem Multicenter Study Group, 2002) and a significant improvement of nocturnal sleep quality ($p = 0.001$) with sodium oxybate 3–9 g , due to increased slow wave sleep (U.S. Xyrem Multicenter Study Group, 2003).

Adverse effects are the same as already listed.

Modafinil (N06BA07)

In the U.S. Modafinil in narcolepsy Multicenter Study Group (2000) a small improvement in sleep consolidation was evidenced through increased sleep efficiency. Thus it is always advisable to wait for the effects of modafinil before prescribing a special treatment for disturbed nocturnal sleep.

Behavioural therapy

No study has been conducted to investigate the effects of behavioural treatments on night sleep in narcoleptic patients in clinically relevant settings.

Parasomnias

Narcoleptic patients often display vivid and frightening dreams and REM sleep behaviour disorder (RBD). Given the beneficial effects of sodium oxybate on disturbed nocturnal sleep, this medication might be of interest in the case of disturbed dreams. However, no systematic study of sodium oxybate on dreams of narcoleptics has ever been conducted.

In the case of RBD its occurrence in narcoleptic patients is remarkable for two aspects: first, the mean age of onset of RBD in narcoleptic patients is young (between 25 and 30 years of age) and RBD may precede narcolepsy in one third of patients; second, RBD events are usually less violent in narcoleptic patients than in other patients.

There is no available report of any prospective, double-blind, placebo-controlled trial of any drug specific for RBD in narcoleptic subjects, but only a few case reports of narcoleptic subjects with RBD. Use of clonazepam was reported as successful in two cases (Schuld et al., 1999; Yeh et al., 2004). In one case (Schuld et al., 1999) clonazepam led to the development of obstructive sleep apnea syndrome. An alternative treatment is needed when patients affected with RBD do not respond or are intolerant to clonazepam. In a recent study involving 14 patients, two of whom had narcolepsy, melatonin was used successfully in 57% of cases at a dose of 3–12 mg per night (Boeve et al., 2003). Adverse effects such as sleepiness, hallucination and headache were recorded in one third of patients.

Associated features

Obstructive sleep apnea/hypopnea syndrome

According to several publications (Baker et al., 1986; Mayer et al., 2002) the prevalence of obstructive sleep apnea/hypopnea syndrome (OSAHS) is larger in narcoleptic patients than in the general population. One potential explanation is the frequency of obesity in narcolepsy, which could predispose to OSAHS. There is no documented effect of OSAHS treatments in narcoleptic patients.

Periodic limb movements in sleep

Periodic limb movements in sleep (PLMS) are more prevalent in narcolepsy than in the general population (Montplaisir et al., 2000; Mayer et al., 2002). This applies particularly to young narcoleptic patients. L-Dopa (Boivin et al., 1989), gammahydroxybutyrate (Bedard et al., 1989), bromocriptine (Boivin et al., 1993) are effective treatments. However, there is no documented effect on excessive daytime sleepiness.

Neuropsychiatric symptoms

No higher rate of psychotic manifestations has been evidenced in narcoleptic patients. On the other hand depression is more frequent in narcoleptic patients than in the general population (Roth and Nevsimalova, 1975; Broughton et al., 1981; Kales et al., 1982; Vourdas et al., 2002).

Antidepressant drugs and psychotherapy are indicated. However, there is no systematic study of these therapeutic procedures in depressed narcoleptic patients.

experience that the majority of patients refuse to continue CPAP therapy because of a lack of clinical improvement. There is usually no need to treat periodic limb movements in sleep in narcoleptic patients. Antidepressants and psychotherapy should be used in depressed narcoleptic patients (Level C) as in non-narcoleptic depressed patients.

Psychosocial support and counselling
Patients' groups
Interaction with those who have narcolepsy is often of great benefit to the patient and his (or her) spouse regarding the recognition of symptoms and possible counter measures. Here are the website addresses of four important patient support groups:

France : http://perso.wanadoo.fr/anc.paradoxal/
Germany : http://dng-ev.org
NL : http://www.narcolepsie.nl
UK : http://www.narcolepsy.org.uk

Social workers
Social workers can provide support and counselling in various important areas such as career selection, adjustments at school or at work, and when financial or marital problems exist.

RECOMMENDATIONS

Interaction with narcoleptic patients and counselling from trained social workers are recommended (Level C).

Good Practice Points
A prerequisite before implementing a potentially life-long treatment is to establish an accurate diagnosis of narcolepsy with or without cataplexy, and to check for possible comorbidity. Following a complete interview the patient should undergo an all-night polysomnography followed immediately by a MSLT. HLA typing is rarely helpful. CSF hypocretin-1 measurement may be of help and is added as diagnostic test in the revised International Classification of Sleep Disorders (2005), particularly if the MSLT cannot be used or provides conflicting information. Levels of CSF hypocretin are only significantly reduced or absent in cases of narcolepsy with cataplexy. In the absence of cataplexy, the value of measuring hypocretin is debatable.

Once diagnosed, patients must be given as much information as possible about their condition (nature of the disorder, genetic implication, medications available and their potential adverse effects) to help them cope with a potentially debilitating condition.

Regular follow-up is essential to monitor response to treatment, adapt the treatment in case of insufficient response or adverse effects, and above all encourage the patient to persist with a management plan. Repeated polysomnographic evaluation of patients should be considered in case of worsening of symptoms or development of other symptoms, but not for evaluating treatment in general.

Future treatments
Current treatments for human narcolepsy are symptomatically based. However, given the major developments in understanding the neurobiological basis of the condition, new therapies are likely to emerge. It is imperative that neurologists remain aware of future developments, not only out of interest but also because of the implications for treating a relatively common and debilitating disease.

There are three focuses for future therapy:

- Symptomatic endocrine/transmitter modulating therapies: selective histamine agonists (H3-antagonists), GHRH antagonists, GHB agonists and GABA-B agonists, most of which have been tried in narcoleptic mice or canines (Shiba et al., 2004).
- Hypocretin-based therapies: hypocretin agonists and cell transplantation (Fujiki et al., 2003; Murillo-Rodriguez et al. 2004).
- Immune-based therapies including steroid therapy, intravenous-immunoglobulins (IVIg) and plasmaphoresis.

The latter are of special interest as several attempts have been made so far in man, the most promising being an association of prednisone and

IVIg near the onset of narcolepsy in a 10-year-old boy (Lecendreux *et al.*, 2003) and IVIg alone in four subjects (Dauvilliers *et al.*, 2004) and in another four subjects (Zuberi *et al.*, 2004) with positive subjective effects mainly on cataplexy.

Conclusion

The recommendations expressed in these guidelines are based on the best currently available knowledge. However, developments in the field of narcolepsy are rapidly advancing and the use of agents such as sodium oxybate may become widespread, largely depending on regulation issues. In addition treatments directed at replacing hypocretin or even preventing the loss of neurons containing the neuropeptide may become a reality in the near future.

Conflicts of interest

Dr. Billiard received honoraria from Orphan Drugs for invited talks and is a member of the Xyrem (UCB Pharma) advisory board.

Dr. Bassetti received honoraria from Orphan Drugs for invited talks and is a member of the Xyrem (UCB Pharma) advisory board. He was involved in clinical trials with Cephalon and Orphan.

Dr. Dauvilliers was involved in a clinical trial with Cephalon and another one with Orphan.

Dr. Lammers is a member of the Narcolepsy advisory group for Organon Nederland BV (licence holder for modafinil in the Netherlands) and a member of the Xyrem (UCB Pharma) advisory board.

Dr, Mayer received honoraria from Cephalon and UCB Pharma for invited talks. He was involved in one trial with Cephalon and two trials with Orphan Drugs, He is a member of the Xyrem advisory board.

Dr, Reading received honoraria from Cephalon for invited talks.

Dr. Sonka was involved in two trials with Orphan and is currently involved in a trial with Cephalon. Dr. Sonka is also a member of the Xyrem advisory board.

Jazz and UCB manufacture and distribute sodium oxybate, respectively.

References

Akimoto H, Honda Y, Takahashi Y (1960). Pharmacotherapy in narcolepsy. *Diseases of the Nervous System* **21**:1–3.

Alvarez B, Dahlitz M, Grimshaw J, Parkes JD (1991). Mazindol in long-term treatment of narcolepsy. *Lancet* **337**:1293–1294.

American Academy of Sleep Medicine (2005). *ICSD-2 - International Classification of Sleep Disorders: Diagnostic and Coding Manual*, 2nd ed, American Academy of Sleep Medicine.

Baker TL, Guilleminault C, Nino-Murcia G, Dement WC (1986). Comparative polysomnographic study of narcolepsy and idiopathic central nervous system hypersomnia. *Sleep* **9**:232–242.

Bedard MA, Montplaisir J, Godbout R, Lapierre O (1989). Nocturnal gamma-hydroxybutyrate. Effect on periodic leg movements and sleep organization of narcoleptic patients. *Clin Neuropharmacol* **12**:29–36.

Beusterien KM, Rogers AE, Walsleben JA, Emsellem HA, Reblando JA, Wang L, Goswami M, Steinwald B (1999). Health-related quality of life effects of modafinil for treatment of narcolepsy. *Sleep* **22**:757–765.

Billiard M, Besset A, Montplaisir J, Laffont F, Goldenberg F, Weill JS, Lubin S (1994). Modafinil: a double-blind multicenter study. *Sleep* **17** (suppl):107–112.

Boeve BF, Silber MH, Ferman TJ (2003). Melatonin for treatment of REM sleep behaviour disorder in neurologic disorders: results in 14 patients. *Sleep Med* **4**:281–284.

Boivin DB, Lorrain D, Montplaisir J (1993). Effects of bromocriptine on periodic limb movements in human narcolepsy. *Neurology* **43**:2134–2136.

Boivin DB, Montplaisir J, Poirier G (1989). The effects of L-Dopa on periodic leg movements and sleep organization in narcolepsy. *Clin Neuropharmacol* **16**:339–345.

Brainin M, Barnes M, Baron JC, Gilhus NE, Hughes R, Selmaj K, Waldemar G (2004). Guidance for the preparation of neurological management guidelines by EFNS scientific task forces -revised recommendations 2004. *Eur J Neurol* **11**:577–581.

Britton T, Hansen A, Hicks J, Howard R, Meredith A, Smith I, Stores G , Wilson S, Zaiwalla Z, Zeman A (2002). Guidelines on the diagnosis and management of narcolepsy in adults and children. Evidence-based guidelines for the UK with graded recommendations. Taylor Patten Communications Ltd, UK. 65 pages.

Broughton RJ, Fleming JAE, George CFP, Hill JD, Kryger MH, Moldofsky H, Montplaisir JY,

Morehouse RL, Moscovitch A, Murphy WF (1997). Randomized, double-blind, placebo-controlled crossover trial of modafinil in the treatment of excessive daytime sleepiness in narcolepsy. *Neurology* **49**:444–451.

Broughton R, Mamelak M (1979). The treatment of narcolepsy-cataplexy with nocturnal gammahydroxybutyrate. *Can J Neurol Sci* **6**:16.

Chen SY, Cloift SJ, Dahlitz MJ, Dunn G, Parkes JD (1995). Treatment in the narcoleptic syndrome : self assessment of the action of dexamphetamine and clomipramine. *J Sleep Res* **4**:113–118.

Dauvilliers Y, Carlander B, Touchon J, Tafti M (2004). Successful management of cataplexy with intravenous immunoglobulins at narcolepsy onset. *Ann Neurol* **56**:905–908.

Dauvilliers Y, Neidhart E, Lecendreux M, Billiard M, Tafti M (2001). MAO-A and COMT polymorphisms and gene effects in narcolepsy. *Molecular Psychiatry* **6**:367–372.

Ferraro L, Tanganelli S, O'Connor WT, Antonelli T, Rambert F, Fuxe K (1996). The vigilance promoting drug modafinil increases dopamine release in the rat nucleus accumbens via the involvement of a local GABAergic mechanism. *Eur J Pharmacol* **306**:33–39.

Frey J, Darbonne C (1994). Fluoxetine suppresses human cataplexy: a pilot study. *Neurology* **44**:707–709.

Fujiki N, Yoshida Y, Ripley, Mignot E, Nishino S (2003). Effects of IV and ICV hypocretin-1 orexin A) in hypocretin receptor-2 gene mutated narcoleptic dogs and IV hypocretin-1 replacement therapy in a hypocretin-ligand-deficient narcoleptic dog. *Sleep* **26**:953–959.

Gelineau J (1880). De la narcolepsie. *Gaz des Hôp (Paris)* **55**:626–628; 635–637.

Guilleminault C (1993). Amphetamines and narcolepsy : use of the Stanford database. *Sleep* **16**:199–201.

Guilleminault C, Carskadon MA, Dement WC (1974). On the treatment of rapid eye movement narcolepsy. *Arch Neurol* **30**:90–93.

Guilleminault C, Mancuso J, Quera Salva MA, Hayes B, Milter M, Poirier G, Montplaisir J (1986). Viloxazine hydrochloride in narcolepsy: a preliminary report. *Sleep* **9**:275–279.

Guilleminault C, Raynal D, Takahashi S, Carkadon M, Dement W (1976). Evaluation of short-term and long-term treatment of the narcolepsy syndrome with clomipramine hydrochloride. *Acta Neurol Scand* **54**:71–87.

Hishikawa Y, Ida H, Nakai K, Kaneko Z (1965). Treatment of narcolepsy with imipramine (tofranil) and desmethylimipramine (pertofran). *Journal of the Neurological Sciences* **3**:453–461.

Honda Y, Hishikawa Y (1980). A long-term treatment of narcolepsy and excessive daytime sleepiness with pemoline (Bentanamin®). *Curr Ther Res* **27**:429–441.

Honda Y, Hishikawa Y, Takahashi Y (1979). Long-term treatment of narcolepsy with methylphenidate (Ritalin®). *Curr Ther Res* **25**:288–298.

Hublin C, Partinen M, Heinonen E, Puuka P, Salmi T (1994). Selegiline in the treatment of narcolepsy. *Neurology* **44**:2095–2101.

Iijima S, Sugita Y, Teshima Y, Hishikawa Y (1986). Therapeutic effects of mazindol on narcolepsy. *Sleep* **9**:265–268.

Kales A, Soldatos CR, Bixler EO, Caldwell A, Cadieux RJ, Verrechio JM, Kales JD (1982). Narcolepsy-cataplexy.II. Psychosocial consequences and associated psychopathology. *Arch Neurol* **39**:169–171.

Lammers GJ, Arends J, Declerck AC, Ferrari MD, Schouwink G, Troost J (1993). Gammahydroxybutyrate and narcolepsy : a double-blind placebo-controlled study. *Sleep* **16**:216–220.

Langdon N, Bandak S, Shindler J, Parkes JD (1986). Fluoxetine in the treatment of cataplexy. *Sleep* **9**:371–372.

Larrosa O, de la Liave Y, Barrio S, Granizo JJ, Garcia-Borreguero D (2001). Stimulant and anticataplectic effects of reboxetine in patients with narcolepsy. *Sleep* **24**:282–285.

Lecendreux M, Maret S, Bassetti C, Mouren MC, Tafti M (2003). Clinical efficacy of high-dose intravenous immunoglobulins near the onset of narcolepsy in a 10-year-old boy. *J Sleep Res* **12**:347–348.

Lieberman HR, Wurtman RJ, Emde GG, Roberts C, Coviella IL (1987). The effects of low doses of caffeine on human performance and mood. *Psychopharmacology* (Berlin) **92**:308–312.

Lin JS, Roussel B, Akaoka H, Fort P, de Billy G, Jouvet M (1992). Role of catecholamines in modafinil and amphetamine induced wakefulness, a comparative pharmacological study. *Brain Res* **591**:319–326.

Mamelak M, Black J, Montplaisir J. (2004) A pilot study on the effects of sodium oxybate on sleep architecture and daytime alertness in narcolepsy. *Sleep* **27**:1327–1334.

Mamelak M, Scharf MB, Woods M (1986). Treatment of narcolepsy with gamma-hydroxybutyrate. A review of clinical and sleep laboratory findings. *Sleep* **9**:285–289.

Mayer G, Kesper K, Peter H, Ploch T, Leinweber T, Peter JH (2002). Comorbidity in narcoleptic patients. *Deutsche Med Wochenschr* **127**:1942–1946.

Mayer G, Meier-Ewert K (1995). Selegiline hydrochloride treatment in narcolepsy. A double-blind, placebo-controlled study. *Clin Neuropharmacol* **18**:306–319.

Mignot E, Nishino S, Guilleminault C, Dement WC (1994). Modafinil binds to the dopamine uptake carrier site with low affinity. *Sleep* **17**:436–437.

Mitler MM, Aldrich MS, Koob GF, Zarcone V (1994). Narcolepsy and its treatment with stimulants (ASDA standards of practice). *Sleep* **17**:352–371.

Mitler MM, Hajdukovic R, Erman M, Koziol JA (1990). Narcolepsy. *J Clin Neurophysiol* **7**:93–118.

Mitler MM, Hajdukovic R, Erman M (1993). Treatment of narcolepsy with methamphetamine. *Sleep* **16**:306–317.

Mitler MM, Hirsh J, Hirshkowitz M, Guilleminault C, for the U.S. Modafinil in Narcolepsy Multicenter Study Group (2000). Long-term efficacy and safety of modafinil (PROVIGIL?) for the treatment of excessive daytime sleepiness associated with narcolepsy. *Sleep Med* **1**:231–243.

Mitler MM, Shafor R, Hajdukovik R, Timms RM, Browman CP (1986). Treatment of narcolepsy : objective studies on methylphenidate, pemoline, and protriptyline. *Sleep* **9**:260–264.

Moldofsky H, Broughton RJ, Hill JD (2000). A randomized trial of the long-term, continued efficacy and safety of modafinil in narcolepsy. *Sleep Med* **1**:109–116.

Montplaisir J, Michaud M, Denesle R, Gosselin A (2000). Periodic leg movements are not more prevalent in insomnia or hypersomnia but are specifically associated with sleep disorders involving a dopaminergic impairment. *Sleep Med* **1**:163–167.

Mullington J, Broughton R (1993). Scheduled naps in the management of daytime sleepiness in narcolepsy-cataplexy. *Sleep* **16**:444–456.

Murillo-Rodriguez E, Arias-Carrion O, Xu M, Blanco-Centurion C, Drucker-Colin R, Shiromani PJ ((2004). Time course of survival of hypocretin neuronal transplantation into the pons of adult rats. *Sleep* **27**:Abtsract Supplement, A238.

Nishino S, Mignot E (1997). Pharmacological aspects of human and canine narcolepsy. *Progr Neurobiol* **52**:27–78.

Palovaara S, Kivisto KT, Tapanainen P, Manninen P, Neuvonen PJ, Laine K (2000). Effect of an oral contraceptive preparation containing ethinylestradiol and gestodene on CYP3A4 activity as measured by midazolam l-hydroxylation. *Br J Clin Pharmacol* **50**: 333–337.

Parkes JD, Dahlitz M (1993). Amphetamine prescription. *Sleep* **16**:201–203.

Parkes JD, Schachter M (1979). Mazindol in the treatment of narcolepsy. *Acta Neurol Scand* **60**:250–254.

Passouant P, Baldy-Moulinier M (1970). Données actuelles sur le traitement de la narcolepsie. Action des imipraminiques. *Concours Médical* **92**:1967–1970.

Poryazova R, Siccoli M, Werth E, Bassetti C (2005). Unusually prolonged rebound cataplexy after withdrawal of fluoxetine. *Neurology* (in press).

Reinish LW, MacFarlane JG, Sandor P, Shapiro CM (1995). REM changes in narcolepsy with selegiline. *Sleep* **18**:362–367.

Rogers AE, Aldrich MS (1993). The effect of regularly scheduled naps on sleep attacks and excessive daytime sleepiness associated with narcolepsy. *Nursing Res* **42**:111–117.

Rogers AE, Aldrich MS, Lin X (2001). Comparison of three different sleep schedules for reducing daytime sleepiness in narcolepsy. *Sleep* **24**:385–391.

Roth B, Nevsimalova S (1975). Depression in narcolepsy and hypersomnia. *Schweiz Arch Neurol Psychiatry* **116**:291–300.

Schachter M, Parkes JD (1980). Fluvoxamine and clomipramine in the treatment of cataplexy. *J Neurol Neurosurg Psychiatry* **43**:171–174.

Schrader H, Kayed K, Bendixen Markset AC, Treidene HE (1986). The treatment of accessory symptoms in narcolepsy : a double-blind cross-over study of a selective serotonin re-uptake inhibitor (femoxetine) versus placebo. *Acta Neurol Scand* **74**:297–303.

Schuld A, Kraus T, Haack M, Hinze-Selch D, Pollmächer T (1999). Obstructive sleep apnea syndrome induced by clonazepam in a narcoleptic patient with REM-sleep-behavior disorder. *J Sleep Res* **8**:321–322.

Schmidt HS, Clark RW, Hyman PR (1977). Protriptyline: an effective agent in the treatment of the narcolepsy-cataplexy syndrome and hypersomnia. *Am J Psychiatry* **134**:183–185.

Schwartz JR, Feldman NT, Bogan RK, Nelson MT, Hughes RJ (2003). Dosing regimen of modafinil for improving daytime wakefulness in patients with narcolepsy. *Clin Neuropharmacol* **26**:252–257.

Scrima L, Hartman PG, Johnson Jr FH, Hiller FC (1989). Efficacy of gamma-hydroxybutyrate versus placebo in treating narcolepsy-cataplexy: double-blind subjective measures. *Biol Psych* **26**:331–343.

Shapiro CM (1975). Treatment of cataplexy with clomipramine. *Arch Neurol* **32**:653–656.

Shiba T, Fujiki N, Wisor JP, Dale EM, Sakurai T, Nishino S (2004). Wake promoting effects of thioperamide, a histamine H3 antagonist in orexin/ataxin-3 narcoleptic mice. *Sleep* **27**: Abstract Supplement:A241.

Shindler J, Schachter M, Brincat S, Parkes JD (1985). Amphetamine, mazindol, and fencamfamin in narcolepsy. *BMJ* **290**:1167–1170.

Smith M, Parkes JD, Dahlitz M (1996). Venlafaxine in the treatment of the narcoleptic syndrome. *J Sleep Res* **5(Suppl 1)**:217.

Standards of Practice Committee of the American Sleep Disorders Association. Practice parameters for the use of stimulants in the treatment of narcolepsy (1994). *Sleep* **17:**348–351.

Standards of Practice Committee. Practice parameters for the treatment of narcolepsy : an update for 2000 (2001). *Sleep* **24:**451–466.

The Xyrem International Study Group. (2005). A double-blind, placebo-controlled study demonstrates sodium oxybate is effective for the treatment of excessive daytime sleepiness in narcolepsy. *J Clin Sleep Med* **1:**391–397.

Thirumalai SS, Shubin RA (2000). The use of citalopram in resistant cataplexy. *Sleep Med* **1:**313–316.

Thorpy MJ, Snyder M, Aloe FS, Ledereich PS, Starz KE (1992). Short-term triazolam use improves nocturnal sleep of narcoleptics. *Sleep* **15:**212–216.

U.S. Modafinil in Narcolepsy Multicenter Study Group (1998). Randomized trial of modafinil for the treatment of pathological somnolence in narcolepsy. *Ann Neurol* **43:**88–97.

U.S. Modafinil in Narcolepsy Multicenter Study Group (2000). Randomized trial of modafinil as a treatment for the excessive daytime somnolence of narcolepsy. *Neurology* **54:**1166–1175.

U.S. Xyrem® Multicenter Study Group (2002). A randomized, double-blind, placebo-controlled multicenter trial comparing the effects of three doses of orally administered sodium oxybate with placebo for the treatment of narcolepsy. *Sleep* **25:**42–49.

U.S. Xyrem® Multicenter Study Group (2003). A 12-month, open-label multi-center extension trial of orally administered sodium oxybate for the treatment of narcolepsy. *Sleep* **26:**31–35

U.S. Xyrem® Multicenter Study Group (2004). Sodium oxybate demonstrates long-term efficacy for the treatment of cataplexy in patients with narcolepsy. *Sleep Med* **5:**119–123.

Vespignani H, Barroche G, Escaillas, M. Weber (1984). Importance of mazindol in the treatment of narcolepsy. *Sleep* **7:**274–275.

Vourdas A, Shneerson JM, Gregory CA, Smith IE, King MA, Morrish E, McKenna PJ (2002). Narcolepsy and psychopathology; is there an association? *Sleep Med* **3:**353–360.

Westphal C (1877). Eigentümliche mit Einschlafen verbundene Anfälle. *Arch Psychiatr Nervenkr* **7:** 631–635.

Wisor JP, Nishino S, Sora I, Uhl GH, Mignot E, Edgar DM (2001). Dopaminergic role in stimulant-induced wakefulness. *J Neurosci* **21:**1787–1794.

Wyatt R, Fram D, Buchbinder R, Snyder F (1971). Treatment of intractable narcolepsy with a monoamine oxidase inhibitor. *N Engl J Med* **285:**987–999.

Xyrem International Study Group (2005). Further evidence supporting the use of sodium oxybate for the treatment of cataplexy: a double -blind, placebo-controlled study in 228 patients. *Sleep Med* **6:**415–421.

Yeh SB, Schenck CH (2004). A case of marital discord and secondary depression with attempted suicide resulting from REM sleep behavior disorder in a 35-year-old woman. *Sleep Med* **5:**151–154.

Yoss RE, Daly D (1959). Treatment of narcolepsy with Ritalin. *Neurology* **9:**171–173.

Zuberi SM, Mignot E, Ling L, Mcarthur I (2004). Variable response to intravenous immunoglobulin therapy in childhood narcolepsy. *J Sleep Res* **13(Suppl 1):**828.

CHAPTER 42

Sleep disorders in neurologic disease

P. Jennum,[a] J. Santamaria Cano,[b] C. Bassetti,[c]
P. Clarenbach,[d] B. Högl,[e] I. Arnulf,[f] R. Poirrier,[g]
K. Sonka,[h] E. Svanborg,[i] L. Dolenc Groselj,[j]
D. Kaynak,[k] M. Kruger,[l] A. Papavasiliou,[m]
P. Reading,[n] Z. Zahariev[o]

Abstract

Background Patients with neurological diseases often have significant sleep disorders accompanied by sleep-related breathing disorders including obstructive sleep apnoea syndrome (OSAS), central sleep apnoea-hypopnoea syndrome (CSAHS), Cheyne-Stokes breathing syndrome (CSBS) and sleep-related hypoventilation/hypoxemic syndromes (SHVS), sleep fragmentation insomnia, sleep-related motor disorders and rapid eye movement (REM) behavioural disorders that may affect both nocturnal sleep and daytime function with increased morbidity and even mortality. Many of these disorders are potentially treatable.

Methods The recommendations were based on review of available guidelines supplemented with articles and graded in accordance to the strength of available scientific evidence.

Increased awareness should be directed to sleep disorders in patient with neurodegenerative, cerebrovascular and neuromuscular diseases. A polysomnography is usually a diagnostic minimum for the diagnoses of the most commonly reported sleep disorders in patients with neurological diseases, eventually supplied with a full video polysomnography PSG/video–electroencephalography-polysomnography (EEG-PSG) that should be considered in patients with nocturnal motor and behaviour manifestations.

Respiratory polygraphy has a moderate sensitivity and specificity in the diagnosis of OSAS without neurological diseases, but its value for diagnosis of sleep breathing disorders (SBD) in patients with neurological diseases has not been evaluated as compared to gold standard PSG. Oximetry has a poor–moderate sensitivity-specificity for the identification of OSAS in patients without neurological diseases.

[a]Department of Clinical Neurophysiology, Glostrup Hospital, University of Copenhagen, Denmark; [b]Servicio de Neurologia, Hospital Clinic of Barcelona, Spain; [c]Department of Neurology, Universitatsspital Zurich, Switzerland; [d]Department of Neurology, Evangelisches Johannes-Krankenhaus, Germany; [e]Department of Neurology, Medical University of Innsbruck, Austria; [f]Federation des Pathologies du Sommeil, Hopital Pitie-Salpetriere, Paris, France; [g]Department of Neurology, CHU Sart Tilman, Liège, Belgium; [h]Department of Neurology, Charles University of Prague, Czech Republic; [i]Department of Neuroscience and Locomotion, Division of Clinical Neurophysiology, Linköping, Sweden; [j]Institute of Clinical Neurophysiology, Division of Neurology, University Medical Centre, Ljubljana, Slovenia; [k]Department of Neurology, Sleep Disorders Unit, Faculty of Medicine, Dokuz Eylu l University, Izmir, Turkey; [l]Department of Neurology, Hôpital de la Ville, Luxembourg; [m]Department of Pediatric Neurology, Palia Pendeli Children's Hospital, Athens, Greece; [n]Department of Neurology, Sunderland Royal Hospital, UK; [o]Department of Neurology, High Medical School – Plovdiv, Bulgaria.

Continuous positive airway pressure (CPAP) is the most effective treatment of OSAS. This probably also includes patients with OSAS and neurological diseases. Bi-level PAP/variable PAP and volumetric ventilation are useful for SBD like CSAHS, CSBS and SHVS, especially in neuromuscular diseases.

There is a need for further studies focusing on the diagnostic procedures and treatment modalities in patients with sleep disorders, degenerative neurological diseases and stroke.

Objectives

To review the different sleep disorders occurring in degenerative neurological diseases and stroke.

To review the different methods of sleep evaluation available in these patients.

To report the evidence supporting that the evaluation and treatment of sleep disorders in patients with degenerative neurological disorders and stroke improves the management of these diseases.

Background

Sleep is an active process generated and modulated in the nervous system subject to a complex set of neural systems located mainly in the hypothalamus, brainstem and thalamus. Sleep is altered in many neurological diseases due to several mechanisms: lesions of the areas that control sleep, lesions or diseases that produce pain, paralysis or poor mobility (due to tremor, rigidity, dystonia or other motor disturbances) or treatments given to control neurologic symptoms. Hypersomnolence, sleep attacks, sleep fragmentation, nocturnal stridor, nocturnal behavioural phenomena like REM sleep behaviour disorder or nocturnal seizures, restless leg syndrome and periodic leg movements in sleep, and the like, are sleep problems that are increasingly recognised as common features of several neurological disorders. Furthermore, obstructive sleep apnoea (OSA) is one of the most common sleep problems, with a prevalence of more than 2–4% of the adult population. In patients with neurological diseases like stroke, dementia, Parkinson's disease and atypical Parkinsonian syndromes, myelopathies, motor neuron diseases, polyneuropathy, diseases related to the motor end-plate and myopathies, OSA and other SBD

occur even more often with prevalences exceeding more than one third of the patients (supplementary table 1 available at the European Journal of Neurology, www.blackwellpublishing.com). OSA is strongly associated with increased cardio- and cerebrovascular risks and causes significant family and social problems. It is also strongly related to increased traffic accidents and work-related accidents. There is increasing evidence that SBD in patients with neurological diseases reduces daytime functioning and increases mortality.

Diagnostic procedures and treatment of sleep disorders have developed considerably in recent years. Digital electroencephalography (EEG), audio-visual recording, ambulatory polysomnography (PSG), abbreviated respiratory recordings and actigraphy represent only a few examples of the different sleep recording strategies available.

Treatment modalities have been proposed for many of these disorders including hypersomnia in Parkinson's disease, abnormal motor activity and behaviour during sleep, and sleep fragmentation. Important developments have also taken place in the treatment of SBD and include continuous positive airway pressure (CPAP)/auto-adjusted CPAP, variable PAP (VPAP), bi-level-PAP for patients with OSA and barometric or volumetric non-invasive ventilation for patients with weak diaphragm. CPAP treatment reduces respiratory abnormalities, normalises sleep abnormalities, and reduces daytime symptoms and cardio- and cerebrovascular risks. In patients with severe neurological deficits like amyotrophic lateral sclerosis (ALS) and multiple system atrophy (MSA) recent data suggest that non-invasive ventilation may increase survival.

The current Guideline will focus on *neurodegenerative disorders* and *stroke* with an emphasis on *sleep breathing disorders* in neurologic disease.

The review will cover three main areas:

1. Taupathies (Alzheimer's disease, progressive supranuclear palsy and corticobasal degeneration).
2. Synucleinopathies (Parkinson's disease, multiple system atrophy and dementia with Lewy bodies).
3. Stroke, ALS, myotonic dystrophy, myasthenia gravis and spinocerebellar ataxias.

Search strategy

Several electronic databases were searched including MEDLINE, PUBMED, EMBASE, WEB OF SCIENCE, Cochrane, Clinical Trials, National Library of Medicine, and National Guideline Clearinghouse. These were searched until October 2004 or as much of this range as possible looking for the different sleep disorders and symptoms in each of the most frequent or relevant degenerative neurological disorders and stroke. Additional articles were sought by handsearching reference lists in standard textbooks and reviews in the field and by contacting academic centres in palliative care and pharmaceutical companies. Language is restricted to European languages.

Selection criteria: Studies considered for inclusion were, when possible, randomised controlled trials of adult patients, in any setting, suffering a neurodegenerative disorder (motor neurone disease, Parkinson's disease, Alzheimer's disease) or stroke. There had to be an explicit complaint of insomnia, parasomnia or hypersomnia in study participants. We also included observational studies. Sleep disorders have been described in several neurodegenerative diseases, but we have decided not to include them in this review because most are small case series and some lack PSG recordings.

Data collection and analysis: Abstracts were selected by the chairmen and independently inspected by individual members of the Task Force; full papers were obtained where necessary. A classification of the different studies according to evidence levels for therapeutic interventions and diagnostic measures will be done in accordance to the guidance (Brainin *et al.*, 2004). The panel will discuss what possible diagnostic tests and health care interventions could be recommended in each particular disease.

Method for reaching consensus

Where there was uncertainty further discussion was sought by the panel. Data extraction and quality assessments were undertaken independently by the panel reviewers.

Sleep disorders

Classification of sleep disorders

The International Classification, version 2 (ICSD-2) lists 95 sleep disorders (2005). The ISCD-2 has eight major categories

1. Insomnias
2. Sleep-related breathing disorders
3. Hypersomnias not due to a sleep-related breathing disorder
4. Circadian rhythm sleep disorders
5. Parasomnias
6. Sleep-related movements disorders
7. Isolated symptoms
8. Other sleep disorders

In the following pages only a selected number of the sleep disorders related to neurological diseases are mentioned.

Insomnia

Insomnias are defined by a repeated difficulty with sleep initiation, duration, consolidation or quality that occurs despite adequate time and opportunity for sleep, and the result in some form of daytime impairment. Insomnia complaints typically include difficulty in initiating and maintaining sleep, and they usually include extended periods of nocturnal wakefulness and insufficient amount of nocturnal sleep.

Typical insomnias are acute insomnia and psychophysiological insomnias. Insomnias are often reported in patients with neurological disorders due to degeneration or dysfunction of the central nervous system areas involved in sleep regulation; motor or sensory symptoms produced by the disease (pain, reduced nocturnal mobility, nocturnal motor activity, etc.) that lower the threshold for arousal from sleep and easily break it and secondary alerting effects of the drugs employed in the treatment of neurological diseases.

Sleep disordered breathing

These disorders are characterised by disordered breathing during sleep. A uniform syndrome recommendation was suggested in 1999 by the American Academy of Sleep Medicine (1999c), which is included in ICSD-2:

1. Obstructive sleep apnoea syndromes (OSAS).
2. Central sleep apnoea-hypopnoea syndrome (CSAHS)
3. Cheyne–Stokes Breathing Syndrome (CSBS) and
4. Sleep-related hypoventilation/hypoxemic syndromes.

Obstructive sleep apnoea syndrome
Obstructive sleep apnoea syndrome (OSAS) is characterised by recurrent episodes of partial (causing hypopnoea) or complete upper airway obstructions (causing apnoea) during sleep, often terminated by arousals. Obstructive sleep apnoea requires at least five obstructive breathing episodes per hour of sleep (Apnoea-Hypopnoea Index, AHI$\geq$5/h). An apnoea is defined by complete cessation of ventilation for a duration exceeding 10 s. A hypopnoea is defined as

1. A clear decrease ($>$50%) from baseline in the amplitude of flow signal during sleep.
2. A clear amplitude reduction that does not reach the above criterion, but is associated with an oxygen desaturation of $\geq$3% or an arousal.
3. The event should last 10 s or longer.

OSAS is characterised by excessive daytime sleepiness, snoring eventually choking and gasping during sleep, recurrent awakenings from sleep, unrefreshing sleep, daytime fatigue, and impaired concentration and insomnia.

OSAS are reported in least 2% of females and 4% of males aged more than 30 years (Young *et al.*, 1993). OSAS increase with age. OSAS are more commonly observed in patients with obesity, upper airway and craniofacial abnormalities, cardiac, pulmonary, endocrine (acromegaly, myxoedema, diabetes) and cerebrovascular diseases.

PSG findings include: oxyhaemoglobin desaturations, sleep fragmentation, reduced REM, non-rapid eye movement (NREM) stage 3 and 4 sleep.

Central sleep apnoea-hypopnoea syndrome
Central sleep apnoea-hypopnoea syndrome (CSAHS) is defined by recurrent apnoeic episodes during sleep with absence of obstructive components. A central apnoea-hypopnoea is defined by:

1. Reduction of airflow of at least 50%.
2. Lack of signs of respiratory drive as determined by respiratory activation.
3. The event should last 10 s or longer.

These episodes may be associated with desaturations, arousals and daytime sleepiness. Central sleep apnoea can be divided into normocapnic (idiopathic central sleep apnoea, Cheyne-Stokes breathing and high altitude induced central sleep apnoea) and hypercapnic (presenting overlap to sleep hypoventilation syndrome).

CSAHS is characterised by excessive daytime sleepiness, frequent nocturnal arousals/awakenings, and overnight monitoring documents number of central apnoeas $\geq$5/h. The patients should be normocapnic while awake.

Predisposing factors are increase in ventilatory response to pCO_2 that may be present in brain stem lesion due to infarction, haemorrhage, demyelination, tumours and the like.

CSAHS is relatively uncommon; precise epidemiological data are not present.

In PSG recording central apnoeas or hypopnoeas without respiratory activation in the abdomino-thoracic movements are observed. These episodes may be associated with arousals. Central apnoeas are more commonly observed in lighter sleep, less frequent in NREM stage 2 and REM, rarely in NREM stage 3 and 4. Central apnoea/mixed apnoeas are sometimes also observed in patients with OSAS.

Cheyne-Stokes breathing syndrome
Cheyne-Stokes breathing syndrome (CSBS) is characterised by cyclic fluctuations in breathing with periods of central apnoeas or hypopnoeas alternating with periods of hyperpnoea. CSBS occurs in approximately 50% of patients with severe congestive heart failure or neurological disease/dysfunction; usually acute cerebrovascular episodes. CSBS occurs mostly during sleep, in more severe cases also during wakefulness.

Associated features: cardiovascular changes, sleep fragmentation, excessive daytime sleepiness, abnormal response to CO_2.

PSG features include typical respiratory pattern especially during NREM sleep.

Sleep-related hypoventilation/hypoxemic syndrome

Sleep-related hypoventilation/hypoxemic syndrome (SHVS) is defined as hypoventilation related to decreased alveolar ventilation that results in increased $PaCO_2$ and hypoxaemia.

Associated features include erythrocytosis, pulmonary hypertension, cor pulmonale, or respiratory failure and excessive daytime sleepiness. Cardiac arrhythmias and systemic hypertension are also observed.

Predisposing factors: morbid obesity (BMI > 35 kg/sqm), chest wall restrictive disorders, neuromuscular weakness or disorders (e.g. amyotrophic lateral sclerosis), brainstem or high spinal cord lesions, phrenic nerve lesions, acute or chronic polyneuropathies including acute inflammatory demyelinating poly-radiculoneuropathy (AIDP), idiopathic central alveolar hypoventilation, obstructive lung disease and myxoedema.

Polysomnographic findings include increase in nocturnal $PaCO_2$ and arterial desaturations. Hypoventilations and hypoxemia are more common and severe during REM than in NREM sleep. Arterial pCO_2 and oxygen saturation during wakefulness does not fully reflect the sleep-induced hypoventilation.

Hypersomnias not due to a sleep-related breathing disorder

Hypersomnias and/or excessive daytime sleepiness are defined as the inability to stay alert and awake during the day, resulting in unintended lapses into sleep. The most common disorders in this group are narcolepsy, idiopathic hypersomnia, restless legs syndrome and periodic limb movements during sleep. Hypersomnia is commonly reported in patients with neurological disease and may be produced by degeneration of sleep/wake centres, sleep fragmentation or, medication.

Circadian-rhythm disorders

Circadian-rhythm disorders are defined as a misalignment between the patient's sleep pattern and the pattern that is desired or regarded as the societal norm. Most of the conditions observed in this group are associated with external factors like social habits, but in relation to neurological diseases, conditions that destruct the neural input to the suprachiasmatic nucleus (e.g. complete bilateral retinal, optic nerve, chiasm or hypothalamic lesions) may induce a condition that resembles circadian disorders.

Parasomnias

Parasomnias are undesirable physical or external events that accompany sleep. Parasomnias are disorders of arousal, partial arousal, and sleep stage transition. These disorders do not primarily cause a complaint of insomnia or excessive sleepiness, but frequently involve abnormal behaviours during sleep. Many of the disorders are common in children, but some are also present in adults. Parasomnias are subdivided into the following groups:

1. Disorders of arousal (from NREM sleep): confusional arousal, sleep walking and sleep terror
2. Parasomnias usually associated with REM sleep: REM sleep behaviour disorder (RBD), recurrent isolated sleep paralysis and nightmare disorder
3. Other parasomnias, e.g. enuresis, sleep-related groaning (Catathrenia).

Of these parasomnias, RBD has a particular relationship to neurodegenerative diseases.

REM sleep behaviour disorder

This disorder is characterised by vigorous movements occurring during REM sleep due to lack of inhibition of muscle tone and activity during REM sleep.

Diagnostic criteria are:

A. Presence of REM sleep without atonia: the electromyography (EMG) finding of excessive amounts of sustained or intermittent elevation of fragmented EMG tone or excessive phasic submental or (upper or lower) EMG twitching.
B. At least one of the following is present:

   a. Sleep-related injuries, potentially injurious or disruptive behaviours by history
   b. Abnormal REM sleep behaviors documented during polysomnographic monitoring

C. Absence of EEG epileptiform activity during REM sleep unless RBD can be clearly distinguished from any concurrent REM sleep-related seizure disorder

D. The sleep disturbance is not better explained by another sleep disorder, medical or neurological disorder, mental disorder, medication use or substance use disorder.

The patient and those sharing the bed can be injured. REM behaviour disorders are observed in a significant proportion of patients with PD (Onofrj *et al.*, 2002). RBD is also commonly observed in multiple system atrophy (MSA) and has been reported in diffuse Lewy body (DLB) (Uchiyama *et al.*, 1995; Boeve *et al.*, 2001, 2004; Turner, 2002) and Machado-Joseph disease (MJD) (Friedman *et al.*, 2003; Iranzo *et al.*, 2003; Syed *et al.*, 2003). Patients with isolated RBD have a significant risk of developing Parkinson's disease, DLB or MSA (Olson *et al.*, 2000). Occurrence of hallucinations in Parkinson's disease is related to the presence of RBD (Onofrj *et al.*, 2002). Reduced striatal dopamine transporters have been observed in these patients (Eisensehr *et al.*, 2003). A confident diagnosis relies on a full PSG recording preferably with synchronised audiovisual recording.

Sleep-related movement disorders

Sleep-related movement disorders are characterised by relatively simple, usually stereotypic movements that disturb sleep. Periodic limb movements (PLM), restless legs syndrome (RLS), bruxism, leg cramps, rhythmic movement disorders and other sleep-related movement disorders are classified under this group. Of these RLS and PLM are of particular interest in patients with neurodegenerative disorders. These disorders will not be discussed here as they are the focus of another chapter.

Sleep disorders associated with neurological disease
Tauopathies

Patients with progressive supranuclear palsy (PSP), Alzheimer's disease (AD) and corticobasal degeneration (CBD) may complain of significant sleep-related circadian disturbances, sleep/wake and daytime problems (Reynolds, III *et al.*, 1985; De Bruin *et al.*, 1996; Pareja *et al.*, 1996; Kimura *et al.*, 1997; Schenck *et al.*, 1997; Janssens *et al.*, 2000; Volicer *et al.*, 2001; Ferman *et al.*, 2004).

1. Sleep/wake disturbances and disruption are commonly observed in AD, with daytime sleep, sleep attack and episodes of micro sleep.
2. Insomnia (sleep fragmentation, difficulties maintaining sleep) is common as are nocturnal wandering, nocturnal confusion, 'Sundowning' psychosis and nocturia.
3. Excessive daytime sleepiness, sleep attacks and episodes of micro sleep during daytime may be associated with cognitive problems.
4. Sleep-related disorders such as RBD, RLS, PLM, nocturnal dystonic movements, cramps may occur in PSP, AD and CBD but are more commonly seen in the Synucleinopathies.
5. Sleep breathing disorders are common in Alzheimer's disease and associated with disease progression and poorer prognosis. OSA is commonly observed in Alzheimer's disease, however the clinical significance is questionable.

RECOMMENDATIONS

Sleep disorders are commonly observed in patients with tauopathies, and there should be increased awareness of these disorders (Level C). Clearly, there is a need for more controlled and intervention studies before definite conclusions can be reached.

Synucleinopathies

Parkinson's disease (PD), multiple system atrophy (MSA) and dementias with Lewy bodies (DLB) are often associated with major sleep disorders. Patients with these disorders often suffer from a number of significant sleep and daytime-related problems (Silber and Levine, 2000; Ferman *et al.*, 2002, 2004; Gilman *et al.*, 2003a,b; Massironi *et al.*, 2003; Yamaguchi *et al.*, 2003; Barone *et al.*, 2004; Boeve *et al.*, 2004):

1. PD-related motor symptoms including nocturnal akinesia, early-morning dystonia, painful cramps, tremor, and difficulties turning in bed.

2. Treatment-related nocturnal disturbances (e.g. insomnia, confusion, hallucinations, and motor disturbances).
3. Sleep-related symptoms such as hallucinations and vivid dreams (nightmares), insomnia (sleep fragmentation, difficulties maintaining sleep), nocturia, psychosis and panic attack.
4. Excessive daytime sleepiness, sleep attacks and episodes of micro sleep during waking hours.
5. Sleep-related disorders including RBD, RLS, PLM, nocturnal dystonic movements, cramps and SBD.
6. Laryngeal stridor and obstructive sleep apnoea are commonly observed in MSA patients. The presence of stridor in MSA patients is associated with a poorer prognosis.

RECOMMENDATIONS

The majority of patients with synucleinopathies experience one or more sleep disorders. Full PSG recording preferably with audiovisual recording is suggested for the diagnosis especially when RBD and/or SBD are suspected (Level C). Clearly, there is a need for more controlled and intervention studies before definite conclusions can be reached.

Stroke

Patients with strokes, primarily infarctions, may suffer from several sleep disorders and disturbances. Their occurrence and manifestations may vary depending on the specific neurological deficits (Bassetti *et al.*, 1996; Harbison *et al.*, 2002b; Cherkassky *et al.*, 2003; McArdle *et al.*, 2003; Nachtmann *et al.*, 2003; Palomaki *et al.*, 2003; Kang *et al.*, 2004; Mohsenin, 2004; Parra *et al.*, 2004; Brown *et al.*, 2005):

1. SBD especially obstructive sleep apnoea and nocturnal oxygen desaturations have been found commonly (>50%) in patients with acute stroke as well as after neurological recovery. SDB may be provoked by stroke, for example, after damage to the respiratory centres in the brain stem or bulbar/pseudobulbar paralysis due to brain stem. It is possible that sleep apnoea prior

to stroke may have predisposed the patient as sleep apnoea has been suggested as a risk factor for stroke. As sleep apnoea is associated with a high incidence of obesity, diabetes, coronary artery disease and hypertension, it remains to be clarified whether it is causative or simply a co-morbidity factor. There are several haemodynamic changes in sleep apnoea that may play a role in the pathogenesis of stroke development. Stroke and SBD are both common and are associated with significant morbidity and mortality.
2. Patients with stroke may present other sleep disorders such as unilateral periodic limb movement in sleep (PLMS).
3. Post-stroke insomnia is commonly reported.
4. Sleepiness and fatigue are commonly reported especially in patients with thalamic stroke.

RECOMMENDATIONS

SDB and other sleep disorders are strongly associated with stroke. The relation to stroke outcome, SDB and effect of treatment is incompletely understood. Increased attention should be addressed in patients with stroke. Specifically identifying SDB and other sleep disorders (Level C). Clearly, there is a need for more controlled and intervention studies before definite conclusions can be reached.

Motor neuron diseases, motor end plate and muscle diseases

Sleep disordered breathing is observed in several neuromuscular diseases including muscular dystrophy, myotonic dystrophy, myasthenia gravis, amyotrophic lateral sclerosis and post-polio syndrome. Although there may be differences, some general observations can be made. Hypoxaemia, especially during REM sleep, is commonly found. Severity is correlated to respiratory strength, and sleep-related hypoventilation is usually non-obstructive (Hukins and Hillman, 2000; Dedrick and Brown, 2004).

Patients with amyotrophic lateral sclerosis (ALS) and other severe motor neuron diseases have progressive motor deterioration with progressive respiratory insufficiency. This may manifest primarily during sleep where the motor drive is reduced. This is especially true for patients with the bulbar form of ALS or involvement of C3-C5 anterior horn (Ferguson *et al.*, 1996; Kimura *et al.*, 1999). The prognosis is closely related to respiratory muscle strength (Lyall *et al.*, 2001). Of note, sudden nocturnal death occurs often during sleep. Respiratory indices such as low nocturnal oxygen saturation are associated with poorer prognosis (Velasco *et al.*, 2002; Pinto *et al.*, 2003). Patients with diaphragmatic involvement may have significantly reduced REM sleep (Arnulf *et al.*, 2000). The primary SBD in patients with ALS – as in other neuromuscular diseases – is therefore a sleep hypoventilation syndrome (SHVS), whereas OSAS are rare (Ferguson *et al.*, 1996).

Management of these patients should therefore include relevant questions regarding symptoms susceptive for SBD. Common symptoms of nocturnal hypoventilations may include insomnia, headache and daytime somnolence (Takekawa *et al.*, 2001).

Oximetry has been suggested for the identification and screening for sleep-related hypoventilation in patients with ALS (Elman *et al.*, 2003; Pinto *et al.*, 2003). Care should be taken because pCO_2 may increase before desaturations are observed, especially in patients with additional chronic obstructive lung disease. Nocturnal oximetry has been suggested valuable for screening and evaluation of the treatment effect (Ferguson *et al.*, 1996; Pinto *et al.*, 2003). However, no studies have compared the diagnostic yield between a full PSG, respiratory polygraphy and nocturnal oximetry in these patients.

RECOMMENDATIONS

PSG with additional CO_2 analysis (transcutaneous or expiratory) should be considered for the identification of sleep-related hypoventilation. The role of oximetry in the identification of sleep-related breathing disorders in neuromuscular diseases is not established (Ferguson *et al.*, 1996; Hayward, 2004) (Level C).

Others

Other neurodegenerative disorders of genetic cause may present several sleep disturbances. Subjects with SCA-3 (Machado-Joseph disease) may also complain of restless legs syndrome, periodic leg movements, vocal cord paralysis and RBD (Schols *et al.*, 1998; Fukutake *et al.*, 2002; Syed *et al.*, 2003; Friedman *et al.*, 2003; Iranzo *et al.*, 2003). In patients with Huntington's disease the involuntary movements tend to diminish during sleep (Fish *et al.*, 1991). Sleep disturbances including disturbed sleep pattern with increased sleep onset latency, reduced sleep efficiency, frequent nocturnal awakenings, and more time spent awake with less slow wave sleep have been reported. These abnormalities correlate in part with duration of illness, severity of clinical symptoms, and degree of atrophy of the caudate nucleus (Wiegand *et al.*, 1991). However, other studies have not reported specific sleep disorders in these patients (Emser *et al.*, 1988).

RECOMMENDATIONS

Some studies suggest sleep disorders occur in genetic neurological diseases (Level C). Clearly, there is a need for more controlled and intervention studies before definite conclusions can be reached.

Diagnostic techniques in sleep disorders

Diagnostic procedures for sleep diagnosis include: polysomnography (PSG), partial time polysomnography, partial polygraphy (or respiratory polygraphy - RP) and limited channel polygraphy: oximetry determining SaO2/pulse and actimetry. Daytime sleep may be evaluated with the multiple sleep latency test (MSLT) or maintenance of wakefulness test (MWT) and standard EEG. An overview of these tests is presented in table 42.1 and more details are available in the web version of this paper.

Table 42.1 Methods for the diagnosis of sleep disorders in neurological diseases.

Type PSG	Definition	Indication	Advantage/disadvantage
Routine PSG	Multi-channels EEG, EOG, submental EMG, ECG, respiration, +/− tibial EMG	Routine screening for sleep disorders: SBD, PLM, chronic insomnia	Golden standard. May be performed in- or outside hospital. Standard method.
Extended PSG	Routine PSG + extra physiolocical channels, e.g., EMG, intraoesophageal pressure, CO_2	Special indications: oesophageal reflux, myoclonias etc. Depends on selected channels	Moderately expensive, time consuming, staff-demanding
Video-PSG	PSG + video recording	Motor and behavioural phenomena during sleep	A video signal is present. Full physiologic recording is obtained. The difference
Full EEG-PSG	Full EEG + PSG	Motor- and behavioural disturbances, differential diagnosis epilepsies	between the methods is primarily the number of EEG channels. Expensive, time consuming, staff-demanding
Partial channel polygraphy			
Respiratory polygraphy	Monitoring of respiration + SaO_2 + / − cardiac measures e.g. pulse	OSAS	Easy, inexpensive. Moderate–good sensitive and specificity for OSAS, the validity for other SBD is not present
Oximetry	Monitoring of SaO_2	Monitoring or screening for severe SBD	Easy, inexpensive. Low sensitive and specificity for SBD
Actigraphy	Determination of motor activity (days–months)	Sleep–wake disturbances	Inexpensive Limited clinical usefulness

Management of sleep disorders

Treatment of SDB in neurological diseases

Treatment of OSAS

1. CPAP is a well-documented treatment for moderate and severe obstructive sleep apnoea (AHI ≥ 15/h) and improves nocturnal respiratory abnormalities, daytime function and cognitive problems (Wright *et al.*, 1997; Douglas, 1998; McMahon *et al.*, 2003) (Level A). There is no significant difference regarding treatment effect or changes in subjective variables between fixed pressure CPAP or auto-adjusted CPAP (Berry *et al.*, 2002) (Level A). In some patients, for example neuromuscular disorder patients, CPAP may be difficult to accept and bi-level PAP may be used (Randerath *et al.*, 2003) (Level B).

2. CPAP and bi-level PAP is potentially useful in patients with SBD in stroke (Harbison *et al.*, 2002), but the evidence whether this influences quality of life, daytime symptoms, rehabilitation, morbidity, mortality is limited (Level C).

3. Severe SBD including laryngeal stridor in patients with MSA may be treated with CPAP/bi-level CPAP. Recent studies suggest that treatment with CPAP in MSA patients with laryngeal stridor showed high CPAP tolerance, no recurrence of stridor, no major side effects, subjective improvement in sleep quality, and increases the survival time to MSA patients without stridor (Iranzo *et al.*, 2000, 2004). CPAP is therefore an effective non-invasive long-term therapy for nocturnal stridor (Level C).

4. There is limited evidence that suggests oral appliance (OA) use improves subjective sleepiness

and sleep-disordered breathing compared with controls in patients with OSAS without neurological diseases (Level B). Nasal continuous positive airway pressure (nCPAP) is apparently more effective in improving sleep-disordered breathing than OA use (Level B). There are no data regarding the use of oral appliances in patients with neurological diseases. Until there is more definitive evidence on the effectiveness of OA, caution should be addressed to the use of OA in patients with OSAS. If used it should only be tried in patients who are unwilling or unable to comply with nCPAP therapy, (Lim *et al.*, 2003; Cohen, 2004) (Level C).

5. Although surgical treatment may be valuable in selected patients there is a limited number of controlled trials documenting an effect of surgery in the upper airway against OSAS (Bridgman and Dunn, 2000) (Level C). There are no studies suggesting that surgery in the upper airway has any effect on OSAS in patients with neurological diseases (Level C).

6. Medical treatments have no positive effect on OSAS (Smith *et al.*, 2002) (Level A). There are no studies available indicating that medication has any treatment effect of OSAS in patients with neurological diseases (Level C).

7. Although some patients with OSAS present increased weight and a negative lifestyle profile (tobacco, alcohol, physical activity), no controlled studies have evaluated the effect of intervention against these factors (Shneerson and Wright, 2001) (Level C). No studies have addressed the effect of lifestyle interventions on OSAS in patients with neurological diseases (Level C).

Treatment of central sleep apnoea-hypopnea syndrome

Case-series have shown that CPAP treatment does not influence the CO_2 response in CSAHS, despite a reduction in apnoeas, increase in PaO_2 and reduction in subjective sleepiness (Yu *et al.*, 1994; Hommura *et al.*, 1997; Verbraecken *et al.*, 2002) (class IV). Probably due to the rareness of the disease, there are no randomised studies regarding CSAHS and treatment. Medical treatment

with acetazolamide and theophyllin have furthermore been suggested (American Thoracic Society, 1999b), but the evidence for their use is poor (Level C).

Treatment of Cheyne-Stokes breathing syndrome

Initially, CPAP was used in patients with central apnoea/CSBS and cardiac insufficiency (Bradley, 1996; Granton *et al.*, 1996; Sin *et al.*, 2000; Krachman *et al.*, 2003), but in recent years adaptive ventilation has been found effective probably by an increased preload in patients with significant cardiac failure and reduce the respiratory abnormalities (Teschler *et al.*, 2001) (class IV). A recent randomised controlled study suggests that the use of non-invasive adaptive ventilation may improve daytime function and respiratory and cardiac measures (Pepperell *et al.*, 2003) (class II). The experience with the use of adaptive ventilation, CPAP or bi-level CPAP in patients with Cheyne-Stokes respiration due to central respiratory failure, for example, brain stem lesions, is sparse and the evidence level is poor (Level C).

Treatment of sleep hypoventilation syndrome

Treatment includes nasal intermittent positive pressure ventilation (NIPPV) with bi-level PAP (Bi-PAP, Variable PAP-VPAP), non-invasive volumetric ventilation, eventually invasive ventilation, under control of nocturnal respiratory parameters (Gonzalez *et al.*, 2002) (class IV). CPAP is not the primary treatment, as the motor effort is mostly reduced in these patients, which may lead to worsening of the SBD. NIPPV may reduce sleep disturbances, increase cognitive function, and prolong the period to tracheostomy (Newsom-Davis *et al.*, 2001; Butz *et al.*, 2003) (class IV). Treatment of these conditions requires a specialised team and ethical aspects should be addressed in the patient's management, especially regarding timing and the need for tracheotomy (Level C).

Follow-up

Although there is no evidence when and how follow-up of treatment with CPAP and NIPPV should be executed, we recommend regular follow-up of the treatment with control of compliance and treatment effect (Level C).

Ethical aspects

Treatment of patients with severe neurological diseases like ALS and MSA with NIPPV include medical and ethical problems that should be addressed. Adequate involvement of the patients and family, and the treatment, its use, limitations should be carefully discussed. It is important to clarify the limitations of the treatment and the discussion should include careful debate regarding whether such treatment should be offered, initiation and discontinuation. There are serious ethical problems; for example, when to initiate, discontinue and whether invasive ventilation should be offered (Bourke and Gibson, 2004; Mast *et al.*, 2004).

Medical treatment

Treatment of excessive daytime sleepiness in neurological diseases

Several groups of patients with neurological diseases commonly complain of excessive daytime sleepiness. The aetiology may be secondary to the disease, medication (dopaminergic or benzodiazepine drugs), sleep disorders such as sleep apnoea, nocturnal motor phenomena and the like. In patients where these factors cannot be modified the wake-promoting agent modafinil may be used. Modafinil was primarily introduced to treat excessive daytime sleepiness (EDS) in narcolepsy (Besset *et al.*, 1996; Narcolepsy Multicenter Study Group, 1998; 2000; Mitler *et al.*, 2000; Moldofsky *et al.*, 2000; Schwartz *et al.*, 2004). Case studies (Rabinstein *et al.*, 2001; Nieves and Lang, 2002) and double-blind controlled studies (Hogl *et al.*, 2002; Adler *et al.*, 2003) suggest that modafinil reduces excessive daytime sleepiness in Parkinson's patients (class B-II). Modafinil has also been suggested in amyotrophic lateral sclerosis (Sternbach, 2002), post-stroke depression (Smith, 2003; Sugden and Bourgeois, 2004) but no controlled studies are present (class IV). Furthermore, modafinil has been used for treatment of hypersomnolence in OSAS without neurological co-morbidity (Kingshott *et al.*, 2001). There are no studies evaluating whether other central acting drugs like methylphenidate may have similar effects.

Other treatment of sleep disorders in neurological diseases

Treatment of sleep disorders in neurodegenerative diseases is often complex and may involve different strategies. Management of some nocturnal disturbances in patients with PD may worsen nocturnal symptoms due to other causes and may increase EDS. PD-related motor symptoms can be treated with long-acting DA agonists to obtain continuous DA receptor stimulation during the night. Both treatment-related nocturnal disturbances and psychiatric symptoms may be related to drug treatment, and therefore, in both cases, drug reduction or discontinuation should be considered.

As patients with tauopathies suffer from a variety of sleep problems and have major motor and cognitive deficits, inpatient polysomnographic assessment is preferable to investigate their sleep symptoms fully. However, this often poses severe practical problems.

Some sleep disorders, such as RLS and PLMS, may be controlled by DA agents, and others, such as insomnia and EDS, may be improved by reducing dopaminergic stimulation (Level C).

Clonazepam or donepezil, possibly prescribed with melatonin have been suggested based on case series for the treatment of REM behaviour disorders. No controlled studies are available (Boeve *et al.*, 2003; Massironi *et al.*, 2003a).

Patients with dementias often present circadian disturbances that may be relieved by melatonin and phototherapy (Mishima *et al.*, 1994, 1998, 2000; Lovell *et al.*, 1995; McGaffigan and Bliwise, 1997; Van Someren *et al.*, 1997; Okumoto *et al.*, 1998; Koyama *et al.*, 1999; Lyketsos *et al.*, 1999; Yamadera *et al.*, 2000; Haffmans *et al.*, 2001; Sheehan and Keene, 2002; Fetveit *et al.*, 2003; Fontana *et al.*, 2003; Luijpen *et al.*, 2003; Skjerve *et al.*, 2004; Sutherland *et al.*, 2004).

In selected cases treatment with hypnotics may be useful, but the evidence is limited and care should be undertaken for chronic use and the additional risk worsening SDB.

Clearly, there is a need for more controlled and intervention studies before definite conclusions can be reached.

GOOD PRACTICE POINTS

1. Patients with neurological diseases often have significant sleep disorders that may affect both nocturnal sleep and daytime function with increased morbidity and even mortality. Many of these disorders are potentially treatable. Therefore, increased awareness should be directed to sleep disorders in patients with neurodegenerative, cerebrovascular and neuromuscular diseases. Despite that, there are practically no Class I or II studies in this area.
2. A PSG is usually a diagnostic minimum for the diagnoses of the most commonly reported sleep disorders in patients with neurological diseases.
3. In patients with nocturnal motor and/behaviour manifestations, a full video-PSG/video-EEG-PSG should be considered.
4. Respiratory polygraphy has a moderate sensitivity and specificity in the diagnosis of OSAS without neurological diseases, but its value for diagnosis of other SBD or in patients with OSAS with neurological diseases has not been evaluated as compared to gold standard PSG.
5. Limited channel polygraphy oximetry has a poor-moderate sensitivity-specificity for the identification of OSAS in patients without neurological diseases. Oximetry cannot differentiate between obstructive and central sleep apnoea or is insufficient to identify stridor. It is possible that oximetry has a role for the screening of hypoventilation in patients with neuromuscular weakness. Furthermore, oximetry may be useful for the control of CPAP treatment.
6. Patients with sleep disordered breathing and muscle weakness and cardiac or pulmonary co-morbidity may present a sleep hypoventilation syndrome, which manifests early as increased CO_2, why $PaCO_2$ should be considered and controlled in such cases during sleep-recordings.
7. Fixed pressure CPAP/auto-adjusted CPAP is the most effective treatment of OSAS. This probably also includes patients with OSAS and neurological diseases. However, there is a need for further evaluation of the effect of CPAP in patients with OSAS and neurological diseases.
1. Bi-level PAP/variable PAP, NIPPV and volumetric ventilation is useful for SBD like central apnoeas, Cheyne-Stokes breathing and alveolar hypoventilation.
2. There is a clear need for further studies focusing on the diagnostic procedures and treatment modalities in patients with sleep disorders and neurological diseases.

Conflicts of interest

None reported.

References

Narcolepsy Multicenter Study Group (1998). Randomized trial of modafinil for the treatment of pathological somnolence in narcolepsy. US Modafinil in Narcolepsy Multicenter Study Group. *Ann Neurol* **43(1):** 88–97.

American Thoracic Society (1999a). Clinical indications for noninvasive positive pressure ventilation in chronic respiratory failure due to restrictive lung disease, COPD, and nocturnal hypoventilation–a consensus conference report. *Chest* **116(2):**521–534.

American Thoracic Society (1999b). Idiopathic congenital central hypoventilation syndrome: diagnosis and management. American Thoracic Society. *Am J Respir Crit Care Med* **160(1):**368–373.

American Academy of Sleep Medicine Task Force (1999c). Sleep-related breathing disorders in adults: recommendations for syndrome definition and measurement techniques in clinical research. The Report of an American Academy of Sleep Medicine Task Force. *Sleep* **22(5):**667–689.

Narcolepsy Multicenter Study Group (2000). Randomized trial of modafinil as a treatment for the excessive daytime somnolence of narcolepsy: US Modafinil in Narcolepsy Multicenter Study Group. *Neurology* **54(5):**1166–1175.

American Academy of Sleep Medicine: International Classification of Sleep Disorders (2005). *Diagnostic and Coding Manual*, 2nd ed. Westchester, Ill, American Academy of Sleep Medicine.

Adler CH, Caviness JN, Hentz JG, Lind M, Tiede J (2003). Randomized trial of modafinil for treating subjective daytime sleepiness in patients with Parkinson's disease. *Mov Disord* **18(3)**:287–293.

Arnulf I, Similowski T, Salachas F, Garma L, Mehiri S, Attali V, Behin-Bellhesen V, Meininger V, Derenne JP (2000). Sleep disorders and diaphragmatic function in patients with amyotrophic lateral sclerosis. *Am J Respir Crit Care Med* **161(3 Pt 1)**:849–856.

Barone P, Amboni M, Vitale C, Bonavita V (2004). Treatment of nocturnal disturbances and excessive daytime sleepiness in Parkinson's disease. *Neurology* **63(8 Suppl 3)**:S35–S38.

Bassetti C, Mathis J, Gugger M, Lovblad KO, Hess CW (1996). Hypersomnia following paramedian thalamic stroke: a report of 12 patients. *Ann Neurol* **39(4)**:471–480.

Berry RB, Parish JM, Hartse KM (2002). The use of auto-titrating continuous positive airway pressure for treatment of adult obstructive sleep apnea. An American Academy of Sleep Medicine review. *Sleep* 25(2):148–173.

Besset A, Chetrit M, Carlander B, Billiard M (1996). Use of modafinil in the treatment of narcolepsy: a long term follow-up study. *Neurophysiol Clin* **26(1)**:60–66.

Boeve BF, Silber MH, Ferman TJ, Lucas JA, Parisi JE (2001). Association of REM sleep behavior disorder and neurodegenerative disease may reflect an underlying synucleinopathy. *Mov Disord* **16(4)**:622–630.

Boeve BF, Silber MH, Ferman TJ (2003). Melatonin for treatment of REM sleep behavior disorder in neurologic disorders: results in 14 patients. *Sleep Med* **4(4)**:281–284.

Boeve BF, Silber MH, Ferman TJ (2004). REM sleep behavior disorder in Parkinson's disease and dementia with Lewy bodies. *J Geriatr Psychiatry Neurol* **17(3)**:146–157.

Bourke SC, Gibson GJ (2004). Non-invasive ventilation in ALS: current practice and future role. *Amyotroph Lateral Scler Other Motor Neuron Disord* **5(2)**:67–71.

Bradley TD (1996). Hemodynamic and sympathoinhibitory effects of nasal CPAP in congestive heart failure. *Sleep* **19(10)**:S232–S235.

Brainin M, Barnes M, Baron JC, Gilhus NE, Hughes R, Selmaj K, Waldemar G (2004). Guidance for the preparation of neurological management guidelines by EFNS scientific task forces–revised recommendations 2004. *Eur J Neurol* **11(9)**:577–581.

Bridgman SA, Dunn KM (2000). Surgery for obstructive sleep apnoea. *Cochrane Database Syst Rev* no. 2, p. CD001004.

Brown DL, Chervin RD, Hickenbottom SL, Langa KM, Morgenstern LB (2005). Screening for obstructive sleep apnea in stroke patients: a cost-effectiveness analysis. *Stroke* **36(6)**:1291–1293.

Butz M, Wollinsky KH, Wiedemuth-Catrinescu U, Sperfeld A, Winter S, Mehrkens HH, Ludolph AC, Schreiber H (2003). Longitudinal effects of noninvasive positive-pressure ventilation in patients with amyotrophic lateral sclerosis. *Am J Phys Med Rehabil* **82(8)**:597–604.

Carvalho BS, Waterhouse J, Edwards B, Simons R, Reilly T (2003). The use of actimetry to assess changes to the rest-activity cycle. *Chronobiol Int* **20(6)**:1039–1059.

Cherkassky T, Oksenberg A, Froom P, Ring H (2003). Sleep-related breathing disorders and rehabilitation outcome of stroke patients: a prospective study. *Am J Phys Med Rehabil* **82(6)**:452–455.

Chesson AL, Jr, Ferber RA, Fry JM, Grigg-Damberger M, Hartse KM, Hurwitz TD, Johnson S, Kader GA, Littner M, Rosen G, Sangal RB, Schmidt-Nowara W, Sher A (1997). The indications for polysomnography and related procedures. *Sleep* **20(6)**:423–487.

Chesson AL, Jr, Wise M, Davila D, Johnson S, Littner M, Anderson WM, Hartse K, Rafecas J (1999). Practice parameters for the treatment of restless legs syndrome and periodic limb movement disorder. An American Academy of Sleep Medicine Report. Standards of Practice Committee of the American Academy of Sleep Medicine. *Sleep* **22(7)**:961–968.

Chesson AL, Jr, Berry RB, Pack A (2003). Practice parameters for the use of portable monitoring devices in the investigation of suspected obstructive sleep apnea in adults. *Sleep* **26(7)**:907–913.

Cohen R (2004). Limited evidence supports use of oral appliances in obstructive sleep apnoea. *Evid Based Dent* **5(3)**:76.

De Bruin VS, Machado C, Howard RS, Hirsch NP, Lees AJ (1996). Nocturnal and respiratory disturbances in Steele-Richardson-Olszewski syndrome (progressive supranuclear palsy). *Postgrad Med J* **72(847)**:293–296.

Dedrick DL, Brown LK (2004). Obstructive sleep apnea syndrome complicating oculopharyngeal muscular dystrophy. *Chest* **125(1)**:334–336.

Douglas NJ (1998). Systematic review of the efficacy of nasal CPAP. *Thorax* **53(5)**:414–415.

Eisensehr I, Linke R, Tatsch K, Kharraz B, Gildehaus JF, Wetter CT, Trenkwalder C, Schwarz J, Noachtar S (2003). Increased muscle activity during rapid eye movement sleep correlates with decrease of striatal presynaptic dopamine transporters. IPT and IBZM SPECT imaging in subclinical and clinically manifest idiopathic REM sleep behavior disorder, Parkinson's disease, and controls. *Sleep* 26(5):507–512.

Elman LB, Siderowf AD, McCluskey LF (2003). Nocturnal oximetry: utility in the respiratory management of amyotrophic lateral sclerosis. *Am J Phys Med Rehabil* **82(11):**866–870.

Emser W, Brenner M, Stober T, Schimrigk K (1988). Changes in nocturnal sleep in Huntington's and Parkinson's disease. *J Neurol* **235(3):**177–179.

Ferguson KA, Strong MJ, Ahmad D, George CF (1996). Sleep-disordered breathing in amyotrophic lateral sclerosis. *Chest* **110(3):**664–669.

Ferman TJ, Boeve BF, Smith GE, Silber MH, Lucas JA, Graff-Radford NR, Dickson DW, Parisi JE, Petersen RC, Ivnik RJ (2002). Dementia with Lewy bodies may present as dementia and REM sleep behavior disorder without parkinsonism or hallucinations. *J Int Neuropsychol Soc* **8(7):**907–914.

Ferman TJ, Smith GE, Boeve BF, Ivnik RJ, Petersen RC, Knopman D, Graff-Radford N, Parisi J, Dickson DW (2004). DLB fluctuations: specific features that reliably differentiate DLB from AD and normal aging. *Neurology* **62(2):**181–187.

Fetveit A, Skjerve A, Bjorvatn B (2003). Bright light treatment improves sleep in institutionalised elderly–an open tria. *Int J Geriatr Psychiatr* **18(6):**520–526.

Fish DR, Sawyers D, Allen PJ, Blackie JD, Lees AJ, Marsden CD (1991). The effect of sleep on the dyskinetic movements of Parkinson's disease, Gilles de la Tourette syndrome, Huntington's disease, and torsion dystonia. *Arch Neurol* **48(2):**210–214.

Fontana GP, Krauchi K, Cajochen C, Someren E, Amrhein I, Pache M, Savaskan E, Wirz-Justice A (2003). Dawn-dusk simulation light therapy of disturbed circadian rest-activity cycles in demented elderly. *Exp Gerontol* **38(1–2):**207–216.

Friedman JH, Fernandez HH, Sudarsky LR (2003). REM behavior disorder and excessive daytime somnolence in Machado-Joseph disease (SCA-3). *Mov Disord* **18(12):**1520–1522.

Fukutake T, Shinotoh H, Nishino H, Ichikawa Y, Goto J, Kanazawa I, Hattori T (2002). Homozygous Machado-Joseph disease presenting as REM sleep behaviour disorder and prominent psychiatric symptoms. *Eur J Neurol* **9(1):**97–100.

Gilman S, Chervin RD, Koeppe RA, Consens FB, Little R, An H, Junck L, Heumann M (2003a). Obstructive sleep apnea is related to a thalamic cholinergic deficit in MSA. *Neurology* **61(1):**35–39.

Gilman S, Koeppe RA, Chervin RD, Consens FB, Little R, An H, Junck L, Heumann M (2003b). REM sleep behavior disorder is related to striatal monoaminergic deficit in MSA. *Neurology* **61(1):**29–34.

Gonzalez MM, Parreira VF, Rodenstein DO (2002). Non-invasive ventilation and sleep. *Sleep Med Rev* **6(1):**29–44.

Granton JT, Naughton MT, Benard DC, Liu PP, Goldstein RS, Bradley TD (1996). CPAP improves inspiratory muscle strength in patients with heart failure and central sleep apnea. *Am J Respir Crit Care Med* **153(1):**277–282.

Haffmans PM, Sival RC, Lucius SA, Cats Q, van Gelder L (2001). Bright light herapy and melatonin in motor restless behaviour in dementia: a placebo-controlled study. *Int J Geriatr Psychiatry* **16(1):**106–110.

Harbison J, Ford GA, Gibson GJ (2002a). Nasal continuous positive airway pressure for sleep apnoea following stroke. *Eur Respir J* **19(6):**1216–1217.

Harbison J, Ford GA, James OF, Gibson GJ (2002b). Sleep-disordered breathing following acute stroke. *QJM* **95(11):**741–747.

Hayward P (2004). News from the European Neurological Society meeting. *Lancet Neurol* **3(8):**449.

Hogl B, Saletu M, Brandauer E, Glatzl S, Frauscher B, Seppi K, Ulmer H, Wenning G, Poewe W (2002). Modafinil for the treatment of daytime sleepiness in Parkinson's disease: a double-blind, randomized, crossover, placebo-controlled polygraphic trial. *Sleep* **25(8):**905–909.

Hommura F, Nishimura M, Oguri M, Makita H, Hosokawa K, Saito H, Miyamoto K, Kawakami Y (1997). Continuous versus bilevel positive airway pressure in a patient with idiopathic central sleep apnea. *Am J Respir Crit Care Med* **155(4):**1482–1485.

Hukins CA, Hillman DR (2000). Daytime predictors of sleep hypoventilation in Duchenne muscular dystrophy. *Am J Respir Crit Care Med* **161(1):**166–170.

Iranzo A, Santamaria J, Tolosa E (2000). Continuous positive air pressure eliminates nocturnal stridor in multiple system atrophy. Barcelona Multiple System Atrophy Study Group. *Lancet* **356(9238):**1329–1330.

Iranzo A, Munoz E, Santamaria J, Vilaseca I, Mila M, Tolosa E (2003). REM sleep behavior disorder and vocal cord paralysis in Machado-Joseph disease. *Mov Disord* **18(10):**1179–1183.

Iranzo A, Santamaria J, Tolosa E, Vilaseca I, Valldeoriola F, Marti MJ, Munoz E (2004). Long-term effect of CPAP in the treatment of nocturnal stridor in multiple system atrophy. *Neurology* **63(5):**930–932.

Janssens JP, Pautex S, Hilleret H, Michel JP (2000). Sleep disordered breathing in the elderly. *Aging (Milano.)* **12(6):**417–429.

Johns MW (2000). Sensitivity and specificity of the multiple sleep latency test (MSLT), the maintenance of wakefulness test and the epworth sleepiness scale: failure of the MSLT as a gold standard *J Sleep Res* **9(1):**5–11.

Kang SY, Sohn YH, Lee IK, Kim JS (2004). Unilateral periodic limb movement in sleep after supratentorial cerebral infarction. *Parkinsonism Relat Disord* **10(7):**429–431.

Kimura K, Tachibana N, Aso T, Kimura J, Shibasaki H (1997). Subclinical REM sleep behavior disorder in a patient with corticobasal degeneration. *Sleep* **20(10):**891–894.

Kimura K, Tachibana N, Kimura J, Shibasaki H (1999). Sleep-disordered breathing at an early stage of amyotrophic lateral sclerosis. *J Neurol Sci* **164(1):**37–43.

Kingshott RN, Vennelle M, Coleman EL, Engleman HM, Mackay TW, Douglas NJ (2001). Randomized, double-blind, placebo-controlled crossover trial of modafinil in the treatment of residual excessive daytime sleepiness in the sleep apnea/hypopnea syndrome. *Am J Respir Crit Care Med* **163(4):**918–923.

Koyama E, Matsubara H, Nakano T (1999). Bright light treatment for sleep-wake disturbances in aged individuals with dementia *Psychiatry Clin Neurosci* **53(2):**227–229.

Krachman SL, Crocetti J, Berger TJ, Chatila W, Eisen HJ, D'Alonzo GE (2003). Effects of nasal continuous positive airway pressure on oxygen body stores in patients with Cheyne-Stokes respiration and congestive heart failure. *Chest* **123(1):**59–66.

Le Bon O, Hoffmann G, Tecco J, Staner L, Noseda A, Pelc I, Linkowski P (2000). Mild to moderate sleep respiratory events: one negative night may not be enough. *Chest* **118(2):**353–359.

Lim J, Lasserson TJ, Fleetham J, Wright J (2003). Oral appliances for obstructive sleep apnoea. *Cochrane Database Syst Rev* no. 4, p. CD004435.

Lovell BB, Ancoli-Israel S, Gevirtz R (1995). Effect of bright light treatment on agitated behavior in institutionalized elderly subjects. *Psychiatry Res* **57(1):**7–12.

Luijpen MW, Scherder EJ, Van Someren EJ, Swaab DF, Sergeant JA (2003). Non-pharmacological interventions in cognitively impaired and demented patients–a comparison with cholinesterase inhibitors. *Rev Neurosci* **14(4):**343–368.

Lyall RA, Donaldson N, Polkey MI, Leigh PN, Moxham J (2001). Respiratory muscle strength and ventilatory failure in amyotrophic lateral sclerosis. *Brain* **124(Pt 10):**2000–2013.

Lyketsos CG, Lindell VL, Baker A, Steele C (1999). A randomized, controlled trial of bright light therapy for agitated behaviors in dementia patients residing in long-term care. *Int J Geriatr Psychiatry* **14(7):**520–525.

Massironi G, Galluzzi S, Frisoni GB (2003). Drug treatment of REM sleep behavior disorders in dementia with Lewy bodies. *Int Psychogeriatr* **15(4):**377–383.

Mast KR, Salama M, Silverman GK, Arnold RM (2004). End-of-life content in treatment guidelines for life-limiting diseases. *J Palliat Med* **7(6):**754–773.

McArdle N, Riha RL, Vennelle M, Coleman EL, Dennis MS, Warlow CP, Douglas NJ (2003). Sleep-disordered breathing as a risk factor for cerebrovascular disease: a case-control study in patients with transient ischemic attacks. *Stroke* **34(12):**2916–2921.

McGaffigan S, Bliwise DL (1997). The treatment of sundowning. A selective review of pharmacological and nonpharmacological studies. *Drugs Aging* **10(1):**10–17.

McMahon JP, Foresman BH, Chisholm RC (2003). The influence of CPAP on the neurobehavioral performance of patients with obstructive sleep apnea hypopnea syndrome: a systematic review. *WMJ* **102(1):**36–43.

Middelkoop H A, van Dam EM, Smilde-van den Doel DA, Van Dijk G (1997). 45-hour continuous quintuple-site actimetry: relations between trunk and limb movements and effects of circadian sleep-wake rhythmicity. *Psychophysiology* **34(2):**199–203.

Mishima K, Okawa M, Hishikawa Y, Hozumi S, Hori H, Takahashi K (1994). Morning bright light therapy for sleep and behavior disorders in elderly patients with dementia. *Acta Psychiatr Scand* **89(1):**1–7.

Mishima K, Hishikawa Y, Okawa M (1998). Randomized, dim light controlled, crossover test of morning bright light therapy for rest-activity rhythm disorders in patients with vascular dementia and dementia of Alzheimer's type. *Chronobiol Int* **15(6):**647–654.

Mishima K, Okawa M, Hozumi S, Hishikawa Y (2000). Supplementary administration of artificial bright light and melatonin as potent treatment for disorganized circadian rest-activity and dysfunctional autonomic and neuroendocrine systems in institutionalized demented elderly persons. *Chronobiol Int* **17(3):**419–432.

Mitler MM, Harsh J, Hirshkowitz M, Guilleminault C (2000). Long-term efficacy and safety of modafinil (PROVIGIL((R))) for the treatment of excessive daytime sleepiness associated with narcolepsy. *Sleep Med* **1(3):**231–243.

Mohsenin V (2004). Is sleep apnea a risk factor for stroke? A critical analysis. *Minerva Med* **95(4):**291–305.

Moldofsky H, Broughton RJ, Hill JD (2000). A randomized trial of the long-term, continued efficacy and safety of modafinil in narcolepsy. *Sleep Med* **1(2):**109–116.

Nachtmann A, Stang A, Wang YM, Wondzinski E, Thilmann AF (2003). Association of obstructive sleep apnea and stenotic artery disease in ischemic stroke patients. *Atherosclerosis* **169(2):**301–307.

Newsom-Davis IC, Lyall RA, Leigh PN, Moxham J, Goldstein LH (2001). The effect of non-invasive positive pressure ventilation (NIPPV) on cognitive function in amyotrophic lateral sclerosis (ALS): a prospective study. *J Neurol Neurosurg Psychiatry* **71(4):**482–487.

Nieves AV, Lang AE (2002). Treatment of excessive daytime sleepiness in patients with Parkinson's disease with modafinil. *Clin Neuropharmacol* **25(2):**111–114.

Okumoto Y, Koyama E, Matsubara H, Nakano T, Nakamura R (1998). Sleep improvement by light in a demented aged individual. *Psychiatry Clin Neurosci* **52(2):**194–196.

Olson EJ, Boeve BF, Silber MH (2000). Rapid eye movement sleep behaviour disorder: demographic, clinical and laboratory findings in 93 cases. *Brain* **123(Pt 2):**331–339.

Onofrj M, Thomas A, D'Andreamatteo G, Iacono D, Luciano AL, Di Rollo A, Di Mascio R, Ballone E, Di Iorio A (2002). Incidence of RBD and hallucination in patients affected by Parkinson's disease: 8-year follow-up. *Neurol Sci* **23(Suppl 2):**S91–S94.

Palomaki H, Berg A, Meririnne E, Kaste M, Lonnqvist R, Lehtihalmes M, Lonnqvist J (2003). Complaints of poststroke insomnia and its treatment with mianserin. *Cerebrovasc Dis* **15(1-2):**56–62.

Pareja JA, Caminero AB, Masa JF, Dobato JL (1996). A first case of progressive supranuclear palsy and pre-clinical REM sleep behavior disorder presenting as inhibition of speech during wakefulness and somniloquy with phasic muscle twitching during REM sleep. *Neurologia* **11(8):**304–306.

Parra O, Arboix A, Montserrat JM, Quinto L, Bechich S, Garcia-Eroles L (2004). Sleep-related breathing disorders: impact on mortality of cerebrovascular disease. *Eur Respir J* **24(2):**267–272.

Pepperell JC, Maskell NA, Jones DR, Langford-Wiley BA, Crosthwaite N, Stradling JR, Davies RJ (2003). A randomized controlled trial of adaptive ventilation for Cheyne-Stokes breathing in heart failure. *Am J Respir Crit Care Med* **168(9):**1109–1114.

Pinto A, de Carvalho M, Evangelista T, Lopes A, Sales-Luis L (2003). Nocturnal pulse oximetry: a new approach to establish the appropriate time for non-invasive ventilation in ALS patients. *Amyotroph Lateral Scler Other Motor Neuron Disord* **4(1):**31–35.

Rabinstein A, Shulman LM, Weiner WJ (2001). Modafinil for the treatment of excessive daytime sleepiness in Parkinson's disease: a case report. *Parkinsonism Relat Disord* **7(4):**287–288.

Randerath WJ, Galetke W, Ruhle KH (2003). Auto-adjusting CPAP based on impedance versus bilevel pressure in difficult-to-treat sleep apnea syndrome: a prospective randomized crossover study. *Med Sci Monit* **9(8):**CR353-CR358.

Reyner LA, Horne JA, Reyner A (1995). Gender- and age-related differences in sleep determined by home-recorded sleep logs and actimetry from 400 adults. *Sleep* **18(2):**127–134.

Reynolds CF, III, Kupfer DJ, Taska LS, Hoch CC, Sewitch DE, Restifo K, Spiker DG, Zimmer B, Marin RS, Nelson J (1985b). Sleep apnea in Alzheimer's dementia: correlation with mental deterioration. *J Clin Psychiatry* **46(7):**257–261.

Ross SD, Allen IE, Harrison KJ, Kvasz M, Connelly J, Sheinhait IA (1999). *Systematic Review of the Literature Regarding the Diagnosis of Sleep Apnea.*

Schenck CH, Mahowald MW, Anderson ML, Silber MH, Boeve BF, Parisi JE (1997). Lewy body variant of Alzheimer's disease (AD) identified by postmortem ubiquitin staining in a previously reported case of AD associated with REM sleep behavior disorder. *Biol Psychiatry* **42(6):**527–528.

Schols L, Haan J, Riess O, Amoiridis G, Przuntek H (1998). Sleep disturbance in spinocerebellar ataxias: is the SCA3 mutation a cause of restless legs syndrome? *Neurology* **51(6):**1603–1607.

Schwartz JR, Nelson MT, Schwartz ER, Hughes RJ (2004). Effects of modafinil on wakefulness and executive function in patients with narcolepsy experiencing late-day sleepiness. *Clin Neuropharmacol* **27(2):**74–79.

Sforza E, Johannes M, Claudio B (2005). The PAM-RL ambulatory device for detection of periodic leg movements: a validation study. *Sleep Med* **6(5):**407–413.

Sheehan B, Keene J (2002). Sunlight levels and behavioural disturbance in dementia. *Int J Geriatr Psychiatry* **17(8):**784–785.

Shneerson J, Wright J (2001). Lifestyle modification for obstructive sleep apnoea. *Cochrane Database Syst Rev* no. 1, p. CD002875.

Silber MH, Levine S (2000). Stridor and death in multiple system atrophy 10. *Mov Disord* **15(4):**699–704.

Sin DD, Logan AG, Fitzgerald FS, Liu PP, Bradley TD (2000). Effects of continuous positive airway pressure on cardiovascular outcomes in heart failure patients with and without Cheyne-Stokes respiration. *Circulation* **102(1):**61–66.

Skjerve A, Bjorvatn B, Holsten F (2004). Light therapy for behavioural and psychological symptoms of dementia. *Int J Geriatr Psychiatry* **19(6):**516–522.

Skjerve A, Holsten F, Aarsland D, Bjorvatn B, Nygaard HA, Johansen IM (2004). Improvement in behavioral symptoms and advance of activity acrophase after short-term bright light treatment in severe dementia. *Psychiatry Clin Neurosci* **58(4):**343–347.

Smith BW (2003). Modafinil for treatment of cognitive side effects of antiepileptic drugs in a patient with seizures and stroke. *Epilepsy Behav* **4(3):**352–353.

Smith I, Lasserson T, Wright J (2002). Drug treatments for obstructive sleep apnoea. *Cochrane Database Syst Rev* no. 2, p. CD003002.

Sternbach H (2002). Adjunctive modafinil in ALS. *J Neuropsychiatry Clin Neurosci* **14(2):**239.

Sugden SG, Bourgeois JA (2004). Modafinil monotherapy in poststroke depression. *Psychosomatics* **45(1):**80–81.

Sutherland D, Woodward Y, Byrne J, Allen H, Burns A (2004). The use of light therapy to lower agitation in people with dementia. *Nurs Times* **100(45):**32–34.

Syed BH, Rye DB, Singh G (2003). REM sleep behavior disorder and SCA-3 (Machado-Joseph disease). *Neurology* **60(1):**148.

Takekawa H, Kubo J, Miyamoto T, Miyamoto M, Hirata K (2001). Amyotrophic lateral sclerosis associated with insomnia and the aggravation of sleep-disordered breathing. *Psychiatry Clin Neurosci* **55(3):**263–264.

Teschler H, Dohring J, Wang YM, Berthon-Jones M (2001). Adaptive pressure support servo-ventilation: a novel treatment for Cheyne-Stokes respiration in heart failure. *Am J Respir Crit Care Med* **164(4):**614–619.

Turner RS (2002). Idiopathic rapid eye movement sleep behavior disorder is a harbinger of dementia with Lewy bodies. *J Geriatr Psychiatry Neurol* **15(4):**195–199.

Uchiyama M, Isse K, Tanaka K, Yokota N, Hamamoto M, Aida S, Ito Y, Yoshimura M, Okawa M (1995). Incidental Lewy body disease in a patient with REM sleep behavior disorder. *Neurology* **45(4):**709–712.

Van Someren EJ, Kessler A, Mirmiran M, Swaab DF (1997). Indirect bright light improves circadian rest-activity rhythm disturbances in demented patients. *Biol Psychiatry* **41(9):**955–963.

Velasco R, Salachas F, Munerati E, Le Forestier N, Pradat PF, Lacomblez L, Orvoen FE, Meininger V (2002). Nocturnal oxymetry in patients with amyotrophic lateral sclerosis: role in predicting survival. *Rev Neurol(Paris)* **158(5 Pt 1):**575–578.

Verbraecken J, Willemen M, Wittesaele W, van de HP, De Backer W (2002). Short-term CPAP does not influence the increased CO_2 drive in idiopathic central sleep apnea. *Monaldi Arch Chest Dis* **57(1):**10–18.

Volicer L, Harper DG, Manning BC, Goldstein R, Satlin A (2001). Sundowning and circadian rhythms in Alzheimer's disease. *Am J Psychiatry* **158(5):**704–711.

Wiegand M, Moller AA, Lauer CJ, Stolz S, Schreiber W, Dose M, Krieg JC (1991). Nocturnal sleep in Huntington's disease. *J Neurol* **238(4):**203–208.

Wright J, Johns R, Watt I, Melville A, Sheldon T (1997). Health effects of obstructive sleep apnoea and the effectiveness of continuous positive airways pressure: a systematic review of the research evidence. *BMJ* **314(7084):**851–860.

Yamadera H, Ito T, Suzuki H, Asayama K, Ito R, Endo S (2000). Effects of bright light on cognitive and sleep-wake (circadian) rhythm disturbances in Alzheimer-type dementia. *Psychiatry Clin Neurosci* **54(3):**352–353.

Yamaguchi M, Arai K, Asahina M, Hattori T (2003). Laryngeal stridor in multiple system atrophy. *Eur Neurol* **49(3):**154–159.

Young T, Palta M, Dempsey J, Skatrud J, Weber S, Badr S (1993). The occurrence of sleep-disordered breathing among middle-aged adults. *N Engl J Med* **328(17):**1230–1235.

Yu L, Huang XZ, Wu Q Y (1994). Management of nocturnal nasal mask continuous positive airway pressure in central hypoventilation in patients with respiratory diseases. *Zhonghua Jie He He Hu Xi Za Zhi* **17(1):**38–40.

CHAPTER 43

Restless legs syndrome and periodic limb movement disorder

L. Vignatelli,[a] M. Billiard,[b] P. Clarenbach,[c]
D. Garcia-Borreguero,[d] D. Kaynak,[e] V. Liesiene,[f]
C. Trenkwalder,[g] P. Montagna[a]

Abstract

Background In 2003, the EFNS Task Force was set up for putting forth guidelines for the management of the restless legs syndrome (RLS) and the periodic limb movement disorder (PLMD).

Methods After determining the objectives for management and the search strategy for primary and secondary RLS and for PLMD, a review of the scientific literature up to 2004 was performed for the drug classes and interventions employed in treatment (adrenergics; antiepileptic drugs; benzodiazepines/hypnotics; dopaminergic agents; opioids; other treatments). Previous guidelines were consulted. All trials were analysed according to class of evidence, and recommendations formed according to the 2004 EFNS criteria for rating.

Results Dopaminergic agents came out as having the best evidence for efficacy in primary RLS. Reported adverse events were usually mild and reversible; augmentation was a feature with dopaminergic agents. No controlled trials were available for RLS in children and for RLS during pregnancy.

The following Level A recommendations can be offered: for primary RLS, cabergoline, gabapentin, pergolide, ropinirole, levodopa and rotigotine by transdermal delivery (the latter two for short-term use) are effective in relieving the symptoms. Transdermal oestradiol is ineffective for PLMD.

Background

Restless legs syndrome (RLS) was first identified by Willis (1685) and reviewed in full monographic form by Ekbom (1945). Accordingly, it is also termed 'Ekbom's Syndrome'. RLS is also known as 'anxietas tibiarum' and by the colloquial term 'leg jitters'. RLS has a significant motor counterpart in the form of recurrent jerking movements termed 'periodic limb movements in sleep' (PLMS, formerly 'nocturnal myoclonus' and 'periodic leg movements in sleep'). Even though PLMS may

---

[a]Department of Neurological Sciences, University of Bologna Medical School, Bologna, Italy; [b]Faculty of Medicine, Gui de Chauliac Hospital, Montpellier, France; [c]Neurologische Klinik, EV Johannes-Krankenhaus, Bielefeld, Germany; [d]Department of Neurology, Fundacion Jimenez Diaz, Sleep Disorders Unit, Universidad Autonoma de Madrid, Madrid, Spain; [e]Istanbul University, Cerrahpasa Faculty of Medicine, Sleep Disorders Unit, Istanbul, Turkey; [f]Faculty of Medicine, University of Kaunas, Lithuania; [g]Department of Clinical Neurophysiology, University of Goettingen, Goettingen, Germany.

occur independently from RLS as an incidental polysomnographic finding, the International Classification of Sleep Disorders recognizes the 'Periodic Limb Movement Disorder' (PLMD) because of its potential impact on sleep quality and a possible source of excessive daytime sleepiness, particularly when PLMS are associated with arousals (PLMS-A) (AASM 2005a). PLMS/PLMD severity is assessed by the PLMS Index (PLMS-I: PLMS per hour of polysomnographic recording).

The International Restless Legs Syndrome Study Group has proposed four minimal clinical diagnostic criteria for RLS (Walters *et al.*, 1995) revised in 2003 (Allen *et al.*, 2003): (1) an urge to move the legs, usually accompanied or caused by uncomfortable and unpleasant sensations in the legs; (2) the urge to move or unpleasant sensations begin or worsen during periods of rest or inactivity such as lying or sitting; (3) the urge to move or unpleasant sensations are partially or totally relieved by movement, such as walking or stretching, at least as long as the activity continues; (4) the urge to move or unpleasant sensations are worse in the evening or night than during the day or only occur in the evening or night.

Severity is measured on the International RLS rating scale that has ten questions for disease severity (Walters *et al.*, 2003). A RLS Quality of Life Instrument measuring quality of life has been recently validated (Atkinson *et al.*, 2004).

RLS may be either primary or secondary (AASM 2005b). Primary RLS often represents a familial disorder. RLS may also be secondary to other pathological conditions, in particular peripheral neuropathies, myelopathies, uraemia, rheumatoid arthritis, Parkinson disease, iron deficiency, attention deficit-hyperactivity disorder in children, and pregnancy. Dysfunction of the endogenous opioid and dopaminergic systems has been implicated in RLS principally based on the favourable effects of pharmacological interventions. The evidence for a central dopaminergic defect is still controversial. A role for iron and iron storage in the pathophysiology has also been derived from studies on iron metabolism in RLS.

The goal of therapy for RLS and PLMD is to control the symptoms. The aim of this guideline is to examine the best evidence available on the effectiveness of any treatment in these disorders.

Objectives

To determine the effectiveness and maintained effect of drugs and physical interventions in the treatment of RLS and PLMD, the following hypotheses were tested:

(1) Any drug is more effective than no treatment or treatment with placebo:
  a. in abolishing or reducing the occurrence of RLS and PLMD;
  b. in improving the quality of life.
(2) One class or one molecule is better than another.
(3) Any physical intervention is more effective than no treatment or treatment with placebo:
  a. in abolishing or reducing the occurrence of RLS and PLMD;
  b. in improving the quality of life.
(4) The side effects of the class or molecules and of the physical treatments proved to be effective do not exceed the therapeutic effects.

Methods and search strategy

The best available evidence to address each question was sought, with the classification scheme by type of study design according to the EFNS Guidance document (Class I to Class IV evidence, Brainin *et al.*, 2004). If the highest class of evidence was not sufficient or required updating the literature search was extended to the lower adjacent class of evidence.

Patients with RLS and PLMD, with any other co-morbidity and co-treatment were considered. Explicit diagnostic criteria of RLS were not required for inclusion.

Therapies with any kind of drugs (any dose, any regimen) and with any kind of physical intervention were included. The following classes of drugs were considered: adrenergic agents; antiepileptic drugs; benzodiazepines/hypnotics; dopaminergic agents (levodopa; ergot-derived; non-ergot derived dopaminergics); opioids; other treatments.

The duration of treatment in every study was divided into short term ($\leq$30 days) or long term (>30 days).

For RLS, types of outcome measures were the following domains:

a. Paraesthesia/Dysaesthesia, or pain (by simple subjective report or subjective validated scales/questionnaires).
b. Polysomnographic indexes of sleep dysfunction (mean PLMS-I in sleep, mean PLMS-A, sleep efficiency, sleep latency, actigraphic activity in sleep).
c. Quality of life.
d. Adverse events; augmentation effect, defined as 'markedly augmented RLS symptoms occurring in the afternoon and the evening prior to the taking the next nightly dose' was rated among adverse events at the latest follow-up.
e. Drop-outs.
f. Rate of patients choosing to remain in treatment after completion of trial.

For PLMD, the outcomes belonged to the following domains:

a. Polysomnographic indexes of sleep dysfunction.
b. Quality of life.
c. Adverse events.
d. Drop-outs.

In the strategy for identification of studies, search terms were generated for searching the following electronic databases (see table 43.1): Cochrane Library, National Library of Medicine's MEDLINE (from 1966), EMBASE (from 1980), CINAHL (from 1982). Existing guidelines were also sought and taken into consideration.

All references until the end of 2004 were reviewed to assess potentially relevant studies for inclusion, and data extraction performed. For every key question, an evidence table was created listing the design and methodological classification of each study. For forming guideline recommendations, the volume of evidence, applicability, generalisability, consistency and clinical impact were summarized by every member of the Task Force. Classes of evidence and rating levels of recommendations were attributed according to the EFNS Task Force Guidance (Brainin *et al.*, 2004). Disagreement was resolved by discussion.

Finally, every member of the guideline group had to declare a potential conflict of interest, if any.

Results

Class I to III studies are reported here, and are referenced in supplementary table 1 available online at *European Journal of Neurology*, www.blackwellpublishing.com. Class IV studies were also considered, but are only referenced in supplementary table 2 (see Vignatelli *et al.*, 2006).

Adrenergic agents

Fifteen reports concerned the use of adrenergic agents (clonidine, phenoxybenzamine, propranolol, talipexole). In primary RLS, in a class II study (Wagner *et al.*, 1996), clonidine (mean dosage 0.5 mg 2 h before onset of symptoms) for 2–3 weeks, improved paraesthesiae and motor restlessness (1.6 and 1.7 points respectively of a non-validated scale) and sleep latency (35.5 min) but PLMS-I, PLMS-A, actigraphy and sleep efficiency were left unchanged. Adverse events (dry mouth, decreased cognition, constipation, decreased libido, light-headedness, sleepiness, headache) during clonidine did not lead to drop-outs. There is a class III evidence (Inoue *et al.*, 1999) that talipexole (an agonist both at dopamine D2 and adrenergic alpha-2 autoreceptors) 0.4–0.8 mg at bedtime improved symptoms and sleep efficiency and reduced PLMS-I and PLMS-A.

In secondary RLS there is a class III evidence (Ausserwinkler and Schmidt, 1989b) that 0.075 mg clonidine, twice daily, showed decrease/relief of symptoms in nine out of ten compared to one out of ten patients treated with placebo, at 3 days, in chronic uraemia.

RECOMMENDATIONS

Clonidine is probably effective in reducing symptoms and sleep latency in primary RLS at short term (Level B). Clonidine had several but tolerated adverse events (dry mouth, decreased cognition and libido, light-headedness, sleepiness, headache) (Level B). There is not sufficient evidence to make a recommendation about talipexole, propranolol and phenoxybenzamine, and about clonidine in secondary RLS.

Table 43.1 Search strategy for identification of studies

Sources

Published papers (Systematic Reviews, Meta-analysis, Randomised Trials, Cohort studies, Case-control studies, Observational non-analytic studies) were identified from the following sources

- Cochrane Database of Systematic Reviews (CSDR) in the Cochrane Library: issue 3, 2004
- Database of Abstract of Reviews of Effects (DARE) in the Cochrane Library: issue 3, 2004
- CENTRAL (Cochrane Central Register of Controlled Trial) in the Cochrane Library: issue 3, 2004
- National Library of Medicine's MEDLINE database: from 1966 to December 2004
- EMBASE database: from 1980 to December 2004
- CINAHL database: from 1982 to December 2004
- Checking Reference Lists: bibliographies of identified articles reviewed to find additional references.

Search terms

All the electronic data base considered were checked with terms focusing only on the condition.
With regard to Restless Legs Syndrome the following terms were used for the search with 'free text':

1 Restless*
2 Leg*
3 Limb*
4 #1 AND #2
5 #1 AND #3
6 Anxiet*
7 Tibia*
8 #6 AND #7
9 jitter*
10 #2 AND #9
11 #3 AND #9
12 Ekbom*
13 #4 OR #5 OR #8 OR #10 OR #11 OR #12

For the search with MeSH terms (MEDLINE, from 1972 to now): 'Restless Legs Syndrome[MeSH]'.
With regard to PLMD the following terms were used for the search with 'free text':

1 Myoclon*
2 Noct*
3 Sleep*
4 #1 AND #2
5 #1 AND 3#
6 Periodic*
7 Movement*
8 #2 AND #6 AND #7
9 #3 AND #6 AND #7
10 Leg*
11 Limb*
12 #6 AND #7 AND #10
13 #6 AND #7 AND #11
14 #4 OR #5 OR #8 OR #9 OR #12 OR #13

For the search with MeSH terms (MEDLINE, from 1999 to now): 'Nocturnal Myoclonus Syndrome'[MeSH]

The search strategy identified 2892 references for RLS and 5291 references for PLMD. After assessing from title, abstract or full text of articles, a total of 281 articles for RLS or PLMD were found eligible. In particular, according to each treatment

Continued

Table 43.1 Continued

category the following articles were included (possible duplicates):
- adrenergic agents: 15
- antiepileptic drugs: 22
- benzodiazepines/hypnotics: 36
- dopaminergic agents:
  - levodopa: 52
  - ergot derivatives: 39
  - non-ergot derivatives: 39
- opioids: 22
- other treatments: 82

Antiepileptic drugs

Twenty-two reports concerned the use of antiepileptic drugs (carbamazepine, gabapentin, lamotrigine, topiramate, valproate). In primary RLS, there is class II evidence (Telstad *et al.*, 1984) that carbamazepine 100–300 mg (median dose 236 mg) at bedtime improved the frequency of RLS symptoms reducing attacks from a mean of 2.9 to 1.5/week in a long-term (5 weeks) trial. Adverse events were reported as 'not serious' in 34 out of 84 patients versus 20 out of 90 with placebo. Another class II evidence (Lundvall *et al.*, 1983) reported a beneficial effect of carbamazepine with respect to placebo, but without calculation of statistical significance. There is class I evidence (Garcia-Borreguero *et al.*, 2002a) that gabapentin at a dose of 1800 mg daily (one third of total dosage at 12 a.m. and two thirds at 8 p.m.) versus placebo reduced RLS symptoms by 8.4 points according to the RLS Rating Scale, improved sleep efficiency by 9.8% and reduced PLMS-I by 9.8 events, at 6 weeks. Adverse events were more frequent with gabapentin (48% vs 20.8%), and commonly included malaise, somnolence and gastro-intestinal symptoms. No adverse events led to discontinuation of treatment. Class III evidence trials with gabapentin (Mellick and Mellick, 1996; Adler 1997; Happe *et al.*, 2001, 2003) reported an improvement in RLS symptoms at long-term follow-up (6–18 months) with minor adverse events (dizziness, drowsiness, enhanced alcohol effect, headache).

In a class II evidence trial with 20 patients (Eisensehr *et al.*, 2004), valproate slow release at an average dose of 600 mg versus placebo significantly reduced RLS symptom intensity by 1.7 points according to a non-validated scale, and RLS symptom duration by 92.3 min/24 h, but not PLMS-I and PLMS-A, at 3 weeks. The most commonly reported adverse event was drowsiness.

In secondary RLS in haemodialysis patients, there is class II evidence (Thorp *et al.*, 2001) that gabapentin at a dose of 200/300 mg after each haemodialysis session versus placebo reduced RLS symptoms by 2.8 points, according to a non-validated scale, at 6 weeks. Two patients dropped out for somnolence and lethargy under gabapentin. In a class III study (Freye *et al.*, 2004), subjects with secondary RLS and heroin abuse during rapid opiate detoxification had symptoms reduced by 2.0 points in a non-validated scale at 1 h, after taking gabapentin at a dose of 1200 mg.

RECOMMENDATIONS

Gabapentin, at 800–1800 mg/day can be considered effective in primary RLS (Level A) and probably effective in secondary RLS after haemodialysis (Level B). Adverse events were usually mild and reversible. Carbamazepine 100–300 mg and valproate slow-release at 600 mg/day can be recommended as probably effective in primary RLS (Level B). There is insufficient evidence to make a recommendation about topiramate and lamotrigine, and about the use of antiepileptic drugs in PLMD.

Benzodiazepines/hypnotics

A total of 36 reports concern the use of ben-
zodiazepines/hypnotics (alprazolam, clonazepam,
diazepam, nitrazepam, oxazepam, temazepam, triazolam and zolpidem).

For primary RLS, there is conflicting class II
evidence (Montagna *et al.*, 1984; Boghen *et al.*,
1986) that clonazepam 0.5–2 mg did or did
not significantly eliminate/reduce paraesthesiae/
dysaesthesiae compared to placebo (a discrepancy
possibly related to different administration schedules: before bedtime versus four doses/throughout
the day). As for polysomnographic indices, only a
14% improvement in sleep efficiency was reported
in a class III short-term trial with clonazepam
1 mg at bedtime (Saletu *et al.*, 2001a). In a
class II trial (Montagna *et al.*, 1984), clonazepam
1 mg at bedtime improved subjective sleep quality. Adverse events were absent in one class II
study but daily sleepiness was found in three
patients (out of six) versus one on placebo in
another class II study of clonazepam 0.5–2 mg
at four doses throughout the day (Boghen *et al.*,
1986).

For PLMD, there is class II evidence that clonazepam, 1 mg was not more effective than
temazepam 30 mg (Mitler *et al.*, 1986) and that
clonazepam 0.5–1.5 mg was not more effective
than cognitive behavioural therapy (Edinger *et al.*,
1996). Several class III trials show that clonazepam
0.5–2 mg at bedtime decreased the PLMS-I and
sometimes the PLMS-A (Ohanna *et al.*, 1985; Mitler
et al., 1986; Peled and Lavie, 1987; Inami *et al.*,
1997; Arens *et al.*, 1998). Adverse events with
clonazepam 0.5 mg at bedtime were increased anxiety leading to drop-out in one patient out of six
(Edinger *et al.*, 1996, class II trial), and somnolence or dizziness in two with one dropout out
of ten patients (Peled and Lavie, 1987; class III
trial). There are two class II studies that triazolam (0.125–0.50 mg) improved sleep efficiency and
daytime sleepiness without any effect on PLMS
at short-term follow-up (Doghramji *et al.*, 1991;
Bonnet and Arand, 1991). There are single class III
trials that temazepam (30 mg) (Mitler *et al.*, 1986)
and nitrazepam (2.5–10 mg) (Moldofsky *et al.*,
1986) improved sleep efficiency, sleep latency and
PLMS-I.

RECOMMENDATIONS

Clonazepam should be considered as probably
effective for improving symptoms in primary RLS
when given at 1 mg before bedtime, but also probably ineffective when given at four doses throughout the day (Level B). In PLMD, clonazepam at
0.5–2 mg/daily is probably effective in ameliorating PLMS-I and PLMS-A (Level B) and triazolam
(0.125–0.50 mg/day) is probably effective in ameliorating sleep efficiency and probably ineffective
in reducing PLMS (Level B). Adverse events with
benzodiazepines (morning sedation, memory dysfunction, daytime somnolence, muscle weakness)
were usually mild, dose-dependent and reversible.
There is insufficient evidence to make a recommendation about alprazolam, nitrazepam, temazepam
and zolpidem. Likewise no recommendation can
be offered for benzodiazepines/hypnotics in secondary RLS.

Dopaminergic agents
Levodopa

Fifty-two reports concerned the use of levodopa.
For primary RLS, at 4 weeks, there is class I evidence
(Benes *et al.*, 1999) that levodopa/benserazide in
a single bedtime dose (mean: 159/40 mg) versus
placebo improved quality of sleep by 0.7 points
on a 1–5 point scale, reduced sleep latency by
26 min, improved quality of life, and reduced
PLMS-I by 27.8 events/h. This study did not
consider improvement in RLS symptoms as outcome. There are class II studies (Akpinar, 1987;
Brodeur *et al.*, 1988; Trenkwalder *et al.*, 1995;
Montplaisir *et al.*, 1996; Collado-Seidel *et al.*, 1999;
Saletu *et al.*, 2003; Eisensehr *et al.*, 2004) that
short-term (1 night/4 weeks) levodopa/benserazide
in a single bedtime dose (100–200 mg) without
or with an extra 100 mg dose 3 h after bedtime reduced RLS symptoms moderately, by 0.5
points on a 4-point scale, 1.9 points on a 10 point
scale, and 29.3 points on a VAS. The same was
not demonstrated in another study. In a class II
study of selected RLS patients of rapid release lev-
odopa/benserazide (from 100/25 to 200/50 mg)
versus rapid release levodopa/benserazide plus

slow release levodopa/benserazide (100/25 mg) at bedtime, the latter was shown to reduce RLS symptoms in the second half of the night, improve subjective sleep quality and reduce sleep latency (Collado-Seidel *et al.*, 1999). Commonly reported adverse events in these studies were diarrhoea, nausea, dyspepsia, reduced general drive, muscle weakness, somnolence and headache. Worsening or augmentation of RLS was reported in 2/37 and 4/20 patients, or 16.7–26.7% of patients.

On long-term (2–24 months), open phase (class III) trials levodopa proved still 'effective' in 70.2% of patients, showed satisfaction with therapy in 29–31% of patients and improved RLS symptoms by 6.0–6.5 points in a 7-point scale and reduced perceived sleep latency by 131 min. Drop-outs were many, 30–70% in these series, and augmentation ranged from 18.6 to 82%.

For secondary RLS, at short-term follow-up, two class II studies (Trenkwalder *et al.*, 1995; Walker *et al.*, 1996) evaluated levodopa (plus benserazide or carbidopa) in a single bedtime dose (100–200 mg) versus placebo in uraemic patients. In one study, RLS symptoms were reduced (0.9 points improvement on a 0–10-point scale). PLMS-I and PLMS-A were also reduced and quality of life improved. In Walker *et al.*'s study (1996) however, only PLMS indexes but not RLS symptoms were improved.

For PLMD, there are class II studies of levodopa (plus benserazide or carbidopa; 200 mg at bedtime or 100 mg five times a day) versus placebo in PLMD with or without RLS (Kaplan *et al.*, 1993), PLMD with narcolepsy (Boivin *et al.*, 1989) and PLMD in complete spinal lesion patients (De Mello *et al.*, 1999): PLMS-I and PLMS-A were reduced.

RECOMMENDATIONS

In primary RLS and at short-term follow-up, levodopa was effective in reducing symptoms of RLS and in improving sleep quality and quality of life and reducing PLMS (Level A). Adverse events were minor but more frequent than placebo (Level A). In long-term follow-up, levodopa was possibly still effective, but 30–70% of patients dropped out because of adverse events or lack of efficacy (Level C). Augmentation probably occurred in 20–82% of treated patients, in a still uncertain number of them leading to treatment discontinuation. In RLS secondary to uraemia, at short-term follow-up, levodopa was probably effective in reducing symptoms, improving quality of life and reducing PLMS-I and PLMS-A (Level B). In PLMD, at short-term follow-up, levodopa was probably effective in improving PLMS-I and PLMS-A (Level B).

Ergot derivatives

Thirty-nine reports concerned the use of ergot derivatives (alpha-dihydroergocriptine, bromocriptine, cabergoline, lisuride, pergolide, terguride).

In primary RLS, Alpha-dihydroergocriptine 10–40 mg gave subjective reduction of RLS symptoms in a class III study; subjective sleep patterns also improved (Tergau *et al.*, 2001). Bromocriptine 7.5 mg in a class II study (Walters *et al.*, 1988) gave partial subjective improvement in restlessness and paresthesiae in five out of six patients, without relevant adverse side effects. For cabergoline (0.5, 1 and 2 mg once daily), a class I trial in 86 patients (Stiasny-Kolster *et al.*, 2004a) showed a change from baseline respectively of −13.1, −13.5 and −15.7 points on the International RLS scale score with respect to −3.3 with placebo at 5 weeks. Abolition of symptoms was observed in 36.4% of the 2 mg cabergoline group with respect to 4.4% with placebo. Long-term (1 year) open label treatment at mean doses of 2.2 mg/day or at 1.5 mg/day for 26 weeks (Benes *et al.*, 2004) remained effective (class III). During long-term treatment, adverse events led to drop-outs in 11 out of 85; in particular augmentation was found in 11% of patients. For pergolide, there are six short-term and five long-term studies. In a class I evidence trial (total number of patients involved was 100) pergolide at dosages from 0.05 upwards to 1.5 mg and at mean dosages of 0.4–0.55 mg daily significantly improved RLS severity, significantly ameliorated subjective quality of sleep and significantly decreased PLMS-I and PLMS-A (Trenkwalder *et al.*, 2004b). The rate of responders ('much improved' or 'very much improved' to Patient Global Impression scale) at 6 weeks was 68% in the pergolide versus 15% in the placebo group. Maintenance for 12 months resulted in a significant reduction of PLMS-I and PLMS-A at a mean dosage of 0.52 mg daily (class III evidence). Adverse events were reported in 40–70% of patients as mild: nausea, headache, nasal congestion, dizziness, orthostatic hypotension, easily controlled in one study with domperidone 20 mg. No rebound or augmentation phenomenon was observed in class I and II trials. A class II comparative trial of pergolide versus levodopa (Staedt *et al.*, 1997) pointed out the better outcome with pergolide treatment: pergolide 0.125 mg daily gave complete relief in 82% of patients as compared with 9% with levodopa 250 mg; moreover pergolide caused a 79% reduction in PLMS-I as compared to 45% with levodopa. Terguride 0.25–0.5 mg/day improved subjective RLS symptoms in a class III trial.

In RLS secondary to uraemia undergoing haemodialysis, pergolide 0.05–0.25 mg in short-term (10 nights) did not modify time to sleep onset, numbers of awakenings and actigraphy for PLMS. Subjective improvement in sleep quality and RLS symptoms in five out of eight patients was not validated by statistical analysis against the placebo (class II study) (Pieta *et al.*, 1998). Adverse events were nausea in one subject and nightmares in another.

In PLMD in narcolepsy, there is class II evidence (Boivin *et al.*, 1993b) that bromocriptine (7.5 mg) was effective.

RECOMMENDATIONS

In primary RLS, pergolide is established as effective at mean dosages of 0.4–0.55 mg/day at short term (Level A) and possibly effective in the long term (Level C). PLMS-I, and PLMS-A are also improved. Cabergoline is also effective at 0.5–2 mg/day at short term (Level A) and possibly effective in the long term (Level C). Bromocriptine 7.5 mg can be recommended as probably effective (Level B). In secondary RLS associated with chronic haemodialysis, pergolide in short-term administration is probably ineffective at 0.25 mg/day (Level B). In PLMD associated with narcolepsy,

bromocriptine is probably effective (Level B). Most frequent adverse events of ergot-derived dopamine agonists (nausea, headache, nasal congestion, dizziness, orthostatic hypotension) were controlled by domperidone. Augmentation was not assessed with pergolide in class I studies. There is insufficient evidence to make a recommendation about alpha-dihydroergocryptine, lisuride and terguride.

Non-ergot derivatives

Thirty-nine reports concerned the use of non-ergot derivatives (pramipexole, ropinirole, rotigotine). At the time of writing ropinirole was the most extensively studied drug for RLS in class I studies. For primary RLS, in a class I trial of 284 patients (Trenkwalder *et al.*, 2004a) treatment with ropinirole at a mean effective dose of 1.9 mg/daily caused a significant reduction in the International RLS scale score (11.04 points versus 8.03 under placebo) and quality of life after 12 weeks. Similar results obtained in two other class I trials, one of 266 patients with ropinirole at 1.5 mg/day mean effective dose (11.2 points reduced International RLS scale score versus 8.7 under placebo) (Walters *et al.*, 2004) and another of 22 patients with ropinirole at a mean dosage of 4.6 mg daily (Adler *et al.*, 2004). Mild and transient adverse events included nausea, headache, fatigue and dizziness. As for polysomnographic indices of sleep disruption, in a class I study with polysomnography (Allen *et al.*, 2004), ropinirole at a mean dose of 1.8 mg/day significantly improved PLMS-I (by 76.2% versus 14% on placebo), PLMS-A and sleep latency. Adverse events were headache and nausea, less commonly dizziness. Worsening of RLS possibly due to augmentation was observed in 4 out of 59 (7%) patients.

As for pramipexole, a class II trial of pramipexole (0.75–1.5 mg 1 h before bedtime) in 10 patients (Montplaisir *et al.*, 1999) demonstrated significantly reduced RLS subjective scores and significant improvements in PLMS-I. Adverse events (nausea, constipation, loss of appetite in 90% of patients; dizziness in 40%, daytime fatigue in 30%) were reported as mild and transient, but persistent nausea was observed in 33% at 1.5 mg/day. Long-term use of pramipexole was effective in class III trials.

Rotigotine continuous transdermal patch delivery (1.125, 2.25 and 4.5 mg/day) improved RLS symptoms (by 10.5–15.7 points compared to 8 on placebo) in a short-term class I trial of 63 patients, significantly so at the 4.5 mg dose (Stiasny-Kostler *et al.*, 2004c). Adverse events and skin tolerability were similar with placebo. As these data were obtained over a 1-week study period, the mid- and long-term efficacy of rotigotine remains to be seen.

For RLS secondary to uraemia undergoing haemodialysis, there is one class II study in 11 patients whereby ropinirole 1.45 mg/day gave better improvement of symptoms than levodopa 190 mg/daily (Pellecchia *et al.*, 2004).

RECOMMENDATIONS

In primary RLS, ropinirole at 1.5–4.6 mg/day has a Level A of efficacy. Rotigotine by transdermal patch delivery is also effective in the short term (Level A), and pramipexole is probably effective (Level B). In RLS secondary to uremia ropinirole is probably effective (Level B). Adverse events were those common to all dopaminergic agents. Augmentation has not been well studied for any of these drugs, and has been reported by 7% of patients with ropinirole (class I evidence). There is insufficient evidence to make recommendations about the use of non-ergot derivatives in PLMD.

Opioids

Twenty-two reports concerned the use of opioids (codeine and dihydrocodeine, dextromethorphan, methadone, morphine, oxycodone, propoxyphene, tilidine and tramadol). For primary RLS, there is class II evidence (Walters *et al.*, 1993) that short-term oxycodone at a mean dose of 11.4 mg daily gave a 52% improvement in subjective rating scales on RLS symptoms. In this study oxycodone also significantly reduced PLMS-I (by 34%) and PLMS-A (by 23%), while improving sleep efficiency (by 25%). Adverse events were minimal

constipation in two out of eleven and daytime lethargy in one out of eleven patients.

For PLMD, there is class II evidence (Kaplan *et al.*, 1993) that short-term propoxyphene 100–200 mg before bedtime did not improve sleep latency, sleep efficiency and PLMS-I, but reduced PLMS-A by 28.6 events/h versus placebo. Adverse events were mild depression, dizziness, nausea and 1/6 patients dropped out because of urticaria and tongue swelling.

RECOMMENDATIONS

For primary RLS, oxycodone at a mean dosage of 11.4 mg can be considered as probably effective in improving RLS symptoms and PLMS-I, PLMS-A and sleep efficiency on a short-term basis (Level B). Adverse events (mild sedation and rare nocturnal respiratory disturbances on long-term use) were usually mild and reversible, problems of addiction being observed only rarely. For PLMD, short-term propoxyphene is probably ineffective in improving sleep quality and PLMS-I (Level B). There is insufficient evidence to make a recommendation about morphine, tramadol, codeine and dihydrocodeine, tilidine, and methadone and about the intrathecal route of administration. There is insufficient evidence to make a recommendation about the use of opioids in secondary RLS.

Other treatments

Eighty-two reports concerned the use of other treatments. Non-pharmacological cognitive or physical agent interventions, and drug treatments with myorelaxants, vitamins/minerals, hormones (oestrogens, melatonin, erythropoietin) and antidepressants were the subjects of these trials. Surgical interventions with deep brain stimulation in Parkinson's disease, venous sclerotherapy and kidney transplant were also available.

For primary RLS, one class II trial of iron sulphate 325 mg given in liquid form per os over 12 weeks (concurrently with other treatments) did not show any significant effect either on RLS symptoms or sleep quality; 7 out of 28 patients dropped out and relevant adverse events were nausea, constipation, tooth discoloration, dark stools, vertebral fracture and RLS worsening (Davis *et al.*, 2000). No effect was noted with vibration in a class II trial (Montagna *et al.*, 1984). Improved RLS severity, sleep efficiency or decreased PLMS-I were reported in class III single trials of iron dextran given intravenous in a single of 1000 mg (Early *et al.*, 2004), magnesium oxide 12.4 mmol (Hornyak *et al.*, 1998) and amantadine 100–300 mg/day (Evidente *et al.*, 2000).

For RLS secondary to uraemia, there is class II evidence (Sloand *et al.*, 2004) for improved RLS symptoms with intravenous iron dextran 1000 mg; efficacy waned however 4 weeks after treatment. In a class III study, kidney transplantation abolished RLS symptoms at short term in all of eleven patients, and in four patients out of the eleven at long term (Winkelmann *et al.*, 2002).

In PLMD, a class I trial with transdermal oestradiol 2.5 g/day gel (or 50 μg/24h for patients older than 55 years) showed no effect on PLMS-I and PLMS-A at 3 months (Polo-Kantola *et al.*, 2001). Single class II trials showed that modafinil 200–440 mg/day in PLMD associated with narcolepsy (Broughton *et al.*, 1997) and one-day nocturnal haemodialysis (Hanly *et al.*, 2003) were ineffective. In PLMD associated with insomnia, a class II trial of cognitive behavioural therapy (sleep education, stimulus control, sleep restriction) found no difference with clonazepam 0.5–1.5 mg/day (Edinger *et al.*, 1996). Several class III trials with nasal continuous airway positive pressure in patients with obstructive sleep apnoeas resulted in conflicting findings of either unchanged, increased or decreased PLMS-I. In PLMD associated with depressive insomnia, trazodone 100 mg did not modify sleep quality or PLMS-I, or on the contrary reduced PLMS-I by 10.8 (two 1-night only class III studies, Saletu-Zyhlarz *et al.*, 2001, 2002). In class III studies, 5-OH-tryptophan 500 mg did not modify PLMS-I/PLMS-A (Guilleminault *et al.*, 1987), while apomorphine, either 0.5 mg single dose subcutaneously or transdermal (Priano *et al.*, 2003; Haba-Rubio *et al.*, 2003) and physical exercise in PLMD patients with complete spinal lesion (De Mello *et al.*, 1996, 1997, 2002) reduced the PLMS-I.

RECOMMENDATIONS

In primary RLS, both iron sulphate per os and vibration are probably ineffective (Level B). There is insufficient evidence to make any recommendation about the use of intravenous iron dextran, magnesium oxide and amantadine. In RLS secondary to uraemia, iron dextran 1000 mg in a single intravenous dose is probably effective in the short term (less than 1 month) (Level B). In PLMD, transdermal oestradiol is established as ineffective (Level A) and modafinil and one-day nocturnal haemodialysis as probably ineffective, while cognitive behavioural therapy is no different than clonazepam (Level B). 5-OH-tryptophan and trazodone are possibly ineffective and apomorphine and physical exercise (in myelopathy) possibly effective (Level C).

Discussion

Before offering final comments, we wish to emphasize that dopaminergic agents are the best studied drugs to date because of the increasing interest of pharmaceutical companies in achieving an official treatment indication for RLS. However, as only a few and small-scale studies have been carried out on non-dopaminergic compounds, and some have shown promising therapeutic effects, it is to be hoped that an increased effort from both industry and investigators to develop further alternatives will be taken. Accordingly, lack of controlled trials for many drug classes should not be construed as implying negative evidence of efficacy. The most frequently observed weak points of the above cited randomised controlled trials were flaws in allocation concealment procedures, the absence of a predefined primary endpoint, the overuse of non-validated or surrogate endpoints instead of clinically relevant patient-oriented endpoints (e.g. rate of remission, quality of life). Such problems are generally, but not only, shared by studies predating the year 2000. The recently validated international scales of disease severity and disease-specific quality of life (Walters *et al.*, 2003; Atkinson *et al.*, 2004) will represent valuable tools to design future trials with clinically relevant primary endpoints. Furthermore, augmentation has not been assessed adequately for most drugs (both dopaminergic and not-dopaminergic) and it is hoped that, as more specific and reliable tools are being developed, they will allow a better assessment of both the long-term efficacy and augmentation.

Recommendation

For primary RLS, ropinirole given at mean dosages of 1.5–4.6 mg/day, and pergolide at 0.4–0.55 mg/day have confirmed Level A efficacy for relieving paraesthesiae and motor restlessness. Cabergoline, levodopa and transdermal delivery rotigotine are also established as effective, the latter two so far only for short-term use (Level A). Among the antiepileptic drugs, gabapentin should be considered as effective in primary RLS (Level A).

For other dopaminergics (pramipexole, bromocriptine) and for valproate, carbamazepine, clonidine and oxycodone there is evidence to consider these drugs as probably effective (Level B), while for clonazepam evidence for probable efficacy (at 1 mg at bedtime) and probable inefficacy (at four doses/day), according to dosage schedule (Level B). Iron sulphate and vibration are probably ineffective (Level B). In long-term use, levodopa is possibly effective (Level C).

For RLS secondary to uraemia, levodopa, ropinirole 1.45 mg/d, gabapentin 200–300 mg/d and iron dextran 1000 mg intravenous are probably effective, the latter on short-term use (Level B). For PLMD, transdermal oestradiol is ineffective (Level A). Clonazepam and levodopa are probably effective while propoxyphene, triazolam, modafinil and 1 night haemodialysis probably ineffective (Level B). Bromocriptine is probably effective in PLMD associated with narcolepsy (Level B). 5-OH-tryptophan and trazodone are possibly ineffective and apomorphine and physical exercise possibly effective (Level C).

As for adverse events, these were reported as usually mild and reversible upon discontinuation of treatment in the generality of the trials. In particular the peripheral adverse events of dopaminergics were easily relieved by domperidone. For this class of drugs, augmentation represents a troublesome adverse event: even though reported particularly with levodopa, it is hard to get reliable comparative data, especially in the absence of an augmentation rating scale. Recently, concern with the ergot derivatives was raised by the discovery of severe multivalvular heart defects and constrictive pericarditis and pleuropulmonary fibrosis after long-term use in Parkinson's Disease (reported with cabergoline, pergolide and bromocriptine). Daily dosages in these cases were equal or greater than 4 mg pergolide for several months. Spontaneous echocardiographic regression of valvular insufficiency along with marked clinical improvement was reported after cessation of the ergot derivatives in some case reports. It was suggested that high doses should be avoided and that patients under dopamine agonists receive a clinical cardiac assessment at 3–6 months intervals and if there is any doubt, to obtain an echocardiogram. However, the cardiopulmonary fibrosis side effects of the ergot derivatives have been described too recently for a meaningful analysis across the different compounds.

Comparison of these versus guidelines already published (Chesson *et al.*, 1999; Hening *et al.*, 1999, 2004) demonstrates minor differences in judgement, in part related to the different sets of evidence utilised. In all guidelines, dopaminergic agents come out as the best recommended agents for the treatment of RLS. Opioids have not been here considered as established, and for iron supplementation we found only class II favourable trials (short term) or even evidence of inefficacy. Iron has been reported as more effective in low ferritin patients. Unfortunately, still partial evidence is overall available for secondary RLS, almost all in RLS secondary to uraemia, and for PLMD. In particular, recommendations cannot be offered for RLS during pregnancy or during childhood, where quality trials are needed.

Finally, it is useful to underline that these guidelines should not be considered as exhausting all methods of care for RLS or PLMD. In consideration of the circumstances presented by any particular patient, the ultimate judgement regarding the type of care need always rest with the attending physician.

RECOMMENDATIONS

Final Level A
For primary RLS:

- Cabergoline (0.5–2 mg once daily) improves RLS scores.
- Gabapentin (dosage 800–1800 mg/daily) reduces RLS scores and improves sleep efficiency and PLMS-I.
- Levodopa/benserazide (mean dose 159/40 mg at bedtime) improves RLS symptoms, quality of sleep, sleep latency, PLMS-I and quality of life.
- Pergolide (mean doses 0.4–0.55 mg/day) is effective in improving RLS severity and ameliorating subjective quality of sleep.
- Ropinirole (mean doses 1.5–4.6 mg/day) is effective in ameliorating RLS scale scores and quality of life, and in improving sleep latency and PLMS-I/PLMS-A.
- Rotigotine by transdermal patch delivery (4.5 mg) and in short-term use improves RLS symptoms.

For PLMD:

- Transdermal oestradiol is ineffective.

Conflicts of interest
Dr Billiard received continuing medical education honoraria from GSK. Dr. Clarenbach was involved in a trial with Schwarz Pharma, and Dr. Montagna was involved in trials with GlaxoSmithKline, Schwarz Pharma and received consultant honoraria from Boehringer-Ingelheim. Dr. Trenkwalder received grants/research support from GlaxoSmithKline, is a consultant for Boehringer-Ingelheim, GlaxoSmithKline and Novartis, and received speakers honoraria for educational symposia from GlaxoSmithKline, Hoffmann La Roche and Pfizer. Dr. Garcia-Borreguero received research grants from Pfizer and is a consultant for Pfizer, GlaxoSmithKline, Schwarz Pharma and Boehringer-Ingelheim.

Acknowledgements
We wish to acknowledge the help of Ms A. Laffi in typing the manuscript and Ms. S. Muzzi for help with the bibliography. Supported by MURST ex 60% grants.

References
Adler CH (1997). Treatment of restless legs syndrome with gabapentin. *Clin Neuropharmacol* **20**:148–151.

Adler CH, Hauser RA, Sethi K, Caviness JN, Marlor L, Anderson WM, Hentz JG (2004). Ropinirole for restless legs syndrome: A placebo-controlled crossover trial. *Neurology* **62**:1405–1407.

Ahmed I (2002). Ropinirole in restless leg syndrome. *Mo Med* **99**:500–501.

Akpinar S (1982). Treatment of restless legs syndrome with levodopa plus benserazide. *Arch Neurol* **39**:739.

Akpinar S (1987). Restless legs syndrome treatment with dopaminergic drugs. *Clin Neuropharmacol* **10**:69–79.

Allen RP, Earley CJ (1996). Augmentation of the restless legs syndrome with carbidopa/levodopa. *Sleep* **19**:205–213.

Allen RP, Picchietti D, Hening WA, Trenkwalder C, Walters AS, Montplaisir J (2003). Restless legs syndrome: diagnostic criteria, special considerations, and epidemiology. A report from the restless legs syndrome diagnosis and epidemiology workshop at the National Institutes of Health. *Sleep Med* **4**:101–19.

Allen R, Becker PM, Bogan R, Schmidt M, Kushida CA, Fry JM, Poceta JS, Winslow D (2004). Ropinirole decreases periodic leg movements and improves sleep parameters in patients with restless legs syndrome. *Sleep* **27**:907–914.

American Academy of Sleep Medicine (2005a). Periodic Limb Movement Disorder. In: *International Classification of Sleep Disorders. Diagnostic and Coding Manual, II Edition*, Westchester, Il, USA, 182–186.

American Academy of Sleep Medicine (2005b). Restless Legs Syndrome. In: *International Classification of Sleep Disorders. Diagnostic and Coding Manual, II Edition*, Westchester, Il, USA, 178–181.

Ancoli-Israel S, Seifert AR, Lemon M (1986). Thermal biofeedback and periodic movements in sleep: patients' subjective reports and a case study. *Biofeedback Self Regul* **11**:177–188.

Arens R, Wright B, Elliott J, Zhao H, Wang PP, Brown LW, Namey T, Kaplan P (1998). Periodic limb movement in sleep in children with Williams syndrome. *J Pediatr* **133**:670–674.

Atkinson MJ, Allen RP, DuChane J, Murray C, Kushida C, Roth T (2004). RLS Quality of Life Consortium.

Validation of the Restless Legs Syndrome Quality of Life Instrument (RLS-QLI): findings of a consortium of national experts and the RLS Foundation. *Qual Life Res* **13:**679–693.

Ausserwinkler M, Schmidt P (1988). Clonidine is effective in the treatment of 'Restless Leg' syndrome in chronic uraemic patients. *Nephrol-Dial-Transplant* **3:**530.

Ausserwinkler M, Schmidt P (1989a). Clonidine is effective in the treatment of 'Restless Leg' syndrome in chronic uraemia patients. *Nephrol-Dial-Transplant* **4:**149.

Ausserwinkler M, Schmidt P (1989b). Erfolgreiche Behandlung des "restless legs"-Syndroms bei chronischer Niereninsuffizienz mit Clonidin. *Schweiz Med Wochenschr* **119:**184–186.

Ayres SJ, Mihan R (1969). Leg cramps (systremma) and "restless legs" syndrome. Response to vitamin E (tocopherol). *Calif Med* **111:**87–91.

Bamford CR, Sandyk R (1987). Failure of clonidine to ameliorate the symptoms of restless legs syndrome. *Sleep* **10:**398–399.

Baran AS, Richert AC, Douglass AB, May W, Ansarin K (2003). Change in periodic limb movement index during treatment of obstructive sleep apnea with continuous positive airway pressure. *Sleep* **26:**717–720.

Bastani B, Westervelt FB (1987). Effectiveness of clonidine in alleviating the symptoms of "restless legs". *Am J Kidney Dis* **10:**326.

Bassetti C, Clavadetscher S, Gugger M, Hess CW (2002). Pergolide-associated 'sleep attacks' in a patient with restless legs syndrome. *Sleep Med* **3:**275–277.

Becker PM, Jamieson AO, Brown WD (1993). Dopaminergic agents in restless legs syndrome and periodic limb movements of sleep: response and complications of extended treatment in 49 cases. *Sleep* **16:**713–716.

Becker PM, Ondo W, Sharon D (1998). Encouraging initial response of restless legs syndrome to pramipexole. *Neurology* **51:**1221–1223.

Bedard MA, Montplaisir J, Godbout R (1987). Effect of L-dopa on periodic movements in sleep in narcolepsy. *Eur Neurol* **27:**35–38.

Bedard MA, Montplaisir J, Godbout R, Lapierre O (1989). Nocturnal gamma-hydroxybutyrate. Effect on periodic leg movements and sleep organization of narcoleptic patients. *Clin Neuropharmacol* **12:**29–36.

Benes H, Kurella B, Kummer J, Kazenwadel J, Selzer R, Kohnen R (1999). Rapid onset of action of levodopa in restless legs syndrome: a double-blind, randomized, multicenter, crossover trial. *Sleep* **22:**1073–1081.

Benes H, Deissler A, Clarenbach P, Rodenbeck A, Hajak G (2000). Lisuride in the management of restless legs syndrome. *Mov Disord* **15:**S134–S135.

Benes H (2001). Idiopathisches Restless-legs-Syndrom: Behandlung mit Lisurid. *Nervenheilkunde* **20:**119–122.

Benes H, Heinrich CR, Ueberall MA, Kohnen R (2004). Long-term safety and efficacy of cabergoline for the treatment of idiopathic restless legs syndrome: results from an open-label 6-month clinical trial. *Sleep* **27:**674–682.

Benz RL, Pressman MR, Hovick ET, Peterson DD (1999). A preliminary study of the effects of correction of anemia with recombinant human erythropoietin therapy on sleep, sleep disorders, and daytime sleepiness in hemodialysis patients (the SLEEPO study). *Am J Kidney Dis* **34:**1089–1095.

Bezerra ML, Martinez JV (2002). Zolpidem in restless legs syndrome. *Eur Neurol* **48:**180–181.

Blattler W, Muhlemann M (1982). Restless legs und nachtliche Beinkrampfe – Vergessenes zur Diagnose – Neues zur Therapie. *Schweiz Med Wochenschr* **112:**115–117.

Boghen D (1980). Successful treatment of restless legs with clonazepam. *Ann Neurol* **8:**341.

Boghen D, Lamothe L, Elie R, Godbout R, Montplaisir J (1986). The treatment of the restless legs syndrome with clonazepam: a prospective controlled study. *Can J Neurol Sci* **13:**245–247.

Boivin DB, Montplaisir J, Poirier G (1989). The effects of L-Dopa on periodic leg movements and sleep organization in narcolepsy. *Clin Neuropharmacol* **12:**339–345.

Boivin DB, Montplaisir J, Lambert C (1993a). Effects of bromocriptine in human narcolepsy. *Clin Neuropharmacol* **16:**120–126.

Boivin DB, Lorrain D, Montplaisir J (1993b). Effects of bromocriptine on periodic limb movements in human narcolepsy. *Neurology* **43:**2134–2136.

Bonnet MH, Arand DL (1990). The use of triazolam in older patients with periodic leg movements, fragmented sleep, and daytime sleepiness. *J Gerontol* **45:**M139–M144.

Bonnet MH, Arand DL (1991). Chronic use of triazolam in patients with periodic leg movements, fragmented sleep and daytime sleepiness. *Aging (Milano)* **3:**313–324.

Botez MI, Cadotte M, Beaulieu R, Pichette LP, Pison C (1976). Neurologic disorders responsive to folic acid therapy. *Can Med Assoc J* **115:**217–223.

Botez MI, Fontaine F, Botez T, Bachevalier J (1977). Folate-responsive neurological and mental disorders: report of 16 cases. Neuropsychological correlates of computerized transaxial tomography and radionuclide cisternography in folic acid deficiencies. *Eur Neurol* **16:**230–246.

Brainin M, Barnes M, Baron JC, Gilhus NE, Hughes R, Selmaj K, Waldemar G (2004). Guidance for the preparation of neurological management guidelines by EFNS scientific task forces – revised recommendations 2004. *Eur J Neurol* **11**:577–581.

Brenning R (1969). [Enantaldehydes and furaldehydes in molimina crurum nocturna including "restless legs". A comparative trial with carbacholine, inositolnicotinate, and placebo]. *Nordisk Medicin* **81**:528–534.

Briellmann RS, Mathis J, Bassetti C, Gugger M, Hess CW (1997). Patterns of muscle activity in legs in sleep apnea patients before and during nCPAP therapy. *Eur Neurol* **38**:113–118.

Brodeur C, Montplaisir J, Godbout R, Marinier R (1988). Treatment of restless legs syndrome and periodic movements during sleep with L-dopa: a double-blind, controlled study. *Neurology* **38**:1845–1848.

Broughton RJ, Fleming JAE, George CFP, Hill JD, Kryger MH, Moldofsky H, Montplaisir JY, Morehouse RL, Moscovitch A, Murphy WF (1997). Randomized, double-blind, placebo-controlled crossover trial of modafinil in the treatment of excessive daytime sleepiness in narcolepsy. *Neurology* **49**:444–451.

Brown LK, Heffner JE, Obbens EA (2000). Transverse myelitis associated with restless legs syndrome and periodic movements of sleep responsive to an oral dopaminergic agent but not to intrathecal baclofen. *Sleep* **23**:591–594.

Bruno RL (1998). Abnormal movements in sleep as a post-polio sequelae. *Am J Phys Med Rehabil* **77**:339–344.

Burns KE (2000). Use of tramadol to control restless legs syndrome after orthopedic surgery. *Hosp Pharm* **35**:673.

Buysse DJ, Reynolds-III CF, Hoch CC, Houck PR, Kupfer DJ, Mazumdar S, Frank E (1996). Longitudinal effects of nortriptyline on EEG sleep and the likelihood of recurrence in elderly depressed patients. *Neuropsychopharmacology* **14**:243–252.

Campos H, Tufik S, Bittencourt L, Haidar M, Baracat EC (2002). Progeston reduces periodic leg movements in menopause (abstract). *Climacteric* **5**:157.

Cavatorta F, Vagge R, Solari P, Queirolo C (1987). Risultati preliminari con clonidina nella sindrome delle gambe senza riposo in due pazienti uremici emodializzati. *Minerva Urol Nefrol* **39**:93.

Chesson AL Jr, Wise M, Davila D, Johnson S, Littner M, Anderson WM, Hartse K, Rafecas J (1999). Practice parameters for the treatment of restless legs syndrome and periodic limb movement disorder. An American Academy of Sleep Medicine Report. Standards of Practice Committee of the American Academy of Sleep Medicine. *Sleep* **22**:961–968.

Christiansen I (1970). Mesionositolhexanikotinat (Hexanicit) og pentaerytritoltetranikotinat (Bufon) ved restless legs. *Ugeskr Laeger* **132**:1475–1476.

Cicolin A, Lopiano L, Zibetti M, Torre E, Tavella A, Guastamacchia G, Terreni A, Makrydakis G, Fattori E, Lanotte MM, Bergamasco B, Mutani R (2004). Effects of deep brain stimulation of the subthalamic nucleus on sleep architecture in parkinsonian patients. *Sleep Med* **5**:207–210.

Collado-Seidel V (1997). Treatment of the restless legs syndrome with a combination of standard and sustained release levodopa/benserazide (Madopar Depot): A double-blind controlled study. *Pharmacopsychiatry* **30**:158.

Collado-Seidel V, Kazenwadel J, Wetter TC, Kohnen R, Winkelmann J, Selzer R, Oertel WH, Trenkwalder C (1999). A controlled study of additional sr-L-dopa in L-dopa-responsive restless legs syndrome with late-night symptoms. *Neurology* **52**:285–290.

Danoff SK, Grasso ME, Terry PB, Flynn JA (2001). Pleuropulmonary disease due to pergolide use for restless legs syndrome. *Chest* **120**:313–316.

Davis BJ, Rajput A, Rajput ML, Aul EA, Eichhorn GR (2000). A randomized, double-blind placebo-controlled trial of iron in restless legs syndrome. *Eur Neurol* **43**:70–75.

de Mello MT, Lauro FAA, Silva AC, Tufik S (1996). Incidence of periodic leg movements and of the restless legs syndrome during sleep following acute physical activity in spinal cord injury subjects. *Spinal Cord* **34**:294–296.

de Mello MT, Silva AC, Rueda AD, Poyares D, Tufik S (1997). Correlation between K complex, periodic leg movements (PLM), and myoclonus during sleep in paraplegic adults before and after an acute physical activity. *Spinal Cord* **35**:248–252.

de Mello MT, Poyares DL, Tufik S (1999). Treatment of periodic leg movements with a dopaminergic agonist in subjects with total spinal cord lesions. *Spinal Cord* **37**:634–637.

de Mello MT, Silva AC, Esteves AM, Tufik S (2002). Reduction of periodic leg movement in individuals with paraplegia following aerobic physical exercise. *Spinal Cord* **40**:646–649.

de Mello MT, Esteves AM, Tufik S (2004). Comparison between dopaminergic agents and physical exercise as treatment for periodic limb movements in patients with spinal cord injury. *Spinal Cord* **42**:218–221.

Derom E, Elinck W, Buylaert W, van der Straeten M (1984). Which beta-blocker for the restless leg? *Lancet* **1**:857.

Dimmitt SB, Riley GJ (2000). Selective serotonin receptor uptake inhibitors can reduce restless legs symptoms. *Arch Intern Med* **160:**712.

Doghramji K, Browman CP, Gaddy JR, Walsh JK (1991). Triazolam diminishes daytime sleepiness and sleep fragmentation in patients with periodic leg movements in sleep. *J Clin Psychopharmacol* **11:** 284–290.

Earley CJ, Allen RP (1996). Pergolide and carbidopa/levodopa treatment of the restless legs syndrome and periodic leg movements in sleep in a consecutive series of patients. *Sleep* **19:**801–810.

Earley CJ, Yaffee JB, Allen RP (1998). Randomized, double-blind, placebo-controlled trial of pergolide in restless legs syndrome. *Neurology* **51:**1599–1602.

Earley CJ, Heckler D, Allen RP (2004). The treatment of restless legs syndrome with intravenous iron dextran. *Sleep Med* **5:**231–235.

Edinger JD, Fins AI, Sullivan RJ, Marsh GR, Dailey DS, Young M (1996). Comparison of cognitive-behavioral therapy and clonazepam for treating periodic limb movement disorder. *Sleep* **19:**442–444.

Ehrenberg BL, Eisensehr I, Corbett KE, Crowley PF, Walters AS (2000). Valproate for sleep consolidation in periodic limb movement disorder. *J Clin Psychopharmacol* **20:**574–578.

Eisensehr I, Ehrenberg BL, Rogge-Solti S, Noachtar S (2004). Treatment of idiopathic restless legs syndrome (RLS) with slow-release valproic acid compared with slow-release levodopa/benserazid. *J Neurol* **251:**579–583.

Ekbom KA (1945). Restless legs. *Acta Med Scand* **158(Suppl):**5–123.

Estivill E, de la Fuente V (1999a). Uso de ropinirol como tratamiento del sindrome de piernas inquietas. *Rev Neurol* **28:**962–963.

Estivill E, de la Fuente V (1999b). Eficacia del ropinirol como tratamiento del insomnio cronico secundario al sindrome de piernas inquietas: datos polisomnograficos. *Rev Neurol* **29:**805–807.

Estivill E, Fuente-Panell V, Segarra-Isern F, Albares-Tendero J (2004). Sindrome de piernas inquietas en un paciente con amputacion de ambas piernas. *Rev Neurol* **39:**536–538.

Evidente VG, Adler CH, Caviness JN, Hentz JG, Gwinn-Hardy K (2000). Amantadine is beneficial in restless legs syndrome. *Mov Disord* **15:**324–327.

Evidente VG (2001). Piribedil for restless legs syndrome: a pilot study. *Mov Disord* **16:**579–581.

Fantini ML, Gagnon J, Filipini D, Montplaisir J (2003). The effects of pramipexole in REM sleep behavior disorder. *Neurology* **61:**1418–1420.

Ferini-Strambi L (2002). Restless legs syndrome augmentation and pramipexole treatment. *Sleep Med* **3:**S23–S25.

Freeman A, Rye DB, Bliwise D, Chakravorty S, Krulewicz S, Watts RL (2001). Ropinirole for Restless Legs Syndrome (RLS): An Open Label and Double Blind Placebo-Controlled Study. *Neurology* **56:**A5.

Freye E, Levy J (2000). Acute abstinence syndrome following abrupt cessation of long-term use of tramadol (Ultram): a case study. *Eur J Pain* **4:**307–311.

Freye E, Levy JV, Partecke L (2004). Use of gabapentin for attenuation of symptoms following rapid opiate detoxification (ROD)–correlation with neurophysiological parameters–. *Neurophysiol Clin* **34:**81–89.

Galvez-Jimenez N, Khan T (1999). Ropinirole and restless legs syndrome. *Mov Disord* **14:**890–892.

Garcia-Borreguero D, Larrosa O, de la Llave Y, Verger K, Masramon X, Hernandez G (2002a). Treatment of restless legs syndrome with gabapentin: a double-blind, cross -over study. *Neurology* **59:**1573–1579.

Garcia-Borreguero D, Larrosa O, Verger K, Masramon X, Hernandez G (2002b). Effects of gabapentin on restless legs syndrome accompanied by nocturnal pain: results of a double-blind, crossover study with polysomnographic control in 24 patients. *Euro J Neurol* **9:**49–50.

Garcia-Borreguero D, Serrano C, Larrosa O, Jose-Granizo J (2004). Circadian effects of dopaminergic treatment in restless legs syndrome. *Sleep Med* **5:**413–420.

Ginsberg HN (1986). Propranolol in the treatment of restless legs syndrome induced by imipramine withdrawal. *Am J Psychiatry* **143:**938.

Grewal M, Hawa R, Shapiro C (2002). Treatment of periodic limb movements in sleep with selegiline HCl. *Mov Disord* **17:**398–401.

Gulden J (1994). Levodopa in the treatment of restless legs syndrome. *Fortschr Med* **112:**61–62.

Guilleminault C, Flagg W (1984). Effect of baclofen on sleep-related periodic leg movements. *Ann Neurol* **15:**234–239.

Guilleminault C, Mondini S, Montplaisir J, Mancuso J, Cobasko D, Dement WC (1987). Periodic leg movement, L-dopa, 5-hydroxytryptophan, and L-tryptophan. *Sleep* **10:**393–397.

Guilleminault C, Crowe C, Quera-Salva MA, Miles L, Partinen M(1988). Periodic leg movement, sleep fragmentation and central sleep apnoea in two cases: reduction with Clonazepam. *Eur Respir J* **1:**762–765.

Guilleminault C, Cetel M, Philip P (1993). Dopaminergic treatment of restless legs and rebound phenomenon. *Neurology* **43:**445.

Haba-Rubio J, Staner L, Cornette F, Lainey E, Luthringer R, Krieger J, Macher JP (2003). Acute low single dose of apomorphine reduces periodic limb movements but has no significant effect on sleep arousals: a preliminary report. *Neurophysiol Clin* **33**:180–184.

Ha HC (1988). Regional intravenous analgesia for restless legs syndrome. *Pain Clinic* **2**:121–123.

Hain C (2002). Development of opioid dependence in a not diagnosed restless legs syndrome. *Psychiatr Prax* **29**:321–323.

Handwerker J-VJ, Palmer RF (1985). Clonidine in the treatment of "restless leg" syndrome. *N Engl J Med* **313**:1228–1229.

Hanly P, Zuberi N (1992). Periodic leg movements during sleep before and after heart transplantation. *Sleep* **15**:489–492.

Hanly PJ, Gabor JY, Chan C, Pierratos A (2003). Daytime sleepiness in patients with CRF: Impact of nocturnal hemodialysis. *Am J Kidney Dis* **41**:403–410.

Hanna PA, Kumar S, Walters AS (2004). Restless legs symptoms in a patient with above knee amputations: a case of phantom restless legs. *Clin Neuropharmacol* **27**:87–89.

Happe S, Klosch G, Saletu B, Zeitlhofer J (2001). Treatment of idiopathic restless legs syndrome (RLS) with gabapentin. *Neurology* **57**:1717–1719.

Happe S, Sauter C, Klosch G, Saletu B, Zeitlhofer J (2003). Gabapentin versus ropinirole in the treatment of idiopathic restless legs syndrome. *Neuropsychobiology* **48**:82–86.

Hening WA, Walters A, Kavey N, Gidro-Frank S, Cote L, Fahn S (1986). Dyskinesias while awake and periodic movements in sleep in restless legs syndrome: treatment with opioids. *Neurology* **36**:1363–1366.

Hening W, Walters AS, Wagner ML, Grasing K, Mills R, Chokroverty S, Kavey N (1993). Successful oxycodone therapy for the restless legs syndrome: a double-blind study. *Canad J Neurol Sci* **20**:S212.

Hening WA, Allen R, Earley C, Kushida C, Picchietti D, Silber M (1999). The treatment of restless legs syndrome and periodic limb movement disorder. An American Academy of Sleep Medicine Review. *Sleep* **22**:970–999.

Hening WA, Allen RP, Earley CJ, Picchietti DL, Silber MH (2004). An update on the dopaminergic treatment of restless legs syndrome and periodic limb movement disorder. *Sleep* **27**:560–583.

Hogl B, Rothdach A, Wetter TC, Trenkwalder C (2003). The effect of cabergoline on sleep, periodic leg movements in sleep, and early morning motor function in patients with Parkinson's disease. *Neuropsychopharmacology* **28**:1866–1870.

Holman AJ, Neiman RA, Ettlinger RE (2004). Preliminary efficacy of the dopamine agonist, pramipexole, for fibromyalgia: The first, open label, multicenter experience. *J Musculoskelet Pain* **12**:69–74.

Horiguchi J, Inami Y, Miyoshi N, Kakimoto Y (1985). [Restless legs syndrome in four parkinsonian patients treated with amantadine]. *Rinsho Shinkeigaku* **25**:153–156.

Horiguchi J, Inami Y, Sasaki A, Nishimatsu O, Sukegawa T (1992). Periodic leg movements in sleep with restless legs syndrome: effect of clonazepam treatment. *Jpn J Psychiatry Neurol* **46**:727–732.

Horiguchi J, Yamashita H, Mizuno S, Kuramoto Y, Kagaya A, Yamawaki S, Inami -Y (1999). Nocturnal eating/drinking syndrome and neuroleptic-induced restless legs syndrome. *Int Clin Psychopharmacol* **14**:33–36.

Hornyak M, Voderholzer U, Hohagen F, Berger M, Riemann D (1998). Magnesium therapy for periodic leg movements-related insomnia and restless legs syndrome: an open pilot study. *Sleep* **21**:501–505.

Hu J (2001). Acupuncture treatment of restless leg syndrome. *J Tradit Chin Med* **21**:312–316.

Hundemer HP, Trenkwalder C, Lledo A, Quail D, Rubin M, Swieca J, Polo O, Wetter TC, Ferini-Ştrambi L, De Groen H (2001). The safety of pergolide in the treatment of restless legs syndrome (RLS): Results of a randomized long-term multicenter trial of pergolide in the treatment of RLS. *Neurology* **56**:A20.

Hurlimann F (1974). [Restless legs and crampi in the night. Double blind study with Circonyl in patients with defective peripheric arterial circulation]. *Schweizerische Rundschau fur Medizin Praxis* **63**:194–195.

Inami Y, Horiguchi J, Nishimatsu O, Sasaki A, Sukegawa T, Katagiri H, Yamawaki S (1997). A polysomnographic study on periodic limb movements in patients with restless legs syndrome and neuroleptic-induced akathisia. *Hiroshima J Med Sci* **46**:133–141.

Inoue Y, Mitani H, Nanba K, Kawahara R (1999). Treatment of periodic leg movement disorder and restless leg syndrome with talipexole. *Psychiatry Clin Neurosci* **53**:283–285.

Ishizu T, Ohyagi Y, Furuya H, Araki T, Tobimatsu S, Yamada T, Kira J (2001). [A patient with restless legs syndrome/periodic limb movement successfully treated by wearing a lumbar corset]. *Rinsho Shinkeigaku* **41**:438–441.

Jakobsson B, Ruuth K (2002). Successful treatment of restless legs syndrome with an implanted pump for intrathecal drug delivery. *Acta Anaesthesiol Scand* **46**:114–117.

Kanter AH (1995). The effect of sclerotherapy on restless legs syndrome. *Dermatol Surg* **21**:328–332.

Kaplan PW, Allen RP, Buchholz DW, Walters JK (1991). Double-blind comparison of L-dopa versus propoxyphene in patients with periodic limb movements in sleep. *Electroencephalogr Clin Neurophysiol* **79**:32P.

Kaplan PW, Allen RP, Buchholz DW, Walters JK (1993). A double-blind, placebo-controlled study of the treatment of periodic limb movements in sleep using carbidopa/levodopa and propoxyphene. *Sleep* **16**:717–723.

Kapur N, Friedman R (2002). Oral ketamine: a promising treatment for restless legs syndrome. *Anesth Analg* **94**:1558–1559.

Kastin AJ, Kullander S, Borglin NE, Dahlberg B, Dyster-Aas K, Krakau CE, Ingvar DH, Miller MC, III, Bowers CY, Schally AV (1968). Extrapigmentary effects of melanocyte-stimulating hormone in amenorrhoeic women. *Lancet* **1**:1007–1010.

Kavey N, Walters AS, Hening W, Gidro-Frank S (1988). Opioid treatment of periodic movements in sleep in patients without restless legs. *Neuropeptides* **11**:181–184.

Kerr PG, van Bakel C, Dawborn JK (1989). Assessment of the symptomatic benefit of cool dialysate. *Nephron* **52**:166–169.

Kotterba S, Clarenbach P, Bommel W, Rasche K (2000). Periodic leg movements in patients with obstructive sleep apnea syndrome during nCPAP therapy. *Somnologie* **4**:93–95.

Kovacevic-Ristanovic R, Cartwright RD, Lloyd S (1991). Nonpharmacologic treatment of periodic leg movements in sleep. *Arch Phys Med Rehabil* **72**:385–389.

Kryger MH, Otake K, Foerster J (2002). Low body stores of iron and restless legs syndrome: A correctable cause of insomnia in adolescents and teenagers. *Sleep Med* **3**:127–132.

Kumar VG, Bhatia M, Tripathi M, Srivastava AK, Jain S (2003). Restless legs syndrome: diagnosis and treatment. *J Assoc Physicians India* **51**:782–783.

Kunz D, Bes F (2001). Exogenous melatonin in Periodic Limb Movement Disorder: An open clinical trial and a hypothesis. *Sleep* **24**:183–187.

Larsen S, Telstad W, Sorensen O, Thom E, Stensrud P, Nyberg-Hansen R (1985). Carbamazepine therapy in restless legs. Discrimination between responders and non-responders. *Acta Med Scand* **218**:223–227.

Laschewski F, Sanner B, Konermann M, Kreuzer I, Horstensmeyer D, Sturm A (1997). Ausgepragte Hypersomnie einer 13jahrigen bei periodic leg movement. *Pneumologie* **51(Suppl 3)**:725–728.

Lauerma H (1991). Nocturnal wandering caused by restless legs and short-acting benzodiazepines. *Acta Psychiatr Scand* **83**:492–493.

Lauerma H, Markkula J, Hyvonen H, Kyyronen K (1997). Idiopathic restless legs syndrome and psychoses. *Nord J Psychiatry* **51**:205.

Lauerma H, Markkula J (1999). Treatment of restless legs syndrome with tramadol: an open study. *J Clin Psychiatry* **60**:241–244.

Lavie P, Nahir M, Lorber M, Scharf Y (1991). Nonsteroidal antiinflammatory drug therapy in rheumatoid arthritis patients: Lack of association between clinical improvement and effects on sleep. *Arthritis Rheum* **34**:655–659.

Lee MS, Choi YC, Lee SH, Lee SB (1996). Sleep-related periodic leg involvements associated with spinal cord lesions. *Mov Disord* **11**:719–722.

Leonhardt M, Abele M, Klockgether T, Dichgans J, Weller M (1999). Pathological yawning (chasm) associated with periodic leg movements in sleep: Cure by levodopa. *J Neurol* **246**:621–622.

Lin SC, Kaplan J, Burger CD, Fredrickson PA (1998). Effect of pramipexole in treatment of resistant restless legs syndrome. *Mayo Clin Proc* **73**:497–500.

Lin Z (2003). How to treat restless leg syndrome with traditional Chinese medicine? *J Tradit Chin Med* **23**:306–307.

Lipinski JF, Zubenko GS, Barreira P, Cohen BM (1983). Propranolol in the treatment of neuroleptic-induced akathisia. *Lancet* **2**:685–686.

Lipinski JF, Sallee FR, Jackson C, Sethuraman G (1997). Dopamine agonist treatment of Tourette disorder in children: results of an open-label trial of pergolide. *Mov Disord* **12**:402–407.

Lundvall O, Abom PE, Holm R (1983). Carbamazepine in restless legs. A controlled pilot study. *Eur J Clin Pharmacol* **25**:323–324.

Malek-Ahmadi P (1999). Bupropion, periodic limb movement disorder, and ADHD. *J Am Acad Child Adolesc Psychiatry* **38**:637–638.

Manconi M, Casetta I, Govoni V, Cesnik E, Ferini-Strambi L, Granieri E (2003). Pramipexole in Restless Legs syndrome. Evaluation by suggested immobilization test. *J Neurol* **250**:1494–1495.

Matthews WB (1979). Treatment of the restless legs syndrome with clonazepam. *Br Med J* **1**:751.

McLean AJ (2004). The use of the dopamine-receptor partial agonist aripiprazole in the treatment of restless legs syndrome. *Sleep* **27**:1022.

Mellick GA, Mellick LB (1996). Management of restless legs syndrome with gabapentin (Neurontin). *Sleep* **19**:224–226.

Merren MD (1998). Gabapentin for treatment of pain and tremor: a large case series. *South Med J* **91**:739–744.

Michalsen A, Schlegel F, Rodenbeck A, Ludtke R, Huether G, Teschler H, Dobos GJ (2003). Effects of short-term modified fasting on sleep patterns and daytime vigilance in non-obese subjects: Results of a pilot study. *Ann Nutr Metab* **47:**194–200.

Micozkadioglu H, Ozdemir FN, Kut A, Sezer S, Saatci U, Haberal M (2004). Gabapentin versus levodopa for the treatment of restless legs syndrome in hemodialysis patients: An open-label study. *Renal Fail* **26:**393–397.

Miranda M, Fabres L, Kagi M, Aguilera L, Alvo M, Elgueta L, Erazo S, Venegas P (2003). Tratamiento del sindrome de piernas inquietas en pacientes uremicos en dialisis con pramipexole: resultados preliminares. *Rev Med Chil* **131:**700–701.

Miranda M, Kagi M, Fabres L, Aguilera L, Alvo M, Elgueta L, Erazo S, Venegas P (2004). Pramipexole for the treatment of uremic restless legs in patients undergoing hemodialysis. *Neurology* **62:**831–832.

Mitler MM, Browman CP, Menn SJ, Gujavarty K, Timms RM (1986). Nocturnal myoclonus: treatment efficacy of clonazepam and temazepam. *Sleep* **9:**385–392.

Moldofsky H, Tullis C, Quance G, Lue FA (1986). Nitrazepam for periodic movements in sleep (sleep-related myoclonus). *Can J Neurol Sci* **13:**52–54.

Montagna P, Sassoli-de-Bianchi L, Zucconi M, Cirignotta F, Lugaresi E (1984). Clonazepam and vibration in restless legs syndrome. *Acta Neurol Scand* **69:**428–430.

Montplaisir J, Godbout R, Boghen D, DeChamplain J, Young SN, Lapierre G (1985). Familial restless legs with periodic movements in sleep: electrophysiologic, biochemical, and pharmacologic study. *Neurology* **35:**130–134.

Montplaisir J, Godbout R, Poirier G, Bedard MA (1986). Restless legs syndrome and periodic movements in sleep: physiopathology and treatment with L-dopa. *Clin Neuropharmacol* **9:**456–463.

Montplaisir J, Lorrain D, Godbout R (1991). Restless legs syndrome and periodic leg movements in sleep: the primary role of dopaminergic mechanism. *Eur Neurol* **31:**41–43.

Montplaisir J, Boucher S, Gosselin A, Poirier G, Lavigne G (1996). Persistence of repetitive EEG arousals (K-alpha complexes) in RLS patients treated with L-DOPA. *Sleep* **19:**196–199.

Montplaisir J, Nicolas A, Denesle R, Gomez-Mancilla B (1998). Pramipexole alleviates sensory and motor symptoms of restless legs syndrome. *Neurology* **51:**311–312.

Montplaisir J, Nicolas A, Denesle R, Gomez-Mancilla B (1999). Restless legs syndrome improved by pramipexole: a double-blind randomized trial. *Neurology* **52:**938–943.

Montplaisir J, Denesle R, Petit D (2000). Pramipexole in the treatment of restless legs syndrome: a follow-up study. *Eur J Neurol* **7(Suppl 1):**27–31.

Morgan LK (1967). Restless limbs: a commonly overlooked symptom controlled by "Valium". *Med J Aust* **2:**589–594.

Morgan LK (1975). Letter: Restless legs: precipitated by beta blockers, relieved by orphenadrine. *Med J Aust* **2:**753.

Mountifield JA (1985). Restless leg syndrome relieved by cessation of smoking. CMAJ **133:**426–427.

Nassr DG (1986). Paradoxical response to nitrazepam in a patient with hypersomnia secondary to nocturnal myoclonus. *J Clin Psychopharmacol* **6:**121–122.

Nishimatsu O, Horiguchi J, Inami Y, Sukegawa T, Sasaki A (1997). Periodic limb movement disorder in neuroleptic-induced akathisia. *Kobe J Med Sci* **43:**169–177.

Noel S, Korri H, Vanderheyden JE (1998). Low dosage of pergolide in the treatment of restless legs syndrome. *Acta Neurol Belg* **98:**52–53.

Nofzinger EA, Fasiczka A, Berman S, Thase ME (2000). Bupropion SR reduces periodic limb movements associated with arousals from sleep in depressed patients with periodic limb movement disorder. *J Clin Psychiatry* **61:**858–862.

Nordlander NB (1953). Therapy in restless legs. *Acta Med Scand* **145:**453–457.

Noseda A, Nouvelle M, Lanquart JR, Kempenaers C, De Maertelaer V, Linkowski R, Kerkhofs M (2002). High leg motor activity in sleep apnea hypopnea patients: efficacy of clonazepam combined with nasal CPAP on polysomnographic variables. *Respir Med* **96:**693–699.

Novelli G, Mediati RD, Casali R, Palermo P (2000). Treatment of 'restless legs syndrome' with gabapentin. *Pain Clinic* **12:**61–63.

Oechsner M (1998). Idiopathic Restless Legs Syndrome: Combination therapy with levodopa and ropinirole. *Aktuel Neurol* **25:**190–192.

Ohanna N, Peled R, Rubin AH, Zomer J, Lavie P (1985). Periodic leg movements in sleep: effect of clonazepam treatment. *Neurology* **35:**408–411.

O'Keeffe ST, Noel J, Lavan JN (1993). Restless legs syndrome in the elderly. *Postgrad Med J* **69:**701–703.

O'Keeffe ST, Gavin K, Lavan JN (1994). Iron status and restless legs syndrome in the elderly. *Age Ageing* **23:**200–203.

Ondo W (1999). Ropinirole for restless legs syndrome. *Mov Disord* **14:**138–140.

Oshtory MA, Vijayan N (1980). Clonazepam treatment of insomnia due to sleep myoclonus. *Arch Neurol* **37:**119–120.

Paradiso G, Khan F, Chen R (2002). Effects of apomorphine on flexor reflex and periodic limb movement. *Mov Disord* **17:**594–597.

Peled R, Lavie P (1987). Double-blind evaluation of clonazepam on periodic leg movements in sleep. *J Neurol, Neurosurg Psychiatry* **50:**1679–1681.

Pellecchia MT, Vitale C, Sabatini M, Longo K, Amboni M, Bonavita V, Barone P (2004). Ropinirole as a treatment of restless legs syndrome in patients on chronic hemodialysis: an open randomized crossover trial versus levodopa sustained release. *Clin Neuropharmacol* **27:**178–181.

Perez-Bravo A (2004). Utilidad del topiramato en el tratamiento del sindrome de piernas inquietas. *Actas Esp Psiquiatr* **32:**132–137.

Petiau C, Zamagni M, Trautmann D, Sforza E, Krieger J (1995). Periodic movements during sleep syndrome. *J Med Strasbourg* **26:**166–169

Picchietti DL, Walters AS (1999). Moderate to severe periodic limb movement disorder in childhood and adolescence. *Sleep* **22:**297–300.

Pieta J, Millar T, Zacharias J, Fine A, Kryger M (1998). Effect of pergolide on restless legs and leg movements in sleep in uremic patients. *Sleep* **21:** 617–622.

Polo-Kantola P, Rauhala E, Erkkola R, Irjala K, Polo O (2001). Estrogen replacement therapy and nocturnal periodic limb movements: a randomized controlled trial. *Obstet Gynecol* **97:**548–554.

Popkin RJ (1971). Orphenadrine citrate (Norflex) for the treatment of "restless legs" and related syndromes. *J Am Geriatr Soc* **19:**76–79.

Priano L, Albani G, Brioschi A, Guastamacchia G, Calderoni S, Lopiano L, Rizzone M, Cavalli R, Gasco MR, Fraschini F, Bergamasco B, Mauro A (2003). Nocturnal anomalous movement reduction and sleep microstructure analysis in parkinsonian patients during 1-night transdermal apomorphine treatment. *Neurol Sci* **24:**207–208.

Read DJ, Feest TG, Nassim MA (1981). Clonazepam: effective treatment for restless legs syndrome in uraemia. *Br Med J (Clin Res Ed)* **283:**885–886.

Reuter I, Ellis CM, Ray-Chaudhuri K (1999). Nocturnal subcutaneous apomorphine infusion in Parkinson's disease and restless legs syndrome. *Acta Neurol Scand* **100:**163–167.

Riemann D, Gann H, Dressing H (1995). Restless legs syndrome and periodic leg movements in sleep. *TW Neurol Psychiatr* **9:**1951.

Rodrigues RN, Silva AA (2002). Sonolencia diurna excessiva pos-traumatismo de cranio: associacao com movimentos periodicos de pernas e disturbio de comportamento do sono REM: relato de caso. *Arq Neuropsiquiatr* **60:**656–660.

Roehrs T, Zorick F, Wittig R, Roth T (1985). Efficacy of a reduced triazolam dose in elderly insomniacs. *Neurobiol Aging* **6:**293–296.

Romano TJ (1999). Pharmacotherapy. Presence of nocturnal myoclonus in patients with fibromyalgia syndrome. *Am J Pain Manage* **9:**85.

Rousseau JJ, Debatisse DF (1985). Etude clinique et polygraphique de deux observations de "nocturnal myoclonus" sensibles au clonazepam. *Acta Neurol Belg* **85:**318–326.

Rye DB, DeLong MR (1999). Amelioration of sensory limb discomfort of restless legs syndrome by pallidotomy. *Ann Neurol* **46:**800–801.

Saletu B, Gruber G, Saletu M, Brandstatter N, Hauer C, Prause W, Ritter K, Saletu-Zyhlarz G (2000). Sleep laboratory studies in restless legs syndrome patients as compared with normals and acute effects of ropinirole. 1. Findings on objective and subjective sleep and awakening quality. *Neuropsychobiology* **41:**181–189.

Saletu M, Anderer P, Saletu B, Hauer C, Mandl M, Oberndorfer S, Zoghlami A, Saletu-Zyhlarz G (2000). Sleep laboratory studies in restless legs syndrome patients as compared with normals and acute effects of ropinirole. 2. Findings on periodic leg movements, arousals and respiratory variables. *Neuropsychobiology* **41:**190–199.

Saletu-Zyhlarz GM, Abu-Bakr MH, Anderer P, Semler B, Decker K, Parapatics -S, Tschida U, Winkler A, Saletu B (2001). Insomnia related to dysthymia: Polysomnographic and psychometric: Comparison with normal controls and acute therapeutic trials with trazodone. *Neuropsychobiology* **44:**139–149.

Saletu M, Anderer P, Saletu-Zyhlarz G, Prause W, Semler B, Zoghlami A, Gruber G, Hauer C, Saletu B (2001a). Restless legs syndrome (RLS) and periodic limb movement disorder (PLMD): acute placebo-controlled sleep laboratory studies with clonazepam. *Eur Neuropsychopharmacol* **11:**153–161.

Saletu M, Anderer P, Saletu B, Hauer C, Mandl M, Semler B, Saletu ZG (2001b). Sleep laboratory studies in periodic limb movement disorder (PLMD) patients as compared with normals and acute effects of ropinirole. *Hum Psychopharmacol* **16:**177–187.

Saletu-Zyhlarz GM, Abu-Bakr MH, Anderer P, Gruber G, Mandl M, Strobl R, Gollner D, Prause W, Saletu B (2002). Insomnia in depression: differences in objective and subjective sleep and awakening quality to normal controls and acute effects of trazodone. *Prog Neuropsychopharmacol Biol Psychiatry* **26**:249–260.

Saletu A, Gritsch F, Mailath-Pokorny G, Gruber G, Anderer P, Saletu B (2002). Objektivierung der Therapieeffizienz eines neuartigen mandibularen Protrusionsbehelfs fur Schnarchen und schlafbezogene Atmungsstorungen mittels Polysomnographie. *Wien Klin Wochenschr* **114**:807–815.

Saletu M, Anderer P, Saletu-Zyhlarz G, Hauer C, Saletu B (2002). Acute placebo-controlled sleep laboratory studies and clinical follow-up with pramipexole in restless legs syndrome. *Eur Arch Psychiatry Clin Neurosci* **252**:185–194.

Saletu M, Anderer P, Hogl B, Saletu-Zyhlarz G, Kunz A, Poewe W, Saletu B (2003). Acute double-blind, placebo-controlled sleep laboratory and clinical follow -up studies with a combination treatment of rr-L-dopa and sr-L-dopa in restless legs syndrome. *J Neural Transm* **110**:611–626.

Salvi F, Montagna P, Plasmati R, Rubboli G, Cirignotta F, Veilleux M, Lugaresi E, Tassinari CA (1990). Restless legs syndrome and nocturnal myoclonus: Initial clinical manifestation of familial amyloid polyneuropathy. *J Neurol Neurosurg Psychiatry* **53**:522–525.

Sandyk R (1986). L-Tryptophan in the treatment of restless legs syndrome. *Am J Psychiatry* **143**:554–555.

Sandyk R, Bernick C, Lee SM, Stern LZ, Iacono RP, Bamford CR(1987a). L-dopa in uremic patients with the restless legs syndrome. *Int J Neurosci* **35**:233–235.

Sandyk R, Bamford CR, Gillman MA (1987b). Opiates in the restless legs syndrome. *Int J Neurosci* **36**:99–104.

Sandyk R, Iacono RP, Bamford CR (1988a). Spinal cord mechanisms in amitriptyline responsive restless legs syndrome in Parkinson's disease. *Int J Neurosci* **38**:121–124.

Sandyk R, Kwo-on-Yuen, Bamford CR (1988b). The effects of baclofen in the restless legs syndrome: evidence for endogenous opioid involvement. *J Clin Psychopharmacol* **8**:440–441.

Santamaria J, Iranzo A, Tolosa E (2003). Development of restless legs syndrome after dopaminergic treatment in a patient with periodic leg movements in sleep. *Sleep Med* **4**:153–155.

Satzger-Harsch U (1998). Current studies: Therapy with L-Dopa/benserazide relieves excruciating symptoms in restless leg syndrome. *Arztlich Prax Neurol Psychiatr* **11**:40.

Scharf MB, Brown L, Hirschowitz J (1986). Possible efficacy of alprazolam in restless leg syndrome. *Hillside J Clin Psychiatry* **8**:214–223.

Schenck CH, Mahowald MW (1996). Long-term, nightly benzodiazepine treatment of injurious parasomnias and other disorders of disrupted nocturnal sleep in 170 adults. *Am J Med* **100**:333–337.

Scherbaum N, Stuper B, Bonnet U, Gastpar M (2003). Transient restless legs-like syndrome as a complication of opiate withdrawal. *Pharmacopsychiatry* **36**:70–72.

Scholle S, Scholle HC, Zwacka G (2001). Periodic leg movements and sleep-disordered breathing in children. *Somnologie* **5**:153–158.

Schwarz J, Trenkwalder C (1996). Restless legs syndrome: Treatment with L-Dopa or L-Dopa slow release preparations. *Aktuel Neurol* **23**:26–29.

Sharif AA (2002). Entacapone in restless legs syndrome. *Mov Disord* **17**:421.

Silber MH, Shepard J-WJ, Wisbey JA (1997). Pergolide in the management of restless legs syndrome: an extended study. *Sleep* **20**:878–882.

Silber MH, Girish M, Izurieta R (2003a). Pramipexole in the management of restless legs syndrome: an extended study. *Sleep* **26**:819–821.

Silber MH, Richardson JW (2003b). Multiple blood donations associated with iron deficiency in patients with restless legs syndrome. *Mayo Clin Proc* **78**:52–54.

Simakajornboon N, Gozal D, Vlasic V, Mack C, Sharon D, McGinley BM (2003). Periodic limb movements in sleep and iron status in children. *Sleep* **26**:735–738.

Sloand JA, Shelly MA, Feigin A, Bernstein P, Monk RD (2004). A double-blind, placebo-controlled trial of intravenous iron dextran therapy in patients with ESRD and restless legs syndrome. *Am J Kidney Dis* **43**:663–670.

Sonka K, Pretl M, Kranda K (2003). Management of restless legs syndrome by the partial D2-agonist terguride. *Sleep Med* **4**:455–457.

Sorensen O, Telstad W (1984). Carbamazepin (Tegretol) ved restless legs syndrom. *Tidsskr Nor Laegeforen* **104**:2093–2095.

Staedt J, Stoppe G, Kogler A, Munz DL, Hajak G, Staedt U, Riemann H, Ruther E (1994). Nachtliches Myoklonie-Syndrom (NMS) und Restless-Legs-Syndrom (RLS)–Ubersicht und Fallbeschreibung. *Fortschr Neurol Psychiatr* **62**:88–93.

Staedt J, Stoppe G, Riemann H, Hajak G, Ruther E, Riederer P (1996). Lamotrigine in the treatment of nocturnal myoclonus syndrome (NMS): two case reports. *J Neural Transm* **103**:355–361.

Staedt J, Wassmuth F, Ziemann U, Hajak G, Ruther E, Stoppe G (1997). Pergolide: treatment of choice in restless legs syndrome (RLS) and nocturnal myoclonus syndrome (NMS). A double-blind randomized crossover trial of pergolide versus L-Dopa. *J Neural Transm* **104**:461–468.

Staedt J, Hunerjager H, Ruther E, Stoppe G (1998). Pergolide: treatment of choice in Restless Legs Syndrome (RLS) and Nocturnal Myoclonus Syndrome (NMS). Longterm follow up on pergolide. Short communication. *J Neural Transm* **105**:265–268.

Stautner A, Stiasny-Kolster K, Collado-Seidel V, Bucher SF, Oertel WH, Trenkwalder C (1996). Comparison of idiopathic and uremic restless legs syndrome: results of data base of 134 patients. *Mov Disord* **11**:S98.

Stiasny K (1999). Restless legs syndrome: Sometimes are hot and cold showers sufficient. *Arztlich Prax Neurol Psychiatr*:38–40.

Stiasny K, Moller JC, Oertel WH (2000). Safety of pramipexole in patients with restless legs syndrome. *Neurology* **55**:1589–1590.

Stiasny K, Robbecke J, Schuler P, Oertel WH (2000). Treatment of idiopathic restless legs syndrome (RLS) with the D2-agonist cabergoline–an open clinical trial. *Sleep* **23**:349–354.

Stiasny K (2001a). Clinical data on restless legs syndrome: a dose-finding study with cabergoline. *Eur Neurol* **46(Suppl 1)**:24–26.

Stiasny K (2001b). Handling the problem of augmentation in restless legs syndrome (RLS). *Eur J Neurol* **8**:15.

Stiasny K, Wetter TC, Winkelmann J, Brandenburg U, Penzel T, Rubin M, Hundemer HP, Oertel WH, Trenkwalder C (2001c). Long-term effects of pergolide in the treatment of restless legs syndrome. *Neurology* **56**:1399–1402.

Stiasny K, Moller JC, Bodenschatz R, Sommer H, Pagalu I, Benes H, Franz P, Clarenbach P, Zotter J, Warmuth R, Schollmayer E, Woltering F, Kohen R, Oertel WH (2002a). Rotigotine CDS in the treatment of moderate to advanced stages of restless legs syndrome: A double-blind placebo-controlled study. *Mov Disord* **17**:S241.

Stiasny K, Uberall M, Oertel WH (2002b). Cabergoline in restless legs syndrome (RLS) - a double-blind placebo-controlled multicenter dose-finding trial. *Eur J Neurol* **9**:50.

Stiasny-Kolster K, Benes H, Peglau I, Hornyak M, Holinka B, Wessel K, Emser W, Leroux M, Kohnen R, Oertel WH (2004a). Effective cabergoline treatment in idiopathic restless legs syndrome. *Neurology* **63**:2272–2279.

Stiasny-Kolster K, Magerl W, Oertel WH, Moller JC, Treede RD (2004b). Static mechanical hyperalgesia without dynamic tactile allodynia in patients with restless legs syndrome. *Brain* **127**:773–782.

Stiasny-Kolster K, Kohen R, Schollmayer E, Moller JC, Oertel WH, Rotigotine Sp 666 Study Group (2004c).

Patch application of the dopamine agoinst rotigotine to patients with moderate to advanced stages of restless legs syndrome: a double-blind, placebo-controlled pilot study. *Mov Discord* **19**:1432–1438.

Stiasny-Kolster K, Oertel WH (2004d). Low-dose pramipexole in the management of restless legs syndrome. An open label trial. *Neuropsychobiology* **50**:65–70.

Strang RR (1967). The symptom of restless legs. *Med J Aust* **1**:1211–1213.

Tagaya H, Wetter TC, Winkelmann J, Rubin M, Hundemer HP, Trenkwalder C, Friess E (2002). Pergolide restores sleep maintenance but impairs sleep EEG synchronization in patients with restless legs syndrome. *Sleep Med* **3**:49–54.

Teive HA, de Quadros A, Barros FC, Werneck LC (2002). Sindrome das pernas inquietas com heranca autossomica dominante piorada pelo uso de mirtazapina: relato de caso. *Arq Neuropsiquiatr* **60**:1025–1029.

Telstad W, Sorensen O, Larsen S, Lillevold PE, Stensrud P, Hansen R (1984). Treatment of the restless legs syndrome with carbamazepine: a double blind study. *Br Med J (Clin Res Ed)* **288**:444–446.

Tergau F, Wischer S, Wolf C, Paulus W (2001). Treatment of restless legs syndrome with the dopamine agonist alpha -dihydroergocryptine. *Mov Disord* **16**:731–735.

Thorp ML, Morris CD, Bagby SP (2001). A crossover study of gabapentin in treatment of restless legs syndrome among hemodialysis patients. *Am J Kidney Dis* **38**:104–108.

Tollefson G, Erdman C (1985). Triazolam in the restless legs syndrome. *J Clin Psychopharmacol* **5**:361–362.

Trenkwalder C, Stiasny K, Pollmacher T, Wetter T, Schwarz J, Kohnen R, Kazenwadel J, Kruger HP, Ramm S, Kunzel M, *et al.* (1995). L-dopa therapy of uremic and idiopathic restless legs syndrome: a double -blind, crossover trial. *Sleep* **18**:681–688.

Trenkwalder C, Seidel VC, Kazenwadel J, Kohnen R, Wetter T, Selzer R, Oertel W (1997). Treatment of the restless legs syndrome with a combination of standard and sustained-release levodopa/benserazide (Madopar Depot(R)): A double-blind controlled study. *J Neurol Sci* **150**:S204.

Trenkwalder C, Brandenburg U, Hundemer HP, Lledo A, Quail D, Wood E, Swieca J, Polo O, Wetter TC, Ferini-Strambi L, De Groen H, PEARLS study group (2001a). A Randomized Long-Term Placebo-Controlled Multicenter Trial of Pergolide in the Treatment of Restless Legs Syndrome with Central Evaluation of Polysomnographic Data. *Neurology* **56**:A5–A6.

Trenkwalder C, Brandenburg U, Hundemer HP, Lledo A, Quail D, Swieca J (2001b). A long-term controlled multicenter trial of pergolide in the treatment of restless legs syndrome with central evaluation of polysomnographic data. *J Neurol Sci* **187:**S432.

Trenkwalder C (2003). Dyskinesia on dopaminergic therapy for restless legs syndrome? *Internist Prax* **43:**99–100.

Trenkwalder C, Collado-Seidel V, Kazenwadel J, Wetter TC, Oertel W, Selzer R, Kohnen R (2003). One-year treatment with standard and sustained-release levodopa: appropriate long-term treatment of restless legs syndrome? *Mov Disord* **18:**1184–1189.

Trenkwalder C, Garcia-Borreguero D, Montagna P, Lainey E, de Weerd A-W, Tidswell P, Saletu-Zyhlarz G, Telstad W, Ferini-Strambi L (2004a). Ropinirole in the treatment of restless legs syndrome: results from the TREAT RLS 1 study, a 12 week, randomised, placebo controlled study in 10 European countries. *J Neurol Neurosurg Psychiatry* **75:**92–97.

Trenkwalder C, Hundemer HP, Lledo A, Swieca J, Polo O, Wetter TC, Ferini-Strambi L, De Groen H, Quail D, Brandenburg U (2004b). Efficacy of pergolide in treatment of restless legs syndrome: The PEARLS Study. *Neurology* **62:**1391–1397.

Trzepacz PT, Violette EJ, Sateia MJ (1984). Response to opioids in three patients with restless legs syndrome. *Am J Psychiatry* **141:**993–995.

Vahedi H, Kuchle M, Trenkwalder C, Krenz CJ (1994). Peridurale Morphiumanwendung bei Restless-Legs-Status. *Anasthesiol Intensivmed Notfallmed Schmerzther* **29:**368–370.

van Dijk JG, Bollen EL, Slootweg J, van der Meer CM, Durian FW, Zwinderman AH (1991). Geen verschil in werkzaamheid tussen hydrokinine en placebo bij het 'restless legs'-syndroom. *Ned Tijdschr Geneeskd* **135:**759–763.

Vaskivskyj M (1973). Vliv hyperemizujici vodolecby na syndrom neklidnych nohou. *Fysiatr Revmatol Vestn* **51:**308–309.

Vignatelli L, Billiard M, Clarenbach P, Garcia-Borreguero D, Kaynak D, Liesiene V, Trenkwalder C, Montagna P (2006). Restless Legs Syndrome and Periodic Limb Movement Disorder. *Eur J Neurology* **13:** in press

von Scheele C (1986). Levodopa in restless legs. *Lancet* **2:**426–427.

von Scheele C, Kempi V (1990). Long-term effect of dopaminergic drugs in restless legs. A 2-year follow-up. *Arch Neurol* **47:**1223–1224.

Wagner ML, Walters AS, Coleman RG, Hening WA, Grasing K, Chokroverty S (1996). Randomized, double-blind, placebo-controlled study of clonidine in restless legs syndrome. *Sleep* **19:**52–58.

Walker SL, Fine A, Kryger MH (1996). L-DOPA/carbidopa for nocturnal movement disorders in uremia. *Sleep* **19:**214–218.

Walters A, Hening W, Cote L, Fahn S (1986). Dominantly inherited restless legs with myoclonus and periodic movements of sleep: a syndrome related to the endogenous opiates? *Adv Neurol* **43:**309–319.

Walters AS, Hening WA, Kavey N, Chokroverty S, Gidro-Frank S (1988). A double-blind randomized crossover trial of bromocriptine and placebo in restless legs syndrome. *Ann Neurol* **24:**455–458.

Walters AS, Wagner ML, Hening WA, Grasing K, Mills R, Chokroverty S, Kavey N (1993). Successful treatment of the idiopathic restless legs syndrome in a randomized double-blind trial of oxycodone versus placebo. *Sleep* **16:**327–332.

Walters AS (1995). Toward a better definition of the restless legs syndrome. The International Restless Legs Syndrome Study Group. *Mov Disord* **10:**634–642.

Walters AS, Mandelbaum DE, Lewin DS, Kugler S, England SJ, Miller M (2000). Dopaminergic therapy in children with restless legs/periodic limb movements in sleep and ADHD. Dopaminergic Therapy Study Group. *Pediatr Neurol* **22:**182–186.

Walters AS, Winkelmann J, Trenkwalder C, Fry JM, Kataria V, Wagner M, Sharma R, Hening W, Li L (2001). Long-term follow-up on restless legs syndrome patients treated with opioids. *Mov Disord* **16:**1105–1109.

Walters AS, LeBrocq C, Dhar A, Hening W, Rosen R, Allen RP, Trenkwalder C (2003). International Restless Legs Syndrome Study Group. Validation of the International Restless Legs Syndrome Study Group rating scale for restless legs syndrome. *Sleep Med* **4:**121–132.

Walters AS, Ondo W, Dreykluft T, Grunstein R, Lee D, Sethi K, TREAT RLS 2 Study Group (2004). Ropinirole is effective in the treatment of restless legs syndrome. TREAT RLS 2: a 12-week, double-blind, randomized, parallel-group, placebo-controlled study. *Mov Disord* **19:**1414–1423.

Ware JC, Blumoff R, Pittard JT (1988). Peripheral vasoconstriction in patients with sleep related periodic leg movements. *Sleep* **11:**182–186.

Watts RL, Freeman A, Rye DB, Bliwise DL, Krulewicz S (2000). Ropinirole for restless legs syndrome. *Mov Disord* **15:**S134–S134.

Wetter TC, Trenkwalder C, Stiasny K, Pollmacher T, Kazenwadel J, Kohnen R, Kunzel M, Oertel WH (1995). Behandlung des idiopathischen und uramischen Restless-legs-Syndrom mit L-Dopa–Eine doppelblinde Cross-over-Studie. *Wien Med Wochenschr* **145:**525–527.

Wetter TC, Stiasny K, Winkelmann J, Buhlinger A, Brandenburg U, Penzel T, Medori R, Rubin M, Oertel WH, Trenkwalder C (1999). A randomized controlled study of pergolide in patients with restless legs syndrome. *Neurology* **52:**944–950.

Willis T. *The London Practice of Physick.* 1st ed. London: Thomas Bassett and William Crooke, 1685:404.

Winkelmann J, Wetter TC, Stiasny K, Oertel WH, Trenkwalder C (1998). Treatment of restless leg syndrome with pergolide–an open clinical trial. *Mov Disord* **13:**566–569.

Winkelmann J, Stautner A, Samtleben W, Trenkwalder C (2002). Long-term course of restless legs syndrome in dialysis patients after kidney transplantation. *Mov Disord* **17:**1072–1076.

Winkelman JW, Johnston L (2004). Augmentation and tolerance with long-term pramipexole treatment of restless legs syndrome (RLS). *Sleep Med* **5:**9–14.

Yamashiro Y, Kryger MH (1994). Acute effect of nasal CPAP on periodic limb movements associated with breathing disorders during sleep. *Sleep* **17:**172–175.

Yasuda T, Nishimura A, Katsuki Y, Tsuji Y (1986). Restless legs syndrome treated successfully by kidney transplantation–a case report. *Clin Transpl* **12:**138.

Yatzidis H, Koutsicos D, Agroyannis B, Papastephanidis C, Plemenos M, Delatola Z (1984). Biotin in the management of uremic neurologic disorders. *Nephron* **36:**183–186.

Zoe A, Wagner ML, Walters AS (1994). High-dose clonidine in a case of restless legs syndrome. *Ann Pharmacother* **28:**878–881.

Zucconi M, Coccagna G, Petronelli R, Gerardi R, Mondini S, Cirignotta F (1989). Nocturnal myoclonus in restless legs syndrome effect of carbamazepine treatment. *Funct Neurol* **4:**263–271.

Zucconi M, Oldani A, Castronovo C, Ferini-Strambi L (2003). Cabergoline is an effective single-drug treatment for restless legs syndrome: clinical and actigraphic evaluation. *Sleep* **26:**815–818.

Full paper not found and data from abstract not available: Brenning, 1969 (possible class III evidence for carbacholine and inositolnicotinate), Christiansen, 1970 (possible class III evidence for meso-inositol hexa-nicotinate and pentaerythritol tetranicotinate), Hurlimann, 1974 (possible class III evidence for Other treatments), Noseda *et al.,* 2002 (possible class III evidence for Benzodiazepines), Sorensen and Telsad, 1984 (possible class II evidence for Carbamazepine).

Unite Text: Gulden, 1994 (possible class IV evidence for levodopa), Hain, 2002 (possible class IV evidence for opioid), Horiguchi *et al.,* 1985 (possible class IV evidence for amantadine), Kastin *et al.,* 1968 (possible class IV evidence for Other treatments), Nassr, 1986 (possible class IV evidence for nitrazepam), Petiau *et al.,* 1995 (possible class IV evidence for dopaminergic drugs), Satzger-Harsch, 1998 (possible class IV evidence for levodopa), Schwarz and Trenkwalder, 1996 (possible class IV evidence for levodopa), Staedt *et al.,* 1994 (possible class IV evidence for levodopa), Stiasny, 1999 (possible class IV evidence for other treatments), Trenkwalder, 2003 (possible class IV evidence for levodopa).

CHAPTER 44

Cognitive rehabilitation

S.F. Cappa,[a] T. Benke,[b] S. Clarke,[c] B. Rossi,[d]
B. Stemmer,[e] C.M. van Heugten[f]

Abstract

Disorders of language, spatial perception, attention, memory, calculation and praxis are a frequent consequence of acquired brain damage (in particular, stroke and traumatic brain injury) and a major determinant of disability. The rehabilitation of aphasia and, more recently, of other cognitive disorders is an important area of neurological rehabilitation. We report here a review of the available evidence about effectiveness of cognitive rehabilitation. Given the limited number and generally low quality of randomized controlled trials (RCTs) in this area of therapeutic intervention, the Task Force considered, besides the available Cochrane reviews, evidence of lower classes that was critically analysed until a consensus was reached. In particular, we considered evidence from small group or single case studies including an appropriate statistical evaluation of effect sizes. The general conclusion is that there is evidence to award a grade A, B or C recommendation to some forms of cognitive rehabilitation in patients with neuropsychological deficits in the post-acute stage after a focal brain lesion (stroke, TBI). These include aphasia therapy, rehabilitation of unilateral spatial neglect (ULN), attentional training in the post-acute stage after traumatic brain injury (TBI), the use of electronic memory aids in memory disorders and the treatment of apraxia with compensatory strategies. There is clearly a need for adequately designed studies in this area, which should take into account specific problems such as patient heterogeneity and treatment standardisation.

Objectives

The rehabilitation of disorders of cognitive functions (language, spatial perception, attention, memory, calculation, praxis), following acquired neurological damage of different aetiology (in particular, stroke and traumatic brain injury), is an expanding area of neurological rehabilitation, and has been the focus of considerable research interest in recent years. In 1999, a Task Force on Cognitive Rehabilitation was set up under the auspices of the European Federation of Neurological Societies (EFNS). The aim was to evaluate the existing evidence for the clinical effectiveness of cognitive rehabilitation in stroke and traumatic brain injury, and provide recommendations for neurological

[a]Departments of Psychology, Neurology and Neuroscience, Vita Salute San Raffaele S. Raffaele University, Milano, Italy; [b]Klinik fuer Neurologie Innsbruck, Austria; [c]Division de Neuropsychologie, Lausanne, Switzerland; [d]Section of Neurology, Department of Neuroscience, University of Pisa, Pisa, Italy; [e]Centre de Recherche, Institut de Geriatrie de Montreal, and Department de Linguistique et Traduction, Universite de Montreal, Montreal Canada; [f]Netherlands Institute of Primary Health Care NIVEL, Utrecht, The Netherlands.

practice. The present guidelines are an update and a revision of the previous work, which was published in 2003 in the *European Journal of Neurology* (Cappa *et al.*, 2003).

Background

For these guidelines, we have limited ourselves to a review of studies dealing with the rehabilitation of non-progressive neuropsychological disorders due to stroke and traumatic brain damage (TBI). As a consequence several important areas of 'cognitive rehabilitation' were excluded such as the rehabilitation of dementia, psychiatric and developmental disorders. In addition, we have not considered pharmacological treatment and rehabilitation.

The prevalence and relevance of cognitive rehabilitation for stroke and TBI patients require the establishment of recommendations for the practice of cognitive rehabilitation, and these have been formally recognized by a subcommittee of the Brain Injury-Interdisciplinary Special Interest Group of the American Congress of Rehabilitation Medicine. The initial recommendations of the Committee were published in 1992 as the Guidelines for Cognitive Rehabilitation (Harley *et al.*, 1992) and were based on the so-called expert opinion that did not take into account empirical evidence on the effectiveness of cognitive rehabilitation. More recently, a review of the scientific literature for cognitive rehabilitation in TBI patients published from January 1988 through August 1998 (including 11 randomised clinical trials – RCTs) noted that data on the effectiveness of cognitive rehabilitation programmes were limited by the heterogeneity of subjects, interventions and outcomes studied (NIH Consensus Development Panel, 1999).

As a preliminary consideration, we wish to underline that the present status of studies on the effectiveness of cognitive rehabilitation is unsatisfactory. We are fully convinced that the standards required for the evaluation of pharmacological and surgical interventions also apply to rehabilitation. In particular, it is necessary to show that rehabilitation is effective not only in modifying the impairment but also in having sustained effects at the disability level. Unfortunately, the majority of

RCTs in this area are of poor methodological quality, have insufficient sample size and fail to assess the outcome at the disability level. Many other studies fail to compare intervention with placebo or sham treatment.

Search strategy

Each member of the Task Force was assigned an area of cognitive rehabilitation (SFC-aphasia; SC-unilateral neglect; BR-attention; BS-memory; CvH-apraxia; TB-acalculia) and systematically searched the EBM Reviews – Cochrane Central Register of Controlled Trials, the Medline and Psych-Info databases using the appropriate key words, and searched textbooks and existing guidelines. The general consensus was to include articles only if they contained data that could be rated according to the grades of recommendation for management, classified in terms of level of evidence following the guidance statement for neurological management guidelines of the EFNS-revised (Brainin *et al.*, 2004).

Method for reaching consensus

Data collection and analysis of evidence were performed independently by each participant according to the assignment mentioned above. On the basis of the single reports, SFC produced a first draft of the guidelines that was circulated several times among the Task Force members until the discrepancies in each topic were solved and a consensus was reached.

Results

Rehabilitation of aphasia

The rehabilitation of speech and language disorders following brain damage is the area of intervention for acquired cognitive deficits with the longest tradition, dating back to the nineteenth century (Howard and Hatfield, 1987). A variety of approaches have been applied to the rehabilitation of aphasia, from stimulation approaches to the recent attempts to establish theory-driven treatment programmes based on the principles of cognitive neuropsychology (Basso, 2003). The need to establish the effectiveness of aphasia rehabilitation has stimulated a number of investigations, dating back to the period after the Second World War, and has been based on a variety of methodologies. A meta-analysis of studies dealing with the effectiveness of language rehabilitation, limited to aphasia as a result of stroke, has been made available by the Cochrane collaboration. The review covers articles about speech and language rehabilitation after stroke up to January 1999 (Greener *et al.*, 2000). The conclusion of the review is that 'speech and language therapy treatment for people with aphasia after a stroke has not been shown either to be clearly effective or clearly ineffective within an RCT. Decisions about the management of patients must therefore be based on other forms of evidence. Further research is required to find out if speech and language therapy for aphasic patients is effective. If researchers choose to do a trial, this must be large enough to have adequate statistical power, and be clearly reported'. This conclusion is based on a limited number of RCTs (12), all of which were considered of poor quality. Another review by Cicerone *et al.* (2000) reached a different conclusion. The conclusion is that 'cognitive-linguistic therapies' can be considered as Practice Standard for aphasia after stroke; similar, positive conclusions for TBI were based on less consistent evidence. The reasons for this discrepancy can be found in the different criteria used in the two reviews. Several studies included by Cicerone *et al.* (2000) were not considered in the Cochrane review for the following reasons. In comparison with an untreated control group, one study by Hagen (1973) was excluded because of the lack of true randomisation (the patients were sequentially assigned to treatment or no treatment). Another study (Katz and Wertz, 1997) was probably excluded because it dealt only with computer-assisted reading rehabilitation. Two small RCTs (Helffenstein and Wechsler, 1982; Thomas-Stonell *et al.*, 1994), which reported positive treatment effects, were excluded from the Cochrane review because they were devoted to communication disorders after TBI.

Some of the RCT comparing therapy with unstructured stimulation were based on a very limited number of treatment sessions. A meta-analysis by Bhogal *et al.* (2003) showed that studies reporting a significant treatment effect provided 8.8 hours of therapy per week for 11.2 weeks, while the negative studies only provided approximately 2 h per week for 22.9 weeks. The total length of therapy was significantly inversely correlated with a mean change in the Porch Index of Communicative Abilities (PICA) scores. The number of hours of therapy provided in a week was significantly correlated to greater improvement on the PICA and the Token Test. These results suggest that an intense therapy programme provided over a short amount of time can improve outcomes of speech and language therapy for stroke patients with aphasia.

By definition, all class II and III evidence is not included in the Cochrane review. This resulted in the exclusion of the three large studies by Basso *et al.* (1979), Shewan and Kertesz (1985) and Poeck *et al.* (1989), all indicating significant benefits of treatment. An additional small class II study by Carlomagno *et al.* (2001) supported the usefulness of writing rehabilitation in patients in the post-acute stage. Additional evidence for treatment effects comes from some recent randomised investigations on small patient samples (class II). A study comparing group communication treatment with 'deferred treatment' indicated positive effects on both linguistic and communication measures (Elman and Bernstein-Ellis, 1999). Another study based on a small sample compared 'massed' with conventional treatment and showed a significant superiority of the 'massed' intervention (Pulvermueller *et al.*, 2000). A recent randomised study compared semantic with phonological treatment of anomia. Both treatments resulted in a significant improvement in functional communication (Doesborgh *et al.*, 2004)

Similarly, single case studies are not considered in the Cochrane reviews. This is particularly relevant because most of the recent treatment studies based on the cognitive neuropsychological approach make use of the single case methodology. A review paper by Robey *et al.* (1999) critically discusses this approach and concludes that generally a large treatment effect has been found in aphasic patients.

RECOMMENDATIONS

The conclusions of the Cochrane review of aphasia rehabilitation after stroke are not compatible with Level A for aphasia therapy. There is, however, considerable evidence from class II and III studies, as well as from rigorous single-case studies indicating its probable effectiveness (Level B). There is clearly a need for further investigations in the field. In particular, the evidence of effectiveness of pragmatic-conversational therapy after TBI is based on a limited number of studies on small samples and is in need of confirmation.

Rehabilitation of ULN

The presence of hemineglect beyond the acute stage is associated with poor outcome in terms of independence (Denes *et al.*, 1982; Stone *et al.*, 1992) and considerable effort is therefore devoted to its rehabilitation. We review here published studies of neglect rehabilitation, and refer also to recently published reviews (Robertson and Hawkins, 1999; Robertson, 1999; Diamond, 2001; Pierce and Buxbaum, 2002; Kerkhoff, 2003; Paton *et al.*, 2004), including the Cochrane review (Bowen *et al.*, 2002). The latter analysed 15 studies and found evidence that cognitive rehabilitation resulted in significant and persisting improvements in performance on impairment level assessments. There was, however, insufficient evidence to confirm or exclude an effect of cognitive rehabilitation at the level of disability or on destination following discharge from hospital. Different types of approaches are currently used for neglect rehabilitation; we review here evidence for these different approaches.

Combined training of visual scanning, reading, copying and figure description yielded statistically significant improvement of neglect symptoms in one class II (Antonucci *et al.*, 1995) and two class III studies (Pizzamiglio *et al.*, 1992; Vallar *et al.*, 1997). Visual scanning training alone was shown to improve neglect significantly in one class I study (Weinberg *et al.*, 1977). *Spatiomotor or visuospatiomotor cueing* improved neglect significantly in one class I (Kalra *et al.*, 1997) and two class III studies (Lin *et al.*, 1996; Frassinetti *et al.*, 2001). *Visual*

cueing with kinetic stimuli was found to bring significant, albeit transient, improvement in three class III studies (Butter *et al.*, 1990; Pizzamiglio *et al.*, 1990; Butter and Kirsch, 1995). However, the use of optokinetic stimulation did not improve neglect in a recent class I study (Pizzamiglio *et al.*, 2004). *Video feedback* (Tham and Tegner, 1997) and *visuomotor feedback* (Harvey *et al.*, 2003) were shown to improve significantly performance on trained tasks in class III and II studies, respectively. *Training of sustained attention, increasing of alertness or cueing of spatial attention* were shown to significantly improve neglect in class III studies (Hommel *et al.*, 1990; Ladavas *et al.*, 1994; Robertson *et al.*, 1995; Kerkhoff, 1998).

Several studies investigated the effects of *influencing multisensory representations*. These studies in general demonstrated transient effects, lasting little longer than the end of the appropriate stimulation. Vestibular stimulation by cold water infusion into the left outer ear canal showed significant effects on different aspects of the unilateral neglect in two class III studies (Rode and Perenin, 1994; Rode *et al.*, 1998). Galvanic vestibular stimulation significantly improved neglect symptoms in one class III study (Rorsman *et al.*, 1999). Transcutaneous electrical stimulation of the left neck muscles showed significant effects in three class III studies (Vallar *et al.*, 1995; Guariglia *et al.*, 1998; Perennou *et al.*, 2001) and neck muscle vibration in one class II study (Schindler *et al.*, 2002). The latter is the only study of this group that showed a persistent effect after 2 months. Changes in trunk orientation had significantly positive effects in one class II study (Wiart *et al.*, 1997).

The use of *prism goggles* deviating by 10 degrees to the right, introduced relatively recently, was shown to improve significantly, in a transient fashion, neglect symptoms in two class II (Rossetti *et al.*, 1998; Angeli *et al.*, 2004) and one class III study (Farne *et al.*, 2002). A class III study applied the prism goggle treatment for a 2-week period and obtained statistically significant improvement in the long term (Frassinetti *et al.*, 2002). *Forced use of left visual hemifield or left eye* showed a relative benefit in neglect in one class II (Beis *et al.*, 1999) and two class III studies (Butter and Kirsch, 1992; Walker *et al.*, 1996).

Computer training yielded mixed results. One class I (Robertson *et al.*, 1990) and one class III study (Bergego *et al.*, 1997) reported absence of significantly positive effects, while a more recent class II study showed statistically significant improvement in wheel chair mobility (Webster *et al.*, 2001).

RECOMMENDATIONS

Several methods of neglect rehabilitation were investigated in Level I or II studies. The present evidence confers Level A recommendation to visual scanning training and to visuo-spatio-motor training, and Level B recommendation to the combined training of visual scanning, reading, copying and figure description; to trunk orientation; to neck vibration; and to forced use of left eye. The use of prism goggles obtains the same level of recommendation for transient effect and Level C for long-term effect if used over longer periods. Level B recommendation exists for video feedback; and Level B-C for training of sustained attention and alertness. Level C of recommendation is valid for transient effects due to caloric or galvanic vestibular stimulations as well as transcutaneous electrical stimulation of neck muscles. Visual cueing with kinetic stimuli and the use of computers in neglect rehabilitation remain controversial.

Rehabilitation of attention disorders

Attention deficits follow many types of brain damage, including stroke and TBI (Bruhn and Parsons, 1971; Van Zomeren and Van DenBurg, 1985). A pioneer study by Ben-Yishay *et al.* (1978) explored the treatment of deficits in focusing and sustaining attention in 40 brain-injured adults. There was not only improvement on the attention- training tasks, but also generalisation to other psychometric measures of attention that were maintained at 6-month follow-up. Using a multiple-baseline design, with patients at 4–6 years after head injury, Wood (1986) found that contingent token reinforcement was effective in increasing patients' ability to sustain attention on a task. Several studies (Ponsford and Kinsella, 1988; Niemann *et al.*, 1990; Novack *et al.*, 1996) have explicitly incorporated and evaluated therapeutic interventions such as feedback, reinforcement and strategy teaching into the attention rehabilitation programmes.

The Cochrane review by Lincoln *et al.* (2000), having searched for controlled trials of attention training in stroke, identified only the study of Schottke (1997) showing the efficacy of attention training in improving sustained attention.

Thirteen studies were reviewed by Cicerone *et al.* (2000), including three prospective RCTs (Niemann *et al.*, 1990; Gray *et al.*, 1992; Novack *et al.*, 1996), four class II controlled studies (Sohlberg and Mateer, 1987; Strache, 1987; Ponsford and Kinsella, 1988; Sturm and Wilmes, 1991); and six class III studies (Wood, 1986; Ethier *et al.*, 1989; Gray and Robertson, 1989; Gansler and McCaffrey, 1991; Wilson and Robertson, 1992; Sturm *et al.*, 1997). Most controlled studies compared attention training with an alternative treatment, without including a no-treatment condition; a very important distinction is between studies conducted in the acute and post-acute stage. Cicerone *et al.* (2000) concluded that evidence from two RCT (Niemann *et al.*, 1990; Gray *et al.*, 1992) with a total of 57 subjects and two controlled studies (Sohlberg and Mateer, 1987; Strache, 1987) with a total of 49 subjects supports the effectiveness of attention training beyond the effects of non-specific cognitive stimulation for subjects with TBI or stroke during the post-acute phase of recovery and rehabilitation. Cicerone *et al.* (2000) recommended such a form of intervention as a practice guideline for these persons. Interventions should include not only training with different stimulus modalities and complexity, but also therapist activities such as monitoring subjects' performance, providing feedback and teaching strategies. Attention training appears to be more effective when directed at improving the subject's performance on more complex, functional tasks. However, the effects of treatment may be relatively small or task-specific, and an additional need exists to examine the impact of attention treatment on activities of daily living (ADL) or functional outcomes.

Acute studies

One class I and two class II studies evaluated the effectiveness of attention treatment during the acute period of rehabilitation. The class I study of Novack (1996) compared the effectiveness of focused treatment consisting of sequential, hierarchical interventions directed at specific attention mechanisms versus unstructured intervention consisting of non-sequential, non-hierarchical activities requiring memory or reasoning skills. Both groups improved, but there were no intergroup differences: the observed improvements are probably due to spontaneous recovery. One class II study (Ponsford and Kinsella, 1988) used a multiple baseline design across subjects and evaluated a programme for the remediation of processing speed deficits in 10 patients with severe TBI (6–34 weeks post-injury). The authors reported no benefit or generalisation of effects of attention training; however, improvement did occur in some patients when practice on attention training tasks was combined with therapist feedback and praise. In the other class II study (Sturm and Wilmes, 1991), 35 subjects with lateralised stroke showed beneficial effects of attention training on .ve of 14 outcome measures, especially on measures of perceptual speed and selective attention in left hemisphere lesions.

Post-acute

Two class I and two class II studies assessed the attention treatment effectiveness during the post-acute period of rehabilitation. Gray et al. (1992) treated 31 patients with attention dysfunction, randomly assigned to receive either computerised attention retraining or an equivalent amount of recreational computer use. Immediately after training, the experimental group showed marked improvement on two measures of attention (but, when pre-morbid intelligence score and time since injury were added as covariates, the treatment effect was no longer significant); at 6-month follow-up, the treatment group showed continued improvement and superior performance compared to the control group on tests involving auditory–verbal working memory. The authors suggested that the improvement,

continuing over the follow-up period, was consistent with a strategy training model as it becomes increasingly automated and integrated into a wider range of behaviours (Gray et al., 1992). In the second post-acute class I study (Niemann et al., 1990) community-dwelling patients with moderate to severe brain injury were screened for orientation, vision, aphasia and psychiatric illness. The experimental attention training group improved significantly more than the alternative (memory) treatment group on four attention measures administered throughout the treatment period, although the effects did not generalise to the second set of neuropsychological measures. Sohlberg and Mateer (1987) employed a class II multiple baseline design with four patients to evaluate the effectiveness of a specific, hierarchical attention training programme. All subjects showed gain on a single attention outcome measure administered after the start of attention training but not after training on visuospatial processing: this improvement also generalised to cognitive and everyday problems. Strache (1987) conducted a prospective class II study on patients with mixed trauma and vascular aetiologies, and compared two closely related interventions for concentration with subjects in an untreated control group receiving general rehabilitation. After 20 treatment sessions, both attention treatments resulted in significant improvement on attention measures in respect of control subjects, with some generalisation to memory and intelligence measures. Rath et al. (2004) in three inter-related class II controlled studies examined the construct of problem solving as it relates to the assessment of deficits in higher level outpatients with TBD. The difference between the groups were significant first for timed attention tasks, then for psychosocial and problem solving self-report inventories, then for patients' self-report problem solving and also in self-report inventory. It means that it is necessary to have a lot of different approaches to the construct of problem solving (multidimensional approach) to obtain good rehabilitation. Several attempts were made to establish the differential role for effectiveness of training of specific components of attention. Rios et al. (2004) in a class II controlled study on traumatic brain injury consider attention as a basic cognitive function, a pre-requisite for other cognitive processes. It is divided into four different sub-processes: cognitive flexibility, speed of processing, interference and working memory, which must be taken into consideration. The results of the work support the view that these different sub-processes of attentional control can be differentiated between high and low level processes and may have implications for neuropsychological assessment and rehabilitation.

Improvements in speed of processing appear to be less robust than improvements on non-speeded tasks (Ponsford and Kinsella, 1988; Ethier *et al.*, 1989; Sturm *et al.*, 1997). Moreover, several studies also suggest greater benefits of attention training on more complex tasks requiring selective or divided attention than on basic tasks of reaction time or vigilance (Sturm and Wilmes, 1991; Gray *et al.*, 1992; Sturm *et al.*, 1997). Wilson and Robertson (1992), implementing a series of individualised interventions intended to facilitate voluntary control over attention during functional activities, effectively decreased the attention lapses that the subject experienced when reading novels and texts.

RECOMMENDATIONS

During the acute period of recovery and inpatient rehabilitation, evidence is insufficient to distinguish the effects of specific attention training from spontaneous recovery or more general cognitive interventions for patients with moderate-to-severe TBI and stroke. Therefore, specific interventions for attention during the period of acute recovery are not recommended. On the other hand, the availability of class I evidence for attention training in the post-acute phase after TBI is compatible with a Level A recommendation.

Rehabilitation of memory

Memory impairment is a well-documented sequel following traumatic brain injury and has also been reported following stroke. Some studies investigating memory rehabilitation are oriented towards alleviating general memory problems such as problems of learning and retrieval or everyday functioning problems. Others focus on specific contents such as orientation, dates, names, faces, routines, appointments. Yet others are oriented towards modality specific impairments such as visual versus verbal memory problems. As memory is not a unitary concept, studies also address different aspects of memory such as working memory or prospective memory.

The studies reviewed fall roughly into three categories: studies targeting techniques without external memory aids, studies targeting techniques with non-electronic external memory aids, and studies focusing on the use of assistive electronic technologies (for a review of the application of external memory aids and computer-based procedures for the enhancement of memory functioning in neurological patients with memory deficits see Kapur *et al.*, 2004).

Studies targeting techniques without external memory aids

The effectiveness of training memory strategies without external aids in memory rehabilitation was investigated by three class III studies. Doornhein and de Haan (1998) (class III) investigated memory impairment in 12 stroke patients. Memory strategy training was performed with the target group for 4 weeks at two sessions per week. The training program consisted of six memory strategies for the target group and non-specific training involving repetitive practice on memory tasks for the control group. At the end of the treatment, a significant difference between the groups on a test of face-name associations was found. However, the weighted mean difference showed that memory strategy training had no significant effects on memory impairment or subjective memory complaints. Berg, Koning-Haanstra, and Deelman (1991) (class III study) investigated memory strategy training versus drill and repetitive practice versus no treatment in 39 TBI patients. Only the strategy training group showed improved memory functions and the largest effect was observed 4 months after therapy. Ryan and Ruff (1988) (class III study) investigated 20 TBI patients using rehearsal and visual imagery strategies on association and chaining tasks versus some alternative treatment. After 6 weeks of training both groups showed improved memory functioning. The training was most beneficial for subjects with mild memory impairment before treatment.

In sum, one class III study did not find positive effects on memory impairment using compensatory strategies, whereas another class III study reported positive effects and yet another class III only found a training effect for mild memory impairment.

Several class III studies have compared errorless learning (people were prevented from making errors) and errorful learning (such as trial-and-error) in people with memory impairments and shown that the participants (stroke and TBI patients with mixed aetiologies) benefited most when learning without errors was encouraged (Baddeley and Wilson, 1994; Squires et al., 1997; Hunkin et al., 1998). A quantitative meta-analysis on implicit learning and memory rehabilitation in TBI, stroke and Alzheimer's patients was performed by Kessels and de Haan (2003) (class IV study). The authors compared the errorless learning and vanishing cues methods. They found errorless learning techniques to be more advantageous than trial-and-error learning. They also observed that the superiority of a learning technique such as errorless learning may depend on the exact task used and the way in which memory is tested. This is exemplified by Riley et al. (2004) (class III) who compared the efficacy of errorless learning without fading (ELWF) and the method of vanishing cues (MVC) debating whether MVC or ELWF produced better implicit or explicit memory performance. MVC led to better performance than ELWF when effortful but successful study-trial recall was elicited suggesting a positive effect of MVC on explicit memory. With respect to implicit memory, MCV was more effective than ELWF when a stem completion task was used but not when a free association task or perceptual identification task was used. The authors concluded that the relative effectiveness of the two methods depended on the way in which memory was tested. In another class III study researchers compared errorless learning and errorful learning with or without pre-exposing the participants (TBI and stroke patients) to the target

stimuli (Kalla et al., 2001). The authors reported a significant advantage for errorless learning compared to errorful learning. Pre-exposure of the target stimuli strongly enhanced the advantage of errorless learning. In a multi-center study, Wilson et al. (2001) performed nine experiments in three study phases comparing 'errorless' and 'trial-and-error (errorful)' learning in patients with different aetiologies including stroke and TBI patients. The authors found that preventing memory impaired patients from making errors (errorless learning) in situations that facilitated retrieval of implicit memory for the learned material (but not in situations that required the explicit recall of novel associations) had a positive effect on learning. Their results also suggested that under certain circumstances errorless learning might be more beneficial for more severely memory impaired patients.

In sum: A series of class III studies reports an advantage of errorless learning techniques over errorful techniques. There is some indication that any benefit of errorless learning may depend on the type of task used, the way in which memory is tested and on the severity of the memory impairment. Pre-exposition to the target stimuli seems to enhance the benefit of errorless learning.

A different learning technique was investigated by Hillary et al. (2003) (class III study). The authors investigated whether learning in moderate to severe TBI is improved by learning a spacing-of-repetitions procedure using consecutive learning trials as a control condition. The spacing-of-repetitions procedure is based on the spacing effect that has been shown to improve learning and memory when repeated trials are distributed over time (spaced repetitions). The authors found that the participants recalled and recognised significantly more spaced words than massed words during the word list learning task. Statistically accounting for the different neuropsychological status of the patients, there remained a significant influence of the spacing effect on recall and recognition performance. These results support findings of an earlier class III study (Schacter et al., 1985) in which the spaced retrieval technique was investigated in four mild to severely memory impaired patients. Better performance for learning new information was reported.

In sum: Two class III studies report an advantageous effect of spaced retrieval techniques on specific memory performance.

Studies targeting techniques with non-electronic external memory aids

The keeping of external aids such as a notebook or a diary has been investigated by two class III studies and a series of single case studies (class IV studies). Schmitter-Edgecombe *et al.* (1995) (class III study) investigated notebook training treatment in TBI patients and reported significantly fewer everyday memory failures in the notebook group compared to a support treatment group. Ownsworth and McFarland (1999) (class III) investigated the efficacy of a diary only (DO) training versus a diary plus self-instructional training (DSIT) approach in patients with different aetiologies including TBI and stroke patients. Compared to the DO group, the DSIT group maintained a more consistent use of the diary strategy over time, reported a lower level of memory difficulties and rated the strategies used as more helpful.

In sum: Two class III studies support the use of external non-electronic memory aids such as a notebook or diary. It seems that a combined treatment of an external memory aid (diary) and internal strategy training increases efficacy.

The effectiveness of external non-electronic memory aids has also been shown by several case studies or uncontrolled studies (class IV studies) (Sohlberg and Mateer, 1989; Zencius *et al.*, 1990; Burke *et al.*, 1994; Squires *et al.*, 1996). There is one class IV study that seems to suggest that not all aids or strategies are beneficial. Evans *et al.* (2003) investigated the use of memory aids or strategies in a large number of participants with brain damage with different aetiologies. The most commonly used memory aids were external aids such as calendars, lists, notebooks, and diaries. However, from the efficacy ratings obtained from the relatives/independent persons the most widely used aids/strategies were not necessarily the most effective.

The use of assistive electronic technologies

The increasing availability of computers, the internet, wireless connections, and other electronic devices opens a wide range of possibilities to incorporate these technologies into memory rehabilitation (for a review on assistive technology for cognition (ATC) devices see LoPresti *et al.*, 2004). It is surprising that despite the relatively low costs and increasing availability there are still relatively few well-controlled studies. An early class III study by Kerner and Acker (1985) (class III study) showed improved memory performance of mild to moderately memory impaired TBI patients after using computer-based memory training software. Support for the efficacy of computer-assisted memory training also comes from some class IV studies (Glisky and Glisky, 2002; Kapur *et al.*, 2004). Another class III study tested the effectiveness of four different computer-assisted memory training strategies (self-pacing, feedback, personalised, visual presentation) in Chinese patients with closed-head injury (Tam and Man, 2004). Comparing the pre-test and post-test memory outcome (computer quiz scores) of the patient and study group showed significant improvement for all four memory tasks but not in an independent memory outcome measure. Besides computers, portable paging systems have been used to enhance memory performance. Wilson *et al.* (2001) (class III) investigated the effectiveness of a portable externally programmed paging system (NeuroPage) in a large number of TBI, stroke, and other patients with memory and planning/organizational problems. More than 80% of the patients who completed the 16-week trial showed a significant improvement in carrying out everyday activities (such as self-care, self-medication, keeping appointments) when using the pager system, and this improvement was maintained when they were evaluated 7 weeks after returning the pager. It is worth mentioning that this research has been extended by Inglis *et al.* (2002) who developed an interactive memory aid using personal digital assistants (PDAs) with data transmission via the mobile phone network. Neuropage can thus also communicate with the carer's computer system who can thus remotely monitor the use and functionality of the PDA. No controlled efficacy study has been published yet. Successful use of an alphanumeric paging system has also been shown in a class IV TBI single case study (Kirsch *et al.*,

2004). Another electronic memory aid device is the portable voice organizer (VO). This device can be trained to recognise a patient's individual speech patterns, store messages dictated by the user and replay messages at pre-specified time periods. Hart *et al.* (2002) investigated the efficacy of such a system in memory impaired TBI patients aimed at facilitating the recall of therapy goals and plans in a controlled within-subject design (class III study). Results showed that recorded goals were recalled significantly better than unrecorded goals in both free and cued recall conditions. The authors point out that caution needs to be applied to generalising the results due to the low number of subjects, the short training time and the lack of independent memory measures. The efficacy of the VO has also been demonstrated in a well-controlled class IV study with patients of different aetiologies including TBI patients (van den Broek *et al.*, 2000). Virtual reality technology has been used in memory assessment to provide more ecologically valid and controlled evaluation than is possible in rehabilitation settings. Its usefulness in memory rehabilitation has been investigated in two class III studies (for a review of the use and possibilities of virtual reality in memory rehabilitation see Brooks and Rose, 2003). Two class III studies investigated the performance of patients when specific memory tasks were performed in a virtual environment. The effect of active and passive participation in a non-immersive virtual environment on spatial memory in stroke patients was investigated Rose *et al.* (1999) (class III study). The participants' performance in spatial and object recognition memory tests was evaluated after active exploration of the virtual environment or passive observation of the spatial layout of the virtual environment. The stroke patients as well as the controls showed better performance in the active than in the passive spatial recognition task. However, whereas passive controls performed better on the object recognition task than active controls, the patients did not show any difference on the active versus passive object recognition task. Grealy *et al.* (1999) (class III) investigated the impact of non-immersive virtual stimulating exercise environments on attention, information processing, learning and memory in TBI patients.

A comparison of the pre- and post-intervention scores showed significant improvements on the tests of attention, information processing, verbal and visual learning. No improvement was found on memory functions tested by the logical memory test and the complex figure test.

The two class III studies indicate that patients can improve on spatial memory performance or verbal and visual learning in a virtual environment.

Cicerone *et al.* (2000) (using a different rating system from the one used here) recommended compensatory memory training for subjects with mild memory impairments as a practice standard. These authors point out that independence in daily function, active involvement in identifying the memory problem to be treated and the capability and motivation to continue active and independent strategy use strongly contribute to effective memory remediation.

RECOMMENDATIONS

Based on the currently available evidence we judge the use of memory strategies without electronic aid as possibly effective (Level C) although it remains unclear to what degree the benefit depends on the severity of the memory impairment. Specific learning strategies such as errorless learning are supported by a series of class III studies and are thus rated as probably effective (Level B). However, some studies suggest that the efficacy of a specific learning technique may depend on the task used, whether implicit or explicit memory is implicated, and the severity of the memory impairment. Two class III studies supported by several class IV studies have shown possible efficacy (Level C) of non-electronic external memory aids such as diary or notebook keeping. Electronic external memory devices such as computers, paging systems or portable voice organizers have been shown to be effective in several class III studies and are thus recommended as probably effective (Level B) aids for improving TBI or stroke patients' everyday activities. The use of virtual environments has shown positive effects on verbal, visual and spatial

continued

learning in stroke and TBI patients in two class III studies. A direct comparison of performing learning and memory training in virtual environments versus non-virtual environments is still lacking and no recommendation can be made as to the specificity of the technique. Currently, memory training in virtual environments is rated as possibly effective (Level C).

Despite the many studies investigating memory rehabilitation, the problems raised in previous reports concerning the heterogeneity of the population studied (in terms of age, aetiology and type of brain damage, severity of brain-damage, severity of functional impairments, time post-onset) and the subsequent difficulty of interpreting the results are still valid. It is conceivable that the type and intensity of training has different effects depending on the neural circuits damaged, the functional impairment profile, the age and gender of the patient, the time of the post-injury, the education level of the patient, and other external factors (such as social and vocational situation). The number of variables involved makes generalisation across individuals difficult and favours training programmes tailored to the individual circumstances. No specific recommendations are made for different diagnostic groups or stages of severity. There is still a lack of studies that directly compare patients with different aetiologies (e.g. stroke versus TBI), type and severity of brain damage, age, gender, or stage of recovery.

Rehabilitation of apraxia

Although the incidence of apraxia after acquired brain damage is considerable, the literature on recovery and treatment is very minimal. Several reasons for this lack of evidence can be identified (Maher and Ochipa, 1997). First, patients with apraxia often seem to be unaware of their deficit and rarely complain; second, many researchers believe that recovery from apraxia is spontaneous and treatment is not necessary; third, some authors believe that apraxia only occurs when performance is requested of patients in testing situations, and

that correct behaviour is displayed in natural settings. By now, however, there is agreement that apraxia hinders ADL independence. Goldenberg et al., (2001) assessed complex activities of daily living in patients with apraxia and controls. They found that apraxic patients had more difficulties than patients with left brain damage without apraxia and healthy controls. In two other studies comparable results were found: Hanna-Paddy et al., (2003) found a significant relationship between apraxia severity and dependency in physical functioning. Walker et al., (2004) studied the impact of cognitive impairments on upper body dressing difficulties after stroke using video analysis; those patients who failed shirt dressing showed neglect and apraxia at follow-up. These results suggest that treatment of apraxia should be part of the overall neuro-rehabilitation programme after brain damage. In this brief summary, studies examining the effectiveness of treating apraxia will be reviewed. The studies are labelled either observational or experimental and the quality of the studies is described.

There are two recent RCTs on the rehabilitation of apraxia. Smania et al. (2000) assessed in an RCT the effectiveness of a rehabilitative training programme for patients with limb apraxia. Thirteen patients with acquired brain injury and limb apraxia (lasting more than 2 months) as a result of lesions in the left cerebral hemisphere participated in the study. The study group underwent an experimental training for limb apraxia consisting of a behavioural training programme with gesture-production exercises. The control group received conventional treatment for aphasia. Assessments involved neuropsychological tests of aphasia, verbal comprehension, general intelligence, oral apraxia, constructional apraxia and three tests concerning limb praxic function (ideational and ideomotor apraxia and gesture recognition). Everyday activities related to each test were used to measure the outcome. The patients in the study group achieved a significant improvement of performance in both ideational and ideomotor apraxia tests. They also showed a significant reduction of errors in ideational and ideomotor apraxia tests. The change in performance was not significant for the control group. The results show the possible effectiveness of a specific training programme for the treatment of limb apraxia. Donkervoort *et al.* (2002) determined in a controlled study the efficacy of strategy training in left hemisphere stroke patients with apraxia. A total of 113 left hemisphere stroke patients with apraxia were randomly assigned to two treatment groups: (1) strategy training integrated into usual occupational therapy and (2) usual occupational therapy only. The primary outcome measure was a standardised ADL observation by a blinded research assistant. Additional ADL measures were used as secondary outcome measures (Barthel ADL index, ADL judgement by occupational therapists and by patients). After 8 weeks of treatment, patients who received strategy training ($n = 43$) improved significantly more than patients in the usual treatment group ($n = 39$) on the ADL observations. This reflects a small-to-medium effect (effect size 0.37) of strategy training on ADL functioning. With respect to the secondary outcome measures a medium effect (effect size 0.47) was found on the Barthel ADL index. No beneficial effects of strategy training were found after 5 months (at follow-up).

Recently, we performed secondary analyses on the data of Donkervoort *et al.* (2002) to examine the transfer of the effects of cognitive strategy training for stroke patients with apraxia from trained to non-trained tasks. The analyses showed that in both treatment groups, the scores on the ADL observations for non-trained tasks improved significantly after 8 weeks of training as compared with the baseline score. Change scores of non-trained activities were larger in the strategy training group as compared with the usual treatment group. These results suggest that transfer of training is possible, although further research should confirm these exploratory findings (Geusgens *et al.*, in press).

Several class II studies also support the efficacy of apraxia rehabilitation. Goldenberg and Hagman (1998) studied a group of 15 patients with apraxia, who made fatal errors in activities of daily living: an error was rated as fatal if the patient could not proceed without help or if the error prohibited the patient from accomplishing the task successfully. The study design was as follows: each week an ADL test was performed; between tests the patient was trained in one of three activities, whereas support, but no therapeutic advice, was given for two other activities. Each week the patient was trained in another activity, while the other activities were performed in daily life. The next week training was done in another activity and in the third week the remaining activity. In case fatal errors were still seen during performance, another cycle of therapy was run. At the end of the therapy, ten patients could perform all three activities without fatal errors. Three patients made only one fatal error. No generalisation of training effects was found from trained to non-trained activities. Seven patients were re-examined after 6 months: only those patients who kept practising the activities in their daily life, still showed the positive results of the training.

Van Heugten *et al.* (1998) performed a study evaluating a therapy programme for teaching patients strategies to compensate for the presence of apraxia. The outcome was studied in a pre-post test design; measurements were conducted at baseline and after 12 weeks of therapy. Thirty-three stroke patients with apraxia were treated at occupational therapy departments in general hospitals, rehabilitation centres and nursing homes. The patients showed considerable improvement in ADL functioning on all measures and slight improvements on the apraxia test and motor functioning test. The effect sizes for the disabilities, ranging from 0.92 to 1.06, were large compared with the effect sizes for apraxia (0.34) and motor functioning (0.19). The significant effect of treatment is also seen when individual improvement and subjective improvement are considered. These results suggest that the programme seems to be successful in teaching patients compensatory strategies that enable them to function more independently, despite the lasting presence of apraxia. Poole (1998) published a study examining the ability of participants with left-hemisphere stroke to learn one-handed shoe tying. Participants with left hemisphere stroke with and without apraxia and control participants were taught how to tie their shoes with one hand. Retention was assessed after a 5-min interval during which participants performed other tasks. All groups differed significantly in regard to the number of trials to learn the task.

However, on the retention task, the control adults and the stroke patients without apraxia required similar numbers of trials whilst the participants with apraxia required significantly more trials than the other two groups. All groups required fewer trials on the retention task than on the learning task.

Further evidence is provided by single case studies. Wilson (1988) studied a female adolescent with extensive damage to the brain following an anaesthetic accident. One of the most disabling consequences of the damage was apraxia, which made her almost completely dependent in daily life. Wilson concluded that the step-by-step programme was successful in teaching the patient some tasks, but generalisation to new tasks was not found at follow-up. Maher *et al.* (1991) studied the effects of treatment on a 55-year-old man with ideomotor apraxia and preserved gesture recognition. One-hour therapy sessions were given daily during a 2-week period. During therapy sessions many cues were offered that were withdrawn systematically while feedback and correction of errors were given as well. The production of gestures improved qualitatively. Ochipa *et al.* (1995) subsequently developed a treatment programme aimed at specific error types. Praxis performance was studied in two stroke patients. It appeared that both patients achieved considerable improvement in performance but the observed effects were treatment specific: treatment of a specific error type did not improve across untreated gestures. Jantra *et al.* (1992) studied a 61-year-old man with a right-sided stroke followed by apraxic gait. After 3 weeks of gait training supplemented with visual cues, the patient became independent with safe ambulating. Pilgrim and Humphreys (1994) presented a case of a left-handed head injured patient with ideomotor apraxia of his left upper limb. The patient's performance on the 10 objects was measured before and after training in three different modalities. A mixed design analysis of variance (ANOVA) was carried out showing a positive effect of therapy, but little carry-over to everyday life. Bulter (1997) presents a case study that explores the effectiveness of tactile and kinaesthetic stimulation as an intervention strategy, in addition to visual and verbal mediation, in the rehabilitation of a man with ideational and ideomotor apraxia following a head injury. The results indicated some improvement after a training period and limited evidence of the effectiveness of additional sensory input.

Goldenberg *et al.* (2001) conducted a therapy study with six apraxic patients in which two methods of treatment were compared: direct training of the activity based on the guided performance of the whole activity and exploration training aimed at teaching the patient structure–function relationships underlying correct performance but which did not involve actual completion of the activity. Exploration training had no effect on performance, whereas direct training of the activity reduced errors and the need for assistance. Training effects were largely preserved at follow-up, but the rate of errors increased when the trained activities were tested with a partially different set of objects. Performance improved with repeated testing of untrained activities during initial baseline, but there was no reduction of errors or amount of assistance required for untrained activities during training of other activities. As therapeutic results were restricted to trained activities and to some degree to trained objects, the authors conclude that therapy should be tailored to the specific needs of the patients and their family and should be linked closely to the normal routines of daily life.

RECOMMENDATIONS

There is Level A evidence for the effectiveness of apraxia treatment with compensatory strategies. Treatment should focus on functional activities that are structured and practised using errorless learning approaches. As transfer of training is difficult to achieve, training should focus on specific activities in a specific context close to the normal routines of the patients. Recovery of apraxia should not be the goal for rehabilitation. Further studies of treatment interventions are needed, which also address if the treatment effects generalise to non-trained activities and situations.

Rehabilitation of acalculia

Disorders of number processing and calculation (DNPC) may occur after many types of brain damage. Depending on the underlying disease and on lesion location, the frequency of calculation disorders in patients with neurological disorders has been estimated to range between 10% and 90% (Jackson and Warrington, 1986).

Two main types of rationales have been applied to DNPC. One, the 'reconstitution' or 're-teaching' approach consists of extensive lost or damaged abilities by way of extensive practice. The other, indirect approach promotes the use of 'back-up' strategies based on the patient's residual resources (Girelli et al., in press). In this case, the treatment would not merely point to restore the functionality of the impaired component but rather to exploit the preserved abilities to compensate for the deficit. Both types of remediation employ step-by-step training consisting in presentation of problems of increasing difficulty, facilitation cues and other types of assistance that eventually fade with progressive recovery; in all cases direct feedback is provided to the patient on his/her accuracy and errors.

Outcome measures typically consist in comparison of individual's pre- and post-treatment performance in transcoding tasks, simple and complex calculation. Most research designs and statistical evaluation procedures are taken from the field of single-subject research (Kratochwill and Levin, 1992; Randall et al., 1999). The amount of functional disability in daily life is rarely assessed or estimated in this corpus of studies.

As a literature search based on data banks resulted unsatisfactory, the authors have reviewed the existing literature themselves and they have used a pre-existing overview related to the topic (Girelli and Seron, 2001).

Studies were mostly 'quasi-experimental' using a single-case or small-group approach guided by the principles of cognitive neuropsychology (Shallice, 1979; Caramazza, 1989; Seron, 1997; Riddoch and Humphreys, 1994) and single-subject research (Kratochwill and Levin, 1992; Randall et al., 1999) (class II, III and IV evidence). Group studies using control groups are considered inadequate by most authors due to known reasons (problems with patient selection, group homogeneity, and heterogeneity of subjacent deficit and pre-morbid functional level). The recent group study of Gauggell

and Billino (2002) deals with the effects of motivation rather than of specific treatment.

Rehabilitation of DNPC may be grouped into several areas of intervention (Girelli and Delazer, 2001). Rehabilitation of *transcoding ability* (the ability to translate numerical stimuli between different formats) has been successfully performed in several studies (Deloche et al., 1989, 1992; Jacquemin et al., 1991; Sullivan et al., 1996), mostly by re-teaching the patient the required set of rules. Impairments of *arithmetical facts* (simple multiplication, addition, subtraction or division solved directly from memory) were the target of several rehabilitation studies (Miceli and Capasso, 1991; Hittmair-Delazer et al., 1994; Girelli and Delazer, 1996; Whetstone, 1998; Girelli et al., 2002; Domahs et al., 2003, 2004). In all studies, extensive practice with the defective domain of knowledge, that is, multiplication tables determined significant improvement. A positive outcome was reached also by a rehabilitation programme based on the strategic use of the patient's residual knowledge of arithmetic (Girelli et al., 2002). This specific case suggests that the integration of declarative, procedural, and conceptual knowledge critically mediates the re-acquisition process. Miceli and Capasso (1991) have successfully rehabilitated a patient with deficient *arithmetical procedures* (the knowledge required to solve multi-digit calculations). Deficient a *rithmetical problem solving* (the ability to provide a solution for complex, multi-step arithmetical text problems) has also been treated in one study (Delazer et al., 1998). The study was rated as partly successful by the authors, as patients benefited from the cueing procedure engaged and generated a higher number of correct solution steps, but did not show a prominent effect on the actual execution process.

RECOMMENDATIONS

Overall, the available evidence suggests that rehabilitation procedures used to treat selected variants of DNPC were successful (Level C). Notably, significant improvements were observed even in severely impaired and chronic patients. Several caveats need to be mentioned in this context. At present, little is known about the prognosis and spontaneous recovery of DNPC; thus, the effects of different interventions in the early stages of numerical disorders may be difficult to evaluate. Moreover, different underlying neurological disorders (e.g. stroke, dementia, and trauma) have only partly been compared as to their specific effects on DNPC. Furthermore, it has not been studied in detail how impairments of attention or executive functions influence the rehabilitation process of DNPC.

General recommendations

In our opinion, there is enough overall evidence to award a grade A, B or C recommendation to some forms of cognitive rehabilitation in patients with neuropsychological deficits in the post-acute stage after a focal brain lesion (stroke, TBI). This general conclusion is based on a limited number of RCTs, and is supported by a considerable amount of evidence coming from class II, III and IV studies. In particular, the use of a rigorous single-case methodology has been considered by the present reviewers as a source of acceptable evidence in this specific field, in which the application of the RCT methodology is difficult for a number of reasons, related to the lack of consensus on the target of treatment, the methodology of the intervention and the assessment of the outcomes.

Future developments

There is clearly a need for large-scale RCTs, evaluating well-defined methodologies of intervention in common clinical conditions (e.g. the assessment of the efficacy of an intervention for ULN after RH stroke on long-term motor disability). The main difficulty of this approach lies in the highly heterogeneous nature of cognitive deficits. For example, it is hard to believe that the same standardised aphasia treatment may be effective for a patient with a fluent neologistic jargon and another with agrammatic nonfluent production. Research in neuropsychology has focused on the assessment of

specific, theoretically driven treatments on well-defined area of impairment, usually by means of single-case methodology (e.g. the effect of a linguistically driven intervention compared with simple stimulation on the ability to retrieve lexical items belonging to a defined class). To the present panel, both approaches represent potentially fruitful avenues for research in this field.

Future studies should also aim at a better clinical and pathological definition of the patients included in the trials. The gross distinction between stroke and TBD used in the present review is clearly insufficient: a separation among the main categories of cerebrovascular pathology, and the subdivision on pathological grounds of survivors of TBD can be expected to improve the quality of rehabilitation studies.

Acknowledgements

A. Bellmann*, C.Bindschaedler*, L. Bonfiglio#, P. Bongioanni#, S. Chiocca#, M. Delazer§, L. Girelli§ contributed to the reviews on ULN (*), attention rehabilitation (#) and on acalculia (§).

References

Angeli V, Benassi MG, Ladavas E (2004). Recovery of oculo-motor bias in neglect patients after prism adaptation. *Neuropsychologia* **42**:1223–1234.

Antonucci A, Guariglia C, Judica A, Magnotti L, Paolucci S, Pizzamiglio L, Zoccolotti P (1995). Effectiveness of neglect rehabilitation in a randomized group study. *J Clin Exp Neuropsychol* **17**:383–389.

Baddeley A, Wilson BA (1994). When implicit learning fails: amnesia and the problem of error elimination. *Neuropsychologia* **32**:53–68.

Basso A, Capitani E, Vignolo LA (1979). Influence of rehabilitation on language skills in aphasic patients. A controlled study. *Arch Neurol* **36**:190–196.

Basso A, Cappa SF, Gainotti G (2000). *Cognitive Neuropsychology and Language Rehabilitation*. Hove, Psychology Press.

Beis J-M, André J-M, Baumgarten A, Challier B (1999). Eye patching in unilateral spatial neglect: efficacy of two methods. *Arch Physical Med Rehab* **80**:71–76.

Ben-Yishay Y, Diller L, Rattok J (1978). A modular approach to optimizing orientation, psychomotor alertness and purposive behaviour in severe head trauma patients. Rehabilitation Monograph n° 59. New York University Medical Centre, 63–67.

Berg I, Koning-Haanstra M, Deelman B (1991). Long term effects of memory rehabilitation. A controlled study. *Neuropsychol Rehab* **1:**97–111.

Bergego C, Azouvi P, Deloche G, Samuel C, Louis-Dreyfus A, Kaschel R, Willmes K (1997). Rehabilitation of unilateral neglect: a controlled multiple-baseline-across-subjects trial using computerised training procedures. *Neuropsychol Rehab* **7(4):**279–293.

Bhogal SK, Teasell R, Speechley M (2003). Intensity of aphasia therapy, impact on recovery. *Stroke* **34:**987–993.

Bowen A, Lincoldn NB, Dewey M (2002). Cognitive rehabilitation for spatial neglect following stroke. The Cochrane Library, Issue **3.**

Brainin MBM, Baron J-C, Gilhus NE, Hughes R, Selmaj K, Waldema G (2004). Guidance for the preparation of neurological management guidelines by EFNS scientific task forces – revised recommendations 2004. *Euro J Neurol* **11:**1–6.

Brooks B, Rose F (2003). The use of virtual reality in memory rehabilitation: current findings and future directions. *Neuro Rehabil* **18(2):**147–157.

Bruhn P, Parsons O (1971). Continuous reaction time in brain damage. *Cortex* **7:**278–291.

Bulter J (1997). Intervention effectiveness: evidence from a case study of ideomotor and ideational apraxia. *Brit J Occup Ther* **60:**491–497.

Burke J, Danick J, Bemis B, Durgin C (1994). A process approach to memory book training for neurological patients. *Brain Injury* **8:**71–81.

Butter CM, Kirsch N (1992). Combined and separate effects of eye patching and visual stimulation on unilateral neglect following stroke. *Arch Phys Med Rehabil* **73:**1133–1139.

Butter CM, Kirsch N (1995). Effect of lateralized kinetic visual cues on visual search in patients with unilateral spatial neglect. *J Clin Exper Neuropsychol* **17:**856–867.

Butter CM, Kirsch NL, Reeves G (1990). The effect of lateralized dynamic stimuli on unilateral spatial neglect following right hemisphere lesions. *Restorative Neurol Neurosci* **2:**39–46.

Cappa SF, Benke T, Clarke S, Rossi B, Stemmer B, van Heugten C (2003) EFNS guidelines on cognitive rehabilitation. *Euro J Neurol* **10:**11–23.

Caramazza A (1989). Cognitive neuropsychology and rehabilitation: an unfulfilled promise? In X. Seron and G. Deloche (eds.) *Cognitive Approach in Neuropsychological Rehabilitation* (Hillsdale, N.J.: Lawrence Erlbaum Associates Ltd).

Carlomagno S, Pandolfi M, Labruna L, Colombo A, Razzano C (2001). Recovery from moderate aphasia in the first year post-stroke: effect of type of therapy. *Arch Phys Med Rehab* **82:**1073–1080.

Carney N, Chesnut RM, Maynard H, Mann NC, Hefland M (1999). Effect of cognitive rehabilitation on outcomes for persons with traumatic brain injury: a systematic review. *J Head Trauma Rehabil* **14:**277–307.

Cicerone KD, Dahlberg C, Kalmar K, Langenbahn DM, Malec JF, Berquist TF, Felicetti T, Giacino J, Harley JP, Harrington DE, Herzog J, Kneipp S, Laatsch L, Morse PA (2000). Evidence-based cognitive rehabilitation: recommendations for clinical practice. *Arch Phys Med Rehab* **81:**1596–1615.

Delazer M, Bodner T, Benke T (1998). Rehabilitation of arithmetical text problem solving. *Neuropsychol Rehab* **8:**401–412.

Deloche G, Seron X, Ferrand I (1989). Reeducation of number transcoding mechanisms: a procedural approach. In X. Seron and G. Deloche (eds.) *Cognitive Approach in Neuropsychological Rehabilitation* (Hillsdale, NJ: Lawrence Erlbaum Associates).

Deloche G, Ferrand I, Naud E, Baeta E, Vendrell J, Claros-Salinas D (1992). Differential effects of covert and overt training of the syntactic component of verbal processing and generalisations to other tasks: a single-case study. *Neuropsychol Rehab* **2:**257–281.

Denes G, Semenza C, Stoppa E, Lis A (1982). Unilateral spatial neglect and recovery from hemiplegia: A follow-up study. *Brain* **105:**543–552.

Diamond PT (2001). Rehabilitative management of post-stroke visuospatial inattention. *Disabil Rehab* **23:**407–412.

Doesborgh SJ, van de Sandt-Koenderman MW, Dippel DW, van Harskamp F Koudstaal PJ, Visch-Brink EG (2004). Effects of semantic treatment on verbal communication and linguistic processing in aphasia after stroke: a randomized controlled trial. *Stroke* **35:**141–146.

Domahs F, Bartha L, Delazer M (2003). Rehabilitation of arithmetical abilities: different intervention strategies for multiplication. *Brain Lang* **87:**165–166.

Domahs F, Lochy A, Eibl G, Delazer M (2004). Adding colour to multiplication: rehabilitation of arithmetical fact retrieval in a case of traumatic brain injury. *Neuropsychol Rehab* **14:**303–328.

Donkervoort M, Dekker J, Stehmann-Saris J, Deelman BG (2002). Efficacy of strategy training in left-hemisphere stroke patients with apraxia: a randomized clinical trial. *Neuropsychol Rehab* (in press).

Doornhein, K, de Haan, EHF (1998). Cognitive training for memory deficits in stroke patients. *Neuropsychol Rehab* **8**:393–400.

Elman RJ, Bernstein-Ellis E (1999). The efficacy of group communication treatment in adults with chronic aphasia. *J Speech Lang Hear Res* **42**:411–419.

Ethier M, Braun CMJ, Baribeau JMC (1989). Computer-dispensed cognitive-perceptual training of closed head injury patients after spontaneous recovery. Study 1: speeded tasks. *Can J Rehabil* **2**:223–233.

Evans JJ, Wilson BA, Needham P, Brentnall S (2003). Who makes good use of memory aids? Results of a survey of people with acquired brain injury. *J Internat Neuropsychol Soc* **9**:925–935.

Farne A, Rossetti Y, Toniolo S, Ladavas E (2002). Ameliorating neglect with prism adaptation: visuo-manual and visuo-verbal measures. *Neuropsychologia* **40**:718–729.

Frassinetti F, Rossi M, Ladavas E (2001). Passive limb movements improve visual neglect. *Neuropsychologia* **39**:725–733.

Frassinetti F, Angeli V, Meneghello F, Avanzi S, Ladavas E (2002). Long-lasting amelioration of visuospatial neglect by prism adaptation *Brain* **125**:608–623.

Freeman MR, Mittenberg W, DiCowden M, Bat-Ami M (1992). Executive and compensatory memory retraining in traumatic brain injury. *Brain Injury* **6**:65–70.

Gansler DA, McCaffrey RJ (1991). Remediation of chronic attention deficits in traumatic brain-injured patients. *Arch Clin Neuropsychol* **6**:335–353.

Gauggel S, Billino J (2002). The effects of goal-setting on arithmetic performance of brain damaged patients. *Arch Clin Neuropsychol* **17**:283–294.

Geusgens C, Heugten CM van, Donkervoort M, Ende E van den, Jolles J, Heuvel W van den (2005). Transfer of training effects in stroke patients with apraxia: an exploratory study. *Neuropsychol Rehab*, in press.

Girelli L, Delazer M (1996). Subtraction bugs in an alcalculic patient. *Cortex* **32**:547–555.

Girelli L, Seron X (2001). Rehabilitation of number processing and calculation skills. *Aphasiology* **15**:695–712.

Girelli L, Bartha L, Delazer M (2002). Strategic learning in the rehabilitation of semantic knowledge. *Neuropsychol Rehab* **12**:41–61.

Glisky EL, Glisky ML (2002). Learning and memory impairments. In PJ Eslinger (ed.), *Neuropsychological Interventions: Clinical Research and Practice* (pp. 137–162). New York, NY: Guilford Press.

Goldenberg G, Hagman S (1998). Therapy of activities of daily living in patients with apraxia. *Neuropsychol Rehabil* **8**:123–141.

Goldenberg G, Daumuller M, Hagman S (2001). Assessment and therapy of complex activities of daily living in apraxia. *Neuropsychol Rehabil* **11(2)**:147–169.

Goldstein G, Beers SR, Longmore S, McCue M (1996). Efficacy of memory training: a technological extension and replication. *Clinical Neuropsychologist* **10**:66–72.

Gray JM, Robertson I (1989). Remediation of attentional difficulties following brain injury: 3 experimental single case studies. *Brain Injury* **3**:163–170.

Gray JM, Robertson I, Pentland B, Anderson S (1992). Microcomputer-based attentional retraining after brain damage: a randomised group controlled trial. *Neuropsychol Rehabil* **2**:97–115.

Grealy MA, Johnson DA, Rushton SK (1999). Improving cognitive function after brain injury: the use of exercise and virtual reality. *Arch Phys Med Rehab* **80**:661–667.

Greener J, Enderby P, Whurr R (2000). Speech and language therapy for aphasia following stroke. The Cochrane Database of Systematic Reviews.

Guariglia C, Lippolis G, Pizzamiglio L (1998). Somatosensory stimulation improves imagery disorders in neglect. *Cortex* **34**:233–241.

Hagen C (1973). Communication abilities in hemiplegia: effect of speech therapy. *Arch Phys Med Rehab* **54**:454–463.

Hanna-Paddy B, Heilman KM, Foundas AL (2003). Ecological implications od ideomotor apraxia: evidence from physical activities of daily living. *Neurology* **60(1)**:487–490.

Harley JP, Allen C, Braciszeski TL, Cicerone KD, Dahlberg C, Evans S (1992). Guidelines for cognitive rehabilitation. *Neuro Rehabil* **2**:62–67.

Hart T, Hawkey K, Whyte J (2002). Use of a portable voice organizer to remember therapy goals in traumatic brain injury rehabilitation: a within-subjects trial. *J Head Trauma Rehabil* **17(6)**:556–570.

Harvey M, Hood B, North A, Robertson IH (2003). The effects of visuomotor feedback training on the recovery of hemispatial neglects symptoms: assessment of a 2-week and follow-up intervention. *Neuropsychologia* **41**:886–893.

Helffenstein D, Wechsler R (1982). The use of interpersonal process recall (IPR) in the remediation of interpersonal and communication skill deficits in the newly brain injured. *Clin Neuropsychol* **4**:139–143.

Hillary FG, Schultheis MT, Challis BH, Millis SR, Carnevale GJ (2003). Spacing of repetitions improves learning and memory after moderate and severe TBI. *J Clin Exper Neuropsychol* **25(1)**:49–58.

Hittmair-Delazer M, Semenza C, Denes G (1994). Concepts and facts in calculation.*Brain* **117:**715–728.

Hommel M, Peres B, Pollack P, Memin B, Besson G, Gaio J-M, Perret J (1990). Effects of passive tactile and auditory stimuli on left visual neglect. *Arch Neurol* **47:**573–576.

Howard D, Hatfield FM (1987). *Aphasia Therapy: Historical and Contemporary Issues.* Hove and London, Lawrence Erlbaum Associates.

Hughes RA, Barnes MP, Baron JC, Brainin M, European Federation of Neurological Societies (2001). Guidance for the preparation of neurological management guidelines by EFNS scientific task forces. *Eur J Neurol* **8:**549–550.

Hunkin NM, Squires EJ, Parkin AJ, Tidy JA (1998). Are the benefits of errorless learning dependent on implicit memory? *Neuropsychologia* **36:**25–36.

Inglis E, Szymkowiak A, Gregor P, Newell AF, Hine N, Wilson NA, Evans J (2002). Issues surrounding the user-centred development of a new interactive memory aid. Keates S, Langdon P, Clarkson PJ, Robinson P (eds.), *Universal Access and Assistive Technology.* Proceedings of the Cambridge Workshop on UA and AT '02 (pp. 171–178), Cambridge.

Jackson M, Warrington EK (1986). Arithmetic skills in patients with unilateral cerebral lesions. *Cortex* **22:**611–620.

Jacquemin A, Calicis F, van der Linden M, Wyns C, Noël MP (1991). Evaluation et prise en charge des déficits cognitifs dans les états démentiels. In de Partz MP, Leclercq M (eds.), *La rééducation neuropsychologique de l'adulte.* (Edition de la Société de Neuropsychologie de Langue Française, Paris).

Jantra P, Monga TN, Press JM, Gervais BJ (1992). Management of apraxic gait in a stroke patient. *Arch Phys Med Rehabil* **73:**95–97.

Kalla T, Downes JJ, van den Broek M (2001). The pre-exposure technique: enhancing the effects of errorless learning in the acquisition of face-name associations. *Neuropsychol Rehabil* **11(1):**1–16.

Kalra L, Perez I, Gupta S, Wittink M (1997). The influence of visual neglect on stroke rehabilitation. *Stroke* **28:**1386–1391.

Kapur N, Glisky EL, Wilson BA (2004). Technological memory aids for people with memory deficits. *Neuropsychol Rehabil* **14(1/2):**41–60.

Katz RC, Wertz RT (1997). The efficacy of computer-provided reading treatment for chronic aphasic adults. *J Speech Lang Hear Res* **40:**493–507.

Kerkhoff G (1998). Rehabilitation of visuospatial cognition and visual exploration in neglect: a cross-over study. *Restorative Neurol Neurosci* **12:**27–40.

Kerkhoff G (2003). Modulation and rehabilitation of spatial neglect by sensory stimulation. *Prog Brain Res* **142:**257–271

Kerner MJ, Acker M (1985). Computer delivery of memory retraining with head injured patients. *Cognitive Rehab* **Nov/Dec:**26–31.

Kessels RPC, de Haan EHF (2003). Implicit learning in memory rehabilitation: a meta-analysis on errorless learning and vanishing cues methods. *J Clin Exp Neuropsychol* **25:**805–814.

Kime S, Lamb D, Wilson G (1996). Use of a comprehensive programme of external cueing to enhance procedural memory in a patient with dense amnesia. *Brain Injury* **10:**17–25.

Kirsch NL, Levine SP, Fallon-Krueger M, Jaros LA (1987). The micro-computer as an "orthotic" device for patients with cognitive deficits. *J Head Trauma Rehab* **2:**77–86.

Kirsch NL, Levine SP, Lajiness-O'Neil R, Schnyder M (1992). Computer-assisted interactive task guidance: facilitating the performance of simulated vocational task. *J Head Trauma Rehab* **7:**13–25.

Kirsch NL, Shenton M, Rowan J (2004). A generic, 'in-house', alphanumeric paging system for prospective activity impairments after traumatic brain injury. *Brain Injury* **18(7):**725–734.

Kratochwill TR, Levin LR (eds.) (1992). *Single-Case Research Design and Analysis.* Hove: Lawrence Erlbaum Associates.

Ladavas E, Menghini G, Umilta C (1994). A rehabilitation study of hemispatial neglect. *Cog Neuropsychol* **11:**75–95.

Lin K-C, Cermark SA, Kinsbourne M, Trombly CA (1996). Effects of left-sided movements on line bisection in unilateral neglect. *J Intern Neuropsychol Soc* **2:**404–411.

Lincoln NB, Majid MJ, Weyman N (2000). Cognitive rehabilitation for attention deficits following stroke (Cochrane Review). In: The Cochrane Library, Issue 4.

LoPresti EF, Mihailidis A, Kirsch N (2004). Assistive technology for cognitive rehabilitation: state of the art. *Neuropsychol Rehabil* **14(1/2):**5–39.

Maher ML, Ochipa C (1997). Management and treatment of limb apraxia. In: Rothi and Heilman (eds.), *Apraxia: The Neuropsychology of Action.* Hove, UK: Psychology Press.

Maher LM, Rothi LJG, Greenwald ML (1991). Treatment of gesture impairment: a single case. *Am Speech Hear Assoc* **33:**195.

Majid MJ, Lincoln NB, Weyman N (2001). Cognitive rehabilitation for memory deficits following stroke (Cochrane Review). *Cochrane Library,* 1.

Miceli G, Capasso R (1991). *I disturbi del calcolo. Diagnosi e riabilitazione.* Milano: Masson.

Morey CE, Cilo M, Berry J, Cusick C (2003). The effect of Aricept in persons with persistent memory disorder following traumatic brain injury: a pilot study. *Brain Injury* **17(9):**809–815.

Niemann H, Ruff RM, Baser CA (1990). Computer assisted attention retraining in head injured individuals: a controlled efficacy study of an out-patient program. *J Consult Clin Psychol* **58:**811–817.

Niermeir JP (1998). The lighthouse strategy: use of a visual imagery technique to treat visual inattention in stroke patients. *Brain Injury* **12:**399–406.

NIH Consensus Development Panel on Rehabilitation of Persons with Traumatic Brain Injury (1999). Rehabilitation of persons with traumatic brain injury. *J Am Med Assoc* **282:**974–983.

Novack TA, Caldwell SG, Duke LW, Bergquist TF (1996). Focused versus unstructured intervention for attention deficits after traumatic brain injury. *J Head Trauma Rehabil* **11:**52–60.

Ochipa C, Maher LM, Rothi LJG (1995). Treatment of ideomotor apraxia. *Int J Neuropsychol Soc* **2:**149.

Ownsworth TL, McFarland K (1999). Memory remediation in long-term acquired brain injury: two approaches in diary training. *Brain Injury* **13:**605–626.

Parente R (1994). Effects of monetary incentives on performance after traumatic brain injury. *Neuro Rehab* **4:**198–203.

Paton A, Malhortra P, Husain M (2004). Hemispatial neglect. *J Neurol Neurosurg Psychiatry* **75:**13–21.

Perennou DA, Leblond C, Amblard B, Micallef JP, Herisson C, Pelissier JY (2001). Transcutaneous electric nerve stimulation reduces neglect-related postural instability after stroke. *Arch Phys Med Rehab* **82:**440–448.

Pierce SR, Buxbaum LJ (2002). Treatments of unilateral neglect: a review. *Arch Phys Med Rehabil* **83:**256–268.

Pilgrim E, Humphreys GW (1994). Rehabilitation of a case of ideomotor apraxia. In Riddoch and Humphreys (eds.), *Cognitive Neuropsychology and Cognitive Rehabilitation*. *Hove*, UK: Erlbaum.

Pizzamiglio L, Frasca R, Guariglia C, Incoccia C, Antonucci G (1990). Effect of optokinetic stimulation in patients with visual neglect. *Cortex* **26:**535–540.

Pizzamiglio L, Antonucci G, Judica A, Montenero P, Razzano C, Zoccolotti P (1992). Cognitive rehabilitation og the hemineglect disorder in chronic patients with unilateral right brain damage. *J Clin Exp Neuropsychol* **14:**901–923.

Pizzamiglio L, Perani D, Cappa SF, Vallar G, Paolucci S, Grassi F, Paulesu E, Fazio F (1998). Recovery of neglect after right hemispheric damage. *Arch Neurol* **55:**561–568.

Pizzamiglio L, Fasotti L, Jehkonen M, Antonucci G, Magnotti L, Boelen D, Asa S (2004). The use of optokinetic stimulation in rehabilitation of the hemineglect disorder. *Cortex* **40:**441–450.

Poeck K, Huber W, Willmes K (1989). Outcome of intensive language treatment in aphasia. *J Speech Hear Dis* **54:**471–479.

Ponsford JL, Kinsella G (1988). Evaluation of a remedial programme far attentional deficits following closed-head injury. *J Clin Exp Neuropsychol* **10:**693–708.

Poole J (1998). Effect of apraxia on the ability to learn one-handed shoe tying. *Occup Ther J Res* **18:**99–104.

Pulvermueller F, Neininger B, Elbert T, Mohr B, Rockstroh B, Koebbel P, Taub E (2000). Constraint-induced therapy of chronic aphasia after stroke. *Stroke* **32:**1621–1626.

Randall RR, Schultz MC, Crawford AB, Sinner CA (1999). Single-subject clinical outcome research: designs, data, effect sizes, and analyses. *Aphasiology* **13:**445–473.

Rath JF, Langenbahn DM, Simon D, Sherr RL, Fletcher J, Diller L (2004). The construct of problem solving in higher level neuropsychological assessment and rehabilitation. *Arch Clin Neuropsychol* **19:**613–635.

Riddoch MJ, Humphreys GW (1994). (eds), *Cognitive Neuropsychology and Cognitive Rehabilitation*. (Hove: Lawrence Erlbaum Associates).

Riley GA, Sotiriou D, Jaspal S (2004). Which is more effective in promoting implicit and explicit memory: the method of vanishing cues or errorless learning without fading? *Neuropsychol Rehabil* **14(3):**257–283.

Rios M, Perianez JA, Munoz-Cespedes JM (2004). Attentional control and slowness of information processing after severe traumatic brain injury. *Brain Injury* **18:**257–272.

Robertson I, Gray J, McKenzie S (1988). Microcomputer-based cognitive rehabilitation of visual neglect: three multiple-baseline single-case studies. *Brain Injury* **2(2):**151–163.

Robertson IH (1999). Cognitive rehabilitation: attention and neglect. *Trends Cog Sci* **3:**385–393.

Robertson IH, Gray J, Pentland B, Waite LJ (1990) Microcomputer-based rehabilitation for unilateral left visual neglect: a randomized controlled trial. *Arch Phys Med Rehab* **71:**663–668.

Robertson IH, Hawkins K (1999). Limb activation and unilateral neglect. *Neurocase* **5:**153–160.

Robertson IH, Tegnér R, Tham K, Lo A, Nimmo-Smith I (1995). Sustained attention training for unilateral neglect: theoretical and rehabilitation implications. *J Clin Exp Neuropsychol* **17:**416–430.

Robertson IH, Hogg K, McMillan TM (1998a). Rehabilitation of unilateral neglect: improving function by contralesional limb activation. *Neuropsychol Rehab* **8(1)**:19–29.

Robey RR, Schultz MC, Crawford AB, Sinner CA (1999). Single-subject clinical-outcome research: designs, data, effect sizes, and analyses. *Aphasiology* **13**:445–473

Rode G, Perenin MT (1994). Temporary remission of representational hemineglect through vestibular stimulation. *Neuro Report* **5**:869–872.

Rode G, Tiliket C, Charopain P, Boisson D (1998). Postural asymmetry reduction by vestibular caloric stimulation in left hemiparetic patients. *Scand J Rehab Med* **30**:9–14.

Rorsman I, Magnusson M, Johansson BB (1999). Reduction of visuo-spatial neglect with vestibular galvanic stimulation. *Scand J Rehab Med* **31**:117–124.

Rose FD, Brooks BM, Attree EA, Parslow DM, Leadbetter AG, McNeil JE, Jayawardena S, Greenwood R, Potter J (1999). A preliminary investigation into the use of virtual environments in memory retraining after vascular brain injury: indications for future strategy? *Disab Rehab* **21**:548–554.

Rossetti Y, Rode G, Pisella L, Farné A, Li L, Boisson D, Perenin M-T (1998). Prism adaptation to rightward optical deviation rehabilitates left hemispatial neglect. *Nature* **395**:166–169.

Ryan TV, Ruff RM (1988). The efficacy of structural memory retraining in a group comparison of head trauma patients. *Arch Clin Neuropsychol* **3**:165–179.

Schacter DL, Rich SA, Stampp MS (1985). Remediation of memory disorders: experimental evaluation of the spaced retrieval techniques. *J Clin Exp Neuropsychol* **7**:79–96.

Schindler I, Kerkhoff G, Karnath HO, Keller I, Goldenberg G (2002). Neck muscle vibration induces lasting recovery in spatial neglect. *J Neurol Neurosurg Psychiatry* **73**:412–419.

Schmitter-Edgecombe M, Fahy J, Whelan J, Long C (1995). Memory remediation after severe closed head injury. Notebook training versus supportive therapy. *J Consult Clin Psychol* **63**:484–489.

Schoettke H (1997). Rehabilitation von Aufmerksamkeitsstörungen nach einem Schlagenfall. Effektivität eines verhaltensmedizinisch-neuropsychologischen Aufmerksamkeitstrainings. *Verhaltenstherapie* **7**:21–23.

Seron X (1997). Effectiveness and specificity in neuropsychological therapies: a cognitive point of view. *Aphasiology* **11**:105–123.

Shallice T (1979). Case-study approach in neuropsychological research. *J Clin Neuropsychol* **1**:183–211.

Shewan CM, Kertesz A (1985) Effects of speech language treatment on recovery from aphasia. *Brain Lang* **23**:272–299.

Smania N, Girardi F, Domenciali C, Lora E, Aglioti S (2000). The rehabilitation of limb apraxia: a study in left brain damaged patients. *Arch Phys Med Rehab* **81**:379–388.

Sohlberg MM, Mateer CA (1989). Training use of compensatory memory books: a three stage behavioral approach. *J Clin Exp Neuropsychol* **11**:871–891.

Squires EJ, Hunkin NM, Parkin AJ (1996). Memory notebook training in a case of severe amnesia: generalzing from paired associate learning to real life. *Neuropsychol Rehab* **6**:55–65.

Squires EJ, Hunkin NM, Parkin AJ (1997). Errorless learning of novel associations in amnesia. *Neuropsychologia* **35**:1103–1111.

Stone SP, Patel P, Greenwood RJ, Halligan PW (1992). Measuring visual neglect in acute stroke and predicting its recovery: the visual neglect recovery index. *J Neurol Neurosurg Psychiat* **55**:431–436.

Strache W (1987). Effectiveness of two modes of training to overcome deficits of concentration. *Int J Rehab Res* **10 S5**:141S–145S.

Sturm W, Wilmes K (1991). Efficacy of a reaction training on various attentional and cognitive functions in stroke patients. *Neuropsychol Rehabil* **1**:259–280.

Sturm W, Wilmes K, Orgass B (1997). Do specific attention deficits need specific training? *Neuropsychol Rehab* **7**:81–103.

Sullivan KS, Macaruso P, Sokol SM (1996). Remediation of Arabic numeral processing in a case of development dyscalculia. *Neuropsychol Rehab* **6**:27–53

Tam S-F, Man W-K (2004). Evaluating computer-assisted memory retraining programmes for people with post-head injury amnesia. *Brain Injury* **18(5)**:461–470.

Tham K, Tegnér R (1997). Video feedback in the rehabilitation of patients with unilateral neglect. *Arch Phys Med Rehabil* **78**:410–413.

Thomas-Stonell NP, Johnson *et al.* (1994). Evaluation of a computer-based program for cognitive-communication skills. *J Head Trauma Rehab* **9**:25–37.

Vallar G, Rusconi ML, Barozzi S, Bernardini B, Ovadia D, Papagno C, Cesarani A (1995). Improvement of left visuo-spatial hemineglect by left-sided transcutaneous electrical stimulation. *Neuropsychologia* **33**:73–82.

Vallar G, Guariglia C, Magnotti L, Pizzamiglio L (1997). Dissociation between position sense and visual-spatial components of hemineglect through a specific rehabilitation treatment. *J Clin Exp Neuropsychol* **19**:763–771.

van den Broek MD, Downes J, Johnson Z, Dayus B, Hilton N (2000). Evaluation of an electronic memory aid in the neuropsychological rehabilitation of prospective memory deficits. *Brain Injury* **14**:455–462.

Van Heugten CM, Dekker J, Deelman BG, van Dijuk AJ, Stehmann-Saris JC, Kinebanian A (1998). Outcome of strategy training in stroke patients: a phase-II study. *Clin Rehab* **2:**294–303.

Van Zomeren AH, Van DenBurg W (1985). Residual complaints of patients two years after severe head injury. *J Neurol Neurosurg Psychiat* **48:**21–28.

Walker R, Young AW, Lincoln NB (1996). Eye patching and the rehabilitation of visual neglect. *Neuropsychol Rehab* **6:**219–231.

Walker CM, Sunderland A, Sharma J, Walker MF (2004). The impact of cognitive impairments on upper body dressing difficulties after stroke: a video analysis of patterns of recovery. *J Neurol Neurosurg Psychiat* **75:**43–48.

Webster JS, McFarland PT, Rapport LJ, Morrill B, Roades LA, Abadee PS (2001). Computer-assisted training for improving wheelchair mobility in unilateral neglect patients. *Arch Phys Med Rehab* **82:**769–775.

Weinberg J, Diller L, Gordon WA, Gerstman LJ, Liebermann A, Lakin P, Hodges G, Ezrachi O (1977). Visual scanning training effect on reading-related tasks in acquired right brain damage. *Arch Phys Med Rehabil* **58:**479–486.

Whestone T (1998). The representation of arithmetic facts in memory: Results from retraining a brain-damaged patient. *Brain Cog* **36:**290–309.

Wiart L, Bon Saint Côme A, Debelleix X, Petit H, Josph PA, Mazaux JM, Barat M (1997). Unilateral neglect syndrome rehabilitation by trunk rotation and scanning training. *Arch Phys Med Rehabil* **78:**424–429.

Wilson B, Robertson IH (1992). A home based intervention for attentional slips during reading following head injury: a single case study. *Neuropsychol Rehabil* **2:**193–205.

Wilson B (1982). Success and failure in memory training following a cerebral vascular accident. *Cortex* **18:**581–594.

Wilson BA (1988). Sarah: rehabilitation of apraxia following an anaesthetic accident. In West and Spinks (eds.), *Case Studies in Clinical Psychology*. Bristol, UK: John Wright.

Wilson BA, Evans JJ, Emslic H, Malinek V (1997). Evaluation of NeuroPage: a new memory aid. *J Neurol Neurosurg Psychiat* **63:**113–115.

Wilson BA, Emslic HC, Quirk K, Evans JJ (2001). Reducing everyday memory and planning problems by means of a paging system: a randomised control crossover study. *J Neurol Neurosurg Psychiat* 477–482.

Wood RL (1986). Rehabilitation of patients with disorders of attention. *J Head Trauma Rehabil* **1:**43–53.

Zencius A, Wesolowski MD, Burke WH (1990). A comparison of four memory strategies with traumatically brain-injured clients. *Brain Injury* **4:**33–38.

Index

Page numbers in *italics* refer to figures and those in **bold** to tables

acalculia 604–6
acetylcholinesterase
    inhibitors 325
acetylsalicylic acid **163**, **166**
acquired pendular nystagmus
    487–8
Actinobacter spp. **21**
acute disseminated
    encephalomyelitis
    18, 398
    neuroimaging 402
acute viral encephalitis 399
acyclovir 406
adenovirus **22**
adolescents, migraine in 169
adrenergic agents 571
adrenleukodystrophy, CSF
    oligoclonal IgG
    bands **20**
Advanced Trauma Life
    Support 217
affinity chromatography 75
aftersensation 113
agitation 149, 270
aggression 270
AIDS, CSF oligoclonal IgG
    bands **20**
airway protection 141
Alberta Stroke Programme Early
    CT Score (ASPECTS) 31
albumin in CSF 16–17
albumin CSF/serum ratio 14,
    16–17
alcohol consumption 134
alcohol-related seizures 451–60
    background 451–2
    biomarkers 453
    diagnosis 452–3
    electroencephalography 454
    history taking 452
    methods 452
    neuroimaging 454
    patient examination and
        observation
        453–4, **453**
    questionnaires 452–3
    treatment 454–7

electrolyte
    disturbances 455
    management of epilepsy
        456–7
    primary prevention 455–6
    prophylaxis 455
    secondary prevention 456
    status epilepticus 456
    thiamine therapy 454–5
allodynia 111
    brush-induced 113
almotriptan **164**
alpha-adrenoceptor
    agonists 496
Alzheimer, Alois 5
Alzheimer's disease 266–98
    activities of daily living 271
    behavioural and
        psychological
        symptoms 270–1
    blood tests 272
    clinical diagnosis 268
    cognitive function
        assessment 269–70
    co-morbidity 271–2
    CSF analysis 275–7
    disclosure of diagnosis 278
    electroencephalography 275
    genetic testing 277
    medical history 268
    neuroimaging 272–5
        CT 272
        MRI 272–4
        SPECT and PET 274
    neurological and physical
        examination 268–9
    treatment 278–81
        cholinesterase inhibitors
            278–9
        memantine 279–80 *see
            also* dementia
amantadine
    Parkinson disease 226, 227,
        235, 246
    post-polio syndrome 325
American Academy of
    Neurology 8, 16

amitriptyline **166**, **415**
amnesia, post-traumatic 211
amphetamine 539–40, 545
amyotrophic lateral sclerosis
    558–9
analgesics in migraine 162
anti-AChR **89**
anti-aggregants 282–3
anti-amphiphysin **89**
Antibody Index 23
anticholinergics 198,
    226–7, **235**
anticoagulation 137, 505–6
anti-CV2/CRMP5 **89**
antidepressants 167, 414, 417,
    419–20
    adverse effects 423–4
anti-dopaminergic drugs 198–9
antiemetics 162, **163**
antiepileptics 166–7, 198,
    415–16, 417, 418–19,
    420, 573
anti-GAD **89**
anti-GD1a (IgG) **89**
anti-GD1b **89**
anti-GM1 **89**
anti-GM1 (IgG/IgM) **89**
anti-GM2 (IgM) **89**
anti-Hu (ANNA-1) **89**
anti-hypertensive treatment
    138, 142, **143**
anti-interferon antibody
    multiple sclerosis 72–86
        background and objectives
            72–3
        binding antibodies 75
        clinical use of antibody
            measurements
            79, **80**
        effect on disease
            progression 81–2
        effect on MRI outcomes 81
        effect on relapses 81
        immunogenicity 73–5, **74**
        neutralizing antibodies
            75–9, **76–8**

anti-interferon antibody
(*Contd.*)
prevention and treatment
of NABs 82–3
recommendations 83
safety issues 82
search strategy and
consensus 73
anti-MAG/SGPG (IgM) **89**
anti-nerve antibodies
87–93, **89**
background 88
Good Practice Points 91
methods 88, 90
objective 88
results 90
antiplatelet therapy 136–7
anti-Ri (ANNA-2) **89**
anti-(TA) Ma2 **89**
antithrombotic therapy 135
anti-Tr **89**
anti-VGCC **89**
anti-VGKC **89**
anti-viral therapy 406
anti-Yo (PCA-1) **89**
anxiety 271
apathy 270
aphasia 593–5
apomorphine **235**
apraxia 602–4
arterial hypertension 132
arterio-venous
malformations 67
Aspergillus fumigatus **22**
aspiration 148
aspirin 136, 146
assistive devices 327
Asymptomatic Carotid
Atherosclerosis Study
35, 136
ataxia-telangiectasia, CSF
oligoclonal IgG
bands **20**
attention disorders 596–8
atypical antipsychotics 253–4
Australian Streptokinase Trial
(ASK) 31
autoimmune neuromuscular
conduction disorders
332–43
background and
objectives 333
consensus methods 333
Lambert-Eaton myasthenic
syndrome 339–40
myasthenia gravis 334–9
neuromyotonia/Isaacs
syndrome 340
search strategy 333

autoimmune polyneuropathy,
CSF parameters **15**
autonomic dysfunction 256–7
erectile dysfunction 257
gastrointestinal motility
problems 257
orthostatic hypotension 256
urinary disturbance 256–7
autonomic tests in non-acute
headache 65–6, 69
azathioprine
CIDP **350**
myasthenia gravis 337–8

baclofen **181**
intrathecal 201
Bacteroides fragilis **21**
barbiturates 448
Beck Depression Scale 114
bed rest 218
bedside examination 111
Behçet's disease, CSF
oligoclonal IgG bands
20
Bell, Charles 4
Bell, John 4
benzodiazepines 545, 574
beta-adrenoceptor
blockers 166
beta-oxidation defects 528–32
binding antibodies 72
measurement 75
affinity
chromatography 75
ELISA 75, **76**
radio-
immunoprecipitation
assay 75
Western blot 75
biopsy 118
nerve 118
punch skin 118
skin *see* skin biopsy
bisoprolol **166**
body temperature 144
Borrelia burgdorferi sensu lato **21**
borreliosis, CSF oligoclonal IgG
bands **20**
botulinum toxins 197–8
brain
imaging 30–4, 37
mild traumatic injury
207–23
ancillary investigations
215–16
background 208
bed rest 218
biochemical markers
216–17
classification 209, **209**

clinical observation
217–18
complications 211, 213–15
duration of loss of
consciousness
209–11, *211*
follow-up 218–19
Glasgow Coma Score on
admission 209
initial patient
management 217
mechanisms 208
post-traumatic
amnesia 211
risk factors 211, **212–13**
search strategy 208
brain metastases 461–71
background 462
consensus method 462–3
diagnosis 463–4
Karnofsky Performance
Status **463**
objectives 462
search strategy 462
supportive care 464
treatment
chemotherapy 466
emerging 466–7
multiple brain
metastases 466
stereotactic
radiosurgery 465
surgery 464–5
whole-brain radiotherapy
465–6
brain oedema 149
brain stem encephalitis **89**
bright-field
immunohistochemistry 99
bromocriptine **235**
Brucella spp. **21**

cabergoline **235**
caffeine **163**
calcium channel blockers 166
Campylobacter fetus **21**
candesartan **166**
CANOMAD 367
capsaicin **415**
captopril **143**
carbamazepine **415**, 424
cardiac care 141–2
CARESS trial 36
carnitine palmytoyl transferase
deficiency 527–8
carnitine transport defects 528
carotid angioplasty 140
carotid artery angioplasty 136
carotid endarterectomy 139
carotid surgery 136

cataplexy 542–5
catechol-O-methyl transferase
        inhibitors 226, 228–9,
        246–7
central nervous system
        infections 521–2
central pain 419–20
central pontine myelinolysis
        519–20
central sleep
        apnoea-hypopnoea
        syndrome 555
    treatment 51
cerebellar degeneration **89**
    paraneoplastic **89**, 476–7
cerebellar infection 150
cerebral toxoplasmosis 388
cerebral vasculitis 510–15
    diagnostic approach *513*
    methods 511
    presentation **512**
    survey results 511–14
    treatment **514**
cerebral venous thrombosis
        501–9
    background and
        objectives 502
    CT 32
    heparin therapy 503–4
    MRI 33
    oral anticoagulation 505–6
    search strategy 503
    symptomatic treatment
        506–7
        elevated intracranial
            pressure 507
        seizure control 506–7
    thrombolysis 504–5
cerebrospinal fluid analysis
        14–27
    Alzheimer's disease 275–6
    cytological examination 19,
        22–3
    glucose concentration, serum
        glucose ratio and
        lactate 19
    immunoglobulin G synthesis
        18–19, *18*
    immunoglobulin synthesis
        17–18, *17*
    infectious agents **21–2**, 23–4
    inflammatory disease **20**
    neurological diseases **15**
    PDN 368
    search strategy 15–16
    total protein and albumin
        16–17
cerebrovascular disorders 521
Charcot, Jean-Martin 4

Charcot Marie Tooth
        disease 101
Cheyne-Stokes breathing
        syndrome 555–6
    treatment 561
children, migraine in 169
cholesterol lowering
        therapy 138
cholinesterase inhibitors
        253, 254
    Alzheimer's disease 278–9,
        281–2
chronic inflammatory
        demyelinating
        polyradiculoneuropathy
        344–53
    background 345
    concomitant disease **349**
    consensus methods 345–6
    diagnostic categories **349**
    diagnostic criteria 346
        clinical **347**
        electrodiagnostic **348**
        supportive **348**
    investigations 346, **350**
    objectives 345
    search strategy 345
    treatment 346–51
        corticosteroids 346–7
        general 351
        immunosuppressants
            348–9, **350**
        initial management 350
        interferons 349–50
        intravenous
            immunoglobulin
            347–8
        long-term management
            350–1
        plasma exchange 347
chronic pseudo-obstruction **89**
ciclosporin
    CIDP **350**
    myasthenia gravis 338
CIDP *see* chronic inflammatory
        demyelinating
        polyradiculoneuropathy
cisapride 257
clomipramine **415**
clonidine **143**
clopidogrel 136
clozapine 253
cluster headache 177–90
    background 178
    clinical syndromes 178
    consensus method 178
    diagnosis **179**
    episodic and chronic 179
    objectives 177–8

    paroxysmal hemicrania
        179–80, **180**
    search strategy 178
    SUNCT syndrome 180, **180**
    treatment 180–6, **181**
Cochrane Central Register of
        Controlled Trials
        (CENTRAL) 443, 444
Cochrane Library 11
coenzyme Q10 **166**
cognitive function assessment
        269–70
cognitive rehabilitation
        592–612
    acalculia 604–6
    aphasia 593–5
    apraxia 602–4
    attention disorders 596–8
    background 593
    consensus method 593
    future developments 606
    memory 598–602
    objectives 592–3
    recommendations 606
    search strategy 593
    unilateral spatial neglect
        595–6
computed tomography *see* CT
Conference on Guideline
        Standardization 10
corticosteroids *see* steroids
Coxiella burnetti **21**
creatine kinase 380
Creutzfeldt, Hand-Gerhardt 5
Creutzfeldt-Jakob disease 276
cryptococcal meningitis 388–9
Cryptococcus neoformans **22**
CSF/serum glucose ratio 19
CT
    Alzheimer's disease 272
    brain 30–2
    clinical decision rules
        215–16
    skull 215
CT angiography 35
cyclophosphamide
    CIDP **350**
    multifocal motor
        neuropathy 358
    myasthenia gravis 338
cyclosporine neurotoxicity
        517–18
cytomegalovirus **22**
    encephalitis 389–90
    polyradiculomyelitis 390

DADS phenotype **366**
data collection 11–13
decompressive surgery 150
decubital ulcer 148

deep brain stimulation
199–200, 248–50
deep vein thrombosis 148
de-fibrinogenating
enzymes 146
dementia 252–3
counselling and support 286
driving 287
HIV 391
legal issues 287
Lewy body 283–4
Parkinson disease 283–4
treatment 281–4
behavioural and
psychological
symptoms 284–6
monitoring 284
vascular 281–3 *see also*
Alzheimer's disease
depression 254–5, 271
desipramine **415**
desmopressin 257, 498
Desmoteplase in Acute Stroke
(DIAS) trial 29
dextromethorphan **415**
diabetes mellitus, and stroke
132, 134
diclofenac **163**
dihydralazin **143**
dihydroergocryptine **235**
dihydroergotamine 256, 498
dihydroxyphenylserine 497
dipyridamole 136–7
disinhibition 271
domperidon **163**
domperidone 257
dopamine agonists 197–8, 226,
230–1, 247–8, 254, 257
downbeat nystagmus 485–6
duloxetine **415**
DVT *see* deep vein thrombosis
dysesthesias 111
dyskinesia, biphasic 252
dystonia 191–206
background 192
brain imaging 196–7
classification 193–4, **193**
consensus method 102
diagnosis 192
genetic testing 194–5
neurophysiological
techniques 195–6
objectives 192
search strategy 102
treatment 197–202
anticholinergic drugs 198
anti-dopaminergic drugs
198–9
antiepileptic drugs 198
botulinum toxins 197–8

dopaminergic drugs 199
neurosurgical procedures
199–202

EFNS *see* European Federation
of Neurological Societies
electrodiagnostic studies 115
electroencephalography 275
alcohol-related seizures 454
non-acute headache 64–5
electrolyte balance 144
eletriptan **164**
ELISA 75
EMBASE 11
encephalitis 396–411
acute viral 399
clinical manifestations
398–9
definitions and scope 397–8
diagnostic investigations
399–405
histopathology 404–5
neuroimaging 400–2
nucleic acid detection
402–3
viral culture 402
virological tests 402
differential diagnosis 405–6
evidence classification
397, **398**
herpes simplex 399–400
infective causes 405–6
methods 397
Rasmussen's 402
therapy 406–8
anti-viral 406
corticosteroids 406–7
preventive measures 407
rehabilitation 407
surgical intervention 407
encephalomyelitis **89**
endovascular treatment 136
entacapone **235**
enteroviruses **21**
ephedrine 498
epilepsy
alcohol consumption in 457
management in patients with
alcohol overuse 456–7
treatment *see* antiepileptics
see also seizures
Epstein-Barr virus **22**, 398
erectile dysfunction 257
ergot alkaloids 162
ergotamine tartrate **181**
ergot derivatives 575–6
erythropoietin 256, 498
Escherichia coli **21**
etanercept, CIDP **350**
etilefrine hydrochloride 256

euphoria 271
European Agency for the
Evaluation of Medicinal
Products 229
European Federation of
Neurological Societies
3, 160
guidelines 7–13
evidence classification scheme
diagnostic measure 9
therapeutic intervention 9
EVIDENCE study 74, 81
evoked potentials, non-acute
headache 65, 68
excessive daytime sleepiness
537–42
executive functions 269–70
extracranial-intracranial
anastomosis 140
extracranial vessels, imaging
34–5, 57

fatty acid mitochondrial
disorders 526–33, *527*
background 526
beta-oxidation defects
528–32
carnitine palmytoyl
transferase deficiency
527–8
carnitine transport defects
528
search strategy 526–7
FK506 *see* tacrolimus
fludrocortisone 256, 496
fluid attenuated inversion
recovery (FLAIR) 33, 67
fluid balance 144
flunarizine **166**
foetal mesencephalic
grafts 250
freezing 252
fronto-temporal lobar
degeneration 273
frovatriptan **164**
Fukutin related protein 379
functional neuroimaging 117
functional neurosurgery
248–50
deep brain stimulation
248–50
pallidotomy 248

gabapentin **166**, **415**, 424–5
Galen 3
gamma-hydroxybutyrate
540–1, 542–3, 545
gastrointestinal motility
problems 257
GD1b (IgM) **89**

gemfibrozil 138
genetic testing 277
Gilles de la Tourette,
        George-Edmund-Albert-
        Brutus 4
Glasgow Coma Score 140
    mild traumatic brain
        injury 209
global cognitive functions 269
Global Impression of
        Change 114
Glucose
    CSF concentration 19
    metabolism 142–4
Good Practice Points 10 *see
        also individual conditions*
Gracely Pain Scale 113
group B streptococci **21**
guidelines 7–8
    aim of 8
    critical review 10–11
    data collection 11–13
    scientific basis 8–10, **9**
Guillain-Barré syndrome 18,
        421–2

HAART 387
haemodilution 136, 146–7
Haemophilus influenzae **21**
hallucinations 545
Harada's meningitis-uveitis,
        CSF oligoclonal IgG
        bands **20**
headache
    cluster 177–90
        background 178
        clinical syndromes 178
        consensus method 178
        diagnosis **179**
        episodic and chronic 179
        episodic and chronic
            paroxysmal
            hemicrania
            179–80, **180**
        objectives 177–8
        search strategy 178
        SUNCT syndrome
            180, **180**
        treatment 180–6, **181**
    non-acute 63–71
        aims and methods 64
        autonomic tests 65–6, 69
        electroencephalography
            64–5
        evoked potentials 65, 68
        neuroimaging 66–7, 69
        pericranial muscle
            tenderness 66
        photic driving 68
        reflex responses 65, 68–9

SPECT and PET 67–8, 69
        transcranial Doppler 68,
            69–70 *see also*
            migraine
heparin therapy 503–4
herpes simplex encephalitis
        399–400
    neuroimaging 401
herpes simplex virus **21**, 398
hippocampal atrophy 273
HIV **21**, 386–95
    background and
            objectives 386
    cerebral toxoplasmosis 388
    cryptococcal meningitis
            388–9
    cytomegalovirus encephalitis
            389–90
    cytomegalovirus
            polyradiculomyelitis
            390
    grading of recommendations
            388–92
    HAART 387
    neuroimaging 401
    neurological complications
            386–7
    primary CNS lymphoma
            390–1
    progressive multifocal
            leukoencephalopathy
            389
    search strategy 387–8
    tuberculous meningitis 390
HIV dementia 391
HIV myelopathy 391–2
HIV polyneuropathy 392
HOPE study 138
hormone replacement therapy
        138–9
Hospital Anxiety and
        Depression Scale 114–15
human immunodeficiency
        virus *see* HIV
human T-cell leukaemia virus
        type I **22**
Huntington, George Summer 4
hyperalgesia 111, 113
hyperdense middle cerebral
        artery sign 31
hyperlipidaemia 134
hypersomnias 556
hypertension
    and stroke 132
    supine 495
hypnotics 574
hypocretin 536
hypomagnesemia 455
hypothermia 149–50

ibuprofen **163**
IgA PDN 366
    DADS phenotype **366**
    treatment 371
IgG PDN 366
    DADS phenotype **366**
    treatment 371
IgM PDN **89**, 366
    antibodies to
            myelin-associated
            glycoprotein 366, **367**
    clinical phenotype 365–6
    electrophysiology 366
    treatment 368–71
        corticosteroids 370
        immunosuppressants 370
        interferon-alpha 370
        intravenous
                immunoglobulin
                370
        plasma exchange 368–70
        rituximab 370
imaging
    stroke 28–44
        brain 30–4
        extracranial vessels 34–5
        intracranial vessels 35–6
        method for reaching
                consensus 30
        search strategy 29–30 *see
                also individual
                modalities*
imipramine **415**
immunofluorescence 100–1
immunoglobulins
    CSF 17–19, **17**, *18*
    intravenous
        CIDP 347–8
        IgM type PDN 370
        multifocal motor
                neuropathy 357
        myasthenia gravis 335–6
        see also Ig
immunosuppressants
    CIDP 348–9, **350**
    IgM type PDN 370
    neurotoxicity 517–18
INCOMIN study 81
indomethacin 256, 498
inertia 270
infectious polyneuropathy, CSF
        parameters **15**
influenza virus **22**
insomnia 554
instrumental functions 270
interferons, CIDP 349–50
interferon-alpha, IgM type
        PDN 370
International Normalised
        Ratio 135

intracerebral haemorrhage 31
intracranial haemorrhage 33
intracranial pressure, elevated 149, 507
intracranial vessels, imaging 35–6
intraepidermal nerve fibres 95
 quantification of 96–9, *97, 98 see also* skin biopsy
Isaacs syndrome 340

Jakob, Alfons Maria 5
JC virus 389

Karnofsky Performance Status **463**
Koch, Robert 5

labetalol **143**
lactate, CSF 19
Lambert-Eaton myasthenic syndrome **89**, 339–40, 478
lamotrigine **415**, 425
laser-evoked potentials 116–17, *116*
leptomeningeal metastases, CSF parameters **15**
Leptospira interrogans **21**
leucocyte antigen antibodies 339
levodopa 226, 229–30, **235**, 247, 254
 controlled release formulations 247
 restless legs syndrome 574–5
Lewy body dementia 283–4
lidocaine **181, 415**
lifestyle modifications 327
Likert scale 114
limb girdle muscular dystrophies 376–85
 background 376–7
 cardiac management 383
 classification **377**
 clinical assessment 378–80
 clinical features **379**
 consensus method 377
 drug treatment 384
 Good Practice Points 378–84
 investigation 380–2
 objectives 376
 respiratory management 382–3
 search strategy 377
limbic encephalitis **89**
 paraneoplastic 474–5
lisinopril **166**

Listeria monocytogenes **21**
lisuride **235**
lithium **181**
liver transplantation 516–25
 background and objectives 516
 central nervous system infections 521–2
 central pontine myelinolysis 519–20
 cerebrovascular disorders 521
 grading of recommendations 517
 immunosuppression neurotoxicity 517–18
 neuromuscular disorders 520–1
 search strategy 516–17
 seizures 518–19
loss of consciousness, duration of 209–11, *211*
Lyme neuroborreliosis, CSF immunoglobulins **17**
lymphocytic chorio-meningitis **22**
lymphoma, CNS 390–1

McGill Pain Questionnaire 113
magnesium **166**
magnetic resonance angiography 35
magnetic resonance imaging
 Alzheimer's disease 272–4
 brain 32–3
 multiple sclerosis 45–62
 aims of EFNS Task Force 46
 at presentation 46–50
 in established disease 50–4
mazindol 541, 544
medium-chain acyl-CoA-dehydrogenase deficiency 530
MEDLINE 11
melatonin **181**
memantine 279–80, 282, **415**
memory
 function 269
 rehabilitation 598–602
Mendel, Gregor Johann 5
meningeal carcinomatosis, CSF immunoglobulins **17**
meningitis
 acute bacterial
 CSF oligoclonal IgG bands **20**
 CSF parameters **15**
 cryptococcal 388–9
 tuberculous 390
menstrual migraine 168

metamizol **163**
methotrexate 338
methylphenidate 540
methylprednisolone 437
methysergide **166, 181**
metoclopramide **163**, 257
metoprolol **166**
microneurography 115
midazolam 448
midodrine 256, 496–7
migraine 4, 159–76
 background 160
 in children and adolescents 169
 classification **161**
 clinical aspects 160–1, **160, 161**
 consensus method 160
 diagnosis **160**, 161
 drug treatment 161–5, **163, 164**
 analgesics 162
 antiemetics 162
 ergot alkaloids 162
 triptans 162–5
 epidemiology 161
 menstrual 168
 in pregnancy 168–9
 prophylaxis 165–8, **166**
 antidepressants 167
 antiepileptic drugs 166–7
 betablockers 166
 calcium channel blockers 166
 NSAIDs 167
 search strategy 160 *see also* headache, non-acute
modafinil 537–8, 545
monoamine oxidase inhibitors 225–6, 227–8, 246, 255, 542, 543–4
monoclonal gammopathy of uncertain significance 364, **365**
motor end plate disease 558–9
motor neuron diseases 558–9
MRC European Carotid Surgery Trial (ECST) 35
MRI *see* magnetic resonance imaging
multifocal motor neuropathy 354–61
 background 355
 consensus methods 355–6
 diagnostic categories **358**
 diagnostic criteria 356, **356**
 Good Practice Points 358, **358**
 investigation 356–7, **357**
 objectives 355

search strategy 355
treatment 357–8
multiple sclerosis 46–50
  acute relapse 433–42
    background 433–4
    consensus method 434
    glucocorticoid and ACTH
      treatment 434–8
    in pregnancy 439–40
    search strategy 434
  anti-interferon antibody
    72–86
    background and objectives
      72–3
    binding antibodies 75
    clinical use of antibody
      measurements
      79, **80**
    effect on disease
      progression 81–2
    effect on MRI outcomes 81
    effect on relapses 81
    immunogenicity 73–5, **74**
    neutralizing antibodies
      75–9, **76–8**
    prevention and treatment
      of NABs 82–3
    recommendations 83
    safety issues 82
    search strategy and
      consensus 73
  CSF oligoclonal IgG bands
    20
  CSF parameters **15**
  magnetic resonance imaging
    45–62
    aims of EFNS Task Force 46
    in established disease 50–4
multiple sleep latency test 536
mumps virus **22**
muscle biopsy 380–1, **381**
muscle carnitine
  deficiency 528
muscular dystrophy *see* limb
  girdle muscular
  dystrophies
muscular training 325–6
MuSK **89**
myasthenia gravis **89**, 334–9
  antibodies against leucocyte
    antigens 339
  azathioprine 337–8
  ciclosporin 338
  corticosteroids 337
  cyclophosphamide 338
  immune-directed treatment
    334–5
  intravenous
    immunoglobulin
    335–6

methotrexate 338
mycophenolate mofetil 338
plasma exchange 335
symptomatic treatment 334
tacrolimus 338–9
thymectomy 336–7
training, weight control
  and lifestyle
  modifications 339
Mycobacterium tuberculosis **21**
mycophenolate mofetil
  CIDP **350**
  myasthenia gravis 338
Mycoplasma pneumoniae **21**
myectomy 200–1
myelopathy, HIV 391–2
myoclonus **89**

NABs *see* neutralizing
  antibodies
naproxen **163**, **166**
naratriptan **164**
narcolepsy 534–51
  background 535–6
  behavioural therapy 538–9,
    543, 545
  cataplexy 542–5
  consensus methods 537
  excessive daytime sleepiness
    and irresistible
    episodes of sleep
    537–42
  Good Practice Points 547
  hallucinations and sleep
    paralysis 545
  methods and search strategy
    536–7
  neuropsychiatric symptoms
    546
  objectives 535
  obstructive sleep
    apnoea/hypopnoea
    syndrome 546
  parasomnias 546
  periodic limb
    movements 546
  poor sleep 545–6
  psychosocial support and
    counselling 547
National Institute of
  Neurological Disorders
  and Stroke (NINDS)
  trial 31
Neisseria meningitides **21**
nerve biopsy, PDN 368
neuroimaging
  alcohol-related seizures 454
  encephalitis 400–2
  non-acute headache
    66–7, 69

neuromuscular disorders 520–1
neuromyotonia/Isaacs
  syndrome 340
neuropathic pain 109–22
  background and objectives
    109–10
  clinical examination and
    psychophysiological
    measures 111–15
    bedside examination
      111, *112*
    pain quality and intensity
      scales 113–14
    quantitative sensory
      testing 111–13, **112**
    treatment efficacy 114
  definitions 110–11
  laboratory tests 115
    biopsy 118
    electrodiagnostic
      studies 115
    functional
      neuroimaging 117
    laser-evoked potentials
      116–17, *116*
    microneurography 115
    nociceptive reflexes
      115–16
  search strategy 110
  treatment 412–32
    adverse events and
      indications for use
      423–5
    background and
      objectives 413
    central pain 419–20
    effects on pain symptoms
      and signs 422
    effects on quality of life
      and comorbidities
      422–3
    future recommendations
      425–7, *426*
    methods 413–14
    painful polyneuropathy
      414–17, **415**
    postherpetic neuralgia
      417–18
    trigeminal neuralgia
      418–19
Neuropathic Pain
  Questionnaire 113
Neuropathic Pain Symptom
  Inventory 113
neuroprotection 147
  Parkinson's disease 225–6
neurosyphilis, CSF oligoclonal
  IgG bands **20**
neutralizing antibodies 72
  dynamics 73–4

neutralizing antibodies (*Contd.*)
measurement 75–9, **76–8**
existing
recommendations 79
validation 76, 79
multiple sclerosis
effect on disease progress
81–2
effect on MRI outcomes 81
effect on relapses 81
NAB-positive patients **74**
prevention and treatment
82–3
immunosuppressants 82
steroids 82
switching prepara-
tions/increasing
dose 82–3
safety issues 82
NIH Stroke Scale 140
nitroglycerin **143**
nitroprusside **143**
Nocardia asteroides **21**
nociceptive reflexes 115–16
norepinephrine uptake
inhibitors 544
nortriptyline **415**
NSAIDs 167
nucleic acid detection 402–3
number needed to treat 114
nystagmus and oscillopsia
484–92
methods 485
nuclear and infranuclear
ocular disorders
489–90
supranuclear ocular motor
disorders 485–9
central vestibular 485–7
non-vestibular 487–9

obstructive sleep
apnoea/hypopnoea
syndrome 546, 555
occupational therapy 232–6,
235
octreotide **181**, 497–8
ocular flutter 488–9
oestrogen-replacement
therapy 134
olanzapine 253
opioids **415**, 416, 417–18, 420,
425, 577
opsoclonus **89**, 488–9
opsoclonus-myoclonus,
paraneoplastic 477–8
optic neuritis 436–7
orthostatic hypotension 256,
493–500
background 493–4

diagnostic strategies 494
management 495
non-pharmacological
treatment 495–6
objectives 494
pharmacological treatment
496–8
oscillopsia *see* nystagmus and
oscillopsia
oxcarbazepine **415**, 424
oxycodone **415**

Pain Anxiety Symptom
Scale 115
painful polyneuropathy
414–17, **415**
pain quality and intensity
scales 113–14
Pain Relief Scale 114
pain thresholds 113
pallidotomy 248
paracetamol **163**
parainfluenza virus **22**
paraneoplastic syndromes
472–82, **473**
background 472–3
cerebellar degeneration **89**,
476–7
CSF immunoglobulins **17**
encephalitis **89**
Lambert-Eaton myasthenic
syndrome **89**, 339–40,
478
limbic encephalitis 474–5
methods 474
opsoclonus-myoclonus
477–8
peripheral nerve
hyperexcitability
479–80
subacute sensory
neuronopathy **89**,
475–6
paraproteinaemic
demyelinating
neuropathy 362–75
background 363
cerebrospinal fluid and nerve
biopsy 368
classification 364, **364**
consensus methods 363
definition 364, **365**
investigation 364, **364**, **365**
objectives 363
relationship between
paraprotein and
neuropathy 368
search strategy 363
syndromes of 364–6
CANOMAD 367

IgA type 366
IgG type 366
IgM type 365–6
POEMS 366–7
Waldenström's
macroglobulinaemia
367
treatment 368–71
IgA type 371
IgG type 371
IgM type 368–71
monitoring of
haematological
disease 368
POEMS 371
parasomnias 546, 556–7
paresthesias 111
Parkinson disease 4
dementia 283–4
early 224–44
background 224–5
consensus method 225
interventions 225–36
search strategy 225
late 245–65
interventions 246–58
methods 245
Parkinson, James 4
paroxetine 255
paroxysmal hemicrania
179–80, **180**
diagnostic criteria **180**
treatment 185
paroxysmal vestibular episodes
489–90
Pasteurella multocida **21**
patent foramen ovale 137
PDN, *see also* paraproteinaemic
demyelinating
neuropathy
pemoline 541
pergolide **235**
pericranial muscle
tenderness 66
periodic alternating
nystagmus 487
periodic limb movements 546
see also restless legs
syndrome
peripheral nerve
hyperexcitability
479–80
peripheral neuropathy
skin biopsy 94–106
consensus 95
correlations 103–4
diagnostic performance 99
diagnostic yield 99–102
EU standards 105

methods and choice of location 95–6
morphological changes 102
new study proposals 105
objectives 95
search strategy 95
skin reinnervation 104–5
sweat gland innervation 102–3
tissue processing and quantification of IENF 96–9, *97*, *98*
PET
  Alzheimer's disease 274
  brain 33–4
  head injury 216
  non-acute headache 65, 68–9
petasites **166**
phantom limb pain 421
phenazon **163**
phenelzine 541, 545
photic driving 68
physical therapy 232–6, **235**
Pick, Arnold 5
piribedil **235**
plasma exchange
  CIDP 347
  IgM type PDN 368–9
  myasthenia gravis 335
plasma expansion 496
pneumonia 148
POEMS 366–7
  treatment 371
poliovirus **22**
poor sleep 545–6
positron emission tomography *see* PET
postherpetic neuralgia 417–18
post-polio syndrome 322–31
  background 323–4
  clinical neurophysiology 324
  national surveys 325
  objectives 323
  scheduled update 328
  search strategy 324
  therapeutic interventions 325–8
  acetylcholinesterase inhibitors, steroids and amantadine 325
  bulbar symptoms 327
  educational interventions 327
  muscular training 325–6
  respiratory aid 326–7
  warm climate and training in water 326

weight control, assistive devices and lifestyle modifications 327
post-traumatic amnesia 211
pramipexole **235**
pregabalin **415**, 424–5
pregnancy, multiple sclerosis 439–40
pressure pain threshold 66
progressive multifocal leukoencephalopathy 389
progressive rubella panencephalitis, CSF oligoclonal IgG bands **20**
PROGRESS trial 138
propofol 448
propranolol **143**, **166**
PROSPER trial 138
psychosis 253
pulmonary embolism 148
pulmonary function 141

quantitative sensory testing 111–13, **112**
quetiapine 253–4

rabies virus **22**
radiating pain 113
radiofrequency lesions 201
radiography, skull 215
radio-immunoprecipitation assay 75
rasagiline **23**, 225–6, 227–8
Rasmussen's encephalitis 402
reboxetine 255
reflex responses, non-acute headache 65, 68–9
REM sleep behaviour disorder 556–7
respiratory aid 326–7
respiratory alkalosis 455
restless legs syndrome 569–91
  adrenergic agents 571
  antiepileptic drugs 573
  background 569–70
  benzodiazepines/hypnotics 574
  dopaminergic agents 574–7
  objectives 570
  recommendations 579
  search strategy 570–1, **572–3**
riboflavin **166**
riboflavin-responsive multiple acyl-CoA-dehydrogenase defects 531
rickettsia **21**
risperidone 254
rituximab

CIDP **350**
  IgM type PDN 370
rivastigmine 253, 254
rizatriptan **164**
ropinirole **235**
rotavirus **22**
rubella virus **22**

sandfly virus **22**
sarcoid, CSF oligoclonal IgG bands **20**
Scandinavian Stroke Scale 140
Scottish Intercollegiate Guidelines Network 10
seesaw nystagmus 486–7
seizures 148–9
  alcohol-related 451–60
  cerebral venous thrombosis 506–7
  post-head injury 214
  post-liver transplantation 518–19
selective peripheral denervation 200–1
selective serotonin reuptake inhibitors 255
selegiline 225–6, 227–8, **235**, 542, 545
serotonin-noradrenaline reuptake inhibitors 424
serotonin specific uptake inhibitors 544
sertraline 255
short-chain acyl-CoA dehydrogenase deficiency 530–1
short tau inversion recovery sequence 47
sildenafil 257
single photon emission computed tomography *see* SPECT
skin biopsy
  peripheral neuropathy 94–106
  consensus 95
  correlations 103–4
  diagnostic performance 99
  diagnostic yield 99–102
  EU standards 105
  methods and choice of location 95–6
  morphological changes 102
  new study proposals 105
  objectives 95
  search strategy 95
  skin reinnervation 104–5
  sweat gland innervation 102–3

skin biopsy (*Contd.*)
    tissue processing and
        quantification of
        IENF 96–9, *97, 98*
skull base fracture 214
sleep disordered breathing
    554–5
sleep disorders 552–68
  background 553
  classification 554–7
  consensus methods 554
  diagnostic techniques
    559–60, **560**
  motor neuron diseases,
    motor end plate and
    muscle diseases 558–9
  objectives 553
  search strategy 554
  stroke 558
  synucleinopathies 557–8
  tauopathies 557
  treatment 560–2
    medical 562–3 *see also*
      narcolepsy
sleep hypoventilation
    syndrome 561
sleep paralysis 545
sleep-related hypoventila-
    tion/hypoxaemic
    syndrome 556
sleep-related movement
    disorders 557
small fibre sensory
    neuropathy 95
smoking 134, 139
sodium oxybate 540–1, 542–3,
    545
SPECT
  Alzheimer's disease 274
  brain 33–4
  head injury 216
  non-acute headache 65,
    68–9
speech therapy 232–6, **235**
spontaneous pain 111
Staphylococcus aureus **21**
State, Trait and Anxiety
    scale 115
statins 281
status epilepticus 443–50
  alcohol-related 456
  anaesthetising
    anticonvulsants 447
  consensus methods 444
  definitions 444–5
  incidence, mortality and
    morbidity 443–4
  initial treatment 445–6
  literature evaluation 444
  mechanisms 444

  non-anaesthetising
    anticonvulsants 447
  refractory 446–7, 448
  search strategy 444
steroids
  CIDP 346–7
  Duchenne muscular
    dystrophy 384
  encephalitis 406–7
  IgM type PDN 370
  multiple sclerosis 434–8, **436**
  myasthenia gravis 337
  neurotoxicity 517–18
  post-polio syndrome 325
  side effects 438
stiff person syndrome **89**
stimulus-evoked pain 111
Streptococcus mitis **21**
Streptococcus pneumoniae **21**
stroke 3, 123–58, 558
  complications 147–50
    agitation 149
    aspiration and
      pneumonia 148
    brain oedema and elevated
      intracranial pressure
      149
    decompressive surgery 150
    decubital ulcer 148
    hypothermia 149–50
    pulmonary embolism and
      DVT 148
    seizures 148–9
    urinary tract infection 148
  diagnostic imaging 129–30
  diagnostic tests **129**
  education 125–6
  general treatment 141–5
    blood pressure
      management 142,
      143
    body temperature 144
    cardiac care 141–2
    fluid and electrolyte
      management 144
    glucose metabolism 142–4
    pulmonary function and
      airway
      protection 141
  imaging 28–44
    brain 30–4
    extracranial vessels 34–5
    intracranial vessels 35–6
    method for reaching
      consensus 30
    search strategy 29–30
  levels of evidence **124**
  monitoring of neurological
    functions 140–5

  quality control of treatment
    131
  referral 126
  rehabilitation 131–2
  specific treatment 145–7,
    147
  stroke care 124–5
stroke prevention 132–40
  primary 132–6
    alcohol consumption 134
    antithrombotic therapy
      135
    arterial hypertension 132
    carotid artery angioplasty
      136
    carotid surgery and
      endovascular
      treatment 136
    cigarette smoking 134
    diabetes mellitus 132, 134
    hyperlipidaemia 134
    life-style modification 134
    oestrogen-replacement
      therapy 134
    relative risk reduction **133**
  secondary 136–40
    acute management 140
    anticoagulation 137
    anti-hypertensive
      treatment 138
    antiplatelet therapy 136–7
    carotid angioplasty and
      stenting 140
    carotid endarterectomy
      139
    cholesterol lowering
      therapy 138
    extracranial-intracranial
      anastomosis 140
    hormone replacement
      therapy 138–9
    smoking 139
stroke units 127–31, **128**, **129**,
    131
subacute sclerosing
    panencephalitis 400
  CSF oligoclonal IgG bands **20**
subacute sensory
    neuronopathy **89**,
    475–6
subarachnoid haemorrhage
  CSF parameters **15**
  CT 31–2
  MRI 33
subthalamic nucleus,
    stimulation 250
sumatriptan **164**, **181**
SUNCT syndrome 180, **180**
  diagnostic criteria **180**
  treatment 185

superior oblique
    myokymia 489
supine hypertension 495
sural nerve
    action potential 103
    biopsy 104
sweat glands, innervation
    102–3
Symptom Score Scale 113
synucleinopathies 557–8
systemic lupus erythematosus,
    CSF oligoclonal IgG
    bands **20**

tacrolimus 338–9
    neurotoxicity 517–18
tanacetum parthenium **166**
tauopathies 557
temporal summation 113
tension headache 66
thalamotomy 250
thalamus, stimulation 250
thiamine 454–5
l-threo-3,4-
    dihydroxyphenylserine
    256
thrombolysis 504–5
thrombolytic therapy 145–7,
    147

thymectomy 336–7
tocapone **235**
tolfenamic acid **163**
topiramate **166**, **181**, **415**
total protein, CSF 16–17
tramadol *see* opioids
transcranial Doppler 35–6
Treponema pallidum **21**
tricyclic antidepressants 255
trifunctional enzyme
    deficiency 529–30
trigeminal neuralgia 418–19
triptans 162–5
Tropheryma whipplei **21**
tuberculous meningitis 390

unilateral spatial neglect 595–6
upbeat nystagmus 496
urapidil **143**
urinary disturbance 256–7
urinary tract infection 148

valproic acid **166**, **181**, **415**
vanlafaxine 255
varicella-zoster virus **21**, 398
    neuroimaging 401
vascular dementia 273
venlafaxine **415**, 544

verapamil **181**
very long-chain acyl-CoA
    dehydrogenase
    deficiency 529
viral culture 402
viral encephalitis, CSF
    oligoclonal IgG bands
    20
virological tests 402
visual analogue scales 113
visually evoked potentials 68

Waldenström's
    macroglobulinaemia
    367
warm climate 326
water-based training 326
weight control 327, 339
Western blot 75
Willis, Thomas 4
Women's Oestrogen for Stroke
    Trial 138–9
Wren, Christopher 4

yohimbine 256, 498

zolmitriptan **164**, **181**

Evidence classification schemes

Evidence classification scheme for a therapeutic intervention

Class I An adequately powered prospective, randomized, controlled clinical trial with masked outcome assessment in a representative population or an adequately powered systematic review of prospective randomized controlled clinical trials with masked outcome assessment in representative populations. The following are required:

(a) randomization concealment;
(b) primary outcome(s) is/are clearly defined;
(c) exclusion/inclusion criteria are clearly defined;
(d) adequate accounting for dropouts and crossovers with numbers sufficiently low to have minimal potential for bias; and
(e) relevant baseline characteristics are presented and substantially equivalent among treatment groups or there is appropriate statistical adjustment for differences.

Class II Prospective matched-group cohort study in a representative population with masked outcome assessment that meets a–e above *or* a randomized, controlled trial in a representative population that lacks one criteria a–e.

Class III All other controlled trials (including well-defined natural history controls or patients serving as own controls) in a representative population, where outcome assessment is independent of patient treatment.

Class IV Evidence from uncontrolled studies, case series, case reports, or expert opinion.

Rating of recommendations

Level A (established as effective, ineffective, or harmful) requires at least one convincing class I study or at least two consistent, convincing class II studies.

Level B (probably effective, ineffective, or harmful) requires at least one convincing class II study or overwhelming class III evidence.

Level C (possibly effective, ineffective, or harmful) rating requires at least two convincing class III studies.

Evidence classification scheme for a diagnostic measure

Class I A prospective study in a broad spectrum of persons with the suspected condition, using a 'gold standard' for case definition, where the test is applied in a blinded evaluation, and enabling the assessment of appropriate tests of diagnostic accuracy.

Class II A prospective study of a narrow spectrum of persons with the suspected condition, or a well-designed retrospective study of a broad spectrum of persons with an established condition (by 'gold standard') compared to a broad spectrum of controls, where test is applied in a blinded evaluation, and enabling the assessment of appropriate tests of diagnostic accuracy.

Class III Evidence provided by a retrospective study where either persons with the established condition or controls are of a narrow spectrum, and where test is applied in a blinded evaluation.

Class IV Any design where test is not applied in blinded evaluation or evidence provided by expert opinion alone or in descriptive case series (without controls).

Rating of recommendations

Level A (established as useful/predictive or not useful/predictive) requires at least one convincing class I study or at least two consistent, convincing class II studies.

Level B (established as probably useful/predictive or not useful/predictive) requires at least one convincing class II study or overwhelming class III evidence.

Level C (established as possibly useful/predictive or not useful/predictive) requires at least two convincing class III studies.